Physical Management for Neurological Conditions

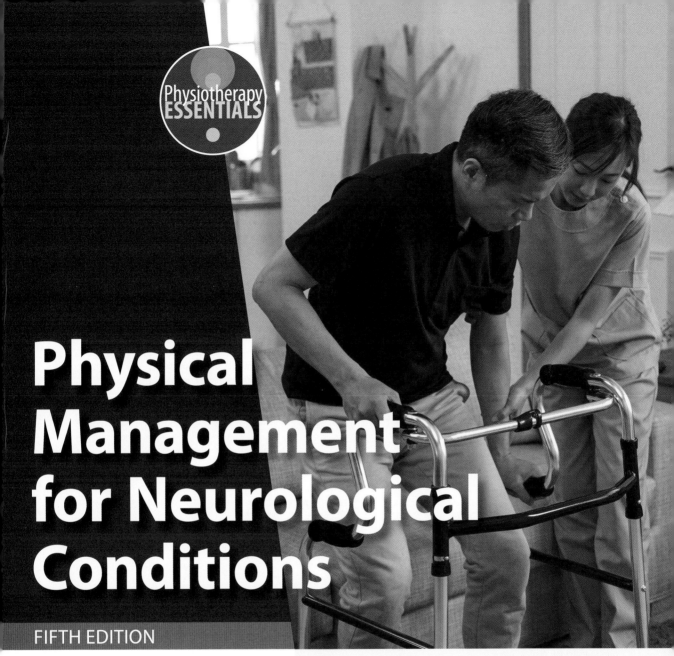

Physiotherapy
ESSENTIALS

Physical Management for Neurological Conditions

FIFTH EDITION

Edited by   **Sheila Lennon,** PhD, MSc, BSc, FCSP
Professor Emerita of Physiotherapy College of Nursing and Health Sciences Flinders University Adelaide, AUS

Gita Ramdharry, PhD, MSc, PG Cert, BSc (Hons)
Consultant Allied Health Professional Queen Square Centre for Neuromuscular Diseases The National Hospital for Neurology and Neurosurgery University College London NHS Foundation Trust London, UK

Honorary Associate Professor Department of Neuromuscular Diseases Institute of Neurology University College London London, UK

Geert Verheyden, PhD
Professor of Rehabilitation Sciences and Physiotherapy Department of Rehabilitation Sciences KU Leuven - University of Leuven Leuven, BEL

ELSEVIER

First edition 1998
Second edition 2004
Third edition 2011
Fourth edition 2018

Notices

ISBN: 978-0-323-88132-6

Content Strategist: Andrae Akeh
Content Project Manager: Fariha Nadeem
Cover Design: Amy Buxton
Illustration Manager: Akshaya Mohan
Marketing Manager: Deborah Watkins

Printed in India

 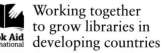

Working together to grow libraries in developing countries

www.elsevier.com • www.bookaid.org

Last digit is the print number: 9 8 7 6 5 4 3 2 1

Abiodun E. Akinwuntan, PT, PhD, MPH, MBA
Dean and Professor
School of Health Professions
University of Kansas Medical Center
Kansas City, KS
USA

Stephen Ashford, PhD, MSc, BSc, PGC Education, PGC Prescribing, PGC Sonography, FCSP, FACPIN
Honorary Reader and Consultant
    Physiotherapist
Regional Hyper-acute Rehabilitation
    Unit
London North West University
    Healthcare NHS Trust
London
UK

Reader (Associate Professor)
Department of Palliative Care, Policy
    and Rehabilitation
King's College London
London
UK

Clare C. Bassile, PT, EdD
Associate Professor
Programs in Physical Therapy
Columbia University Irving Medical
    Center
New York, NY
USA

Paolo Bonato, PhD
Associate Professor
Department of Physical Medicine and
    Rehabilitation
Harvard Medical School
Spaulding Rehabilitation Hospital
Boston, MA
USA

(Elizabeth) Caroline Brown, MSc, BSc (Hons)
Quality Improvement Academy
    Manager
University Hospitals of North
    Midlands NHS Trust
Stoke on Trent
Staffordshire
UK
Associate Physiotherapist
PhysioVitality
Newcastle-under-Lyme
UK

Lisa May Bunn, PhD
Associate Professor of Neurological
    Rehabilitation
Associate Head of School for
    Postgraduate Study
School of Health Professions
University of Plymouth
Plymouth
UK

Lisa Burrows, BSc (Hons), MSc, IP
Consultant Vestibular Physiotherapist
Mersey Care NHS Foundation Trust
Liverpool
UK

Monica Busse, BSc, BSc (Hons), MSc, PhD
Professor
Centre for Trials Research
Cardiff University
Cardiff
UK

Joseph Buttell, PT, BSc (Hons), PG Dip, PGC Prescribing, PGC Injection Therapy
Consultant Physiotherapist and Clinical
    Lead Adult Focal Spasticity Service
Clinical Specialist Physiotherapist
    and Head of Department Regional
    Neurological Rehabilitation Unit
Homerton Healthcare
Homerton Hospital
London
UK

Ailsa Carmichael, BSc (Hons)
Highly Specialist Physiotherapist
Neurocritical Care, Therapy and
    Rehabilitation Services
The National Hospital for Neurology
    and Neurosurgery
University College London NHS
    Foundation Trust
London
UK

Aisling Carr, MD, PhD
Consultant Neurologist
University College London
Queen Square Centre for
    Neuromuscular Diseases
London
UK

Elizabeth Cassidy, MSc, PhD
Retired Physiotherapy Lecturer
UK

Chih-Chung Chen, PhD, MPhil, BSc (Hons
Assistant Professor
Department of Physical Therapy
College of Medicine
Chang Gung University
Taoyuan
TW

Vanina Dal Bello-Haas, PT, PhD
Professor
School of Rehabilitation Science
McMaster University
Hamilton, Ontario
CAN

Helen Dawes, PhD
Professor of Clinical Rehabilitation
College of Medicine and Health
University of Exeter Medical School
St Luke's Campus
Exeter
UK

Liesbet De Baets, PT, PhD
Doctor-assistant
Department Rehabilitation Sciences
 and Physiotherapy
Hasselt University
Diepenbeek
BEL
Doctor-assistant
Pain in Motion Research Group (PAIN)
Department of Physiotherapy, Human
 Physiology and Anatomy
Faculty of Physical Education &
 Physiotherapy
Vrije Universiteit Brussel
Brussels
BEL

Hannes Devos, PT, PhD, FACRM
Associate Professor
Department of Physical Therapy,
 Rehabilitation Science, and Athletic
 Training
University of Kansas Medical Center
Kansas City, KS
USA

Camilla Erwee, MSc, BSc (Hons
Clinical Specialist Occupational
 Therapist
Head of Department Regional
 Neurological Rehabilitation Unit
Homerton Healthcare
Homerton Hospital
London
UK

**Jennifer A. Freeman, BAppSci
(Physiotherapy), PhD**
Professor in Physiotherapy and
 Rehabilitation
Faculty of Health
School of Health Professions
University of Plymouth
Plymouth
UK

**Jill Patricia Garner, Grad Dip Phys,
MClinRehab**
Department of Physiotherapy
Caring Futures Institute
College of Nursing and Health Sciences
Flinders University
Adelaide
AUS

Mariella Graziano, BSc (Hons)
Neuro Physiotherapy Practice
Esch-sur-Alzette
LUX

**Hilary Gunn, PhD, MSc, Grad Dip
Phys**
Associate Professor in Physiotherapy
Faculty of Health
School of Health Professions
University of Plymouth
Plymouth
UK

**Alexandra Henson, SLT, MSc, BA
(Hons)**
Professional Lead Adult SLT
Homerton Healthcare
Homerton Hospital
London
UK

**David Herdman, BSc (Hons), PhD,
MCSP**
Principal Vestibular Physiotherapist
St George's University Hospital NHS
 Foundation Trust
London
UK

Benita Hexter, BSc (Hons)
Clinical Specialist and Lead
 Physiotherapist
London Spinal Cord Injury Centre
The Royal National Orthopaedic
 Hospital NHS Trust
Stanmore
UK
Honorary Clinical Teaching Fellow
University College
London
UK
Chair
Multidisciplinary Association of Spinal
 Cord Injury Professionals
UK

Carlee Holmes, PT, PhD
Senior Physiotherapist
Young Adult Complex Disability Service
St. Vincent's Hospital
Melbourne
AUS
Postdoctoral Research Fellow,
 CP-Achieve
Murdoch Children's Research Institute
Royal Children's Hospital
Melbourne
AUS

Kate Holt (Ms), BSc (Physiotherapy)
Clinical and Research Physiotherapist
Neurosciences Research Centre
Molecular & Clinical Sciences Research
 Institute
St George's University of London
London
UK

Noit Inbar, BPT, PhD
Movement Disorders Unit
Tel Aviv Sourasky Medical Center
Tel Aviv
ISR

Meredith James, PhD, BAppSc
Clinical Specialist Neuromuscular
    Physiotherapist
John Walton Centre for Muscular
    Dystrophy Research
Newcastle University
Newcastle upon Tyne
UK

Mark I. Johnson, PhD, BSc
Professor
Centre for Pain Research
School of Health
Leeds Beckett University
Leeds
UK

Fiona Jones, PhD, MSc, FCSP, MBE
Professor of Rehabilitation Research
Population Health Research Institute
St George's University of London
London
UK

Dorit Kunkel, PhD
Senior Research Fellow in Long-Term
    Conditions
School of Health Sciences
University of Southampton
Southampton
UK

**Belinda Lange, BSc, BPhysio
(Hons), GCertBA, PhD, FAIDH**
Associate Professor
Caring Futures Institute
College of Nursing and Health Sciences
Flinders University of South Australia
Adelaide
AUS

Matilde Laurá, MD, PhD
Consultant Neurologist
University College London
Queen Square Centre for
    Neuromuscular Diseases
London
UK

Fiona Leggat, PhD, MSc
Research Associate
Population Health Research Institute
St George's University of London
London
UK

Sheila Lennon, PhD, MSc, BSc, FCSP
Professor Emerita of Physiotherapy
College of Nursing and Health Sciences
Flinders University
Adelaide
AUS

**Professor William Mark Magnus
Levack, PhD, MHealth Sci, BPhty**
Dean and Head of Campus
University of Otago, Wellington
Wellington
NZ

Jonathan Marsden, BSc, MSc, PhD
Professor
School of Health Professions
Faculty of Health and Human Sciences
University of Plymouth
Plymouth
UK

**Charlotte Massey, BSc (Hons)
Physiotherapy, MCSP**
Specialist Neuromuscular and
    Respiratory Physiotherapist
Queen Square Centre for
    Neuromuscular Diseases
The National Hospital for Neurology
    and Neurosurgery
University College London NHS
    Foundation Trust
London
UK
Sheffield Institute for Translational
    Neuroscience (SITraN)
University of Sheffield
Sheffield
UK

Anna Mayhew, PhD
Consultant Research Physiotherapist
The John Walton Muscular Dystrophy
    Research Centre
Newcastle University
Newcastle upon Tyne
UK

**Rory McConn-Walsh, MA, MD,
FRCSI, FRCS (ORLHNS), FFSEM**
Consultant Otolaryngologist
Beaumont Hospital
Dublin
IRL

**James Vincent McLoughlin, BAppSc,
MSc, PhD**
Director
Advanced Neuro Rehab
Royston Park
Adelaide
AUS
Co-Director
Your Brain Health
Adelaide
AUS
Lead Educator
Advanced Neuro Education,
Adelaide
AUS
Associate Professor
Flinders University
Adelaide
AUS

Dara Meldrum, PhD
Associate Professor
School of Medicine
Trinity College
Dublin
IRL

Prue Morgan, PT, PhD
Professor of Physiotherapy
Specialist Neurological Physiotherapist
Head of Physiotherapy, Monash
    University
Frankston, Victoria
AUS

Jane Newman, Grad Dip Phys, PhD, MCSP
Research Advanced Physiotherapist
Newcastle upon Tyne Hospitals NHS
    Foundation Trust
Wellcome Centre for Mitochondrial
    Research
NIHR Biomedical Research Centre
Newcastle University
Newcastle upon Tyne
UK

Glenn Nielsen, BSc (Physiotherapy) Hons, PhD
Senior Lecturer in Neurological
    Physiotherapy
Neurosciences Research Centre
Molecular & Clinical Sciences Research
    Institute
St George's University of London
London
UK

Sue Paddison, Grad Dip Phys
Clinical Specialist and Lead
    Physiotherapist
London Spinal Cord Injury Centre
Royal National Orthopaedic Hospital
    Trust
Stanmore
Middlesex
UK
Honorary Clinical Teaching Fellow
University College London
London
UK

Aleksandra Pietrusz, MRes, BSc (Hons), MCSP
Specialist Neuromuscular Physiotherapist
Research Physiotherapist
Adult DMD NorthStar Network
    Coordinator
Department of Neuromuscular Diseases
UCL Queen Square Institute of
    Neurology
The National Hospital for Neurology
    and Neurosurgery
University College London NHS
    Foundation Trust
London
UK

Louise Platt, MSc, BSc (Hons), BA (Hons)
Therapy Team Lead Neurosurgery
Therapy and Rehabilitation
The National Hospital for Neurology
    and Neurosurgery
London
UK

José Eduardo Pompeu, PhD
Professor of Physical Therapy Course
School of Medicine
University of Sao Paulo
Sao Paulo
BR

Lori Quinn, PT, EdD, FAPTA
Professor
Department of Biobehavioral Sciences
Teachers College
Columbia University
New York, NY
USA

Bhanu Ramaswamy, OBE, FCSP, DProf, MSc, Grad Dip Phys
Honorary Visiting Fellow
Sheffield Hallam University
Sheffield
UK

Gita Ramdharry, PhD, MSc, PG Cert, BSc (Hons)
Consultant Allied Health Professional
Queen Square Centre for
    Neuromuscular Diseases
The National Hospital for Neurology
    and Neurosurgery
University College London NHS
    Foundation Trust
London
UK
Honorary Associate Professor
Department of Neuromuscular Diseases
Institute of Neurology
University College London
London
UK

Sarah F. Tyson, PhD, MSc, FCSP
Professor of Rehabilitation
Stroke Research Group
School of Health Sciences
University of Manchester
Manchester
UK

Digna van de Bovenkamp-de Kam, PhD, PT
Saxion University of Applied Sciences
Enschede
NED

Janne M. Veerbeek, PhD
Researcher, Physical Therapist
Neurocenter
Luzerner Kantonsspital
Lucerne
CH

Geert Verheyden, PhD
Professor of Rehabilitation Sciences and
    Physiotherapy
Department of Rehabilitation Sciences
KU Leuven - University of Leuven
Leuven
BEL

Amanda C. Wallace, PhD, BSc
Senior Lecturer in Advanced Clinical
    Practice, University of Plymouth
Senior Lecturer in Clinical Research,
    University of Exeter
Devon
UK

Gavin Williams, PhD, Grad Dip, BAppSci, FACP
Professor of Physiotherapy Research
Department of Physiotherapy
Epworth Healthcare & The University
    of Melbourne
Melbourne
AUS

F. Colin Wilson, BSc, MMedSc, DClinPsych, AFBPsS
Consultant Clinical Neuropsychologist
Regional Acquired Brain Injury Unit
Belfast
UK

We are delighted to present the 5th edition of this popular textbook on *Physical Management for Neurological Conditions*. This revised edition includes up-to-date chapters on the physical management of common and less common neurological conditions by internationally renowned clinicians and researchers. We hope these collaborative efforts appeal to all members of the healthcare team, with a special focus on physiotherapy.

This book continues to be organised in three sections starting with background knowledge presenting an overview of guiding principles underlying neurological rehabilitation with a new chapter on clinical reasoning, followed by chapters on neurological conditions, then concluding with specific aspects of management such as technologies for neurorehabilitation, physical activity and exercise and clinical neuropsychology. Many of the authors have stayed on board for this new edition, and we believe to have constructed a textbook that attracts physiotherapy students, newly graduated colleagues as well as more experienced therapists. For students, the comprehensive overview of foundational material in the neurorehabilitation domain should provide first learning material; for new colleagues,

the wealth of topics covered in this book will broaden the understanding of the complex neurorehabilitation domain; and for experienced therapists, the depth of coverage and the updated chapters deliver a new and contemporary evidence base for practice and reflection. Many chapters include lessons learned from the Covid-19 pandemic for their domain, for example, through discussing telerehabilitation. We have also retained the self-assessment questions and answers to enable the reader to test their understanding.

We hope this 5th edition continues to provide clinically relevant theories and tools backed up by the current evidence base to help clinicians deliver high quality, evidence-based care in partnership with people with neurological conditions.

Sheila Lennon
Adelaide, Australia
Gita Ramdharry
London, United Kingdom
Geert Verheyden
Leuven, Belgium

We the editors have all worked at some point in the United Kingdom, and we have shared ideas at many international conferences. It truly has been such an easy and collegiate experience to collaborate as editors on this book, despite our now far-spread locations and different time zones! Fitting it into our busy clinical, academic, research and administrative workloads (and for one of us, retirement) has been rather more challenging!

We thank all the students, clinicians and academic colleagues who have provided invaluable feedback on the previous 4th edition. We thank the team at Elsevier for keeping us on track in such a supportive way, with special thanks to our content editor Fariha Nadeem.

We are grateful to all our authors for generously sharing their updated knowledge and expertise. Last but not least, we thank the patients who have informed our own practice and have also been willing to share their stories in the chapter case studies.

Sheila Lennon
Adelaide, Australia
Gita Ramdharry
London, United Kingdom
Geert Verheyden
Leuven, Belgium

CONTENTS

Section 1 Background Knowledge

1 **Guiding Principles in Neurological Rehabilitation** 3
Clare C. Bassile and Sheila Lennon

2 **Clinical Reasoning in Neurological Physiotherapy: Assessment and Treatment Principles** 33
Jill Patricia Garner, Sheila Lennon, and James Vincent McLoughlin

3 **Common Impairments and the Impact on Activity** 53
James Vincent McLoughlin

4 **Observation and Analysis of Movement** 71
Amanda C. Wallace, Lisa May Bunn, and Elizabeth Cassidy

5 **Measurement Tools** 113
Geert Verheyden and Sarah F. Tyson

6 **Goal Setting in Rehabilitation** 129
William Mark Magnus Levack

Section 2 Management of Specific Conditions

7 **Stroke** 151
Janne M. Veerbeek and Geert Verheyden

8 **Traumatic Brain Injury** 177
Gavin Williams

9 **Spinal Cord Injury** 197
Sue Paddison and Benita Hexter

10 **Multiple Sclerosis** 235
Jennifer A. Freeman and Hilary Gunn

11 **Parkinson's** 265
Bhanu Ramaswamy and Mariella Graziano

12 **Inherited Neurological Conditions** 293
Monica Busse, Jonathan Marsden, Noit Inbar, and Lori Quinn

13 **Motor Neurone Disease** 327
Caroline Brown and Vanina Dal Bello-Haas

14 **Polyneuropathies** 355
Gita Ramdharry, Aisling Carr, and Matilde Laurá

15 **Neuromuscular Disorders** 383
Anna Mayhew, Gita Ramdharry, Aleksandra Pietrusz, Meredith James, Jane Newman, and Charlotte Massey

16 **Functional Motor Disorders** 413
Glenn Nielsen and Kate Holt

17 **Vestibular Rehabilitation** 437
Dara Meldrum, Lisa Burrows, David Herdman, and Rory McConn-Walsh

Section 3 Specific Management

18 **Respiratory Management** 473
Louise Platt and Ailsa Carmichael

19 **Self-Management** 495
Fiona Jones and Fiona Leggat

20 **Neurorehabilitation Technologies** 517
Belinda Lange, José Eduardo Pompeu, and Paolo Bonato

21 **Falls and Their Management** 545
Dorit Kunkel and Digna de Kam

22 **Physical Activity and Exercise in Neurological Rehabilitation** 571
Helen Dawes

23 **Pain Management** 583
Mark I. Johnson and Chih-Chung Chen

24 **Clinical Neuropsychology in Rehabilitation** 611
F. Colin Wilson

25 **Selected Topics in Physical Management for Neurological Conditions** 627
Liesbet De Baets, Stephen Ashford, Hannes Devos, Abiodun E. Akinwuntan, Joseph Buttell, Camilla Erwee, Alexandra Henson, Prue Morgan, and Carlee Holmes

Appendix: Answers to Self-Assessment Questions 673
Abbreviations 689
Index 693

Background Knowledge

Guiding Principles in Neurological Rehabilitation

Clare C. Bassile and Sheila Lennon

OUTLINE

Introduction, 3
Why is a Theoretical Framework Important?, 4
  Key Points, 5
Guiding Principles for Neurological Rehabilitation, 5
  Principle 1: The ICF, 6
    The Value of Participation, 6
  Principle 2: Team Work, 7
  Principle 3: Person-Centred Care, 7
  Principle 4: Prognosis, 9
  Principle 5: Neural Plasticity, 10
    What Type of Training Drives Neural Plasticity and
    Recovery of Function? 10
  Principle 6: Motor Control: A Systems Model, 11
  Principle 7: Functional Movement Reeducation, 12
  Principle 8: Skill Acquisition, 13
    Intrinsic Motivation and Attentional Focus, 13

Task Practice Issues, 15
Role of Feedback, 16
Amount of Practice, 16
Variable Practice, 16
Modelling/Action–Observation, 17
Mental Practice, 17
Principle 9: Exercise Prescription, 17
Principle 10: Health Promotion, 18
Principle 11: Self-Management, 19
Principle 12: Mindset, 19
  Motivation, 20
  Resilience and Hope, 21
Principle 13: Behaviour Change, 22
  Habit Formation, 23
Conclusion, 25

INTRODUCTION

Various neurological conditions such as stroke, multiple sclerosis (MS) or Parkinson's change cognitive, sensory and/or motor capacities and alter the physical, psychological and emotional well-being of those affected, leading to disability in their everyday lives (Platz & Sandrini 2020). The Global Burden of Disease Study 2019 has identified 255 million people worldwide living with the consequences of these neurological conditions who may benefit from rehabilitation (Cieza et al 2020). Neurological rehabilitation has been defined as a process that assists individuals who experience disability to achieve and maintain optimal function and health in interaction with their environment (World Health Organization [WHO] 2017). It requires an active partnership between the patient, their family and a whole range of health and social care professionals. Effective rehabilitation depends on an expert multidisciplinary team, working within the biopsychosocial model of illness and working collaboratively towards agreed goals (Wade 2020). This book provides an explanation of the theories, tools and techniques that underpin the physical, psychological and emotional well-being of people with neurological conditions in rehabilitation practice.

Health professionals use a clinical reasoning (CR) approach to plan management across any neurological condition. There is a broad array of components deemed important for CR and limited reference to any evidence-based conceptual frameworks (Brentnall et al 2022). There are five essential components in the CR process: (1) assessment, (2) interpretation, (3) treatment planning, (4) intervention and (5) reassessment (+ outcomes) (adapted from

Atkinson & Nixon-Cave 2011, Garner & Lennon 2018, Lexell & Brogardh 2015; see Chapter 2 for more detailed discussion). These five essential components are also influenced by other contributory components, such as the *International Classification of Functioning, Disability and Health* (ICF), prognosis, the client problem list, goal setting and reflection within a person-centred care model of healthcare. The choice of interventions is influenced by what we know about prognosis, therapy aims and the goals and preferences of the client, as well as other contextual factors such as healthcare setting, healthcare funding and policy. Cultural frameworks also influence how patients and healthcare providers understand health and illness, and the expectations and values that they bring to their clinical interactions (Horvat et al 2014).

Assessment is always the starting point for CR. The assessment process is used to guide intervention by identifying clinical problems categorised according to the ICF. The rehabilitation team together with patients and their families collaboratively agree on joint treatment goals before devising a treatment plan. Developing a treatment plan is not easy; therapy is a complex intervention composed of multiple components that are combined to tailor the intervention to each patient's needs and preferences. A treatment plan is essential to provide appropriate interventions, which should be based on the best available evidence. Standardised measurement tools with published reliability, validity and sensitivity should be used to establish a baseline of performance before rehabilitation and then at key strategic points to document change as a result of rehabilitation interventions (see Chapter 5 on measurement tools). The assessment, interventions and measurement tools specific to each neurological condition are discussed in subsequent separate chapters.

Since the late 1980's there has been an explosion of knowledge in neurological rehabilitation providing sound evidence upon which to base healthcare interventions, yet to date incorporating evidence into practice has remained challenging. Therefore, it is also important to identify effective implementation interventions that enhance the uptake and use of evidence in clinical practice (Oral 2022), as well as contextual factors such as health systems and service organisations including health insurance availability, its coverage of interventions, and availability of technical equipment and qualified personnel for its use (Gutenbrunner & Nugraha 2020). The beliefs, attitudes and culture of both patients and health professionals may impose barriers to implementing evidence-based interventions in practice (Holmes et al 2020). This chapter will explain why theory and evidence-based practice (EBP) are important, and discuss a theoretical framework for neurological rehabilitation

comprising 13 key principles derived from neuroscience, skill acquisition and motor learning, psychological and behavioural principles.

WHY IS A THEORETICAL FRAMEWORK IMPORTANT?

Theories can be used to understand and explain health behaviour and to guide the identification, development and implementation of interventions. The beliefs of health professionals influence how they deliver intervention, as well as the techniques they select in their intervention plans (Lennon 2003, Lennon et al 2006). Theory provides the explanation for the actions and decisions of the healthcare team (Carr & Shepherd 2006), enabling hypotheses to be formulated and tested. Understanding the theoretical framework to which therapists subscribe can also lead to the development of new treatment strategies (Carr & Shepherd 2006). The explicit application of theory could shorten the time needed to design novel interventions, improve existing interventions and identify conditions of context necessary for their success (Davidoff et al 2015).

Physical management in neurological conditions needs to be based on beliefs that are substantiated by evidence, bearing in mind that the theoretical explanation underlying intervention may have to change as the evidence evolves. Historically, specific treatment approaches such as the Bobath concept have influenced the content, structure and aims of physical therapies based on therapist preference. Although such approaches remain popular today, to date there is no evidence to suggest that adopting a treatment approach such as the Bobath concept is more effective than other approaches (Kollen et al 2009). In fact, some systematic reviews have confirmed that other interventions may be superior to traditional treatment approaches such as the Bobath concept in regaining mobility and upper limb and lower limb activities after stroke (Diaz-Arribas et al 2020, Scrivener et al 2020). Current evidence supports the application of training parameters that enhance the effects of neuroplasticity and functional gains, including specificity, amount, intensity and saliency of task practice (Scheets et al 2021). These training parameters and the adjunct use of technology appear to be critical factors in improving outcomes, providing further support to the statement that neurological rehabilitation should not be limited to named approaches, but rather should be composed of evidenced-based physical techniques, regardless of historical or philosophical origin (Pollack et al 2014).

The evidence base underlying physical interventions is expanding year upon year. The challenge for clinicians is to keep up to date with that evidence, to transfer/implement that evidence into practice, but also to be prepared to change their preferred practice when the evidence clearly identifies that their preferred intervention is not effective or that a different intervention would be more appropriate. There are many examples of specific training strategies, such as strength training or task-specific practice, which are effective at improving movement and function (French et al 2016; Verbeek et al 2014; see http://www.cochrane.org for relevant systematic reviews). There are also many clinical guidelines that provide a comprehensive review of all the available evidence to date for the management of people after stroke (Stroke Foundation 2022, Winstein & Stein 2016), with Parkinson's (http://www.parkinsonnet.com) and with MS (National Institute for Health and Care Excellence 2022). These guidelines, developed by a multidisciplinary panel and subjected to peer review, provide a useful starting point for busy clinicians, when available.

Components selected within therapy sessions should be evidence based rather than based on therapist preference for a specific treatment approach. However, it is also important to realise that there are still many key areas of clinical practice with no evidence or conflicting evidence; therefore, therapists will always need to rely on their clinical reasoning skills to select treatment techniques appropriate to the needs, wishes and goals of patients and their carers. Since the turn of the 21st century, EBP has attempted to replace tradition and anecdote with high-quality randomised controlled trials to guide neurological rehabilitation; getting this research adopted in practice has proved problematic. Complex patients do not easily map to a single evidence-based guideline. EBP should respect professional knowledge and apply appropriate research evidence to inform dialogue with our patients and families about what best to do and why at each point in the patient's illness in a more personalised way with sensitivity to context and individual goals (Greenhalgh et al 2014).

Key Points

- Understanding the beliefs that guide practice helps explain the content, structure and delivery of therapy.
- A theoretical framework is essential to enable clinicians to determine their assessment and intervention strategies.
- Components selected within rehabilitation sessions should be evidence based rather than based on therapist preference for a specific treatment approach.
- Evidence needs to be individualised through shared decision making within the context of the clinician–patient relationship.

GUIDING PRINCIPLES FOR NEUROLOGICAL REHABILITATION

Neurological rehabilitation requires that health professionals keep up to date with evidence across many practice fields. A theoretical framework is essential to enable clinicians to determine their assessment and intervention strategies. This framework should integrate neurophysiological, kinesiological, skill acquisition and motor learning, as well as psychological, emotional and behavioural perspectives to focus on both physical and psychological recovery. We propose 13 key principles for consideration in our framework to guide clinicians working in neurological rehabilitation: the WHO ICF, team work, patient-centred care, prognosis (prediction), neural plasticity, a systems model of motor control, functional movement reeducation, skill acquisition, exercise prescription, health promotion, self-management (self-efficacy), mindset and behaviour change (Fig. 1.1).

These principles have evolved from our shift away from a biomedical to a biopsychological model of health in neurological rehabilitation by embracing the ICF and person-centred care (Barnes 2003, WHO 2017). As the evidence base underlying neurological rehabilitation has strengthened, there has been a focus on unpacking the active ingredients in the black box of rehabilitation interventions that have contributed to improved outcomes initially recognised from stroke unit care such as team work, specialist

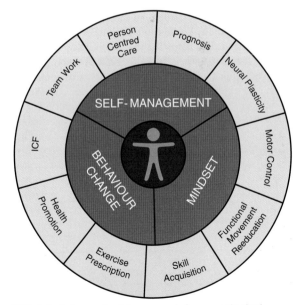

FIG. 1.1 A theoretical framework for neurological rehabilitation.

expertise, service organisation and setting (Langhorne et al 2020). Emerging research has confirmed that there is more to a successful intervention than a single element such as type, dose, specificity, and setting to drive recovery; thus, it is important to evaluate the combination of critical elements that account for change in our clients (Ward et al 2019, Wingfield et al 2022). This research supports our underpinning principles of neural plasticity, prognosis, motor control, functional movement reeducation, skill acquisition and exercise prescription. Lessons learned as we emerge from the Covid-19 global pandemic have reinforced how important the principles of health promotion, self-management and self-efficacy, mindset and behaviour change are to both physical and psychological well-being.

Principle 1: The ICF

In 2001 the WHO developed the ICF (http://www.who.int/classifications/icf) with the aim of shifting the focus from disability and impairments to health (Fig. 1.2). The ICF has become accepted as a universal framework for describing neurological disability, composed of five categories: body functions and structures, activities, participation, environmental factors and personal factors. The ICF provides a systematic way of understanding the problems faced by patients, illustrating the multiple levels at which neurological rehabilitation may act. The activities dimension covers the range of activities performed by an individual. The participation dimension classifies the areas of life in which for each individual there are societal opportunities or barriers.

Impairment is defined as a deficit in body structure or function. Following a stroke, an example of impairment would be weakness, leading to a limitation in the activity of walking and thus requiring the use of a wheelchair for mobility. Being in a wheelchair may restrict that individual from resuming their job, a limitation in participating in that individual's previous role in society. Environmental and personal factors are the contextual factors that enable the rehabilitation team to identify facilitators and barriers for the neurorehabilitation process such as having a house that is wheelchair accessible without stairs.

Within the ICF framework, physical interventions may directly target both impairment (a loss or abnormality of body structure) and activity (performance in functional activities) with the overall aim of improving quality of life and participation in desired life roles. Lexell and Brogardh (2015) have reviewed how the ICF can be used to enhance the clinical reasoning process by facilitating assessment and goal setting, as well as selecting appropriate interventions and outcome tools. However, further research is required to determine the benefits of using the ICF within clinical practice.

The Value of Participation

Changes at the level of impairment and activity are really meaningful for the patient and their carers only if they enable them to participate in their family and community life by resuming, albeit in a different way, their desired life roles. That is why health professionals need to measure the effects of their interventions at different levels of the ICF; they should use standardised measurement tools that have been shown to have meaningful clinically important differences (see Chapter 5 on measurement tools).

The concept of person-centred care is fundamental to ensuring that patient and family preferences and priorities are central to the clinical reasoning process of team members. Although it is important to identify the main clinical problems that can be modified by our intervention, assessment should also identify strengths, interests and desires that are specific to the achievement of a patient's goals. Goal setting also needs to be adapted to different stages in the

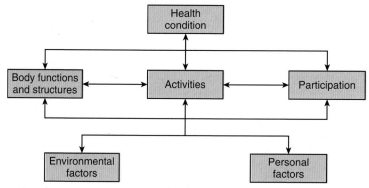

FIG. 1.2 Interactions between components of *International Classification of Functioning, Disability and Health* (WHO 2001, p. 18)

rehabilitation process (see Chapter 6 on goal setting). For example, more consideration needs to be given to community-based training in context to enable people with neurological disability to gain confidence and skills in their own environments. Innovative strategies such as wearable and assistive technologies may also help to translate gains in rehabilitation departments to the home and community environment (Kimberley et al 2017). The influence of assistive technology in neurorehabilitation is discussed in Chapter 20.

An optimal treatment plan will use a range of measurement tools that will evaluate whether improvements in impairments and function (activity) translate into improved participation such as quality of life and improved health status. It is not sufficient to choose measures that mainly measure impairment or function (see Chapter 5 and the pathology-specific chapters for selected measurement tools).

Government and society have a responsibility to develop policies, systems and services to ensure inclusion and access to health services, education, work and leisure opportunities for people with neurological disability in the global health agenda (Tomlinson et al 2009). A WHO (2017) report entitled 'Rehabilitation 2030: A Call for Action' has called for global action by all key stakeholders to upscale rehabilitation services worldwide. Clinicians are mostly concerned about the impact of their interventions at an individual level, but they also need to consider how they can influence and improve practice at the policy and service delivery level.

Principle 2: Team Work

Neurological rehabilitation requires an active partnership between the patient, the family and a whole range of healthcare and social care professionals; thus, team work is a critical element of care. Zajac et al (2021) have proposed a comprehensive framework for team effectiveness, identifying common challenges to team work in healthcare along with evidence-based strategies for overcoming them. The current evidence base distinguishes teams who are multidisciplinary versus interdisciplinary in their way of working. Teams have been defined as multidisciplinary where there is sharing of information on assessments and interventions, whereas team members have been defined as interdisciplinary where there is a high level of communication, mutual goal planning and evaluation. It should be emphasised that it is really important not just to share information, but rather to collaborate as a team in goal setting, care planning and decision making in partnership with the patient and their carers. The evidence in support of the best model of team work remains unclear (Clarke & Forster 2015). There is moderate quality evidence that

patients who receive organised inpatient care are more likely to be alive, independent and living at home 1 year after stroke (Langhorne et al 2020). Studies suggest that team work is generally associated with better outcome (Wade 2020).

Developing an appropriate plan of care revolves around collaborative goal setting within the team. Team goal setting is recognised as a core component of neurorehabilitation. Setting goals aims to motivate the team and the patient, coordinate activities, and ensure that all important goals are identified (see Chapter 6 for a review of goal setting). Team goals need to be based on the patient's wishes, expectations, priorities and values; one way of facilitating appropriate goal planning is to use the SMART acronym, which recommends that goals should be specific, measurable, achievable/ambitious, relevant and timed (Playford et al 2009; see Bovend'Eerdt et al 2009 for some practical guidance on how to set SMART goals).

Clarke and Forster (2015) offer the following recommendations for improving team working in stroke survivors during the rehabilitation phase:

- Have written protocols and pathways that help remove organisational and professional barriers.
- Have specialist training and knowledge.
- Agree on a consistent approach for clinical problems.
- Share treatment sessions.
- Understand the thinking and beliefs of different disciplines.
- Have an information provision strategy with consistent messages and access to further information when required.

These recommendations may also benefit people with other long-term neurological conditions (e.g., MS, Parkinson's). After the initial rehabilitation phase, patients will continue to need long-term follow-up, with collaboration between different disciplines remaining important; supported self-management may be a more appropriate mode of care at this later review stage of care.

Principle 3: Person-Centred Care

Person-centred care can be defined as a philosophy of care that encourages and supports patients and their carers to develop the knowledge, skills and confidence they need to effectively manage and make decisions about health (Health Foundation 2016). Person-centred care can be viewed as a partnership from the perspective of the patient, the family and the healthcare professional. Person-centred care not only is about working in partnership and sharing decision making with individual patients and their families within the rehabilitation process, but also it means using that patient and carer experience to plan, deliver and evaluate healthcare to improve care; this is often referred to in the literature as coproduction (Batalden et al 2015). Thus, active involvement should be encouraged at all levels and at all stages of the rehabilitation process, including research and service development and design. The Picker Institute, which focuses on using patient experience to improve health and social care, has identified eight principles of person-centred care (see The Picker Principles of Patient-Centred Care box).

THE PICKER PRINCIPLES OF PERSON CENTRED CARE (HTTP://WWW.PICKER.ORG)

1. Fast access to reliable healthcare advice
2. Effective treatment by trusted professionals
3. Continuity of care and smooth transitions
4. Involvement and support for family and carers
5. Clear information, communication and support for self-care
6. Involvement and shared decision making with respect for patient preferences
7. Emotional support, empathy and respect
8. Attention to both physical and environmental needs

Having a team approach is a key step to promoting person-centred care, where the team discusses and explains treatment options; patients and their carers then use this information to share decisions about their goals and choose treatment solutions. The process of goal setting provides a mechanism for patient-centred care by enabling autonomy and appropriate pacing of information and responsibility (Playford et al 2009).

Growing evidence links patient experience to health outcomes and adherence to recommended clinical practice and safety (Doyle et al 2013). Parish et al (2015) offer the following suggestions for getting person-centred care into practice:

- Ensure that services are well coordinated.
- Support and empower people to take charge of their health.
- Adopt a coproduction approach to healthcare.
- Produce a cultural change within policy and practice.

Emphasis on involving family members, and their preferences and needs, in the rehabilitation planning process is important, especially when the family carers may be the only ones providing ongoing support for patients after they leave the health service (Tang Yan et al 2014). Caring for people with neurological conditions can be very challenging; the healthcare team needs to also focus on the health and well-being of the carer to reduce caregiver burden and burnout (Krishnan et al 2017). Key strategies to help relieve

caregiver stress and burden include education, effective communication, maintaining physical and psychological well-being and building a local support system (Krishnan et al 2017). Getting involved with voluntary organisations and peer and caregiver support groups can also reduce feelings of isolation and provide additional support.

Health professionals are encouraged to listen to the perspectives of both patients and carers. The personal experience of Fuller (2016), who cared for her husband for 21 years after a devastating stroke at age 50 years, sends some strong messages on understanding the carer experience to help the patient live as full a life as possible (Table 1.1):

*'From day one of Clive's stroke, my family stepped out of a life we once knew and took for granted and stepped into an alien world; a world which we knew we would have to embrace to move forward with our lives. Our lives, especially mine, revolved around Clive's therapy sessions, as I was very aware how important therapy was in an endeavour to regain any sort of movement; always at the back of my mind was the golden rule: "**if you don't use it, you lose it**." The only way I could give Clive the support he needed, was to step into his shoes; try to feel what he was feeling and continually ask myself: "What would I want if the tables were turned and it was I who had experienced the stroke?"'*

Fuller, personal communication, with permission

One of Fuller's key messages is 'to never rule out hope, as hope is the only "positive" they can aim toward to create a change in their life.' Hope supports adjustment, perseverance and positive outcomes; it can reflect expectations, goals and optimism, as well as act as a motivator and source of strength (Bright et al 2011). There can be a tendency among health professionals to emphasise the importance of being 'realistic' in the early stages of recovery or being worried about giving false hope to patients and their families. However, hope is not just about physical improvement; it can represent the possibility of returning to activities that are important and meaningful to a patient's past self (Soundy et al 2014). The meaning of hope in neurological rehabilitation requires further exploration. Amati et al (2019) explored the role of hope with health professionals in rehabilitation identifying three strategies to maintain hope while avoiding false hope: (1) giving space for self-evaluation, (2) tailoring the communication of prognostic information and (3) supporting the person in dealing with the prognosis. These three strategies support person-centred care while emphasising the need for strengthening communication skills. Getting and maintaining the right type of hope may be the first sign that the patient is taking control towards managing their own recovery and

TABLE 1.1 Key Messages from a Carer on the Rehabilitation Process (adapted from Fuller 2016 with permission)

Overwhelming disbelief, shock and grief	• Give patients time to absorb that **they** have suffered a life-threatening illness.
Fear of the unknown, depression	• Evoke negative thoughts – is the effort worthwhile?
Take into consideration the extent of the stroke, the hidden disabilities: aphasia/dysphasia and dyspraxia	• Language barriers may impede the process of understanding a directive thereby sending an erroneous message to the patient and resulting in misinterpretation by the therapist (e.g., the client has plateaued)
Chronic fatigue	• Inhibits clients to work at their full capacity
Medication and side effects may play a negative role	• Affects comprehension
Changes regarding rehabilitation centres: closures/reallocation	• Client having to travel longer distances to access therapy causing disorientation – intensifies fatigue and/or anxiety
Limited parking or car parks situated some distance from venue	• Difficult for carers and clients who require the use of wheelchairs – increases anxiety
Do not discourage, give the client the chance to prove themself	• They all want to improve – they want to be the best they can be
Give encouragement, even if the session is a non event	• Some will do better than others – there may be an underlying issue
Listen to the client and/or carer	• They may have experienced/witnessed some significant gain
Introduce achievable hobbies	• All work and no play is not a good balance
Never, ever rule out **HOPE**	• For some, hope is the only 'positive' they can aim towards to create a change in their life

rehabilitation by identifying their own goals and developing their own strategies to pursue these goals (Soundy et al 2010). This can in fact be viewed as self-management, another guiding principle of rehabilitation that will be discussed later in this chapter.

Research highlights the importance of the patient's and the carer's voice and representing their expectations in clinical decisions (Trede 2012). Dialogue between the patients and their carers can be dominated by professional authority; thus, another important aspect of person-centred care is training healthcare professionals to be more person centred. A Cochrane Review by Dwamena et al (2012) has confirmed that training healthcare professionals to promote person-centred care in clinical consultations is successful in improving person-centred skills, with some evidence that person-centred care has beneficial effects on patient satisfaction, health behaviour and health status in general medical conditions. Person-centred care is a cornerstone of the rehabilitation process. Yet despite emerging literature on the benefits of person-centred care in healthcare settings and government legislation and policies to support person-centred care, little is known on how to practically embed person-centred care in different settings (Burgers et al 2021, Frakking et al 2020). Changing workplace

culture remains challenging. Innovative frameworks and models to embed person-centred care are evolving, but critical changes are required to how care is delivered and how patients and health professionals interact (Santana et al 2018). Achieving person-centred care remains challenging especially since the onset of the global Covid-19 pandemic in 2020 with accessibility and cost cited as significant areas for improvement (Dawda et al 2022).

Principle 4: Prognosis

Therapists are being asked to prognosticate about patient recovery every day, regardless of practice setting. In the acute care hospital setting in the USA, the team must make a discharge recommendation soon after initial assessment of the patient with an acute stroke. What forms the basis of that recommendation? Embedded along with the home situation, previous and current level of functioning and the severity of the neurological injury is the therapist's prediction bias about recovery for the patient (Bland et al 2015, Magdon-Ismail et al 2016, Mees et al 2016, Stein et al 2015). Will recovery be fast and attainable in the home or outpatient department setting, or will it be slow and possibly not full so that a subacute setting is more appropriate, or will recovery be fast enough to be attained in a 2- to 3-week stay on an acute inpatient rehabilitation unit? Finally, is there a difference in the timeline of recovery for those individuals with a hemorrhagic versus an ischemic stroke? Recent work differentiating the three discharge destinations after acute stroke hospitalisation in the USA has highlighted the significance that current level of functioning plays in the prediction model (Casertano et al 2022) and a therapist's recommendation (Rakesh et al 2019).

We are also asked by our patients: 'Will I walk again?' 'Will I be able to use my hand again, move my arm, run again?' These queries reflect the patient's focus on mobility along with task-specific activities that promote return to participation. Having knowledge of the prediction literature allows the therapist to be realistic with the patient and carer while also using their clinical judgement (Pelletier-Roy et al 2021), knowing the limitations of the research literature with reference to populations investigated and outcome assessments used.

Much research has been performed to identify predictors of recovery for arm and walking function for a variety of neurological diagnoses. For example, as early as 72 hours after ischaemic stroke, slight shoulder abduction and minimal digit extension predicts good arm recovery (Kwah & Herbert 2016, Nijland et al 2010). Ambulation recovery after ischaemic stroke has also been linked to early static sitting attainment in the acute hospital setting (Kwah & Herbert 2016, Verheyden et al 2006) and Berg Balance Scale scores on admission in the inpatient rehabilitation setting (Louie & Eng 2018). Predictors for ambulation recovery after nontraumatic and traumatic spinal cord injuries using key lower extremity muscle grades from the American Spinal Cord Injury Association Impairment Scale along with age and sensation sparing have yielded promising results (AlHuthaifi et al 2017, Jean et al 2021, Sturt 2020).

Prediction is never 100% accurate, and there will always be those patients who defy the odds. However, having this knowledge allows us to express optimism to those patients who exhibit the positive predictors. It also encourages us to intervene to promote the exhibition of these motor responses, and thereby enhance recovery. Thus, EBP requires therapists to know and use the prediction literature to influence their assessments and interventions. Prediction of outcomes will lead to clearer patient expectations and better selection of interventions (Kimberley et al 2017). All EBP practitioners must be aware of the limitations of prediction models with respect to the patient populations not investigated in the original studies and the outcome measures used to assess recovery.

Principle 5: Neural Plasticity

Advances in neuroimaging have confirmed that plasticity (defined as enduring changes in structure, function and connections) does occur after damage to the central nervous system as a result of experience and therapy. Spontaneous recovery is now understood to be a period of heightened neural plasticity that is occurring both through depression of contralesional corticospinal activity and enhancement of ipsilesional corticospinal activity (Hordacre et al 2021, McDonnell & Stinear 2017). The brain responds to injury by adaptation aimed at restoring function. Thus, cortical maps can be modified by a variety of inputs, such as sensory inputs, experience, learning and therapy, as well as in response to injury (Nudo et al 2013). This is also the case after incomplete spinal cord injury (Brown & Martinez, 2019; Mount & Monje 2017). Rehabilitation is likely to be most effective when principles of neuroplasticity are considered (see Principles of Neuroplasticity for Clinicians box).

PRINCIPLES OF NEUROPLASTICITY FOR CLINICIANS (FROM HORDACRE & MCCAMBRIDGE, 2018 WITH PERMISSION)

- Neuroplasticity is use dependent and specific.
- Repetition (practice) and greater intensity induce neural changes.
- Neuroplasticity is time sensitive; early intervention may be better.
- Neuroplasticity is influenced by salience, motivation, feedback and attention.
- Neuroplasticity is strongly influenced by features of the environment.
- Enhanced sensory, cognitive, motor and social stimulation facilitate increased neuroplasticity and learning (Nithianantharajah & Hannan 2006).
- Adjunct therapies prime the motor system to facilitate greater neuroplastic response (Ackerley et al 2014, Byblow et al 2012) [e.g., mirror therapy (Deconinck et al 2015), aerobic exercise before intervention (El-Sayes et al 2019, Ploughman & Kelly 2016)].
- Neuroplasticity is influenced by patient characteristics such as age, genetics and stress levels (Ploughman & Kelly 2016).
- Pharmacology influences neuroplasticity.

What Type of Training Drives Neural Plasticity and Recovery of Function?

Task-specific training facilitates functional and neural plasticity (Dayan & Cohen 2011, Dobkin et al 2004, Hornby et al 2016, Livingston-Thomas et al 2016). Task-specific training should be relevant to the patient and to the context (Hubbard et al 2009). When patients practice tasks that are meaningful, their focus is on achieving success of the task. It is the therapist's expertise that structures the task in such a way as to get the movements they wish to encourage and to have the task be challenging yet achievable to enhance self-efficacy, but also varied enough to encourage generalisation. This environmental enrichment/experience dependency allows for the practice of actual tasks, which enhances positive transfer of training principles both on a musculoskeletal level and by repetitively activating pathways that are engaged in the activity being practiced (Dayan & Cohen 2011, Dean & Shepherd 1997, Dean et al 2000, Dobkin et al 2004). In the spinal cord injury literature, the proposed mechanism for plasticity brought about through body weight support (BWS) downhill treadmill walking is thought to be through activity-dependent myelination via the oligo-dendrocytes (Hordacre et al 2021, Fields 2015, Mount and Monje 2017).

Activity-dependent aerobic exercise enhances neural plasticity by increasing blood flow to the brain, facilitating the release of neurotrophic factors (e.g., brain-derived neurotrophic factor) and improving brain health (brain volume) (Griffin & Bradke 2020, Ploughman & Kelly 2016). A minimum of 30 minutes of moderate intensity aerobic exercise has been associated with neurotrophic factor release (Ploughman & Kelly 2016). A variety of individuals with neurological diseases have been shown to lack aerobic conditioning as a result of either their impairments interfering in physical activity or adoption of a sedentary lifestyle (Brazzelli et al 2012, English et al 2016). This puts them at risk for further comorbidities, including hypertension, diabetes mellitus and stroke. Thus, activity-dependent aerobic conditioning should be part of every patient's programme for reasons beyond increasing exercise capacity (Ploughman & Kelly 2016). The recent clinical practice guideline on improving locomotor function following chronic stroke and incomplete spinal cord injury found strong evidence supporting the implementation of a moderate to high intensity walking programme (>60% heart rate [HR] reserve or 70% HR_{max}) (Hornby et al 2020).

Actively engaging patients in problem solving when relearning motor tasks also influences neural plasticity. Enhancement and diminution of neural activation within the brain is dependent on the stage of skill acquisition (Dayan & Cohen 2011). The early stage of learning has shown enhanced excitation of multiple regions of the brain, including cerebellum and visual and prefrontal cortices, where the learner is identifying the relevant features of the task to pay attention to and attempting to organise a movement pattern that is successful at accomplishing the goal. During the later stage of skill acquisition, there is a diminution of activity in the aforementioned areas and an

enhancement in the motor cortices, where the learner is modifying the successful movements to become efficient and less effortful. There is recent behavioural evidence to support actively engaging patients in ambulation training with increasing task difficulty that induces errors during walking practice. These investigations have been shown to generalise to better upright dynamic balance and reduced fall risk (Mansfield et al 2018).

Most behavioural studies on early versus later intervention after stroke have supported early intervention (Liu et al 2014, Momosaki et al 2016). Emerging neurophysiological evidence in humans supports this critical time period for rehabilitation poststroke, where early intervention promotes greater functional gains (Hordacre et al 2021, McDonnell et al 2015). The 2- to 4-week window after stroke demonstrated the period of greatest neural plasticity, which then declined over the next 6 months. Thus, it is also important to consider when best to deliver rehabilitation to maximise any critical time windows to promote neural plasticity and to optimise functional recovery.

A current clinical practice model whereby all the neuroplasticity principles are put into clinical practice is the use of variable high intensity early walking task practice after stroke. Hornby and colleagues have successfully used the converging evidence from both the neuroplasticity and motor learning literature to promote walking recovery after stroke as measured by walking speeds (self-selected and fast) and 6-minute walk distance (Hornby et al 2016, Hornby et al 2020).

Principle 6: Motor Control: A Systems Model

Motor control is an area of science that explores how the nervous system interacts with other body parts and the environment to produce purposeful, coordinated actions (Muratori et al 2013); thus, it is critical for therapists involved in neurorehabilitation to understand how different systems within the nervous system interact to produce movement and perform tasks. For example, when patients are learning to dress themselves, they must use the movement they can reproduce in terms of personal available range, strength, pain level, and so on, as well as their cognitive ability to plan the task alongside external factors in the environment, for example, bed surface, clothing type and location and environmental distractors, to perform the functional task.

There are many different models of motor control. A dynamic systems theory (synonymous names – systems theory, dynamic action theory) considers that solutions to patient problems change according to the interaction between the individual, the task and the environment (Shumway-Cook et al 2022, pp. 11–17). Although it is important to understand the role of major circuits and pathways of the central nervous system, the effects of lesions on these structures and circuits, and how the many subsystems and multiple connections within the nervous system work in hierarchy and in parallel to generate movement, the nervous system is not the only contributor to the movement. The body is a mechanical system operating in a physical world, so the biomechanical factors affecting a multijointed system and the external environment (e.g., gravity, friction, object distance and orientation) also play a role in the ultimate executed movement. Finally, the individual's goal or intention plays a role in shaping the outcome as well. Thus, it is important to understand that movement emerges from the interaction of the individual's systems (intentions, biomechanical and neuromotor processes) with their environment to successfully accomplish a task (Shumway-Cook et al 2022, pp. 30–34). This means in clinical practice it is essential to work on functional tasks rather than mainly focusing on movement patterns to improve quality of movement and recognising that the both the patient and the external environmental setup of the tasks need to be factored into the functional task practice.

The actions of a person with damage to the nervous system are the result of an individual's best effort at that time to organise a movement to achieve a successful task (A.M. Gentile 1991, personal communication). It is a consequence of the impairments caused by the damage, the compensatory strategies that enable function to be achieved in the presence of impairments, the effects of the environment the person has been experiencing since the lesion and the person's confidence in their ability to achieve success (Shumway-Cook et al 2022, pp. 11–17). Scapular elevation with shoulder abduction and trunk lateral flexion is an example of a compensatory strategy that may be seen in a patient after a stroke performing a seated reaching task to an anterior target. Because of weakness in the scapulohumeral complex, this stereotypical compensatory movement may be effective in accomplishing the reaching task because it is available to the individual at that time. The therapist can promote recovery of reaching ability with flexible movement pattern development by altering the task constraints to facilitate emergence of other movement solutions. If the reach task is now performed at elbow height while providing forearm support and adjusting the target location to a position that requires shoulder abduction and external rotation, the therapist is considering the individual's biomechanical and neural constraints by altering the environmental constraints. The individual is practicing reaching to objects (functional task) with more flexible movement pattern development while also working on weakness of the scapulohumeral complex.

The key points to remember when designing therapy programmes are that therapists can reduce impairments and compensatory movement strategies by promoting functional recovery and return to participation. This can occur through structuring the environment or the task in a way that enables the patient to elicit or practice both the desired movement and the tasks required to achieve their goals. As previously stated, changes to the task instruction and increasing a person's confidence can also enhance goal attainment.

Principle 7: Functional Movement Reeducation

Normative data for everyday activities help therapists to understand motor performance and the impact of impairments on these everyday activities (Carr & Shepherd 2006; see Chapter 4 for an overview of how therapists observe and analyse movement). Therapists place an emphasis on training control of muscles and promoting learning of relevant actions and tasks. Therapists aim to optimise movement and function; however, with the majority of neurological conditions, recovery of normal movement and function is not achievable for many patients; this depends to some extent on whether the patient has a progressive, deteriorating condition or a stable condition (Edwards 2002, p. 256).

One of the key roles of the therapist working in neurology is to help the patient experience and relearn optimal movement and function in everyday life within the constraints imposed by the disease process and presenting impairments. Therapists are not only interested in which functional activities patients can or cannot perform but also in how the patient moves (the quality of movement) to execute these activities in order to optimise movement. The aims of neurological physiotherapy can be summed up using the acronym RAMP — recovery, adaptation, maintenance and prevention.

Therapists ideally aim to restore movement and function in people with neurological pathology, but this may not always be possible. Adaptation (compensation) refers to the use of alternative movement strategies to complete a task, that is, performing an old movement in a new way (Levin et al 2009). For many patients with degenerative and progressive neurological disorders, adaptation is critical to living well with their disorder. When restoring movement is a possibility, therapists may focus on promoting compensatory strategies that are necessary for function and discouraging those that may be detrimental to the patient, for example, promoting musculoskeletal damage such as knee hyperextension (Levin et al 2009). Interventions aimed at recovery of function need to be emphasised over compensation if the patient has the potential to change. Maintenance of function is just as important as recovery and should be viewed as a positive achievement; several reviews have now confirmed that functional ability can be maintained despite deteriorating impairments in progressive neurological disease (Keus et al 2014). However, in progressive diseases, therapists may focus on goals of maintaining activities longer term and problem-solving strategies to facilitate adaptation. Maintaining physical function is not possible if a condition declines in its natural history, and therapists need to be wary of setting unrealistic expectations that can have a detrimental effect on the person's psyche if they consider decline a personal failure (Ramdharry & Andersson 2022).

Therapy also aims to prevent the development of complications such as sedentary behaviour/physical inactivity, contracture, swelling and disuse atrophy. There are different stages in patient management, where these aims may have differential priorities. Understanding the nature of the pathology and the prognosis for recovery in collaboration with patients and caregivers to establish desired goals will help determine which of these aims should be emphasised in physical interventions.

Therapists use an array of techniques in their tool kit to optimise movement. It is always preferable to prioritise the practice of functional activities selected in collaboration with the patient; however, if the patient has impairments that make it difficult to practice these tasks directly, therapists also need to address impairments or practice specific movements either before or during a modified version of functional task practice. For example, a patient may not have any signs of motor activity in the lower limb to practice the task of walking. In this case, the patient may require either hands-on assistance from therapists or support from assistive technologies, for example, a partial body weight system to practice the task of walking.

Principle 8: Skill Acquisition

Evidence from motor learning and skill acquisition can provide some guiding principles about how to structure practice within therapy sessions to improve these aspects of skilled performance (Marley et al 2000, Muratori et al 2013, Winstein et al 2014). Both Fitts & Posner's theory and Bernstein's theory of motor skill learning can be divided into three phases: an early phase, an intermediate associative or advanced phase and an autonomous or expert phase (Bernstein 1967 and Fitts & Posner 1967, cited in Shumway-Cook et al 2022, pp. 30–32). When subjects are in the early stage of learning, individuals should be encouraged to actively explore the environment through trial and error. It is a cognitive heavy phase, where the subject is figuring out what are the important things in the environment to attend to, how to plan a movement and then execute a movement that emphasises controlling the body's degrees of freedom to successfully accomplish the task. During this early phase, movement strategies such as freezing of the limbs and cocontraction of agonist and antagonist muscles may be seen (Guimaraes et al 2020). In the intermediate

associative or advanced phase, the learner has gained some control over what makes for a successful solution and has begun to allow for more joints to move during movement execution. However, errors are still notable during this phase. Consistency in goal attainment and efficiency of movements are accomplished in the autonomous or expert phase. Here the well-learned task no longer requires the cognitive focus of 'what to do' to accomplish the task. The emphasis is on refining the movement solution(s) to accomplish the task consistently. (Schmidt & Lee 2005, pp. 357–383). Some tips for structuring therapy sessions are outlined in Table 1.2.

When working with individuals with neurological disorders, principles of motor learning cannot be separated from those of neural plasticity because learning is a stage-related process that simultaneously yields changes in neuromotor processes as well. Thus, physical therapists promoting recovery in their patients must seek to use the principles that promote both learning and plasticity. Maier and colleagues have expanded their initial meta-analysis (2019a) where motor learning principles used in neurorehabilitative literature were identified to include an analysis and expansion of these principles (2019b). In the following section, a consensus on the motor learning principles that all therapists should use to promote motor learning is discussed.

Intrinsic Motivation and Attentional Focus

Wulf and Lewthwaite (2016), through their 'Optimal Theory of Motor Learning,' provide a template by which enhanced learning may be achieved in individuals. The theory proposes that optimising the intrinsic motivation of the learner and providing verbal cues to enhance the attentional focus of the learner enhances learning on multiple levels of analysis: (1) enhance the learner's expectation, (2) enhance the learner's autonomy and (3) provide an external focus of attention for the learner.

To enhance the learner's expectation and increase their confidence level, the therapist must find ways that reinforce the learner's ability to achieve success. By providing positive feedback, confidence levels are increased, thereby creating the learner's expectation that they will achieve success (self-efficacy). Both achieving success and the patient's perception on this success are associated with dopamine release in the brain (Schultz 2013). Dopaminergic systems are involved in motor, cognitive and motivational functioning (Nieoullon & Coquerel 2003). Ways to enact this in the clinic are:

1. Provide feedback after good trials, e.g., 'That was a good one,' 'Do that again.'
2. Reduce perceived task difficulty: Define success liberally so the criterion for a successful performance is not too difficult.

TABLE 1.2 Key Motor Learning Variables for Neurological Rehabilitation

Key Variables	Issues to Consider (adapted mainly from Muratori et al 2013, Winstein et al 2014, Wulf & Lewthwaite 2016)
Practice	• Amount (intensity or dose) (Hornby et al 2016, Kwakkel 2006, Lang et al 2015) • Frequency (number of repetitions) • Duration (number of minutes per session) • Variety (alter regulatory features) (Gentile 2000), e.g., transfers from different height chairs and different surface types • Practice schedule (e.g., blocked practice, five reps at each seat height) versus random practice (e.g., different seat heights each time) (Gilmore & Spaulding 2001, Muratori et al 2013) • Choosing the practice schedule depends on a number of patient-centred issues such as experience, age, memory and task. However, there are insufficient data on which sequence works best for which patient (Boyd & Winstein 2001, Muratori et al 2013, Wulf & Lewthwaite 2016)
Specificity of training	• Functional task practice must be both task and context specific; therefore, whenever possible, practice the task (Kwakkel et al 2006, Verbeek et al 2014) • Consider critical requirements for each task (Carr & Shepherd 2003), as well as the impairments being targeted (Muratori et al 2013, Winstein et al 2014)
Transfer of training (generalisability)	• Impairment-focused training such as strength, range, symmetry and postural sway may improve the parameters being trained, but these changes do not generalise to the activity or participation level (Kwakkel et al 2004, Muratori et al 2013, Verbeek et al 2014) • Consider two types of transfer of training (Winstein 1991): (a) part task training: break the task down into simple steps, then put the steps back together again by practising the whole task; and (b) adaptive training: simplify the task by controlling a particularly difficult part, e.g., using a body weight support system that gradually adds the body weight into gait • Task-related practice: some transferability will occur to a task which incorporates the components of transferring the centre of mass from the trunk to the lower extremities (e.g., practice of reaching greater than arm's length in sitting transfers to the sit to stand transitional activity) (Dean & Shepherd 1997, Dean et al 2000).
Feedback	• Frequency (How often? All or some of the time?) Do not give feedback on every trial (Muratori et al 2013, Winstein 1994) • Timing (when to deliver the information: before, during or after?) • Delivery mode (visual, verbal, manual) • Consider using extrinsic feedback or feedback with an external focus (Wulf 2013); e.g., for a sit-to-stand task, the focus should be on 'pushing into the floor' rather than 'push your feet into the floor' or 'stand tall' rather than 'straighten your spine/back'
Modelling	• Demonstrate what you want the patient to do • Consider delivery mode, e.g., live versus videotaped versus written instruction (Reo & Mercer 2004, Laguna 2000, Williams & Hodges 2004, pp. 145–174)

TABLE 1.2	**Key Motor Learning Variables for Neurological Rehabilitation**—Cont'd
Key Variables	**Issues to Consider (adapted mainly from Muratori et al 2013, Winstein et al 2014, Wulf & Lewthwaite 2016)**
Mental practice	• Defined as the act of repeating imagined movements several times with the intention of improving motor performance (Jackson et al 2001); an adjunct to physical practice, it is not better than physical practice (Braun et al 2006, Malouin & Richards 2010, Nilsen et al 2010) • Consider when to use it, e.g., when patient needs additional personnel to set up environment for independent practice, during rest periods or when patient is not safe to practice independently • Reference point for imaging – 'seeing' themselves or 'feeling' themselves (Nilsen et al 2010)

3. Alleviate the learner's concerns.
4. When using self-modelling, show their best performance.

The learning literature supports enhancing learner autonomy. Allowing the patient to have choices, even if these choices are incidental, has a positive effect on learning. Using autonomy-supported language (e.g., 'I've placed you in the parallel bars for this balance activity; if you wish to use the rail to stabilise yourself after a loss of balance, you may' [even though the therapist knows that if a loss of balance occurs, the patient will most likely reach for the rail]. 'Here is your cane; you may place it wherever you wish while we work on this activity.') and linking the environmental effect with the learner's intention to produce it has been shown to enhance learning (Sanli et al 2013).

Most of Wulf's (2013) research on attentional focus during learning of motor skills has supported an external focus of attention to achieve the desired movement result rather than an internal focus on body movements regardless of the phase of learning that the learner is in. Cues should be as external from the person as possible (e.g., for a golf swing, focus on club tip swing, not the arms/body; for a sit-to-stand task, the focus should be on 'pushing into the floor' rather than 'push your feet into the floor' and 'stand tall' rather than 'straighten your spine/back'). The movement patterns that emerge from using an external focus have been shown to be smoother, more coordinated and achieve success earlier when compared with those using an internal focus. Wording of instructions for an external focus requires a change from what is most often used by therapists and may present a difficult challenge.

Task Practice Issues

Task-specific or task-oriented practice is an approach to rehabilitation that focuses on performance of functional tasks that are meaningful to the individual and arise from the patient's specific goals. For this type of practice to be successful, a therapist must be able to accurately assess their patient and identify their strengths, limitations and deficits. The therapist then alters the task (e.g., simplifying) and/or the environment to allow for repetitive successful practice while achieving the task and reducing the impairment(s). The task difficulty is progressed as the patient's success increases. Both the initial task alteration and the progression are done on an individual basis. Movement errors are permissible as long as flexible movement patterns are observed and the safety of the patient is not compromised.

Different techniques may work better with different patients; sometimes it will be necessary to practice the components of movement that comprise an activity, such as pelvic tilting, before placement in the functional activity. Sometimes it will work best to break tasks down and repeatedly practice the different temporal sequences before getting the patient to practice the whole sequence of activity in a functional task, such as getting the legs off the bed before elevating the trunk in a supine-to-sit task or scooting forward in the chair before attempting to stand up. This is an example of a transfer of training variable referred to as part–whole practice. Carr and Shepherd (2010) recommend that for successful transfer of the part into the whole task, the patient must understand how the piece fits into the whole task and the whole task must be practiced in conjunction with the part (e.g., temporal sequence or interspersed with the part practice).

On other occasions, it may work best to practice the functional task in its entirety by simplifying the task. If the patient is unable to assume standing from a standard height chair (19 inches), increasing the seat height (22 inches) may enable the practice without the therapist's physical assistance, or the compensatory shift of the body weight onto the stronger leg. This is an example of adaptive transfer of training.

Role of Feedback

Feedback is defined as augmented information produced by an external source, not an inherent part of the task. Feedback's uses are many; it can motivate the performer, orient the learner to the goal, control the degrees of freedom for the patient and provide information to the learner about their performance so they can improve the next attempt. Stanton and colleagues (2015) demonstrated that most of the physical therapist feedback provided to the patient was of the motivational type. Feedback can be delivered in many modes (visual, verbal or manual) at various times (prescriptive [before], concurrent [during] or terminal [after]) and in varying quantities from continuous to intermittent fashion (absolute, relative, bandwidth or faded) (Muratori et al 2013, Shumway-Cook et al 2022, pp. 34–35). Feedback can also be categorised into two types: knowledge of results (KR) and knowledge of performance (KP). KR answers the question what was done. It is linked to the behaviour and can be objectively measured (e.g., success, failure, number of errors, time and distance). KP is about how the task was accomplished. It is linked to the movement and can be objectively measured in the clinic by identifying the movement strategies used or the specific errors made (e.g., gait deviations). Most often therapists provide feedback to their patients using their clinical observation skills. For example, a patient is performing a sit-to-stand activity and does not flex forward enough during the flexion momentum phase of the task, which causes the patient during the extension phase of standing to lose their balance and fall back into the chair. Providing feedback relating to the inadequate trunk/hip flexion should occur. This is an example of terminal KP feedback.

Certain modes and amounts of feedback may be beneficial at different points in skill acquisition. For example, manual guidance, an example of controlling the degrees of freedom, should mainly be used at the early cognitive stage of motor learning, especially when safety is a concern, to give the patient the idea of the movement or to control a degree of freedom. However, during the later associative and autonomous stages of skill acquisition, it is preferable for the learner to actively problem solve without relying on the therapist for feedback (Schmidt & Lee 2005, pp. 357–383, Sidaway et al 2008). Fading the amount of feedback as the learning process occurs is particularly common when working with individuals with neurological disorders.

Amount of Practice

Both type of practice (e.g., what the patient does) and amount of practice (e.g., performing many repetitions) are important. Using the evidence to prescribe the most appropriate dose of task-specific practice for individual patients is a challenge because the literature is replete with confounding factors: controlling for repetitions or duration of practice, timing post injury of the study, recovery level of the study subjects and function being studied (Maier et al. 2019a; Maier et al. 2019b). Amount has been quantified as the *number of repetitions* or the *number of minutes of active therapy*. Early research suggested the critical amount of task-specific practice required for meaningful upper extremity recovery was largely based on the constraint-induced movement therapy (CIMT) literature, which used a massed practice paradigm of 6 hours of therapy a day over an intensive 2-week period (Kwakkel et al 2015). The general consensus was that more was better. However, some recent studies have indicated that timing may interact with dose (Bernhardt et al 2015); for example, more therapy *may not* be better in the first few hours and days after stroke and *could* lead to slower recovery. The VECTORS study (Dromerick et al 2009) demonstrated that an increased dose of CIMT during acute inpatient rehabilitation was less effective when compared with a lesser dosage or conventional therapy. Lang et al (2016) showed that gains in upper limb function did not improve as a function of dose for task-specific therapy in patients, beginning 6 months or more poststroke. Current best practice suggests a dosage threshold may be required with a minimum of 300–400 repetitions of upper extremity actions or tasks per session to demonstrate gains (Birkenmeier et al 2010, Dean & Shepherd 1997), or 90 hours across 3 weeks to demonstrate clinically meaningful gains (Ward et al 2019), and a minimum of 30 minutes of walking practice over 12 sessions at moderate to high intensities is needed improve gait in stroke survivors (Hornby et al 2020). Remember to enhance neuroplastic changes and promote brain-derived neurotrophic factor release, a minimum of 20 minutes of moderate intensity aerobic training three times per week for 3 months is recommended (El-Sayes et al 2019, Ploughman & Kelly 2016).

Variable Practice

The variability of practice hypothesis states that variable practice is better than constant practice. It leads to greater flexibility in the motor plan development and allows for greater transferability and generalisation (Shumway-Cook et al 2022, Chapter 2, p 36-37). In the healthy adult population, practicing variable tasks has yielded better learning as measured by retention and transfer tasks (Shumway-Cook et al 2022, Chapter 2, p 36-37). Variable task practice has also been used successfully in investigations with neurological populations, but always in conjunction with other learning principles (Hornby et al 2016). Questions to answer when using variable practice with a patient population are:

1. Will you provide the variable tasks in a blocked (e.g., all of one variation before you move onto another variation of the task) or random order (e.g., deliver the variations

in a mixed-up order)? This may be related to the memory capabilities of the patient and their cognitive development/cognitive ability. A random practice schedule has been advocated but may not always be better.
2. How similar or dissimilar are the tasks that you are having the patient practice? You can change an environmental feature of task (e.g., using chairs of different heights for sit-to-stand practice) or have a variety of similar tasks (e.g., various locomotion tasks).

Modelling/Action–Observation

Modelling or action–observation is the use of observation in learning a motor skill. When using modelling to enhance motor skill acquisition, it is important to show the whole body even if you want to focus on a particular segment or joint (Scully & Newell 1985). It is also important to choose the best viewing angle (McCullagh et al 1989) for the demonstration. From the literature, a meta-analysis elucidating the types of tasks and outcome measures amenable to the positive effects of demonstration in the healthy population (Ashford et al 2006) can be applied when working with a neurological population. The correct movement strategy must be visible to the patient while observing the whole task, irrespective of whether that task is a discrete, serial or continuous task. Demonstrations are used to acquire movement patterns, so outcome measures should include measures of movement outcomes (e.g., accuracy, speed) and movement dynamics (e.g., gait deviations, kinematic analysis). Physical practice should be interspersed with the demonstrations. Therapists frequently accompany their verbal instructions to patients by demonstration of the task they wish the patient to practice. Functional magnetic resonance imaging (fMRI) research on movement observation has shown similar activations of premotor and parietal areas noted during movement execution (Hardwick 2018). An early study by Ertelt and colleagues (2007) supported the hypothesis that action–observation with physical practice was more effective in upper limb recovery than the conventional practice group for the Wolf Motor Function Test (WMFT), the Frenchay Arm Test (FAT), the Stroke Impact Scale (SIS) and increased cerebral activation in the fMRI data.

Mental Practice

The imagining of a motor task without its execution is motor imagery, and mental practice is the symbolic repetition or rehearsal of the imagined motor task. The neurophysiological evidence supports similar brain activations during imagined and actual movements (subcortical, premotor and somatosensory areas, cingulate gyrus) (Hardwick 2018). Mental practice should be interspersed with actual physical practice. Using mental practice to

increase practice time during a therapeutic session (e.g., when the patient is resting) or outside of therapy (e.g., when it is not safe for the patient to practice the task on their own) should be encouraged. Systematic reviews of the mental practice literature for upper extremity (Nilsen et al 2010) and walking recovery (Malouin & Richards 2010) have explored the ratio of physical to mental practice and examined the mental practice perspective (kinesthetic/feeling themselves versus visual/seeing themselves).

Principle 9: Exercise Prescription

Whether the aim is to improve cardiorespiratory (aerobic) endurance, muscular fitness or flexibility, all therapists prescribe exercise for their patients with neurological disorders. It is imperative that therapists follow the general principles put forth by the American College of Sports Medicine (ACSM) when working with their patients who have neurological disorders (ACSM's Guidelines for Exercise Testing & Prescription 2021, Chapter 6). The FITT principle (frequency, intensity, time, type) can guide healthcare professionals to prescribe appropriate exercise in rehabilitation (Billinger et al 2015). However, the literature suggests these FITT principles are underused, incomplete and inconsistently reported by rehabilitation professionals (Amman et al 2014). Therapists should pay more attention to using all components of the FITT principle when prescribing and promoting exercise in neurological rehabilitation. However, this is not often the case. In a review of therapeutic interventions to enhance the aerobic capacity or strength of patients with inflammatory myopathies, Baschung Pfister and colleagues (2015) found that only half of the studies included in their review indicated progression and overload principles. In a survey exploring barriers to promoting aerobic exercise in their patients, physical therapists identified knowledge gaps not only in the ACSM guidelines for exercise prescription but also in safe delivery skills for this population (Moncion et al 2020).

Assuming that the exercises are functional in nature, the challenge becomes clear when working with individuals who cannot perform these functional activities independently (e.g., locomotion, reach and grasping, sit to stand and standing activities). The therapist must answer the following questions:
1. What adaptation(s) are required to allow their patient to perform the functional task exercise safely and yet be sufficiently challenging to the muscular or cardiovascular system? (e.g., when working on locomotion use, an overhead harness system to reduce the load through the weakened legs and prevent falls).
2. How should their patient perform this functional task exercise while following the guidelines for aerobic exercise prescription (frequency, intensity, exercise time, type, exercise volume and rate of progression)? (e.g.,

when working on locomotion with the overhead harness system, the duration of exercise should be a minimum of 30 minutes of moderate level activity; however, this may require 10 minute interval bouts of exercise with accompanying rest periods).

3. How should their patient perform this functional task exercise while following the guidelines to improve muscular fitness (resistance frequency, type, sets and reps, exercise technique and progression/maintenance) (e.g., when working on the seated reach task that was modified in the earlier motor control section, the number of repetitions should be between 8 and 12 per set with an aim of three sets for each location. Initially the load of the limb is sufficient resistance. The patient may progress to being able to perform these repetitions with an additional load [resistance band or cuff weight] placed around the forearm or reaching further distances [increasing the load at the shoulder by the longer lever arm] or heights [>90° after scapular and shoulder muscles >3/5 strength]. However, the exercise stops when the therapist observes changes that are associated with muscle fatigue).

4. It is not uncommon for patients with neurological disorders to also have other comorbidities (e.g., diabetes mellitus, hypertension or coronary artery disease) that require specific exercise prescription modification (ACSM Guidelines 2021, Chapters 9 & 10). How should the therapist incorporate these disease limitations as well into their patient's exercise prescription, modification and monitoring? (e.g., the patient has atrial fibrillation and their medication blocks heart rate response to aerobic exercise). The Borg rate of perceived exertion scale can be used, along with monitoring for any breakthrough cardiac arrythmias, and blood pressure monitoring with clear maximum parameters for both systolic and diastolic pressures should be incorporated.

The final challenge for therapists when prescribing exercises for their patients is knowing when to modify. Is something too hard? Then it needs to be made easier by regression. Is something too easy? Then it needs to be progressed. Here again, we must use the learning literature to guide us in recognising which should occur. If an individual is in the early stages of skill acquisition, you will see errors, and it will take the patient longer to initiate and execute the solution. However, these errors need to be accompanied by some successes. If there are only failures in the repetition set, then it is too hard. The patient runs the risk of losing confidence or self-efficacy in their ability to attain the skill. The opposite is true for the patient who performs all the repetitions easily without any errors. Now it is too easy, and the exercise should be progressed. The therapist is looking to work the patient in the middle phase of learning, where

it is challenging but not overwhelming, where success is occurring more often, and the patient is gaining control over what is to be done and the degrees of freedom to do it.

Principle 10: Health Promotion

Promoting health is of critical importance to the field of neurological rehabilitation. The WHO (2017) has emphasised that accessible and affordable rehabilitation plays a fundamental role in ensuring healthy lives and promoting well-being for all ages (sustainable development goal). Promoting health can be considered on three levels: primary, secondary and tertiary prevention. Primary prevention seeks to prevent the onset of disease through healthy living. It is achieved by health education, lifestyle and behavioural changes. Secondary prevention aims to stop or slow disease progression and prevent complications through early diagnosis and adequate treatment. Tertiary prevention is focused on reducing impairments and activity restrictions. All members of the rehabilitation team have a role to play in enabling people to return towards meaningful roles in the wider community with a focus on health and wellness, rather than a focus mainly on ill health and disability (Cott et al 2007, Dean 2009). Ultimately this means that rehabilitation involves changing behaviour.

Neurological rehabilitation has to date focused on tertiary prevention, delivering short bursts of physical therapies to restore function after acute events or declines in function resulting in a loss of the initial gains, resumption of sedentary lifestyles and worsening levels of disability over time (Ellis & Motyl 2013). The goals of physical interventions must extend beyond impairments and function to include health promotion with an emphasis on physical activity and exercise. There is growing evidence that rehabilitation can prevent secondary complications if we intervene early to delay onset of motor symptoms in progressive disease (Kimberley et al 2017).

Physical therapists should encourage fitness through participation in enjoyable activities that follow ACSM guidelines for regular physical activity and exercise (see Chapter 22 on physical activity for further guidance). Diseases like hypertension and diabetes mellitus may be prevented (1° prevention) or if present may be controlled (2° prevention) through regular exercise, thus preventing other diseases (stroke or heart attack). For instance, in the event of a stroke, the medical team will use 2° prevention measures to stop or slow the progression of the stroke (e.g., give tissue plasminogen activator for ischemic stroke if in time window, remove blood for intracerebral hemorrhage) and to prevent a recurrence (e.g., lower blood pressure, correct cardiac arrhythmias). Physical therapists are well equipped to promote health and participation across all levels of prevention through identifying, modifying and encouraging appropriate enjoyable exercises and physical activities for patients.

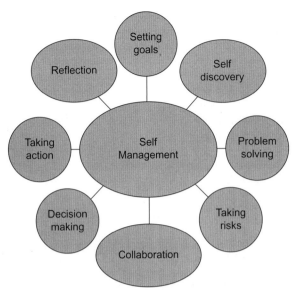

FIG. 1.3 Key components involved in effective self-management. (Adapted from Jones & Leggat 2023)

TABLE 1.3	Key Components of Self-Management (based on Chapter 19 by Jones & Leggat with permission)
Problem solving by the patient	• Deciding on the problem • Breaking it down into small steps • Thinking of various solutions • Selecting a course of action • Trying out the action or strategy • Evaluating success • Choosing an alternative action if necessary
Target or goal setting	• Translating thoughts into actions • Providing mastery experiences
Resource utilisation	• Accessing local self-help group • Seeking expert advice • Using friends or family for support
Collaboration	• Working together with a healthcare professional • Sharing expertise

Principle 11: Self-Management

A report by National Health Service England (2016) defines self-management as 'any form of formal education or training for people with long-term conditions that focuses on helping people to develop the knowledge, skills and confidence to manage their own health and care effectively.' Self-management is not just about complying with advice of health professionals or following their instructions. The client's motivation for change and ability to cope and adapt to a changed lifestyle following diagnosis with a neurological condition also needs to be considered when developing self-management skills. Other key strategies that health professionals use in rehabilitation are education about the effects of practice and exercise that are relevant to the person, goal setting, identification of possible barriers, problem solving, feedback about performance, tailored instruction, decision making and ongoing personal or social support (Dobkin 2016).

In Chapter 19, Jones and Leggat have outlined the key components involved in effective self-management (Fig. 1.3). They propose that self-management is best defined as 'enhancing a person's knowledge, skills and confidence in their condition through personalised support from a healthcare professional.' These components are highlighted in more detail in Table 1.3.

Self-efficacy is a cornerstone of self-management; it is defined as people's beliefs about their capabilities to influence key events that affect their lives (Bandura 1997). People with a strong sense of efficacy set themselves challenging goals and maintain strong commitment to them; they continue to sustain their efforts in the face of failure or setbacks (Bandura 1997). A review specific to physiotherapy by Barron et al (2007) has shown that self-efficacy can be related to better health, higher achievement, more social integration and higher motivation to act. Growing evidence provides support for the importance of self-efficacy as a correlate of adherence to therapy (Rhodes & Fiala 2009); however, evidence is still emerging regarding the most effective ways of supporting and enabling individuals with neurological problems to manage ways of living with their chronic disability (Jones 2006).

Health professionals need to consider how they can promote self-efficacy and enhance their patients' self-management skills. Tailoring self-management support requires an appreciation of factors that act as barriers to or enablers of behaviour change. Two systematic reviews have found that self-management programmes improve quality of life and self-efficacy for stroke survivors in the community, but further research is required to identify key features of effective programmes (Fryer et al 2016, Lennon et al 2013). The therapist–patient relationship and rehabilitation setting play significant roles in nurturing self-efficacy and motivation in patients (Gangwani et al 2022).

Principle 12: Mindset

Mindset is a critical component of rehabilitation. Mindset refers to the *thoughts, beliefs and expectations* that influence adaptation and recovery on the part of the clients and the health professionals leading to improved mental health (Crum et al 2017). Adopting a positive mindset has been identified as a major determinant of mental health, well-being and self-efficacy in positive psychology and educational psychology research; however, these elements have not yet been widely investigated or adopted in rehabilitation services and disability research (Simpson et al 2021).

The PERMA (Positive emotion, Engagement, Relationships, Meaning and Accomplishment) theory of well-being identifies these five elements required for individuals to flourish (Seligman 2011). Adapting to and coping with living with a chronic illness has the potential to profoundly affect these multiple components of well-being. Health professionals who promote a positive mindset through positive expectations and who facilitate hope can influence both physical and psychological well-being. Traditionally, health professionals have always supported individuals to learn and to gain confidence in dealing with their neurological condition without specifically focusing on embedding critical psychosocial elements into rehabilitation practice. Many clinical guidelines now specifically recommend the promotion of self-efficacy within the rehabilitation process, yet there are many other psychological concepts such as motivation, resilience and hope that merit further exploration as key ingredients critical to optimising recovery and adjustment. Likewise, sociocultural context, environment and client–provider relationship also influence optimal rehabilitation outcomes. The evidence base to support this approach can be found in the sociological, psychological and public health literature. There is growing evidence about the influence of patient mindset and social context on response to healthcare that can improve outcomes (Crum et al 2017). Tools and resources for clients and health professionals are readily accessible via organisations such as Action for Happiness and Smiling Minds, freely available at https://actionforhappiness.org/ and https://www.smilingmind.com.au/.

Mindset, the foundation of all thoughts, behaviours, beliefs and action (Dweck & Yeager 2019), embodies psychological and emotional well-being leading to mental health; therefore, it needs to be embraced as a stand-alone key principle in neurological rehabilitation, although it is also embedded in many other principles, such as person-centred care, team work and self-management. Crum et al (2017) have explored the impact of the placebo response, evoked by people's mindset, which can account for clinically significant benefit in an estimated 60%–90% of various conditions; for example, the physical benefits of exercise may depend on the degree to which someone perceives a specific physical activity to be beneficial. The qualities of the patient–provider relationship, also known as therapeutic alliance, like empathy and understanding, can also produce measurable physiological improvements beyond the effects of actual treatment by boosting patient expectations, lowering anxiety, increasing psychological support and improving patient mood. The way in which health professionals communicate can determine how much or how little an individual will feel consulted and involved in their care. Crum et al (2017) have proposed that the client–provider relationship and the context or environment, rather than being incidental to treatment (e.g., a placebo response), are crucial psychosocial elements in determining clinical outcomes.

'By motivating care teams to recognize patient mindsets that may be hindering health behavior change (such as "this illness is a catastrophe") or medication adherence (such as "this medication is going to cause side effects"), care providers become better equipped to help their patients adopt more useful mindsets (such as "this treatment will work," "this illness is manageable," "my body is capable" and "I am in good hands").'

From Medicine Plus Mindset Training Overview (https://mbl.stanford.edu./)

Motivation

Motivation is closely related to self-efficacy; motivation refers to an individual's will to perform a certain behaviour towards achieving their goal (Gangwani et al 2022). Through interviews with clients in a rehabilitation hospital following stroke, Yoshida et al (2021) have identified seven core factors for influencing motivation in stroke rehabilitation. Clients highlighted that the variation and appropriateness of the exercises, sharing goal setting and understanding the purpose of the exercise positively influenced their motivation. Core factors for motivation in stroke rehabilitation adapted from Yoshida et al (2021) are:

- Patients' goals
- Experiences of success and failure
- Physical condition and cognitive function
- Resilience
- Influence of rehabilitation professionals
- Relationships between patients
- Conversations with patients' supporters

From the provider perspective, a survey of health professionals (n = 362) has identified 15 strategies used by more than 75% of respondents to motivate their patients (Oyake et al, 2020), including active listening, praise, respect for self-determination, control of task difficulty and provision of a goal-oriented practice, as well as also explaining the necessity of practice and exercise (Fig. 1.4).

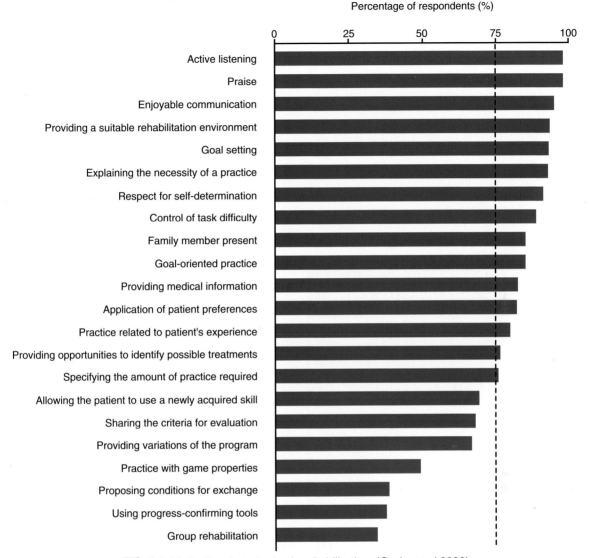

FIG. 1.4 Motivational strategies in rehabilitation. (Oyake et al 2020)

Resilience and Hope

Resilience has been defined as the capacity for successful adaptation despite challenging circumstances (Masten 2018). Hope is defined as the expectation that there will be improvement in the future; hope enables the adaptive coping with adversity involved in resilience. The promotion of optimism, motivation, self-efficacy and interpersonal connectedness can enhance resilience. These psychosocial skills can be integrated into rehabilitation sessions, especially by focusing on how we engage with our patients to deliver therapy, and how our patients engage in their recovery (Rothbart and Sohlberg 2021). However, clinicians require training in developing and coaching these skills, such as motivational interviewing (MI) to promote optimism, enhance self-efficacy and bolster resilience. In MI, practitioners focus on encouraging patients to explore their reasons for behaviour change and help them to develop their own strategies to enable this change (Lundell et al 2013). MI is useful for improving compliance with therapeutic activities and increasing readiness to change (McGrane et al 2015, Medley & Powell 2010).

All members of the rehabilitation team need to acquire knowledge and practice of psychosocial skills to help their clients with neurological conditions to thrive. Improving psychological and emotional well-being should be a common aim, which may require rehabilitation professionals to broaden their focus beyond their discipline (Simpson et al 2021). Health professionals should ensure they are implementing the positive behaviours and mindsets that support these critical psychosocial variables of motivation, resilience and hope. To date there is limited research in health psychology related to neurorehabilitation. A recent perspectives article by Rothbart and Sohlberg (2021) has illustrated how speech and language therapists can intentionally embed resilience and hope into their neurorehabilitation practice (see Strategies for Promoting Resilience and Hope box).

Although a biopsychosocial perspective is supported by physiotherapy practice guidelines and physiotherapists

---

STRATEGIES FOR PROMOTING RESILIENCE AND HOPE (ADAPTED FROM ROTHBART & SOHLBERG 2021)

- Promotion of optimism and acceptance using MI to enable clients to make autonomous choices and identify gains throughout the recovery process.
- Promotion of motivation and self-efficacy using MI to decrease ambivalence about compliance with therapeutic activities and increasing readiness to change.
- Using collaborative goal setting to provide patients with an opportunity to predict and reflect on their performance to improve outcomes.
- Establishing interconnectedness through the development of social support systems and an effective therapeutic alliance to improve patient engagement and adherence.

---

have positive attitudes towards using a variety of psychosocial strategies in practice, barriers such as lack of knowledge, time constraints, role clarity and the need to prioritise biomedical factors over psychosocial factors affect practice behaviours (Driver et al 2017). Many physiotherapists are choosing to incorporate psychosocial strategies such as goal setting, relaxation and positive reinforcement, and only a small percentage are using more advanced strategies such as cognitive behavioural therapy and motivational interviewing (Driver et al 2019a,b).

Engagement can be defined as an increased motivation, attention and active participation in rehabilitation, grounded in and supported by the interaction and relationship between the client and clinician (Danzl et al 2012). Applying principles of active engagement through

concepts such as rapport building, attention, motivation and enriched environments may also yield greater neuroplastic changes and functional outcomes (Danzl et al 2012). The greater the understanding and comprehension that clients have in terms of the rehabilitation process, goals, diagnosis and healing process, the more invested and empowered they will be in their own recovery. It can be viewed as the responsibility of all health professionals to deliver supportive care and promote self-care, as we are in an ideal position to help our clients develop their skill sets and nurture their personal strengths and resources to deal with the challenges of living well with a neurological condition. Adopting a positive mindset as health professionals and fostering a positive mindset in our clients based on the neuroscience of positive psychology for mental health has been well-examined over the past decade, yet to date these ideas have not been widely implemented as a critical ingredient in neurological rehabilitation.

All health professionals can promote lifestyle factors that our clients may need to modify to affect their mental and physical health. A starting point could be for us all to encourage our clients to also take their other MEDS, where M stands for Mood/Mindfulness (promoting a positive mindset and activating the parasympathetic nervous system via breathing techniques), E is for Exercise and physical activity (30 minutes of moderate to high intensity exercise and physical activity), D is for Diet (eating well to reduce inflammation) and S is for Sleep (aiming for 6–8 hours per night), minimising Stress and building Social Support networks.

Principle 13: Behaviour Change

Facilitating behaviour change is critical to our work as healthcare professionals from clinical work to policy change and guideline implementation. The goals of physical interventions must extend beyond impairments and function to include health promotion with an emphasis on physical activity and exercise. However, behaviour change is not only about health promotion, for example, helping our clients to change their behaviours that pose significant health risks; it is also about improving client adherence and engagement within our therapy programmes and on an everyday basis. Behaviour change needs to be embraced as a stand-alone key principle in neurological rehabilitation, although it is also embedded in many other principles, such as functional movement reeducation, skill acquisition, exercise prescription, health promotion, mindset and self-management. As rehabilitation professionals, we have a unique opportunity to enable individuals to manage their symptoms and to develop a range of skills and strategies to live in an optimum way with their neurological condition.

Using behaviour change techniques (BCTs) for habit formation enables us to coach our clients in behaviour change. All health professionals need to feel confident promoting modifiable lifestyle factors, although there will be specific members of the multidisciplinary team who will be required to prescribe, monitor and problem solve these lifestyle factors according to their area of expertise (Casey et al 2018). Understanding behaviour change would seem to be critically important especially related to principles of self-efficacy, mindset and health promotion, for example, getting clients to engage in 30 minutes of moderate to intensive exercise and/or physical activity in compliance with clinical guidelines.

Adherence (synonymous with compliance) is the extent to which patients' behaviours align with the recommendations of healthcare providers regarding education and advice, medication intake, diet observance or lifestyle changes (WHO 2016). There is a sound evidence base for promoting lifestyle changes in people after stroke relating to smoking, body mass index, physical activity, alcohol consumption and diet because these combined factors reduce the risk of ischaemic stroke by up to 80% (Lennon et al 2021). Yet levels of adherence to modifiable lifestyle guidelines remain suboptimal, for example, rates of participation in exercise and physical activity remain low in people after stroke and many other neurological conditions where clients reduce their activity levels and adopt a sedentary lifestyle over time.

Research has highlighted that patient education alone has very little impact on behaviour change. Tailoring interventions to suit our clients requires an appreciation of barriers and enablers of behaviour change and action. Health professionals integrate patient education into their practice, yet they report that they are often unable to prioritise this in their clinical practice because of resource issues (Donkers et al 2020). Behaviour change underpins how our clients cope with and adapt to their new life following diagnosis of a neurological condition. Our clients need to understand not only how they may modify their symptoms but also how to take small steps to work towards achieving their goals. However, behaviour change is hard, especially when engaging in modifying lifestyle factors to promote health and well-being when dealing with a life-changing neurological condition. Some excellent resources on behaviour change can be found at the Centre for Behaviour Change at UCL led by Susan Michie.

The Behaviour Change Wheel (BCW) framework by Michie et al (2011) (see Fig. 1.5) is based on elements from 19 theoretical frameworks of behaviour change centred on three core elements that are needed for a behaviour to occur: Capability, Opportunity and Motivation (see inner circles in the COM-B model). Therapists have always assessed client capability to devise treatment plans that provide opportunities to practice tasks and exercises in a meaningful way. This COM-B model provides a systematic way for us to consider

not only our clients' capabilities but also their potential barriers and enablers of behaviour change that may affect their motivation (Levy et al 2021). Additional 'active' ingredients of rehabilitation intervention for consideration are the BCTs (see middle circle within Fig. 1.5), which work to change these three elements.

Many authors have proposed that using behaviour change theory and including BCTs in the design and implementation of interventions may improve adherence to guidelines and improve participation rates in specific lifestyle factors such as exercise and physical activity (Dobkin 2016, Ellis & Motyl 2013, Hassett et al 2022, Morris et al 2022, Motl et al 2018) (see BCT Strategies box), yet to date these ideas have not been widely implemented in neurological rehabilitation. Evidence is now starting to emerge to design, test and implement interventions based on behaviour change theory and techniques. Hassett et al (2022) are conducting a cluster randomised controlled trial testing the implementation and effectiveness of delivering brief physical activity counselling by physiotherapists across five hospitals within a Sydney health district to promote physical activity. Morris et al 2022 used the BCW framework to design and develop an outdoor 12-week period walking intervention with a friend to increase physical activity after stroke in community dwellers. Adherence to exercise programmes has been shown to be especially challenging after stroke, with between 30% and 50% of patients ceasing their exercise programmes within the first year (Levy et al 2021). Levy et al (2021) have developed a useful clinician guide to promote exercise after stroke based on stroke survivors' experiences of participating in an intensive exercise programme using the BCW framework and the COM-B model.

Key BCTs adapted from Dobkin (2016) and Morris et al (2022)
- Education about the effects of practice and exercise
- Goal setting
- Identification of possible barriers
- Problem solving
- Feedback about performance
- Tailored instruction
- Person-centred decision making
- Ongoing personal or social support

Habit Formation

A change in habits leads to a change in behaviour, and understanding how habit forms can help people change their behaviour in ways that make them happier and healthier. Recent years have seen growing interest among social psychologists in promoting habit formation to encourage people to adopt and maintain actions that are good for their health

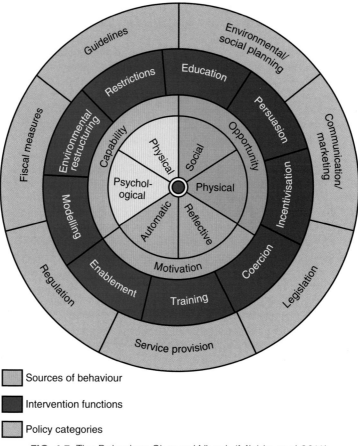

Sources of behaviour

Intervention functions

Policy categories

FIG. 1.5 The Behaviour Change Wheel. (Michie et al 2011)

or well-being (Gardner et al 2022). Changes in motivation, capability or opportunity may be brought about by the individual: forming an intention to take up a new action (e.g., resolving to exercise every morning), which enhances motivation; mobilising self-regulatory resources (e.g., watching instructional exercise videos), which increases the capability to act; or seeking or creating new possibilities for action (e.g., waking up earlier than normal to allow more time to exercise), which boosts opportunity (Gardner et al 2022).

Health professionals can encourage their clients to adopt healthy behaviours by understanding and applying the science underlying habit formation. James Clear, an author and ideas advocate, categorises the creation of all habits (whether good or bad) as a result of the three Rs: Reminder (the cue or trigger that starts the habit), Routine (the action you take), and Reward (the benefits gained). If you are rewarded in some way and have a desire to repeat the action, eventually this action will become a habit (see Strategies for Creating Healthy Habits box).

STRATEGIES FOR CREATING HEALTHY HABITS ADAPTED FROM CLEAR (2018)

1. Decide on a goal.
2. Choose a simple action you can take every day.
3. Plan when and where you will take your action: Choose a time and place that you encounter every day of the week.
4. Every time you encounter that time and place, take the action.
5. Congratulate yourself when you find yourself doing the action.
6. It gets easier with time, and within 10 weeks you should find you are doing it without even thinking. It can take a minimum of 21 days up to 66 days to form a new habit.

BJ Fogg, a behavioural psychologist at Stanford University, has also developed a system to promote healthy habits that fits well with the COM-B model and provides coaching tips to promote healthy habits (Fogg 2019). His model is called the B=MAP model (Change in Behaviour = Motivation, Ability to Do and Prompting) where the client needs to consider:

- Behaviour: What is the behaviour you are trying to start?
- Motivation: What bigger goals in your life is this activity connected to?
- Ability: Are you able to do it?
- Prompt: How will you remind yourself to do this?

Fig. 1.6 illustrates if a habit is hard to do and your motivation is low, prompts from a coach or therapist are unlikely to encourage you to stop a bad habit and create a new habit. Fogg (2019) recommends always starting small (tiny habits) by tagging the new habit you want to develop onto a habit that is already well-established, for example, every time you stand up, practice a few mini squats to improve your sit to stand. This approach of embedding movement moments throughout the day to accumulate 30 minutes of physical activity in small bouts is referred to in the research literature as incidental exercise and is well-suited to people with neurological conditions who suffer from many symptoms such as fatigue, weakness and pain that interfere with their ability to block exercise (Saunders et al 2021).

A habit is a process whereby situational cues automatically trigger an impulse to act (Gardner et al 2022).

Therefore, habit is also an important determinant of behaviour brought about by changes to one or more of the three elements within the COM-B model: motivation, capability and opportunity (Michie et al 2011). Since 2013, there is an emerging body of literature that supports using BCTs to modify lifestyle factors by targeting self-efficacy, outcome expectations, goals, facilitators and barriers. Developing healthy habits and behaviours is critical for people with neurological conditions to live well, yet the science underlying habit formation and behaviour change has yet to be extensively applied in the field of neurological rehabilitation.

CONCLUSION

Health professionals have a key role to play in promoting both mental and physical health. Neurological rehabilitation enables our clients to experience and relearn optimal movement and function in everyday life within the constraints imposed by neurological disease and presenting impairments. Neurophysiological, kinesiological, motor learning and behavioural principles need to be considered in the theoretical framework underlying neurorehabilitation. This chapter has discussed 13 principles to guide current clinical practice in neurorehabilitation: the ICF, team work, patient-centred care, prognosis, neural plasticity, a systems model of motor control, functional movement reeducation, skill acquisition, exercise promotion and prescription, health promotion, self-management (self-efficacy), mindset, and behaviour. The concept of person-centred care is fundamental to ensuring that patient and family preferences and priorities are central to the CR process of the rehabilitation team. Developing an appropriate plan of care revolves around collaborative goal setting with the patient and carers within the interdisciplinary team. This process of goal setting provides a key mechanism for patient-centred care. As well as focusing on the physical activities required to reeducate movement and promote skill acquisition, health professionals need to consider the importance of client mindset in adherence to rehabilitation and engagement in collaborative goal setting for optimal rehabilitation outcomes. Facilitating behavioural change is critical by enhancing self-efficacy and patients' self-management skills. Components selected within therapy sessions should be evidence based rather than based on therapist preference for a specific treatment approach. It is crucial to link clinical practice to quality research, then to ensure that research findings are translated into practice. More research is required to understand which patient responds best to which interventions and to determine optimal dose, intensity and timing. It is crucial to link clinical practice to quality research.

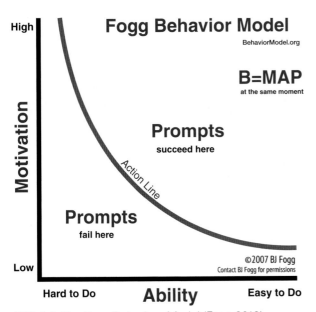

FIG. 1.6 The Fogg Behaviour Model (Fogg 2019)

SELF-ASSESSMENT QUESTIONS

1. How can the ICF enhance clinical reasoning by the rehabilitation team?
2. What factors can improve team work with stroke survivors during rehabilitation?
3. Which eight principles related to person-centred care can improve healthcare and social care services?
4. What are the three principles underlying Wulf and Lewthwaite's 'Optimal Theory of Motor Learning?' Explain with the clinical example of the sit-to-stand task how you would integrate them into practice.
5. When do therapists make predictions about functional recovery for their patients? How is the prediction literature useful for clinicians?
6. What are the three types of prevention for health promotion? Explain how physical therapy can influence both 1° and 2° prevention of some neurological disorders.

REFERENCES

Ackerley, S.J., Stinear, C.M., Barber, P.A., Byblow, W.D., 2014. Priming sensorimotor cortex to enhance task-specific training after subcortical stroke. Clin. Neurophysiol. 125, 1451–1458.

AlHuthaifi, F., Krzak, J., Hanke, T., Vogel, L.C., 2017. Predictors of functional outcomes in adults with traumatic spinal cord injury following inpatient rehabilitation: a systematic review. J. Spinal Cord. Med 40, 282–294.

Amati, M., Grignoli, N., Rubinelli, S., Amann, J., Zanini, C., 2019. The role of hope for health professionals in rehabilitation: a qualitative study on unfavorable prognosis communication. PLoS One. 14, e0224394.

American College of Sports Medicine, 2021. ACSM's Guidelines for Exercise Testing & Prescription, 11th ed. Wolters Kluwer, Philadelphia.

Ammann, B.C., Knols, R.H., Baschung, P., et al., 2014. Application of principles of exercise training in sub-acute and chronic stroke survivors: a systematic review. BMC Neurol. 14, 167.

Ashford, D., Bennett, S.J., Davids, K., 2006. Observational modeling effects for movement dynamics and movement outcome measures across differing task constraints: a meta-analysis. J. Mot. Behav 38, 185–205.

Atkinson, H.L., Nixon-Cave, K., 2011. A tool for clinical reasoning and reflection using the International Classification of Functioning, Disability and Health (ICF) framework and patient management model. Phys. Ther. 91, 416–430.

Bandura, A., 1997. The nature and structure of self-efficacy. In: Bandura, A. (Ed.), Self-Efficacy: The Exercise of Control. W.H. Freeman and Company, New York, pp. 36–78.

Barnes, M., 2003. Principles of neurological rehabilitation. J. Neurol. Neurosurg. Psychiatry. 74 (Supp. 4), iv3–iv7.

Barron, C.J., Klaber Moffett, J.A., Potter, M., 2007. Patient expectations of physiotherapy: definitions, concepts and theories. Physiother. Theory Pract. 23, 37–46.

Baschung Pfister, P., de Bruin, E.D., Tobler-Ammann, 2015. The relevance of applying exercise training principles when designing therapeutic interventions for patients with inflammatory myopathies: a systematic review. Rheumatol. Int. 35, 1641–1654.

Batalden, M., Batalden, P., Margolis, P., et al., 2015. Coproduction of health care service. BMJ Qual. Saf. 25, 509–517.

Bernhardt, J., Raffelt, A., Churilov, L., et al., 2015. Efficacy and safety of very early mobilization within 24 hours of stroke onset (AVERT): a randomized controlled trial on behalf of the AVERT Trial Collaboration group. Lancet. 386, 46–55.

Billinger, S.A., Boyne, P., Coughenour, E., Dunning, K., Mattlage, A., 2015. Does aerobic exercise and the FITT principle fit into stroke recovery? Curr. Neurol. Neurosci. Rep. 15, 519.

Birkenmeier, R.L., Prager, E.M., Lang, C.E., 2010. Translating animal doses of task-specific training to people with chronic stroke in one hour therapy sessions: a proof of concept study. Neurorehabil. Neural Repair. 24, 620–635.

Bland, M.D., Whitson, M., Harris, H., 2015. Descriptive data analysis examining how standardized assessments are used to guide post-acute discharge recommendations for rehabilitation services after stroke. Phys. Ther. 95, 710–719.

Bovend'Eerdt, T.J.H., Botell, R.E., Wade, D.T., 2009. Writing SMART rehabilitation goals and achieving goal attainment scaling: a practical guide. Clin. Rehabil. 23, 352–361.

Boyd, L., Winstein, C.J., 2001. Implicit motor-sequence learning in humans following unilateral stroke: the impact of practice and explicit knowledge. Neurosci. Lett 298, 65–69.

Brazzelli, M., Saunders, D.H., Greig, S.A., 2012. Physical fitness training for patients with stroke: updated review. Stroke. 43, e39–e40.

Brentnall, J., Thackray, D., Judd, B., 2022. Evaluating the clinical reasoning of student health professionals in placement and simulation settings: a systematic review. Int. J. Environ. Res. Public Health 19, 936.

Bright, F.A.S., Kayes, N.M., McCann, C.M., McPherson, K.M., 2011. Understanding hope after stroke: a systematic review of the literature using concept analysis. Top Stroke Rehabil. 18, 490–508.

Braun, S.M., Beurskens, A.J., Borm, P.J., Schack, T., Wade, D.T., 2006. The effects of mental practice in stroke rehabilitation: a systematic review. Arch. Phys. Med. Rehabil 87, 842–852. https://doi.org/10.1016/j.apmr.2006.02.034

Brown, A.R., Martinez, M., 2019. From cortex to cord: motor circuit plasticity after spinal cord injury. Neural Regen. Res. 14, 2054–2062.

Burgers, J.S., van der Weijden, T., Bischoff, E.W.M.A., 2021. Challenges of research on person-centered care in general practice: a scoping review. Front. Med. 8, 669491.

Byblow, W.D., Stinear, C.M., Smith, M.C., et al., 2012. Mirror symmetric bimanual movement priming can increase corticomotor excitability and enhance motor learning. PLoS ONE. 7, e33882.

Carr, J., Shepherd, R., 2000. Movement Science Foundations for Physical Therapy in Rehabilitation, 2nd ed. Aspen Publishers, Inc, Gaithersburg, Maryland.

Carr, J.H., Shepherd, R.B., 2003. Stroke Rehabilitation: Guidelines for Exercise and Training to Optimise Motor Skills. Butterworth Heinemann, Oxford.

Carr, J.H., Shepherd, R.B., 2006. Neurological rehabilitation. Disabil. Rehabil. 28, 811–812.

Carr, J.H., Shepherd, R.B., 2010. Chapter 2: Training motor control, increasing strength and fitness and promoting skill acquisition. Neurologic Rehabilitation: Optimizing Motor Performance, 2nd ed. Churchill Livingstone Elsevier, London.

Casertano, L.O., Bassile, C.C., Pfeffer, J.S., et al., 2022. Utility of the AM-PAC "6 clicks" basic mobility and daily activity short forms to determine discharge destination in an acute stroke population. Am. J. Occup. Ther. 76, 7604205060

Casey, B., Coote, S., Hayes, S., et al., 2018. Changing physical activity behavior in people with multiple sclerosis: a systematic review and meta-analysis. Arch. Phys. Med. Rehabil. 99, 2059–2075.

Cieza, A., Causey, K., Kamenov, K., et al., 2020. Global estimates of the need for rehabilitation based on the Global Burden of Disease study 2019: a systematic analysis for the Global Burden of Disease Study 2019. Lancet. 396, P2006–2017.

Clarke, D.I., Forster, A., 2015. Improving post recovery: the role of the multi-disciplinary health care team. J. Multidiscip. Health. 8, 433–442.

Clear, J., 2018. Atomic Habits: An Easy & Proven Way to Build Good Habits & Break Bad Ones. Penguin, Random House, New York.

Cott, C.A., Wiles, R., Devitt, R., 2007. Continuity, transition and participation: preparing clients for life in the community post-stroke. Disabil. Rehabil. 29, 1566–1574.

Crum, A.L., Leibowitz, K.A., Verghese, A., 2017. Making mindset matter. BMJ. 356, j674.

Danzl, M.M., Etter, N.M., Andreatta, R.D., Kitzman, P.H., 2012. Facilitating neurorehabilitation through principles of engagement. J. Allied Health. 41, 35–41.

Davidoff, F., Dixon-Woods, M., Leviton, L., et al., 2015. Demystifying theory and its use in improvement. BMJ Qual. Saf. 24, 228–238.

Dawda, P., Janamian, T., Wells, L., 2022. Creating person-centred health care value together. Med. J. Austral. 216 (Suppl), S3–S4.

Dayan, E., Cohen, L.G., 2011. Neuroplasticity subserving motor skill learning. Neuron. 72, 443–454.

Dean, C.M., Richards, C.L., Malouin, F., 2000. Task-related circuit training improves performance of locomotor tasks in chronic stroke: a randomized, controlled pilot trial. Arch. Phys. Med. Rehabil. 81, 409–417.

Dean, C.M., Shepherd, R.B., 1997. Task-related training improves performance of seated reaching tasks after stroke. A randomized controlled trial. Stroke. 28, 722–728.

Dean, E., 2009. Foreword from the special issue editor of 'Physical Therapy Practice in the 21st Century: a new evidence-informed paradigm and implications'. Physiother. Theory Pract. 25, 328–329.

Deconinck, F.J.A., Smorenburg, A.R.P., Benham, A., et al., 2015. Reflections on mirror therapy: a systematic review of the effect of mirror visual feedback on the brain. Neurorehabil. Neural. Repair. 29, 349–361.

Díaz-Arribas, M.J., Martín-Casas, P., Cano-de-la-Cuerda, R., Plaza-Manzano, G., 2020. Effectiveness of the Bobath concept in the treatment of stroke: a systematic review. Disabil. Rehabil. 42, 1636–1649.

Djajamihardja, Stephens, K., 2016. The Little Book of Hope. Affirm Press, Melbourne, Australia.

Dobkin, B.H., Firestine, A., West, M., 2004. Ankle dorsiflexion as an fMRI paradigm to assay motor control for walking during rehabilitation. NeuroImage. 23, 370–381.

Dobkin, B.H., 2016. Behavioural self-management strategies for practice and exercise should be included in neurologic rehabilitation trials and care. Curr. Opin. Neurol. 29, 693–699.

Donkers, S.J., Oosman, S., Milosavljevic, S., Musselman, K.E., 2020. Addressing physical activity behavior in multiple sclerosis management: a qualitative account of health care providers' current practices and perspectives. Int. J. MS. Care. 22, 178–186.

Doyle, C., Lennox, L., Bell, D., 2013. A systematic review of evidence on the links between patient experience and clinical safety and effectiveness. BMJ Open. 3, e001570.

Driver, C., Kean, B., Oprescu, F., Lovell, G.P., 2017. Knowledge, behaviors, attitudes and beliefs of physiotherapists towards the use of psychological interventions in physiotherapy practice: a systematic review. Disabil. Rehabil. 39, 2237–2249.

Driver, C., Lovell, G.P., Oprescu, F., 2019a. Physiotherapists' views, perceived knowledge, and reported use of psychosocial strategies in practice. Physiother. Theory Pract. 1–14.

Driver, C., Oprescu, F., Lovell, G.P., 2019b. Exploring physiotherapists' considerations regarding the use of psychosocial strategies in practice. Physiother. Res. Int. 24, e1783.

Dromerick, A.W., Lang, C.E., Birkenmeier, R.L., et al., 2009. Very early constraint-induced movement during stroke rehabilitation. Neurology. 73, 195–201.

Dwamena, F., Holmes-Rovner, M., Gaulden, C., et al., 2012. Interventions for providers to promote a patient-centred approach in clinical consultations (review). Cochrane Database Syst. Rev 12, CD003267.

Dweck, C.S., Yeager, D.S., 2019. Mindsets: a view from two eras. Perspect. Psychol. Sci. 14, 481–496.

Edwards, S., 2002. Neurological Physiotherapy. Churchill Livingstone, Edinburgh.

Ellis, T., Motyl, R.W., 2013. Physical activity behavior change in persons with neurologic disorders: overview and examples from Parkinson disease and multiple sclerosis. J. Neurol. Phys. Ther. 37, 85–90.

El-Sayes, J., Harasym, D., Turco, C.V., et al., 2019. Exercise-induced neuroplasticity: a mechanistic model and prospects for promoting plasticity. Neuroscientist. 25, 65–85.

English, C., Healy, G.N., Coates, A., et al., 2016. Sitting and activity time in people with stroke. Phys. Ther. 96, 193–201.

Ertelt, D., Small, S., Solodkin, A., et al., 2007. Action observation has a positive impact on rehabilitation of motor deficits after stroke. NeuroImage. 36, T164–T173.

Fields, R.D., 2015. A new mechanism of nervous system plasticity: activity-dependent myelination. Nat. Rev. Neurosci. 16, 756–767.

Fogg, B.J., 2019. Tiny Habits: The Small Changes That Change Everything. Houghton Mifflin Harcourt, Philadelphia.

Frakking, T., Michaels, S., Orbell-Smith, J., et al., 2020. Framework for patient, family-centred care within an Australian Community Hospital: development and description. BMJ Open Qual. 9, e000823.

French, B., Thomas, L.H., Coupe, J., et al., 2016. Repetitive task training for improving functional ability after stroke (review). Cochrane Database Syst. Rev 11, CD006073.

Fryer, C.E., Luker, J.A., McDonnell, M.N., Hillier, S., 2016. Self-management programmes for quality of life in people with stroke. Cochrane Database Syst. Rev 8, CD010442.

Fuller, C.R., 2016. Echoes of a Closed Door: A Life Lived Following a Stroke. Self-published. Available at: www.carolrfuller.com.

Gangwani, R., Cain, A., Collins, A., Cassidy, J.M., 2022. Leveraging factors of self-efficacy and motivation to optimize stroke recovery. Front. Neurol. 13, 823202.

Gardner, B., Rebar, A.L., Lally, P., 2022. How does habit form? Guidelines for tracking real-world habit formation. Cogent. Psychol. 9, 2041277.

Garner, J., Lennon, S., 2018. Chapter 4: Neurological assessment: the basis of clinical decision-making. In: Lennon, S., Ramdharry, G., Verheyden, G. (Eds.), Neurological Physiotherapy Pocketbook. Elsevier Science, London.

Gentile, A.M., 1991. Personal communication between CC Bassile and AM Gentile during video presentation of patient after stroke observed ambulating overground and over obstacles of varying heights/widths.

Gentile, A.M., 2000. Skill acquisition: action, movement and neuromotor processes. In: Carr, J., Shepherd, R. (Eds.), Movement Science Foundations for Physical Therapy in Rehabilitation, 2nd ed. Aspen Publishers, Maryland.

Gilmore, P.E., Spaulding, S.J., 2001. Motor control and motor learning: implications for treatment in individuals post stroke. Phys. Occup. Ther. Geriatr. 20 (1), 1–15.

Greenhalgh, T., Howlick, J., Maskrey, N., et al., 2014. Evidence based medicine: a movement in crisis? BMJ. 348, g3725.

Griffin, J.M., Bradke, F., 2020. Therapeutic repair for spinal cord injury: combinatory approaches to address a multifaced problem. EMBO Mol. Med. 12, e11505.

Guimaraes, A.N., Ugrinowitsch, H., Dascal, J.B., et al., 2020. Freezing degrees of freedom during motor learning: a systematic review. Motor Control. 24, 457–471.

Gutenbrunner, C., Nugraha, B., 2020. Decision-making in evidence-based practice in rehabilitation medicine: proposing a fourth factor. Am. J. Phys. Med. Rehabil. 99, 436–440.

Hardwick, R.M., Caspers, S., Eickhoff, S.B., Swinnen, S.P., 2018. Neural correlates of action: comparing meta-analyses of imagery, observation, and execution. Neurosci. Biobehav. Rev. 94, 31–44.

Hassett, L., Jennings, M., Brady, B., et al., 2022. Brief physical activity counselling by physiotherapists (BEHAVIOUR): protocol for an effectiveness-implementation hybrid type II

cluster randomised controlled trial. Implement. Sci. Commun. 3, 39.

Health Foundation, 2016. Person-Centred Care Made Simple. Available at: http://personcentredcare.health.org.uk.

Holmes, J.A., Logan, P., Morris, R., Radford, K., 2020. Factors affecting the delivery of complex rehabilitation interventions in research with neurologically impaired adults: a systematic review. Syst. Rev. 9, 268.

Hordacre, B., Austin, D., Brown, K.E., et al., 2021. Evidence for a window of enhanced plasticity in the human motor cortex following ischemic stroke. Neurorehabil. Neural. Rep. 35, 307–320.

Hordacre, B., McCambridge, A., 2018. Motor control: structure and function of the nervous system. In: Lennon, S., Ramdharry, G. (Eds.), Verheyden G. Pocketbook of Neurological Physiotherapy, 2nd ed. Elsevier Science, London.

Hornby, G.T., Holleran, C.L., Hennessy, P.W., et al., 2016. Variable Intensive Early Walking Poststroke (VIEWS): a randomized controlled trial. Neurorehabil. Neural Repair. 30, 440–450.

Hornby, T.G., Reisman, D.S., Ward, I.G., et al., 2020. Clinical practice guideline to improve locomotor function following chronic stroke, incomplete spinal cord injury, and brain injury. JNPT. 44, 49–100.

Horvat, L., Horey, D., Romios, P., et al., 2014. Cultural competence education for health professions (review). Cochrane Database Syst. Rev. 5, 1–98.

Hubbard, I.J., Neil, C., Carey, L.M., 2009. Task-specific training: evidence for and translation into clinical practice. Occup. Ther. Int. 16, 175–189.

Jackson, P.L., Lafleur, M.F., Malouin, F., Richards, C., Doyon, J., 2001. Potential role of mental practice using motor imagery in neurologic rehabilitation. Arch. Phys. Med. Rehabil. 82, 1133–1141. https://doi.org/10.1053/apmr.2001.24286

Jean, S., Mac-Thiong, J.M., Marie-Christine, J., et al., 2021. Early clinical prediction of independent outdoor functional walking capacity in a prospective cohort of traumatic spinal cord injury patients. Am. J. Phys. Med. Rehabil. 100, 1034–1041.

Jones, F., 2006. Strategies to enhance chronic disease self-management: how can we apply this to stroke? Disabil. Rehabil. 28, 841–847.

Keus, S., Munneke, M., Graziano, M., et al., 2014. European Physiotherapy Guidelines for Parkinson's Disease. KNGf/ParkinsonNet, The Netherlands.

Kimberley, T.J., Novak, I., Boyd, L., et al., 2017. Stepping up to rethink the future of rehabilitation: IV STEP considerations and inspirations. Pediatr. Phys. Ther. 41, S63–S72.

Kollen, B.J., Lennon, S., Lyons, B., et al., 2009. The effectiveness of the Bobath concept in stroke rehabilitation: what is the evidence? Stroke. 40, e89–e97.

Krishnan, S., York, M.K., Bacchus, D., Heyn, P.C., 2017. Coping with caregiver burnout when caring for a person with neurodegenerative diseases: a guide for caregivers. Arch. Phys. Med. Rehabil. 98, 805–807.

Kwah, L.K., Herbert, R.D., 2016. Prediction of walking and arm recovery after stroke: a critical review. Brain. Sci. 6, 53.

Kwakkel, G., 2006. Impact of intensity of practice after stroke: issues for consideration. Disabil. Rehabil 28, 823–830.

Kwakkel, G., Veerbeek, L.M., van Wegen, E.E., Wolf, S.L., 2015. Constraint-induced movement therapy after stroke. Lancet Neurol. 14, 224–234.

Laguna, P.L., 2000. The effect of model observation versus physical practice during motor skill acquisition and performance. J. of Hum. Mov. Stud 39, 171–191.

Lang, C.E., Lohse, K.E., Birkenmeier, R.E., 2015. Dose and timing in neurorehabilitation: prescribing motor therapy after stroke. Curr. Opin. Neurol 28 (6), 549–555.

Lang, C.E., Strube, M.J., Bland, M.D., et al., 2016. Dose response of task-specific upper limb training in people at least 6 months post stroke: a phase II, single-blind, randomized, controlled trial. Ann. Neurol. 80, 342–354.

Langhorne, P., Ramachandra, S., 2020. Organised inpatient (stroke unit) care for stroke: network meta-analysis. Cochrane Database Syst. Rev. 4, CD000197.

Lennon, S., 2003. Physiotherapy practice in stroke rehabilitation: a survey. Disabil. Rehabil. 25, 455–461.

Lennon, S., Ashburn, A., Baxter, G.D., 2006. Gait outcome following outpatient physiotherapy based on the Bobath concept in people post stroke. Disabil. Rehabil. 28, 873–881.

Lennon, S., McKenna, S., Jones, F., 2013. Self-management programmes for people post stroke: a systematic review. Clin. Rehabil. 27, 867–878.

Lennon, O., Hall, P., Blake, C., 2021. Predictors of adherence to lifestyle recommendations in stroke secondary prevention. Int. J. Environ. Res. Public. Health. 18, 4666.

Levin, M.F., Kleim, J.A., Wolf, S.L., 2009. What do motor recovery and compensation mean in patients following stroke? Neurorehabil. Neural. Rep. 23, 313–319.

Levy, T., Christie, L.J., Killington, M., et al., 2021. "Just that four letter word, hope": stroke survivors' perspectives of participation in an intensive upper limb exercise program; a qualitative exploration. Physiother. Theory Pract. 38, 1624–1638.

Lexell, J., Brogardh, C., 2015. The use of the ICF in the neurorehabilitation process. Neurorehabilitation 36, 5–9.

Liu, N., Cadilhac, D.A., Andrew, N.E., et al., 2014. Randomized controlled trial of early rehabilitation after intracerebral hemorrhage stroke: difference in outcomes within 6 months of stroke. Stroke. 45, 3502–3507.

Livingston-Thomas, J., Nelson, P., Karthikeyan, S., et al., 2016. Exercise and environmental enrichment as enablers of task-specific neuroplasticity and stroke recovery. Neurotherapeutics. 13, 395–402.

Louie, D.R., Eng, J.J., 2018. Berg balance scale score at admission can predict walking suitable for community ambulation at discharge from inpatient stroke rehabilitation. J. Rehabil. Med. 50, 37–44.

Lundahl, B., Moleni, T., Burke, B.L., et al., 2013. Motivational interviewing in medical care settings: a systematic review and meta-analysis of randomized controlled trials. Patient. Educ. Couns. 93, 157–168.

Magdon-Ismail, Z., Sicklick, A., Hedeman, R., et al., 2016. Selection of postacute stroke rehabilitation facilities: a survey of discharge planners from the Northeast Cerebrovascular Consortium (NECC) region. Medicine (Baltimore). 95, e3206.

Maier, M., Ballester Rubio, B., Duff, A., et al., 2019a. Effect of specific over nonspecific VR-based rehabilitation on poststroke motor recovery: a systematic meta-analysis. Neurorehabil. Neural. Rep 33, 112–129.

Maier, M., Ballester, B.R., Verschure, P.F.M.J., 2019b. Principles of neurorehabilitation after stroke based on motor learning and brain plasticity mechanisms. Front. Syst. Neurosci. 13, 74.

Malouin, F., Richards, C.L., 2010. Mental practice for relearning locomotor skills. Phys. Ther. 90, 240–251.

Mansfield, A., Aqui, A., Danells, C.J., et al., 2018. Does perturbation-based balance training prevent falls among individuals with chronic stroke? A randomised controlled trial. BMJ. Open. 8, e021510.

Marley, T.L., Ezekiel, H.J., Lehto, N.K., et al., 2000. Application of motor learning principles: the physiotherapy client as a problem solver. II. Scheduling practice. Physiother. Can. 52, 315–320.

Masten, A.S., 2018. Resilience theory and research on children and families: past, present, and promise. J. Fam. Theory. Rev 10, 12–31.

McCullagh, P., Weiss, M.R., Ross, D., 1989. Modelling considerations in motor skill acquisition and performance: an integrated approach. Exerc. Sports. Sci. Rev. 14, 475–513.

McDonnell, M.N., Stinear, C.M., 2017. TMS measures of motor cortex function after stroke: a meta-analysis. Brain Stimul. 10, 721–734.

McDonnell, M.N., Koblar, S., Ward, N.S., et al., 2015. An investigation of cortical neuroplasticity following stroke in adults: is there evidence for a critical window for rehabilitation? BMC. Neurol. 15, 109.

McGrane, N., Galvin, R., Cusack, T., Stokes, E., 2015. Addition of motivational interventions to exercise and traditional physiotherapy: a review and meta-analysis. Physiotherapy. 101, 1–12.

Medley, A.R., Powell, T., 2010. Motivational interviewing to promote self-awareness and engagement in rehabilitation following acquired brain injury: a conceptual review. Neuropsychol. Rehabil. 20, 481–508.

Mees, M., Klein, J., Yperzeele, L., et al., 2016. Predicting discharge destination after stroke: a systematic review. Clin. Neurol. Neurosurg. 142, 15–21.

Michie, S., van Stralen, M.M., West, R., 2011. The behaviour change wheel: a new method for characterising and designing behaviour change interventions. Implement. Sci. 6, 42.

Momosaki, R., Yasunaga, H., Kakuda, W., et al., 2016. Very early versus delayed rehabilitation for acute ischemic stroke patients with intravenous recombinant tissue plasminogen activator: a nationwide retrospective cohort study. Cerebrovasc. Dis. 42, 41–48.

Moncion, K., Biasin, L., Jagrooop, D., et al., 2020. Barriers and facilitators to aerobic exercise implementation in stroke rehabilitation: a scoping review. J. Neurol. Phys. Ther 44, 179–187.

Morris, J.H., Irvine, L.A., Dombrowski, S.U., et al., 2022. We Walk: a person-centred, dyadic behaviour change intervention to promote physical activity through outdoor walking after stroke—an intervention development study. BMJ Open. 12, e058563.

Motl, R.W., Pekmezi, D., Wingo, C.B., 2018. Promotion of physical activity and exercise in multiple sclerosis: importance of behavioral science and theory. Mult. Scler. J. Exp. Transl. Clin. 4 2055217318786745

Mount, C.W., Monje, M., 2017. Wrapped to adapt: experience-dependent myelination. Neuron. 95, 743–756.

Muratori, L.M., Lamberg, E.M., Quinn, L., Duff, S.V., 2013. Applying principles of motor learning and control to upper extremity rehabilitation. J. Hand. Ther. 26, 94–103.

National Health Service England, 2016. Realising the Value. Ten Key Actions to Put People and Communities at the Heart of Health and Wellbeing. NHS England, London.

National Institute for Health and Care Excellence (NICE), 2022. Multiple Sclerosis: Management of Multiple Sclerosis in Primary and Secondary Care. Clinical Guidelines CG8, NICE Available at: http://www.nice.org.uk.

Nieoullon, A., Coquerel, A., 2003. Dopamine: a key regulator to adapt action, emotion, motivation and cognition. Curr. Opin. Neurol. 16 (Suppl 2), S3–S9.

Nithiananthrajah, J., Hannan, A.J., 2006. Enriched environments, experience-dependent plasticity and disorders of the nervous system. Nat. Rev. Neurosci. 7, 697–709.

Nijland, R.H.M., van Wegen, E.E.H., Harmeling-van der Wel, B.C., 2010. Presence of finger extension and shoulder abduction within 72 hrs after stroke predicts functional recovery: early prediction of functional outcome after stroke: the EPOS cohort study. Stroke. 41, 745–750.

Nilsen, D.M., Gillen, G., Gordon, A.M., 2010. Use of mental practice to improve upper limb recovery after stroke: a systematic review. Am. J. Occup. Ther. 64, 695–708.

Nudo, R.J., 2013. Recovery after brain injury: mechanisms and principles. Front. Hum. Neurosci. 7, 887.

Oral, A., 2022. Are implementation interventions effective in promoting the adoption of evidence-based practices in stroke rehabilitation? A Cochrane Review summary with commentary. NeuroRehabilitation. 50, 255–258.

Oyake, K., Suzuki, M., Otaka, Y., Tanaka, S., 2020. Motivational strategies for stroke rehabilitation: a descriptive cross-sectional study. Front. Neurol. 11, 553.

Parish, E.B.M.J., 2015. Roundtable debate: how can we get better at providing person-centred care? BMJ. 350, h412.

Parkinsons Guidelines Europe. Available at: www.parkinsonnet.com.

Pelletier-Roy, R., Richard-Denis, A., Jean, S., et al., 2021. Clinical judgment is a cornerstone for validating and using clinical prediction rules: a head-to-head study on ambulation outcomes for spinal cord injured patients. Spinal Cord. 59, 1104–1110.

Platz, T., Sandrini, G., 2020. Specialty grand challenge for neurorehabilitation research. Front. Neurol. 11, 349.

Playford, E.D., Siegert, R., Levack, W., Freeman, J., 2009. Areas of consensus and controversy about goal setting in rehabilitation: a conference report. Clin. Rehabil. 23, 334–344.

Ploughman, M., Kelly, L.P., 2016. Four birds with one stone? Reparative, neuroplastic, cardiorespiratory and metabolic benefits of aerobic exercise poststroke. Curr. Opin. Neurol. 29, 684–692.

Pollock, A., Baer, G., Campbell, P., et al., 2014. Physical rehabilitation approaches for the recovery of function and mobility following stroke. Cochrane Database Syst. Rev. 2014, CD001920

Rakesh, N., Boiarsky, D., Athar, A., et al., 2019. Post-stroke rehabilitation: factors predicting discharge to acute versus subacute rehabilitation facilities. Medicine. 98, e15934.

Ramdharry, G.M., Anderson, A., 2022. Exercise in myositis: what is important, the prescription or the person? Best Pract. Res. Clin. Rheumatol. 36, 101722.

Reo, J.A., Mercer, V.S., 2004. Effects of live, videotaped or written instruction on learning an upper-extremity exercise program. Phys. Ther. 84 (7), 622–633.

Rhodes, R.E., Fiala, B., 2009. Building motivation and sustainability into the prescription and recommendations for physical activity and exercise therapy: the evidence. Physiother. Theory. Pract. 25, 424–441.

Rothbart, A., Sohlberg, M., Moore, 2021. Resilience as a mainstream clinical consideration for speech-language pathologists providing post–acquired brain injury neurorehabilitation. Perspect. ASHA. Spec. Inter. Grp 6, 1026–1032.

Sanders, J.P., Stuart, J.H., Biddle, J.H., et al., on behalf of the Snacktivity Study Team., 2021. Snacktivity™ to increase physical activity: time to try something different? Prev. Med. 153, 106851.

Sanli, E.A., Patterson, J.T., Bray, S.R., et al., 2013. Understanding self-controlled motor learning protocols through self-determination theory. Front. Psychol. 3, 611.

Santana, M.J., Manalili, K., Jolley, R., et al., 2018. How to practice person-centred care: a conceptual framework. Health Expect. 21, 429–440.

Scheets, P.L., Hornby, G., Perry, S.B., et al., 2021. Moving forward. JNPT. 45, 46–49.

Schmidt, R.A., Lee, T., 2005. Chapter 13: The Learning Process Motor Control and Learning: A Behavioural Emphasis, 4th ed. Human Kinetics. Champaign, Illinois, 257–383.

Schultz, W., 2013. Updating dopamine reward signals. Curr. Opin. Neurobiol. 23, 229–238.

Scrivener, K., Dorsch, S., McCluskey, A., et al., 2020. Bobath therapy is inferior to task-specific training and not superior to other interventions in improving lower limb activities after stroke: a systematic review. J. Physiother. 66, 225–235.

Scully, D.M., Newell, K.M., 1985. Observational learning and the acquisition of motor skills: toward a visual perception perspective. J. Hum. Movement Stud. 11, 169–186.

Seligman, M., 2011. Flourish: A Visionary New Understanding of Happiness and Well-being. Simon & Schuster, New York.

Shumway-Cook, A., Woollacott, M.H., Rachwani, J., Santamaria, V., 2022. Motor Control Translating Research into Clinical Practice, 6th ed. Williams & Wilkins, Baltimore.

Sidaway, B., Ahn, S., Boldeau, P., et al., 2008. A comparison of manual guidance and knowledge of results in the learning of a weight-bearing skill. J. Neurol. Phys. Ther. 32, 32.

Simpson, B., Villeneuve, M., Clifton, 2021. Exploring well-being services from the perspective of people with SCI: a scoping review of qualitative research. Int. J. Qual. Stud. Health Well-being 16, 1986922.

Soundy, A., Liles, C., Stubbs, B., Roskell, C., 2014. Identifying a framework for hope in order to establish the importance of a generalised hopes for individuals who have suffered a stroke. Adv. Med. 2014, 471874.

Soundy, A., Smith, B., Butler, M., et al., 2010. A qualitative study in neurological physiotherapy and hope: beyond physical improvement. Physiother. Theory Pract. 26, 79–88.

Stanton, R., Ada, L., Dean, C.M., Preston, E., 2015. Feedback received while practicing everyday activities during rehabilitation after stroke: an observational study. Physiother. Res. Int. 20, 166–173.

Stein, J., Prvu Bettger, J., Sicklick, A., et al., 2015. Use of a standardized assessment to predict rehabilitation care after acute stroke. Arch. Phys. Med. Rehabil. 96, 210–217.

Stroke Foundation. 2022. Clinical Guidelines for Stroke Management, Australia. Available at: www.informme.org.au.

Sturt, R., Hill, B., Holland, A., 2020. Validation of a clinical prediction rule for ambulation outcome after non-traumatic spinal cord injury. Spinal Cord. 58, 609–615.

Tang Yan, H.S., Clemson, L.M., Jarvis, F., Laver, K., 2014. Goal setting with caregivers of adults in the community: a mixed methods systematic review. Disabil. Rehabil. 36, 1943–1963.

Tomlinson, M., Swartz, L., Officer, A., et al., 2009. Research priorities for health of people with disabilities: an expert opinion exercise. Lancet. 374, 1857–1862.

Trede, F., 2012. Emancipatory physiotherapy practice. Physiother. Theory Pract. 28, 466–473.

Verbeek, J.M., Van Wegen, E.E.H., Van Peppen, R., et al., 2014. KNGF Clinical Practice Guideline for Physical Therapy in Patients with Stroke. Royal Dutch Society for Physical Therapy, The Netherlands.

Verheyden, G., Vereeck, L., Truijen, S., et al., 2006. Trunk performance after stroke and the relationship with balance, gait and functional ability. Clin. Rehabil. 20, 451–458.

Wade, D.T., 2020. What is rehabilitation? An empirical investigation leading to an evidence-based description. Clin. Rehabil. 34, 571–583.

Ward, N.S., Brander, F., Kelly, K., 2019. Intensive upper limb neurorehabilitation in chronic stroke: outcomes from the Queen Square programme. J. Neurol. Neurosurg. Psychiatry. 90, 498–506.

Williams, M., Hodges, N.J., 2004. Skill acquisition in sport: research, theory and practice. Routledge, London.

Wingfield, M., Fini, N.A., Brodtmann, A., et al., 2022. Upper-limb motor intervention elements that drive improvement in biomarkers and clinical measures post-stroke: a systematic review in a systems paradigm. Neurorehabil. Neural Rep. 36, 726–739.

Winstein, C.J., 1991. Knowledge of results and motor learning: Implications for physical therapy. Phys. Ther 71, 140–149.

Winstein, C., Lewthwaite, R., Blanton, S.R., et al., 2014. Infusing motor learning research into neurorehabilitation practice: a historical perspective with case exemplar from the accelerated skill acquisition program. J. Neurol. Phys. Ther. 38, 190–200.

Winstein, C.J., Stein, J., 2016. Guidelines for adult stroke rehabilitation and recovery. A guideline for healthcare professionals from the American Heart Association/American Stroke Association. Stroke. 47, e98–e169.

World Health Organization., 2001. International Classification of Functioning, Disability and Health (ICF). World Health Organization, Geneva. Available at: http://www.who.int/classification/icf.

World Health Organization., 2016. Adherence to Long-Term Therapies: Evidence for Action. World Health Organization, Geneva. Available at: https://www. who.int/chp/knowledge/publications/adherence_report/en/.

World Health Organization., 2017. Rehabilitation 2030: A Call for Action. Available at: http://www.who.int/disabilities/care/rehab-2030/en/.

Wulf, G., 2013. Attentional focus and motor learning: a review of 15 years. Int. Rev. Sport. Exerc. Psychol. 6, 77–104.

Wulf, G., Lewthwaite, R., 2016. Optimizing performance through intrinsic motivation and attention for learning: the OPTIMAL theory of motor learning. Psychol. Bull. Rev. 23, 1382–1414.

Yoshida, T., Otaka, Y., Osu, R., et al., 2021. Motivation for rehabilitation in patients with subacute stroke: a qualitative study. Front. Rehabil. Sci. 2, 664758.

Zajac, S., Woods, A., Tannenbaum, S., et al., 2021. Overcoming challenges to teamwork in healthcare: a team effectiveness framework and evidence-based guidance. Front. Commun. 6, 606445.

2

Clinical Reasoning in Neurological Physiotherapy: Assessment and Treatment Principles

Jill Patricia Garner, Sheila Lennon, and James Vincent McLoughlin

OUTLINE

Introduction, 33
    Evidence for Clinical Reasoning Frameworks, 34
A CR Framework for Neurological Physiotherapy, 34
Primary CR Components, 34
    Assessment, 34
    Interpretation, 35
        The ICF-Based Problem List, 35
        Prognosis, 36
        Collaborative Goal Setting, 36
    Treatment Planning, 36
        Defining Therapy Aims Using RAMP, 37
        Developing a Treatment Plan, 37
    Intervention, 38
        Implementing the Treatment Plan, 38

    Reflection, 38
    Reassessment (+Outcomes), 39
Putting It All Together in Case Scenarios, 39
    Clinical Case 1 Developed by Jill Garner, 39
    Clinical Case 2 Developed by James McLoughlin, 46
        CR During Session 1, 46
        Intervention, 48
        CR During Session 2, 48
        CR During Session 3, 49
        Summary Reflection, 49
Conclusion, 50

INTRODUCTION

Clinical reasoning (CR) is an essential component of any health professional's practice. CR is the sum of the thinking and decision-making processes associated with clinical practice (Jones et al 2018). It has been defined as 'a process in which the therapist, interacting with significant others (e.g., family and other healthcare team members), structures meaning, goals and health management strategies based on clinical data, client choices and professional judgement and knowledge' (Jones & Rivett 2004).

One of the key roles of the therapist working in neurology is to help the patient experience and relearn optimal movement and function in everyday life within the constraints imposed by the disease process and presenting impairments to enable clients to participate in their desired life roles (see Chapter 1 on principles of neurological rehabilitation). During the CR process, the therapist analyses multiple variables contributing to the client's cognitive and/or physical capacity (the ability to execute a task or action in a standard

environment) and performance (what the client can do in their own current environment). Cultural frameworks also influence how patients and therapists understand health and illness, and the expectations and values that they bring to their clinical interactions (Horvat et al 2014).

CR is a complex process that focuses on making the therapist's thinking processes explicit to explain to clients, students, other healthcare team members and novice practitioners why we assess and treat clients in the way that we do. CR is difficult to define and challenging to assess in both the academic and practice setting. Ways of CR have been shown to differ between students and experts. Students and novice physiotherapists tend to apply a hypotheticodeductive reasoning strategy with clients. This has been defined as a process of gathering information from clients to construct a hypothesis, which is then tested to confirm it or to develop a further hypothesis. Expert therapists often rely on pattern recognition drawing on previous experiences of similar cases (Jones et al 2018, May et al 2010).

33

Evidence for Clinical Reasoning Frameworks

The evidence base underlying how health professionals use the CR process in practice is limited. A systematic review by Brentnall et al (2022) aimed to evaluate the attainment of CR skills in health professionals on clinical placement and in simulation settings. Only 4 of the 61 studies reviewed were specific to physiotherapy; there was limited reference to any conceptual frameworks.

Elven and Dean (2017) published a systematic review of 10 studies aiming to identify CR components specific to physiotherapy. They identified that a lack of consensus on essential components of CR is leading to variable and inconsistent teaching, assessment and research. Another systematic review of the evidence base for neurological physiotherapy assessment has identified six studies that explored clinical reasoning in neurological physiotherapy (Garner et al, 2023). This review highlighted that experienced physiotherapists often used a 'form of pattern recognition' to assess for certain deficits such as neglect rather than a specific assessment tool or a consensus of essential domains. They also used their in-depth understanding of movement behaviours to assist in prognostication.

There is a broad array of components deemed important for CR and limited reference to any evidence-based conceptual frameworks (Brentnall et al 2022). The American Physical Therapy Association (2020) identified clinical reasoning as one of seven core domains expected of a postgraduate physiotherapist, defining CR as an ability to organise, synthesise, integrate and apply sound clinical rationale for patient management. At a postgraduate level, CR can be tested across four domains: knowledge generation, knowledge application, justification of clinical decision-making and anticipating outcomes (APTA 2020). Furze et al (2022) have proposed that CR is a complex cycle of cognitive and metacognitive processes requiring the integration of knowledge, psychomotor skills and reflection within the situational context of clinical practice. More research is required to standardise the use of terminology and components essential to the development of CR.

As the physiotherapy profession has yet to reach consensus on the essential components underpinning an optimal CR framework, this chapter will focus on our understanding and application of essential assessment and treatment principles within the CR cycle using case scenarios to illustrate how experienced clinicians apply these principles in the clinical setting.

A CR FRAMEWORK FOR NEUROLOGICAL PHYSIOTHERAPY

We have identified five primary components within the CR cycle: (1) assessment, (2) interpretation, (3) treatment planning, (4) intervention and (5) reassessment (+outcomes) [see rectangles in Fig. 2.1 adapted from Atkinson & Nixon-Cave (2011), Garner and Lennon (2018, p. 68), Lexell & Brogardh (2015)]. These components are also influenced by other important components, such as the *International Classification of Functioning, Disability and Health* (ICF), prognosis, the problem list, goal setting and reflection within a person-centred care model of healthcare. RAMP is an acronym (Recovery, Adaptation, Maintenance and Prevention) related to the main aims of therapy intervention. RAMP influences how therapists reflect on the client prognosis, interpret assessment and discuss treatment options with clients during treatment planning. Person-centred care can be viewed as a partnership from the perspective of the patient, the family and the healthcare professional; thus, active involvement should be encouraged at all stages of the CR cycle (Fig. 2.1).

In practice, the components of CR may be considered in isolation or may all occur in the same session at the same time. For example, our client may be discussing an aspect of their health condition as we are observing their movement behaviours; we may be assessing their ability to balance while considering what person-centred factors may be influencing balance (e.g., sensation, strength, vision, vestibular system, postural alignment) and how our client is responding to increasing demands on their balance during the assessment. The additional components of a problem list, prognosis, collaborative patient-centred goal setting and reflection are important considerations after assessment has begun.

PRIMARY CR COMPONENTS

Assessment

Assessment in neurological physiotherapy is always the starting point for CR. Physiotherapy assessment describes a process that includes history taking (subjective examination) and the objective examination that consists of observation and physical examination including standardised tests and measures (Garner & Lennon 2018, p. 55).

Measurement is a core component of physical therapy practice. Measurement tools can be used for (Fulk & Field-Fote 2011):

- Diagnosis
- Prognosis
- Care planning
- Assessing patient progress
- Evaluating the effectiveness of interventions

Assessment consists of two parts: a subjective exploration of the person's perspective of an issue and an objective examination of performance. The objective assessment includes observation, physical examination and the use of

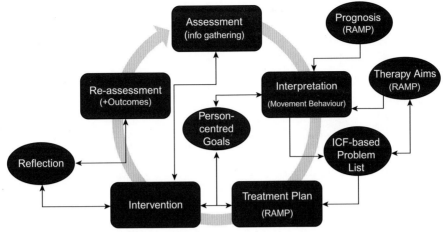

FIG. 2.1 Key components of clinical reasoning in neurological physiotherapy.

TABLE 2.1	**Key Assessment Components**
Subjective	**Objective**
• Information gathering from the patient's medical record/chart • Liaison with the care team • Interviewing the patient and family	• Observation • Examination • Standardised measurement tools

standardised measurement tools with published reliability and validity (Garner & Lennon 2018, p. 56) (Table 2.1).

Background knowledge of neurological conditions, reading the medical records and discussions with other health professionals gives the therapist ideas for questions to ask the patient. During the subjective interview, the therapist aims to find out about the patient's current symptoms and their understanding of why they have been admitted to hospital or referred for physiotherapy, their past medical history and social history that involves family, work, hobbies and accommodation, as well as to gain an idea of their general mobility and function.

The interview provides an opportunity to build rapport with the client and family/carers and explore psychosocial factors that may affect movement and function. Factors that may have a negative impact on movement and function are mood, increased anxiety levels, disruptions at home and low socioeconomic status (Dimitriadis et al 2015).

For those people attending outpatient physiotherapy appointments, it also important to determine why they are attending, what are their main concerns and what are their preconceived expectations about neurological physiotherapy. A detailed symptom history and its impact on activities of daily living is important, as is establishing what other health professionals are involved in their care.

During the objective examination, the therapist identifies the tasks and components within the task that require assistance (see Chapter 4 on observation and movement analysis for more detail). The choice of activities usually depends on the subjective report and goals.

Bland et al (2015) state that a comprehensive assessment:
- Facilitates decision-making and treatment planning.
- Helps determine patient prognosis.
- Helps therapists to design and select appropriate interventions.
- Helps therapists to understand the need for referral to other members of the interdisciplinary team, and additional services.

Although it is essential to assess range, weakness and functional performance like any other type of assessment, there are several impairments that are unique and important in neurological assessment (see Chapter 3 for a review of common impairments in neurology and their impact on activity).

Interpretation
The ICF-Based Problem List

The ICF framework for rehabilitation enables the therapist to classify underlying impairments, activity limitations and participation restrictions (World Health Organization 2001). The ICF provides a systematic way of understanding the problems faced by clients and their carers, illustrating the multiple levels at which neurological rehabilitation may act. Following assessment, this leads the therapist to develop a problem list based on the ICF. This framework represents a biopsychosocial model of health that enables

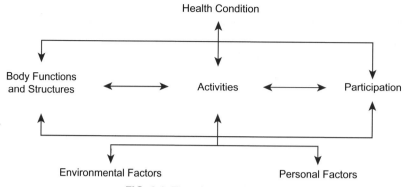

FIG. 2.2 The ICF (WHO 2001)

therapists to holistically understand and manage their clients (Fig. 2.2).

The neurological physiotherapist generates a hypothesis of how impairments affect movement dysfunction, function (activity) and participation to come up with a movement diagnosis (Deutsch et al 2022, Lexell & Brogardh 2015). Therapists must also consider and reflect on their own values, beliefs, assumptions and biases when interpreting assessment findings to derive the most appropriate problem list in partnership with the client (O'Donoghue et al 2021).

The problem list is not a list of every impairment noted in the assessment; rather, the therapist, having analysed the client's movement behaviours, signs and symptoms, develops a hypothesis based on the relevant impairments linked to the appropriate activity limitations that will become the focus of goal setting and rehabilitation intervention strategies to affect motor performance, activity and participation (Shumway-Cook & Woollacott 2017, p. 142).

Prognosis

Regarding prognosis, therapists consider the evidence base for potential recovery to influence their assessments and interventions. Therapists consider in the first instance the type of neurological condition that the client presents with, for example, whether the client is likely to spontaneously recover, make a full recovery, be left with any residual disability or likely to experience progressive deterioration. Ideally, prediction of outcomes will lead to clearer patient expectations and better selection of interventions (Kimberley et al 2017).

A key part of assessment is prognostication to help determine the client's rehabilitation potential. This potential can be fluid and subject to change depending on intrinsic patient factors, such as medical stability, motivation and progress, and extrinsic factors, such as their environment/ home situation. Therapists must consider their own professional culture, institutional culture and the culture of the individual when collecting information to make clinical decisions with the client to ensure that incorrect assumptions are not made about rehabilitation potential that may be because of misunderstandings of that person's values and health beliefs.

Collaborative Goal Setting

Our choice of interventions is influenced by what we know about prognosis, therapy aims, and the goals and preferences of the client, as well as other contextual factors such as healthcare setting, healthcare funding and policy. Working with the client to collaboratively set goals helps focus the development of a treatment plan (Siegert & Levack 2014).

Developing an appropriate plan of care revolves around collaborative goal setting with the patient and/or the caregiver as well as the rehabilitation team (see Chapter 6 for a review of goal planning). Person-centred goals need to be based on patient's wishes, expectations, priorities and values; one way of facilitating appropriate goal planning is to use the SMART acronym, which recommends that goals should be specific, measurable, achievable/ambitious, relevant and timed (Playford et al 2009; see Bovend'Eerdt et al 2009 for some practical guidance on how to set SMART goals).

Treatment Planning

The therapist together with the client and their family agree joint treatment goals before collaboratively devising a treatment plan. The findings derived from the history and physical examination enable clinicians to use the prediction literature (prognosis) to influence their intervention plan, thus helping therapists to establish short- and long-term goals in partnership with the person with a neurological condition and their carer(s) (Dimitriadis et al 2015).

Defining Therapy Aims Using RAMP

Therapists aim to optimise movement and function; however, for many neurological conditions, recovery of normal movement and function is not achievable. This depends to some extent on whether the patient has a progressive, deteriorating condition or a stable condition (Edwards 2002, p. 256).

The aims of neurological physiotherapy initially considered under prognosis and interpretation can be summed up using the acronym RAMP (Recovery, Adaptation, Maintenance and Prevention) (see Chapter 1, Principle 7) (Fig. 2.3).

The therapist needs to reflect about the aims of therapy in terms of RAMP defined as:

Recovery: Interventions are aimed at enhancing recovery and restitution of previous movement skills as much as possible, especially when the person still has the potential to change.

Adaptation: Adaptation is a key strategy for living well with neurological conditions. Compensatory movements can develop as an adaptation to remain functional. The type and variation of movement compensations can be influenced by training to encourage optimal adaptations to real-world goals for each individual. Sometimes compensatory movements may be discouraged if they do not allow new or preferred movement strategies an opportunity to be practiced (Levin et al 2009). These new and preferred movements need careful justification based on ability, potential, disease trajectory, performance goals and treatment progress.

Maintenance: Maintenance of function despite deteriorating impairments should be viewed as a positive achievement, with plans to mitigate decline as much as possible. Therapists focus on optimising activities and problem-solving strategies to facilitate adaptation in progressive diseases. Expectations and goal setting in progressive conditions such as multiple sclerosis (MS) and Parkinson's need to take into consideration an up-to-date knowledge of the condition and the factors that determine physical decline in any individual. However, in some progressive diseases, maintaining physical function is not possible if a condition declines in its natural history, and therapists need to be wary of setting unrealistic expectations that can have a detrimental effect on the person's psyche if they consider decline a personal failure (Ramdharry & Andersson 2022).

Prevention: The prevention of the development of complications such as weakness, physical inactivity, falls, injury, pain, pressure areas, contracture and swelling is important.

Developing a Treatment Plan

A structured treatment plan is essential to provide appropriate interventions, which should be based on the best available evidence. Evidence about the disease(s), symptomatic management, treatment options and clinical effectiveness can all be incorporated in the decision-making process. A clinical reasoning form (CRF) that integrates the ICF can help by providing a detailed list of important problem, goals and treatment plans in relation to body function/impairments, activities, and participation. It also brings in contextual, personal and environmental considerations that influence decision making. This form enables the therapist to sum up their thinking (see examples of a CRF presented later in the case scenarios).

Physiotherapists identify the movement system as the key focus of our expertise (Deutsch et al 2022). It is important to understand that the neurological physiotherapist's CR is not focused on differential diagnosis, as often the client's neurological condition has already been confirmed. The physiotherapist synthesises information and generates hypotheses with an emphasis on the analysis of movement behaviour within a biopsychosocial model of health (Gilliland & Wainwright 2020).

Treatment planning is also influenced by other factors such as the beliefs, attitudes and culture of both patients and health professionals (Holmes et al 2020). Contextual factors such as health systems and service organisation including health insurance availability, its coverage of interventions, as well as availability of technical equipment and qualified personnel for its use, also influence healthcare delivery (Gutenbrunner & Nugraha 2020).

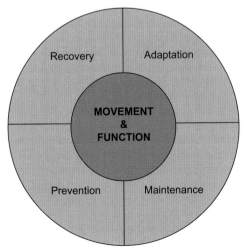

FIG. 2.3 Aims of neurological rehabilitation – RAMP.

Tips for developing a treatment plan:

- Consider the client's signs and symptoms in the context of relevant anatomy and physiology, e.g., in terms of the ascending/descending pathways affected, and pathology related to neurological conditions.
- Consider the client's mindset (Crum et al 2017), capabilities, opportunities, motivation to change (see Michie et al 2011 for more detail on the COM-B model of behaviour change) and ability to self-manage and importance of promoting self-efficacy (Gangwani et al 2022) (see Chapter 19).
- Develop a hypothesis of how impairments affect function (activity) and participation for the patient problems.
- Form a plan from your assessment collaboratively with your patient.
- Consider possible treatment options and time frames available in each setting, e.g., acute, rehabilitation and outpatient settings.
- Consider movement training principles to be considered within your chosen interventions (Kleynen et al 2020, Maier et al 2019, McLoughlin 2020).
- Use the prediction literature about recovery or disease progression to inform your client expectations and guide your choice of interventions (Kimberley et al 2017).
- Communicate closely with the caregivers and other members of the rehab team.

Intervention

Neural plasticity is the rationale for the process of learning and relearning movement and is often exploited within physiotherapy interventions (Maier et al 2019). The structure and the function of the nervous system can be changed through use, experience and therapy in many neurological conditions. However, in some conditions (e.g., in progressive neuromuscular diseases), maintaining physical function is not possible if a condition declines in its natural history; therapists will focus on goals of maintaining activities longer term and problem-solving strategies to facilitate adaptation. Thus, it is important not to overemphasise neural plasticity in every person with a neurological condition.

Therapists provide an opportunity to optimise physical function and reduce disability associated with a neurological condition. Our interventions can include task practice, exercise prescription, manual therapy, education, support, prescription of aids or orthotics, assessment, reports and referrals. The principles of neuroplasticity underpin many of our movement-based therapies that focus on relearning important skills for function (Maier et al 2019). Education, problem-solving strategies and plans for improving health, activity levels and quality of life are also important in the context of all neurological conditions including progressive neuromuscular conditions.

Implementing the Treatment Plan

The neurological physiotherapist's role is to:

- Reeducate movement and function.
- Prescribe exercises, monitor and update.
- Prescribe aids, splints and rehabilitation technology.
- Coach movement through education, support, motivation and empowerment.
- Treat, manage and advise about injuries.
- Support patients and their families.
- Liaise with the healthcare team.
- Refer to other members of the team or other relevant health professionals.
- Advocate for services, equipment, treatments and accessibility.
- Prevent deterioration and promote healthy lifestyles by encouraging physical activity and exercise.

Reflection

Reflection is an important part of the CR process. Physiotherapists use reflective practice to critically evaluate themselves, their beliefs and attitudes related to patient assessment and management (Donaghy and Moss 2000). They reflect on existing and new knowledge, making connections between both. This reflection enables the clinician to manage uncertainty, which in turn supports development of expertise and metacognition, which are also important elements for CR (Murphy 2004). Reflection can help clinicians understand the purpose of the questions they ask and the assessments they do. Reflection can encourage clinicians to think more broadly beyond the immediate diagnosis. Finally, reflection can encourage the creation of frameworks to organise clinical knowledge in ways that allow good decisions to be made (Jones et al 2018, Ziebart & MacDermid 2019).

Tips for Intervention:

- Intervention should occur as early as feasible. Remember intensity and repetition matter! Early and higher doses of exercises and movements are often encouraged. Consider frequency, intensity and time and type of exercise depending on phase of the patient's condition, types of learning, physical capacity, fatigability and/or any pathology or injuries. Consider neuroplasticity principles.
- Remember that although many of our interventions are aimed at improving impairments, the therapist is always

seeking carryover from impairment-focused intervention into functional activity and participation.

- Always prioritise task-specific practice whenever possible; however, if the patient has impairments that make it difficult to practice these tasks directly, you may also need to address impairments or practice specific movements either before or during a modified version of functional task practice.
- Choose exercises and activities that are meaningful for the patient.
- Consider exercise programs for independent practice wherever possible.
- Consider how you can support self-efficacy (confidence) and self-management in your patients (see Chapter 19 for some examples).
- Promote a positive mindset of encouragement, hope, resilience, adaptability and perseverance (Crum et al 2017).
- Focus also on health promotion through lifestyle modifications and behaviour change with your patients whenever possible. Encourage fitness with a focus on health and well-being through participation in enjoyable physical activity.
- Focus also on the health and well-being of the carer to reduce caregiver burden and burnout by providing information, education and skills training (Krishnan et al 2017).

Reassessment (+Outcomes)

The therapist reflects on the patient's responses to the intervention and conducts periodic reassessments to evaluate the effectiveness of treatment to decide to continue with treatment, periodically review or discharge the patient.

Measurement tools should be selected to establish a baseline of performance before physiotherapy and then at key strategic points to further document any change.

Objective measures can inform treatment planning and decision making by enabling members of the healthcare team to quantify certain movements, skills or functions relevant to the goals of rehabilitation and effectively monitor progress (see Chapter 5 for further reading on measurement tools).

The choice of measures used to monitor performance may also be guided by policy, audit, research or funding requirements. Although therapy time may be limited, therapists need to use a range of tools that will evaluate if improvements in impairments and function (activity) translate into improved participation such as quality of life and improved health status.

Online Sources of Standardised Measurement Tools From Verheyden & Tyson (2023) with permission

- Academy of Neurologic Physical Therapy Outcome Measures Recommendations (EDGE): http://www.neuropt.org/professional-resources/neurology-section-outcome-measures-recommendations Recommendations for stroke, multiple sclerosis, traumatic brain injury, spinal cord injury, Parkinson's, and vestibular disorders.
- Stroke-specific databases and evidence-based review of stroke rehabilitation: http://www.ebrsr.com/evidence-review/20-outcome-measures-stroke-rehabilitation; and StrokeEngine: http://www.strokengine.ca/find-assessment/
- Moore, J.L., Potter, K., Blankshain, K., et al., 2018. A core set of outcome measures for adults with neurologic conditions undergoing rehabilitation: a clinical practice guideline. J. Neurol. Phys. Ther. 42, 174–220. https://doi.org/10.1097/NPT.0000000000000229.

PUTTING IT ALL TOGETHER IN CASE SCENARIOS

Clinical Case 1 Developed by Jill Garner

Sarah, 1 week poststroke transferred from the acute stroke unit to the inpatient rehabilitation unit of a major metropolitan hospital

My CR process for Sarah is based on two sessions that focused on conducting a comprehensive physiotherapy assessment and completing my CR form. Sarah's full assessment is presented in Table 2.2.

Sarah is a 59-year-old woman who has had a right middle cerebral artery (MCA) cerebrovascular accident (CVA) resulting in a left-sided hemiplegia. She expressed her goals during my subjective examination as: 'I really want to get home by the end of the week, and I need to go outside somehow for a smoke.'

Sarah was someone who was preadmission managing her life independently with her husband and working part time in a school. Her hobbies included taking her dog for long walks, and she smoked 10 cigarettes a day.

Most inpatient rehabilitation units have discharge planning as the top priority during admission, ensuring safety for discharge for the client and the environment to which she was being discharged to. Often when a patient is admitted to rehabilitation, we have only parts of the picture of

TABLE 2.2 Sarah's Physiotherapy Assessment

History of present complaint	59-year-old woman admitted from an acute hospital to inpatient rehabilitation unit. History of code stroke activated after falling from her bed due to **left-sided weakness** upon waking. Diagnosis of right MCA infarct with left hemiplegia CT head showed large right MCA infarct Medical plan: For cardiac monitoring whilst still an inpatient. Commenced on Asasantin **Medications:** Asasantin Citalopram Perinodopril Atrovastain
Past medical history	Nil of note
Social history and environment	• Works 2 days a week at local preschool • Living in her own home with her husband in a 2-storey home with 9 stairs • She has 2 grownup children who do not live at home • Smoker (10 cigarettes a day) • Hobbies: walking her dog • No history of falls before this episode
Previous mobility	• Previously independently mobile unaided with nil issues • Usually fit and active, taking the dog for an hour-long walk every day • Attends local gym 3 times a week
Expressed goals	• I really want to get home by the end of the week. • I need to go outside somehow for a smoke.
Cognition and communication	• Alert, orientated, motivated to participate • Consent: YES • Limited insight into her functional abilities, appears to understand all information given to her • Expresses herself well • Poor concentration on task at present
Pain	• Nil at rest • Reports some pain on moving arm: 3/10 VAS
General observations	• Left lower facial paralysis • Lying asymmetrically in bed • Note lack of spontaneous movements on left
Right upper limb	• Full range of movement • Muscle power 5/5 • Sensation intact • Coordination: NAD
Left upper limb	• On palpation: no GHJ subluxation, head of humerus internally rotated and sitting anterior in glenoid fossa • Full passive ROM of GHJ, elbow, RUJs, wrist and fingers • Some activity all muscle groups, not full range antigravity • Poor proximal stability when moving distally, especially shoulder girdle and GHJ • In sitting, poor shoulder girdle stability while raising arms and reaching; shoulder hitches into elevation, shoulder flexion (60°) abduction (20°), elbow flexion (30°). Minimal movement of wrist/fingers noted. No selective movement at wrist or fingers. All movements slow and effortful. • When arms supported on table, patient able to supinate half range, no active pronation, wrist extension with forearm support. Minimal finger flexion/extension with sensory facilitation. • Tone: hypotonia throughout • Sensation light touch R = L, sensory inattention to left Proprioception R = L • Coordination: not tested as limited activity

TABLE 2.2   Sarah's Physiotherapy Assessment—Cont'd

Right lower limb	• Full range of movement • Muscle power 5/5 • Sensation intact • Coordination: NAD

Left lower limb	• ROM, reduced external rotation left hip compared with right; hip extension is limited by hip flexor muscle tightness. Note dorsiflexion −5° limited by plantar flexor muscle tightness.
	Motor control
	Sitting
	• Lifts leg in flexor pattern through half range. Ankle dorsiflexion with supination noted during lift of leg. Able to extend knee 50° with ankle plantarflexion. Minimal ability to isolate active knee or ankle flexor movements.
	Supine
	• Active hip and knee synergistic flexor and extensor movements through available range.
	• Unable to place or maintain foot on bed in bridging position. Left leg assisted to flexion by therapist, able to 'bridge', needs manual cueing to maintain level pelvis and left knee stable.
	  • Tone: decreased compared with right
	  • Sensation light touch R = L, sensory inattention to left Proprioception R = L
	  • Coordination: dysmetric

Bed mobility	• Independently rolls to L side, initiates with R arm and head • Independently moves up the bed mostly using right leg • Able to bridge with assistance, uses R leg mainly and weight shift to L only • Able to roll onto R side with verbal cueing and minimal assistance for L leg; patient can activate leg muscles to assist movement to side lying
Lying to sitting	• Overactive R and limited use of left upper limb and lower limb to assist • Sits up by pulling up with R arm and sitting straight up in bed; able to perform with one person assisting via side lying
Sitting on edge of bed	• Observation: head slightly rotated, and side flexed to right • Trunk side flexed to right, with elongated, low tone trunk on left, decreased postural control in sitting. Uneven weight bearing in sitting. L foot not fully in contact with the floor. Sitting on bed with R arm support • Able to initiate forward flexion/extension, needs manual and verbal cueing to maintain position • Able to reach out of base of support to right with R arm, decreased ability to return to midline. When attempting to reach to left displaces trunk posteriorly.
Vision	• Visual fields intact • Horizontal or vertical gaze: no saccadic eye movements • Visual inattention to left
Sit to stand	• Tending to pull up to stand, overusing R side • One-person assistance needed to position foot • Verbal cueing to bring trunk forward to stand. Unable to maintain weight through L foot as standing. • Stands with two-person assistance and verbal cueing. Unable to maintain knee in extension once standing; knee gives way, needs one-person support. • Arm postures in 20° elbow flexion during attempt to stand, no posturing during sitting
Standing balance	• Poor lower limb control on left in standing, • pulling with right hand • Unable to stand without support of one- or two-person assist.
Transfers bed to chair	• Transfer to right with assistance of one person behind to assist in weight transfer and another person in front to brace left knee • When fatigued may require stand lifter
Gait	Unable to assess
Stairs and running	Unable to assess

CT, Computed tomography; *GHJ*, glenohumeral joint; *L*, left; *NAD*, no abnormality detected; *R*, right; *RUJs*, radial-ulnar joints; *VAS*, Visual Analogue Scale.

the patient's condition and circumstances, and it may take a few days of assessment and discussion with the patient, carers, family members, and team with information on home setup to develop a provisional plan. This plan may be modified or change depending on intrinsic and extrinsic patient factors and the progress of the patient. It is normal practice in the rehabilitation setting to have regular discussions with the patient and family and regular team meetings with the treating team to review progress and challenges to discharge planning.

Fig. 2.4 presents some of the key factors that neurological physiotherapists may want to consider when interpreting their assessment findings and developing a treatment plan. The therapist considers the aim of therapy using RAMP as well as organisational and therapist factors.

My CRF for Sarah is presented in Table 2.3. As part of her management, I looked at her goals and impairments and function and worked out collaboratively with Sarah and the inpatient team what would be needed to help her reach the goals. I considered her mood, motivation, cardiovascular fitness and anything else affecting her recovery and progression.

I hypothesised that the loss of sitting balance, difficulty within ability to transfers and move from sitting to standing was due to:

1. Weakness and loss of control in trunk.
2. Loss of voluntary and selective movement in the leg – insufficient hip–knee extension and inability to depress the leg into the supporting surface.
3. Ankle–foot weakness and loss of ankle joint range of motion.
4. Impaired lower leg proprioception.
   My key observations for treatment planning were as follows:
- In sitting: Head not in midline, trunk side flexed to right, uneven weight bearing (WB) in sitting, needs manual and verbal cues to maintain midline, unable to reach out of base of support and return to midline. Left foot supinated.
- Sit to stand uses right upper limb to initiate all functional activities; left foot supinated and in front of left when attempting to stand. Using right leg and arm to initiate standing. Needs two people to assist standing with each holding the patient' hand, facilitate pelvic tilt, gluteal activity, foot placement and verbal using. May need wedge under left heel to facilitate WB on left, as foot is tending into plantarflexion. Once standing, decreased motor control in left gluteals, quads, dorsiflexors and joint position sense affects her ability to use left leg and stack trunk over WB limb.

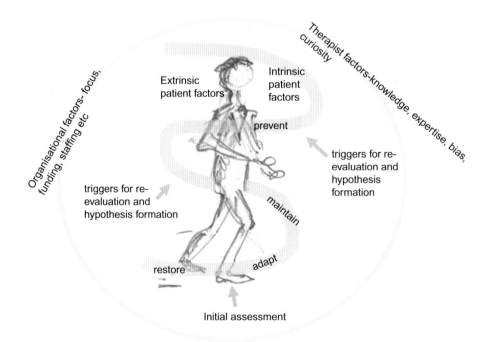

FIG. 2.4 Clinical reasoning considerations for neurological physiotherapists.

TABLE 2.3 Clinical Reasoning Form for Sarah

Body Structure and Function

Problem list	Causes	Goals	Interventions
Left UL • Pain in left arm on movement 7/10 • GHJ sitting anterior in glenoid fossa • Unable to stabilise scapular when reaching with arm • Sensory inattention on testing	Poor resting position of GHJ: decreased management strategies for UL in lying, sitting and standing Low muscle tone	Decrease pain on movement from 7/10 to 3/10 GHJ sitting in anatomical position 2–3 weeks Able to stabilise scapular when reaching with arm supported on plinth 1 week	Education to patient/staff regarding positioning and use of available muscles Discussion with nursing staff regarding adequate pain relief before therapy session Repositioning techniques Realign left GHJ before beginning ROM activities FES, bilateral techniques Scapular setting exercises in sideling, sitting and while reaching Therapy sessions to include therapist sitting on left side to bring attention to left and encouraging patient to look at arm during functional activities Functional strengthening using activity that she has in a functional way, mirror therapy, motor imagery Hydrotherapy for facilitating UL activation Use of gaming/robotics to facilitate activity Programme of exercise in her room, encouraging independent practice
Left LL • Muscle tightness: hip, foot; hip held in flexion, hip extension only to neutral, foot not in plantigrade • LL moving in synergies when rolling and sit to stand	Decreased activation muscles in left LL Low muscle tone	Full passive range hip extension, full range dorsiflexion in 1 week Full active range in 2 week	Gastrocnemius/soleus/hip flexor stretches in supine, sitting and standing Active gluteal activation in side lying Bridging Sit-to-stand practice with equal weight bearing, starting with wedge under heel Standing practice with trunk aligned over stance leg to stretch hip flexors and DF Encouraging weight bearing out of synergistic pattern: abduction and extension of LL Progress to body weight support treadmill training/robotics Hydrotherapy for gait practice and activation Programme of exercises in her room for independent practice

(Continued)

TABLE 2.3   Clinical Reasoning Form for Sarah—Cont'd

Body Structure and Function

Problem list	Causes	Goals	Interventions
Trunk • Overactive right side with poor activity and elongation on left with loss of control • Uneven weight bearing in standing • Able to stand feet apart eyes open 10 seconds with standby • Poor ability to reach out of BOS and return to midline	Right side overactive to assist in keeping up against gravity Mostly using right leg while standing: poor activation left LL, decreased weight bearing and activity left trunk LL especially inactive foot: poor acceptance of BOS	Able to elongate trunk on left when reaching 2 weeks Sit unsupported, hands on lap 1–2 weeks in midline Able to reach out of BOS to both sides 3 weeks Use change in Trunk Impairment Scale as measure	Sitting practice: use of towel to get even weight bearing and midline awareness Pelvic tilting: anterior and lateral Reaching out of base of support Head turning and interacting with the environment Exercises from Trunk Impairment Scale to facilitate trunk activation Sit to stand with support Standing with support
Low postural tone	Right CVA and prolonged bed rest		To sit out of bed after breakfast: a tabled sitting regimen Incorporate standing with support during ADL tasks as able Engage in activities on ward Encourage support and activities from family members Remember use of voice for facilitation of activity and engagement
Visual inattention to left	Right CVA	To scan to left without external cueing 3 weeks	Practice scanning environment when sitting and supported standing and later when walking/moving around the ward
Activity Limitations Function • Overactive right side throughout functional activities • Poor activation on left, decreased awareness of midline • Needs assistance to move from lying to sitting to standing • Transfers to right needing assistance of 2 helpers	Decreased activity and function on left Prolonged bed rest: deconditioning and poor initiation of functional tasks	Rolling in bed independently 1 week Lie to sit and sit to lie independently 3 weeks Sit to stand with close standby 2–3 weeks Standing with close standby for a few seconds 2–3 weeks Transfer to right and left with one-person assist 2–3 weeks	UL and LL strengthening and balance Cardiovascular training Practice task daily facilitating normal movement Practice safe transfer techniques with nursing staff and carers as able Discussion with patient as able regarding neuroplasticity principle and focus the importance of focusing on the left

TABLE 2.3 Clinical Reasoning Form for Sarah—Cont'd

Body Structure and Function

Problem list	Causes	Goals	Interventions
Decreased cardiovascular fitness	Prolonged bed rest	To be active achieving moderate exertion on the (BORG) perceived rate of exertion scale	UL and LL arm and leg cycle: increase repetitions of practice This can happen in the first part of the therapy session as priming for function
Does not continue with independent practice in her room	Impacted by severe impairments so limited choice of exercises to practice Does not understand why she should be exercising or what the exercises are helpful for Has a low mood and does not want to engage with exercises	Daily independent practice of 20 minutes per day achieved in 1 week	Collaboratively work on independent exercise program, including exercises that are relevant to the patient recovery and that are salient to her, use of graphs or iPad to monitor adherence, check repetitions and gain feedback from the patient regarding progression of exercises

Contextual Factors

Problem list	Causes	Goals	Interventions
Limited family involvement in patient therapy	Time poor, lack of therapists' discussion	Family members to attend therapy sessions as able and be involved in encouraging independent practice	Family members to attend therapy sessions as able and be involved in encouraging independent practice
Cognition • Decreased insight • Concentration span of 1–2 minutes at present and easily distracted	Right CVA	Early family meeting to support patient's goal regarding discharge Over next 2–3 weeks, increase time spent focused on activity from 2 minutes to 20 minutes	Work with client, staff and carers to keep patient safe, discuss abilities/limitations Keep therapy sessions short Timetable all sessions Possible use of private spaces to assist with focus
Smoker (10 cigarettes a day)	Premorbid addiction	Involve councillors specifically trained regarding this. Use motivational interviewing skills to help decrease or stop smoking because this will affect cardiovascular fitness and addresses secondary prevention	
Limited engagement in therapy, reluctant to attend therapy, only able to participate for 10 minutes at a time and then wants to return to her room	Diagnosis of stroke linked to depression	Patient to be able to attend full therapy sessions and work collaboratively with therapist on her goals	Discuss with team regarding motivation strategies Involvement of social worker or psychologist Possible assessment for diagnosis of anxiety/depression

(Continued)

TABLE 2.3	**Clinical Reasoning Form for Sarah**—Cont'd		
Body Structure and Function			
Problem list	**Causes**	**Goals**	**Interventions**
Participation Restrictions			
Unable to return home at present Has 9 stairs at home that she is unable to negotiate	Currently not enough activity on left side to stand, walk or use stairs	To discuss situation with occupational therapist, case workers, social workers, patient and family regarding use of upstairs and assess needs for day leave To discuss with occupational therapist regarding review of home situation and possible need for home modification	Involve family members and carers in discussing home options Work collaboratively with occupational therapist regarding home modifications If using downstairs of home only: Simulate home setup and practice with family and carers regarding transfers and activities from home

ADL, Activities of daily living; *BOS*, base of support; *BWS*, body weight support; *DF*, dorsiflexion; *FES*, functional electrical stimulation; *GHJ*, glenohumeral joint; *LL*, lower limb; *UL*, upper limb.

Regarding treatment options, priorities at this stage would be to increase awareness and activity on the left side to enable less dependency in functional tasks and so work towards discharging Sarah home. Regarding my choice of standardised outcome measures, I used the Functional Independence Measure to measure level of dependency with functional tasks, the Trunk Impairment Scale to measure trunk activation and function, the Modified Clinical Test of Sensory Integration of Balance and functional reach in standing for balance assessment.

For any changes in Sarah's motor control and function, my expectation would be to see some gains of function initially within the first session, although there may not initially be carryover between sessions. I would expect her function to change from light assist to standby within 1–2 weeks dependent on time in therapy, patient motivation and no other limiting factors.

Clinical Case 2 Developed by James McLoughlin

Ms M is a 38-year-old woman with relapsing-remitting MS, diagnosed 8 years ago, who is attending a private clinic for assessment treatment and advice.

Ms M lives at home with husband and three young children, ages 5, 8, and 12 years. She is independently mobile over small distances and is still driving. Ms M has had a stable neurological presentation since starting ocrelizumab in 2020, with no relapses or new neurological symptoms. There has been a slow progression of disability since diagnosis, but exercise and her medications have helped over the past 2 years. The National Insurance Disability Scheme in Australia funds monthly physiotherapy reviews.

Ms M stopped attending the gym for over 5 months because of Covid-19. Ms M fell two times in the past 2 months. Both times she caught left her foot and tripped forward; previously the last fall was more than 2 years ago. Her score on the Patient Disease Steps is 2, indicating moderate disability with visibly abnormal gait, without use of ambulation aids. The CRF for Ms M is presented in Table 2.4.

CR During Session 1

Reflection. The main concerns in this session were falls (n = 2 over 2 months), potential injury and loss of confidence. Ms M stopped attending the gym for over 5 months because of Covid-19. Reduced physical activity and exercise during lockdown, with worsening mobility levels and the pain from a right ingrown toenail with clawing of great toe may be adding to more recent changes in gait pattern, balance and falls. After a discussion with Ms M about her main concerns and goals, balance and falls took priority for this session, with a focus on selecting and practicing the key home exercises. Exercise self-efficacy (ESE) indicated low confidence in being able to do exercises when fatigued, down/depressed or busy. The Timed Up and Go (TUG)

TABLE 2.4   Ms M's Clinical Reasoning Form

ICF Framework	Problem list	Goals	Treatment plan/progress
Body function and impairments	**Upper motor neurone weakness bilaterally** Left power, generally 4 Right power, generally 4+ **Bilateral spasticity** Left knee extension MAS = 0; knee flex = 1 Ankle clonus at 10 DF Right knee extension MAS = 1, knee flex = 1 Ankle clonus -10 mild unsustained **Gait observations** Slow cadence Reduced push-off Minimal knee flexion, ankle PF midswing Occasional footdrop/catch either foot **(Note: has had two falls)** **Right ingrown toenail** Foot, right, ingrown toenail, painful Right great toe claw: flexor hallucis longus, reduce ROM, tone, pressure area **Balance** Slower and ineffective left balance step **Fatigue** **Bladder frequency and urgency** **Emotional lability (mild)**	**Increase and maintain lower limb strength** **Monitor spasticity and spasms** **Reduce pain and spasticity** from toe clawing **Improve walking speed** **Improve walking safety/ balance** **Treat/remove ingrown toenail** **Reduce pain** from ingrown toenail **Reduce risk of falls** **Improve balance** when out of the house and in crowds of other people **Monitor general fatigue** **Reduce motor fatigue and weakness** linked to strength and endurance performance **Monitor** **Impact on ADLs** **Signs of infection** **Manage and monitor with GP**	Incorporate progressive strengthening to lower limbs Incorporate with balance and functional movement as much as possible Intermittent assessment and outcome measures of spasticity Refer to spasticity clinic for possible future adjunct botulinum toxin Specific gait exercises to increase push-off, knee flexion and balance Functional exercises to increase strength and coordination through early knee flexion Refer to podiatrist Improve balance strategies and strength with less toe clawing Balance exercises focus on fast and effective stepping strategies, mainly forward, dynamic stepping and gait Subjective questioning Endurance training: intermittent treadmill walking at gym Possible future FES Subjective questioning with GP or physiotherapist GP prescribed SSRI medication in 2021; monitor effects and any side effects
Activities	**Walking small distances** **Dynamic balance and falls risk** **Walking longer distances**	**Improve balance and mobility levels, self-efficacy** **Reduce falls risk, improve confidence** **Increase walking capacity and physical activity levels**	Recommence treadmill training Increase HEP for balance three times a week Treadmill training for 6–8 weeks; then introduce further overground walks
Participation	**Walking when other people present,** e.g., school drop-off, pick-up **Play with kids and dog** inside and outside **Social gatherings,** family, parties	**Keep independent walking in the community with people and social engagements** **Continue safe active play at home** **Increase balance and confidence in gatherings, such as family gatherings, school drop-off/pick-up**	

(Continued)

TABLE 2.4	Ms M's Clinical Reasoning Form—Cont'd		
ICF Framework	**Problem list**	**Goals**	**Treatment plan/progress**
Contextual personal environmental	MS is a chronic progressive condition Gym stopped now due to Covid-19 (included treadmill training) Finding time to exercise at home difficult Reduced activity with pandemic lockdowns, home schooling Fallen two times in past month (more than usual): tripped as left foot scuffed the floor Busy with three young children and a puppy HEP needs to be safe as often home alone	**Prevent, mitigate progression of disability** **Return to supervised gym** **Increase confidence** **Increase physical activity** **Reduce falls risk**	Education about brain health and physical activity in MS Support, praise and reinforce to help with motivation to begin gym session again Reinforce importance of HEP in relation to balance, mobility and confidence plus health benefits long term, encouragement, motivation Monitor number and type/context of falls Focus first on balance aspect of mobility > distance – Stance ML control – Stepping reactions – Response to perturbations – Footwear (home agility, vs treadmill, longer walks) Ms M to demonstrate and practice HEP carefully Check safety, give choice for autonomy and ability to adjust for fatigue and confidence Write report recommending smartwatch for falls detection, activity tracker with National Disability Insurance Scheme (Australia)

ADL, Activities of daily living; *DF*, dorsiflexion; *FES*, functional electrical stimulation; *GP*, general practitioner; *HEP*, home exercise program; *MAS*, Modified Ashworth Scale; *ML*, medial-lateral; *PF*, plantarflexion; *SSRI*, selective serotonin reuptake inhibitor.

speed of 10.22 seconds indicated a slightly higher risk of falls.

Intervention

Balance home exercise prescription focused on lateral weight transfer and momentary single leg stance balance with light touch at a wall, and forward lean with quick stepping daily for 5 minutes per exercise. Both balance exercises were deliberately chosen as only slightly challenging with an emphasis on adherence and becoming more confident and consistent with performance. Emphasis was on getting exercise back into a routine, if possible, before prescribing more specific exercise doses. Walking advice focused on slowly increasing walking capacity again on flat paths using running shoes with greater forefoot–toe rocker support for

longer walks. Referral and an appointment were made for the podiatrist in 2 weeks for right ingrown toenail on right side.

CR During Session 2

Reassessment. Two months later, there had been no falls since last visit. The podiatrist operated 6 weeks ago on the right ingrown toe successfully. Walking and physical activity levels had reduced. Covid-19 rules had resulted in intermittent home schooling for her children, as well as gym closure, making exercising more difficult. The TUG had improved to 12.12 seconds.

Her 10-meter walk speed was 11.89 seconds with 16 steps. Her gait symmetry and weight shift had improved compared with 2 months earlier. Cadence remained slow.

Balance reactions remained slowed with forward stepping, with improved balance control on landing compared with the last session. The toe was healing well, with some pain under the right toe in stance, with velocity-dependent tone increase in her right great toe with slightly reduced passive range of motion in great toe extension.

Treadmill assessment (holding on): Treadmill performance had deteriorated since last assessment 9 months ago. At a speed of 1.8 km/h, 0 incline, there was a reduced push-off bilaterally, with subsequent reduced knee flexion at this terminal phase in stance. We trialled various combinations and found speed of 2.2 km/h, 2 incline, with perceived exertion on Borg at 12 (between light and somewhat hard), which was much preferred by Ms M, improved plantarflexion, observed push-off and knee flexion angles.

Reflection. Walking speed was included as a measurement tool at this assessment. Treadmill walking was assessed to enable some preparation, guidance and confidence when returning to the gym. The idea was to build confidence by providing some achievable parameters to begin training. These treadmill training parameters will be discussed with the exercise physiologist for Ms M's return to the gym. The ESE revealed worsening confidence in ability to exercise at home during this most recent home-schooling period. No falls, improved balance with exercises and reduced toe pain were pleasing, and Ms M was clear about her desire to focus on walking. This resulted in this session focusing on gait pattern and treadmill training.

Interventions. Reactive stepping forward for balance was progressed to more random steps by using the Clock Yourself phone application at 30 steps per minute using the top half clock face to give some variation and practice at a level of challenge to encourage learning.

I contacted her general practitioner to recommend referral to the spasticity clinic for an assessment of suitability for botulinum toxin injection to reduce clawing and associate pain in the right great toe, and a trial of the Bioness L300 (functional electrical stimulation) device, which may be an option to help gait and mobility for Ms M when considering dorsiflexion and catching the foot has caused recent falls.

CR During Session 3

Reassessment. Three weeks later, Ms M attended the gym and has booked in for two times per week. It was important to encourage and support this decision and congratulate Ms M on this important step. Gait observation showed improved bilateral push-off, knee flexion and symmetry with slight improvement in speed; however, intermittent lateral pelvic drop in early swing phase, especially on the left, was identified as contributing to unreliable toe clearance and therefore a movement to practice in gait training.

Ms M subjectively felt tight in both hamstring regions with walking and hips felt 'stiff' and 'heavy'. Objectively, hip range of motion (ROM) was full, with some minor stiffness and guarding in passive flexion beyond 80°. There were slight improvements with TUG of 10.64 seconds and 10-meter walk speed of 10.38 seconds with 15 steps.

Interventions. Exercise started as self-mobilising hip flexion ROM by reaching down with one foot up on step providing a mild hamstring stretch while simultaneously gaining some practice control and stabilise stance on the grounded leg behind. This was followed by step-ups onto a 10-cm step in front to encourage hip flexion with pelvic stability and trunk in more neutral extension. The aim was to become familiar and confident with this type of movement using practice and feedback via a combination on knowledge of result (by being able to complete the type of stance successfully without loss of balance) and knowledge of performance (where it enables faster and higher hip flexion). Stair climbing and walking were also mentioned as functional tasks that will benefit from these skills.

Progression ideas were shared with Ms M to ensure she has an idea of where this kind of exercise was leading to and allowing Ms M to progress safely between sessions. This was an important educational part of the session. Ideas and variations by Ms M were invited and actively encouraged to allow for a greater sense of ownership and autonomy.

The last part of the session ran through the Clock Yourself stepping. The exercise was progressed by adding the full Clock yourself stepping app, with an extra 30 seconds for three sets of 2 minutes, 30 seconds every 'non-gym' day. The Intermittent Treadmill program at the gym twice per week was continued as planned at the last session.

Summary Reflection

This case demonstrated the need to provide a comprehensive assessment that may extend over multiple sessions, with further brief reassessments in follow-up sessions. Monitoring both physical performance and self-efficacy with suitable outcome measures helped guide the interventions, and clinical experience about MS, fatigue, exertion, spasticity, balance and gait analysis helped fine-tune the interventions selected.

Listening skills, empathy and flexibility were needed to adapt physiotherapy sessions and exercise planning. The ESE added information not gained otherwise; this influenced prioritisation of exercises. The TUG and 10-meter walk speed test allowed for measures of objective data over time and to use as feedback and motivation for Ms M. Video analysis also allowed for some feedback and coaching education about what movement we are focusing on.

There are many training principles to consider when designing a physical rehabilitation program. The 10 guiding movement training principles (McLoughlin 2020) were used to categorise principles that were considered and the level of importance within each of the three sessions. The most important principles identified for this client were beliefs and self-efficacy (especially confidence with balance and mobility after recent falls, and return to the gym), biomechanics (large focus on treadmill speed for desired gait pattern with optimal ankle plantarflexion and knee flexion at push-off, while minimising exertion), feedback (tactile and verbal cues used to gain effective balance positions), error-based learning (important for balance stepping and to maintain desired walk speed and pattern on treadmill) and attentional focus (external focus on speed and rhythm to induce performance change in gait).

This case also demonstrates that the neurological physiotherapist in the community plays an important role in referring to other health professionals for symptomatic management and additional rehabilitation interventions.

CONCLUSION

We have identified five primary components within the CR cycle: assessment, interpretation, treatment planning, intervention and reassessment (+outcomes). These primary components are also influenced by other important components such as the prognosis based on RAMP aims of therapy, the ICF-based problem list, person-centred goals, and reflection within a person-centred care model of healthcare. Two case scenarios were presented to illustrate how experienced clinicians apply these principles in the clinical setting. A CRF was completed for each case that enabled the therapists sum up their thinking in a more explicit way.

Both cases emphasised the many factors that influence CR within neurological physiotherapy sessions. The ICF problem list provided a detailed framework to identify many relevant issues in the specific context of the clients' lives. The interventions selected were influenced by prognosis, therapy aims in terms of RAMP, the goals and preferences of the client, as well as other contextual factors such as social situation, healthcare setting, healthcare funding and policy. Both cases demonstrated how treatment plans are modified depending on intrinsic and extrinsic patient factors and the progress of the patient. Monitoring therapy with suitable outcome measures helped guide the therapist interventions. Knowledge from research evidence, as well as reflection about what movement training principles to prioritise, helped with clinical decision making to design an individualised exercise program and plan for its progression over time. Liaising and linking with other relevant health professionals ensured a more comprehensive plan to support and advocate for both clients. Both cases discussed the importance of considering mood, motivation and self-efficacy to optimise recovery and progression.

SELF-ASSESSMENT QUESTIONS

1. Define clinical reasoning.
2. What are the main components within the clinical reasoning cycle?
3. What is the meaning of the RAMP acronym?
4. What is the advantage of using the ICF framework to identify problems lists, goals and treatment plans/progress? Case Study 1
5. How would some of Sarah's intrinsic factors such as general health, mood, motivation and fitness affect her treatment?
6. What would you as a therapist need to consider when discharging Sarah from inpatient rehabilitation? Case Study 2
7. How might low scores on the ESE influence your reasoning in relation to how challenging the types of home exercises prescribed?
8. What factors were considered when selecting the speed and incline for treadmill training?

REFERENCES

American Physical Therapy Association (APTA), 2020. Core Competencies of a Physical Therapist Resident. Accessed November 4, 2021. Available at: https://www.apta.org/content assets/89db00a8ab01418c844ced87e401563e/core-competencies-pt-resident.pdf.

Atkinson, H.L., Nixon-Cave, K., 2011. A tool for clinical reasoning and reflection using the international classification of functioning, disability, and health (ICF) framework and patient management model. Phys. Ther. 91, 416–430.

Bland, M.D., Whitson, M., Harris, H., et al., 2015. Descriptive data analysis examining how standardized assessments are used to guide post–acute discharge recommendations for rehabilitation services after stroke. Phys. Ther. 95, 710–719.

Bovend'Eerdt, T.J.H., Botell, R.E., Wade, D.T., 2009. Writing SMART rehabilitation goals and achieving goal attainment scaling: a practical guide. Clin. Rehabil. 23, 352–361.

Brentnall, J., Thackray, D., Judd, B., 2022. Evaluating the clinical reasoning of student health professionals in placement and simulation settings: a systematic review. Int. J. Environ. Res. Public. Health 19, 936.

Crum, A.L., Leibowitz, K.A., Verghese, A., 2017. Making mindset matter. BMJ. 356, j674.

Deutsch, J.E., Gill-Body, K.M., Schenkman, M., 2022. Updated integrated framework for making clinical decisions across the lifespan and health conditions. Phys. Ther. 102, pzab281

Dimitriadis, Z., Skoutelis, V., Tsipra, E., 2015. Clinical reasoning in neurological physiotherapy. Arch. Hellenic. Med. 33, 447–457.

Donaghy, M.E., Morss, K., 2000. Guided reflection: a framework to facilitate and assess reflective practice within the discipline of physiotherapy. Physiother. Theory Pract. 16, 3–14.

Edwards, S., 2002. Neurological Physiotherapy. Edinburgh, Churchill-Livingstone.

Elvén, M., Dean, E., 2017. Factors influencing physical therapists' clinical reasoning: qualitative systematic review and meta-synthesis. Phys. Ther. Rev. 22, 60–67.

Fulk, G., Field-Fote, E.C., 2011. Measures of evidence in evidence-based practice. J. Neurol. Phys. Ther. 35, 55–56.

Furze, J.A., Black, L., McDevitt, A.W., Kobal, K.L., Durning, S.J., Jensen, G.M., 2022. Clinical reasoning: the missing core competency in physical therapist education and practice. Phys. Ther. 102, pzac093.

Gangwani, R., Cain, A., Collins, A., Cassidy, J.M., 2022. Leveraging factors of self-efficacy and motivation to optimize stroke recovery. Front. Neurol. 13, 823202.

Garner, J., Lennon, S., 2018. Chapter 4. Neurological assessment: the basis of clinical decision-making. In: Lennon, S., Ramdharry, G., Verheyden, GNeurological Physiotherapy Pocketbook. Elsevier Science, London.

Garner, J, Van der Berg, M, Lange, B, Vuu, S, Lennon, S., 2023. Physiotherapy assessment in people with neurological conditions—Evidence for the most frequently included domains: a mixed-methods systematic review. J Eval Clin Pract. 1–23.

Gilliland, S., Wainwright, S.F., 2020. Perspectives and practice: physical therapist students' clinical reasoning. J. Phys. Ther. Educ. 34, 150–159.

Gutenbrunner, C., Nugraha, B., 2020. Decision-making in evidence-based practice in rehabilitation medicine: proposing a fourth factor. Am. J. Phys. Med. Rehabil. 99, 436–440.

Holmes, J.A., Logan, P., Morris, R., Radford, K., 2020. Factors affecting the delivery of complex rehabilitation interventions in research with neurologically impaired adults: a systematic review. Syst. Rev. 9, 268.

Horvat, L., Horey, D., Romios, P., et al., 2014. Cultural competence education for health professions (review). Cochrane Database Syst. Rev. 5, 1–98.

Jones, M., Rivett, D., 2004. Clinical Reasoning for Manual Therapists. Butterworth Heinemann, Edinburgh.

Jones, Edwards, Jensen, 2018. Clinical reasoning in physiotherapy. In: Higgs, J., Jensen, G.M., Loftus, S., Christensen, N. (Eds.), Clinical Reasoning in the Health Professions, 4th Ed. Elsevier Science, London.

Kimberley, T.J., Novak, I., Boyd, L., Fowler, E., 2017. Stepping up to rethink the future of rehabilitation: IV STEP considerations and inspirations. Paediatr. Phys. Ther. S76–S85.

Kleynen, M., Beurskens, A., Olijve, H., Kamphuis, J., Braun, S., 2020. Application of motor learning in neurorehabilitation: a framework for health-care professionals. Physiother. Theory Pract. 36, 1–20.

Krishnan, S., York, M.K., Backus, D., Heyn, P.C., 2017. Coping with caregiver burnout when caring for a person with neurodegenerative disease: a guide for caregivers. Arch. Phys. Med. Rehabil 98, 805–807.

Levin, M.F., Kleim, J.A., Wolf, S.L., 2009. What do motor recovery and compensation mean in patients following stroke? Neurorehabil. Neural. Repair. 23, 313–319.

Lexell, J., Brogårdh, C., 2015. The use of ICF in the neurorehabilitation process. Neurorehabilitation. 36, 5–9.

Maier, M., Ballester, B.R., Verschure, P.F.M.J., 2019. Principles of neurorehabilitation after stroke based on motor learning and brain plasticity mechanisms. Front. Syst. Neurosci. 13, 74.

May, S., Withers, S., Reeve, S., Greasley, A., 2010. Limited clinical reasoning skills used by novice physiotherapists when involved in the assessment and management of patients with shoulder problems: a qualitative study. J. Manual Manipul. Ther. 18, 84–88.

McLoughlin, J., 2020. Ten guiding principles for movement training in neurorehabilitation. Openphysio J. Available at: https://www.openphysiojournal.com/article/ten-guiding-principles-for-movement-training-in-neurorehabilitation/.

Michie, S., van Stralen, M.M., West, R., 2011. The behaviour change wheel: a new method for characterising and designing behaviour change interventions. Implement. Sci. 6, 42.

Murphy, J.I., 2004. Using focused reflection and articulation to promote clinical reasoning: an evidence-based teaching strategy. Nurs. Educ. Perspect. 25, 226–231.

O'Donoghue, G., McMahon, S., Holt, A., Nedai, M., Nybo, T., Peiris, C.L., 2021. Obesity bias and stigma, attitudes, and beliefs among entry-level physiotherapy students in the Republic of Ireland: a cross sectional study. Physiotherapy. 112, 55–63.

Playford, E.D., Siegert, R., Levack, W., Freeman, J., 2009. Areas of consensus and controversy about goal setting in rehabilitation: a conference report. Clin. Rehabil. 23, 334–344.

Ramdharry, G.M., Anderson, M., 2022. Exercise in myositis: what is important, the prescription or the person? Best Pract. Res. Clin. Rheumatol., 36.

Shumway-Cook, A., Woollacott, M.M., 2017. Motor Control: Translating Research Into Clinical Practice, 4th Ed. Lippincott Williams & Wilkins, Baltimore.

Siegert, R.J., Levack, W.M. (Eds.), 2014. Rehabilitation Goal Setting: Theory, Practice, and Evidence. CRC Press, Boca Raton.

Verheyden, G., Tyson, S., 2023. Chapter 4: Standardised measurement tools. In: Lennon, S., Ramdharry, G., Verheyden, G. (Eds.), Physical Management for Neurological Conditions. Elsevier Science, London.

World Health Organization, 2001. International Classification of Functioning, Disability and Health (ICF). World Health Organization, Geneva, http://www.who.int/classification/icf.

Ziebart, C., MacDermid, J.C., 2019. Reflective practice in physical therapy: a scoping review. Phys. Ther. 99, 1056–1068.

Common Impairments and the Impact on Activity

James Vincent McLoughlin

OUTLINE

Introduction, 53
Weakness, 54
    Upper Motor Neurone Weakness, 54
    Lower Motor Neurone Weakness, 55
Fatigue, 55
    General Fatigue, 55
    Motor Fatigue, 55
Disorders of Muscle Tone, 56
    Hypertonus, 56
    Hypotonus, 57
    Dystonia, 57
    Involuntary Muscle Spasms, 58
    Dyskinesias, 58
Key Points, 58
Disorders of Coordination, 58
    Cerebellar Ataxia, 58
    Sensory Ataxia, 59
    Resting Tremor, 59
    Intention Tremor, 59
    Loss of Dexterity, 59
Disorders of Motor Planning, 60
    Apraxia, 60

Bradykinesia/Akinesia, 60
Freezing of Gait, 60
Functional Movement Disorders, 60
Vestibular Disorders, 61
    Peripheral Vestibular Disorders, 61
    Central Vestibular Disorders, 61
Visuospatial Disorders, 62
    Hemianopia, 62
    Unilateral Spatial Neglect, 62
    Contraversive Pushing, 62
    Cognitive Dysfunction, 62
Sensory Disorders, 63
    Sensory Loss, 63
    Paraesthesia and Dysaesthesia, 63
    Pain, 63
Secondary Complications, 64
    Contracture, 64
    Physical Inactivity and Deconditioning, 64
    Learned Non-Use, 65
Conclusion, 65

INTRODUCTION

It is important for any clinician working in neurological rehabilitation to become familiar with common neurological impairments. The knowledge and ability to identify and assess many neurological impairments is crucial, in addition to a clear understanding of how these impairments affect movement and activity. Many of the impairments discussed in this chapter relate directly to neurological injury or pathology, whereas other issues relate to secondary physical, cognitive and behavioural adaptations. In clinical practice, most people with neurological conditions present with a complex mixture of impairments that affect activity levels in many different ways. Optimal clinical reasoning begins with an ability to identify all relevant neurological impairments. The next major challenge facing the neurotherapist is the ability to tease out the many overlapping impairments affecting physical performance and function, and select the most appropriate evidence-based rehabilitation strategies based on all this information.

A common example of overlapping impairments is the spectrum of signs that can exist in a stroke survivor presenting with upper limb hemiparesis. Within the upper motor neurone (UMN) syndrome, impairments include negative features of weakness, slowness and loss of skill, in addition to positive features of increased muscle tone and hyperreflexia. Both features might be addressed with various interventions, depending on the level of function and individual goals of therapy. Often in this situation, rapid secondary changes as result of reduced activity will contribute to weakness and contracture, which will further affect the overall impairment of movement. In addition to this, pain, motor fatigue and balance impairments can influence movement adaptations. Coexisting impairments in motor planning, visuospatial awareness and cognition often also affect movement behaviour. A skilled neurotherapist will assess the degree of each impairment, consider the overall situation and develop strategies based on the individual's presentation.

This chapter will outline some of the most common impairments seen in neurological practice (Table 3.1) and will highlight clinical presentations, possible causes, impact on function and briefly indicate current directions for managing these issues within neurological rehabilitation.

WEAKNESS

Upper Motor Neurone Weakness

Weakness in muscle will occur following a lesion to descending UMNs. An UMN lesion can occur at any level above the anterior horn of the spinal cord, in either the spinal cord itself, brainstem or brain. UMN weakness is therefore present in many congenital or acquired central nervous system (CNS) neurological conditions, including stroke, traumatic brain injury (TBI), cerebral palsy (CP), multiple sclerosis (MS) or spinal cord injury (SCI).

Without adequate descending control of movement, UMN lesions can lead to a number of clinical signs often referred to as the 'UMN syndrome', which includes weakness, fatigability and reduced skill/dexterity of movement (Ivanhoe & Reistetter 2004). In addition, there can be an overlay of additional 'hyperreflexive' responses to muscle stretch and cutaneous sensory stimulation such as velocity-dependent 'hypertonus' (increases in muscle tone), hyperreflexia, clonus and Babinski sign (exaggerated cutaneomuscular reflexes). Collectively, the increases in muscle tone and hyperreflexive responses are often termed 'spasticity' (Stevenson 2010).

Although the UMN syndrome can lead to several limitations to active movement, it is the underlying UMN

TABLE 3.1 Common Neurological Impairments

Weakness	Upper motor neurone weakness
	Lower motor neurone weakness
Fatigue	General fatigue
	Motor fatigue
Disorders of muscle tone	Hypertonus
	Hypotonus
	Involuntary muscle spasms
	Dystonia
Disorders of coordination	Cerebellar ataxia
	Sensory ataxia
	Resting tremor
	Loss of dexterity
Disorders of motor planning	Apraxia
	Bradykinesia
	Akinesia
	Freezing of gait
	Functional movement disorders
Vestibular disorders	Peripheral vestibular disorders
	Central vestibular disorders
Cognitive dysfunction	Memory
	Attention
	Executive function
	Language aphasia
	Spatial cognition
	Delirium
Disorders of visuospatial perception	Hemianopia
	Unilateral spatial neglect
	Contraversive pushing
Disorders of sensation	Sensory loss
	Paraesthesia/dysaesthesia
	Pain
Secondary complications	Contracture
	Physical inactivity and deconditioning
	Learned non-use

weakness that has the most impact on overall performance of functional activities such as mobility and upper limb use. Physical therapy therefore aims to improve muscle recruitment and control, and then develop strength and endurance in key functional movements. Contemporary practice recognises that, whenever possible, functional strengthening of muscles affected by UMN weakness is an important part of physical rehabilitation. Previous ideologies concerned about the influence of effort and exertion increasing unwanted muscle tone have now taken a step back because of an increasing recognition of the importance in the relationship between strength and function. However, the neurotherapist should identify optimal ways to both teach movement performance and design functional strengthening programmes to maximise the rehabilitation of motor control (Guadagnoli & Lee 2004).

Lower Motor Neurone Weakness

Lesions at the level of the anterior horn in the spinal cord or the lower motor neurone (LMN) output below this level will result in weakness plus may include additional clinical signs. In addition to weakness, the 'LMN syndrome' may include signs of 'hyporeflexia' with reduced or absent tendon or cutaneous reflexes, reduced muscle tone, flaccid weakness and muscle fasciculations. These additional signs become important from a diagnostic point of view.

LMN weakness can be caused by trauma to the peripheral nervous system or as a result of congenital or infectious disease affecting the LMNs such as peripheral motor neuropathy. Amyotrophic lateral sclerosis, otherwise known as motor neurone disease or Lou Gehrig's disease, can result in both UMN and LMN signs (Kiernan et al 2011). LMN signs in motor neurone disease, including progressive weakness, are the result of premature death to anterior horn cells in the spinal cord and subsequent degeneration of descending motor tracts.

The resulting weakness that occurs with the LMN syndrome has the largest impact on function. Depending on which muscle groups are affected, weakness can lead to difficulty with mobility, respiratory function, speech or upper limb use. Physical therapy aims to limit any decline and maintain or increase muscle strength where possible. The peripheral nervous system has some ability to repair, so many conditions presenting with LMN weakness, such as Guillain–Barré syndrome (Willison et al 2016) and peripheral nerve injury (Li et al 2014), can improve slowly with time and specific physical rehabilitation. Assisting longer-term support and control through splinting or an orthosis can limit instability and enable active movements while also preventing secondary complications such as musculoskeletal injury, pain and deformity.

FATIGUE

General Fatigue

Chronic fatigue is common in people with neurological disorders (Khan & Amataya 2018). It is one of the most common self-reported symptoms after stroke (Kuppuswamy et al 2015) and TBI (Mollayeva et al 2014), and it is often rated as the most disabling symptom by people with MS (Bakshi 2003). The subjective feelings of general fatigue affect physical, cognitive and psychological dimensions of life. For example, poststroke fatigue is described as 'a feeling of early exhaustion with weariness, lack of energy and aversion to effort that develops during physical or mental activity and is not usually ameliorated by rest' (Staub & Bogousslavsky 2001). Fatigue permeates all facets of life and can have a severe impact on employment and quality of life. It is this impact that distinguishes the fatigue from that experienced in healthy people. Over the years, there have been varying definitions for fatigue experienced by people with neurological conditions. Kluger and colleagues (2013) have recently proposed a definition that defines perceived fatigue 'as a subjective sensation of weariness, increasing sense of effort, mismatch between effort expended and actual performance, or exhaustion.' For all conditions, a multidimensional approach to managing fatigue is recommended. Sleep, pain and depression can have a strong relationship with fatigue, as well as the side effects of many medications (Ponchel et al 2015). Although physical performance can deteriorate with fatigue, the neurotherapist must also consider the additional effects of fatigue on cognitive function. This may have important implications when considering the important role of cognition on balance, gait (Morris et al 2016) and falls risk (Hoang et al 2016). The impact of fatigue can also affect processing speed (Barr et al 2014, Claros-Salinas et al 2012), which may have implications for activities such employment and safe driving (Yang 2015). Cognitive behavioural therapy has been shown to be an effective intervention in poststroke fatigue (Su et al 2020). Graded exercise and physical activity to address deconditioning need to be approached in different ways depending on the condition and clinical evidence. For example, myalgic encephalomyelitis or chronic fatigue syndrome (ME/CFS) is a complex chronic condition with fatigue as one of the most debilitating aspects. Postexertional malaise is a characteristic sign and can lead to severe fatigue. Consequently, graded exercise can be detrimental for some. Physical activity diaries, pacing and supervised symptom management are usually the best ways to start physical rehabilitation. The use of graded exercise and cognitive behavioural therapy for people with ME/CFS remains controversial at this time (Flottorp et al 2022).

Motor Fatigue

The decremental motor performance observed as weakness with the repetition of physical tasks is often labelled 'motor fatigue'. Evidence suggests that in CNS disorders such as MS and stroke, motor fatigue is caused by both peripheral and central mechanisms (Kuppuswamy et al 2015, Schwid et al 1999). Understanding the physical decline with performance has important implications for physiotherapy because it affects issues such as gait (Abasıyanık et al 2022, McLoughlin et al 2016), balance, strength (McLoughlin et al 2014) and walking performance (Hutchinson et al 2009). Exercise interventions should monitor motor fatigue with performance (Dawes et al 2014), and therapists should design programmes that incorporate frequent rests and consider the risk of falls and injury. This may allow for increased participation as fatigue is often a major barrier in important exercise programmes that aim to increase activity levels (Smith et al 2015).

DISORDERS OF MUSCLE TONE

Hypertonus

Hypertonus or increased muscle tone associated with the UMN syndrome can influence movement in many ways. Historically, there has been considerable debate regarding 'tone' and its relevance to therapeutic intervention. Most of this debate stems from difficulties and differences in defining 'hypertonus' in the context of the entire package of movement impairments associated with the UMN syndrome. In the area of rehabilitation, it is difficult to find definitions that satisfy both researchers (definitions that can be measured) and clinicians (definitions that describe movement performance). Explaining hypertonus is also difficult because it can be observed during both active and passive movements. Unfortunately, 'spasticity' and 'hypertonus' are often used interchangeably, despite some important key differences in definition. The clinical term 'spasticity' has been previously defined as 'a motor disorder characterised by a velocity-dependent increase in tonic stretch reflexes (muscle tone) with exaggerated tendon jerks, resulting from hyperexcitability of the stretch reflex, as one component of the upper motor neurone syndrome' (Lance 1980). This definition was then revised to include a greater emphasis on sensory inputs 'disordered sensory-motor control, resulting from an upper motor neurone lesion, presenting as intermittent or sustained involuntary activation of muscles' (Burridge et al 2005). Spasticity is measured in the laboratory by examining the electromyographic reflexive muscle response to stimulation of 1a afferent sensory nerves, and is thought to arise from both neural and biomechanical adaptations following UMN lesions.

Most clinical outcomes measures assess 'hypertonus' by the passive resistance to movement at different velocities, which represents part of the hyperreflexive response that occurs to muscle stretch (Pandyan et al 1999). In a clinical context, hypertonus can also be described during active movement and may well be influencing movement quality. Examples of

this might be velocity-dependent hypertonus in knee extensors limiting rapid knee flexion in swing phase of gait, or clonus in plantar flexors destabilising balance, or driving the knee back into hyperextension in stance phase of gait. Hypertonus in elbow flexors may also contribute to muscle imbalance and limitations in elbow extension. It is therefore important that neurotherapists assess and monitor hypertonus actively and passively, and under different postural demands.

Neurotherapists have long realised that hypertonus can be temporarily reduced by providing additional sensory inputs, such as hands-on facilitation. Hypertonus can also be reduced by actively or passively improving postural stability with either tactile hands-on input or passive assistance such as seating systems and supports (Kheder & Nair 2012). This indicates that hypertonus is influenced by sensory input, effort and other more global postural demands on movement (Stevenson 2010).

When learning movement, altering sensory inputs may be used to enhance the exploration of movements with reduced tone. Some simple 'bottom-up' methods of reducing hypertonus can include:

- Electrical stimulation (Mills & Dossa 2016);
- Botulinum toxin injections (Stevenson 2010); and
- Positional supports, seating and bed systems and postural changes (Herman & Lange 1999).

These methods of reducing hypertonus can influence not only movement but also can aid with pain and hygiene care, which can both be directly affected by hypertonic muscles. It is also critical to identify hypertonic muscles that remain in a shortened position because this can quickly lead to contracture. Contracture prevention and management are covered later in this chapter in the Secondary Complications section.

Other interventions used by neurotherapists that provide hands-on sensory inputs include neuromuscular facilitation techniques, such as those used within proprioceptive neuromuscular facilitation (Voss et al 1990) or the Bobath concept (Mayston 2016, Raine et al 2013). There is considerable debate about the effectiveness of these treatment approaches. Evidence for physical rehabilitation approaches for recovery of function and mobility following stroke suggests that rehabilitation should comprise evidence-based techniques regardless of historical or philosophical origin (Pollock et al 2014). Labels aside, providing additional hands-on sensory stimulation has been shown to guide movement, reduce associated tone, provide feedback and allow exploration and experience of both stability and mobility (Raine et al 2013). Neurotherapists often chose these techniques taught within these treatment approaches to improve muscle alignment and recruitment, and to explore a greater repertoire of movement performance, which can be incorporated into functional movements.

The muscle imbalances seen with active movement in people with spasticity also reflect deficits in whole body motor control that influence stretch reflex thresholds (Levin et al 2000). Subsequent compensations can sometimes limit the opportunity for muscles to adapt and change with exercise, which supports the need to monitor movement performance carefully in some situations (Subramanian et al 2020). In addition, as mentioned earlier in this chapter (see Upper Motor Neurone Weakness section), the negative consequence of reduced strength also needs to be addressed to also change movement quality in the longer term. As active control improves, task-specific practice is an effective form of functional exercise that does not specifically target hypertonus (French et al 2007). Active interventions shown to reduce muscle tone in stroke include:

- Task-specific training such as constraint-induced movement therapy (CIMT) (Kagawa et al 2013) and
- Body weight support treadmill training (Manella & Field-Fote 2013).

The other advantage of task-specific practice is that it allows for greater autonomy and dose, particularly for those capable of practicing of tasks outside of closely supervised therapy sessions.

The neurotherapist should also be aware that other external triggers such as painful, noxious stimuli and infection usually increase hypertonus. These increases in tone can help identify hidden complications such as pressure sores or urinary tract infections. In some circumstances, hypertonus that emerges as part of the UMN syndrome may provide stability. A common example of this is increased lower limb extensor tone in standing, which becomes part a functional movement strategy. For some patients, a large proportion of stability is provided by hypertonus. Care must therefore be taken if considering reducing tone with antispasmodic medications because this may unintentionally lead to further weakness and instability in some patients.

If hypertonus is targeted with therapy interventions, it will be influenced by sensory inputs, postural control and functional strengthening programmes. The interventions selected by the neurotherapist will depend on the severity of the impairment, the patient's capacity for active practice, access to direct treatments, skill level and training of therapists, and the resource availability for relevant medications and rehabilitation equipment.

Hypotonus

Hypotonus or 'low tone' also becomes difficult to define because it again can be observed and assessed with both passive and active movements. Many neurological populations present with hypotonus as measured by reduced resistance to passive movement. Hypotonus can be seen in cerebellar ataxic patients and in CP. Even early after stroke UMN lesions, paresis presents as 'low tone' possibly because of changes in supplementary motor areas of the cortex, before activity-dependent adaptations lead to a hypertonic presentation (Florman et al 2013). In a relaxed state, patients with hypotonus may have difficulty in generating muscle activity because of reduced tension and 'readiness' in the muscle. Hypotonus can result in slower movements and changes in joint stability and flexibility. Patients with hypotonic postural muscles often use more inactive, stable postures against gravity. Splints and supports can be useful to enable more activity and, whenever possible, close working with an orthotist will ensure these are custom fitted and align with the goals of an existing physical rehabilitation programme.

As with hypertonus, hypotonus should never be considered in isolation when designing intervention strategies. Again, hypotonia can be difficult to define, despite its role in movement performance. Part of the difficulty is that even within the normal population, degrees of hypotonus can be observed. Secondary weakness is a key factor, and interventions that aim to increase muscle tone through tactile stimulation and quick stretch could be paired with faster muscle activity with strength and power training. As with hypertonus, hypotonia can affect posture and movement, yet it may not need to be specifically targeted in therapy. Strength, power and neuromuscular control may therefore be key targets when hypotonia is present.

Dystonia

Dystonia is defined as a movement disorder characterised by sustained or intermittent muscle contractions causing abnormal, often repetitive, movements, postures or both (Albanese et al 2013). A number of dystonia types have been classified and can occur throughout the life span as either inherited, acquired or idiopathic dystonia. Specific muscles groups commonly affected may include cervical (spasmodic torticollis) wrist and hand (writer's cramp) and around the eyelid (blepharospasm). Dystonia can be present in any focal muscle group and can be triggered by either postural or task-specific specific functional activities, or can even occur spontaneously. Dystonia can be seen as a primary disorder, or with other common neurological conditions such as Parkinson's. A form of spastic dystonia can also occur in stroke as part of the UMN syndrome (Nair & Marsden 2014). The underlying physiological cause is not well understood but is believed to associated with maladaptive neuroplastic changes in areas of the CNS that integrate somatosensory input for movement, such as the basal ganglia, cerebellum, thalamus and cerebral cortex. Some of these maladaptive neuroplastic changes may be triggered by long-term intense movement practice in genetically susceptible individuals, and may partly explain writer's cramp and musician's dystonia (Stahl & Frucht 2017).

Dystonia can have an impact on many facets of daily life, including chronic pain, balance/mobility, employment and driving. Mobile dystonia can cause tremor, which can lead to severe embarrassment in social situations. Recent research also highlights other important functional limitations to consider because people with cervical dystonia also show reduced balance, slower choice stepping reaction times and increased fear of falls (Barr et al 2017) (Table 3.2).

Involuntary Muscle Spasms

Sudden involuntary movements in muscle groups can occur spontaneously or more often are triggered by some sensory or visceral stimuli (Nair & Marsden 2014). This can be common in any neurological condition with UMN lesions such as MS, SCI and TBI. The identification of any triggers is very important, such as skin lesions, pressure ulcers, musculoskeletal pains, ill-fitting splints or infections (especially urinary tract infections). Positioning and postural triggers have implications for lying postures, which affect sleep and sexual relationships. Seating systems can be designed to minimise spasms and improve comfort and control. Unexpected spasms can limit standing mobility and can contribute to unexpected falls. Physical management needs to explore postural control, injury management and other biomechanical influences that are commonly targeted within specific neurological physiotherapy. Direct communication with medical colleagues is also needed to explore the medical options that may target spasms, pain and/or sleep.

Dyskinesias

Dyskinesias are another form of abnormal involuntary choreiform or athetoid movements. Tardive dyskinesias often involve movement of the tongue and jaw, and are strongly associated with antipsychotic medication side effects (Aquino & Lang 2014). A more common dyskinesia observed within neurorehabilitation is associated with Parkinson's (Pilleri & Antonini 2015). Onset of dyskinesias in Parkinson's is due to a combination of chronic levodopa use and disease-related degenerative factors leading to postsynaptic changes to dopamine receptor sensitivity. Although treatment focuses on adjustments to type and dose of Parkinson's medical management, the neurotherapist plays a key role in identification and advice, liaising with the medical team and providing reinforcement about medication dose and timing over the 24-hour cycle.

TABLE 3.2 Interventions for Dystonia	
Medical management consists mainly of botulinum toxin injection into the affected muscles, and there is growing evidence for neurosurgical deep brain stimulation to the internal globus pallidus as an effective option for many.	Castelão et al 2015
The addition of specific exercise-based physiotherapy may further improve symptoms and possibly allow for lower doses of botulinum toxin and more effective management.	Ramdharry 2006
Exercises may focus on recruitment and strengthening of muscles that oppose the dystonic movement. Aims of this approach are to improve voluntary range and control of movement, reduce tension and relieve pain.	Bleton 2010
The identification and use of somatosensory facilitation to relieve dystonic postures with 'sensory tricks' or 'geste antagoniste' may help with self-management.	Franco & Rosales 2015
Graded sensorimotor training has also shown benefit with focal hand dystonia.	Byl et al 2003

KEY POINTS

- Weakness in muscle will occur following a lesion to descending UMNs or LMNs.
- Fatigue is one of the most common self-reported symptoms in neurological conditions (Kluger and colleagues 2013).
- Disorders of tone can affect posture and movement, yet tone may not need to be targeted in therapy. Strength, power and neuromuscular control are the key targets for therapy intervention.
- Abnormal tone is influenced by sensory input, effort and other more global postural demands on movement (Stevenson 2010).

DISORDERS OF COORDINATION

Cerebellar Ataxia

Lesions to the cerebellum or its incoming or outgoing connections can lead to difficulties in the coordination of movement. Because of the theorised role of cerebellum in the feedforward sensorimotor control, damage can lead to problems with the temporal and spatial control of movement (Therrien & Bastian 2015). Depending on the site of lesion, these changes can influence limb movement, balance and/or changes oculomotor control. Coordination changes with cerebellar ataxia can be described as jerky, slow and inaccurate, or may be observed as tremor with active limb or postural muscle activity. Clinical terms used to describe these signs include:

- Dyssynergia: decomposition of multijoint movements
- Dysmetria: variable speed, path and accuracy of movement
- Dysdiadochokinesia: slow, alternating rate of movement
- Tremor: kinetic, intentional or postural tremor of varying amplitude and frequency

Oculomotor changes may include gaze-evoked nystagmus, reduced fixation, saccadic or broken smooth pursuit, slow or dysmetric saccades and abnormal vestibulo-ocular reflex reducing gaze stability. Cerebellar signs can also include changes to the coordination of mouth and tongue movements for speech, which is termed 'dysarthria' (Table 3.3).

TABLE 3.3 Interventions for Cerebellar Ataxia

Rehabilitative treatments can focus on compensatory aids to simplify and dampen the effects of ataxia. Example of this may include: • External weights • Tight garments	Gracies et al 1997, Morgan 1975
Counterbalance weights to alter directional balance stability.	Gibson-Horn 2008, Widener et al 2009
Cooling can also reduce cerebellar tremor temporarily.	Feys et al 2005
Restorative approaches may include exercises for strength, and to practice control and accuracy of limb, balance or visual gaze with the use of sensory feedback.	Crowdy et al 2002
Speech therapy that focuses on loudness of phonation often used with people with Parkinson's can also be of benefit for dysarthria.	Sapir et al 2003
The influence of postural control needs to also be explored because postural training may also reduce limb ataxia.	Stoykov et al 2005

Sensory Ataxia

Reduced sensation can lead to the loss of important proprioceptive awareness and feedback need for well-coordinated movement and balance. Rehabilitation approaches may seek to increase additional alternative sensory feedback through vision (Hamman et al 1992) and tactile cues (such as textures insoles) (Dixon et al 2014, Kelleher et al 2010) to improve motor control. Training techniques that encourage sensory integration can help to improve balance and mobility. It is not uncommon for people with MS to have a combination of cerebellar and sensory ataxia. In this instance, a thorough assessment of sensation and coordination may help design individualised exercises that combine restorative and compensatory approaches to maximise adaptation and functional independence.

Resting Tremor

Resting tremor is the most common form of tremor seen in Parkinson's that can be observed at rest or with an unchanging posture. As it can occur with postural activity, it is best termed 'classic tremor' in Parkinson's (Hallett 2014). At present, the aetiology of classical tremor is unknown but may involve changes within the oscillatory networks of basal ganglia and cerebello-thalamo-cortical motor circuits (Dirkx et al 2016).

Intention Tremor

Intention tremor can involve dyssynergia and dysmetria often with increased oscillations or tremor as limb actively approaches the intended target. This perhaps indicates the key role the cerebellum plays in the feedforward anticipatory control of movement, with dysfunction leading difficulties with temporal and spatial control, reduced skill and reduced accuracy of movement because of a reliance on slower feedback control. Essential tremor can be familial and can involve any number of muscle groups, but it commonly involves involuntary intention tremor of the hands or neck/head.

Tremor can have enormous impact on an individual, especially when considering the importance of hand function. It is also worth considering that all forms of tremor can be extremely embarrassing, affecting all aspects of social and working life (Table 3.4).

Loss of Dexterity

Many of the neurological impairments already mentioned can result in a loss of important fine motor control of the hand, fingers and thumb. Sensory loss, UMN and LMN weakness, tremor, dystonia and motor fatigue can all result in impaired motor dexterity. Dexterity can be defined as the ability to find a motor solution for any external situation, that is, to adequately solve any emerging motor problem

TABLE 3.4 Interventions for Intention Tremor	
Some medications can sometimes be helpful for many types of tremor.	Connolly & Lang 2014
Deep brain stimulation to subcortical structures such as subthalamic nucleus, globus pallidus or thalamus can also show beneficial effects.	Okun 2014
Innovative technology such as vibration absorbers may emerge as effective ways of reducing tremor and improving function.	Gebai et al 2016
External weights, peripheral cooling.	Feys et al 2005
Botulinum toxin injections have been shown to have benefit for tremor.	Kim et al 2014

(Gray 2021). Dexterity often refers to reduced individualised and selective control of each digit of the hand, reduced ability in the complex shaping of the palm/fingers to manipulate objects and reduced fine motor control (Backman et al 1992). Loss of dexterity can have a dramatic effect on hand function with a major impact on overall activities of daily living. Interventions used to improve dexterity will depend greatly on the capacity for active practice. Unilateral loss of dexterity can quickly lead to 'learned non-use' of the limb (discussed later under Noteworthy Complications), where behaviour modification and intense practice such as CIMT are recommended for those with adequate active movement. Particular aspects of impairments may be targeted to improve dexterity such as sensory discrimination/sensorimotor training (Byl et al 2003, Carey et al 2011) and part practice of a task (Carr & Shepherd 2003).

DISORDERS OF MOTOR PLANNING

Apraxia

Apraxia is defined as the lack of ability to understand an action or perform an action on command or imitation. When partial effects of apraxia are present, it can be termed 'dyspraxia' (Koski et al 2002). Various subtypes have been defined based on where the dysfunction to movement planning may be occurring in relation to the cognitive,

perceptual and execution of movements – for example, ideomotor apraxia, ideational apraxia and conceptual apraxia. Other subtypes are defined by the actual task – for example, gait apraxia, dressing apraxia and speech apraxia. Dyspraxia can therefore be very frustrating for those presenting with this disorder, and can be very difficult for family and friends to fully comprehend. Identification, education and support become very important before addressing movement dyspraxia with various rehabilitation strategies.

Interventions for apraxia include the following:
- There is very limited evidence to guide interventional training for apraxia (West et al 2008), such as pantomime and imitation gesturing and compensatory strategy training (Smania et al 2000).
- Errorless learning, forward or backward chaining, sensory stimulation/cueing, and instructional approaches for cognitive rehabilitation may all be considered helpful with motor planning.

Bradykinesia/Akinesia

Bradykinesia is described as an overall slowness of movement with a reduction in the amplitude and speed as the movement is continued (Postuma et al 2015). It is a very common feature of Parkinson's, partly caused by a reduction in the neurotransmitter dopamine within the basal ganglia (Bologna et al 2016). Bradykinesia can affect all movements and postures in upper limb and hands, facial expression and speech, as well as lower limb and gait. It can respond well initially to levodopa or dopamine agonist medications (Gao et al 2017), but the neurotherapist needs to be aware of the many nonpharmacological strategies used to reduce the effects of bradykinesia (Tomlinson et al 2014) (Table 3.5).

Freezing of Gait

Freezing of gait (FOG) is common in Parkinson's and occurs as brief episodes of an absence or marked reduction of the forward progression of the feet despite the intention to walk (Heremans et al 2013). FOG has an enormous impact on function and quality of life (Walton et al 2015) and is strongly linked to falls (Moore et al 2007). It is also linked to cognition, such as executive and visuospatial dysfunction (Peterson et al 2016), and is thought to involve disorders in both cognitive and motor processes (Nutt et al 2011). As with bradykinesia, FOG may be managed with medical adjustments, external cueing strategies, education and support (Nonnekes et al 2015), although the responsiveness to these strategies remains mixed, making FOG often very difficult to manage.

Functional Movement Disorders

Functional movement disorders are common signs found in many functional neurological disorders (FNDs). FND is

TABLE 3.5	**Nonpharmacological Interventions for Bradykinesia/Akinesia**
Movement strategies that focus on increasing movement amplitude can help speech and mobility.	Fox et al 2012
Aerobic exercise has the potential to further enhance these neuroplastic training effects by enhancing brain function.	Petzinger et al 2013
Specific exercise regimes focus on high-speed or forced high-velocity cycling exercise, which may also improve some of the motor signs associated with Parkinson's.	Ni et al 2016, Ridgel et al 2009
External auditory or visual cues have been long known to help with bradykinesia with tasks such as gait by possibly bypassing dysfunctional automatic movement planning pathways in the brain.	Lu et al 2017, Spaulding et al 2013
Various genres of dance show benefit and should be considered alongside all of these strategies.	Shanahan et al 2015, Sharp & Hewitt 2014

a common condition that can occur on its own or in combination with other neurological conditions. More recent research is gaining insight into the pathophysiology of FND, which can be found at the intersection of neurology and psychiatry, with likely dysfunction in brain networks that control attention, predictive motor control, agency and emotional processing (Drane et al 2020). Weakness, tremor and dystonia are common signs. Diagnosis, education and a structured rehabilitation approach that explores various types of attentional focus and structured practicing in movement training can be effective (Nielsen et al 2015). See Chapter 16 on Functional Motor Disorders.

VESTIBULAR DISORDERS

Peripheral Vestibular Disorders

Vestibular dysfunction and management are discussed fully in Chapter 17. Peripheral vestibular disorders such as benign paroxysmal positional vertigo (BPPV), vestibular neuronitis and vestibular hypofunction are common disorders seen in the general population, but can also be commonly seen secondary to many neurological conditions. For example, BPPV can occur following TBI (Ahn et al 2011, Motin et al 2005) and can be the most common cause of vertigo seen in MS (Frohman et al 2000). Vertigo associated with peripheral vestibular disorders can be severe and can have enormous impact on all aspects of life.

Very effective treatments for BPPV and individualised vestibular rehabilitation (VR) exercises for those with unilateral and bilateral vestibular hypofunction show benefit for enhancing early vestibular adaptation and multisensory compensation to reduce dizziness and improve balance (Hall et al 2016). VR has shown to be of benefit for peripheral vestibular dysfunction such as:

- Vestibular neuronitis,
- Labyrinthitis,
- Meniere's disease and
- Bilateral hypofunction (Hillier & McDonnell 2011).

Central Vestibular Disorders

Central lesions that involve vestibular inputs and key integrative pathways in the brainstem and cerebellum can also lead to oculomotor dysfunction, signs and symptoms of imbalance, disequilibrium and vertigo. Approximately 5% to 10% of all strokes occur in the brainstem/cerebellum (Karatas 2008), and lesions in this region are very common in MS (Prosperini et al 2011). Diffuse axonal injury is also common following TBI (Johnson et al 2013), and vestibular symptoms can be associated with certain types of migraine (Stolte et al 2015). Many of the balance impairments observed following stroke may result in diaschisis, with an interruption to important corticobulbar pathways from the cortex to vestibular nuclei in the brainstem (Marsden et al 2005).

In the acute setting, careful assessment to differentiate both peripheral and central vestibular signs is important when considering the possibility of stroke (Kattah et al 2009). Often both peripheral and central vestibular signs coexist (Frohman et al 2000, Pula et al 2013) and influence the optimal rehabilitation strategies used (see Chapter 17 for a comprehensive overview of VR).

Signs of vestibular dysfunction include oculomotor dysfunction such as gaze evoked and/or nystagmus, reduced gaze stability because of altered vestibular-ocular reflex, reduced balance and sensitivity to various types of motion.

Vestibular signs and symptoms can have enormous impact on activity levels and balance confidence. It can contribute to reduced mobility levels, increased anxiety, reduced quality of life and falls risk. Training in vestibular assessment and VR has been recognised as an important part of specialist training within neurological physiotherapy (Cohen et al 2011).

VR has shown to be of benefit for central disorders such as:

- MS (Hebert et al 2011),
- Stroke (Brown et al 2006),
- Brain injury/concussion (Kleffelgaard et al 2015, Murray et al 2016) and
- Vestibular migraine (Vitkovic et al 2013).

VISUOSPATIAL DISORDERS

Hemianopia

Homonymous hemianopia (HH) is common after stroke and results in visual field loss on the same side of both eyes. It is caused by any lesion along the retrochiasmal visual pathway (Zhang et al 2006). Monitoring and encouraging early compensatory head turning is important. HH can lead to reduced functioning and quality of life (Gray et al 1989) and increase risk of falls (Ramrattan et al 2001). The impact of HH on activities of daily living may be further reduced with specific visual field training (Pollock et al 2011).

Unilateral Spatial Neglect

Unilateral neglect (UN) is a perceptual disorder commonly seen in stroke, more often with lesion in the right hemisphere. Pathways within the perisylvian neural network include superior/middle temporal, inferior parietal and ventrolateral frontal cortices (Karnath & Rorden 2012). Patients with UN fail to respond to any stimuli from the contralateral space (often left), with characteristic ipsilesional bias of head and eye gaze. Additional deficits in internal body schema are also common, in addition to problems 'disengaging' from visual stimuli in the ipsilesional space (Morrow & Ratcliff 1988). It is also common for a person with UN to not be aware of these deficits (anosognosia) (Dai et al 2014), which creates a further challenge with rehabilitation. UN can have a marked effect on functional recovery (Jehkonen & Laihosalo 2006) and can be difficult to manage (Kwasnica 2002). Interventions for neglect that have shown some benefit include prism adaptation, eye patching, visual scanning, neck muscle vibration and brain stimulation (Yang et al 2013).

Contraversive Pushing

Contraversive pushing, often referred to as 'pusher syndrome' or 'lateropulsion', is another perceptual disorder following stroke that leads to a postural bias toward the hemiplegic side. This disorder can be difficult to manage because of the characteristic 'pushing' or resistance to postural correction to vertical upright in either sitting or standing. It is thought to be caused by an altered perception of postural verticality. This altered perception may underlie the pushing behaviour, resulting in a reorientation to an altered sense of gravity (Karnath et al 2000) or a balance response to correct perceived vertical (Perennou et al 2008). Because this pushing behaviour is thought to be a perceptual problem, the neurotherapist should consider a multisensory approach to integrate correct feedback from visual, tactile and vestibular feedback regarding postural vertical. Theoretically, the more intact systems, the better prognosis with therapy (Babyar & Peterson 2015).

Cognitive Dysfunction

Cognitive disorders in neurological rehabilitation are covered in detail in Chapter 24. Many people with neurological disorders are affected by cognitive dysfunction, including people with stroke, TBI, MS and Parkinson's. Cognitive impairments can affect employment, social functioning and all activities of daily living. Memory can be affected and can influence immediate, short-term and long-term memory recall. Working memory used to hold and manipulate information for brief periods (i.e., seconds to minutes) can affect many important problem-solving tasks, which can also make learning and relearning tasks more difficult. Perseveration can be observed when people are unable to move on and remain stuck on a topic of conversation or perform the same movement over and over.

Difficulties with attention can also be affected, including sustained, selective and divided attention needed for many functional tasks. People can have difficulty with concentration and lose interest. Language and communication can also be affected with difficulty understanding or making sense of written or verbal language due to receptive aphasia. Expressive aphasia refers to difficulty selecting the correct word to say or write. Aphasia can often be a combination of both expressive and receptive brain networks (Fridriksson et al 2018). Agnosias are disorders of recognition with difficulty identifying objects, faces, voices or even a lack of insight about problems associated with a person's own illness. This is called anosognosia. This presents major challenges in self-regulated behaviour, judgement and decision making, which can lead to risky behaviour, impulsiveness, falls and injury. It can also make the goal-setting process in rehabilitation difficult (Orfei et al 2009). Spatial awareness and spatial cognitive deficits can impair visual perception and are functionally important for planning, navigation and balance. Executive dysfunction is very common across many neurological disorders (O'Callaghan & Lewis 2017, Oreja-Guevara et al 2019) and refers to difficulty with planning, monitoring, multitasking and flexible thinking used in many activities of daily living. It can make employment more challenging. Delirium is a temporary syndrome that leads to a fluctuating state of confusion and can include disorientation, fluctuating levels of attention, hallucinations and reduced consciousness (Wilson et al 2020). It is most often seen in older people with underlying cognitive dysfunction and can occur postoperatively, during an infection, as a side effect of medications, intoxication and malnutrition.

Physical rehabilitation sessions can be planned to prepare for the fact that people with cognitive impairments may require more time and be given opportunities to try various strategies to learn. Cognitive challenges can be increased or decreased depending on the type of task and the environment in which it is performed. Cognitive dysfunction can link closely with fatigue and depressive symptoms, and neurotherapists will need to be aware of how these issues affect both rehabilitation and daily life. There are promising effects of exercise on many aspects of cognitive function. It is a matter of 'watch this space' as research helps us determine what type and dose of exercise might help important cognitive functions (Sanders et al 2019).

SENSORY DISORDERS

Sensory Loss

Sensory loss can be associated with both CNS and peripheral nervous system pathology, and can have considerable impact on movement and function. Lower limb sensory loss can contribute to problems with balance and mobility. Lower limb peripheral sensory neuropathies can be congenital, acquired or complications associated with poorly controlled diabetes. Lower limb proprioceptive loss is common in MS and is often caused by demyelinating lesions to the long dorsal column tracts of the spinal cord (Zackowski et al 2009). Sensory loss can contribute to an increase in postural sway and falls risk (Cameron et al 2008). Rehabilitation that uses sensory reweighting can help with adaptation of balance, as well as novel ways to enhance lower limb proprioceptive feedback such as vibration (Claerbout et al 2012) and textured insoles (Dixon et al 2014, Hatton et al 2016).

Sensory loss to the upper limbs and hands can have a dramatic effect on dextrous, skilled hand movements for both perception and action. Light touch, discriminatory, proprioceptive and vibration sensations can be tested and mapped by the neurotherapist and should be taken into consideration when observing how a patient explores, recognises and interacts with both self and the surrounding environment. Although there is little research to date on somatosensory impairments on activity and participation following stroke, these deficits are likely to play an important role, with potential for research into targeted therapies (Meyer et al 2014). Sensory training programmes that seek to provide additional sensory information in the context of perceptual learning provide the basis for many old

(Champion et al 2009) and new (Carey et al 2011) rehabilitation strategies. The addition of sensory priming such as electrical stimulation or vibration can also assist with improving upper limb function (Stoykov & Madhavan 2015).

Paraesthesia and Dysaesthesia

Paraesthesia can often be hard for patients to describe, but common descriptions may be 'pins and needles' and 'tingling'. If these sensations become uncomfortable, they can be termed '*dysaesthesia*'. These sensations may be described as burning or hypersensitive and can be associated with change in sensory pathways in both the peripheral nervous system and CNS. Mapping out the areas of paraesthesia or dysaesthesia can help pinpoint areas of nerve injury, particularly in the peripheral nervous system. There are common areas where a peripheral nerve can be compromised by direct impact or compression at either distal or proximal sites. Disc bulges or osetoathritic changes where nerve roots exit the foramen can cause proximal compression. In the periphery, external pressure, muscle tension changes or oedema can also lead to compression such as carpal tunnel syndrome. This information becomes an important part of the diagnostic clinical examination. Disease states and long-term compression can lead to nerves being more sensitive to pressure or mechanical stretch (Choi & Kuntz 2015). Lhermitte's sign is one example where neck flexion can lead to strong paraesthesia sensations in arms and/or the legs in people with MS (Al-Araji & Oger 2005). This unusual symptom is thought to be due to mechanosensitivity in spinal sensory tracts in demyelinated and remyelinating lesions of the cervical cord.

Pain

Pain is defined as 'an unpleasant sensory and emotional experience associated with actual or potential tissue damage, or described in terms of such damage' (Loeser & Treede 2008). Pain is a personal experience, influenced not only by biological factors but also by psychological and social factors. Injury or disease affecting peripheral and central nerves can lead to many forms of pain. Terminology of these pain states can vary, with common terms such as neuropathic pain and neuralgia used. Other terms that describe nerve root involvement might include 'radicular pain' or 'sciatica'. Nerve pain diagnosis can be important because the medical management may be more effective with medications that alter CNS responsiveness such as anticonvulsant and antidepressant drugs, as opposed to strong analgesic medications, which may have limited effects. Various forms of peripheral injury and impaired motor control can contribute to pain syndromes in the neurological population. In many situations, pain is caused by a combination of peripheral and central mechanisms, such is often the case in shoulder pain following stroke (Roosink et al 2012). When pain becomes persistent and chronic, it can lead to maladaptive brain and immune responses. This may result in a cluster of other symptoms controlling temperature, blood supply, swelling and sweating. In addition, altered movement behaviour and fear of movement can reinforce poor movement and lead to secondary problems such as ongoing pain, weakness, inactivity and reduced independence. Previously, there was a major underestimation of prevalence and impact of pain in people with stroke, MS and Parkinson's. The neurotherapist interventions should involve education, self-management and sensorimotor learning exercises to develop new strategies that aim to gain a greater repertoire of functional movement. In patients who are unable to communicate verbally, it is important to remember the pain experienced may be expressed in other ways. Pain management in neurological rehabilitation is covered in detail in Chapter 23.

SECONDARY COMPLICATIONS

Contracture

UMN or LMN weakness can quickly lead to structural changes within the muscle. Loss of sarcomeres can occur within hours, and rapid muscle atrophy can take place. Muscles left in a shortened position can quickly lead to more permanent muscle shortening. Contracture develops when the shortened muscle tissue changes structurally, losing its contractile and elastic properties. Contracture can lead to unwanted biomechanical changes that can lead to musculoskeletal deformity and reduced function. Secondary complications can include joint capsule and ligament changes, pain and pressure areas (Farmer & James 2001).

Increased tone in UMN syndrome can lead to muscles developing tension in shortened positions for long periods. This can be caused by the muscle resting in shortened positions either passively or associated increased muscle tone holding muscles in shortened posture during active movements. Common examples of contracture can be:

- Ankle plantar flexors, during prolonged periods of lying or sitting with the ankles left in plantarflexed position.
- Shoulder internal rotators, subscapularis/pectoralis minor when the upper limb is maintained internally rotated when resting on the lap, resting in a sling or as part of an associated posture developed with sitting or standing mobility.
- Wrist and finger flexors resulting from resting position, increased in tone in these muscles and inactivity of extensors.

Physical therapy management focuses on prevention, through careful assessment monitoring and encouraging active and passive movement through range for at-risk muscle groups. Careful positioning with preventative splinting, postural changes, tilt tables and standing frames are all treatments that aim to prevent contracture. Because of the permanent structural changes associated with contracture, there is limited effect of interventions such as prolonged stretching (Harvey et al 2017), botulinum toxin or splinting, and they should not be considered without an additional active rehabilitation programme in place. Aims of rehabilitation may be to improve active range of motion with function, or to help with improved passive range to assist with hygiene and/or pain. Serial casting and some orthopaedic surgical procedures may assist with gaining some increased range (Pidgeon et al 2015). Strengthening antagonistic muscle groups through range with or without electrical stimulation and eccentric training of agonist muscles may be appropriate in some patient groups. For the neurotherapist, preventive strategies that reduce the development of contractures become the highest priority. Contractures can develop within days, or even hours, so education about positioning to the patient, family, carers and the entire multidisciplinary team (including orthotists) is critical. Future research should help understand the structural changes to muscle, identify triggers that might make people susceptible to contracture and guide clinicians on the effectiveness of a range of interventions (Nuckolls et al 2020).

Physical Inactivity and Deconditioning

People living with neurological conditions are faced with many barriers that make it difficult to remain physically active. Secondary deconditioning leads to an increase in risk of lifestyle disease, such as heart disease, diabetes and forms of cancer (Mulligan et al 2012). In stroke, for example, increasing activity in addition to other lifestyle changes can have dramatic results in terms of improving mortality (Towfighi et al 2012). Over the past two decades, research has led to an increased understanding of the important link between inactivity and disability in conditions such as stroke (English et al 2014), MS (Motl 2010), Parkinson's (LaHue et al 2016), SCI (Williams et al 2014), TBI (Hamilton et al 2015) and others (Mulligan et al 2012). Exercises that focus on strength and cardiovascular fitness have therefore become an essential part of neurological rehabilitation and have the potential to make an enormous impact on improved health. Future challenges will include addressing the many barriers to physical activity. This may include engaging in behaviour modification strategies and bridging the gap between inpatient and community rehabilitation services. Future evaluation of rehabilitation technologies such as virtual reality, robotics, exergaming and telerehabilitation may help develop cost-effective methods of proving ongoing exercise within community rehabilitation. Physical activity and exercise are discussed fully in Chapter 22.

Learned Non-Use

Moderate to severe sensorimotor impairments of the upper and lower limb can quickly lead into a cascade of compensatory movement behaviours that favour use of the less affected limb with functions. This results in 'learned non-use' of the hemiparetic extremity. Most research has investigated this behaviour in the upper extremity in patients with hemiparetic stroke (Corbetta et al 2015) and cerebral palsy (Hoare et al 2007). Learned non-use behaviour may well reduce the potential for recovery of the hemiparetic upper extremity. Evidence shows that in those people with some functional movement of the affected extremity, forced use of this limb can improve function. Strongest evidence to date supports the CIMT regimen (Wolf et al 2006), or a modified version (mCIMT) (Page et al 2013). CIMT addresses 'learned non-use' using a number of principles, including constraint of the less affected arm/hand for 90% of waking hours, repetitive task-specific practice or practicing graded segments of tasks (shaping) for up to 6 hours, and a transfer package of repeated behavioural reflection to enhance real-world use of the extremity (Taub et al 2013). It is common for upper extremity rehabilitation to receive little attention in both the inpatient (Serrada et al 2016) and community rehabilitation settings (Rand & Eng 2015), despite growing evidence for these interventions. Learned non-use is a key concept that must be explored by the neurotherapist, including the challenges of addressing the overall behaviour while creating opportunity for more intense practice.

CONCLUSION

This chapter summarises some of the common impairments that can affect the lives of people with neurological conditions. It is essential for the neurotherapist to identify these impairments and appreciate the enormous impact they have on function and quality of life. Sometimes impairments can improve with targeted, restorative rehabilitation strategies, while at other times these impairments will need to be monitored and managed with compensatory strategies. Most importantly, a neurotherapist who is familiar with these issues has an increased capacity to provide much needed education and support to people with neurological conditions. Neurotherapists need to use emerging best evidence, as well as direct future research toward the issues that have the most impact on individuals with these conditions.

SELF-ASSESSMENT QUESTIONS

1. What is the key difference between general fatigue experienced by people with neurological conditions compared with fatigue experience by healthy people?
2. What neurological condition often presents with a combination of cerebellar and sensory ataxia?
3. What neurological conditions might benefit from individualised VR?
4. How might sensory training be used in a person presenting with sensory loss?
5. What muscle groups often lead to contracture, and what secondary complications can occur because of this?

REFERENCES

Abasıyanık, Z., Kahraman, T., Veldkamp, R., Ertekin, Ö., Kalron, A., Feys, P., 2022. Changes in gait characteristics during and immediately after the 6-minute walk test in persons with multiple sclerosis: a systematic review. Phys. Ther. 102, pzac036.

Ahn, S.-K., Jeon, S.-Y., Kim, J.-P., et al., 2011. Clinical characteristics and treatment of benign paroxysmal positional vertigo after traumatic brain injury. J. Trauma. 70, 442–446.

Al-Araji, A.H., Oger, J., 2005. Reappraisal of Lhermitte's sign in multiple sclerosis. Mult. Scler. 11, 398–402.

Albanese, A., Bhatia, K., Bressman, S.B., et al., 2013. Phenomenology and classification of dystonia: a consensus update. Mov. Disord. 28, 863–873.

Aquino, C.C.H., Lang, A.E., 2014. Tardive dyskinesia syndromes: current concepts. Parkinsonism Relat. Disord. 20 (Suppl. 1), S113–S117.

Babyar, S.R., Peterson, M., 2015. Time to recovery from lateropulsion dependent on key stroke deficits a retrospective analysis. Neurorehabil. Neural Repair. 29, 207–213.

Backman, C., Gibson, S.C.D., Parsons, J., 1992. Assessment of hand function: the relationship between pegboard dexterity and applied dexterity. Can. J. Occup. Ther. 59, 208–213.

Bakshi, R., 2003. Fatigue associated with multiple sclerosis: diagnosis, impact and management. Mult. Scler. 9, 219–227.

Barr, C., Barnard, R., Edwards, L., Lennon, S., Bradnam, L., 2017. Impairments of balance, stepping reactions and gait in people with cervical dystonia. Gait. Posture. 4, 55–61.

Barr, C., McLoughlin, J., Lord, S.R., Crotty, M., Sturnieks, D.L., 2014. Walking for six minutes increases both simple reaction time and stepping reaction time in moderately disabled people with multiple sclerosis. Mult. Scler. Relat. Disord. 3, 457–462.

Bleton, J.-P., 2010. Physiotherapy of focal dystonia: a physiotherapist's personal experience. Eur. J. Neurol. 17 (Suppl. 1), 107–112.

Bologna, M., Leodori, G., Stirpe, P., et al., 2016. Bradykinesia in early and advanced Parkinson's disease. J. Neurol. Sci. 369, 286–291.

Brown, K.E., Whitney, S.L., Marchetti, G.F., Wrisley, D.M., Furman, J.M., 2006. Physical therapy for central vestibular dysfunction. Arch. Phys. Med. Rehabil. 87, 76–81.

Burridge, J.H., Wood, D.E., Hermens, H.J., et al., 2005. Theoretical and methodological considerations in the measurement of spasticity. Disabil. Rehabil. 27, 69–80.

Byl, N.N., Nagajaran, S., McKenzie, A.L., 2003. Effect of sensory discrimination training on structure and function in patients with focal hand dystonia: a case series. Arch. Phys. Med. Rehabil. 84, 1505–1514.

Cameron, M.H., Horak, F.B., Herndon, R.R., Bourdette, D., 2008. Imbalance in multiple sclerosis: a result of slowed spinal somatosensory conduction. Somatosens. Mot. Res. 25, 113–122.

Carey, L., Macdonell, R., Matyas, T.A., 2011. SENSe: study of the effectiveness of neurorehabilitation on sensation a randomized controlled trial. Neurorehabil. Neural Repair. 25, 304–313.

Carr, J.H., Shepherd, R.B., 2003. Stroke Rehabilitation: Guidelines for Exercise and Training to Optimize Motor Skill. Butterworth-Heinemann Medical, London.

Castelão, M., Marques, R., Duarte, G., Rodrigues, F.B., Ferreira, J.J., Moore, P., Costa, J., 2015. Botulinum toxin type A therapy for cervical dystonia—an update of a Cochrane systematic review and meta-analysis. Mov. Disord. 30, S201–S202.

Champion, J., Barber, C., Lynch-Ellerington, M., 2009. Recovery of upper limb function. In: Lynch-Ellerington, M., Meadows, L., Raine, S. (Eds.), The Bobath Concept: Theory and Clinical Practice in Neurological Rehabilitation. Wiley-Blackwell, Chicester, U.K, pp. 154.

Choi, H.W., Kuntz, N.L., 2015. Hereditary neuropathy with liability to pressure palsies. Pediatr. Neurol. Briefs. 29, 83.

Claerbout, M., Gebara, B., Ilsbroukx, S., Verschueren, S., Peers, K., Van Asch, P., Feys, P., 2012. Effects of 3 weeks' whole body vibration training on muscle strength and functional mobility in hospitalized persons with multiple sclerosis. Mult. Scler. 18, 498–505.

Claros-Salinas, D., Dittmer, N., Neumann, M., et al., 2012. Induction of cognitive fatigue in MS patients through cognitive and physical load. Neuropsychol. Rehabil. 23, 1–20.

Cohen, H.S., Gottshall, K.R., Graziano, M., Malmstrom, E.-M., Sharpe, M.H., Whitney, S.L., 2011. International guidelines for education in vestibular rehabilitation therapy. J. Vestib. Res. 21, 243–250.

Connolly, B.S., Lang, A.E., 2014. Pharmacological treatment of Parkinson disease: a review. JAMA. 311, 1670–1683.

Corbetta, D., Sirtori, V., Castellini, G., Moja, L., 2015. Constraint-induced movement therapy for upper extremities in people with stroke. Cochrane Database Syst. Rev, CD004433.

Crowdy, K.A., Kaur-Mann, D., Cooper, H.L., Mansfield, A.G., Offord, J.L., Marple-Horvat, D.E., 2002. Rehearsal by eye movement improves visuomotor performance in cerebellar patients. Exp. Brain. Res. 146, 244–247.

Dai, C.-Y., Liu, W.-M., Chen, S.-W., Yang, C.-A., Tung, Y.-C., Chou, L.-W., Lin, L.-C., 2014. Anosognosia, neglect and quality of life of right hemisphere stroke survivors. Eur. J. Neurol. 21, 797–801.

Dawes, H., Collett, J., Meaney, A., et al., 2014. Delayed recovery of leg fatigue symptoms following a maximal exercise session in people with multiple sclerosis. Neurorehabil. Neural Repair. 28, 139–148.

Dirkx, M.F., den Ouden, H., Aarts, E., Timmer, M., Bloem, B.R., Toni, I., Helmich, R.C., 2016. The cerebral network of Parkinson's tremor: an effective connectivity fMRI study. J. Neurosci. 36, 5362–5372.

Dixon, J., Hatton, A.L., Robinson, J., et al., 2014. Effect of textured insoles on balance and gait in people with multiple sclerosis: an exploratory trial. Physiotherapy. 100, 142–149.

Drane, D.L., Fani, N., Hallett, M., Khalsa, S.S., Perez, D.L., Roberts, N.A., 2020. A framework for understanding the pathophysiology of functional neurological disorder. CNS Spectr. 1–7.

English, C., Manns, P.J., Tucak, C., Bernhardt, J., 2014. Physical activity and sedentary behaviors in people with stroke living in the community: a systematic review. Phys Ther. 94, 185–196.

Farmer, S.E., James, M., 2001. Contractures in orthopaedic and neurological conditions: a review of causes and treatment. Disabil. Rehabil. 23, 549–558.

Feys, P., Helsen, W., Liu, X., Mooren, D., Albrecht, H., Nuttin, B., Ketelaer, P., 2005. Effects of peripheral cooling on intention tremor in multiple sclerosis. J. Neurol. Neurosurg. Psychiatry. 76, 373–379.

Florman, J.E., Duffau, H., Rughani, A.I., 2013. Lower motor neuron findings after upper motor neuron injury: insights from postoperative supplementary motor area syndrome. Front. Hum. Neurosci. 7, 85–110.

Flottorp, S.A., Brurberg, K.G., Fink, P., Knoop, H., Wyller, V.B., 2022. New NICE guideline on chronic fatigue syndrome: more ideology than science? Lancet. 399, 611–613.

Fox, C., Ebersbach, G., Ramig, L., Sapir, S., 2012. LSVT LOUD and LSVT BIG: behavioral treatment programs for speech and body movement in Parkinson disease. Parkinson. Dis. 2012, 391946.

Franco, J.H., Rosales, R.L., 2015. Neurorehabilitation in dystonia. In: Kanovsky, P., Bhatia, K.P., Rosales, R.L. (Eds.), Dystonia and Dystonic Syndromes. Springer Verlag, Vienna, pp. 209–226.

French, B., Thomas, L.H., Leathley, M.J., et al., 2007. Repetitive task training for improving functional ability after stroke. Cochrane Database Syst. Rev 4, CD006073.

Fridriksson, J., den Ouden, D.-B., Hillis, A.E., et al., 2018. Anatomy of aphasia revisited. Brain. 141, 848–862.

Frohman, E.M., Zhang, H., Dewey, R.B., Hawker, K.S., Racke, M.K., Frohman, T.C., 2000. Vertigo in MS: utility of positional and particle repositioning maneuvers. Neurology. 55, 1566–1569.

Gao, L.-L., Zhang, J.-R., Chan, P., Wu, T., 2017. Levodopa effect on basal ganglia motor circuit in Parkinson's disease. CNS Neurosci.Ther. 23, 76–86.

Gebai, S., Hammoud, M., Hallal, A., Shaer, A.A., Khachfe, H., 2016. Biomechanical treatment for rest tremor of Parkinson's patient 2016 IEEE International Multidisciplinary Conference on Engineering Technology (IMCET). Beirut. 32–36.

Gibson-Horn, C., 2008. Balance-based torso-weighting in a patient with ataxia and multiple sclerosis: a case report. J. Neurol. Phys. Ther. 32, 139–146.

Gracies, J.M., Fitzpatrick, R., Wilson, L., Burke, D., Gandevia, S.C., 1997. Lycra garments designed for patients with upper limb spasticity: mechanical effects in normal subjects. Arch. Phys. Med. Rehabil. 78, 1066–1071.

Gray, C.S., French, J.M., Bates, D., Cartlidge, N.E., Venables, G.S., James, O.F., 1989. Recovery of visual fields in acute stroke: homonymous hemianopia associated with adverse prognosis. Age Ageing. 18, 419–421.

Gray, R., 2021. How we learn to move: a revolution in the way we coach & practice sports. Skills Perception Action Consulting & Education LLC.

Guadagnoli, M.A., Lee, T.D., 2004. Challenge point: a framework for conceptualizing the effects of various practice conditions in motor learning. J. Mot. Behav. 36, 212–224.

Hall, C.D., Herdman, S.J., Whitney, S.L., et al., 2016. Vestibular rehabilitation for peripheral vestibular hypofunction: an evidence-based clinical practice guideline: from the American Physical Therapy Association neurology section. J. Neurol. Phys. Ther. 40, 124–155.

Hallett, M., 2014. Tremor: pathophysiology. Parkinsonism Relat. Disord. 20 (Suppl. 1), S118–S122.

Hamilton, M., Michelle, K., Williams, G., 2015. Predictors of physical activity levels of individuals following traumatic brain injury (TBI) remain unclear: a systematic review. Brain. Inj. 30, 819–828.

Hamman, R.G., Mekjavic, I., Mallinson, A.I., Longridge, N.S., 1992. Training effects during repeated therapy sessions of balance training using visual feedback. Arch. Phys. Med. Rehabil. 73, 738–744.

Harvey, L.A., Katalinic, O.M., Herbert, R.D., et al., 2017. Stretch for the treatment and prevention of contracture: an abridged republication of a Cochrane Systematic Review. J. Physiother. 63, 67–75.

Hatton, A.L., Dixon, J., Rome, K., Brauer, S.G., Williams, K., 2016. The effects of prolonged wear of textured shoe insoles on gait, foot sensation and proprioception in people with multiple sclerosis: protocol for a randomised controlled trial. Trials. 17, 208.

Hebert, J.R., Corboy, J.R., Manago, M.M., Schenkman, M., 2011. Effects of vestibular rehabilitation on multiple sclerosis-related fatigue and upright postural control: a randomized controlled trial. Phys. Ther. 91, 1166–1183.

Heremans, E., Nieuwboer, A., Vercruysse, S., 2013. Freezing of gait in Parkinson's disease: where are we now? Curr. Neurol. Neurosci. Rep. 13, 350.

Herman, J.H., Lange, M.L., 1999. Seating and positioning to manage spasticity after brain injury. NeuroRehabilitation. 12, 105–117.

Hillier, S.L., McDonnell, M., 2011. Vestibular rehabilitation for unilateral peripheral vestibular dysfunction. Cochrane Database Syst. Rev. 2.

Hoang, P.D., Baysan, M., Gunn, H., et al., 2016. Fall risk in people with MS: a physiological profile assessment study. Mult. Scler. J. 2, 2055217316641130

Hoare, B., Imms, C., Carey, L., Wasiak, J., 2007. Constraint-induced movement therapy in the treatment of the upper limb in children with hemiplegic cerebral palsy: a Cochrane systematic review. Clin. Rehabil. 21, 675–685.

Hutchinson, B., Forwell, S.J., Bennett, S., Brown, T., Karpatkin, H., Miller, D., 2009. Toward a consensus on rehabilitation outcomes in MS: gait and fatigue. Int. J. MS. Care. 11, 67–78.

Ivanhoe, C.B., Reistetter, T.A., 2004. Spasticity: the misunderstood part of the upper motor neuron syndrome. Am. J. Phys. Med. Rehabil. 83 (Suppl. 10), S3–S9.

Jehkonen, M., Laihosalo, M., Kettunen, J.E., 2006. Impact of neglect on functional outcome after stroke: a review of methodological issues and recent research findings. Restor. Neurol. Neurosci. 24, 209–215.

Johnson, V.E., Stewart, W., Smith, D.H., 2013. Axonal pathology in traumatic brain injury. Exp. Neurol. 246, 35–43.

Kagawa, S., Koyama, T., Hosomi, M., Takebayashi, T., Hanada, K., Hashimoto, F., Domen, K., 2013. Effects of constraint-induced movement therapy on spasticity in patients with hemiparesis after stroke. J. Stroke Cerebrovasc. Dis. 22, 364–370.

Karatas, M., 2008. Central vertigo and dizziness: epidemiology, differential diagnosis, and common causes. Neurologist. 14, 355–364.

Karnath, H.O., Ferber, S., Dichgans, J., 2000. The origin of contraversive pushing: evidence for a second graviceptive system in humans. Neurology. 55, 1298–1304.

Karnath, H.-O., Rorden, C., 2012. The anatomy of spatial neglect. Neuropsychologia. 50, 1010–1017.

Kattah, J.C., Talkad, A.V., Wang, D.Z., Hsieh, Y.-H., Newman-Toker, D.E., 2009. HINTS to diagnose stroke in the acute vestibular syndrome three-step bedside oculomotor examination more sensitive than early MRI diffusion-weighted imaging. Stroke. 40, 3504–3510.

Kelleher, K.J., Spence, W.D., Solomonidis, S., Apatsidis, D., 2010. The effect of textured insoles on gait patterns of people with multiple sclerosis. Gait. Posture. 32, 67–71.

Khan, F., Amatya, B., 2018. Management of fatigue in neurological disorders: implications for rehabilitation. J. Int. Soc. Phys. Rehabil. Med. 1, 9–36.

Kheder, A., Nair, K.P.S., 2012. Spasticity: pathophysiology, evaluation and management. Pract. Neurol. 12, 289–298.

Kiernan, M.C., Vucic, S., Cheah, B.C., et al., 2011. Amyotrophic lateral sclerosis. Lancet. 377, 942–955.

Kim, S.D., Yiannikas, C., Mahant, N., Vucic, S., Fung, V.S.C., 2014. Treatment of proximal upper limb tremor with botulinum toxin therapy. Mov. Disord. 29, 835–838.

Kleffelgaard, I., Soberg, H.L., Bruusgaard, K.A., Tamber, A.L., Langhammer, B., 2015. Vestibular rehabilitation after traumatic brain injury: case series. Phys. Ther. 96, 839–849.

Kluger, B.M., Krupp, L.B., Enoka, R.M., 2013. Fatigue and fatigability in neurologic illnesses: proposal for a unified taxonomy. Neurology. 80, 409–416.

Koski, L., Iacoboni, M., Mazziotta, J.C., 2002. Deconstructing apraxia: understanding disorders of intentional movement after stroke. Curr. Opin. Neurol. 15, 71–77.

Kuppuswamy, A., Clark, E.V., Turner, I.F., Rothwell, J.C., Ward, N.S., 2015. Post-stroke fatigue: a deficit in corticomotor excitability? Brain. 138 (Pt. 1), 136–148.

Kwasnica, C.M., 2002. Unilateral neglect syndrome after stroke: theories and management issues. Crit. Rev. Phys. Rehabil. Med. 14, 16.

LaHue, S.C., Comella, C.L., Tanner, C.M., 2016. The best medicine? The influence of physical activity and inactivity on Parkinson's disease. Mov. Disord. 31, 1444–1454.

Lance, J.W., 1980. Symposium synopsis. Spasticity: Disordered Motor Control. Symposia Specialists, Chicago. Distributed by Year Book Medical Publishers, Miami, FL.485–500.

Levin, M.F., Selles, R.W., Verheul, M.H., Meijer, O.G., 2000. Deficits in the coordination of agonist and antagonist muscles in stroke patients: implications for normal motor control. Brain. Res. 853, 352–369.

Li, R., Liu, Z., Pan, Y., Chen, L., Zhang, Z., Lu, L., 2014. Peripheral nerve injuries treatment: a systematic review. Cell. Biochem. Biophys. 68, 449–454.

Loeser, J.D., Treede, R.-D., 2008. The Kyoto protocol of IASP Basic Pain Terminology. Pain. 137, 473.

Lu, C., Amundsen Huffmaster, S.L., Tuite, P.J., Vachon, J.M., MacKinnon, C.D., 2017. Effect of cue timing and modality on gait initiation in Parkinson Disease with freezing of gait. Arch. Phys. Med. Rehabil. 98, 1291–1299.

Manella, K.J., Field-Fote, E.C., 2013. Modulatory effects of locomotor training on extensor spasticity in individuals with motor-incomplete spinal cord injury. Restor. Neurol. Neurosci. 31, 633–646.

Marsden, J.F., Playford, D.E., Day, B.L., 2005. The vestibular control of balance after stroke. J. Neurol. Neurosurg. Psychiatry. 76, 670–679.

Mayston, M., 2016. Bobath and NeuroDevelopmental Therapy: what is the future? Dev. Med. Child. Neurol. 58, 994.

McLoughlin, J.V., Barr, C.J., Crotty, M., Sturnieks, D.L., Lord, S.R., 2014. Six minutes of walking leads to reduced lower limb strength and increased postural sway in people with multiple sclerosis. NeuroRehabilitation. 35, 503–508.

McLoughlin, J.V., Barr, C.J., Patritti, B., Crotty, M., Lord, S.R., Sturnieks, D.L., 2016. Fatigue induced changes to kinematic and kinetic gait parameters following six minutes of walking in people with multiple sclerosis. Disabil. Rehabil. 38, 535–543.

Meyer, S., Karttunen, A.H., Thijs, V., Feys, H., Verheyden, G., 2014. How do somatosensory deficits in the arm and hand relate to upper limb impairment, activity, and participation problems after stroke? A systematic review. Phys. Ther. 94, 1220–1231.

Mills, P.B., Dossa, F., 2016. Transcutaneous electrical nerve stimulation for management of limb spasticity: a systematic review. Am. J. Phys. Med. Rehabil. 95, 309–318.

Mollayeva, T., Kendzerska, T., Mollayeva, S., Shapiro, C.M., Colantonio, A., Cassidy, J.D., 2014. A systematic review of fatigue in patients with traumatic brain injury: the course, predictors and consequences. Neurosci. Biobehav. Rev. 47, 684–716.

Moore, O., Peretz, C., Giladi, N., 2007. Freezing of gait affects quality of life of peoples with Parkinson's disease beyond its relationships with mobility and gait. Mov. Dis. 22, 2192–2195.

Morgan, M.H., 1975. Ataxia and weights. Physiotherapy. 61, 332–334.

Morris, R., Lord, S., Bunce, J., Burn, D., Rochester, L., 2016. Gait and cognition: mapping the global and discrete relationships in ageing and neurodegenerative disease. Neurosci. Biobehav. Rev. 64, 326–345.

Morrow, L.A., Ratcliff, G., 1988. The disengagement of covert attention and the neglect syndrome. Psychobiology. 16, 261–269.

Motin, M., Keren, O., Groswasser, Z., Gordon, C.R., 2005. Benign paroxysmal positional vertigo as the cause of dizziness in patients after severe traumatic brain injury: diagnosis and treatment. Brain. Inj. 19, 693–697.

Motl, R.W., 2010. Physical activity and irreversible disability in multiple sclerosis. Exerc. Sport. Sci. Rev. 38, 186–191.

Mulligan, H.F., Hale, L.A., Whitehead, L., Baxter, G.D., 2012. Barriers to physical activity for people with long-term neurological conditions: a review study. Adapt. Phys. Activ. Q. 29, 243–265.

Murray, D.A., Meldrum, D., Lennon, O., 2016. Can vestibular rehabilitation exercises help patients with concussion? A systematic review of efficacy, prescription and progression patterns. Br. J. Sports Med. 51, 442–451.

Nair, K.P., Marsden, J., 2014. The management of spasticity in adults. BMJ. 349, g4737.

Ni, M., Signorile, J.F., Mooney, K., et al., 2016. Comparative effect of power training and high-speed yoga on motor function in older patients with Parkinson disease. Arch. Phys. Med. Rehabil. 97, 345–354.

Nielsen, G., Stone, J., Matthews, A., et al., 2015. Physiotherapy for functional motor disorders: a consensus recommendation. J. Neurol. Neurosurg. Psychiatry. 86, 1113–1119.

Nonnekes, J., Snijders, A.H., Nutt, J.G., Deuschl, G., Giladi, N., Bloem, B.R., 2015. Freezing of gait: a practical approach to management. Lancet. Neurol. 14, 768–778.

Nuckolls, G.H., Kinnett, K., Dayanidhi, S., et al., 2020. Conference report on contractures in musculoskeletal and neurological conditions. Muscle. Nerve. 61, 740–744.

Nutt, J.G., Horak, F.B., Bloem, B.R., 2011. Milestones in gait, balance, and falling. Mov. Disord. 26, 1166–1174.

O'Callaghan, C., Lewis, S.J.G., 2017. Cognition in Parkinson's disease. Int. Rev. Neurobiol. 133, 557–583.

Okun, M.S., 2014. Deep-brain stimulation—entering the era of human neural-network modulation. N. Engl. J. Med. 371, 1369–1373.

Oreja-Guevara, C., Ayuso Blanco, T., Brieva Ruiz, L., Hernández Pérez, M.Á., Meca-Lallana, V., Ramió-Torrentà, L., 2019. Cognitive dysfunctions and assessments in multiple sclerosis. Front. Neurol. 10, 581.

Orfei, M.D., Caltagirone, C., Spalletta, G., 2009. The evaluation of anosognosia in stroke patients. Cerebrovasc. Dis. 27, 280–289.

Page, S.J., Boe, S., Levine, P., 2013. What are the "ingredients" of modified constraint-induced therapy? An evidence-based review, recipe, and recommendations. Restor. Neurol. Neurosci. 31, 299–309.

Pandyan, A.D., Johnson, G.R., Price, C., Curless, R.H., Barnes, M.P., Rodgers, H., 1999. A review of the properties and limitations of the Ashworth and modified Ashworth Scales as measures of spasticity. Clin. Rehabil. 13, 373–383.

Perennou, D.A., Mazibrada, G., Chauvineau, V., Greenwood, R., Rothwell, J., Gresty, M.A., Bronstein, A.M., 2008. Lateropulsion, pushing and verticality perception in hemisphere stroke: a causal relationship? Brain. 131, 2401–2413.

Peterson, D.S., King, L.A., Cohen, R.G., Horak, F.B., 2016. Cognitive contributions to freezing of gait in Parkinson disease: implications for physical rehabilitation. Phys. Ther. 96, 659–670.

Petzinger, G.M., Fisher, B.E., McEwen, S., Beeler, J.A., Walsh, J.P., Jakowec, M.W., 2013. Exercise-enhanced neuroplasticity targeting motor and cognitive circuitry in Parkinson's disease. Lancet Neurol. 12, 716–726.

Pidgeon, T.S., Ramirez, J.M., Schiller, J.R., 2015. Orthopaedic management of spasticity. R. I. Med. J 98, 26–31.

Pilleri, M., Antonini, A., 2015. Therapeutic strategies to prevent and manage dyskinesias in Parkinson's disease. Expert. Opin. Drug. Saf. 14, 281–294.

Pollock, A., Baer, G., Campbell, P., et al., 2014. Physical rehabilitation approaches for the recovery of function and mobility after stroke: major update. Stroke. 45, e202.

Pollock, A., Hazelton, C., Henderson, C.A., et al., 2011. Interventions for disorders of eye movement in patients with stroke. Cochrane Database Syst. Rev. 10, CD008389.

Ponchel, A., Bombois, S., Bordet, R., Hénon, H., 2015. Factors associated with poststroke fatigue: a systematic review. Stroke. Res. Treat. 2015, 347920.

Postuma, R.B., Berg, D., Stern, M., et al., 2015. MDS clinical diagnostic criteria for Parkinson's disease. Mov. Disord. 30, 1591–1601.

Prosperini, L., Kouleridou, A., Petsas, N., Leonardi, L., Tona, F., Pantano, P., Pozzilli, C., 2011. The relationship between infratentorial lesions, balance deficit and accidental falls in multiple sclerosis. J. Neurol. Sci. 304, 55–60.

Pula, J.H., Newman-Toker, D.E., Kattah, J.C., 2013. Multiple sclerosis as a cause of the acute vestibular syndrome. J. Neurol. 260, 1649–1654.

Raine, S., Meadows, L., Lynch-Ellerington, M., 2013. Bobath Concept: Theory and Clinical Practice in Neurological Rehabilitation. Wiley-Blackwell, London.

Ramdharry, G., 2006. Physiotherapy cuts the dose of botulinum toxin. Physiother. Res. Int. 11, 117–122.

Ramrattan, R.S., Wolfs, R.C., Panda-Jonas, S., et al., 2001. Prevalence and causes of visual field loss in the elderly and associations with impairment in daily functioning: the Rotterdam Study. Arch. Ophthalmol. 119, 1788–1794.

Rand, D., Eng, J.J., 2015. Predicting daily use of the affected upper extremity 1 year after stroke. J. Stroke Cerebrovasc. Dis. 24, 274–283.

Ridgel, A.L., Vitek, J.L., Alberts, J.L., 2009. Forced, not voluntary, exercise improves motor function in Parkinson's disease patients. Neurorehabil. Neural Repair. 23, 600–608.

Roosink, M., Renzenbrink, G.J., Geurts, A.C.H., Ijzerman, M.J., 2012. Towards a mechanism-based view on post-stroke shoulder pain: theoretical considerations and clinical implications. NeuroRehabilitation. 30, 153–165.

Sanders, L.M.J., Hortobágyi, T., la Bastide-van Gemert, S., van der Zee, E.A., van Heuvelen, M.J.G., 2019. Dose-response relationship between exercise and cognitive function in older adults with and without cognitive impairment: a systematic review and meta-analysis. PloS One. 14, e0210036.

Sapir, S., Spielman, J., Ramig, L.O., Hinds, S.L., Countryman, S., Fox, C., Story, B., 2003. Effects of intensive voice treatment (the Lee Silverman Voice Treatment [LSVT]) on ataxic dysarthria: a case study. Am. J. Speech Lang. Pathol. 12, 387–399.

Schwid, S.R., Thornton, C.A., Pandya, S., et al., 1999. Quantitative assessment of motor fatigue and strength in MS. Neurology. 53, 743–750.

Serrada, I., McDonnell, M.N., Hillier, S.L., 2016. What is current practice for upper limb rehabilitation in the acute hospital setting following stroke? A systematic review. NeuroRehabilitation. 39, 431–438.

Shanahan, J., Morris, M.E., Bhriain, O.N., Saunders, J., Clifford, A.M., 2015. Dance for people with Parkinson disease: what is the evidence telling us? Arch. Phys. Med. Rehabil. 96, 141–153.

Sharp, K., Hewitt, J., 2014. Dance as an intervention for people with Parkinson's disease: a systematic review and meta-analysis. Neurosci. Biobehav. Rev. 47, 445–456.

Smania, N., Girardi, F., Domenicali, C., Lora, E., Aglioti, S., 2000. The rehabilitation of limb apraxia: a study in left-brain–damaged patients /4. Arch. Phys. Med. Rehabil. 81, 379–388.

Smith, C.M., Fitzgerald, H.J.M., Whitehead, L., 2015. How fatigue influences exercise participation in men with multiple sclerosis. Qual. Health Res. 25, 179–188.

Spaulding, S.J., Barber, B., Colby, M., Cormack, B., Mick, T., Jenkins, M.E., 2013. Cueing and gait improvement among people with Parkinson's disease: a meta-analysis. Arch. Phys. Med. Rehabil. 94, 562–570.

Stahl, C.M., Frucht, S.J., 2017. Focal task specific dystonia: a review and update. J. Neurol. 264, 1536–1541.

Staub, F., Bogousslavsky, J., 2001. Fatigue after stroke: a major but neglected issue. Cerebrovasc. Dis. 12, 75–81.

Stevenson, V.L., 2010. Rehabilitation in practice: spasticity management. Clin. Rehabil. 24, 293–304.

Stolte, B., Holle, D., Naegel, S., Diener, H.-C., Obermann, M., 2015. Vestibular migraine. Cephalalgia. 35, 262–270.

Stoykov, M.E., Madhavan, S., 2015. Motor priming in neurorehabilitation. J. Neurol. Phys. Ther. 39, 33–42.

Stoykov, M.E.P., Stojakovich, M., Stevens, J.A., 2005. Beneficial effects of postural intervention on prehensile action for an individual with ataxia resulting from brainstem stroke. NeuroRehabilitation. 20, 85–89.

Su, Y., Yuki, M., Otsuki, M., 2020. Non-pharmacological interventions for post-stroke fatigue: systematic review and network meta-analysis. J. Clin. Med. 9, 621.

Subramanian, S.K., Baniña, M.C., Sambasivan, K., Haentjens, K., Finestone, H.M., Sveistrup, H., Levin, M.F., 2020.

Motor-equivalent intersegmental coordination is impaired in chronic stroke. Neurorehabil. Neural Repair. 34, 210–221.

Taub, E., Uswatte, G., Mark, V.W., et al., 2013. Method for enhancing real-world use of a more affected arm in chronic stroke: transfer package of constraint-induced movement therapy. Stroke. 44, 1383–1388.

Therrien, A.S., Bastian, A.J., 2015. Cerebellar damage impairs internal predictions for sensory and motor function. Curr. Opin. Neurobiol. 33, 127–133.

Tomlinson, C.L., Herd, C.P., Clarke, C.E., et al., 2014. Physiotherapy for Parkinson's disease: a comparison of techniques. Cochrane Database Syst. Rev. 6, CD002815.

Towfighi, A., Markovic, D., Ovbiagele, B., 2012. Impact of a healthy lifestyle on all-cause and cardiovascular mortality after stroke in the USA. J. Neurol. Neurosurg. Psychiatry. 83, 146–151.

Vitkovic, J., Winoto, A., Rance, G., Dowell, R., Paine, M., 2013. Vestibular rehabilitation outcomes in patients with and without vestibular migraine. J. Neurol. 260, 3039–3048.

Voss, D.E., Ionta, M.K., Myers, B.J., 1990. Proprioceptive Neuromuscular Facilitation, PNF: Patterns & Techniques. Rehabilitation Institute of Chicago.

Walton, C.C., Shine, J.M., Hall, J.M., et al., 2015. The major impact of freezing of gait on quality of life in Parkinson's disease. J. Neurol. 262, 108–115.

West, C., Bowen, A., Hesketh, A., Vail, A., 2008. Interventions for motor apraxia following stroke. Cochrane Database Syst. Rev. 23, CD004132.

Widener, G.L., Allen, D.D., Gibson-Horn, C., 2009. Balance-based torso-weighting may enhance balance in persons with multiple sclerosis: preliminary evidence. Arch. Phys. Med. Rehabil. 90, 602–609.

Williams, T.L., Smith, B., Papathomas, A., 2014. The barriers, benefits and facilitators of leisure time physical activity among people with spinal cord injury: a meta-synthesis of qualitative findings. Health. Psychol. Rev. 8, 404–425.

Willison, H.J., Jacobs, B.C., van Doorn, P.A., 2016. Guillain-Barré syndrome. Lancet. 388, 717–727.

Wilson, J.E., Mart, M.F., Cunningham, C., et al., 2020. Delirium. Nat. Rev. Dis. Primers. 6, 90. Erratum in: Nat. Rev. Dis. Primers. 2020; 6, 94.

Wolf, S.L., Winstein, C.J., Miller, J.P., et al., 2006. Effect of constraint-induced movement therapy on upper extremity function 3 to 9 months after stroke: the EXCITE randomized clinical trial. JAMA. 296, 2095–2104.

Yang, C.P., 2015. Post stroke fatigue and return to driving. Int. J. Stroke. 10, 105.

Yang, N.Y.H., Zhou, D., Chung, R.C.K., Li-Tsang, C.W.P., Fong, K.N.K., 2013. Rehabilitation interventions for unilateral neglect after stroke: a systematic review from 1997 through 2012. Front. Hum. Neurosci. 7, 187.

Zackowski, K.M., Smith, S.A., Reich, D.S., et al., 2009. Sensorimotor dysfunction in multiple sclerosis and column-specific magnetization transfer-imaging abnormalities in the spinal cord. Brain. 132, 1200–1209.

Zhang, X., Kedar, S., Lynn, M.J., Newman, N.J., Biousse, V., 2006. Homonymous hemianopia in stroke. J. Neuroophthalmol. 26, 180–183.

4

Observation and Analysis of Movement

Amanda C. Wallace, Lisa May Bunn, and Elizabeth Cassidy

OUTLINE

Walking, 71
    The Gait Cycle, 72
    Walking Kinematics and Muscle Activity, 72
    Walking Kinetics, 77
    Spatiotemporal Characteristics, 77
    Clinical Focus: Walking for People With
        Parkinson's, 77
Sit To Stand, 77
    Typical Phases of Sit to Stand, 78
    Muscle Action During Sit to Stand, 82
    Contextual Factors Influencing Sit to Stand, 82
    Clinical Focus on Sit to Stand for People
        After Stroke, 82
Rolling and Getting Out of Bed, 82
    Clinical Focus on Getting Out of Bed for People with
        Parkinson's, 83

Reach and Grasp, 83
    Essential Components of Reach and Grasp, 87
    Kinematics, 87
    Muscle Activity, 89
    Clinical Focus on Reach and Grasp for People With
        Stroke, 91
Posture and Balance, 91
    Sensorimotor Control of Balance, 93
        Essential Sensory Components, 94
        Essential Motor Components of Balance, 94
    Movement Analysis Strategies to Quantify Posture, 95
    Movement Analysis Strategies to Quantify Balance, 96
    Clinical Foci of Posture and Balance, 97
Key Messages, 102

All voluntary movement including walking, sit to stand (STS), reach and grasp, rolling and the underlying postural control that accompanies these actions involves the complex integration of cognitive, neuronal and biomechanical factors. Movement analysis is the systematic study of the movement produced during human action using skilled observational assessment, augmented by instruments that measure key aspects of performance.

This chapter will describe the analysis of movement of particular functions and illustrate deviations that are observed with specific neurological conditions.

WALKING

Walking refers to a means of locomotion involving the use of two legs where at least one foot is always in contact with the ground, and each leg alternately provides support and propulsion (Whittle et al 2012a). Successful walking satisfies three essential requirements (Patla 1991, 1997) (Table 4.1). Walking is an inherently unstable activity that demands a high degree of neural control (Patla 1991, Winter et al 1991). Whilst acting within the biomechanical constraints afforded by the human body, the central nervous system is required to generate a locomotor pattern, modulate propulsive forces, overcome the effects of gravity and integrate visual, proprioceptive and vestibular afferent information in a matter of milliseconds, on an ongoing basis, usually whilst the individual is involved in doing something else (Leonard 1998). Despite its complexity, it is possible to understand the essential components of walking and to apply this understanding to clinical

TABLE 4.1	**The Essential Components of Walking (Patla 1991, 1997)**
Component	**Explanation**
Propulsion	The generation, maintenance and termination of a basic locomotor cycle using patterned activation and coordination of the legs and trunk to propel the body in the intended direction
Postural control	Maintenance of dynamic stability of the moving body through the appropriate postural orientation of body segments relative to each other and environmental conditions, to overcome gravity and to respond to expected and unexpected perturbations
Adaptation	Modulation of the locomotor pattern to achieve goals in real-world environments, e.g., through changing speed and direction to meet the demands of variable terrain or to avoid obstacles; the focus on adaptability underscores the importance of understanding human walking as a skilled behaviour rather than as simply the generation of basic locomotor patterns

practice. This section offers an overview of the key constituents of walking, with a clinical focus on the impact of Parkinson's on walking.

The Gait Cycle

An analysis of walking involves the observation and measurement of relevant components of the gait cycle (Fig. 4.1). One complete gait cycle occurs from the point when one foot makes contact with the ground to the next occasion when the same foot touches the ground again. Simple gait analysis involves the observation of a person walking continuously over a period during which multiple gait cycles are observed.

The gait cycle is divided into stance phase when one foot is in contact with the ground (~60% of the cycle), swing phase when the foot is not in contact with the ground (~20% of the cycle) and two short periods during each full cycle when both feet are in contact with the ground (double support).

In stance phase, the lower limb extensors and biomechanical alignments bear the weight and prevent the limb from collapsing. During this phase and through double support, the trunk not only crosses the midline but also the body mass is propelled forwards over the lead leg beyond anterior stability limits. Postural adjustments are required as the body moves over the small and changing base of support, and the subsequent forwards step in front of the centre of mass (CoM) prevents falling forwards (Winter et al 1990).

In swing phase, the de-weighted trailing leg moves forwards and the foot swings through, clear of the ground. At the same time, the limb trajectory is prepared to enable accurate and safe foot placement at initial contact. Gaze control is critical for tasks that require accurate foot placement, as well as for activities that include turning (Earhart 2013). Up to 50% of everyday tasks are composed of turning steps (Glaister et al 2007).

The terms used for assessment purposes to describe the phases of the gait cycle and foot placements are shown in Fig. 4.1 and are defined in Table 4.2.

Walking Kinematics and Muscle Activity

Kinematic analysis measures average joint movement profiles (e.g., using video cameras) independent from forces acting internally and externally on the body. These studies suggest that most people use similar movement strategies to accomplish the task of walking. Knowledge of average joint angles at given stages of the gait cycle provides useful information for observational assessment. During walking, movement occurs in the sagittal, transverse and frontal planes, but the largest angular changes occur in the sagittal plane (Whittle et al 2012a). Fig. 4.2A shows the successive positions of the right leg at 40-ms intervals measured over one complete gait cycle, and Fig. 4.2B shows the corresponding sagittal plane angles at the hip, knee and ankle.

Fig. 4.3 shows notable short bursts of contraction of the ankle plantar flexors at push-off, hip extensor concentric contraction at heel strike and the hip flexor contraction at preswing (Whittle et al 2012a). In addition to active motor control, evidence also exists to suggest that propulsion is effectively catalysed by a release of stored energy from the combination of contractile and noncontractile structures, coupled with contractions within the triceps surae at push-off, to sharply plantarflex the ankle and almost 'catapult' the shank forward (Ishikawa et al 2005, Lichtwark & Wilson 2006). Within the complex foot and ankle structure, there is potential for the triceps surae to contract isometrically from preswing to toe off to control the release of stored energy in structures such as the Achilles tendon and plantar fascia (Lichtwark & Wilson 2006). Indeed plantar fascia tautness

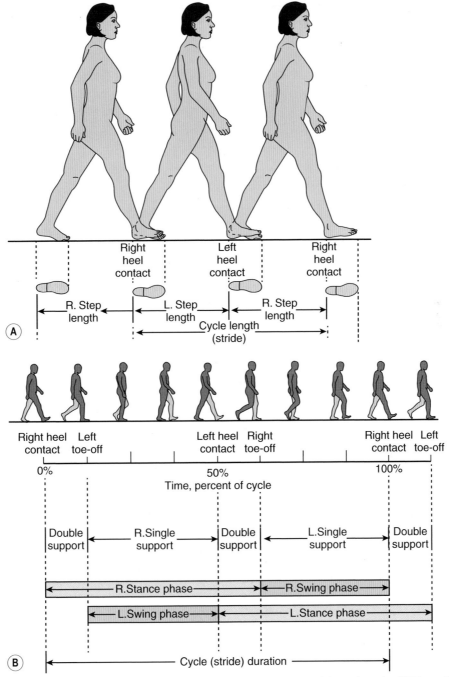

FIG. 4.1 Dimensions of the walking cycle. (A) Spatial dimensions of the gait cycle. (B) Time dimensions of the gait cycle. (From Inman, V.T., Ralston, H.J., Todd, F., 1981. Human Walking. Baltimore, Williams & Wilkins, p. 26, with permission.)

TABLE 4.2	Key Phases of the Gait Cycle and Related Terminology[a]

Stance Phase

Initial contact	The point in the gait cycle when the lead foot makes contact with the ground; this marks the beginning of stance phase
Loading response	The initial double support stance period which occurs from initial contact through to the first 10% of the gait cycle (this subsection is also known as 'weight acceptance')
Mid-stance	The first half of single support; when the trailing limb leaves the floor until body weight is aligned over the forefoot of the supporting lead limb
Terminal stance	About 40% of the stance phase when the lead limb is in single support
Preswing (push-off)	The last 10% of stance, in double support, from the time of initial contact of the opposite limb to toe-off of the observed limb

Swing Phase

Initial swing	The first third of the swing phase, defined as toe-off to the point when the swing limb is opposite the stance limb
Mid-swing	Middle phase of the swing phase, from the time the swing foot is opposite the stance limb to when the tibia is vertical
Terminal swing	The final third of the swing phase, the point when the tibia is vertical to initial contact

Other Commonly Used Terms

Double support	The period when both feet are in contact with the floor. This short phase occurs at the beginning of stance phase and again at the end of stance phase (when observing one limb). It is a critical point for transferring weight from one limb to the other. The two episodes of double support in one complete gait cycle respectively represent ~10% of the full cycle
Single support	The period when only one foot is in contact with the ground (equal to the swing phase of the other leg)
Terminal contact	The point in the gait cycle when the foot leaves the ground (the end of stance phase or the beginning of swing phase)
Toe-off	When terminal contact is made with the toe as the foot leaves the ground at the end of stance phase
Foot flat	The point in time in stance phase when the foot is in plantar grade
Heel-off (heel rise)	The point in time in stance phase when the heel leaves the ground
Heel strike	In typical gait 'heel strike' may be used instead of 'initial contact'; in pathological gait heel strike is often absent and therefore initial contact is a more accurate term, but absence of heel strike should be noted
Push-off	The period in late stance where an ankle plantar flexor moment and power generated by the plantar flexors help to advance the limb into swing phase
Step length	The distance between the first contact point of one foot and the first contact point of the next foot
Stride length	The distance between successive points of contact of one foot and the next point of contact with the same foot
Stride width	Measured from the midpoint of each heel; this is the side-to-side distance between the two feet
Cadence	The number of steps taken in a given time (steps/min)
Velocity	The distance covered in a given time (m/s)
Lead leg	The leg that is in front, e.g., the leg that goes first in walking over obstacles
Trail leg	The leg that follows, e.g., the leg that goes last over obstacles

[a]For further details refer to Whittle et al (2012a).

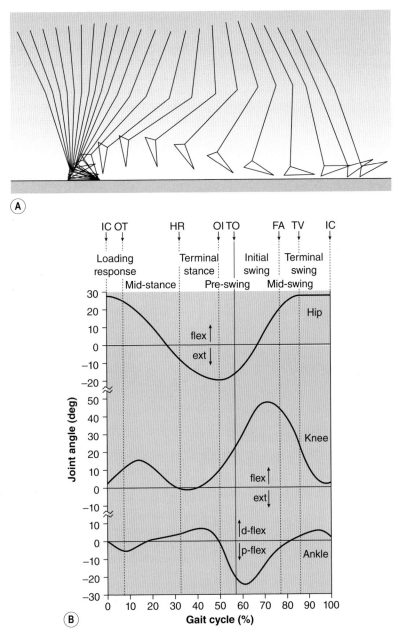

FIG. 4.2 (A) Position of the right leg in the sagittal plane at 40-ms intervals during a single gait cycle. (B) Sagittal plane joint angles (degrees) during a single gait cycle of right hip (flexion positive), knee (flexion positive), and ankle (dorsiflexion positive). IC, initial contact; OT, opposite toe off; HR, heel rise; OI, opposite initial contact; TO, toe off; FA, feet adjacent; TV, tibia vertical. Flex, flexion; ext, extension; d-flex, dorsiflexion; p-flex, plantarflexion. (From Figs. 2.4 and 2.5, p. 35 Levine, D., Richards, J., Whittle, M.W. (eds). Whittle's gait analysis: an introduction, 5th ed. Churchill Livingstone, Elsevier, Edinburgh, with permission.)

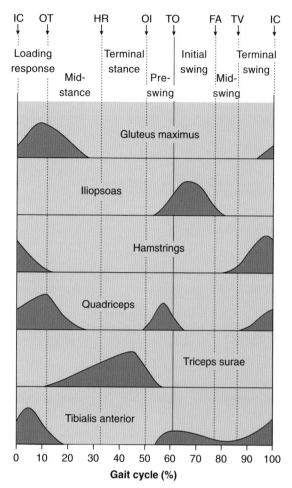

FIG. 4.3 Typical activity of major muscle groups during the gait cycle. IC, initial contact; OT, opposite toe off; HR, heel rise; OI, opposite initial contact; TO, toe off; FA, feet adjacent; TV, tibia vertical. (From Fig 2.10, Typical activity of major muscle groups during the gait cycle, p. 39, Levine, D., Richards, J., Whittle, M.W. (eds). Whittle's gait analysis: an introduction, 5th ed. Churchill Livingstone, Elsevier, Edinburgh, with permission.)

et al 2012a). Muscles contract and relax in carefully coordinated, repeatable, on-off bursts of patterned activation (Shiavi 1985), but a reasonable degree of flexibility exists to engage different muscles if necessary (Lacquaniti et al 2012). This means that there is considerable redundancy in the system that allows other muscles or muscle groups to take over the function of a muscle that is no longer working (Whittle et al 2012a). The following section summarises the key kinematic and typical muscle activity of walking in healthy adults. For more detailed information, see Levine et al (2012).

At *initial contact*, at the beginning of stance phase, the trunk is about half a stride length behind the leading leg and crosses the midline moving towards the leading leg as the foot on that side contacts the ground (Whittle et al 2012a). With reference to Whittle et al (2012a), the hip is flexed but is moving into extension through the concentric action of the hip extensors, gluteus maximus and the hamstrings. The knee moves through from close to full extension at initial contact to slight knee flexion during the loading response ('stance phase flexion'). Eccentric contraction of the quadriceps limits the speed and magnitude of the knee flexion. The ankle starts close to its neutral position (0°) and moves into plantarflexion through the eccentric action of tibialis anterior to bring the forefoot in contact with the ground.

At *mid-stance*, the hip continues to extend approaching 0° through gravity and inertia. Lateral pelvic horizontal movement (4–5 cm) towards the stance leg is controlled by contraction of the hip abductors, especially gluteus medius and tensor fascia lata. The knee reaches its peak of stance phase flexion and starts to extend through concentric action of the quadriceps. With the foot flat on the floor, the ankle moves from plantarflexion into dorsiflexion as the tibia moves forwards over the stationary foot through the isometric action of the plantar flexors (Whittle et al 2012a).

At *terminal stance*, the hip continues to extend, reaching maximum extension (10–20°) just as the opposite leg achieves initial contact. The abductors continue to work to stabilise the pelvis, but this activity is no longer maintained once the opposite foot makes initial contact. The knee begins to flex. Movement into plantarflexion occurs late in terminal stance. At preswing, hip flexion is initiated in preparation to swing the leg forwards, the knee moves rapidly into flexion in preparation for toe clearance with eccentric contraction of rectus femoris to prevent knee flexion occurring too fast. The ankle continues to move into plantarflexion through the concentric action of the plantar flexors. The toes extend at the metatarsophalangeal joints (Whittle et al 2012a).

Swing phase is precisely calibrated to produce an average toe clearance of ~1 cm (Murray 1967). According to

may in turn be finely controlled by metacarpal flexors (involving a 'windlass system') and peronei to convert the foot from a structure able to accommodate a changing underfoot support surface to one that assists with propulsion of the shank over the foot (Gu & Li 2012, Shah et al 2020). Whilst a typical walking pattern appears relatively stable in kinematic studies, the underlying muscle activity may vary between individuals and within one individual with respect to, for example, speed and fatigue (Whittle

Whittle et al (2012a), rectus femoris, adductor longus, tension in the hip ligaments and gravity enable the hip to continue to flex as the foot leaves the ground. The knee continues to flex (effectively shortening the leg), reaching peak flexion just more than halfway through the initial swing; as the hip flexes, the lower leg is left behind because of inertia, resulting in knee flexion. The ankle reaches peak plantarflexion just after toe-off, tibialis anterior contracts during mid-swing to dorsiflex the foot during the rest of swing. The hamstrings contract at the end of swing phase, effectively applying a break to prevent knee hyperextension. This contraction continues into the start of the stance phase.

During walking, the upper body moves forwards, the shoulder girdle and pelvic girdle rotate in opposite directions, and the arms swing out of phase with the legs (left arm and shoulder forwards, right leg and pelvis forwards) in a coordinated manner. Further research is required to consider the role of the upper limb in the coordination of gait, given the understanding that alteration in arm movements during walking affect gait efficiency, coordination and dynamic postural control (Earhart 2013, Meyns et al 2013).

Walking Kinetics

Kinetics is the study of forces, moments, masses and accelerations using equipment such as force platforms (Whittle et al 2012b). During walking, the dominant forces acting at a joint do not necessarily reflect the movement of the joint as revealed by kinematic studies. In stance phase, the combined moments acting at the hip, knee and ankle are far less variable than their individual components and provide a net extensor moment that prevents the knee from collapsing under the weight of the body (Winter 1980). The forces used to generate this net extensor moment are variable from stride to stride and person to person (Whittle et al 2012a).

Propulsion of the body results in the generation of forces on the ground, called ground reaction forces (GRFs). GRFs reflect the horizontal and vertical acceleration and deceleration of the CoM during weight bearing (Winter 1987). In quiet standing (Fig. 4.4A), the GRF is equal and opposite to the weight of an individual and acts only in a vertical direction. However, during walking, there are both vertical and horizontal GRFs. In late stance (Fig. 4.4B), an unopposed horizontal force (F_x) propels the body forwards, whilst a vertical GRF, which is greater than the weight of the person, causes an acceleration of the body upwards (Whittle et al 2012b).

Spatiotemporal Characteristics

Walking speed is one of the most important variables for determining functional competence in the community,

and it may be used to predict functional outcomes (Fritz & Lusardi 2009). For example, following stroke, gait speed is an important predictor of outcome and discharge destination, independent of age and functional status on admission (Rabadi & Blau 2005).

Normative spatiotemporal data synthesised from the recorded gait speed of more than 23,000 individuals over distances of 3–30 metres provide age and gender standards against which individuals can be compared (Bohannon & Williams Andrews 2011) (Table 4.3).

Clinical Focus: Walking for People With Parkinson's

Gait impairment is associated with increased activity limitations (Tan et al 2011) and may make a significant contribution to reduced quality of life among people living with Parkinson's (Soh et al 2011, Walton et al 2015). Gait impairment is a significant feature of Parkinson's, present in early stages of the disease (Rehman et al 2019, Zanardi et al 2021). Recent research involving 'machine learning' approaches has quantified gait characteristics to reveal strong associations between key parameters, such as self-selected walking speed, stride length, cadence, double support and swing time, and traditional disease severity scale measures such as the Hoehn and Yahr scale, the score of the Unified Parkinson's disease Rating Scale or disease duration. The use of wearable inertial sensors is proposed to provide an option for continuous monitoring to inform clinicians of disease progression (Balaji et al 2021, Rehman et al 2020). Inertial sensors as wearables may soon also contribute to the diagnosis of Parkinson's (di Biase et al 2020). People with Parkinson's adopt slower walking speeds, lower cadence, shorter strides and more mediolateral head and pelvis motion, which appears linked to a high risk of falling but could possibly be part of a compensatory strategy to prevent a fall (Creaby & Cole 2018). Freezing of gait (FOG) can affect all stages of Parkinson's and the incidence increases as Parkinson's progresses; up to 80% of people in the later stages of Parkinson's are reportedly affected (Tan et al 2011, Zhang et al 2021). FOG increases the likelihood of falling and nursing home placement (Kerr et al 2010). Table 4.4 presents the common problems associated with walking in Parkinson's and provides evidence-based explanations for these difficulties.

SIT TO STAND

STS is a transitional movement to the upright posture brought about by moving the CoM from a stable to a less stable position over extended lower limbs (Vander Linden et al 1994). As a crucial component of daily living, healthy adults undertake this complex skill on average 60 times a

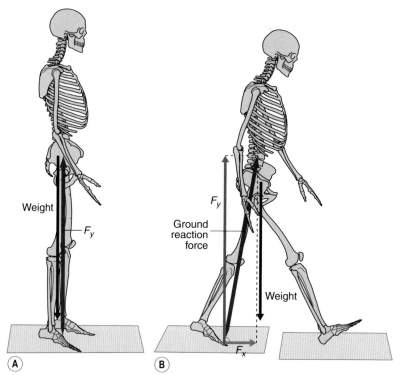

FIG. 4.4 (A) Standing still, the ground reaction force is equal and opposite to the weight of the person, acting in a vertical direction with no horizontal component. (B) Late stance phase: there is a horizontal force Fx which is unopposed and will cause acceleration or propulsion of the body forwards. The vertical force Fy is greater than the weight of the person causing an acceleration of the body forwards. (From Fig 1.19a and b, p. 22, Levine, D., Richards, J., Whittle, M.W. (eds). Whittle's gait analysis: an introduction, 5th ed. Churchill Livingstone, Elsevier, Edinburgh, with permission.)

day (Dall & Kerr 2010). Effective execution of STS is an important goal of neurological rehabilitation. Analyses of STS have focused on understanding the biomechanical, kinetic and kinematic components of this action as it is typically produced and when performed by people living with a range of health conditions. Insights from these studies offer an understanding of the invariant features of STS (the signature or fundamental pattern of the action that determines the order of events), as well as the critical movement parameters (the adjustable quantities of an action such as the timing, scale, force, direction, velocity and acceleration). Any or several of these components of STS may need to be targeted to successfully retrain individuals who have difficulty with this critical functional activity.

Typical Phases of Sit to Stand

Schenkman et al (1990) identified four distinct phases of STS which provide a useful guide for observational analysis

in the clinic (Fig. 4.5). In healthy adults, the phases unfold in a smooth, continuous, curvilinear path which traces a forwards and upwards trajectory (Carr & Shepherd 2010). The key components of each phase are summarised in Table 4.5.

Using simultaneous force plate readings taken from the buttocks and feet, Hirschfeld et al (1999) identified anticipatory actions that occurred before observable STS movements, that is, before the first phase observed by Schenkman et al (1990). Based on these readings, Hirschfeld et al (1999) divided STS into two phases (Table 4.6). While Schenkman et al (1990) provided a clinically useful analysis of STS, Hirschfeld et al (1999) identified the importance of the preparatory forces required for STS, and the precise timing and coordination of muscle force needed to produce a smooth and mechanically efficient movement pattern. Both analyses have relevance for clinical practice. More detailed analyses of STS may be required for research purposes (e.g., see Etnyre & Thomas 2007).

TABLE 4.3 Normative Walking Speed (Results of a Meta-analysis)

Strata Gender (Age in Years)	Source Articles (n)	Subjects (n)	Gait Speed (cm/s)	Grand Mean (95% CI) range	Homogeneity Q (p)
Men (20–29)	10	155	135.8 (127.0–144.7)	121.7–147.4	3.255 (0.953)
Men (30–39)	5	83	143.3 (131.6–155.0)	132.0–153.8	1.169 (0.883)
Men (40–49)	4	96	143.4 (135.3–151.4)	127.0–147.0	2.609 (0.625)
Men (50–59)	6	436	143.3 (137.9–148.8)	112.2–149.1	4.721 (0.580)
Men (60–69)	12	941	133.9 (126.6–141.2)	103.3–159.0	15.217 (0.294)
Men (70–79)	18	3671	126.2 (121.0–132.2)	95.7–141.8	12.848 (0.914)
Men (80 to 99)	10	1091	96.8 (83.4 to 110.1)	60.8 to 122.1	4.159 (0.940)
Women (20–29)	11	180	134. 1 (123.9–144.3)	108.2–149.9	5.307 (0.870)
Women (30–39)	5	104	133.7 (119.3–148.2)	125.6–141.5	0.785 (0.940)
Women (40–49)	7	142	139.0 (133.9–141.1)	122.0–142.0	5.666 (0.579)
Women (50–59)	10	456	131.3 (122.2–140.5)	110.0–155.5	12.291 (0.266)
Women (60–69)	17	5013	124.1 (118.3–130.0)	97.0–145.0	11.515 (0.932)
Women (70–79)	29	8591	113.2 (107.2–119.2)	83.0–150.0	16.775 (0.998)
Women (80–99)	17	2152	94.3 (85.2–103.4)	55.7–117.0	11.428 (0.954)

CI, Confidence interval.
Modified with permission from Table 2 in Bohannon, R.W., Williams Andrews, A., 2011. Normal walking speed: a descriptive meta-analysis. Physiotherapy. 97, 182–189.

TABLE 4.4 Commonly Observed Problems With Walking in Parkinson's

Commonly Observed Problems	Explanations From Gait Analyses
Shuffling steps	The foot continues to move forwards at the point of initial contact, causing shuffling, with little if any heel strike; scuffing of the foot mid-swing may also be observed and cadence is reduced (Baker et al 2012).
Bradykinesia	People with Parkinson's walk with reduced speed (bradykinesia), short stride length [hypokinesia: a scaling down of the size of the movement (Morris et al 2008)] and increased double support time (Švehlik et al 2009). Reduced gait speed may also work as a self-selected compensation in response to fear of falling (Creaby & Cole 2018, Maki 1997).
Freezing of gait (FOG): a sudden or gradual inability to take steps during walking and to initiate subsequent steps despite having the intention to walk (Morris et al 2008); FOG is experienced as a motor block where the feet feel as if they are stuck to the floor (Giladi et al 1992)	FOG may be observed at the initiation of gait, during straight line walking and turning, and may be triggered by environmental cues and spatial constraints such as thresholds and obstacles (Nieuwboer & Giladi 2013). People with FOG have difficulty maintaining a stable rhythm, controlling cadence, and regulating stride-to-stride variations (Hausdorff et al 2003). Although FOG is transient and observed as an episodic phenomenon, the underlying disruption is thought to be continuous (Hausdorff et al 2003, Weiss et al 2015). The exact mechanism underlying FOG is yet to be determined but may involve environmental, cognitive, emotional and motor factors (Nieuwboer & Giladi 2013).
Festination	Festination describes an involuntary progressive reduction in stride length, an increase in cadence during a walking task and a reduction in walking speed (m/s). Freezing may eventually occur (Iansek et al 2006, Morris et al 2008).

(Continued)

TABLE 4.4	Commonly Observed Problems With Walking in Parkinson's—Cont'd
Commonly Observed Problems	**Explanations From Gait Analyses**
Difficulty turning	People with Parkinson's turn slowly, take more steps, have poor foot clearance and may pause before executing a turn (Stack & Ashburn 2008). These alterations to normal movement patterns may preserve postural stability by reducing neuromuscular demands through the reduction of movement amplitude (centre of mass displacement and velocity) (Song et al 2012), but also increase the number of steps that must be controlled and coordinated (Stack & Ashburn 2008). Similar difficulty in motor sequencing, observed as a decoupling of the sequential components of linked tasks, are evident in sit-to-walking transfers (Buckley et al 2008). In people with early-stage/mild Parkinson's, difficulty executing turns may occur before other walking difficulties are evident and may be independent of disturbances that effect straight-line walking (Crenna et al 2007, Song et al 2012). Axial rigidity and impaired intersegmental coordination, where the head and trunk turn at the same time rather than the head turning first followed by the trunk, are indicative of task-specific movement impairment (Crenna et al 2007).
Reduced arm swing	Arm swing is generally reduced and asymmetrical in Parkinson's (Huang et al 2012). The most affected arm has less arm swing. Unlike people after stroke, the less affected arm does not seem to compensate by increasing the swing range (Meyns et al 2013).
Weakness	Muscle strength and power are reduced in people with Parkinson's (Allen et al 2009), resulting in reduced motor unit recruitment and muscle weakness (David et al 2012).

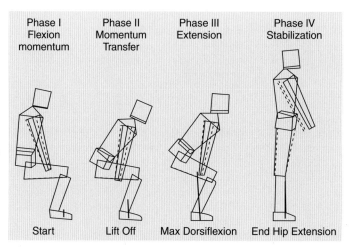

FIG. 4.5 Typical phases of sit to stand. (Reprinted from Schenkman, M. Interrelationship of neurological and mechanical factors in balance control. In: Duncan, P., ed. Balance: Proceedings of the American Physical Therapy Association Forum. Alexandria, VA: American Physical Therapy Association; 1989:29–41, with permission of the American Physical Therapy Association. © 1989 American Physical Therapy Association.)

TABLE 4.5   The Four Phases and Key Characteristics of Sit to Stand (Schenkman et al 1990)

Phase	Key Characteristics
I. Flexion momentum	• From the start of the movement to seat-off (when the buttocks leave the base of support and just the feet are in contact with the ground[a]) • Horizontal linear momentum is generated to move the body mass forwards over the feet • The trunk and pelvis rotate anteriorly as the hips flex • The head, spine and pelvis are usually considered to behave as one segment, with the spine erect as the whole segment rotates forwards (Carr & Shepherd 2010)
II. Momentum transfer	• From seat-off[b] to maximum dorsiflexion (the knees move forwards over fixed feet) • Upper body flexion momentum is transferred into extension as body displacement shifts from the anterior direction of phase I to a forwards and upwards displacement in phase II
III. Extension	• From maximum dorsiflexion to full hip extension • The body is brought into a fully upright posture
IV. Stabilisation	• From the end of hip extension until all motion associated with rising has stopped • The completion of this phase is difficult to determine because of the observable normal postural sway associated with quiet stance (Lomaglio & Eng 2005)

[a]Before seat-off 85% of body weight is distributed on the buttocks and thighs, and 15% on the feet (Hirschfeld et al 1999).
[b]Seat-off usually occurs at approximately 34% of the total movement time (Cheng et al 2004, Kralj et al 1990).

TABLE 4.6   The Two Phases and Key Characteristics of Sit to Stand (Hirschfeld et al 1999)

Phase	Key Characteristics
Preparatory phase	• From the onset of backwards-directed (anteroposterior) propulsive forces beneath the buttocks to seat-off • Before visible STS movements, anticipatory isometric forces occur around the feet and the hip, trunk and pelvis to prepare the body for forwards acceleration • These forces are coordinated in advance of movement to match an individual's weight, and the distance between the feet and buttocks • The ground reaction forces generated against the seat and the ground under the feet enable the body mass to be propelled horizontally • Horizontal momentum is then primarily brought about by the head-arm-trunk segment through angular rotation at the hip (Pai & Rogers 1991) • Forwards momentum of the trunk reaches a peak and then decelerates because of braking actions, before the rising phase, suggesting tight control of the transition from one phase to the next • Precise timing and scaling of braking forces before seat-off is crucial to control equilibrium during weight transfer
Rising phase	• From seat-off until the vertical velocity of the centre of mass decreases to zero • Vertical momentum is brought about by extension at the hips, knees and ankles (Pai & Rogers 1991) • Large vertical ground reaction forces under the feet peak at seat-off (Carr & Shepherd 2010)

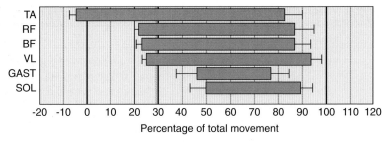

FIG. 4.6 Mean and standard error of time normalised onsets and durations of six lower limb muscles during sit to stand at a preferred speed. *BF*, Biceps femoris; *GAST*, gastrocnemius; *RF*, rectus femoris; *SOL*, soleus; *TA*, tibialis anterior; *VL*, vastus lateralis; 0%, movement onset, 31%, thighs off; 100%, movement end. (From Khemlani, M.M., Carr, J.H., Crosbie, W.J., 1999. Muscle synergies and joint linkages in sit-to-stand under two initial foot positions. Clin. Biomech. 14, 236–246.)

Muscle Action During Sit to Stand

Electromyogram (EMG) recordings demonstrate that key lower limb muscle groups are activated in sequence during STS in healthy adults (Khemlani et al 1999). Tibialis anterior is one of the first muscles to be activated, followed by the quadriceps and hamstrings, with soleus coming in last (Fig. 4.6). Table 4.7 summarises the action and purpose of key muscle groups during STS.

Contextual Factors Influencing Sit to Stand

Several determinants of STS performance and their influence on kinematic and kinetic outcomes have been reported and summarised in the literature (Frykberg & Häger 2015, Janssen et al 2002). Key determinants are listed in Table 4.8. Many diverse environmental, psychological and sensorimotor factors are likely to influence the performance of STS and should be considered in the clinical assessment of this action. A recent review by van der Kruk et al (2020) explores compensatory strategies in STS with altered physical ability and makes recommendations for future research.

Clinical Focus on Sit to Stand for People After Stroke

Independence in STS is often lost in the acute phase after stroke (Bohannon 2007). Most stroke survivors will gain independence in STS, usually in the first 12 weeks post-stroke, with improved performance characterised by increased speed and increased STS events (Janssen et al 2010). Table 4.9 provides evidence-based explanations of commonly observed problems in STS after stroke.

ROLLING AND GETTING OUT OF BED

Rolling over and getting out of bed are important functional skills for independent living; however, the characteristic features of the underlying movement patterns in adults have been less well investigated when compared with STS, walking, and reach and grasp. Videotaped analysis of getting out of bed suggests that adults use a wide variety of strategies (Alexander et al 1995, Ford-Smith & VanSant 1993, Mount et al 2006, Richter et al 1989). For example, Mount et al (2006) identified 75 different combinations of movement patterns of the upper limbs, lower limbs, and the head and trunk from a video analysis of more than 170 trials of older adults (aged 65–90 years) getting out of bed in a bedroom environment closely resembling the home situation.

In these studies, some participants were asked to start in supine with their arms by their side (Alexander et al 1995, Ford-Smith & VanSant 1993), whilst others selected a preferred start position (Mount et al 2006). Regarding possible task constraints, participants were asked to roll into prone (Richter et al 1989), or to get up from the bed and walk to a chair (Mount et al 2006), or to rise from supine to sitting on the edge of the bed, with and without using the upper limbs (Alexander et al 1995). Participants were also asked to either move as fast as possible (Ford-Smith & VanSant 1993, Richter et al 1989) or to move as they would at home (Mount et al 2006). Such differences in the experimental setup may account for some of the variability seen across studies.

The strategies used to move from a lying position also vary with age (Alexander et al 1995, Ford-Smith & VanSant 1993, Mount et al 2006). Older adults who lack the capacity to generate force may use multiple pushes with both arms to initiate trunk flexion, or may grasp one leg to compensate for weak abdominal muscles or weak hip flexors, or drop the legs over the side as a counterweight to help raise the trunk (Mount et al 2006). Table 4.10 provides guidance for the observational analysis of rolling and lying to sitting.

TABLE 4.7 Action and Purpose of Key Muscle Groups During Sit to Stand

Muscle/Muscle Group	Action and Purpose
Tibialis anterior	• One of the first muscles to be activated before the beginning of the movement (anticipatory postural activity) (Cheng et al 2004) • Works to secure the foot to the floor as the trunk moves forwards (Cheng et al 2004, Khemlani et al 1999) • Stabilises the foot as the shank moves forwards over the fixed foot (Cheng et al 2004, Khemlani et al 1999)
Iliopsoas	• Hip flexion; bringing the erect trunk and pelvis forwards at the hips (Carr & Shepherd 2010)
Quadriceps	• Rectus femoris contributes to hip flexion before seat-off (Carr & Shepherd 2010, Khemlani et al 1999); quads stabilise the knee before knee extension (Khemlani et al 1999) • Contributes to knee extension after seat-off with the rest of the quadriceps (Carr & Shepherd 2010, Khemlani et al 1999)
Biceps femoris	• Flexes the knee to bring the feet back in position before flexion momentum • Acts as a breaking force at the end of flexion momentum to stabilise the knee in preparation for extension (Carr & Shepherd 2010, Cheng et al 2004, Khemlani et al 1999)
Trunk muscles, rectus abdominis, paraspinals	• Stabilise the erect trunk (Carr & Shepherd 2010)
Lumbar paraspinals, hip and knee extensors	• Reach peak activity together at seat-off to achieve the upright posture
Knee and hip extensors and plantar flexors	• Knee extension starts the extensor activity to achieve the upright posture followed by hip extension and finally plantarflexion (shank moves backwards over the fixed foot) (Khemlani et al 1999) • Soleus is the last muscle to be activated because it works to decelerate and stabilise at the end of STS (Carr & Shepherd 2010, Cheng et al 2004)
Anticipatory and ongoing postural adjustments	• Occur before and during STS to control the complex multisegmental action required when moving from a relatively large and stable base of support to a less stable position with a small base of support (Goulart & Valls-Solé 1999) with the goal of keeping the centre of gravity within the base of support (Carr & Shepherd 2010)

Clinical Focus on Getting Out of Bed for People with Parkinson's

People with Parkinson's frequently get out of bed because of nocturia (Bhidayasiri et al 2014, Sringean et al 2016), and yet they frequently struggle with impaired bed mobility (Stack & Ashburn 2006), nocturnal hypokinesia (Bhidayasiri et al 2014, Louter et al 2012), early morning akinesia, tremor and dystonia, as well as light-headedness, dizziness and weakness when standing up from lying or sitting (Bhidayasiri et al 2014, Louter et al 2012). These difficulties may also be present in the early stages of this condition (Louter et al 2015). Table 4.11 identifies and provides explanations for several difficulties that contribute to impaired bed mobility.

REACH AND GRASP

Successful use of the upper limb is an essential component of most activities of daily living from feeding and self-care to leisure pursuits such as music, art and sports. This section will concentrate on reach and grasp as one part of upper limb function. The upper limb also participates in other important activities that are beyond the scope of this chapter, such as throwing, striking, balance (including protective mechanisms when balance reactions fail) and weight bearing.

Reach to grasp strategies have been extensively investigated in the motor control research literature. Early work by Jeannerod (1984) described the characteristics of reach to grasp and prehension in healthy subjects as invariant,

TABLE 4.8   Contextual Factors That Influence Sit to Stand

Contextual Factors	Influence on STS	Explanation
Foot position	Standing up with the feet placed about 10 cm behind the knee (75° ankle dorsiflexion) is more efficient than neutral (feet below knees) or forwards foot placement (Kawagoe et al 2000)	• Posterior foot placement requires less forwards displacement of the centre of gravity (Kawagoe et al 2000). • Tibialis anterior is active for a shorter time before seat-off (Kawagoe et al 2000). • The feet usually take up a symmetrical position and are equally loaded at seat-off. Asymmetrical foot placement increases the loading of the most posterior foot (Lecours et al 2008).
Seat height	The lower the seat, the harder it is to stand (seat heights measured either as the distance from the floor to the seat or as a percentage of lower leg length)	Rising from a low chair requires: • simultaneous acceleration and braking for a long time after seat-off (Kawagoe et al 2000); • greater hip, knee and ankle flexion (Rodosky et al 1989); • increased knee maximum flexion moment (Rodosky et al 1989) and required knee extension moment (Hughes et al 1996); and • increased trunk flexion angular velocity to overcome mechanical difficulties (Schenkman et al 1996).
Arm rests	Use of arm rests may reduce the lower limb work of STS	• Using arm rests reduces hip and knee moments (Janssen et al 2002).
Age	Young adults, mean age 41 years, perform the FTSST faster (8.2 s) than older adults (13.4 s), mean age 73 years (Whitney et al 2005) Functionally independent older adults demonstrate greater postural sway during both raising and stabilization phases (Piano et al 2020)	• Quadriceps muscle strength may be the most important variable to explain variance in STS time in older community-dwelling adults, but other psychological and physiological factors also impact performance (Lord et al 2002). • Because of age-related decline in maximal leg strength, older adults may use twice as much of their available leg strength compared with younger adults, and work close to their maximum capacity (Hortobágyi et al 2003). • Older adults may place a high importance on achieving acceptable postural stability which slows STS performance (Schultz et al 1992).
Strength	Lower limb weakness adversely impacts on STS performance (Hughes et al 1996)	• FTSST times reflect knee extension strength across the age span (Bohannon et al 2010). • Knee extension, knee flexion and ankle dorsiflexion strength are significant predictors of STS performance and make independent contributions to STS performance in older adults (Lord et al 2002)
Balance	People with balance disorders perform the FTSTT slower than those without balance disorders (Lord et al 2002)	• People with balance disorders have difficulty with transitional actions such as STS and may move more slowly to avoid provoking dizziness (Whitney et al 2005).

TABLE 4.8   Contextual Factors That Influence Sit to Stand—Cont'd

Contextual Factors	Influence on STS	Explanation
Range of movement	Restricted range of motion at key joints alters biomechanical components of STS	• <100° of knee flexion requires a higher angular velocity of the hip to move the trunk forwards (Hokazu et al 1998).
Body weight	Body weight has an independent effect on STS performance in older adults (Janssen et al 2002)	• More work is required to raise heavier bodies from a seated position (Lord et al 2002). • Heavier people minimise forwards trunk movement which reduces hip joint torque and lower back loading but significantly increases knee joint torque (Sibella et al 2003).
Vision	Contrast sensitivity has an independent effect on STS performance in older adults (Lord et al 2002)	• Good vision (contrast sensitivity and depth perception) may provide an additional cue for safety (Lord et al 2002).
Sensation	Lower limb sensation has an independent effect on STS performance in older adults (Lord et al 2002)	• Effective tactile sensation and proprioception may assist with reacting quickly and maintaining balance control during transition (Lord et al 2002).
Pain	Pain has an independent effect on STS performance in older adults (Lord et al 2002)	• Pain may affect motivation and apprehension during STS (Lord et al 2002).
Psychological status	Anxiety and vitality are significant and independent predictors of STS performance in older adults (Lord et al 2002)	• Anxiety and vitality may affect motivation and apprehension during STS (Lord et al 2002).

FTSST, Five times sit to stand test; *STS*, sit to stand.

TABLE 4.9   Commonly Observed Difficulties in the Execution of Sit to Stand After Stroke

Commonly Observed Problems	Explanations From Analyses of Sit to Stand
Slow STS performance	• Stroke survivors execute STS more slowly than healthy control subjects (Arcelus et al 2009, Baillieul et al 2015, Cameron et al 2003, Cheng et al 1998, 2004, Hesse et al 1994), taking approximately 1 s longer, ~3.3 versus 2.3 s (Arcelus et al 2009, Baillieul et al 2015), at least in part because of slow muscle activation and recruitment. • Major muscle groups of the paretic lower limb (tibialis anterior, quadriceps, hamstrings and soleus) are weaker than those in the nonparetic limb (Cameron et al 2003, Lomaglio & Eng 2005, Prudente et al 2013), suggesting that the overall capacity to generate sufficient force to overcome gravity and to control stability during STS is impaired (Bohannon 2007). • Weakness of the knee extensors, and the ankle dorsiflexors and plantar flexors in the paretic limb, is associated with slower FTSST (Lomaglio & Eng 2005).

(Continued)

TABLE 4.9	Commonly Observed Difficulties in the Execution of Sit to Stand After Stroke—Cont'd
Commonly Observed Problems	**Explanations From Analyses of Sit to Stand**
Anterior posterior instability	• Alterations in the neuromuscular control and coordination of activity at the knee and ankle in the paretic limb may compromise anteroposterior stability during STS and may be associated with excessive (compensatory) activation of muscles in the nonparetic limb (Cheng et al 2004, Prudente et al 2013). • Balance, rather than strength or endurance, may be the most important determinant of FTSST performance in community-dwelling stroke survivors (Ng 2010). Although both balance and knee extensor muscle strength have been sown to independently contribute to FTSST performance. • Anticipatory postural activity is disrupted by delayed onset of tibialis anterior activity, as well as early activation of soleus (Cheng et al 2004, Silva et al 2013), which may occur in both the paretic and nonparetic lower limbs (Silva et al 2013).
Weight-bearing asymmetry	• Approximately one-third of body weight is taken through the paretic leg before and during STS in individuals after stroke, compared with an even distribution observed in healthy control subjects (Baillieul et al 2015, Cheng et al 1998, Engardt & Olsson 1992, Lecours et al 2008). • Compared with patients with mild knee extensor weakness, individuals with moderate and severe knee extensor weakness are more likely to adopt an asymmetrical loading strategy during STS (Brière et al 2013). • Individuals are less able to accurately judge their weight distribution during STS compared with healthy control subjects and perceive themselves as more symmetrical than they really are (Brière et al 2010, Nadeau et al 2016). • Kinematic reorganisation of this task happens before seat-off (Duclos et al 2008) with the centre of pressure moving towards the nonparetic side in advance of and during STS (Cheng et al 1998, Duclos et al 2008, Lecours et al 2008).
Asymmetrical foot placement	• Bilateral backwards placement of both feet by 10 cm from 90° knee flexion significantly decreases the time taken for the FTSST when compared with a start position of 90° knee flexion, irrespective of arm position, in individuals in the chronic phase after stroke (Kwong et al 2014). • Symmetrical foot placement provides more evenly distributed limb loading during sit to stand than posterior placement of the nonparetic limb (Camargos et al 2009, Roy et al 2006). • Backwards placement of the nonparetic foot from the neutral starting position increases weight-bearing asymmetry (Roy et al 2006), increases movement time and delays activation of soleus during STS (Camargos et al 2009). Backward placement of the paretic limb increases muscle activation in that limb (Nam et al 2015). • Elevation (e.g., on a step) or forwards placement of the nonparetic foot from a neutral starting position increases muscle activity in the paretic limb, reduces muscle activity in the nonparetic limb (Brunt et al 2002) and reduces trunk asymmetry (Duclos et al 2008, Lecours et al 2008).
Arm position	• The impact of arm position on STS performance after stroke has not been extensively investigated.
Other factors	• Trunk muscle weakness (Silva et al 2015), impaired generation and transfer of trunk flexion momentum (Silva et al 2017) and asynchronous trunk muscle recruitment (Lee et al 2015) may also contribute to poor STS performance. • Body weight alone does not have an independent effect on STS poststroke, but it is relevant when considered with knee extension strength and may therefore contribute to the independent achievement of STS for some individuals (Bohannon 2007).

FTSST, Five times sit-to-stand test; *STS*, sit to stand.

TABLE 4.10 Observational Analysis of Lying to Sitting/Getting Out of Bed

Component	Explanation
Timing	The average movement time for getting out of bed for healthy individuals older than 65 years is 5.3 s (SD 2.9 s, range 2.3–17.3 s) (Mount et al 2006). The lie-to-sit-to-stand-to-walk test (Reicherz et al 2011) is a timed test that is valid for quantifying difficulty with this transfer in elderly populations.
Environment	Match the test and practice environment to conditions in the home situation including the availability of assistive equipment and caregiver assistance.
Instructions	Record whether patients are asked to undertake the task in their own time, or to try to move as fast as possible.
Task	Standardise instructions because different patterns may be observed depending on the task, e.g., whether patients are asked to get up to sit on the edge of the bed, or to get up to walk to a chair.
Movement analysis	Record movement patterns with respect to four body segments: head and trunk, the far upper limb (farthest away from the direction of travel), the near arm (closest to the side of the bed of the direction of travel) and the lower limbs (look for synchronous or asynchronous movement). For further details (up to eight movement strategies have been observed for each body segment), refer to Mount et al (2006).

characterised by a straight-line path to the object and a smooth, bell-shaped velocity profile, with velocity slowing in the last 25% of reach and digits completing their final closure adjustment to grip the object in that same phase of movement. These characteristics were consistently present with different movement amplitudes and regardless of whether visual feedback from the moving limb was available (Jeannerod 1984). The emergence of a cost-efficient and consistent movement strategy demonstrates that the nervous system deals with multiple possible combinations of movement by applying a motor plan strategy which can then be adapted to constraints placed by the individual, the task and the environment. Both feed-forward (anticipatory) and feedback mechanisms are used during reach and grasp (Shumway-Cook & Woollacott 2012). This section offers an overview of the essential components of reach and grasp.

Essential Components of Reach and Grasp

There are four essential parts to reach and grasp (Table 4.12). Object location and identification, plus anticipatory postural adjustments occur before the actual movement. The major action of the arm is to reach towards a target (transport phase), whereas the major purpose of the hand is interaction with the environment (manipulation phase). Postural adjustments continue to occur throughout the action. Despite the multiple degrees of freedom, the arm and hand act as a single functional unit. In many activities the single functional unit also includes the upper body

or the entire body where this is required to position the hand for efficient interaction with the task or environment.

Kinematics

Reaching within arm's length involves the shoulder, elbow and wrist joints. Beyond arm's length the trunk and hip are also involved (Dean et al 1999). Upper limb segments have multiple degrees of freedom (three at the shoulder, one at the elbow, one in the forearm and two at the wrist, as well as multiple joints within the scapulohumeral complex) giving an infinite number of movement solutions to reach to a specific target. Despite this in-built flexibility, movement strategy has been shown to be similar for given targets and constraints across a healthy population (Jeannerod 1984, Marteniuk et al 1987). Wang & Stelmach (1998) investigated reach kinematics in healthy subjects using arm movements only, trunk movements only and a combination of both. They demonstrated that parameters related to reach (peak velocity, time to peak velocity) varied across conditions, but that parameters related to grasp (peak aperture, time to peak aperture, closing distance) were strikingly invariant (Wang & Stelmach 1998).

Palmar arch and finger joint movement to shape the hand for grasp are initiated almost simultaneously and occur early in the transport phase (within 125 ms of onset), which suggests that prehensile configuration is planned as early as intent to grasp (Sangole & Levin 2008b). Anatomically, the hand is described as having three palmar arches (transverse, longitudinal and oblique), but work by

TABLE 4.11 Common Difficulties With Bed Mobility Experienced by People With Parkinson's

Commonly Observed Problems	Explanation From Analyses of Rolling and Getting Out of Bed
Execution of movement patterns	Stack & Ashburn (2006) found that approximately 20% of people with Parkinson's were unable to turn in bed and 82% reported having difficulty with turning. Mount et al (2009) identified 80 different combinations of movement patterns from 166 trials with people with Parkinson's. The most common movement patterns occurred in only 5.2% of the trials in this study, indicating a high variability across participants. Only 3 of 39 participants used the same movement pattern combination across five trials. Coming up to sit rather than rolling whilst horizontal was found to be a frequently adopted head and trunk strategy (Mount et al 2009, Stack & Ashburn 2006).
Bradykinesia (slow movement)	The mean time for people with Parkinson's to get out of bed (from horizontal to full standing) is 8.2 s (SD 7.8 s, range 1.9–65.1 s) (Mount et al 2009).
Difficulty turning	People with Parkinson's roll over in bed less frequently and more slowly, turn through a smaller range, and produce less axial acceleration when compared with their spouses (Sringean et al 2016).
Weakness	Muscle strength and power are reduced in people with Parkinson's (Allen et al 2009). Robichaud et al (2004) found that in Parkinson's the extensors exhibited a more profound activation impairment than the flexors. A movement strategy that involves sitting up to roll has been commonly observed for the head and trunk component in people with Parkinson's (Mount et al 2009, Stack & Ashburn 2006). This strategy may reduce the need for trunk rotation and allows use of the trunk and hip flexors to elevate the trunk rather than using the elbow extensors to push the trunk upwards from side lying (Mount et al 2006). Taniguchi et al (2022) found that weakness in hip adductors (and to a lesser extent hip flexors) was correlated with impaired bed mobility in people with Parkinson's. They suggest this may be because hip adduction and flexion are often used by people with Parkinson's to create the momentum to bring the legs out of bed when trunk rotation is restricted.
Upper limb rigidity	In one small study (n = 16) arm rigidity statistically explained 75% of the variance in movement time to get out of bed (Taniguchi et al 2022).

Sangole and Levin (2008a) described a biomechanical arch that they named the 'kinematic transverse arch', considering the actions of the thenar and hypothenar eminences in arch formation and hand shaping (Sangole & Levin 2008a). They found that during transport phase there was relatively more thenar contribution to hand shape modulation, whereas the hypothenar contribution was more evident during preshaping and contact shaping.

A detailed understanding of the typical kinematics of reach and grasp in the healthy population (Table 4.13) can help clinicians to identify where deficits are occurring in the clinical population. Reach and grasp are distinct components which seem to be controlled by different neural mechanisms giving the potential for either or both to be affected in a clinical population (see Shumway-Cook & Woollacott 2012, pp. 481–490, for a more detailed discussion of motor control).

Reach and grasp parameters are influenced by features of the task such as object size, fragility, size of contact surface, texture and weight. For a recent review, see Castiello (2005). The location of the object to be reached for with reference to body axis (i.e., ipsilateral or contralateral to the reach arm) influences visual and motor processing times in that ipsilateral reaches are faster and simpler to achieve (Fisk & Goodale 1985). The goal of the task also has an effect where actions that require more accuracy lengthen the time required for reach and grasp (Marteniuk et al 1987). These factors can be used to vary therapeutic interventions to grade difficulty of rehabilitation intervention.

TABLE 4.12 Key Phases of Reach and Grasp

Phase	Key Elements
Object location and identification	• Object location and identification: There are two distinct routes in the brain: a ventral stream that is active in object identification and a dorsal stream for visual control of object-oriented actions. Information from these streams interact for complex tasks that require skilled grasp (van Polanen & Davare 2015) • Visual information about the characteristics of the object is used to preprogramme the forces required (Jenmalm et al 2000) and to improve accuracy of grasp scaling for object size (Borchers & Himmelbach 2012)
Postural control	• Anticipatory postural adjustments occur before movement onset and allow movement of the arm(s) without destabilising the body (Horak et al 1984) • Trunk stabilisation activity is ongoing throughout an activity, is task and context specific, and can include lower limb activity particularly when an object is beyond arm's reach (Dean et al 1999) • Trunk or body movement occurs with the aim of efficiently orienting the arm and hand to the task and environment, and controlling the centre of mass relative to the base of support
Transport	• Acceleration and deceleration, with a smooth, bell-shaped velocity curve • Hand shaping occurs throughout • Trajectory is determined by the relative position of the target and hand with a straight path to the target when there are no obstacles to overcome
Manipulation	• Stabilisation and movement of an object in space or with reference to another object • Within hand manipulation includes three major movement types: translation (moving objects from palm to fingertips and vice versa), shift (linear movement along an object, e.g., the shaft of a pencil) and rotation (includes simple and complex movements)

For a more detailed description of kinematics, see Table 4.13.

Muscle Activity

Prange et al (2009) investigated muscle activity during reach and retrieval in healthy elderly subjects. They found that most muscles had persistent levels of muscle activity throughout the reach and retrieval movements, except for triceps activity, which was low (see Fig. 4.7 for an example subject). Biceps was active to lift and hold the arm above the table and aid in forwards flexion of the shoulder. Muscle activity of triceps was very low but did contribute minimally to extension of the elbow towards the target in some subjects. Anterior and medial deltoid were active to maintain some shoulder abduction and to assist forwards flexion of the shoulder during reach. Activity of posterior deltoid decelerated forwards flexion of the shoulder towards the end of reach. Trapezius was active to elevate the arm at the start of reach and to stabilise and position the scapula appropriately. Activity increased towards the end of the reach phase most likely because of the larger torques acting on the arm as it moved farther from the body. Muscle patterns and coordination were similar when gravity was reduced by adding support for the arm (Prange et al 2009).

This tonic activation of muscles is thought to counteract gravity and may be particularly important in controlling the many degrees of freedom available for upper extremity movement. Appropriate cocontraction in agonist and antagonist muscles stabilises joints and controls interaction torques during movements. Superimposed phasic muscle activity then produces increases and decreases in velocity for purposeful movement (Flanders & Herrmann 1992, Prange et al 2009). There is a suggestion in human kinematic studies that most of the variation in grasp posture comes from hand shaping during reach, and that refinements in finger and thumb position are introduced just before contact to produce unique hand shapes for grasping different objects (Mason et al 2001).

Animal studies measuring EMG activity in 10–12 hand muscles suggest that specific complex patterns of EMG activation achieve distinct hand postures for grasping different objects. These patterns were consistent within one animal and distinctive enough to identify the object grasped from EMG patterns alone, but showed some differences between animals (Brochier 2004). Human cadaveric studies have

TABLE 4.13	**Essential Components of Transport and Manipulation Phases**
Component	**Invariant Features and Influences of Task and Environment**

Transport Phase

Object location
- Eye movement only when object is in central visual field; eye then head movement when it is in peripheral visual field; eye, head and trunk for far visual field (Jeannerod 1990)
- Muscles are activated synchronously but because of different inertial latencies and movement speeds, eye movement occurs first (shortest latency) and completes first (fast saccades), followed by head and then hand to the target (Jeannerod 1990)
- Vision defines the location of an object for planning motor control and monitors changes in its location, size and orientation but is not required for the final shaping of the hand to the object (Jeannerod 1986, Johansson et al 2001, Santello et al 2002); in fact, visual fixation on the object stops before the critical period for final hand shape and is redirected to subsequent landmarks required for action with the grasped object (Johansson et al 2001)
- Studies with congenitally blind participants provide additional evidence that vision is not required to establish reach to grasp coordination: blind subjects appropriately scale aperture, prolong deceleration phase where accuracy is required (precision versus power grip) and demonstrate temporal coupling similar to sighted participants (Castiello et al 1993)

Acceleration
- This fast movement takes the hand close to the vicinity of the object
- Hand aperture starts opening at the start of the transport phase (Jeannerod 1984)
- Aperture increases throughout the acceleration phase, reaching peak at the end of acceleration around 50%–60% of transport phase (Jeannerod 1984)
- The size of maximal grip opening is proportional to the size of the object (Jeannerod 1986)
- There is precise spatial positioning of the thumb with a straight path to the object, and this is established well before maximum hand aperture (Haggard & Wing 1997)

Deceleration
- Aperture decreases during the deceleration phase (Jeannerod 1984)
- Aperture size is controlled mainly by finger movement, with the thumb tending to be held stable and therefore making a smaller contribution (Cole & Abbs 1986, Wing & Fraser 1983)
- Digit tip motion follows a stereotypical trajectory for grasping different objects, and is largely unaffected by initial digit posture (Kamper 2003)
- Digit position is modulated throughout reach, is only partially formed at peak aperture and completes its shaping in the deceleration phase reaching final position only after contact with the object (Santello et al 2002, Santello & Soechting 1998)
- Visual feedback during movement does not alter final hand posture, which does not change if vision is occluded during reach (Santello et al 2002, Winges et al 2003)

Manipulation Phase

Object contact
- Tactile cues and mechanical object interaction influence final hand posture as the hand contacts the object (Santello et al 2002)

Action
- Hand orientation is according to task rather than size or shape of the object (Napier 1956)
- Grip force is closely coupled to load force with a narrow safety margin sufficient to prevent slippage; very precise control with near-constant ratio between grip and load force for different weights; surface material, shape and inclination alter the minimum grip force required (Johansson & Westling 1984, Westling & Johansson 1984)
- Fast-acting mechanoreceptors are likely to be important for scaling grip force control during object lift and manipulation (Park et al 2016)
- Guidance from visual and tactile receptors provides feed-forward information to control fingertip forces and grasp kinematics during manipulation; rotational forces are corrected for by cutaneous afferent input, but in the absence of this input, visual feedback of object movement can allow adaptation (Jenmalm et al 2000)
- In hand manipulation, this includes translation, shift and rotation. For more detailed explanation of digit patterns used for each of these actions, see the review by Elliott and Connolly (1984)

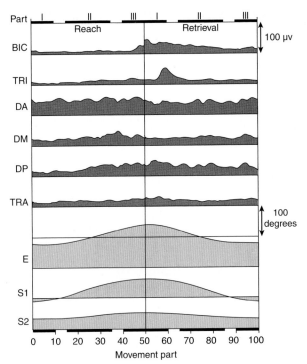

FIG. 4.7 Example muscle activation pattern (MAP) of six muscles and corresponding joint angles during reach and retrieval of an object (time in % of averaged cycle duration) of one subject, including definition of movement parts by black bars. *BIC*, Long head of biceps; *DA*, anterior deltoid; *DM*, medial deltoid; *DP*, posterior deltoid; *E*, elbow flexion/extension angle; *I*, initiation; *II*, steady state; *III*, termination of movement; *S1*, shoulder plane of elevation; *S2*, shoulder angle of elevation; *TRA*, upper trapezius; *TRI*, long head of triceps. (From Prange, G.B., Kallenberg, L.A.C., Jannink, M.J.A., et al., 2009. Influence of gravity compensation on muscle activity during reach and retrieval in healthy elderly. J. Electromyogr. Kinesiol. 19, e40–e49, with permission.)

identified that intrinsic muscle activity provides stability in the shaping of the hand and fingers whilst allowing flexor digitorum to control finger aperture (Arnet et al 2013).

Clinical Focus on Reach and Grasp for People With Stroke

In the acute stage of hemiparesis, grasp and reach are equally disrupted (Lang et al 2005). In one longitudinal study, most recovery of reach and grasp occurred in the first 90 days after stroke with very little further improvement over the course of a year. Speed and accuracy improved for proximal control (reach), but distal deficits in grasp efficiency did not recover as well (Lang et al 2006).

Longitudinal studies of recovery after stroke suggest that less than 40% of patients with significant initial arm paresis recover useful function (Heller et al 1987, Wade et al 1983). More than 60% of stroke survivors in one study reported loss of arm function as a major problem at 4-year follow-up evaluation (Broeks et al 1999), with studies on well-being after stroke indicating that arm motor impairment may have the strongest independent influence on measures of well-being (Wyller et al 1997).

Deficits vary extensively depending on the location and extent of damage after stroke. Table 4.14 identifies some common reach and grasp deficits identified in the literature.

POSTURE AND BALANCE

Posture is the outcome of the overall position of joints adopted to balance skeletal segments against gravity. It serves as a basis for movement and nonverbal communication, maintained by connective tissue and muscles under the control of the nervous system (Rosario 2017). Traditionally, posture has been thought to include the relative position of body segments during rest or activity (Twomey & Taylor 1987). Posture describes the relative position or configuration of body segments during rest or activity, whilst balance (or stability) describes the process through which posture is achieved (Latash et al., 2016).

To maintain any upright posture against gravity, external and internally generated forces acting upon the body, which can be continually changing in terms of magnitude and direction, must be opposed (i.e., balanced). Fundamentally, according to Newton's first law, every object will remain at rest or in uniform motion in a straight line unless compelled to change its state by the action of an external force. The human body could be thought of as such an object and has traditionally been viewed as an inverted pendulum during quiet standing (Smith 1957). However, the human body intrinsically contains numerous internal perturbations with the potential to affect balance (volitional movement, automated reflexes such as coughing, respiration and to a lesser degree blood flow) (Fitzpatrick & Gandevia 2005). Even 'quiet standing' is therefore not quiet but rather involves oscillating and meandering sway around a central position with ankle motor effectors (gastrocnemius and soleus) working ballistically in conjunction with structures around the ankle providing stiffness to maintain balance (Loram et al 2005a, 2005b, Winter et al 2001).

Control of balance is, at least on face value, associated with three broad activities: the maintenance of posture, such as sitting or standing; voluntary movement (the movement between postures); and the reaction to external

TABLE 4.14　Common Reach and Grasp Deficits After Stroke

Commonly Observed Problems	Evidence
Difficulty with object location and/or identification	• Homonymous hemianopia, visual neglect and visual extinction all may affect object location on the contralesional side (Jeannerod 1990) • Visual perception and/or action may also be affected if processing of information from the ventral or dorsal stream is interrupted (Goodale et al 1991)
Variable transport phase	• Prolonged transport time, longer deceleration phase, more segmented and variable movements, and larger movement errors (Cirstea & Levin 2000, Lang et al 2006, Levin 1996, van Vliet & Sheridan 2007) • Temporal characteristics of muscle activation are often impaired in stroke patients with delays in initiation and termination of activity, difficulty with interjoint coordination and higher levels of cocontraction (Beer et al 2000, Chae et al 2002a, 2002b, Dewald & Beer 2001, Dewald et al 1995, Levin 1996, Levin et al 2000, Micera et al 2005) • One paper investigating the cause of reach impairments found that impaired joint individuation explained most of the variance in reach path and endpoint error, whereas strength explained most of the variance in reaching velocity (Zackowski 2004) • Deficits in timing and spatial coordination of arm and trunk have been described for beyond arm's reach movements (Shaikh et al 2014) • In one paper investigating reach direction, no one direction was particularly problematic, but reach farthest away from the torso (independent of direction) was most affected (Kamper et al 2002); the most severely affected were more constrained demonstrating only two gross, stereotypical muscle coactivation patterns for reaching control (Reinkensmeyer et al 2002)
Compensatory use of the trunk in those moderately to severely affected	• Disrupted elbow/shoulder coordination and reduced active range of movement resulted in use of compensatory trunk movements for forwards transport and hand orientation (Cirstea & Levin 2000) • Trunk movement started early in the transport phase and contributed to the final position even for targets placed within arm's reach (Levin et al 2002) • Trunk restraint showed immediate improvement in active range of movement and interjoint coordination suggesting a problem with movement control (Michaelsen et al 2001) • Short- and long-term beneficial effects of restraint over training with verbal cues in chronic stroke have been demonstrated, but effects of treatment are variable (Greisberger et al 2016, Michaelsen & Levin 2004, Michaelsen et al 2001, 2006, Pain et al 2015, Thielman et al 2008, Woodbury et al 2008)
Aperture formation and hand orientation	• Those less affected tend to exaggerate the typical pattern (Roby-Brami et al 2003) with grip aperture size, temporal coordination between hand transport and aperture formation, and timing of grip aperture all relatively preserved (Michaelsen et al 2004) • Those more severely affected used trunk movements to help orient the hand, and adopted a completely different type of grasp approaching the object from above with their forearm pronated and wrist flexed to allow passive placement of the hand around the object with little or no active finger extension present (Roby-Brami et al 2003)

TABLE 4.14 Common Reach and Grasp Deficits After Stroke — Cont'd

Commonly Observed Problems	Evidence
Digit configuration for grasp	• Increased variability (Lang et al 2006, van Vliet & Sheridan 2007) • Limited ability to volitionally extend fingers and thumb is an important factor in deficits in hand shaping (Lang et al 2009) • Motor cortex lesion leads to fingers remaining fully extended until after object contact (i.e., no modulation of grasp before contact) (Jeannerod 1986) • Sensory input or processing (posterior parietal) lesions demonstrated absent grasp formation if visual input was removed, suggesting vision can be used to compensate for sensorimotor processing problems (Jeannerod 1986)
Somatosensory disturbance	• Reduced afferent input with concurrent loss of visual feedback caused increased duration of aperture opening with increased maximum aperture, increased path variability and increased duration of task overall, and finger closure was poorly modified (Gentilucci et al 1997) • Preserved temporal grip force/load force relationship for cyclical movement (feed-forward mechanism); however, impaired sensation and/or cortical sensory processing led to excessive grip force for all types of manipulations (Hermsdörfer et al 2003) • Poor grip force control leads to crushing of fragile objects or instability of grip (slip or drop which may be caused by reduced somatosensory feedback or processing, or lack of strength secondary to reduced descending motor signals and insufficient motor unit firing)
Manipulation	• Finger force magnitude and direction demonstrated large deviation from normal in stroke survivors with severe hand impairment regardless of pinch grip size or force and object stability. Altered grip force direction was associated with altered hand muscle activation patterns (Seo et al 2010) • Poor individuation of fingers may contribute to difficulty with hand manipulation (Raghavan 2005)
Other	• Time taken to relax the finger flexor muscle activity to release grasp may be prolonged in some people after stroke (Seo & Kamper 2008, Seo et al 2009)

perturbing forces, for example, disturbances, such as trips, slips or a push (Pollock et al 2000). No evidence exists to suggest that balance control discriminates between these activities, and it is likely that sensorimotor control of balance and posture is governed by common central nervous system processes. Clinical definitions of balance typically refer to standing balance or balance in sitting, and it is important to appreciate that posture and balance are interdependent. Collectively, posture and balance can be termed 'stability', 'postural control', 'postural sway', 'postural behaviour' or 'postural equilibrium' (Horak 2006, Rosario 2017).

Sensorimotor Control of Balance

Balance is 'no longer considered a summation of static reflexes but rather a complex interaction of dynamic sensorimotor processes' (Horak 2006, p. 1). To control balance, multisensory information is used online or as feedback of postural and positional changes (Day et al 2002). Vision is an important contribution to balance control, but optical flow arising from self-motion needs to be differentiated from external object motion (Guerraz et al 2001, Lee & Lishman 1975) before optical flow can be relied upon as feedback of postural change.

Vestibular, visual and proprioceptive systems provide information regarding the body's position and motion in external space (Day et al 2002). For balance control to be successful, the availability, correct processing and integration of sensory information is essential, and motor execution as a response to the sensory information must be spatially and temporally accurate (i.e., correctly planned in terms of direction, magnitude and timing). The essential sensory and motor control components of balance are highlighted in the following subsections.

Essential Sensory Components

Vestibular System. Vestibular apparatus (otoliths and semicircular canals) provides head-referenced signals of the head's orientation and motion in space. Translation is detected by the utricle and saccule (otolith) signals, and rotation is detected by anterior, posterior and horizontal canal (semicircular canal) signals, all based on acceleration signals (Day & Fitzpatrick 2005).

Proprioceptive System. Proprioceptive end organ afferents from muscles, tendons, joints and skin signal stretch of muscle and connective tissues, and changes in pressure of body parts in contact with the support surface. This in turn signals range-of-motion changes and overall threats to equilibrium. Muscle spindles and Golgi tendon organs appear to have major contributions to this role where increased firing rates correspond with muscle and soft tissue stretch, and in some cases also rate of change of stretch. To construct these signals relative to whole body control, knowledge of how static or moving body parts (or segments) connect and interact is necessary, along with knowledge of the support surface as the close of the kinetic chain (Lackner 1988, Lackner & DiZio 2005). The relation of body parts can be referred to as the 'body schema' or 'dynamic posture'. The human cerebellum is theorised to be responsible for the synthesis of the body schema via sensory integration of somatosensory afferents (Apps & Garwicz 2005).

Dense distributions of mechanoreceptors in the cutaneous tissue of the foot detecting pressure and vibration are able to detect external perturbations (such as a tilt in the underfoot support surface) or changes in static underfoot surfaces during locomotion (e.g., walking on uneven ground). The third and perhaps most significant role of underfoot mechanoreceptors is to detect pressure changes during quiet stance, indicating centre of pressure (CoP) motion where this is the resultant point (vector) of GRFs resisting the gravitational load that the human body effects on the support surface (Kavounoudias et al 1999, 2001). The CoP is widely used in balance research and is further described later in this chapter.

Vision. The visual system translates light patterns intercepted by the retina into a three-dimensional (3D) world (Wurtz & Kandel 2000a). The primary visual cortex receives output signals from retinal flow to deduce object-related pattern, colour and texture (ventral stream) and spatially, object localisation and motion (Wurtz & Kandel 2000a).

However, vision is fundamentally egocentric, and for optic flow to be meaningful for balance control this needs to be whole body referenced. Self-motion–generated optic flow and output modulated by vestibular (head-referenced) input evident in the primary visual cortex suggest visual–vestibular integration could play a role in control of whole body motion (Fetsch et al 2010, Wurtz & Kandel 2000b).

Oculomotor. The eyes are moved in the socket to enable capture of the target image on the area of sharpest resolution, the fovea (Wurtz & Kandel 2000a). This is achieved by extraocular muscles contracting isometrically to fixate an object, smoothly to pursue (smooth pursuit) or sharply to jerk the eye towards a new fixation point (saccade) (Gaymard & Pierrot-Deseilligny 1999). It is theorised that an efference copy of eye movements or reafferent signals from extraocular muscles could contribute to balance control, via integration with vestibular and proprioceptive signals at the level of the superior colliculus and cerebellum (Glasauer et al 2005, Guerraz & Bronstein 2008). This is effectively like the concept of vision guiding balance, set out earlier, in that head motion needs to be integrated with other sensory signals to represent whole body motion. Some evidence suggests that suppression of abnormal eye movements may improve balance in pathologies involving nystagmus (Jahn et al 2002). Additionally, extraocular feedback can be assumed to reflect self-motion from body sway only if the whole visual field moves, and thus some form of object versus self-motion recognition system needs to be in place.

Sensory Integration and Weighting. Balance requires visual, vestibular and proprioceptive sensory afferent signals to guide motor control. Effective integration and weighting of these signals is required to best plan a motor response. Adjustment of motor patterns, sequencing and gain of motor output (e.g., magnitude of contraction) of each motor contributor is required to provide appropriately sequenced, scaled, directed and timed responses. Sensory integration describes the combining of initial afferent signals to sequence efferent motor commands (Assländer & Peterka 2016, Nashner & Berthoz 1978). Sensory weighting describes the extent to which each sensory system is relied upon to direct a motor response. Quiet stance typically weights proprioceptive and visual contributions over that of vestibular, but the absolute weighting remains reliant on the nature of the balance task and sensory afferents available.

Essential Motor Components of Balance

Quiet Stance. In quiet stance, the principal motor effectors are bilateral triceps surae (gastrocnemius and soleus) at the ankle and gluteus medius at the hip. The degree of instability in standing and the motor control sequencing depend on factors such as foot splay and stance width (Day et al 1993). As stance width and foot splay increases, so too does the mechanical stability of bipedal stance, and lateral sway as a measure of instability and contraction of hip abductors reduce.

Overall levels of instability can affect anteroposterior (AP) instability, but widening of stance does not directly mechanically improve stability. Control of AP stability takes place predominantly around the ankle with the triceps surae muscles contracting in a ballistic fashion to slow acceleration of forwards leans (anterior sway) about the ankle joint (and thus prevent falling). Motor control of backwards leans (posterior sway) is mechanically possible by concentric contraction of the tibialis anterior. However, maintenance of the CoM anterior of the ankle joint reduces the need for such motor control. The collective term for this strategy with ballistic activity of triceps surae muscles is the 'ballistic bias theory' (Loram et al 2005a).

Anticipatory Postural Adjustments. Anticipatory postural adjustments take place during predictive control of balance. These involve predictive contraction of muscles either isometrically or concentrically to resist whole body movement secondary to either an external or internally generated perturbation. This was first described by Woollacott and colleagues (1984) when exploring balance responses after push-pull perturbations to the arm (one example of an external perturbation).

Postural Adjustments. Should acceleration of body sway exceed the capacity of typical motor control strategies for quiet stance, secondary strategies are used. Deceleration of backwards sway, for example, can be achieved by contracting ankle dorsiflexors, but if weakened, this is biomechanically achieved by bending the torso forwards at the hips or outstretching arms anteriorly. If the CoM moves towards the limits of stability and further exceeds the capacity of typical motor control strategies for quiet stance, this then precipitates a step to prevent falling (Zettel et al 2002). The 'protective stepping mechanism' has been investigated in people across the life span, and dysfunction of this mechanism has been proposed as a risk factor for falling (Mille et al 2005).

Adaptation. The theory of adaptation typically refers to change in motor responses after repetitive exposure to a task. Adaptation of gait has been explored after systematic changes to spatiotemporal treadmill parameters, showing the ability for those without balance dysfunction to 'adapt' rapidly to changing parameters and 'de-adapt' when the parameters are reset (Choi & Bastian 2007).

Adaptation of sway balance responses to moving visual scenery is well established after repeated stimuli. This artificial moving visual scenery is 'at odds' with unperturbed and unaffected vestibular and proprioceptive channel afferents. The sequential reduction in response to artificial stimuli that perturb balance is better known as habituation.

Sway balance responses to platform perturbations (artificial but more comparable with stepping onto a moving platform, e.g., escalator) also show adaptation in healthy persons (Horak & Nashner 1986).

Motor behaviour and adaptation are influenced by perception of the task. An example of this is the 'broken escalator phenomenon', where people initially overstep onto a stationary escalator but quickly adapt to accurately scale the motor task with practice (Reynolds & Bronstein 2003).

Compensation. If primary ballistic bias activity is ineffective in the control of balance, compensatory strategies may be adopted such as widening of stance, forwards leaning, arm and head movement strategies and use of external stabilisers, such as light touch, furniture or conventional balance aids (Clapp & Wing 1999, Dickstein et al 2003). These compensatory balance strategies inherently promote postural changes, and therefore care is needed to advocate appropriate strategies to people with long-term balance dysfunction. Walking poles, for example, may be a better option for those who require a stability aid but not weight bearing because biomechanically they promote a more upright posture compared with conventional walking stick handles.

Movement Analysis Strategies to Quantify Posture

Ideal posture has been described as symmetrical and having no deviations, using plumb lines as an aid for inspection of posture (Kendall et al 2010). A standardised one-size-fits-all posture is notional given the many factors that exist affecting 'normal' posture at any given time. However, Table 4.15 sets out measurement recommendations as a benchmark for practice. Efficiency of posture has long been accepted as involving minimal stress on joints and minimal muscle energy whilst maintaining balance (Kappler 1982). However, increased muscle activity is difficult to determine clinically and without the use of electromyography; joint stress is similarly difficult to quantify before injury occurs. Assessment of posture therefore still relies on observation, with two-dimensional or 3D technologies supplementing the clinical examination where feasible.

Average joint positions defined by anatomical surface marking over specified timeframes using 3D motion analysis techniques (some with offline human modelling using virtual joints relative to fixed segmental markers) are generally accepted as gold standard measures of quantifying posture. Clinically feasible methods aim to optimise standardisation of procedure using video analysis, photography or goniometry measurement. Traditional 'matching' of typical patterns of posture to described postural syndromes (with observation) is also used.

Similar techniques have been used to define sitting posture. Gold standard methods of 3D analysis and video analysis (static and dynamic) have been found to correlate

TABLE 4.15	'Ideal Posture': Anatomical Surface Marking as a Postural Benchmark	
Frontal Plane View Plumb-Line Bisection (Kuchera 1995)	**Sagittal Plane View Plumb-Line Alignment (Kendall et al 2010)**
Glabella frenulum	Slightly posterior to the apex of the coronal suture
Episternal notch	External auditory canal
Xiphoid process	Bodies of most cervical vertebrae
Symphysis pubis	Shoulder joint
Point midway between the medial malleoli of the ankle joints	Lumbar vertebral bodies
Symmetry of head, neck, trunk, pelvis and limbs is expected around this line	Slightly posterior to the axis of the hip joint
Standardisation of anatomical landmarks for the purpose of quantifying posture is set out by Cappozzo et al (1995)	Slightly anterior to the axis of the knee joint
	Slightly anterior to the lateral malleolus
	With notably some lordosis in the cervical, kyphosis in the thoracic and lordosis in the lumbar spines (Troyanovich et al 1998)

with subjective measures of sitting posture, validated for use with children with cerebral palsy (Sanchez et al 2017). Sanchez et al (2017) suggest that video footage methods may provide a clinically feasible option of objective quantification of posture. Recently smartphone approaches to postural assessment have begun to be developed (Moreira et al 2020), and innovative methods to identify workers at risk for musculoskeletal injuries using software for 3D postural analysis combined with Microsoft Kinect hardware or mobile phone video footage have been explored (Ho et al 2016, Lin et al 2022), which could in future be applied to neurological populations.

Factors that affect posture assessment include environmental conditions (e.g., where someone is directed to look), conscious control (e.g., consciously adopting an 'open' or 'closed' posture) and mood. Increased amplitudes of hip, shoulder, elbow, pelvis and trunk flexion are associated with anger and joy, whereas neck and thoracic flexion are associated with sadness (Gross et al 2012). Gender can also affect posture, namely women tend to possess more genu valgus at the hip, resulting in associated pes planus (owing to a typically wider pelvis), and they possess greater lumbar lordosis and increased trunk extension (Chung et al 2010).

Regardless of the method of postural assessment used, key factors to consider are standardisation of procedure and environment between testing sessions. If fatigue, mood or behaviour relative to medication is known to fluctuate within a day, then a standardised time relative to daily activity or medication is recommended.

Movement Analysis Strategies to Quantify Balance

Body sway is a popular choice of measurement when attempting to quantify balance (Raymakers et al 2005, Winter et al 1996). Gold standard 3D motion analysis has traditionally involved specialist equipment: designated computer hubs connected to multiple cameras or force plates with requirements for space, meaning that this approach has not always been a feasible option for clinicians. Data are typically sampled using these systems at a rate of approximately 200 Hz, meaning that even for simple measures of standing balance, there is a requirement to manage vast datasets and process these data before calculating average measures of body sway. Once again, the technical skills required for these tasks limit feasibility of use in a clinical setting. Body sway measures are derived from velocity or acceleration of markers (sited on top of anatomical landmarks) or GRFs of underfoot contact with force plates. These are continuous quantitative measures with the potential to be sensitive to balance performance (small changes in amplitude and direction), whilst potentially sensitive measures of balance 3D motion analysis methods have been criticised as lacking specificity (Błaszczyk 2016). This can be because of either poor standardisation of procedure or electrical noise between digital systems, and risks reliability of results and poor comparability between different laboratories (Błaszczyk 2016).

Kinematic recording of body sway from trunk markers in 3D space may most accurately reflect body sway but could be altered depending on whether an inverted pendulum model of quiet standing is under consideration or whether an 'ankle and hip strategy' is in use (Winter et al 1996).

Kinematic force plate measurement also is limited in a similar respect. GRFs are monitored across a force plate to derive vector measurements of CoP or combined with anthropometrics to calculate a measure of CoM. Whilst the CoP or CoM can reflect the meandering nature of body sway, this measure can also reflect a measure of motor control at the ankle, namely reflecting ankle torques.

Wearable inertial sensors or devices containing accelerometers and gyroscopes and, most recently, mobile phone and watches have offered an alternative to specialist motion laboratory approaches and offer potentially improved feasibility of use for clinicians (Abou et al 2021a, 2021b, 2021c, Cheng et al 2021, Del Din et al 2016, Mancini & Horak 2010, Midaglia et al 2019, Peters et al 2022, Rashid et al 2022). Abou and colleagues' (2021a) systematic review of smartphone applications for balance and gait assessment covered 31 published studies for assessment of Parkinson's alone. These tend to involve accompanying software packages, with algorithms for analysis, for easier interpretation by clinicians and patients alike. They typically offer measures of angular rate of change of position over time (angular velocities) and accelerations, which are reported as body sway speeds or simply 'measures of balance'. Most report measures of gait alongside balance assessment and some measures of U-turn test ability, all examples of functional balance (Abou et al 2021a, 2021b, 2021c, Cheng et al 2021, Midaglia et al 2019, Peters et al 2022). Similar to the marker placement methods, they could remain susceptible to digital noise and are dependent on standardisation of measurement procedures but have begun to be validated for use with healthy older adults and people with Parkinson's, multiple sclerosis (MS) and stroke (Abou et al 2021a, 2021b, 2021c, Del Din et al 2016, Midaglia et al 2019, Peters et al 2022). Until rigorous validation and feasibility testing of these algorithm-based options are well-established for use with people with neurological conditions, it is important to use these options alongside traditional feasible and validated assessment measures.

Clinically validated analyses of balance are feasible in clinical settings. At an impairment level, a swaymeter provides a feasible and valid alternative to motion analysis (Fig. 4.8). These have been designed to: (a) identify whether a balance problem exists, and (b) determine the underlying cause of the balance problem (Mancini & Horak 2010). Mancini and Horak (2010) review clinical measures according to whether they are assessments of function, sensory systems or objective. Table 4.16 outlines and expands upon these clinical balance assessment tools.

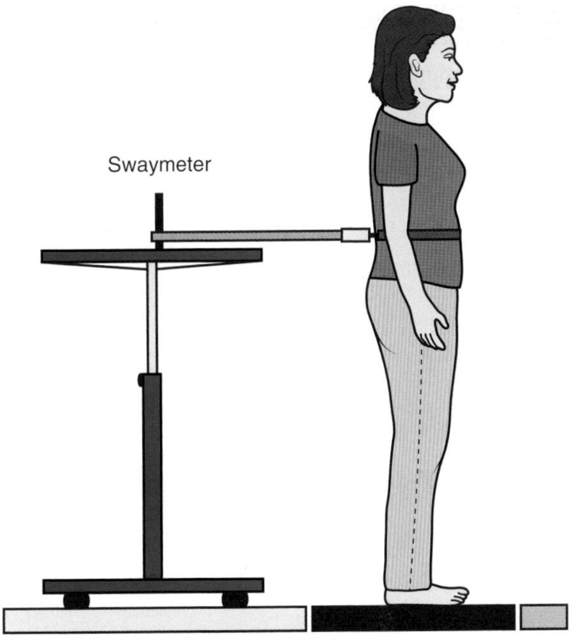

FIG. 4.8 The physiological profile approach's swaymeter: a low-cost, clinically feasible method of recording standing body sway. (From Sturnieks et al., 2011. Validity and reliability of the Swaymeter device for measuring postural sway. BMC Geriatrics. 11, 63.)

Clinical Foci of Posture and Balance

Problems with posture and balance feature in common neurological disorders that affect the cerebellum, diencephalon and cerebral cortices. To provide a simplified and potentially generalisable comparison, posture and balance in models of relatively pure cerebellar ataxia will be explored and compared against Parkinson's and hemiplegic stroke (an overview is provided in Table 4.17).

Ataxia can be caused by either an inherited condition or a cerebellar lesion (such as a cerebellar stroke or multiple sclerosis pathology). In both inherited and acquired types of ataxia, instability is a dominant feature (inherited: Bunn et al 2013, Mauritz et al 1979; multiple sclerosis: Daley & Swank 1983, Nelson et al 1995). For inherited types, instability is typically a presenting feature (Schmitz-Hübsch et al 2008). Instability in ataxia is randomly directed (Bunn et al 2013), and falls tend to be unpredictable (Fonteyn et al 2013). Unlike those with Parkinson's or hemiplegic stroke, people with ataxia tend to demonstrate standing balance with increased entropy; that is, they have a more irregular CoP motion over time, reflecting an upscaling of automatic postural corrections (Bunn et al 2013). Intensive balance exercise with an emphasis on sensorimotor balance

TABLE 4.16   **Balance Assessment Tools**

Classification	Assessment Tools	References	Brief Description
Functional	Activities of Balance Confidence questionnaire	Myers et al 1998	A questionnaire evaluating self-perceived balance confidence while attempting 16 different activities of daily living
	Tinetti Balance and Gait Test	Tinetti 1986	A traditional rating scale involving both balance and gait tasks
	Functional (Berg) Balance Scale	Berg et al 1992	A traditional rating scale involving a range of functional balance activities
	Timed Up and Go Test (TUG)	Mathias et al 1986	A stopwatch-timed standardised stand from a chair, walk, return and sit
	One-leg stance	Fregly & Graybiel 1968	Stopwatch-timed eyes open single-leg stance
	Functional reach test	Duncan et al 1990	A measured forwards reach (as far forwards as possible while standing independently); reaching in the lateral and backwards directions has also been added
	Brunel Balance Assessment	Tyson & DeSouza 2004a	Rating of 12 functional balance activities in a hierarchy of difficulty (valid and reliable for use after stroke; Tyson & DeSouza 2004b)
	Balance subcategories of the scale for assessment and rating of ataxia (Bal-SARA)	Bunn et al 2013, Schmitz-Hübsch et al 2006	This rates balance during sitting, standing and walking against an ordinal scale
Systems	Balance Evaluation Systems Test (BESTest)	Horak et al 2009	Evaluation of six different balance control systems
	Physiological profile approach (PPA)	Lord & Clark 1996	A series of simple tests of vision, cutaneous sensation on the feet, leg muscle force, reaction time and postural sway in stance (see Fig. 4.1); a short or long version is available
Objective	Goniometry or distance measurements: universal goniometer, electrogoniometer and inclinometer	See Fortin et al (2011) for a review	Traditional methods of measuring joints or intersegmental angles or distance of an anatomical landmark relative to another/support surface
Nonclinical options used/in development	Static posturography	Fortin et al (2011) Example: Bunn et al (2013)	Assessment is of balance in a static position such as sitting or standing. This can be achieved using photography, X-ray or with 3D motion analysis systems
	Dynamic posturography	Fortin et al (2011) Example: Cowie et al (2012)	Assessment of balance with gait or other forms of movement (dynamic). This can be achieved using video footage or with 3D motion analysis systems

TABLE 4.16	Balance Assessment Tools—Cont'd		
Classification	**Assessment Tools**	**References**	**Brief Description**
	Wearable inertial sensors, inclusive of accelerometry embedded within smartphones and watches	Godfrey et al 2015, Hansson et al 2001 Examples: Abou et al 2021a,b,c, Bunn et al 2015,Rashid et al 2022 (Parkinson's, stroke, MS); Peters et al 2022 (stroke); Midaglia et al 2019 (MS)	Assessment of static balance with the use of a wearable accelerometer/ gyroscope. Further refinement of gait algorithms is needed to improve reliability with dynamic balance/gait assessment
	Virtual reality optical cameras	Clark et al 2015 Example: Galna et al 2014	Optical motion sensors that can measure 3D motion of a person, e.g., Microsoft Kinect
	Stereophotogrammetry	Example: described by Cappozzo et al 2005	Assessment of balance (static or dynamic). 3D reconstruction of bodies using optoelectric sensors, force plate integration, electromyography integration and indirect calorimetry. Anthropometric quantities also measured with tape measure/ callipers/3D scanners

training has been proposed to improve stability in people with inherited types of ataxia, suggesting an underlying sensorimotor target responsible for the presentation (Bunn et al 2015, Ilg et al 2009).

Instability within Parkinson's, however, develops gradually as the disease progresses and is rarely a cardinal presenting feature (Muller et al 2000). A 'stooped simian' appearance in later stages of Parkinson's is typically described: flexion of the hips and knees and rounding of the shoulders (Doherty et al 2011). This posture appears associated with rigidity and akinesia (Kashihara et al 2006). Mechanisms underpinning balance dysfunction and postural abnormalities could be associated with dystonia, rigidity and proprioceptive disintegration and through secondary peripheral changes, namely myopathy and skeletal and soft tissue changes (Doherty et al 2011). Balance exercises combining lower limb muscle training with visual and vestibular integration exercises have been proposed to improve stability compared with balance exercises alone for people with Parkinson's, suggesting an underlying sensorimotor target responsible for the presentation (Keus et al 2007). In addition to rehabilitation, the use of braces and weighting (e.g., use of a backpack) has been suggested to mechanically compensate for forwards leaning, but caution is advocated given that sudden or uncompensated change to sagittal balance could increase the risk for falling backwards (Bloem et al 1999).

Balance problems after hemiplegic stroke, unlike ataxia and Parkinson's, are potentially caused by impairments in either interpretation of sensory afferents or synthesis of motor efferents, but also by primary impairments of cognitive processing or perception of verticality (De Oliveira et al 2008). Alternatively, secondary complications can lead to altered movement strategies and biomechanical constraints (De Oliveira et al 2008). Motor control for posture and balance can, for example, be affected secondary to weakness or spasticity affecting balance-related muscle groups (e.g., triceps surae for standing balance). Rehabilitation packages combining balance exercise with muscle strengthening and spasticity management can be effective in relearning of movement and improvement of functional balance (de Haart et al 2004, Geiger et al 2001). The different profile in the presentation of balance problems after hemiplegic stroke is outlined in Table 4.17. This provides context for a focus on functional strength training in stroke rehabilitation (such as the training of weight-bearing symmetry or taking compensatory steps to preserve stability) compared with more of a sensorimotor focus for ataxia or Parkinson's balance training programmes (Kollen et al 2009, Pollock et al 2007).

TABLE 4.17 Commonly Observed Balance-Related Features of Ataxia, Parkinson's and Hemiplegic Stroke

Ataxia	Parkinson's	Hemiplegic Stroke
Symmetry		
• Preferred widened stance (van de Warrenburg et al 2005) • No axial asymmetry of posture in frontal or sagittal planes (Bunn et al 2013)	• Postural asymmetry noted (Beretta et al 2015, Geurts et al 2011) with a mean CoP backwards (less severe Parkinson's) or forwards (severe Parkinson's) of the 'typical' position (Schieppati & Nardone 1991); a potentially compensatory forwards lean (Benatrua et al 2008, Mikami et al 2017) • A forwards head position with chin 'poke' extension of the upper cervical spine. In some (5%–6%) a 'dropped head position' (antecollis) is reported. This relates to dystonia of flexor neck muscles or weakness of extensor neck muscles (Doherty et al 2011, Fujimoto 2006, Kashihara et al 2006) • Protracted shoulder girdles and abducted arms (Carpenter et al 2004, Doherty et al 2011) • Flexed hips and knees (Doherty et al 2011) • Scoliosis (a deformity of the spine) is thought to affect 16%–91% of people with Parkinson's. This involves a lateral curve of the spine with a rotation of the vertebrae. A lateral tilt to the side in either sitting or upright stance can also affect people with Parkinson's. When exceeding 15° (thought to affect just 2%), this is classified as Pisa syndrome (Bonanni et al 2007, Doherty et al 2011, Khallaf & Fayed 2015, Tabamo et al 2000)	• Postural changes with reduced efficiency of posture, asymmetry (Peurala et al 2007) and forwards lean in standing (Marigold et al 2004). Sitting posture notably incorporates exaggerated lumbar lordosis, thoracic kyphosis and a forwards head position (Iyengara et al 2014) • Asymmetry typically involves a deviation in mean CoP of up to 40%, generally in the direction of the unaffected side (de Haart et al 2004, Mansfield et al 2013, Piereira et al 2010)
Motion		
• Increased multidirectional instability (Mauritz et al 1979, van de Warrenburg et al 2005), disease severity related (Bunn et al 2013) but notably larger than that of Parkinson's and stroke comparative groups (Catteneo et al 2016) • Postural tremor (Bunn et al 2013, Mauritz et al 1979, van de Warrenburg et al 2005) • Upscaling of automatic postural corrections (an increase in CoP irregularity) observed in normal quiet standing (Bunn et al 2013)	• General standing instability but predominantly in the sagittal plane (Catteneo et al 2016, Frenklach et al 2009) • Postural tremor (Catteneo et al 2016) • Down-scaling of automatic postural corrections (an increase in CoP regularity) observed in normal quiet standing (Catteneo et al 2016) • Reduced axial intersegmental movements are noted with accompanying high axial tone (Wright et al 2007). Stiffness of postural muscles (Cattano et al 2016, Schieppati & Nardone 1991) along with reduced arm swing (Carpenter et al 2004, Doherty et al 2011) potentially affecting body sway	• General standing instability but predominantly in the frontal plane (between 1.5 and 5 times increase). The severity of spasticity is associated with increased instability in the frontal plane (de Haart et al 2004, Khiabani et al 2017) • Reduced ballistic motor control at the ankle is reported and ascribed to weakness and increased tone (de Niet et al 2013, Marigold et al 2004)

TABLE 4.17 Commonly Observed Balance-Related Features of Ataxia, Parkinson's and Hemiplegic Stroke—Cont'd

Ataxia	Parkinson's	Hemiplegic Stroke
Motion		
• Multijoint movement throughout the body for postural control and balance in standing is largely preserved (Bunn et al 2013, Horak & Diener 1994) with the exception of increased ankle excursion (Bunn et al 2013)	• For less severe stages of Parkinson's, reduced ballistic activity of the ankle in anteroposterior direction (pitch) but increased in mediolateral (roll) is observed, but for more severe stages increased body sway is multidirectional (Błaszczyk & Orawiec 2011, Fernandes et al 2015a,b, Mitchell et al 1995). Proprioceptive loss is thought to additionally affect postural stability, namely axial motor control in a transverse plane (Carpenter & Bloem 2011)	• Even in quiet standing there is an increased dependency on visual cues for posture and balance (Weerdesteyn et al 2008). Control of balance can be further challenged by the loss of visual vertical (Bonan et al 2007)
Perturbed Standing Conditions		
• Dysregulation of trunk alignment in standing following a slow underfoot balance perturbation (Paquette et al 2016) • Responses to balance perturbations are increased in magnitude and last longer to result in an overshoot of the preperturbation standing posture (Bunn et al 2015, Horak & Diener 1994) • Increased magnitudes of motor response follow both predictable and unpredictable balance perturbations (Bunn et al 2013, Timmann & Horak 1998)	• Instability may increase with cognitive load (dual tasking) under eyes open conditions (Fernandes et al 2015a,b, Holmes et al 2010) • Abnormal anticipatory postural adjustments and loss of protective stepping mechanism (Bloem et al 1999, Latash et al 1995) • Protective mechanisms of standing balance (e.g., leaning, stepping, reaching, etc. to prevent a fall) are slower, of reduced magnitude and more variable in direction (Carpenter et al 2004, Dimitrova et al 2004, Horak et al 2005)	• Proprioceptive dysfunction affecting control of balance via sensory weighting of impaired visuoproprioceptive and vestibuloproprioceptive mechanisms can affect quiet standing and control of balance following balance perturbations (Marigold & Eng 2006, Marigold et al 2004, Tyson et al 2006). Visual neglect, although a common impairment after stroke, does not appear to be directly associated with balance impairment (Tyson et al 2006) • Lower limb motor responses as protective mechanisms of standing balance are slower, of reduced magnitude and more variable in direction (Mansfield et al 2011, Roerdink et al 2009, van Asseldonk et al 2006)
• Loss of accuracy of protective stepping mechanism (Timmann & Horak 1998) • Increased hip and knee compensatory strategy with reciprocal activation of tibialis anterior and quadriceps with triceps surae and hamstring muscle groups (Horak & Diener 1994) • Notably increased magnitudes of motor responses to visual perturbations, with associations observed between response magnitudes and overall disease severity (Bunn et al 2015)		• This could be arising from weakness, increased tone (de Niet et al 2013, Marigold et al 2004) or reduced lower limb muscle synchronisation for balance control (Mansfield et al 2011) • Loss of anticipatory postural adjustments and protective stepping mechanisms are reported (Mansfield et al 2013), and in some with frontal lobe lesions this is further exacerbated by loss of cognitive balance control strategies (Peurala et al 2007)

Regardless of clinical condition, movement analysis of posture and balance is fundamentally affected by multiple factors such as validity and reliability of tools and procedures, individual anthropometrics, visual environmental conditions and underfoot conditions, including footwear (Chiari et al 1911). Within a clinical setting, feasibility will most commonly dictate the movement analysis method selected, but regardless of the approach, we advise remaining mindful of standardisation of assessment where possible. Fatigue is known to affect all conditions within this focus (ataxia: Brusse et al 2011; Parkinson's: de Groot et al 2003; and stroke: de Groot et al 2003, Duncan et al 2014), and medications could additionally interact with movement analysis outcomes, requiring consistency of assessment time. Foot splay positions and stance width positions need controlling where possible and distraction during assessment minimised (Kirby et al 1987, McIlroy & Maki 1997).

KEY MESSAGES

Movement analysis forms a fundamental component of the assessment process because it helps physiotherapists to understand some of the factors that contribute to the problems people may face in undertaking valued everyday activities and in participating in social roles. Without an adequate assessment of these key components of everyday movement repertoires, hypotheses derived from movement analyses may be incomplete and, when used to inform interventions, may contribute to ineffective practice.

Each section of this chapter has provided an overview of the main factors that should be considered when undertaking an observational assessment using a movement analysis approach. The impact of neurological pathologies on movement, balance and posture has also been briefly outlined and will be further discussed in other chapters of this book. The patient's voice is on the whole absent from this chapter, but patients' experiences of their movement, their views about how and why they move in a particular way, and what they find difficult in their social, psychological and cultural world also form a crucial guide to the assessment process. Only by combining all assessment components will physiotherapists be able to understand how they might make a positive contribution to their patients' lives.

SELF-ASSESSMENT QUESTIONS

Walking

1. What are the three essential components of walking?
2. What are the eight phases of the gait cycle?
3. Although gait analysis usually involves observation of walking in a straight line, why should your assessment also include observation of changes in direction?
4. What is the average speed (in m/s) during self-paced walking for (a) healthy men aged 60–69 years and (b) healthy women aged 60–69 years?

Sit to Stand

1. On average how often do healthy adults undertake STS in a normal day?
2. According to Schenkman et al (1990), what are the four phases of STS?
3. What is the optimal angle of ankle dorsiflexion for the execution of STS?
4. What 12 contextual factors may influence the performance of STS?

Rolling and Getting Out of Bed

1. What is the average movement time for getting out of bed for healthy individuals older than 65 years?
2. Unlike gait and STS, a 'typical' way of getting out of bed has not been identified. This being the case, what should be observed and measured during an observational assessment of getting out of bed?
3. Rolling and getting out of bed is particularly difficult for people with Parkinson's. State five specific difficulties that people with Parkinson's may have with bed mobility.

Reach and Grasp

1. What are the four key phases of reach and grasp?
2. What factors might influence hand shape and orientation? (b) Which factor is thought to override all others?
3. When does aperture formation (a) begin, and (b) when does it reach its maximum?
4. What is the role of vision in reach and grasp?

Posture and Balance

1. What is the difference between posture and balance?
2. What are the main sensory contributions to balance control?
3. What are the principal motor effectors in quiet stance, and what is the name of the theory of motor behaviour exhibited?
4. State three key differences between features of posture and balance for a patient with ataxia compared with a healthy person of a similar age.

REFERENCES

Abou, L., Peters, J., Wong, E., et al., 2021a. Gait and balance assessments using smartphone applications in Parkinson's disease: a systematic review. J. Med. Syst. 45, 87.

Abou, L., Peters, J., Wong, E., et al., 2021b. Smartphone applications to assess gait and balance among stroke survivors. Arch. Phys. Med. Rehabil. 102, e116.

Abou, L., Peters, J., Wong, E., et al., 2021c. Smartphone applications to assess gait and postural control in people with multiple sclerosis: a systematic review. Mult. Scler. Relat. Disord. 51, 102943.

Alexander, N.B., Fry-Welch, D.K., Marshall, L.M., et al., 1995. Healthy young and old women differ in their trunk elevation and hip pivot motions when rising from supine to sitting. J. Am. Geriatr. Soc. 43, 338–343.

Allen, N.E., Canning, C.G., Sherrington, C., Fung, V.S.C., 2009. Bradykinesia, muscle weakness and reduced muscle power in Parkinson's disease. Mov. Disord. 24, 1344–1351.

Apps, R., Garwicz, M., 2005. Anatomical and physiological foundations of cerebellar information processing. Nat. Rev. Neurosci. 6, 297–311.

Arcelus, A., Herry, C.L., Goubran, R.A., et al., 2009. Determinants of sit-to-stand transfer duration using bed and floor pressure sequences. IEEE. Transact. Biomed. Eng. 56, 2485–2492.

Arnet, U., Muzykewicz, D.A., Fridén, J., Lieber, R.L., 2013. Intrinsic hand muscle function, part 1: creating a functional grasp. J. Hand. Surg. 38, 2093–2099.

Assländer, L., Peterka, R.J., 2016. Sensory reweighting dynamics following removal and addition of visual and proprioceptive cues. J. Neurophysiol. 116, 272–285.

Baillieul, S., Fatimi, El, Nadeau, A., Perennou, D., S., 2015. Is the total vertical ground reaction force time-amplitude profile an invariant during sit-to-stand movements following stroke? Ann. Phys. Rehabil. Med. 58S, e117–e122.

Baker, R., Fell, N., Richards, J., Smith, C., 2012. Gait assessment in neurological disorders. In: Levine, D., Richards, J., Whittle, M.W. (Eds.), Whittle's Gait Analysis: An Introduction, 5th ed. Elsevier, Edinburgh, Churchill Livingstone, pp. 127–149.

Balaji, E., Brindha, D., Elumalai, V.K., Umesh, K., 2021. Data-driven gait analysis for diagnosis and severity rating of Parkinson's disease. Med. Eng. Phys. 91, 54–64.

Beer, R.F., Dewald, J.P.A., Rymer, W.Z., 2000. Deficits in the coordination of multijoint arm movements in patients with hemiparesis: evidence for disturbed control of limb dynamics. Exp. Brain Res. 131, 305–319.

Benatru, I., Vaugoyeau, M., Azulay, J.P., 2008. Postural disorders in Parkinson's disease (Anomalies de la posture dans la maladie de Parkinson). Neurophysiol. Clin. 38, 459–465.

Beretta, V.S., Gobbi, L.T.B., Lirani-Silva, E., et al., 2015. Challenging postural tasks increase asymmetry in patients with Parkinson's disease. PLoS One. 10, e0137722.

Berg, K.O., Wood-Dauphinee, S.L., Williams, J.I., Maki, B., 1992. Measuring balance in the elderly: validation of an instrument. Can. J. Pub. Health. 83 (Suppl. 2), S7–S11.

Bhidayasiri, R., Mekawichai, P., Jitkritsadakul, O., et al., 2014. Nocturnal journey of body and mind in Parkinson's disease: the manifestations, risk factors and their relationship to daytime symptoms. Evidence from the NIGHT-PD study. J. Neural Transm. 121 (Suppl. 1), S59–S68.

Błaszczyk, J.W., 2016. The use of force-plate posturography in the assessment of postural instability. Gait Posture. 44, 1–6.

Błaszczyk, J.W., Orawiec, R., 2011. Assessment of postural control in patients with Parkinson's disease: sway ratio analysis. Hum. Mov. Sci. 30, 396–404.

Bloem, B.R., Beckley, D.J., van Dijk, J.G., 1999. Are automatic postural responses in patients with Parkinson's disease abnormal due to their stooped posture? Exp. Brain Res. 124, 481–488.

Bohannon, R.W., 2007. Knee extension strength and body weight determine sit-to-stand independence after stroke. Physiother. Theory. Pract. 23, 291–297.

Bohannon, R.W., Bubela, D.J., Magasi, S.R., et al., 2010. Sit-to-stand test: performance and determinants across the age-span. Isokinet. Exerc. Sci. 18, 235–240.

Bohannon, R.W., Andrews, A., Williams, 2011. Normal walking speed: a descriptive metaanalysis. Physiotherapy. 97, 182–189.

Bonan, I.V., Hubeaux, K., Gellez-Leman, M.C., et al., 2007. Influence of subjective visual vertical misperception on balance recovery after stroke. J. Neurol. Neurosurg. Psychiatry. 78, 49–55.

Bonanni, L., Thomas, A., Varanese, S., et al., 2007. Botulinum toxin treatment of lateral axial dystonia in Parkinsonism. Mov. Disord. 22, 2097–2103.

Borchers, S., Himmelbach, M., 2012. The recognition of everyday objects changes grasp scaling. Vision. Res. 67, 8–13.

Brière, A., Lauzière, S., Gravel, D., Nadeau, S., 2010. Perception of weight-bearing distribution during sit-to-stand tasks in hemiparetic and healthy individuals. Stroke. 41, 1704–1708.

Brière, A., Nadeau, S., Lauzière, S., et al., 2013. Knee efforts and weight bearing asymmetry during sit to stand tasks in individuals with hemiparesis and healthy controls. J. Electromyogr. Kinesiol. 23, 508–515.

Brochier, T., 2004. Patterns of muscle activity underlying object-specific grasp by the macaque monkey. J. Neurophysiol. 92, 1770–1782.

Broeks, J.G., Lankhorst, G.J., Rumping, K., Prevo, A.J., 1999. The long-term outcome of arm function after stroke: results of a follow-up study. Disabil. Rehabil. 21, 357–364.

Brunt, D., Greenberg, B., Sharmin Wankadia, M.H.S., Trimble, M.A., 2002. The effect of foot placement on sit to stand in healthy young subjects and patients with hemiplegia. Arch. Phys. Med. Rehabil. 83, 924–929.

Brusse, E., Brusse-Keizer, M.G.J., Duivenvoorden, H.J., van Swieten, J.C., 2011. Fatigue in spinocerebellar ataxia: patient self-assessment of an early and disabling symptom. Neurology. 76, 953–959.

Buckley, T.A., Pitsikoulis, C., Hass, C.J., 2008. Dynamic postural stability during sit-to-walk transitions in Parkinson's disease patients. Mov. Disord. 23, 1274–1280.

Bunn, L.M., Marsden, J.F., Giunti, P., Day, B.L., 2013. Stance instability in spinocerebellar ataxia type 6. Mov. Disord. 28, 510–516.

Bunn, L.M., Marsden, J.F., Voyce, D.C., et al., 2015. Sensorimotor processing for balance in spinocerebellar ataxia type 6. Mov. Disord. 30, 1259–1266.

Camargos, A.C.R., Rodrigues-de-Paula-Goulart, F., Teixeira-Salmela, L.F., 2009. The effects of foot position on the performance of the sit-to-stand movement with chronic stroke subjects. Arch. Phys. Med. Rehabil. 90, 314–319.

Cameron, D.M., Bohannon, R.W., Garrett, G.E., et al., 2003. Physical impairments related to kinetic energy during sit-to-stand and curb-climbing following stroke. Clin. Biomech. 18, 332–340.

Cappozzo, A., Catani, F., Della Croce, U., Leardini, A., 1995. Position and orientation in space of bones during movement: anatomical frame definition and determination. Clin. Biomech. 10, 171–178.

Cappozzo, A., Della Croce, U., Chiari, L., 2005. Human movement analysis using stereophotogrammetry. Part 1: theoretical background. Gait Posture. 21, 186–196.

Carpenter, M.G., Allum, J.H., Honegger, F., et al., 2004. Postural abnormalities to multidirectional stance perturbations in Parkinson's disease. J. Neurol. Neurosurg. Psychiatry. 75, 1245–1254.

Carpenter, M.G., Bloem, B.R., 2011. Postural control in Parkinson patients: a proprioceptive problem? Exp. Neurol. 227, 26–30.

Carr, J.H., Shepherd, R.B., 2010. Neurological Rehabilitation: Optimizing Motor Performance, 2nd ed. Elsevier, Edinburgh.

Castiello, U., 2005. The neuroscience of grasping. Nat. Rev. Neurosci. 6, 726–736.

Castiello, U., Bennett, K.M.B., Mucignat, C., 1993. The reach to grasp movement of blind subjects. Exp. Brain Res. 96, 152–162.

Catteneo, D., Carpinella, I., Aprile, I., et al., 2016. Comparison of upright balance in stroke, Parkinson and multiple sclerosis. Acta. Neurol. Scand. 113, 346–354.

Chae, J., Yang, G., Park, B.K., Labatia, I., 2002a. Delay in initiation and termination of muscle contraction, motor impairment, and physical disability in upper limb hemiparesis. Muscle Nerve. 25, 568–575.

Chae, J., Yang, G., Park, B.K., Labatia, I., 2002b. Muscle weakness and cocontraction in upper limb hemiparesis: relationship to motor impairment and physical disability. Neurorehabil. Neural Repair. 16, 241–248.

Cheng, P.T., Chen, C.L., Wang, C.M., Hong, W.H., 2004. Leg muscle activation patterns of sit to stand movement in stroke patients. Am. J. Phys. Med. Rehabil. 83, 10–16.

Cheng, P.T., Liaw, M.-Y., Wong, M.-K., et al., 1998. The sit-to-stand movement in stroke patients and its correlation with falling. Arch. Phys. Med. Rehabil. 79, 1043–1046.

Cheng, W., Bourke, A.K., Lipsmeier, F., et al., 2021. U-turn speed is a valid and reliable smartphone-based measure of multiple sclerosis-related gait and balance impairment. Gait Posture. 84, 120–126.

Chiari, L., Rocchi, L., Capello, A., 1911. Stabilometric parameters are affected by anthropometry and foot placement. Clin. Biomech. 17, 666–677.

Choi, J.T., Bastian, A.J., 2007. Adaptation reveals independent control networks for human walking. Nat. Neurosci. 10, 1055–1062.

Chung, C.Y., Park, M.S., Lee, S.H., et al., 2010. Kinematic aspects of trunk motion and gender effect in normal adults. J. Neuroeng. Rehabil. 7, 9.

Cirstea, M.C., Levin, M.F., 2000. Compensatory strategies for reaching in stroke. Brain. 123, 940–953.

Clapp, S., Wing, A.M., 1999. Light touch contribution to balance in normal bipedal stance. Exp. Brain Res. 125, 521–524.

Clark, R.A., Pua, Y.H., Oliveira, C.C., et al., 2015. Reliability and concurrent validity of the Microsoft Xbox One Kinect for assessment of standing balance and postural control. Gait Posture. 42, 210–213.

Cole, K.J., Abbs, J.H., 1986. Coordination of three-joint digit movements for rapid finger-thumb grasp. J. Neurophysiol. 55, 1407–1423.

Cowie, D., Limousin, P., Peters, A., et al., 2012. Doorway-provoked freezing of gait and its treatment in Parkinson's disease. Mov. Disord. 27, 492–499.

Creaby, M.W., Cole, M.H., 2018. Gait characteristics and falls in Parkinson's disease: a systematic review and meta-analysis. Parkinsonism Relat. Disord. 57, 1–8.

Crenna, P., Carpinella, I., Rabuffetti, M., et al., 2007. The association between impaired turning and normal straight walking in Parkinson's disease. Gait Posture. 26, 172–178.

Daley, M.L., Swank, R.L., 1983. Changes in postural control and vision induced by multiple sclerosis. Agressologie. 1983, 327–329.

Dall, P.M., Kerr, A., 2010. Frequency of the sit to stand task: an observational study of free-living adults. Appl. Ergon. 41, 58–61.

David, F.J., Rafferty, M.R., Robichaud, J.A., et al., 2012. Progressive resistance exercise and Parkinson's disease: a review of potential mechanisms. Parkinson. Dis. 2012, 124527.

Day, B.L., Fitzpatrick, R.C., 2005. The vestibular system (Primer). Curr. Biol. 15, R583–R586.

Day, B.L., Guerraz, M., Cole, J., 2002. Sensory interactions for human balance control revealed by galvanic vestibular stimulation. In: Gandevia, S.C. Proske, U. Stuart, D.G. (Eds.),. In: Sensorimotor Control of Movement and Posture. Advances in Experimental Medicine and Biology, vol. 508. Springer, Boston.

Day, B.L., Steiger, M.J., Thompson, P.D., Marsden, C.D., 1993. Effect of vision and stance width on human body motion when standing: implications for afferent control of lateral sway. J. Physiol. 469, 479–499.

de Groot, M.H., Phillips, S.J., Eskes, G.A., 2003. Fatigue associated with stroke and other neurologic conditions: implications for stroke rehabilitation. Arch. Phys. Med. Rehabil. 84, 1714–1720.

de Haart, M., Geurts, A.C., Huidekoper, S.C., et al., 2004. Recovery of standing balance in postacute stroke patients:

a rehabilitation chort study. Arch. Phys. Med. Rehabil. 86, 886–895.

de Niet, M., Weerdesteyn, V., de Bot, S.T., et al., 2013. Does calf muscle spasticity contribute to postural imbalance? A study in persons with pure hereditary spastic paraparesis. Gait Posture. 38, 304–309.

de Oliveira, C.B., de Medeiros, I.R.B., Ferreira Frota, N.A., et al., 2008. Balance control in hemiparetic stroke patients: main tools for evaluation. J. Rehabil. Res. Dev. 45, 1215–1226.

Dean, C., Shepherd, R., Adams, R., 1999. Sitting balance I: trunk–arm coordination and the contribution of the lower limbs during self-paced reaching in sitting. Gait Posture. 10, 135–146.

Del Din, S., Godfrey, A., Rochester, L., 2016. Validation of an accelerometer to quantify a comprehensive battery of gait characteristics in healthy older adults and Parkinson's disease: toward clinical and at home use. IEEE J. Biomed. Health. Inform. 20, 838–847.

Dewald, J., Beer, R.F., 2001. Abnormal joint torque patterns in the paretic upper limb of subjects with hemiparesis. Muscle Nerve. 24, 273–283.

Dewald, J.P., Pope, P.S., Given, J.D., et al., 1995. Abnormal muscle coactivation patterns during isometric torque generation at the elbow and shoulder in hemiparetic subjects. Brain. 118, 495–510.

di Biase, L., Di Santo, A., Caminiti, M.L., et al., 2020. Gait analysis in Parkinson's disease: an overview of the most accurate markers for diagnosis and symptoms monitoring. Sensors. 20, 3529.

Dickstein, R., Peterka, R.J., Horak, F.B., 2003. Effects of light fingertip touch on postural responses in subjects with diabetic peripheral neuropathy. J. Neurol. Neurosurg. Psychiatry. 74, 620–626.

Dimitrova, D., Horak, F.B., Nutt, J.G., 2004. Postural muscle responses to multidirectional translations in patients with Parkinson's disease. J. Neurophysiol. 91, 489–501.

Doherty, K.M., van de Warrenburg, B.P., Peralta, M.C., et al., 2011. Postural deformities in Parkinson's disease. Lancet Neurol. 10, 538–549.

Duclos, C., Nadeau, S., Lecours, J., 2008. Lateral trunk displacement and stability during sit-to-stand transfer in relation to foot placement in patients with hemiparesis. Neurorehabil. Neural Repair. 22, 715–722.

Duncan, F., Greig, C., Lewis, S., et al., 2014. Clinically significant fatigue after stroke: a longitudinal cohort study. J. Psychosom. Res. 77, 368–373.

Duncan, P.W., Weiner, D.K., Chandler, J., Studenski, S., 1990. Functional reach: a new clinical measure of balance. J. Gerontol. 45, M192–M197.

Earhart, G.M., 2013. Dynamic control of posture across locomotor tasks. Mov. Disord. 28, 1501–1508.

Elliott, J.M., Connolly, K.J., 1984. A classification of manipulative hand movements. Dev. Med. Child. Neurol. 26, 283–296.

Engardt, M., Olsson, E., 1992. Body weight-bearing while rising and sitting down in patients with stroke. Scand. J. Rehabil. Med. 24, 67–74.

Etnyre, B., Thomas, D.Q., 2007. Event standardization of sit-to-stand movements. Phys. Ther. 87, 1651–1666.

Fernandes, A., Coelho, T., Vitoria, A., et al., 2015a. Standing balance in individuals with Parkinson's disease during single and dual-task conditions. Gait Posture. 42, 323–328.

Fernandes, A., Sousa, A.S.P., Couras, J., et al., 2015b. Influence of dual-task on sit-to-stand-to-sit postural control in Parkinson's disease. Med. Eng. Phys. 37, 1070–1075.

Fetsch, C.R., DeAngelis, G.C., Angelaki, D.E., 2010. Visual-vestibular cue integration for heading perception: applications of optimal cue integration theory. Eur. J. Neurosci. 31, 1721–1729.

Fisk, J.D., Goodale, M.A., 1985. The organization of eye and limb movements during unrestricted reaching to targets in contralateral and ipsilateral visual space. Exp. Brain Res. 60, 159–178.

Fitzpatrick, R.C., Gandevia, S.C., 2005. Paradoxical muscle contractions and the neural control of movement and balance. J. Physiol. 564, 2.

Flanders, M., Herrmann, U., 1992. Two components of muscle activation: scaling with the speed of arm movement. J. Neurophysiol. 67, 931–943.

Fonteyn, E.M., Schmitz-Hübsch, T., Verstappen, C.C., et al., 2013. Prospective analysis of falls in dominant ataxias. Eur. Neurol. 69, 53–57.

Ford-Smith, C.D., VanSant, A.F., 1993. Age differences in movement patterns used to rise from a bed in subjects in the third through fifth decades of age. Phys. Ther. 73, 300–309.

Fortin, C., Ehrmann Feldman, D., Cheriet, F., Labelle, H., 2011. Clinical methods for quantifying body segment posture: a literature review. Disabil. Rehabil. 33, 367–383.

Fregly, A.R., Graybiel, A., 1968. An ataxia test battery not requiring rails. Aerosp. Med. 39, 277–282.

Frenklach, A., Louie, S., Koop, M.M., Bronte-Stewart, H., 2009. Excessive postural sway and the risk of falls at different stages of Parkinson's disease. Mov. Disord. 24, 377–385.

Fritz, S., Lusardi, M., 2009. White paper: 'walking speed: the sixth vital sign'. . J. Geriatr. Phys. Ther. 32, 2–5.

Frykberg, G.E., Häger, C.K., 2015. Movement analysis of sit-to-stand – research informing clinical practice. Phys. Ther. Rev. 20, 156–167.

Fujimoto, K., 2006. Dropped head in Parkinson's disease. J. Neurol. 253 (Suppl. 7), VII21–VII26.

Galna, B., Barry, G., Jackson, D., et al., 2014. Accuracy of the Microsoft Kinect sensor for measuring movement in people with Parkinson's disease. Gait Posture. 39, 1062–1068.

Gaymard, B., Pierrot-Deseilligny, C., 1999. Neurology of saccades and smooth pursuit. Curr. Opin. Neurol. 12, 13–19.

Geiger, R.A., Allen, J.B., O'Keefe, J., Hicks, R.R., 2001. Balance and mobility following stroke: effects of physical therapy interventions with and without biofeedback/forceplate training. Phys. Ther. 81, 995–1005.

Gentilucci, M., Toni, I., Daprati, E., Gangitano, M., 1997. Tactile input of the hand and the control of reaching to grasp movements. Exp. Brain Res. 114, 130–137.

Geurts, A.C.H., Boonstra, T.A., Voermans, N.C., et al., 2011. Assessment of postural asymmetry in mild to moderate Parkinson's disease. Gait Posture. 33, 143–145.

Giladi, N., McMahon, D., Przedborski, S., et al., 1992. Motor blocks in Parkinson's disease. Neurology. 42, 333–339.

Glaister, B.C., Bernatz, G.C., Klute, G.K., Orendurff, M.S., 2007. Video task analysis of turning during activities of daily living. Gait Posture. 25, 289–294.

Glasauer, S., Schneider, E., Jahn, K., Strupp, M., Brandt, T., 2005. How the eyes move the body. Neurology. 65, 1291–1293.

Godfrey, A., Del Din, S., Barry, G., et al., 2015. Instrumenting gait with an accelerometer: a system and algorithm examination. Med. Eng. Phys. 37, 400–407.

Goodale, M.A., Milner, A.D., Jakobson, L.S., Carey, D.P., 1991. A neurological dissociation between perceiving objects and grasping them. Nature. 349, 154–156.

Goulart, F.R., Valls-Solé, J., 1999. Patterned electromyographical activity in the sit-to-stand movement. Clin. Neurophysiol. 110, 1634–1640.

Greisberger, A., Aviv, H., Garbade, S.F., Diermayr, G., 2016. Clinical relevance of the effects of reach-to-grasp training using trunk restraint in individuals with hemiparesis post-stroke: a systematic review. J. Rehabil. Med. 48, 405–416.

Gross, M.M., Crane, E.A., Fredrickson, B.L., 2012. Effort-Shape and kinematic assessment of bodily expression of emotion during gait. Hum. Mov. Sci. 31, 202–221.

Gu, Y., Li, Z., 2012. Mechanical information of plantar fascia during normal gait. Phys. Procedia. 33, 63–66.

Guerraz, M., Bronstein, A.M., 2008. Ocular versus extraocular control of posture and equilibrium. Clin. Neurophysiol. 38, 391.

Guerraz, M., Thilo, K.V., Bronstein, A.M., Gresty, M.A., 2001. Influence of action and expectation on visual control of posture. Cogn. Brain Res. 11, 259–266.

Haggard, P., Wing, A., 1997. On the hand transport component of prehensile movements. J. Mot. Behav. 29, 282–287.

Hansson, G.A., Asterland, P., Homer, N.G., Skerfving, S., 2001. Validity and reliability of triaxial accelerometers for inclinometry in posture analysis. Med. Biol. Eng. Comput. 39, 405–413.

Hausdorff, J.M., Schaafsma, J.D., Balash, Y., et al., 2003. Impaired regulation of stride variability in Parkinson's disease subjects with freezing of gait. Exp. Brain Res. 149, 187–194.

Heller, A., Wade, D.T., Wood, V.A., et al., 1987. Arm function after stroke: measurement and recovery over the first three months. J. Neurol. Neurosurg. Psychiatry. 50, 714–719.

Hermsdörfer, J., Hagl, E., Nowak, D.A., Marquardt, C., 2003. Grip force control during object manipulation in cerebral stroke. Clin. Neurophysiol. 114, 915–929.

Hesse, S., Schauer, M., Malezic, M., et al., 1994. Quantitative analysis of rising from a chair in healthy and hemiparetic subjects. Scand. J. Rehabil. Med. 26, 161–166.

Hirschfeld, H., Thorsteinsdottir, M., Olsson, E., 1999. Coordinated ground forces exerted by buttocks and feet are adequately programmed for weight transfer during sit-to-stand. J. Neurophysiol. 82, 3021–3029.

Ho, E., Chan, J., Chan, D., et al., 2016. Improving posture classification accuracy for depth sensor-based human activity monitoring in smart environments. Comput. Vis. Image. Underst. 148, 97–110.

Hokazu, M., Uemura, S., Aoki, T., Takatsu, T., 1998. Analysis of rising from a chair after total knee arthroplasty. Bull. Hosp. Joint Dis. N.Y. 57, 88–92.

Holmes, J.D., Jenkins, M.E., Johnson, A.M., et al., 2010. Dual-task interference: the effects of verbal cognitive tasks on upright postural stability in Parkinson's disease. Parkinson. Dis. 2010, 696492.

Horak, F.B., 2006. Postural orientation and equilibrium: what do we need to know about neural control of balance to prevent falls. Age Ageing. 35 (Suppl. 2), ii7–ii11.

Horak, F.B., Diener, H.C., 1994. Cerebellar control of postural scaling and central set in stance. J. Neurophysiol. 72, 479–493.

Horak, F.B., Dimitrova, D., Nutt, J.G., 2005. Direction-specific postural instability in subjects with Parkinson's disease. Exp. Neurol. 193, 504–521.

Horak, F.B., Esselman, P., Anderson, M.E., Lynch, M.K., 1984. The effects of movement velocity, mass displaced, and task certainty on associated postural adjustments made by normal and hemiplegic individuals. J. Neurol. Neurosurg. Psychiatry. 47, 1020–1028.

Horak, F.B., Nashner, L.M., 1986. Central programming of postural movements: adaptation to altered support-surface configurations. J. Neurophysiol. 55, 1369–1381.

Horak, F.B., Wrisley, D.M., Frank, J., 2009. The Balance Evaluation Systems Test (BESTest) to differentiate balance deficits. Phys. Ther. 89, 484–498.

Hortobágyi, T., Mizelle, C., Beam, C., DeVita, P., 2003. Old adults perform activities of daily living near their maximal capabilities. J. Gerontol. 58A, 453–460.

Huang, X., Mahoney, J.M., Lewis, M.M., et al., 2012. Both coordination and symmetry of arm swing are reduced in Parkinson's disease. Gait Posture. 35, 373–377.

Hughes, M.A., Myers, B.S., Schenkman, M., 1996. The role of strength in rising from a chair in the functionally impaired adult. J. Biomech. 29, 1509–1513.

Iansek, R., Huxham, F., McGinley, J., 2006. The sequence effect and gait festination in Parkinson's disease: contributors to freezing of gait? Mov. Disord. 21, 1419–1424.

Ilg, W., Synofzik, M., Brötz, D., et al., 2009. Intensive coordinative training improves motor performance in degenerative cerebellar disease. Neurology. 73, 1823–1830.

Ishikawa, M., Komi, P.V., Grey, M.J., et al., 2005. Muscle-tendon interaction and elastic energy usage in human walking. J. Appl. Physiol. 99, 603–608.

Iyengara, Y.R., Vijayakumara, K., Abrahama, J.M., et al., 2014. Relationship between postural alignment in sitting by photogrammetry and seated postural control in post-stroke subjects. NeuroRehabilitation. 35, 181–190.

Jahn, K., Strupp, M., Krafczyk, S., et al., 2002. Suppression of eye movements improves balance. Brain. 125, 2005–2011.

Janssen, W.G.M., Bussmann, H.B.J., Stam, H.J., 2002. Determinants of the sit-to-stand movement: a review. Phys. Ther. 82, 866–879.

Janssen, W.G.M., Bussmann, H.B.J., Selles, R., et al., 2010. Recovery of the sit-to-stand movement after stroke: a longitudinal cohort study. Neurorehabil. Neural Repair. 24, 763–769.

Jeannerod, M., 1984. The timing of natural prehension movements. J. Mot. Behav. 16, 235–254.

Jeannerod, M., 1986. The formation of finger grip during prehension. A cortically mediated visuomotor pattern. Behav. Brain Res. 19, 99–116.

Jeannerod, M., 1990. The Neural and Behavioural Organization of Goal-directed Movements. Clarendon Press, Oxford.

Jenmalm, P., Dahlstedt, S., Johansson, R.S., 2000. Visual and tactile information about object-curvature control fingertip forces and grasp kinematics in human dexterous manipulation. J. Neurophysiol. 84, 2984–2997.

Johansson, R.S., Westling, G., 1984. Roles of glabrous skin receptors and sensorimotor memory in automatic control of precision grip when lifting rougher or more slippery objects. Exp. Brain Res. 56, 550–564.

Johansson, R.S., Westling, G., Bäckström, A., Flanagan, J.R., 2001. Eye–hand coordination in object manipulation. J. Neurosci. 21, 6917–6932.

Kamper, D.G., 2003. Stereotypical fingertip trajectories during grasp. J. Neurophysiol. 90, 3702–3710.

Kamper, D.G., McKenna-Cole, A.N., Kahn, L.E., Reinkensmeyer, D.J., 2002. Alterations in reaching after stroke and their relation to movement direction and impairment severity. Arch. Phys. Med. Rehabil. 83, 702–707.

Kappler, R.E., 1982. Postural balance and motion patterns. J. Am. Osteopath. Assoc. 81, 69–77.

Kashihara, K., Ohno, M., Tomita, S., 2006. Dropped head syndrome in Parkinson's disease. Mov. Disord. 21, 1213–1216.

Kavounoudias, A., Roll, R., Roll, J.P., 1999. Specific whole-body shifts induced by frequency-modulated vibrations of human plantar soles. Neurosci. Lett. 266, 181–184.

Kavounoudias, A., Roll, R., Roll, J.P., 2001. Foot sole and ankle muscle inputs contribute jointly to human erect posture regulation. J. Physiol. 532, 869–878.

Kawagoe, S., Tajima, N., Chosa, E., 2000. Biomechanical analysis of effects of foot placement with varying chair height on the motion of standing up. J. Orthopaed. Sci. 5, 124–133.

Kendall, F.P., Kendall McCreary, E., 2010. Geise Provance, P. In: Rodgers, M., Romani, W. (Eds.), Muscles: Testing and Function, With Posture and Pain, 5th ed. Lippincott Williams & Wilkins, Baltimore.

Kerr, G.K., Worringham, C.J., Cole, M.H., et al., 2010. Predictors of future falls in Parkinson's disease. Neurology. 75, 116–124.

Keus, S.H.J., Bloem, B.R., Hendriks, E.J.M., et al., 2007. Evidence-based analysis of physical therapy in Parkinson's disease with recommendations for practice and research. Mov. Disord. 22, 451–460.

Khallaf, M.E., Fayed, E.E., 2015. Parkinson's disease early postural changes in individuals with idiopathic Parkinson's disease. Parkinson. Dis. 2015, 369454.

Khemlani, M.M., Carr, J.H., Crosbie, W.J., 1999. Muscle synergies and joint linkages in sit-to-stand under two initial foot positions. Clin. Biomech. 14, 236–246.

Khiabani, R.R., Mochizuki, G., Ismail, F., et al., 2017. Impact of spasticity on balance control during quiet standing in persons after stroke. Stroke Res. Treat. 2017, 6153714.

Kirby, R.L., Price, N.A., MacLeod, D.A., 1987. The influence of foot position on standing balance. J. Biomech. 20, 423–427.

Kollen, B.J., Lennon, S., Lyons, B., et al., 2009. The effectiveness of the Bobath concept in stroke rehabilitation: what is the evidence? Stroke. 40, e89–e97.

Kralj, J.A., Jaeger, R.J., Munih, M., 1990. Analysis of standing up and sitting down in humans: definitions and normative data presentation. J. Biomech. 23, 1123–1138.

Kuchera, M., 1995. Gravitational stress, musculoligamentous strain, and postural alignment. Spine State Art Rev. 9, 463–489.

Kwong, P.W.H., Ng, S.S.M., Chung, R.C.K., Ng, G.Y.F., 2014. Foot placement and arm position affect the five times sit-to-stand test time of individuals with chronic stroke. Biomed. Res. Int. 2014, 636530.

Lackner, J.R., 1988. Some proprioceptive influences on the perceptual representation of body shape and orientation. Brain. 111, 281–297.

Lackner, J.R., DiZio, P., 2005. Vestibular, proprioceptive and haptic contributions to spatial orientation. Ann. Rev. Psychol. 56, 115–147.

Lacquaniti, F., Ivanenko, Y.P., Zago, M., 2012. Patterned control of human locomotion. J. Physiol. 590, 2189–2199.

Lang, C.E., DeJong, S.L., Beebe, J.A., 2009. Recovery of thumb and finger extension and its relation to grasp performance after stroke. J. Neurophysiol. 102, 451–459.

Lang, C.E., Wagner, J.M., Bastian, A.J., et al., 2005. Deficits in grasp versus reach during acute hemiparesis. Exp. Brain Res. 166, 126–136.

Lang, C.E., Wagner, J.M., Edwards, D.F., et al., 2006. Recovery of grasp versus reach in people with hemiparesis poststroke. Neurorehabil. Neural Repair. 20, 444–454.

Latash, M.L., Aruin, A.S., Neyman, I., Nicholas, J.J., 1995. Anticipatory postural adjustments during self inflicted and predictable perturbations in Parkinson's disease. J. Neurol. Neurosurg. Psychiatry. 58, 326–334.

Latash, M.L., Zatsiorsky, V.M., 2016. Posture Biomechanics and Motor Control. Academic Press, San Diego. 305–333.

Lecours, J., Nadeau, S., Gravel, D., Teixera-Salmela, L., 2008. Interactions between foot placement, trunk frontal position, weight-bearing and knee moment asymmetry at seat-off during rising from a chair in healthy controls and persons with hemiparesis. J. Rehabil. Med. 40, 200–207.

Lee, D., Lishman, J.R., 1975. Visual proprioceptive control of stance. J. Hum. Movement Stud. 1, 87–95.

Lee, T.-H., Choi, J.-D., Lee, N.-G., 2015. Activation timing patterns of the abdominal and leg muscles during the sit-to-stand movement in individuals with chronic hemiparetic stroke. J. Phys. Ther. Sci. 27, 3593–3595.

Leonard, C.T., 1998. The Movement Science of Human Movement. Mosby, London.

Levin, M.F., 1996. Interjoint coordination during pointing movements is disrupted in spastic hemiparesis. Brain. 119, 281–293.

Levin, M.F., Selles, R.W., Verheul, M.H., Meijer, O.G., 2000. Deficits in the coordination of agonist and antagonist muscles in stroke patients: implications for normal motor control. Brain Res. 853, 352–369.

Levin, M.F., Michaelsen, S.M., Cirstea, C.M., Roby-Brami, A., 2002. Use of the trunk for reaching targets placed within and beyond the reach in adult hemiparesis. Exp. Brain Res. 143, 171–180.

Levine, D., Richards, J., Whittle, M.W., 2012. Whittle's Gait Analysis: An Introduction, 5th ed. Elsevier, Edinburgh, Churchill Livingstone.

Lichtwark, G.A., Wilson, A.M., 2006. Interactions between the human gastrocnemius muscle and the Achilles tendon during incline, level and decline locomotion. J. Exp. Biol. 209, 4379–4388.

Lin, P.C., Chen, Y.J., Chen, W.S., et al., 2022. Automatic real-time occupational posture evaluation and select corresponding ergonomic assessments. Sci. Rep. 12, 2139.

Lomaglio, M.J., Eng, J.J., 2005. Muscle strength and weight bearing symmetry relate to sit-to-stand performance in individuals with stroke. Gait Posture. 22, 126–131.

Loram, I.D., Maganaris, C.N., Lakie, M., 2005a. Active, non-spring-like muscle movements in human postural sway: how might paradoxical changes in muscle length be produced? J. Physiol. 564, 281–293.

Loram, I.D., Maganaris, C.N., Lakie, M., 2005b. Human postural sway results from frequent, ballistic bias impulses by soleus and gastrocnemius. J. Physiol. 564, 295–311.

Lord, S.R., Clark, R.D., 1996. Simple physiological and clinical tests for the accurate prediction of falling in older people. Gerontology. 42, 199–203.

Lord, S.R., Murray, S.M., Chapman, K., et al., 2002. Sit-to-stand performance depends on sensation, speed, balance, and psychological status in addition to strength in older people. J. Gerontol. 57A, M539–M543.

Louter, M., Munneke, M., Bloem, B.R., Overeem, S., 2012. Nocturnal hypokinesia and sleep quality in Parkinson's disease. J. Am. J. Geriatr. Soc. 60, 1104–1108.

Louter, M., Maetzler, W., Prinzen, J., et al., 2015. Accelerometer-based quantitative analysis of axial nocturnal movements differentiates patients with Parkinson's disease, but not high-risk individuals, from controls. J. Neurol. Neurosurg. Psychiatry. 86, 32–37.

Maki, B.E., 1997. Gait changes in older adults: predictors of falls or indicators of fear? J. Am. Geriatr. Soc. 45, 313–320.

Mancini, M., Horak, F.B., 2010. The relevance of clinical balance assessment tools to differentiate balance deficits. Eur. J. Physiol. Rehabil. Med. 46, 239–248.

Mansfield, A., Danells, C., Inness, E., Mochizuki, G., McIlroy, W.E., 2011. Between-limb synchronisation for control of standing balance in individuals with stroke. Clin. Biomech. 26, 312–317.

Mansfield, A., Inness, E.L., Wong, J.S., Fraser, J.E., McIlroy, W.E., 2013. Is impaired control of reactive stepping related to falls during inpatient stroke rehabilitation? Neurorehabil. Neural Repair. 27, 526–533.

Marigold, D.S., Eng, J.J., 2006. The relationship of asymmetric weight-bearing with postural sway and visual reliance in stroke. Gait Posture. 23, 249–255.

Marigold, D.S., Eng, J.J., Tokuno, C.D., Donnelly, C.A., 2004. Contribution of muscle strength and integration of afferent input to postural instability in persons with stroke. Neurorehabil. Neural Repair. 18, 222–229.

Marteniuk, R.G., MacKenzie, C.L., Jeannerod, M., et al., 1987. Constraints on human arm movement trajectories. Can. J. Psychol. 41, 365.

Mason, C.R., Gomez, J.E., Ebner, T.J., 2001. Hand synergies during reach-to-grasp. J. Neurophysiol. 86, 2896–2910.

Mathias, S., Nayak, U.S., Isaacs, B., 1986. Balance in elderly patients: the "Get-up and Go" test. Arch. Phys. Med. Rehabil. 14, 387–389.

Mauritz, K.H., Dichgans, J., Hufschmidt, A., 1979. Quantitative analysis of stance in late cortical cerebellar atrophy of the anterior lobe and other forms of cerebellar ataxia. Brain. 102, 461–482.

McIlroy, W.E., Maki, B.E., 1997. Preferred placement of the feet during quiet stance: development of a standardized foot placement for balance testing. Clin. Biomech. 12, 66–70.

Meyns, P., Bruijn, S.M., Duysens, J., 2013. The how and why of arm swing during human walking. Gait Posture. 38, 555–562.

Micera, S., Carpaneto, J., Posteraro, F., et al., 2005. Characterization of upper arm synergies during reaching tasks in able-bodied and hemiparetic subjects. Clin. Biomech. 20, 939–946.

Michaelsen, S., Jacobs, S., Roby-Brami, A., Levin, M., 2004. Compensation for distal impairments of grasping in adults with hemiparesis. Exp. Brain Res. 157, 162–173.

Michaelsen, S.M., Dannenbaum, R., Levin, M.F., 2006. Task-specific training with trunk restraint on arm recovery in stroke: randomized control trial. Stroke. 37, 186–192.

Michaelsen, S.M., Levin, M.F., 2004. Short-term effects of practice with trunk restraint on reaching movements in patients with chronic stroke: a controlled trial. Stroke. 35, 1914–1919.

Michaelsen, S.M., Luta, A., Roby-Brami, A., Levin, M.F., 2001. Effect of trunk restraint on the recovery of reaching movements in hemiparetic patients. Stroke. 32, 1875–1883.

Midaglia, L., Mulero, P., Montalban, X., et al., 2019. Adherence and satisfaction of smartphone- and smartwatch-based remote active testing and passive monitoring in people with multiple sclerosis: nonrandomized interventional feasibility study. J. Med. Int. Res. 21, e14863. Erratum in: J. Med. Int. Res. 21, e16287

Mikami, K., Shiraishi, M., Kawasaki, T., Kamo, T., 2017. Forward flexion of trunk in Parkinson's disease patients is affected by subjective vertical position. PLoS One. 12, e0181210.

Mille, M.L., Johnson, M.E., Martinez, K.M., Rogers, M.W., 2005. Age-dependent differences in lateral balance recovery through protective stepping. Clin. Biomech. 20, 607–616.

Mitchell, S.L., Collin, J.J., De Luca, C.J., et al., 1995. Open-loop and closed-loop postural control mechanisms in Parkinson's disease: increased mediolateral activity during quiet standing. Neurosci. Lett. 197, 133–136.

Moreira, R., Teles, A., Fialho, R., et al., 2020. Mobile applications for assessing human posture: a systematic literature review. Electronics. 9, 1196.

Morris, M.E., Iansek, R., Galna, B., 2008. Gait festination and freezing in Parkinson's disease: pathogenesis and rehabilitation. Mov. Disord. 23 (Suppl. 2), S451–S460.

Mount, J., Kresge, L., Klaus, G., et al., 2006. Movement patterns used by the elderly when getting out of bed. Phys. Occup. Ther. Geriatr. 24, 27–43.

Mount, J., Cianci, H., Weiman, R., et al., 2009. How people with Parkinson's disease get out of bed. Phys. Occup. Ther. Geriatr. 27, 333–359.

Muller, J., Wenning, G.K., Jellinger, K., et al., 2000. Stages in Parkinsonian disorders: a clinicopathologic study. Neurology. 55, 888–891.

Murray, M.P., 1967. 'Gait as a total pattern of movement'. Am. J. Phys. Med. 46, 290–333.

Myers, A.M., Fletcher, P.C., Myers, A.H., Sherk, W., 1998. Discriminative and evaluative properties of the Activities-specific Balance Confidence (ABC) scale. J. Gerontol. 53A, M287–M294.

Nadeau, S.M., Boukadida, A., Piotte, F., Mesure, S., 2016. Weight bearing perception during standing and sit to stand tasks in subacute post-stroke individuals undergoing intensive rehabilitation. Ann. Phys. Rehabil. Med. 59S, e67–e79.

Nam, I., Shun, J., Lee, Y., et al., 2015. The effect of foot position on erector spinae and gluteus maximus activation during sit-to-stand performed by chronic stroke patients. J. Phys. Ther. Sci. 27, 571–573.

Napier, J., 1956. The prehensile movements of the human hand. J. Bone Joint Surg. Br. 38–B, 902–913.

Nashner, L., Berthoz, A., 1978. Visual contribution to rapid motor responses during postural control. Brain Res. 150, 403–407.

Nelson, S.R., Di Fabio, R.P., Anderson, J.H., 1995. Vestibular and sensory interaction deficits assessed by dynamic platform posturography in patients with multiple sclerosis. Ann. Otol. Rhinol. Laryngol. 104, 62–68.

Ng, S., 2010. Balance ability, not muscle strength and exercise endurance determines the performance of hemiparetic subjects on the timed-sit-to-stand test. Am. J. Phys. Med. Rehabil. 89, 497–504.

Nieuwboer, A., Giladi, N., 2013. Characterizing freezing of gait in Parkinson's disease: models of an episodic phenomenon. Mov. Disord. 28, 1509–1519.

Pai, Y.-C., Rogers, M.W., 1991. Segmental contributions to total body momentum in sit-to-stand. Med. Sci. Sport. Exerc. 23, 225–230.

Pain, L.M., Baker, R., Richardson, D., Agur, A.M.R., 2015. Effect of trunk-restraint training on function and compensatory trunk, shoulder and elbow patterns during post-stroke reach: a systematic review. Disabil. Rehabil. 37, 553–562.

Paquette, C., Franzen, E., Horak, F., 2016. More falls in cerebellar ataxia when standing on a slow up-moving tilt of the support surface. Cerebellum. 15, 336–342.

Park, S.B., Davare, M., Falla, M., et al., 2016. Fast-adapting mechanoreceptors are important for force control in precision grip but not sensorimotor memory. J. Neurophysiol. 115, 3156–3161.

Patla, A.E., 1991. Understanding control of human locomotion: a prologue. In: Patla, A.E. (Ed.), Adaptability of Human Gait. Elsevier Science Publishers BV, Oxford, North Holland.

Patla, A.E., 1997. Understanding the roles of vision in the control of human locomotion. Gait Posture. 5, 54–69.

Peters, J., Abou, L., Wong, E., et al., 2022. Smartphone-based gait and balance assessment in survivors of stroke: a systematic review. Disabil. Rehabil. Assist. Technol. 18, 1–11.

Peurala, S.H., Könönen, P., Pitkänen, K., et al., 2007. Postural instability in patients with chronic stroke. Restor. Neurol. Neurosci. 25, 101–108.

Piano, L., Geri, T., Testa, M., 2020. Raising and stabilization phase of the sit-to-stand movement better discriminate healthy elderly adults from young subjects: a pilot cross-sectional study. Arch Physiother. 10, 7.

Pieriera, L.C., Botelho, A.C., Martins, E.F., 2010. Relationships between body symmetry during weight bearing and functional reach among chronic hemiparetic patients. Rev. Bras. Fisioter. 14, 229–266.

Pollock, A., Baer, G., Pomeroy, V., Langhorne, P., 2007. Physiotherapy treatment approaches for the recovery of postural control and lower limb function following stroke. Cochrane Database Syst. Rev. 1, CD001920.

Pollock, A.S., Durward, B.R., Philip, J., et al., 2000. What is balance? Clin. Rehabil. 14, 402–406.

Prange, G.B., Kallenberg, L.A.C., Jannink, M.J.A., et al., 2009. Influence of gravity compensation on muscle activity during reach and retrieval in healthy elderly. J. Electromyogr. Kinesiol. 19, e40–e49.

Prudente, C., Rodrigues-de-Paula, F., Faria, C.D., 2013. Lower limb muscle activation during the sit-to-stand task in subjects who have had a stroke. Am. J. Phys. Med. Rehabil. 92, 666–675.

Rabadi, M.H., Blau, A., 2005. Admission ambulation velocity predicts length of stay and discharge disposition following stroke in an acute rehabilitation hospital. Neurorehabil. Neural Repair. 19, 20–26.

Raghavan, P., 2005. Patterns of impairment in digit independence after subcortical stroke. J. Neurophysiol. 95, 369–378.

Rashid, U., Barbado, D., Olsen, S., et al., 2022. Validity and reliability of a smartphone app for gait and balance assessment. Sensors. 22, 124.

Raymakers, J.A., Samson, M.M., Verhaar, H.J.J., 2005. The assessment of body sway and the choice of the stability parameter(s). Gait Posture. 21, 48–58.

Rehman, R.Z.U., Buckley, C., Micó-Amigo, 2020. Accelerometry-based digital gait characteristics for classification of Parkinson's disease: what counts? IEEE Open J. Eng. Med. Biol. 1, 65–73.

Rehman, R.Z.U., Del Din, S., Guan, Y., et al., 2019. Selecting clinically relevant gait characteristics for classification of early Parkinson's disease: a comprehensive machine learning approach. Sci. Rep. 9, 17269.

Reicherz, A., Brach, M., Cerny, J., et al., 2011. Development of the Lie-to-Sit-to-Stand-to-Walk Transfer (LSSWT) test for early mobilization in older patients in geriatric rehabilitation. Z. Gerontol. Geriatr. 44, 262–267.

Reinkensmeyer, D.J., Cole, A.M., Kahn, L.E., Kamper, D.G., 2002. Directional control of reaching is preserved following mild/moderate stroke and stochastically constrained following severe stroke. Exp. Brain Res. 143, 525–530.

Reynolds, R.F., Bronstein, A.M., 2003. The broken escalator phenomenon. Aftereffect of walking onto a moving platform. Exp. Brain Res. 151, 301–308.

Richter, R.R., VanSant, A.F., Newton, R.A., 1989. Description of adult rolling movements and hypothesis of developmental sequences. Phys. Ther. 69, 63–71.

Robichaud, J.A., Pfann, K.D., Comella, C.L., et al., 2004. Greater impairment of extension movements as compared to flexion movements in Parkinson's disease. Exp. Brain Res. 156, 240–254.

Roby-Brami, A., Jacobs, S., Bennis, N., Levin, M.F., 2003. Hand orientation for grasping and arm joint rotation patterns in healthy subjects and hemiparetic stroke patients. Brain Res. 969, 217–229.

Rodosky, M.W., Andriacchi, T.P., Andersson, G.B.J., 1989. The influence of chair height on lower limb mechanics during rising. J. Orthop. Res. 7, 266–271.

Roerdink, M., Geurts, A.C.H., De Haart, M., Beek, P.J., 2009. On the relative contribution of the paretic leg to the control of posture after stroke. Neurorehabil. Neural Repair. 23, 267–274.

Rosario, J.-L., 2017. What is posture? A review of the literature in search of a definition. ECOR 6, 111–133.

Roy, G., Nadeau, S., Gravel, D., et al., 2006. The effect of foot position and chair height on the asymmetry of vertical forces during sit-to-stand and stand-to-sit tasks in individuals with hemiparesis. Clin. Biomech. 21, 585–593.

Sanchez, M., Loram, I., Darby, J., Holmes, P., Butler, P., 2017. A video-based method to quantify posture of the head and trunk in sitting. Gait Posture. 51, 181–187.

Sangole, A.P., Levin, M.F., 2008a. Arches of the hand in reach to grasp. J. Biomech. 41, 829–837.

Sangole, A.P., Levin, M.F., 2008b. Palmar arch dynamics during reach-to-grasp tasks. Exp. Brain Res. 190, 443–452.

Santello, M., Flanders, M., Soechting, J.F., 2002. Patterns of hand motion during grasping and the influence of sensory guidance. J. Neurosci. 22, 1426–1435.

Santello, M., Soechting, J.F., 1998. Gradual molding of the hand to object contours. J. Neurophysiol. 79, 1307–1320.

Schenkman, M., Berger, R.A., Riley, P.O., et al., 1990. Whole-body movement during rising to standing from sitting. Phys. Ther. 70, 638–648.

Schenkman, M., Riley, P.O., Pieper, C., 1996. Sit to stand from progressively lower seat heights – alterations in angular velocity. Clin. Biomech. 11, 153–158.

Schieppati, M., Nardone, A., 1991. Free and supported stance in Parkinson's disease: the effect of posture and 'postural set' on leg muscle responses to perturbation, and its relation to the severity of the disease. Brain. 114, 1227–1244.

Schmitz-Hübsch, T., Coudert, M., Bauer, P., et al., 2008. Spinocerebellar ataxia types 1, 2, 3, and 6: disease severity and nonataxia symptoms. Neurology. 71, 982–989.

Schmitz-Hübsch, T., Tezenas du Montcel, S., Baliko, L., et al., 2006. Scale for the assessment and rating of ataxia: development of a new clinical scale. Neurology. 66, 1717–1720.

Schultz, A.B., Alexander, N.B., Ashton-Miller, J.A., 1992. Biomechanical analysis of rising from a chair. J. Biomech. 25, 1383–1391.

Seo, N.J., Kamper, D.G., 2008. Effect of grip location, arm support, and muscle stretch on sustained finger flexor activity following stroke. Annu Int Conf IEEE Eng Med Biol Soc. 2008, 4170–4173.

Seo, N.J., Rymer, W.Z., Kamper, D.G., 2009. Delays in grip initiation and termination in persons with stroke: effects of arm support and active muscle stretch exercise. J. Neurophysiol. 101, 3108–3115.

Seo, N.J., Rymer, W.Z., Kamper, D.G., 2010. Altered digit force direction during pinch grip following stroke. Exp. Brain Res. 202, 891–901.

Shah, K., Solan, M., Dawe, E., 2020. The gait cycle and its variations with disease and injury. Orthopaed. Trauma. 34, 153–160.

Shaikh, T., Goussev, V., Feldman, A.G., Levin, M.F., 2014. Arm-trunk coordination for beyond-the-reach movements in adults with stroke. Neurorehabil. Neural Repair. 28, 355–366.

Shiavi, R., 1985. Electromyographic patterns in adult locomotion: a comprehensive review. J. Rehabil. Res. Dev. 22, 85–98.

Shumway-Cook, A., Woollacott, M.H., 2012. Motor Control: Translating Research into Clinical Practice, 4th ed. Lippincott Williams & Wilkins, Philadelphia.

Sibella, F., Galli, M., Romei, M., et al., 2003. Biomechanical analysis of sit-to-stand movement in normal and obese subjects. Clin. Biomech. 18, 745–750.

Silva, A., Sousa, A.S.P., Oinheiro, R., et al., 2013. Activation timing of soleus and tibialis anterior muscles during sit-to-stand and stand-to-sit in post-stroke vs healthy subjects. Somatosens. Mot. Res. 30, 48–55.

Silva, P., Franco, J., Gusmão, A., et al., 2015. Trunk strength is associated with sit-to-stand performance in both stroke and healthy subjects. Eur. J. Phys. Rehabil. Med. 51, 717–724.

Silva, P.F., de, S., Quintino, L.F., Franco, J., et al., 2017. Trunk kinematics related to generation and transfer of the trunk flexor momentum are associated with sit-to-stand performance in chronic stroke survivors. NeuroRehabil 40, 57–67.

Smith, J.W., 1957. The forces operating at the human ankle joint during standing. J. Anat. 91, 545–564.

Soh, S.E., Morris, M., McGinley, J.L., 2011. Determinants of health-related quality of life in Parkinson's disease: a systematic review. Parkinsonism. Relat. Disord. 17, 1–9.

Song, J., Sigward, S., Fisher, B., Salem, G.J., 2012. Altered dynamic postural control during step turning in persons with early-stage Parkinson's disease. Parkinson Dis. 2012, 386962.

Sringean, J., Taechalertpaisarn, P., Thanawattano, C., Bhidayasiri, R., 2016. How well do Parkinson's disease patients turn in bed? Quantitative analysis of nocturnal hypokinesia using multisite wearable inertial sensors. Parkinsonism. Relat. Disord. 23, 10–16.

Stack, E., Ashburn, A., 2008. Dysfunctional turning in Parkinson's disease. Disabil. Rehabil. 30, 1222–1229.

Stack, E.L., Ashburn, A.M., 2006. Impaired bed mobility and disordered sleep in Parkinson's disease. Mov. Disord. 21, 1340–1342.

Švehlík, M., Zwick, E.B., Steinwender, G., et al., 2009. Gait analysis in patients with Parkinson's disease off dopaminergic therapy. Arch. Phys. Med. Rehabil. 90, 1880–1886.

Tabamo, R.E., Fernandez, H.H., Friedman, J.H., Lucas, P.R., 2000. Spinal surgery for severe scoliosis in Parkinson's disease. Med. Health. R. I 83, 114–115.

Tan, D.M., McGinley, J.L., Danoudis, M.E., et al., 2011. Freezing of gait and activity limitations in people with Parkinson's disease. Arch. Phys. Med. Rehabil. 92, 1159–1165.

Thielman, G., Kaminski, T., Gentile, A.M., 2008. Rehabilitation of reaching after stroke: comparing 2 training protocols utilizing trunk restraint. Neurorehabil. Neural Repair. 22, 697–705.

Taniguchi, S., D'cruz, N., Nakagoshi, M., et al, 2022. Determinants of impaired bed mobility in Parkinson's disease: Impact of hip muscle strength and motor symptoms. NeuroRehabil. 50, 445-452.

Timmann, D., Horak, F.B., 1998. Perturbed step initiation in cerebellar subjects 1. Modifications of postural responses. Exp. Brain Res. 119, 73–84.

Tinetti, M.E., 1986. Performance-oriented assessment of mobility problems in elderly patients. J. Am. Geriatr. Soc. 34, 119–126.

Troyanovich, S.J., Harrison, D.E., Harrison, D.D., 1998. Structural rehabilitation of the spine and posture: rationale for treatment beyond the resolution of symptoms. J. Manipulative Physiol. Ther. 21, 37–50.

Twomey, L., Taylor, J., 1987. Lumbar posture, movement and mechanics Physical Therapy of the Low Back. Churchill Livingstone, London.

Tyson, S., DeSouza, L., 2004a. Development of the Brunel Balance Assessment: a new measure of balance disability post-stroke. Clin. Rehabil. 18, 801–810.

Tyson, S., DeSouza, L., 2004b. Reliability and validity of functional balance tests post-stroke. Clin. Rehabil. 18, 916–923.

Tyson, S.F., Hanley, M., Chillala, J., et al., 2006. Balance disability after stroke. Phys. Ther. 86, 30–38.

van Asseldonk, E.H., Buurke, J.H., Bloem, B.R., et al., 2006. Disentangling the contribution of the paretic and non-paretic ankle to balance control in stroke patients. Exp. Neurol. 201, 441–451.

van de Warrenburg, B.P., Bakker, M., Kremer, B.P., et al., 2005. Trunk sway in patients with spinocerebellar ataxia. Mov. Disord. 20, 1006–1013.

van der Kruk, E., Silverman, A.K., Reilly, P., et al. 2021. Compensation due to age-related decline in sit-to-stand and sit-to-walk. J Biomechanics. 122, 110411.

van Polanen, V., Davare, M., 2015. Interactions between dorsal and ventral streams for controlling skilled grasp. Neuropsychologia. 79, 186–191.

van Vliet, P.M., Sheridan, M.R., 2007. Coordination between reaching and grasping in patients with hemiparesis and healthy subjects. Arch. Phys. Med. Rehabil. 88, 1325–1331.

Vander Linden, D.W., Brunt, D., McCulloch, M.U., 1994. Variant and invariant characteristics of the sit-to-stand task in healthy elderly adults. Arch. Phys. Med. Rehabil. 5, 653–660.

Wade, D.T., Langton-Hewer, R., Wood, V.A., et al., 1983. The hemiplegic arm after stroke: measurement and recovery. J. Neurol. Neurosurg. Psychol. 46, 521–524.

Walton, C.C., Shine, J.M., Hall, J.M., et al., 2015. The major impact of freezing of gait on quality of life in Parkinson's disease. J. Neurol. 262, 108–115.

Wang, J., Stelmach, G.E., 1998. Coordination among the body segments during reach-to-grasp action involving the trunk. Exp. Brain Res. 123, 346–350.

Weerdesteyn, V., de Niet, M., van Duijnhoven, H.J., Geurts, A.C., 2008. Falls in individuals with stroke. J. Rehabil. Res. Dev. 45, 1195–1213.

Weiss, A., Herman, T., Giladi, N., Hausdorff, J.M., 2015. New evidence for gait abnormalities among Parkinson's disease patients who suffer from freezing of gait: insights using a body-fixed sensor worn for 3 days. J. Neural Transm. 122, 403–410.

Westling, G., Johansson, R.S., 1984. Factors influencing the force control during precision grip. Exp. Brain Res. 53, 277–284.

Whitney, S., Wrisley, D.M., Marchetti, G.F., et al., 2005. Clinical measurement of sit-to-stand performance in people with balance disorders: validity of data for the five-times-sit-to-stand test. Phys. Ther. 85, 1034–1045.

Whittle, M.W., Levine, D., Richards, J., 2012a. Normal gait. In: Levine, D., Richards, J., Whittle, M.W. (Eds.), Whittle's Gait Analysis: An Introduction, 5th ed. Elsevier, Edinburgh, Churchill Livingstone, pp. 29–63.

Whittle, M.W., Levine, D., Richards, J., 2012b. Basic sciences. In: Levine, D., Richards, J., Whittle, M.W. (Eds.), Whittle's Gait Analysis: An Introduction, 5th ed. Elsevier, Edinburgh, Churchill Livingstone, pp. 1–28.

Wing, A.M., Fraser, C., 1983. The contribution of the thumb to reaching movements. Q. J. Exp. Psychol. A. 35, 297–309.

Winges, S.A., Weber, D.J., Santello, M., 2003. The role of vision on hand preshaping during reach to grasp. Exp. Brain Res. 152, 489–498.

Winter, D.A., 1980. Overall principle of lower limb support during stance phase of gait. J. Biomech. 13, 923–927.

Winter, D.A., 1987. The Biomechanics and Motor Control of Human Gait. University of Waterloo Press, Waterloo, Ontario.

Winter, D.A., McFadyen, B.J., Dickey, J.P., 1991. Adaptability of the CNS in human walking. In: Patla, A.E. (Ed.), Adaptability of Human Gait. Elsevier, North Holland.

Winter, D.A., Patla, A.E., Frank, S.J., Walt, S.E., 1990. Biomechanical walking pattern changes in the fit and healthy elderly. Phys. Ther. 70, 340–347.

Winter, D.A., Patla, A.E., Rietdyk, S., Ishac, M.G., 2001. Ankle muscle stiffness in the control of balance during quiet standing. J. Neurophysiol. 85, 2630–2633.

Winter, D.A., Prince, F., Frank, J.M., et al., 1996. Unified theory regarding A/P and M/L balance in quiet stance. J. Neurophysiol. 75, 2334–2343.

Woodbury, M.L., Howland, D.R., McGuirk, T.E., et al., 2008. Effects of trunk restraint combined with intensive task practice on poststroke upper extremity reach and function: a pilot study. Neurorehabil. Neural Repair. 23, 78–91.

Woollacott, M.H., Bonnet, M., Yabe, K., 1984. Preparatory process for anticipatory postural adjustments: modulation of leg muscles reflex pathways during preparation for arm movements in standing man. Exp. Brain Res. 55, 263–271.

Wright, W.G., Gurfinkel, V.S., Nutt, J., et al., 2007. Axial hypertonicity in Parkinson's disease: direct measurements of trunk and hip torque. Exp. Neurol. 208, 38–46.

Wurtz, R.H., Kandel, E.R., 2000a. Central Visual Pathways, 4th ed. In: Kandel, E.R., Schwartz, J.H., Jessell, T.M. (Eds.), McCraw Hill, New York, 543–547, 548–571.

Wurtz, R.H., Kandel, E.R., 2000b. Perception of motion, depth and form, 4th ed. In: Kandel, E.R., Schwartz, J.H., Jessell, T.M., (Eds.), McCraw Hill, New York, pp. 548–571.

Wyller, T.B., Sveen, U., Sodring, K.M., et al., 1997. Subjective well-being one year after stroke. Clin. Rehabil. 11, 139–145.

Zackowski, K.M., 2004. How do strength, sensation, spasticity and joint individuation relate to the reaching deficits of people with chronic hemiparesis? Brain. 127, 1035–1046.

Zanardi, A.P.J., da Silva, E.S., Costa, R.R., et al., 2021. Gait parameters of Parkinson's disease compared with healthy controls: a systematic review and meta-analysis. Sci. Rep. 11, 752.

Zettel, J.L., McIlroy, W.E., Maki, B., 2002. Can stabilising features of rapid triggered stepping reactions be modulated to meet environmental constraints? Exp. Brain Res. 145, 297–308.

Zhang, W.S., Gao, C., Tan, Y.Y., et al., 2021. Prevalence of freezing of gait in Parkinson's disease: a systematic review and meta-analysis. J. Neurol. 268, 4138–4150.

Measurement Tools

Geert Verheyden and Sarah F. Tyson

OUTLINE

Introduction, 113
    Impairments, 114
    Activity Limitations, 115
Types of Measurement Tools, 117
Psychometric Properties, 119
    Reliability, 119
        Assessing Reliability for Nominal and Ordinal Data
        with Two Scoring Categories, 119
        Assessing Reliability for Ordinal Data with Three or
        More Categories, 120
        Assessing Reliability for Interval and Ratio Data, 120

Validity, 121
    Content Validity, 121
    Construct Validity, 121
    Criterion-Related Validity, 122
    Responsiveness, 123
Applied Measurement Science: Towards Clinical
    Implementation, 124
Conclusion, 125

INTRODUCTION

> *"To Measure is to Know."*
>
> **—Lord Kelvin**

Professional organisations such as World Physiotherapy (https://world.physio/) provide definitions and guidelines to standardise professional practice and mandate the use of measurement tools as a core component of clinical practice. However, measurement using objective tools should not be confused with assessment. Patient assessment is a much broader process that also includes, but is not limited to, anamnesis, clinical inspection and observation, interpretation and goal setting. However, using measurement tools can contribute to assessment as well as other aspects of practice, such as monitoring progress and assessing outcome. To achieve this, therapists should not only be familiar with measurement tools but also be able to select and apply them appropriately and understand the underlying principles to evaluate their quality and their application in therapeutic diagnosis, prognosis, care planning, assessing patient progress and evaluating the effectiveness of interventions (Fulk & Field-Fote 2011).

Measurement tools can address the previously mentioned list, but not all tools serve all purposes. It is important to have a clear objective for using a tool and to know whether the tool selected can address the therapist's aim.

You may have noticed that this chapter is entitled 'Measurement Tools', rather than the more commonly used term *outcome measures*. Many clinicians use outcome measures as a generic term for all things related to measurement. Yet measuring outcome is just one contribution that measurement tools can make to clinical practice. Strictly speaking, an outcome measure is a tool used before and after treatment; the scores are compared and then one makes a judgement about the outcome of the treatment, that is, whether the scores (and thus the patient) improved. But as stated earlier, there are other ways that tools can be applied in clinical practice besides measuring treatment outcome, and hence we prefer to refer to the term *measurement tools*, which more accurately reflects the purposes for which tools are used and their potential benefits (Burton et al 2013).

This chapter will firstly discuss why and how measurement tools are used in clinical practice; then the psychometric properties of measurement tools will be explained. These are the statistical components defining the quality of a measurement tool and the accuracy of the information it provides. Understanding the psychometrics is a core element of selecting an appropriate measurement tool for your practice. Finally, we will make recommendations about which measurement tools to use for neurological physiotherapy.

Firstly, how are measurement tools used? A few years ago, Tyson and coworkers undertook an observational study looking at how measurement tools were used in clinical practice. We compared two neurorehabilitation units. In one, measurement tools were embedded into the everyday practice of the multidisciplinary team, but the other unit did not use measurement tools. We found that, although challenging, using the tools supported and informed (rather than replaced) clinical reasoning and judgement. They facilitated communication within the team by providing a 'common language' to define and describe patients' problems, which promoted joint decision making and treatment planning. They also promoted patient-centred care by focusing on the patients' difficulties rather than the professionals' contribution (Greenhalgh et al 2008a, 2008b; Tyson et al 2010, 2012). Importantly, staff noted that not everything in neurological rehabilitation can be, or should be, measured and reduced to numbers! However, using standardised objective measurement tools quickly and effectively dealt with the straightforward, standardisable, measurable aspects of rehabilitation, leaving more time to the complex, multifaceted subjective and personal aspects of care.

In a later project, measurement tools were introduced into stroke rehabilitation units and incorporated into the multidisciplinary team meetings in which patients' difficulties and progress were discussed and their care coordinated (Tyson et al 2015). Through nonparticipant observations and interviews with the participating staff, we found that, although it took a while to become familiar with the tools and 'fluent' in their use, like the earlier study, their introduction was feasible and enabled more accurate problem identification, effective (objective) progress monitoring, and timely decision making, and promoted more effective communication and staff relationships. Staff believed that objective measures enabled them to have a clearer understanding of the patients' difficulties, identify and define goals, develop treatment plans and effectively monitor progress. This, in turn, informed planning and decision making by providing structure and prompting staff to think holistically, comprehensively and proactively.

The next consideration when selecting a measurement tool is what one wants to measure. All too often physiotherapists (and other professionals) seek a single measurement tool to cover all aspects of their input with all patients. This is simply unrealistic. Our patients are rather more complex and their problems more multifaceted than that, and so is the physiotherapy provided!

The *International Classification of Functioning, Disability and Health* (ICF) (World Health Organization 2001) provides a useful framework to define and understand this complexity. It classifies patients' difficulties as *impairments* (or dysfunction of body structure or function), *activity limitations* and *restrictions to participation* in life roles and society. It also considers the social and environmental factors that might facilitate or limit function. The problems that neurological therapy aims to treat are covered within this classification and can be used as a basis to understand the patients' difficulties and identify appropriate measurement tools. This is not without its challenges, however. Neurological therapists' terminology to describe patients' problems and their interventions is often imprecise and inconsistent. The same term is often used to describe different things, or multiple terms are used to describe the same thing. For example, early work to identify the domains of neurological physiotherapy uncovered 10 different terms used in everyday practice for weakness and nine different ways of describing posture (Tyson et al 2007). One of the big benefits of using standardised measurement tools is that they provide a common language to conceptualise, define and describe patients' problems. It takes much of the uncertainty out of clinical communication so that more people are talking about the same thing in the same way at the same time. Taking this approach has produced a consensus framework that identifies and defines the important aspects of neurological therapy that are candidates for objective measurement (Tyson et al 2007).

Impairments

- Ataxia/coordination
- Balance and posture impairment (includes alignment, weight distribution and postural sway)
- Fatigue
- Muscle tone/spasticity
- Muscle weakness/strength (includes active [range of] movement and other terms regarding 'movement')
- Oedema
- Pain
- (Passive) Range of movement/contracture
- Sensation
- Shoulder subluxation
- Walking impairment (includes speed, endurance, step length cadence, etc).

Activity Limitations

- Balance disability (includes sitting, standing, dynamic, supported and assisted balance)
- Falls
- Mobility disability (includes bed mobility, sit-to-stand, transfers, walking, stairs/steps)
- Upper limb (includes grips/grasps, dexterity, activities of everyday life)
- Walking disability (includes indoor/outdoor, assistance, use of equipment, independence).

Recommended measurement tools for these aspects are presented in Table 5.1.

Interestingly (and somewhat controversially), the participating physiotherapists did not identify participation (roles and activities within society) as part of their remit. Also, those working in acute care and early-stage rehabilitation tended to focus on impairments, whereas those working in the community and working with long-term conditions tended to focus more on activity limitations (Burton et al 2013).

TABLE 5.1   Measurement Tools Recommended for Use in Neurological Physiotherapy

Domain	Recommended Measure(s) and Source or Instruction Manual
Ataxia/coordination	• Scale for the assessment and rating of ataxia (SARA): http://www.ataxia-study-group.net/html/about/ataxiascales/sara/SARA.pdf • Finger-nose test: Gagnon et al (2004), also included in SARA
Balance impairment (posture)	Although many instrumented measures of posture and several observational measures are available, their reliability, validity and clinical utility are limited, such that an evidence-based recommendation cannot be made (Tyson 2003). Professionals may be better served by focusing on measures of muscle strength and balance disability/activity.
Fatigue	• Neurological Fatigue Index (NFI) for multiple sclerosis (available from the authors; Mills et al 2010) • Neurological Fatigue Index for motor neurone disease (NFI-MND) (available from the authors; Gibbons et al 2011) • Neurological Fatigue Index for stroke (NFI-Stroke) (available from the authors; Mills et al 2012) Note: Although the Fatigue Severity Scale and Fatigue Impact Scale are widely reported in the research literature, many versions are used, and no standardised operating instructions are available.
Muscle tone/spasticity	• Arm Activity Measure: https://www.kcl.ac.uk/cicelysaunders/resources#ArmA • Leg Activity Measure: https://www.kcl.ac.uk/cicelysaunders/resources#LegActivityMeasure Note: The Modified Ashworth Scale is widely used, but it measures resistance to passive movement, rather than spasticity, and its validity and responsiveness are very limited; therefore, it is not recommended. Other instrumented measures of spasticity are available, but they are infeasible for use in clinical practice.
Muscle strength/weakness	• Motricity Index (Demeurrisse et al 1980, Wade 1992) (https://www.sralab.org/rehabilitation-measures/motricity-index) • Grip strength using a handheld dynamometer: http://www.neuropt.org/docs/stroke-sig/strokeedge_taskforce_summary_document.pdf (pp. 91–93)
Oedema	There is insufficient evidence to make an evidence-based recommendation. The most feasible method appears to be measuring the circumference of the oedematous body part, but careful application regarding the position and force of tape measure application is needed to ensure reliability.
Pain	There is insufficient evidence to make an evidence-based recommendation, but a vertically orientated visual analogy scale or numerical rating scale supplemented with visual images for people with communication, cognitive or visual difficulties is the best bet.

(Continued)

TABLE 5.1	Measurement Tools Recommended for Use in Neurological Physiotherapy—Cont'd
Domain	**Recommended Measure(s) and Source or Instruction Manual**
(Passive) Range of movement/ contracture	Handheld goniometers are often recommended, but no standardised operating instructions are available. Although test-retest reliability can be reasonable, interrater reliability is often poor. This method is often more effective for measuring contractures/limitations of passive range than when measuring people with full or normal range. In this case, an informal estimate of whether range is normal may suffice.
Sensation	• Rivermead Assessment of Somatosensory Perception (RASP) is recommended, but the manual and equipment required are no longer available. However, the most important tests (tactile sensation and proprioception) can be completed without equipment. Instructions are found in Tyson and Busse (2009). • Stereognosis section of Nottingham Sensory Assessment (Connell 2007; http://eprints.nottingham.ac.uk/10247/) • Erasmus version of Nottingham Sensory Assessment (Stolk-Hornsveld et al 2006)
Shoulder subluxation	There is insufficient evidence to make an evidence-based recommendation. However, using manual palpation (the number of finger widths that the subluxation encompasses) or length discrepancy test (difference in distance between the acromial arc and lateral humeral epicondyle on the weak and sound sides) is valid and may be reliable with careful standardised operating instructions. Ultrasound has stronger psychometrics, but the clinical utility is limited.
Walking impairment	• 5- or 10-metre walk test: Brunel Balance Assessment User's Manual (https://www.escholar.manchester.ac.uk/uk-ac-man-scw:188226) • 6-minute (or 2-minute) walk test (https://www.sralab.org/rehabilitation-measures/6-minute-walk-test)
Balance	• Forward Reach and Arm Raise Tests (in sitting and standing): Brunel Balance Assessment User's Manual (https://www.escholar.manchester.ac.uk/uk-ac-man-scw:188226) • Step/Tap, Weight Shift and Step-Up Tests: Brunel Balance Assessment User's Manual (https://www.escholar.manchester.ac.uk/uk-ac-man-scw:188226) • Brunel Balance Assessment: Brunel Balance Assessment User's Manual (https://www.escholar.manchester.ac.uk/uk-ac-man-scw:188226) • Sitting Balance: Trunk Impairment Scale (see Verheyden et al 2004 for scoring sheet; see https://www.youtube.com/watch?v=-9tiR-V2UTM for instruction video) Note: The well-known Berg Balance Scale is not recommended because it is not hierarchical and there is much redundancy in items. The recommended measures demonstrate stronger psychometrics and better clinical utility.
Mobility	• Rivermead Mobility Index (https://www.sralab.org/rehabilitation-measures/rivermead-mobility-index) • High Level Mobility Assessment Tool (http://www.tbims.org/combi/himat/HiMAT.pdf) • Timed Up and Go (https://www.sralab.org/rehabilitation-measures/timed-and-go)
Balance and mobility combined	• Postural Assessment Scale for Stroke (https://www.sralab.org/rehabilitation-measures/postural-assessment-scale-stroke)
Upper limb activity in everyday life	• Motor Activity Log (MAL-14) (Uswatte et al 2005; https://www.sralab.org/rehabilitation-measures/motor-activity-log)

TABLE 5.1	Measurement Tools Recommended for Use in Neurological Physiotherapy—Cont'd
Domain	**Recommended Measure(s) and Source or Instruction Manual**
Grips/grasps and dexterity	• Action Research Arm Test (ARAT) (https://www.sralab.org/rehabilitation-measures/action-research-arm-test) • Box and Block Test (https://www.sralab.org/rehabilitation-measures/box-and-block-test) • Nine Hole Peg Test (https://www.sralab.org/rehabilitation-measures/nine-hole-peg-test)
Reaching	• No evidence-based recommendation can be made, but reaching is encompassed in the measures of grips and grasps recommended earlier.
Fall risk	• Forward Reach and Arm Raise Tests (in sitting & standing): Brunel Balance Assessment User's Manual (https://www.escholar.manchester.ac.uk/uk-ac-man-scw:188226) • Timed Up and Go (https://www.sralab.org/rehabilitation-measures/timed-and-go)
Walking disability	• Functional Ambulation Category (FAC) (https://www.sralab.org/rehabilitation-measures/functional-ambulation-category) Note: The FAC is well-known with good utility and validity. However, evidence about other psychometric properties is limited.

TYPES OF MEASUREMENT TOOLS

Using measurement tools is a core component of clinical practice with identified benefits, recognising that tools can measure different aspects of the ICF. This section will explain which type of data arises from measurement tools – nominal, ordinal, interval and ratio data – with each having different strengths and uses.

A *nominal* tool is a scale with two or more response categories (i.e., possible scores) but without an order between the categories, which means that one category is not better than the other. Examples of nominal scales are colour of the eyes, gender, race and type of stroke (ischaemic or haemorrhagic).

Ordinal tools are scales where each item has two or more possible responses and the items are ordered from worse to better, or vice versa. However, an important feature of an ordinal scale is that the difference between items and different scores is not equal. For example, the Rivermead Mobility Index (Collen et al 1991) is a widely used, robust ordinal scale that measures functional mobility. The higher someone scores, the more mobile they are, but the difference in mobility between items is not all the same. For example, item 4 is 'sit-to-stand' and item 6 is 'transfers'. The difference in performance demand between these two activities is relatively low, and so the patient will not need to improve a great deal to increase their score. In contrast, item 7 is 'walking indoors with an aid (if needed)' and item 8 is 'stairs'. Managing stairs independently is a much more demanding task than walking indoors with an aid, but the

transition from one task to another will score only one extra point.

The items on the Rivermead Mobility Index are dichotomous (i.e., each have a yes/no answer). An alternative design is to have a range of scores for each item. The most common way to do this is to use a Likert scale, which has a range of responses (typically 5, but sometimes 3 or 7) that are given a descriptor. The Barthel Index (Mahoney & Barthel 1965) is an example of an ordinal scale that uses Likert subscales. Each of 10 activities of daily living are scored on a 2-, 3- or 4-point scale assessing independence where, for instance, a 3-point scale uses 0 = dependent, 1 = needs assistance, and 2 = independence (although the wording changes with each item).

Likert scales can also be used as a single item when they are also referred to as numeric rating scales. This approach is often used to measure pain, where pain severity is often categorised as no pain (scores 0), mild (scores 1), moderate (scores 2), severe (scores 3), or very severe (scores 4) (Tyson & Brown 2014b). Sometimes facial expressions or other images and visual cues are added to aid for people with communication difficulties.

Ordinal scales are particularly useful to define, describe and classify patients' difficulties. Their strengths lie in assessment, goal setting, treatment and discharge planning and promoting communication between professionals and with patients and families. They are generally of adequate statistical quality. Most (particularly those recommended in Table 5.1) are quick and simple to perform, cover a wide range of abilities and are relevant to clinical practice.

However, some ordinal scales can be long-winded, complicated to complete and/or divorced from clinical practice, which makes them unsuitable for clinical use. So do not assume that all ordinal scales are useful. The disadvantage of ordinal scales is that they are relatively insensitive to change, particularly the small changes that may be observed over a short treatment period. Although they may pick up the changes between admission and discharge (for example), they are less likely to pick up changes over a shorter period (e.g., day to day) unless the patient is improving rapidly. So they are less useful to monitor progress; functional performance tests (see later) are preferred measurement tools should that be the aim.

An *interval* tool is one in which the difference between different scoring categories is the same. However, for an interval tool, the zero value does not mean the absence of the element that is measured. An example of an interval measurement is temperature measured in degrees Celsius. Zero degrees Celsius does not mean that there is no temperature, it means that it is cold. Scales that adhere to the Rasch model (detailed later in the Validity section) are interval scales. Examples of interval scales are the Trunk Impairment Scale (TIS; Verheyden & Kersten 2010) and Motricity Index (Demeurrisse et al 1980).

A *ratio* tool includes a range of scoring categories where differences between different scoring categories are the same and where the zero means an absence of the element that is measured. Functional performance tests are examples of ratio tools.

Functional performance tests, as the title suggests, measure patients' performance on a functional task. Examples include the 10-metre walk test (time taken to walk 10 metres, a measure of walking speed; Green et al 2002), the Box and Block test (number of wooden blocks that can transferred from one box to another in 2 minutes, a measure of manipulation ability; Platz et al 2005) and the Forward Reach test (the distance a patient can reach their outstretched arm forward while sitting or standing, a measure of balance ability; Duncan et al 1990).

The data produced by these measures are continuous and ratio. This means that scores start at zero, have no upper limit and the difference between scores is uniform at all points of the range. For example, a forward reach of 10 cm is the same whether it is between 2 and 12 cm or 22 and 32 cm. This means that fractions of scores can be used (e.g., 10.5 cm), which makes them much more sensitive to change than ordinal scales, and their strength is in measuring and monitoring performance and progress.

Functional performance tests are generally quick, easy to perform (although some simple equipment may be needed, such as a tape measure or stopwatch), and because the tests are functional, they are relevant to everyday life

and clinical practice. Statistical quality is usually good if they are delivered accurately. It is important that these tests are undertaken in a consistent, standardised manner; otherwise, changes in score may be merely a reflection of differences in doing the test, rather than changes in patients' performance. The other downside is that each test is suitable for only a relatively narrow range of patient ability. For example, the 10-metre walk test is suitable only for people who can walk. A way around this is to arrange a collection of tests into a hierarchy that together cover a wide range of ability, such as used in the Brunel Balance Assessment (Tyson & DeSouza 2004).

Instrumented measures also produce interval data. These are devices used to make objective measurements, usually of movement, producing continuous ratio level data, usually of the patients' impairments. Examples include isokinetic dynamometers, accelerometers, weight distribution, and postural sway monitors and gait analysis systems.

There is often an assumption that using a device to measure something must be better than using 'clinical level' data (i.e., the relatively insensitive and subjective ordinal scales and functional performance tests detailed earlier). Also, there is often an expectation that information from machines provide 'better' data than that produced manually, and that this will better inform clinical decision making. The data obtained from instrumented measures are, indeed, often sensitive; in fact, too sensitive in some cases. Variability of performance is a feature of people relearning a motor activity, and many instrumented measures detect patients' variable performance too sensitively, producing low reliability scores when tested formally. The validity can also be questionable because often the actions patients need to perform when measured are too demanding, or the device does not detect their abnormal movement patterns (a common problem for pedometers and accelerometers). Also, the devices often measure specific aspects of impairment, which, although technically easy to measure, are not strongly related to functional performance or clinical practice, and therefore of little relevance to clinical practice.

There are a few exceptions that prove the rule, however; the use of clinical gait analysis to inform multilevel surgery for people with cerebral palsy is an example where instrumented measures demonstrably contribute to neurological rehabilitation, but there are not many others. Furthermore, the equipment is often expensive, cumbersome and time consuming to use, and suitable for only a narrow range of patients. Unsurprisingly, there are no instrumented measures in the tools recommended for use in clinical practice presented in Table 5.1. Technology continues to develop, however, so it is possible that effective, clinically feasible tools will be produced in the future, particularly if a user-centred approach is applied to their design and development. Nevertheless, in our view, a neurological therapist can currently gather the data needed for everyday clinical practice with simple equipment such as a tape measure, stopwatch, ordinal scales and patient self-report (see Table 5.1 for details).

PSYCHOMETRIC PROPERTIES

When considering a measurement tool, typically reliability, validity, sensitivity and responsiveness are the psychometric properties that need to be considered. Each of these elements is detailed below, after which you should be able to interpret the results of psychometric testing to decide whether a measurement tool is a suitable choice for your practice.

Before considering each property in detail, it is important to note that these properties should be seen as a continuum (Rothstein 2001), and all properties should be viewed together to get an overall view of whether a measurement tool is suitable for clinical use and to acknowledge its strengths and weaknesses. Nevertheless, in the following sections, we will provide guidelines concerning interpretation of the values obtained from psychometric testing.

Reliability

Reliability refers to the stability of the scores obtained when a tool is used to take a measurement more than once. Reliability when two raters evaluate the same group of patients is considered as interrater reliability. This is important in clinical practice because it is probable that a neurological patient will be assessed by more than one person during their patient journey. To make a sensible interpretation of the scores from a measurement tool, one needs to know a change of score (or how big a change in score) indicates change in the patient's ability, rather than merely that a different person has used the tool.

Reliability when one rater evaluates the same group of patients twice is referred to as intrarater, or test-retest, reliability. This is important to make a judgement about whether a patient's ability has changed over time, or whether any change in score is merely arising from the normal day-to-day variation in score.

When a measurement tool is used, the score obtained includes a true score (i.e., the patient's level of ability) and a degree of measurement error (or normal variability in score) (Stokes 2011). Sources of error are inaccuracy by the person carrying out the test (the rater) and natural variability in the patient's performance or ability. Knowledge of the degree of measurement error of a tool is crucial to correctly interpret the score. For instance, when measuring a patient

before and after a series of therapy sessions, if the change in score is lower than the measurement error, then it is caused by variability in the rater's or patient's performance rather than an actual change in the patient's performance. Similarly, if a randomised controlled trial presents a statistically significant change between the experimental and control groups, but the actual difference is smaller than the measurement error of the tool, the difference between both groups is caused by error rather than a true difference in ability between the groups. Thus, although the differences found may be statistically significant, they are unimportant clinically. Sometimes, as part of reliability analysis, the standard error of measurement (SEM) is reported, which is a form of measurement error. It is defined as the absolute error expressed in terms of the actual unit of the original instrument (Stratford 2004). From the SEM, the minimal detectable change (MDC) can be calculated. This is an important psychometric property because it represents the minimal amount of change required before one can say a true change in the patient's performance, overcoming the measurement error. The 95% MDC is calculated as SEM $\times$ $1.96 \times \sqrt{2}$, providing a value that represents with 95% certainty the limit above which a change should be observed, which represents a true change in performance (see the Bland and Altman plots later in this chapter for further details). The reported MDC for many measurement tools is 10% or higher.

The type of analysis used to test reliability depends on the type of data they produce, that is, whether they are nominal, ordinal, interval or ratio scales (see earlier descriptions of types of measurement tools).

Assessing Reliability for Nominal and Ordinal Data with Two Scoring Categories

For nominal and ordinal data (also called *categorical data*), Kappa (κ) coefficients and percentages of agreement are reported. If there are only two scoring categories, the κ coefficient is calculated, which is a number representing the level of agreement between two observations. Percentage agreement (between the two observations) is typically reported as well, but by itself is insufficient to evaluate reliability because it does not consider the chance of any agreement occurring by pure luck or change. This chance is considered in a κ coefficient, hence the choice of κ statistic as the gold standard. A κ coefficient ranges from -1 to 1, with a higher coefficient representing higher agreement or reliability. Landis and Koch (1977) presented useful categories for interpreting the κ coefficient: values from 0.61 until 0.8 indicate 'substantial agreement', which is often seen as the minimum level for establishing reliability. κ values greater than 0.8 imply 'almost perfect' agreement.

Assessing Reliability for Ordinal Data with Three or More Categories

For ordinal data, let us consider an example of a 3-point ordinal scale for sitting balance where:
- 0 means when a patient cannot stay seated, they fall when trying to sit upright;
- 1 means a patient can stay in a seated position but would lose balance and fall over when pushed to the back, front or sideways; and
- 2 means a patient can stay in a seated position and would be able to remain seated when pushed to the back, front or sideways.

Reliability analysis could be performed by means of κ coefficients, but with ordinal data with three or more categories the degree of difference between raters is important. Using a weighted κ coefficient takes into account the degree of agreement/disagreement between raters; raters who score 0 and 1 will receive a higher score than those who score 0 and 2, for example. This weighted κ value thus accommodates the order in scoring and recognises that some disagreement between observations is better or worse than others. The numeric value of a weighted κ statistic is also between −1 and 1, and the same interpretation of scores applies as for the standard κ coefficient (Landis & Koch 1977). It remains important to consider the (weighted) κ coefficient and the percentage of agreement. In certain analyses, a very low κ value can be observed together with a high percentage of agreement (>80%). This is a well-known phenomenon, and although the underlying cause of this discrepancy is outside the scope of this chapter, it is sufficient to know that in the case of low κ but high percentage of agreement, arising from the high percentage of agreement, reliability is believed to be sufficient.

Assessing Reliability for Interval and Ratio Data

For interval and ratio type of data (also called *continuous data*), intraclass correlation coefficients (ICCs) are calculated, which take into account the variance between and within observations, as well as the error. There are several different types of ICC, and the type used should be reported (Rankin & Stokes 1998, Shrout & Fleiss 1979). The ICC value is also between −1 and 1, and higher values indicate higher agreement. A value of 0.8 or higher is used as a cutoff point to establish reliability.

More recently, in addition to ICC values, Bland and Altman plots have been adopted as a further analysis of reliability in continuous data (Bland & Altman 1995). Here the difference between two observations is plotted against the mean of both observations (Fig. 5.1). In addition, the mean difference is calculated and represented in the plot (see Fig. 5.1, solid horizontal line), and the 95% interval of

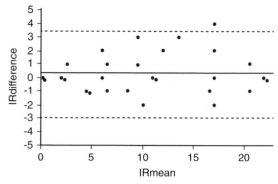

FIG. 5.1 Bland–Altman plot of the total range of differences of total Trunk Impairment Scale scores (IRdifference) against the total range of mean scores (IRmean) for interrater agreement. The solid line represents the mean of the differences. The dashed lines define the limits of agreement (mean of the difference ± 2 SD). (Reproduced with permission from Verheyden, G., Nuyens, G., Nieuwboer, A., Van Asch, P., Ketelaer, P., De Weerdt, W., 2006. Reliability and validity of trunk assessment for people with multiple sclerosis. Phys. Ther. 86, 66–76.)

the mean difference is calculated and added to the plot (see Fig. 5.1, dotted horizontal lines).

When interpreting a Bland and Altman plot, the following information is considered:
- What is the mean difference between the observations? Is it close to zero? This would be expected, otherwise there is a systematic difference/error in the scoring in favour of one observation and so one could obtain a large difference between scores if using the measurement tools on different occasions (or with different people) in practice. In Fig. 5.1, the mean difference is close to zero, indicating the scores are in relative agreement.
- What is the variability of scores? How big a change in score is needed to indicate a 'true' change in the patient's ability (and overcome the measurement error), which involves a score exceeding the 95% confidence interval of the mean difference? The larger the confidence interval, the greater the variation in scoring one can expect if using the tool in practice, and thus the larger the change in score needed to overcome this measurement error to indicate a true change in the patient's ability. In the example provided in Fig. 5.1, the 95% interval for the TIS ranges from −3 to slightly greater than 3, which is a 6-point interval. The TIS has a scoring range from 0 to 23; thus 6 points (about 25% of the scoring interval) is a considerable interval. This is an example

of the relative insensitivity of ordinal scales and why they are very good for assessment and description but less good as a short-term outcome measure or to monitor progress.

- How is the spread of the observations in the 95% interval? For Fig. 5.1, the TIS's scoring range (0 to 23 points) is presented on the x-axis. Looking at the distribution of data, the full range of the scale was examined in this reliability analysis. This is important to know because it implies that reliability for the whole scale has been examined. Furthermore, the shape of the data cloud in Fig. 5.1 indicates whether certain scoring ranges show more agreement. In Fig. 5.1, lower (<5 points) and higher (>20 points) scores show data points closer to the mean difference (zero value on the y-axis). This shows better agreement for these scoring ranges, which also makes clinical sense because patients with very poor or very good trunk control/sitting balance are often more consistent and thus produce more reliable scores.

For reliability analysis, calculation of the regular Pearson or Spearman correlation coefficient must be avoided, as they assess linear association or correlation, thus indicating the relation between two measurements and not the agreement. Imagine two series of measurements are systematically scored 5 units higher than a second series. A Pearson correlation coefficient would give a coefficient of 1, indicating a perfect relationship, which is indeed the case. But in terms of reliability, if one rater would systematically score patients 5 points more than a second rater (on a 10-point scale), then this would mean no agreement between observations.

A final type of reliability is applied to questionnaires that produce nominal or ordinal data. Here, the Cronbach α coefficient is often reported. This coefficient represents the homogeneity (also known as *uni-dimensionality* or *internal consistency*) of a tool (Stokes 2011) that reflects the relation between the items and the overall result. This is also sometimes described as whether the questionnaire addresses a single construct. One would expect a strong relation between the overall result and the underlying items, and a Cronbach α score of 0.90 or higher (1 is maximum) is required to indicate a reliable tool (Stokes 2011).

Finally, we note that reliability analysis needs to consider the total score as well as those of individual items. Often the scores of individual items are added together (or summed) to give an overall total score. Statistically this is an accurate thing to do if the items have equal weighting (i.e., produce interval or ratio data). However, most questionnaires and many clinical tests produce ordinal data and thus summating the items is inaccurate or unreliable because the value of the total score created depends on the weight of the items included. Conducting a Rasch analysis transforms an ordinal scale into an interval scale and is one solution to this issue.

Validity

The term *validity* refers to consideration of whether (or to what extent) a measurement tool measures the construct (or issue/idea) it intends to measure. This is sometimes referred as 'Does it do what it says on the label?' There are three main types of validity: content, construct and criterion-related validity.

Content Validity

Content, or face, validity relates to whether the content of the measurement tool is relevant to the construct the tool intends to measure. There is no statistical test for content validity; it involves making a judgement about how relevant the items are to the aim of the measurement tool. Let us consider the TIS again as an example (Verheyden et al 2004). Its aim is to measure sitting balance for people with stroke. It consists of three subscales: static sitting balance, dynamic sitting balance and coordination. The items in the scale test whether the patient can maintain their balance while sitting still, with legs crossed (smaller base of support), bending sideways (lateral flexion) and turning (rotation). These are clearly strongly connected to sitting balance, indicating that it has content validity. When developing the TIS, the authors completed a thorough process to identify items that represented important aspects of sitting balance. This involved:

- A literature review, searching for other scales evaluating trunk performance and considering their content, or lack of content;
- Observing stroke patients, interpreting deficits in their trunk performance and considering how these deficits could be scored; and
- Clinical experience and discussion with expert clinicians, as well as experts in scale development.

This informed a rationale for the choice of items that were included in the tool, and thus demonstrates its content validity (Verheyden et al 2004). In tools such as patient-reported outcomes, this type of validity should consider patients' opinions as well.

Construct Validity

Construct validity investigates whether the underlying idea, or construct, of the measurement tool is reasonable and whether it produces accurate, robust information. For the TIS, the underlying construct is that the scale measures sitting balance and that people with higher scores have better trunk performance and are likely to achieve better overall abilities than those with a low score. As you can imagine, evaluating this aspect of construct validity is largely a theoretical argument. However, measurable aspects of it are (if an ordinal scale) uni-dimensionality, redundancy, hierarchy and floor and ceiling effects.

As explained in the earlier Reliability section, *uni-dimensionality* (or internal consistency) is a measure of the homogeneity of the items of the tool, that is, whether they all measure the same construct, and is assessed using the Cronbach α coefficient.

Redundancy refers to whether there is overlap between items in the tool. If so, the items are essentially measuring the same attribute (but often described in a slightly different way). This would not only inflate the time and effort required for testing, but also the scores. If there is redundancy between items, a patient who passes one item would also pass the other redundant item(s) measuring the same attribute. So the score they achieve will indicate that they have 'passed' several items. However, they will have passed the same thing several times, rather than passed several different items. Redundancy is assessed using item-item and item-total correlations (Tyson & DeSouza 2004). A score more than $r = 0.9$ indicates redundancy between items, and they can be reduced to just one item.

Hierarchy is another important construct when it comes to using measurement tools in clinical practice. It refers to a formal assessment of whether the items of a scale increase (or decrease) in difficulty in a stepwise fashion. Using a hierarchical scale can save a great deal of time and effort for both tester and subject. If using a hierarchical scale, a patient who is unable to complete an item can be assumed to fail all the subsequent (more difficult) items. However, if they pass an item, it can be assumed that they will pass all the preceding items (Wade 1992). This means that not all the items need to be tested each time the patient is assessed. Testing can stop once the subject has failed an item. Alternatively, it can start at a level the patient would find reasonably challenging. If using a nonhierarchical scale, then all items need to be attempted.

Another advantage of a hierarchical scale is that it gives information about what a patient can or cannot do, rather than merely how many items the patient passes (Eakin 1989). For example, the Brunel Balance Assessment is a hierarchical scale measuring balance disability (Tyson & DeSouza 2004), so each item or level on the scale corresponds with a level of balance ability. If, for example, a patient scores 6, you know that the patient has sitting balance, static and dynamic standing balance, but cannot weight transfer, step or walk. In contrast, the Berg Balance Scale (Berg et al 1989) is a nonhierarchical balance assessment. When using it, one needs to attempt all items and then simply sum the scores. So a patient may score 28/56, for example, but one has no idea which items were passed or failed, merely that they obtained half of the available

score. Hierarchy is assessed by tabulating the pass rates of individual items and using the coefficients of scalability and reproducibility (Guttman 1944, Streiner & Norman 1997).

Finally, *floor and ceiling* effects are measures of whether the measurement tool covers the full range of patients' abilities. A floor effect indicates the lowest scoring items are not low or easy enough and there is a bulge of patients who achieve the lowest scores. The tool needs further lower scoring or easier items to differentiate the abilities of the least able patients. Conversely, a ceiling effect indicates that there is a bulge of patients scoring the highest marks, and further more challenging items are required. Floor and ceiling effects are assessed by plotting the patients' scores and assessing the numbers (or percentage) passing each item.

A more recent form of examining construct validity is through Rasch analysis, also called *internal validity*, which also encompasses all the properties mentioned earlier. It also looks at the mathematics of the tool and how the items can be used. As mentioned in the reliability section earlier, it can be used to transform an ordinal scale into an interval scale; then summed scores can be used to perform and report parametric statistics with confidence. The actual analysis and steps taken to complete a Rasch analysis, however, are beyond the scope of this chapter.

Criterion-Related Validity

Finally, criterion-related validity investigates further aspects of validity such as concurrent, discriminant and predictive validity. Criterion-related validity examines the relation between a measurement tool and a gold standard. However, there are very few truly gold standards in neurorehabilitation; thus, criterion-related validity is assessed by comparing the scores from a measurement tool with those from a well-known and accepted measurement tool of the same (or related) domain/construct. This relationship can be investigated by calculating a correlation coefficient. Using the example of the TIS, if it was a valid measure of sitting balance, scores on the TIS would be expected to show a good correlation with the Trunk Control Test. This is the case, as a correlation of $r = 0.83$ is reported (Verheyden et al 2004). One of the reasons that sitting balance is a key element of neurological rehabilitation is that it is an important stage in gaining independence in activities of daily living. Independence can be measured using the Barthel Index. Thus, if the TIS is a good measure of sitting balance, a patient's scores on the TIS will show a correlation with those on the Barthel Index. Again, this is the case, with a correlation of $r = 0.86$ reported (Verheyden et al 2004).

A further element of the validity is whether the tool can distinguish between important groups or categories of users. This is called *discriminant validity*. For the TIS this was investigated by assessing whether people with stroke had impaired trunk control compared with healthy age- and sex-matched controls (Verheyden et al 2005). Results showed significant differences for TIS subscale and total scores with people with stroke obtaining consistently lower scores than controls, confirming discriminant validity. This type of analysis is conducted by means of t tests or non-parametric between-group comparisons of independent samples or groups.

Predictive validity examines whether a measurement tool has prognostic ability, that is, whether it can predict a result or event in the (near) future. The analysis uses a regression analysis, with two approaches depending on whether outcome is a continuous scale (linear regression) or dichotomous scale (logistic regression). For the TIS, predictive validity was assessed by investigating whether the TIS score on admission to an inpatient stroke rehabilitation centre could predict independence in activities of daily living (measured with the Barthel Index) 6 months post-stroke. Results showed that the total TIS score on admission was a highly significant predictor of Barthel Index score at 6 months (Verheyden et al 2007). Typically for a linear regression model, the R^2 value indicates the amount of variance observed in the outcome measure (in our example, the Barthel Index) explained by the intake variable (in our example, the TIS). In our study, the R^2 was 52%; thus, 52% of the variance of Barthel Index score at 6 months was explained by the TIS score on admission, which establishes the predictive validity of the TIS early after stroke for functional outcome at 6 months.

A different type of predictive validity analysis is used if the outcome is dichotomous (i.e., has a yes/no answer, or whether something is/is not present). In this case, a logistic regression model is used. The relation between the prognostic and outcome tool can be presented in a 2×2 table including four different groups (Stokes 2011):

- True positives: if the prognostic tool predicts that the condition would be present and the outcome tool showed that indeed the condition is present
- False positives: if the prognostic tool predicts that the condition would be present but the outcome tool showed that the condition is not present
- False negatives: if the prognostic tool predicts that the condition would not be present but the outcome tool showed that the condition is in fact present
- True negatives: if the prognostic tool predicts that the condition would not be present and the outcome tool showed that indeed the condition is not present

Based on these four groups, the predictive strength of a measurement tool can be established by calculating sensitivity, specificity and positive and negative predictive value (Stokes 2011):

- Sensitivity is the ability of a tool to correctly predict whether a diagnosis, outcome or event is present (i.e., the number of true positives).
- Specificity is the ability of a tool to correctly predict whether a diagnosis, outcome or event is not present (i.e., the number of true negatives).
- Positive predictive value is the proportion of evaluated subjects with a positive test result and who have the disease, outcome or event (i.e., the proportion of true positives).
- Negative predictive value is the proportion of evaluated subjects with a negative test result and who do not have the disease, outcome or event (i.e., the proportion of true negatives).

These calculations are expressed as percentages with higher values representing better predictive value. As an example, let us consider an imagined measurement tool to predict falls among community-living people with multiple sclerosis with a reported sensitivity of 75% and a specificity of 80%. Based on the sensitivity, 3 out of 4 falls (75%) will be detected, but 1 out of 4 (the remaining 25%) will not, and based on the specificity, 8 out of 10 (80%) of those categorised as fallers will have experienced a fall, whereas 2 out of 10 categorised fallers (the remaining 20%) will not. In this case, the limited sensitivity is the important issue from a clinical perspective. A tool that accurately predicts an event only three-quarters of the time is not very useful. If one used the test in practice and it showed that a patient was at risk for falling, you could be only reasonably (75%) confident that they were really at risk and treat them accordingly. However, if the score indicated that the patient was not at risk, there is a 25% risk that this was a false negative and the person may actually fall. So it would be inadvisable to dismiss fall prevention measures. Thus, understanding these concepts and their underlying interpretation is important for clinical practice.

Responsiveness

Responsiveness is the ability to measure clinically meaningful or important change (Liang 1995). Confusingly, responsiveness is often also referred to as sensitivity to change but is a different concept to the sensitivity of prediction described earlier. The ability of a measurement tool to detect change is a key element if it is to be used to evaluate the effectiveness of an intervention. However, responsiveness is the least frequently investigated aspect of psychometric evaluation.

Different study designs can be used when evaluating responsiveness, but most commonly a longitudinal design with at least two measurement points is used; then the change in scores is analysed to assess whether a change in the patient's level of ability has been detected, usually using effect sizes and receiver operating characteristic (ROC) curves (Stokes 2011). The effect size is the ratio of the change that occurs because of an intervention divided by the variability of the measurement (Stokes 2011). Interpretation of effect sizes is provided by Cohen (1977), with effect sizes >0.8 indicating the measurement tool is responsive to change. Effect sizes <0.2 are to be interpreted as 'unresponsive' and between 0.5 and 0.8 as moderate. The same interpretation applies for the standardised response mean (SRM), which is another value evaluating responsiveness, calculated from the mean difference in scores at two time points, divided by the standard deviation of the differences (Liang 1995).

ROC curves plot sensitivity against specificity (as described in the previous section) of the tool and drawing a best fit curve. The area under the curve is then considered the probability of correctly identifying patients/participants who improve (Stratford et al 1996). The values for the area under the curve range from 0.5 (no accuracy in detecting improved from unimproved) to 1.0 (perfect accuracy) (Deyo & Centor 1986); generally a value of 0.9 is considered a minimum cutoff point for clinical use.

Beninato and Portney (2011) considered responsiveness in terms of the measurement error and minimal clinically important difference, as explained earlier in the Reliability section. Using the TIS as an example, the 95% interrater measurement error is 2 (Verheyden et al 2004). This means that when a patient's score changes by two points (increase or decrease), there is 95% certainty that this change is not arising from error or chance, and that the patient's sitting balance truly has changed.

It is important to bear in mind that this refers to the statistical importance of the changes in score. It does not refer to the functional or clinical importance of the change observed. This final psychometric property is referred to as clinical significance. There is no statistical test for it. It involves considering how important any changes observed are in real life. For example, what is the patient able to do that they could not do at the start, or how well can the patient do something? It is not unusual to find a change that is statistically significant but of little clinical/functional importance, and occasionally vice versa.

APPLIED MEASUREMENT SCIENCE: TOWARDS CLINICAL IMPLEMENTATION

Having considered a measure's psychometric properties to ensure it provides robust (i.e., reliable, valid and responsive) information, the next obvious question is which measurement tool to choose.

Several organisations have compiled information with regard to measurement tools in neurological therapy/ rehabilitation which provides useful listings and oversight of measurement tools and their psychometric properties. Examples of overviews that can be accessed online are:

- The Academy of Neurological Physical Therapy outcome measures recommendations section of the American Physical Therapy Association (http://www.neuropt.org/professional-resources/neurology-section-outcome-measures-recommendations): provides recommendations for stroke, multiple sclerosis, traumatic brain injury, spinal cord injury, Parkinson's and vestibular disorders.
- Shirley Ryan AbilityLab online Rehabilitation Measures Database (https://www.sralab.org/rehabilitation-measures): provides an overview of more than 500 tools for a wide variety of conditions requiring rehabilitation.
- Stroke-specific database: evidence-based review of stroke rehabilitation (http://www.ebrsr.com/evidence-review/20-outcome-measures-stroke-rehabilitation)

Furthermore, in a series of systematic reviews, Tyson, Connell, and colleagues appraised the psychometrics and clinical utility of the tools that measure the domains that are important to neurological physiotherapy, summarise information in a useful synopsis format and make recommendations about which tools to use, where possible. These cover posture (Tyson 2003), walking and mobility (Tyson & Connell 2009a), balance (Tyson & Connell 2009b), upper limb function (Connell & Tyson 2012a), sensation (Connell & Tyson 2012b), fatigue (Tyson & Brown 2014a) and pain (Tyson & Brown 2014b).

Clinical utility refers to how feasible it is to use the measurement tool in everyday clinical practice. The issues raised by physiotherapists as being crucial factors determining whether a tool was implemented in clinical practice were cost (as inexpensive as possible, preferably free), time taken to complete (as quick as possible, preferably less than 5–10 minutes), as easy as possible to use (with no need for specialist training or equipment) and portability (so the tool could be taken to, and used with, the patient wherever the patient is).

Recent and rigorous work from Moore and colleagues (Moore et al 2018) has resulted in a clinical practice guideline presenting a core set of outcome measures for adults with neurological conditions undergoing rehabilitation. Their action statements indicating clinical field and measurement tool to be used are:

- For static and dynamic sitting and standing balance assessment: Berg Balance Scale (BBS)
- For walking balance assessment: Functional Gait Assessment (FGA)
- For balance confidence assessment: Activities-specific Balance Confidence (ABC) Scale

- For walking speed assessment: 10-metre walk test (10-MWT)
- For walking distance assessment: 6-minute walk test (6-MWT)
- For transfer assessment: document type of transfer, level of required assistance, equipment or context adaptations, and time to complete, at least on admission and at discharge; 5 times sit-to-stand (5TSTS) may be used for sit-to-stand domain
- For documentation of patient goals: use of a measurement tool such as Goal Attainment Scale, reporting the task, performance conditions, and time to complete or level of independence desired, at least on admission and at discharge
- Use of the core set (BBS, FGA, ABC, 10-MWT, 6-MWT, 5TSTS, and patient goal assessment) for evaluating change over time in patients who have the goal and capacity to improve transfers, balance, and/or gait, at least on admission and at discharge
- Discuss as clinician the purpose and results from measurement tools, and how the results influence treatment options; through shared decision-making, clinician and patient should decide how results inform the therapy plan

The focus of the work by Moore and colleagues is on balance and walking. A similar clinical practice guideline with a core set for the upper limb in neurorehabilitation does not exist; however, for specific conditions like stroke, work from, for instance, Pohl and colleagues can be consulted (Pohl et al 2020).

Table 5.1 presents an extended overview of measurement tools recommended for clinical practice.

CONCLUSION

The use of measurement tools is a fundamental component of evidence-based practice. Using standardised measurement tools can improve communication with colleagues and patients; enhance the effectiveness of assessment, goal setting and monitoring progress; and speed clinical decision making and planning. Many, probably too many, measurement tools are available, which makes it difficult to decide which tool is most appropriate for a patient. But summary websites and systematic reviews provide useful overviews with recommendations of the plethora of ordinal scales, functional performance tests and instrumented measures available in neurological rehabilitation.

Understanding psychometric evaluation of measurement tools is a key component of clinical practice to evaluate statistical appropriateness of a measurement tool. New evidence will undoubtedly be published continuously, so summary websites and published systematic reviews will become out of date, unless regularly updated. Thus, clinicians should be able to consider independently whether reported reliability, validity and responsiveness of a measurement tool are appropriate.

SELF-ASSESSMENT QUESTIONS

1. Which four types of measurement data exist? Explain briefly the difference between them and give an example for each type.
2. Reliability of the 10-metre walk test when assessed by two therapists (a) is called *test-retest reliability*, and (b) can be examined by calculating the Pearson correlation coefficient between both assessments. Indicate for (a) and (b) whether this is true or false. Why?
3. Which two main types of predictive validity are frequently reported in the literature? What is the difference between these types, and how can we interpret the value of the prediction model?
4. Explain the difference between the concept of 'measurement error' and 'minimal clinically important difference' (MCID). What is their importance in clinical practice?
5. What impact would using standardised measurement tools have on your practice? What advantages might they bring? What would be the barriers to using them? And how might you overcome them?

REFERENCES

Beninato, M., Portney, L.G., 2011. Applying concepts of responsiveness to patient management in neurological physical therapy. J. Neurol. Phys. Ther. 35, 75–81.

Berg, K., Wood-Dauphinee, S., Williams, J.I., Gayton, D., 1989. Measuring balance in the elderly: preliminary development of an instrument. Physiother. Can. 41, 304–331.

Bland, J.M., Altman, D.G., 1995. Statistics notes Cronbach's alpha. BMJ. 314, 572.

Burton, L., Tyson, S.F., McGovern, A., 2013. Staff perceptions of using outcome measures in stroke rehabilitation. Disabil. Rehabil. 35, 828–834.

Cohen, J., 1977. Statistical Power Analysis for the Behavioural Sciences. Academic Press, New York.

Collen, F.M., Wade, D.T., Robb, G.F., Bradshaw, C.M., 1991. The Rivermead Mobility Index: a further development of the Rivermead Motor Assessment. Int. Disabil. Stud. 13, 50–54.

Connell, L.A., 2007. Sensory impairment and recovery after stroke. University of Nottingham. http://eprints.nottingham.ac.uk/10247/.

Connell, L.A., Tyson, S.F., 2012a. The clinical reality of measuring upper-limb ability in neurologic conditions: a systematic review. Arch. Phys. Med. Rehabil. 93, 221–228.

Connell, L.A., Tyson, S.F., 2012b. Measures of sensation in neurological conditions: a systematic review. Clin. Rehabil. 26, 68–80.

Demeurrisse, G., Demol, O., Robaye, E., 1980. Motor evaluation in vascular hemiplegia. Eur. Neurol. 1980, 382–389.

Deyo, R.A., Centor, R.M., 1986. Assessing the responsiveness of functional scales to clinical change: an analogy to diagnostic test performance. J. Chronic. Dis. 39, 897–906.

Duncan, P., Weiner, D., Chandler, J., 1990. Functional reach: a new clinical measure of balance. J. Gerontol. 45, M192–M197.

Eakin, P., 1989. Assessment of activities of daily living; a critical review. Br. J. Occup. Ther. 52, 11–15.

Fulk, G., Field-Fote, E.C., 2011. Measures of evidence in evidence-based practice. J. Neurol. Ther. 35, 55–56.

Gagnon, C., Mathieu, J., Desrosiers, J., 2004. Standardized finger-nose test validity for coordination assessment in an ataxic disorder. Can. J. Neurol. Sci. 31, 484–489.

Gibbons, C.J., Mills, R.J., Thornton, E.V., et al., 2011. Development of a patient reported outcome measure for fatigue in motor neurone disease: the Neurological Fatigue Index (NFIMND). Health Qual. Life Outcomes. 9, 101.

Green, J., Forster, A., Young, J., 2002. Reliability of gait speed measured by a timed walking test in patients one year after stroke. Clin. Rehabil. 16, 306–314.

Greenhalgh, J., Flynn, R., Long, A.F., Tyson, S., 2008a. Tacit and encoded knowledge in the use of standardised outcome measures in multidisciplinary team decision making: a case study of in-patient neurorehabilitation. Soc. Sci. Med. 67, 183–194.

Greenhalgh, J., Long, A.F., Flynn, R., Tyson, S., 2008b. "It's hard to tell." The challenges of scoring patients on standardised outcome measures by multidisciplinary teams: a case study of neurorehabilitation. BMC Health Serv. Res. 8, 217.

Guttman, L., 1944. A basis for scaling quantitative data. Am. Soc. Rev. 139–150.

Landis, J.R., Koch, G.G., 1977. The measurement of observer agreement for categorical data. Biometrics. 33, 159–174.

Liang, M.H., 1995. Evaluating measurement responsiveness. J. Rheumatol. 22, 1191–1192.

Mahoney, F.I., Barthel, D.W., 1965. Functional evaluation: the Barthel index. Md. State. Med. J. 14, 61–65.

Mills, R.J., Young, C.A., Pallant, J.F., et al., 2010. Development of a patient reported outcome measure scale for fatigue in multiple sclerosis: The Neurological Fatigue Index (NFI-MS). Health Qual. Life Outcomes. 8, 22.

Mills, R.J., Pallant, J.F., Koufali, M., et al., 2012. Validation of the Neurological Fatigue Index for stroke (NFI-Stroke). Health Qual. Life Outcomes. 10, 51.

Moore, J.L., Potter, K., Blankshain, K., et al., 2018. A core set of outcome measures for adults with neurologic conditions undergoing rehabilitation: a clinical practice guideline. J. Neurol. Phys. Ther. 42, 174–220.

Platz, T., Pinkowski, C., van Wijck, F., Kim, I.H., di Bella, P., Johnson, G., 2005. Reliability and validity of arm function assessment with standardized guidelines for the Fugl-Meyer Test, Action Research Arm Test and Box & Block Test: a multicentre study. Clin. Rehabil. 19, 404–411.

Pohl, J., Held, J., Verheyden, G., et al., 2020. Consensus-based core set of outcome measures for clinical motor rehabilitation after stroke—a Delphi study. Front. Neurol. 11, 875.

Rankin, G., Stokes, M., 1998. Reliability of assessment tools in rehabilitation: an illustration of appropriate statistical analyses. Clin. Rehabil. 12, 187–199.

Rothstein, J., 2001. Sick and tired of reliability. Editor's note. Phys. Ther. 81, 774–776.

Shrout, P.E., Fleiss, J.L., 1979. Intraclass correlations: uses in assessing rater reliability. Psychol. Bull. 86, 420–428.

Stokes, E.K., 2011. Rehabilitation Outcome Measures. Churchill Livingstone Elsevier, London, UK.

Stolk-Hornsveld, F., Crow, J.L., Hendriks, E.P., van der Baan, R., Harmeling-van der Wel, B.C., 2006. The Erasmus MC modifications to the (revised) Nottingham Sensory Assessment: a reliable somatosensory assessment measure for patients with intracranial disorders. Clin. Rehabil. 20, 160–172.

Stratford, P.W., 2004. Getting more from the literature: estimating the standard error of the measurement from reliability studies. Physiother. Can. 56, 27–30.

Stratford, P.W., Binkley, J.M., Riddle, D.L., 1996. Health status measures analytic methods for assessing change scores. Phys. Ther. 76, 1109–1123.

Streiner, D., Norman, G., 1997. Health Measurement Scales: a Practical Guide to Their Development and Use, 2nd ed. Oxford Medical Publications, Oxford.

Tyson, S., 2003. A systematic review of methods of measuring posture. Phys. Ther. Rev. 8, 45–50.

Tyson, S., Burton, L., McGovern, A., 2015. The impact of an assessment toolkit on use of objective measurement tools in stroke rehabilitation. Clin. Rehabil. 29, 926–934.

Tyson, S., Busse, M., 2009. How many body locations need to be tested when assessing sensation after stroke? An investigation of redundancy in the Rivermead Assessment of Somatosensory Perception. Clin. Rehabil. 23, 91–95.

Tyson, S., DeSouza, L., 2004. Reliability and validity of functional balance tests post-stroke. Clin. Rehabil. 18, 916–923.

Tyson, S., Watson, A., Moss, S., et al., 2007. Development of an evidence based framework for the physiotherapy assessment of neurological conditions? Disabil. Rehabil. 30, 142–144.

Tyson, S.F., Brown, P., 2014a. How to measure fatigue in neurological conditions? A systematic review of psychometric properties and clinical utility. Clin. Rehabil. 28, 804–816.

Tyson, S.F., Brown, P., 2014b. How to measure pain in neurological conditions? A systematic review of psychometric properties and clinical utility. Clin. Rehabil. 28, 669–686.

Tyson, S.F., Connell, L.A., 2009a. The psychometric properties and clinical utility of measures of walking and mobility in neurological conditions: a systematic review. Clin. Rehabil. 23, 1018–1033.

Tyson, S.F., Connell, L.A., 2009b. How to measure balance in clinical practice. A systematic review of the psychometrics and clinical utility of measures of balance activity for neurological conditions. Clin. Rehabil. 23, 824–840.

Tyson, S.F., Greenhalgh, J., Long, A.F., Flynn, R., 2010. The use of measurement tools in clinical practice; an observational study of neurorehabilitation. Clin. Rehabil. 24, 74–81.

Tyson, S.F., Greenhalgh, J., Long, A.F., Flynn, R., 2012. The influence of objective measurement tools on communication and clinical decision-making in neurological rehabilitation. J. Eval. Clin. Pract. 18, 216–224.

Uswatte, G., Taub, E., Morris, D., Vignolo, M., McCulloch, K., 2005. Reliability and validity of the upper-extremity Motor Activity Log-14 for measuring real-world arm use. Stroke 36, 2493–2496.

Verheyden, G., Kersten, P., 2010. Investigating the internal validity of the Trunk Impairment Scale (TIS) using Rasch analysis: the TIS 2.0. Disabil. Rehabil. 32, 2127–2137.

Verheyden, G., Nieuwboer, A., De Wit, L., et al., 2007. Trunk performance after stroke: an eye catching predictor of functional outcome. J. Neurol. Neurosurg. Psychiatry. 78, 694–698.

Verheyden, G., Nieuwboer, A., Feys, H., Thijs, V., Vaes, K., De Weerdt, W., 2005. Discriminant ability of the Trunk Impairment Scale: a comparison between stroke patients and healthy individuals. Diabil. Rehabil. 27, 1023–1028.

Verheyden, G., Nieuwboer, A., Mertin, J., Preger, R., Kiekens, C., De Weerdt, W., 2004. The Trunk Impairment Scale: a new tool to measure motor impairment of the trunk after stroke. Clin. Rehabil. 18, 326–334.

Wade, D.T., 1992. Measurement in Neurological Rehabilitation. Oxford University Press, Oxford.

World Health Organization, 2001. International Classification of Functioning, Disability and Health: ICF. World Health Organization, Geneva.

Goal Setting in Rehabilitation

William Mark Magnus Levack

OUTLINE

Introduction, 129
Definitions and Assumptions, 130
  Rehabilitation Goals and Goal Setting, 130
  Activities to Enhance Goal Pursuit, 130
Pragmatic Person-Centred Goal Setting, 131
  Goal Selection, 131
  Goal Documentation, 132
  Family Involvement in Goal Setting, 133
  Should Goals Be Measurable? 134
Goal Setting in Stroke Rehabilitation – Addressing the Changing Needs from Acute Care to Community Life, 134
  Acute Rehabilitation, 134
    Case Description, 134

Hospital-Based Early Subacute Rehabilitation, 136
  Case Description, 136
Community-Based Late Subacute Rehabilitation, 138
  Case Description, 138
Ongoing Life After Stoke, 139
  Case Description, 139
Goal Achievement As an Outcome Measure – Challenging Current Assumptions, 141
  The Appeal of Goal Attainment As an Outcome, 141
  An Overview of Goal Attainment Scaling, 141
    Problems with Goal Attainment As an Outcome, 142
Conclusion, 144

INTRODUCTION

Since the late 1990's there has been a proliferation of papers on goal setting in rehabilitation. Some of these papers have provided a user's guide to different approaches to goal setting championed by various rehabilitation services (e.g., McMillan & Sparkes 1999, Turner-Stokes 2009, Wade 1999a). Others have examined the impact of goal setting as a strategy to enhance patient engagement in therapy or to improve health outcomes following a period of rehabilitation intervention (e.g., Knutti et al., 2020, McPherson et al 2009, Taylor et al 2012). Researchers have also become interested in the perspectives and experiences of patients regarding goal setting (e.g., Baird et al 2010, Baker et al 2001, Brown et al 2014, Holliday et al 2007, Meyer & Pohontsch 2015). Often findings from these studies have challenged assumptions held by health professionals about how important goals are to patients, how much they want

to publicly share their goals or how involved they have been in the goal selection process. Systematic reviews of all of this quantitative and qualitative literature have arisen (Levack et al 2006c, 2015b, Lloyd et al 2018, Maribo et al 2020, Plant et al 2016; Rosewilliam et al 2011), although arguably these have tended to raise more questions about the practice of goal setting in rehabilitation than they have provided answers.

As research on goal setting in rehabilitation has progressed, it has become increasingly clear that goal setting is perhaps not as simple as we once thought (Levack & Siegert 2015). Goal setting is a complex intervention that requires behaviour changes from both health professionals and patients (Levack et al 2015a). Rehabilitation patients do not necessarily understand or agree with the concept of goal setting in the way intended by health professionals (Brown et al 2014). There is also a range of different reasons underpinning the use of goal setting in rehabilitation

129

(e.g., to enhance patient motivation, to support patient self-determination, to demonstrate the effectiveness of interventions on the basis of goal achievement and to improve teamwork), and although these reasons often can align, they can also at times conflict (Levack et al 2006a, 2006b, 2011). For instance, if goal achievement is being used primarily to demonstrate the effectiveness of a rehabilitation programme (i.e., as an outcome measure), then health professionals will be less inclined to agree to goals that a patient might value (i.e., supporting patient self-determination) if those goals are considered difficult to achieve from a clinical perspective.

It is becoming increasingly clear that one approach to goal setting is unlikely to be suitable in all possible rehabilitation scenarios. Instead, health professionals and health services need to become more sophisticated in their application of goal setting to rehabilitation, tailoring their whole approach to goals to the individual needs of the patient and adapting this at each stage of the recovery process. Goal setting (or even goal achievement) should not be viewed as an endpoint of rehabilitation. A rehabilitation service should not be evaluated on the 'quality' of its goals. Rather, goal setting should be viewed as a tool that health professionals use in different ways to achieve different effects, with the ultimate aim of maximising the best possible rehabilitation outcomes for patients and their families.

This chapter provides an overview of perspectives and research on goal setting in neurological rehabilitation. The chapter begins with a description of one pragmatic goal-setting approach for use in rehabilitation, focusing on person-centred goal identification and documentation, and on a method that can be used by all interdisciplinary team members. Following this, the notion of different approaches to goal setting in different clinical contexts is discussed. To illustrate this, examples are provided on the possible adaptation of goal setting to best meet the needs of patients and their families in different stages of recovery after stroke. Finally, a critique of the use of goal achievement as an outcome measure is offered, raising questions about whether the growing dominance of this concept is justified in neurological rehabilitation.

DEFINITIONS AND ASSUMPTIONS

Before any in-depth discussion of goal setting in rehabilitation, it is important to first clarify what is meant by key terms. This is because the word *goal* means many things to many people. Patients may retrospectively call any achievement that is made in rehabilitation a goal, even if these achievements were not the specific targets of interventions to begin with (Brown et al 2014) – because from the patient's perspective the real goal of rehabilitation is just

to get better. However, in the context of rehabilitation, the term *goal* is usually used to refer to a specific type of behavioural target, which is intended as the object of therapeutic intervention. Drawing on past work, the following subsections offer definitions.

Rehabilitation Goals and Goal Setting

A rehabilitation goal is 'a desired future state to be achieved by a person with a disability as a result of rehabilitation activities' with the additional criteria that rehabilitation goals are 'actively selected, intentionally created, have purpose and are shared (wherever possible) by the people participating in the activities and interventions designed to address the consequences of acquired disability' (Levack et al 2015b, p. 9). Rehabilitation goals also often describe desired achievements at the level of activity or participation as defined by the *International Classification of Functioning, Disability, and Health* (ICF) (World Health Organization 2001). For instance, a rehabilitation goal might be about a person's ability to walk, to speak, to return to living at home, to return to prior social roles, to return to paid employment, to use public transport and so forth. However, it may also be appropriate to set a goal around body structure and function. For instance, for a patient with severe spasticity affecting personal care, a goal around a specific increase in range of movement in a particularly problematic joint might be more clinically meaningful than an indirect goal describing that person's ability to be the passive recipient of washing.

The term *goal setting* can be used to refer to 'the establishment or negotiation of rehabilitation goals' (Levack et al 2015b, p. 9–10). Goal setting therefore focuses primarily on how goals are selected and agreed on. The term *goal planning* can be considered a synonym of 'goal setting' (Wade 1998).

Activities to Enhance Goal Pursuit

Activities around rehabilitation goals do not just stop at goal selection, however. 'Activities to enhance goal pursuit' can be described as 'activities related to how rehabilitation goals are communicated, used or shared in ways that enhance how effective or successful people are in working towards those goals' (Levack et al 2015b, p. 10). This includes activities to develop a documented plan to work towards achievement of stated rehabilitation goals. It might also include the use or discussion of goals in team meetings, family meetings or clinical consultation with the patient in question. Once set, rehabilitation goals ought not be left forgotten in a patient's clinical notes, but used in some way to guide clinical decision making, to encourage patients in their efforts or to help patients, family members and health professionals reflect on process or progress. For instance, some studies have successfully demonstrated the effectiveness of information technology (e.g., regular communication of goals via text messaging or electronic media) as a tool for helping people with brain injury in the community remember their goals of therapy (Culley & Evans 2010, Hart et al 2002).

PRAGMATIC PERSON-CENTRED GOAL SETTING

The process of goal setting can be separated into two key activities: (a) goal selection and (b) goal documentation. Goal selection involves the identification of an area of health, function or life that is a meaningful target for rehabilitation interventions, and the targeted level of performance in that area. Goal documentation involves the translation of that target into a statement that can be reported in a patient's clinical notes and used in discussion with the patient, their family and other team members.

Goal Selection

To set useful, person-centred goals in rehabilitation, health professionals need to know about:
- The patient's current and past health status;
- The patient's current and past functional abilities and limitations;
- The patient's prognosis from a biomedical perspective;
- The patient's past life context and social role;
- The social and physical environment in which the patient lives or hopes to return;
- The patient's personal strengths and resources (including internal factors such as resilience, creativity and self-belief, as well as external ones like social support, financial support and so forth); and
- The patient's values, priorities and ambitions for their recovery.

Some of this information (e.g., health status, functional abilities and prognosis) can be gathered from traditional methods for assessment of a person's health condition. Much of the rest of this information can be gathered only by talking to patients and/or their close family and friends. At times, it can feel difficult for health professionals to prioritise 'just talking' to patients and their family over the seemingly more practical task of actually delivering therapeutic interventions. However, the value of time spent on getting to know patients as people, understanding how they each make sense of their health and impairments and the contexts of their lives outside of the rehabilitation service should not be underestimated.

In the context of an interprofessional team, it is often sensible to have one person (usually a senior nurse or therapist) be a primary point of contact for the patient and family when it comes to rehabilitation planning – that is, a key worker. This person can be responsible for gathering person-centred information from the patient and sharing it with the rest of the team. A structured questionnaire like

> ### EXAMPLES OF KEY QUESTIONS: GOAL SELECTION
>
> - What do you hope to get out of rehabilitation?
> - Where do you see yourself in one month? One year? Five years?
> - What can't you do now that you want to be able to do?
> - Before your injury/illness, what was a typical day like for you? What did you do?
> - Tell me about your home. What is it like? Who lives there with you?
> - Tell me about your work/hobbies. What are your responsibilities? What do you do?
> - What can I help you with?
> - What are your main strengths? What is going to most help you through your recovery?
> - What is most important to you in your life now? What do you need to be able to do to achieve this/have this?
> - Tell me about what you know about your current health/illness/injury.
> - Do you have any concerns about your recovery that you have not talked about to anyone yet?

the Rivermead Life Goals Questionnaire (Nair 2003) can be useful to ensure that health professionals do not miss asking about an important area of someone's life or make incorrect assumptions about the patient's values and priorities.

Once this information is gathered, long-term goals are typically selected for the patient and team to work towards achieving at some point in the foreseeable future (sometimes by discharge; sometimes after discharge from the service in question), with short-terms goals being selected as the steps to be achieved on the path towards these long-term goals. Some services may prefer to use different terms to refer to long- and short-term goals, for example, aims, objectives and targets (Wade 1999b), but the key concept here is identifying short-term steps that need to be achieved to make progress towards some much longer-term, desired outcome.

Recently, technology has been increasingly used to support the involvement of patients in goal selection for rehabilitation. A scoping review identified 16 new technologies, including mobile apps and websites – some connected to wearable devices – that either included goal setting as a component of a digital self-management program or which were designed to support rehabilitation professionals and their clients engage in collaborative, person-centred goal setting (Strubbia et al 2020). One example of this type of new technology is the Aid for Decision Making in Occupational Choice (ADOC). ADOC is a Japanese iPad application that was originally design solely for use by occupational therapists (Tomori et al 2012, 2013a), but which has since been modified for use in English-speaking countries (Levack et al 2018) and tested for use by interprofessional teams (Strubbia et al 2021). ADOC differs from past approaches to goal setting by using a catalogue of text and images to help patients identify meaningful goals at the level of activity and participation that they would like to work towards, and by separating out goals selected by patients from those selected by health professionals before supporting a shared discussion of the objectives of rehabilitation. Early evidence on ADOC suggests that it helps patients understand the breadth of goals that can be considered as part of a rehabilitation programme and helps health professionals gain a more in-depth understanding about things that matter to patients (Strubbia et al 2021). ADOC has also been successfully used with people who have mild to moderate cognitive impairment (Tomori et al 2013b).

Goal Documentation

After selecting areas of health and functioning to feature as goals, the next job is to document these goals in some standardised way that all members of the interprofessional team – as well as the patient, their family and supporters – can understand. One approach to this, proposed by Randall and McEwen (2000), is to write a goal statement in such a way as to provide answers to five key questions.

A couple of points need to be explained regarding this approach to goal setting. Firstly, the answer to the first question 'Who?' should almost always be the patient. Writing all goal statements with the patient as the subject of the goals helps rehabilitation teams avoid documenting objectives that actually describe tasks for health professionals (or others) to perform rather than outcomes for the patient to achieve. For example, 'The occupational therapist will complete a home visit within 2 weeks' is not a goal for the patient to achieve as a result of therapy; it is a task that occupational therapists knows they will complete because it is part of their job. In comparison, 'Juan will walk up his path into his house with assistance of a stick and noncontact supervision of one person within 2 weeks' is a goal to be achieved by Juan (the patient), provided this is something he is not able to achieve at the time of writing.

KEY QUESTIONS: GOAL STATEMENT (RANDALL & MCEWEN 2000)

- Who?
- Will do what?
- Under what conditions?
- How well?
- By when?

The answer to the question 'Will do what?' should describe the function or activity that the patient is aiming to achieve at the end of therapy. In the earlier example, the activity in question, to be completed by Juan, is walking up a path into a house. To encourage health professionals and patients to be more specific regarding the nature of this task or activity, answers to the questions 'Under what conditions?' and 'How well?' provide prompts to specify the environmental context in which the function or activity is to be performed and the quality of performance, respectively. From the earlier example, the environmental conditions include the use of stick as a mobility aid (an environmental factor from the perspective of the ICF). The quality of performance in this case is indicated by reference to this activity being performed with non-contact supervision. An alternative approach to quality of performance might be to specify how long it should take Juan to safely navigate up his path into his house.

As noted earlier, this approach to goal documentation can be usefully adapted by all health professionals in an interprofessional rehabilitation team. To illustrate this, Table 6.1 provides examples of several goals relevant to the work of an interprofessional team in a brain injury rehabilitation unit.

A similar approach to goal documentation is the SMART approach (Bovend'Eerdt et al 2009). SMART is an acronym used to refer to the recommended components of any goal statement. Randall and McEwen's (2000) approach has several advantages over the SMART approach when it comes to guidelines for goal documentation, however. Firstly, there are a variety of interpretations as to what the SMART acronym actually stands for (McPherson et al 2015). The A, for instance, has been used to refer to goals that are achievable, acceptable, ambitious, activity-related, actionable and so forth (McPherson et al 2015). Doran (1981), who originally published the SMART acronym, stated that the A was for 'Assignable – specifically who will do it' (p. 36). Secondly, there is often redundancy in the SMART acronym. For example, goals that are 'measurable' are already 'specific' – both of these terms do not need to be stated.

Thirdly, although the SMART acronym encourages the setting of 'specific' (and/or 'measurable') goals, it provides little guidance on how to make a goal specific. Randall and McEwen's (2000) approach addresses this gap by giving more direction regarding the actual components of a goal statement. Fourthly, elements of the SMART acronym (depending on how it is interpreted) are not well substantiated by research evidence (Swann et al 2022). For example, one common interpretation of the A and R in SMART is that they refer to goals that are 'achievable' and 'realistic'. However, there is no evidence to suggest that achievable or realistic goals result in better outcomes for the patient or better engagement in their therapy (Levack et al 2015b). Indeed there is extensive evidence from behavioural

TABLE 6.1 Case Study Example of Interprofessional Rehabilitation Goals

Background

Sakura is an 18-year-old woman who suffered a serious traumatic brain injury when her bike collided with a car. She was in a coma for 2 weeks but began recovering rapidly after waking up. A month after her injury, Sakura is in an inpatient rehabilitation unit. She is able to walk independently, but has very low cardiovascular fitness and tires easily. She needs assistance from one person to wash herself in the shower because of fatigue, balance and coordination problems. Her stay in the intensive care unit, coupled with loss of appetite, has resulted in significant weight loss such that she is now underweight according her body mass index. She also has had difficulty communicating since she was extubated. Her speech is quiet and slurred to the point that she is resorting almost entirely to gestures to indicate her basic needs. Sakura is also experiencing difficulties with managing her frustration and is lashing out physically at staff and other patients a couple of times a day, which according to her family is completely out of character for her.

Breakdown of Goals

Who?	Will Do What?	Under What Conditions?	How Well?	By When?	Health Professionals Likely to Be Involved?
Sakura	Gain 5 kg	Following a structured dietary plan	—	Within 10 weeks	Nurse, dietician, physiotherapist
Sakura	Complete a 6-minute walk test	Indoors	Walking 450 m	Within 3 weeks	Physiotherapist
Sakura	Wash herself	In the shower, using a shower stool for fatigue	Independently	Within 2 weeks	Occupational therapist, nurse
Sakura	Communicate her basic needs	Verbally	With minimal slurring of words	Within 3 weeks	Speech language therapist
Sakura	Have no episodes of physical aggression	During ordinary, everyday social interactions	With no relapses over a 1-week period	By 4 weeks	Nurse, clinical psychologist

Formulation of Sakura's Goals for Her Rehabilitation Plan

- Sakura will gain 5 kg following a structured dietary plan within 10 weeks.
- Sakura will walk at least 450 m indoors on the 6-minute walk test within 3 weeks.
- Sakura will independently wash herself in the shower, using a shower stool to manage fatigue, within 2 weeks.
- Sakura will communicate her basic needs verbally, with minimal slurring of words, within 3 weeks.
- Sakura will have no episodes of physical aggression during ordinary, everyday social interactions, with no relapses for a 1-week period, within 4 weeks.

psychology to suggest that highly ambitious, potentially unachievable goals result in a greater level of engagement in tasks compared with easily achievable or self-set goals (Locke and Latham 2002, Swann et al 2022), although further research is required to examine the application of these ideas in the context of neurorehabilitation.

Family Involvement in Goal Setting

In general, family members are considered an important group of people to involve in rehabilitation planning. (Here, the term *family* is used in its widest possible sense to include anyone who is considered family from the perspective of the patient rather than just biological relatives.) In the context of adult rehabilitation, the involvement of family in goal setting can be challenging for health professionals. Although often family members are viewed as a valuable source of information about a patient before their injury or illness, or even a surrogate for the patient's voice if a patient has significant cognitive or communicative impairments (Law et al 2014, McClain 2005, McGrath et al 1995, Randall & McEwen 2000), their involvement in the goal-setting process can be contested. Health professionals may be reluctant to involve some family members if they think the family members have expectations for rehabilitation that they cannot address or if they believe the family members are negatively affecting their clinical relationship with the patient (Levack et al 2009, Sherratt et al 2011). Nonetheless, families need to be involved in conversations around the objectives of rehabilitation if they are going to be the ones who are providing ongoing support for the people with the injuries or illnesses after they leave the health service (Tang Yan et al 2014). A family-centred approach to goal setting may also be important for cultural reasons (Foster et al 2012, Harwood 2010).

Also contested is the idea about whether family members should be the subject of a rehabilitation goal (i.e., the 'Who' in the rehabilitation goal statement). Indeed, Randall and McEwen (2000) explicitly stated that family members should never be the focus of a goal, taking a position similar to others on the topic (McMillan & Sparkes 1999). An alternative perspective is that neurological conditions such as stroke, spinal cord injury or traumatic brain injury should be considered family illnesses (i.e., affecting the well-being of all members of a family). As such, it is appropriate for rehabilitation interventions to focus on their needs as well as those of the patient – although of course the extent to which this can happen will depend in part on funding availability. Examples of topics for family-oriented goals of therapy when one member of the family has a traumatic brain injury have been provided by Kreutzer et al (2010). These include objectives such as addressing feelings of guilt, loss of intimacy in relationships or being able to take physical care of oneself when also being a primary caregiver to another person with a disability.

Should Goals Be Measurable?

One common recommendation in rehabilitation literature is that all rehabilitation goals ought to be measureable. Indeed, Randall and McEwen's (2000) approach is one way that a behavioural target can be converted into an operationalised goal, which can be objectively evaluated by a third party as either 'achieved' or 'not achieved'. However, not all things that are important to people are simple to measure. Goals around intimate relationships or spirituality, for instance, are not easily quantifiable. If a man, after a traumatic brain injury, wants to set the goal 'to be a better husband', it would be tempting for a rehabilitation team to reduce this complex (and important) life goal to a simple, measureable activity, such as 'Juan will remember to buy his wife flowers on their anniversary'. This kind of goal is tokenistic and fails to encapsulate the intent of the man's actual aim. To return to a point made at the beginning of this chapter, goal setting ought to be considered a tool that health professionals can use to further the objectives of therapy; it is not an endpoint in itself. At times, it is appropriate to deviate from a standardised approach to goal setting to document and acknowledge goals that are meaningful to the people at the centre of the rehabilitation service.

GOAL SETTING IN STROKE REHABILITATION – ADDRESSING THE CHANGING NEEDS FROM ACUTE CARE TO COMMUNITY LIFE

To illustrate the concept of needing to adapt one's approach to goal setting to a specific clinical condition and stages of rehabilitation, consider the example of rehabilitation for moderate to severe stroke. For the purposes of this example, recovery after stroke is divided into four broad phases: (a) acute (1–7 days after stroke); (b) hospital-based early subacute (7 days to 3 months after stroke), (c) community-based late subacute (3–6 months after stroke), and (d) ongoing life after stroke (6+ months after stroke) (Bernhardt et al 2017).

Figure 6.1 provides a visual representation of these phases of recovery mapped onto life goals, programme goals, weekly goals (within each programme of rehabilitation) and therapy session goals. The programme goals and weekly goals in this case are used to represent the long-term and short-term goals of the rehabilitation programmes in various stages of the recovery process.

Life goals and therapy session goals are not 'rehabilitation goals' in the usual sense of the term (as defined earlier in this chapter). The term *life goals* is a psychological concept that refers to 'the desired states that people seek to obtain, maintain or avoid' (Nair 2003, p. 193). It includes the concept of an 'idealised self-image' – the person an individual spends their lifetime striving to be. Life goals can be interrupted by sudden trauma, illness or injury, but span the time well before rehabilitation and continue long after health professional input ceases. Conversely, the term *therapy session goals* is being used here to refer to the informal targets that a therapist might set a person to reach (or that patients might set themselves) during individual therapy sessions (e.g., 'I want you to stand up and sit down 10 times in a row without pushing up with your hands. Can you do that in less than 2 minutes?').

The following information is intended to illustrate the point that different approaches to goal setting are probably needed in different clinical situations – even within the context of a single health condition.

Acute Rehabilitation
Case Description

Mrs Wilson is admitted to the emergency department after being found on the floor in her bedroom by her daughter. She

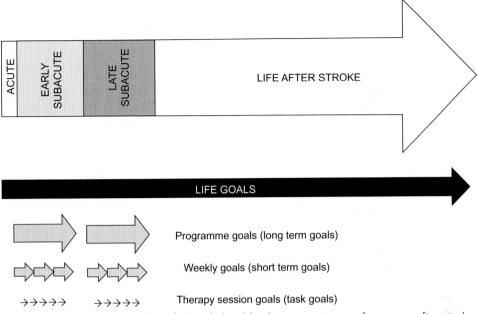

FIG. 6.1 Visual representation of the relationships between stages of recovery after stroke and types of rehabilitation goals.

is dehydrated and hungry after being unable to move from the floor for most of the day. In the emergency department, she is unable to sit upright independently and cannot get from lying to sitting without maximal assistance of two people. She has dense left-sided hemiplegia. A brain scan reveals a large ischemic stroke involving the right middle cerebral artery. Mrs Wilson and her daughter are very worried. Before being found by her daughter, Mrs Wilson had been wondering if she was going to die. She is transferred to an acute stroke unit for management.

In the acute phase of illness after a moderate to severe stroke, the thing that patients and families need most is strong, confident and competent health professional leadership. What most patients generally do not need at this point in recovery (immediately after a life-threatening event) is to be asked open-ended questions about their desired outcomes from rehabilitation a year hence. Indeed, some have argued that person-centred care during acute medical events comes with risks of significantly worse health outcomes that need to be considered before person-centredness is unquestioningly adopted in all clinical contexts (Heidenreich 2013). This is because patients with acute medical events usually do not yet have a comprehensive understanding of their health condition, what therapies they are actually likely to benefit from or what they should expect in terms of outcomes.

Thus, many people who have experienced their first stroke need time to adjust to the impact of the condition on their lives, and time to learn about stroke as a disease and its consequences (Lloyd et al 2014). In this context, a fiduciary model of care is justifiable (Blackmer 2000, Levack et al 2015c). Fiduciary care involves health professionals taking charge of decision making over a patient's health, well-being and treatment during this time of adjustment (without, of course, overtly coercing a patient or acting against their wishes). What distinguishes fiduciary care from medical paternalism is the notion that this authority over clinical decision making is only temporary, with the health professional actively assessing the patient's readiness, over time, to retake charge of the decisions about their health and well-being once again. In situations where patients have significant problems with communication or cognition (particularly orientation to time, place and person), it may be appropriate for health professionals to retain fiduciary care (with appropriate input from family members) longer than is otherwise normally needed.

Regardless of a patient's capacity for decision making, in the acute stages of stroke, one thing that all patients and families need is hope (Bright et al 2011, Snyder et al 2006). There can be a tendency among health professionals to emphasise the importance of being 'realistic' in the early stages of stroke recovery. In this and other clinical contexts, health professionals can worry about the possible negative consequences of instilling false hope. Health professionals working in neurological rehabilitation can be concerned about setting up patients with unrealistic expectations, and so encourage patients to focus instead on the small, achievable next step.

Contrary to this position, Snyder et al (2006) argued that there is no such thing as false hope in rehabilitation, and contended that this view has been empirically demonstrated. In a review of studies on patients' hopes, they report that 'people with high hope may aspire to some goals that are moderately unlikely' and that 'people with high hope recognise that some of their goals are improbable, but they use this knowledge as motivation to more vigorously pursue the goals and to gain a more positive perspective on their situation' (Snyder et al 2006, p. 94).

A good example of the interrelationships between goals, hope, motivation and expectations in acute stroke rehabilitation is the issue of early retraining of mobility. Consider the following:

- All stroke patients, who were independently mobile before their stroke, begin with the goal 'to walk again'. Health professionals may wish to dilute this goal – perhaps setting a goal around other forms of mobility first (sitting balance, standing, transfers); perhaps avoiding formally setting walking as a goal if they are unsure about the time frame that might be needed to achieve it (Levack et al 2011) – but regardless, this goal will be at the forefront of most, if not all, patients' minds during acute and subacute rehabilitation.
- Early mobilisation within 1 or 2 days of stroke onset is now standard rehabilitation practice (Bernhardt et al 2015, Rethnam et al 2022). As such, all rehabilitation teams have independent mobility as a key objective to achieve during the first weeks or months of therapy, even if this is not documented in a patient's notes as a formal goal of therapy.
- The ability for health professionals to predict who is actually likely to walk or not walk after stroke, based on early presentation, is far from completely accurate. Even the best predictive models (based on factors such as age, early functional ability and sitting balance) fail to correctly predict future mobility or immobility in all patients (Kollen et al 2006). Predictive models like this work well at a population level, but provide only probabilistic information at the level of individual patients.

Given all this, a question worth considering is why all patients do not automatically have independent mobility as a documented rehabilitation goal during the acute stage of stroke rehabilitation, even if this goal is considered highly ambitious? Health professionals' concern about setting up patients with unrealistic expectations by documenting overly ambitious goals can be ameliorated by separating discussion of goals from discussion of expectations. A health professional can communicate with patients an ambitious goal while at the same time making it clear what the likelihood is of achieving that goal. The conversation to separate out goal setting from expectations could go something like this:

> 'So, Mrs Wilson, you've had a really bad stroke. Now, I'm not going to mislead you – most people who have a stroke as severe as yours are not always able to leave hospital walking independently. However, people do often surprise us. How about we work on getting you to be one of those people who surprise us? It's going to take a lot of effort on both our parts, but what do you think about us setting a goal of you being able to walk independently, maybe with a frame or a stick, in 2 months? I can't promise how far we might get, but I don't see why we shouldn't be ambitious to begin with. What do you think?'

Another reason why health professionals might be reluctant to set a goal around independent walking for a person after a severe stroke is if they are also using goals to demonstrate the effectiveness of their therapy. This means that goal setting cannot be used to instil hope in patients and encourage motivation in this way at the same time as being used as an outcome measure. Health professionals need to decide which purpose for goal setting is more important in their clinical practice, and structure their approach to goal setting accordingly. Similar arguments can be made around health professional leadership in goal setting for other aspects of basic functioning and well-being in the early days of stroke recovery (e.g., communication, self-cares and toileting).

In summary, goal setting in the acute stage (1–7 days) of stroke probably ought to be specific, therapist-led and ambitious. Goals at this stage should focus on the best possible outcomes to instil hope, rather than focusing on conservative outcomes that are easy or highly likely to be achieved. Discussion of these rehabilitation goals with patients ought to include information about the health professionals' expectations regarding how difficult a particular goal might be, while at the same time encouraging patients to think that they are capable of rising to the challenge of giving their recovery the best possible shot.

Hospital-Based Early Subacute Rehabilitation
Case Description

After a week in the acute stroke unit, Mrs Wilson is medically stable and is transferred to a general rehabilitation ward, which has expertise in early subacute stroke rehabilitation.

She is assigned a keyworker on the ward, who reviews her medical file from the acute stroke unit and meets with her to discuss plans for the remainder of her stay in hospital. Early on, the keyworker introduces the notion of planning for discharge, and spends time with Mrs Wilson and her daughter finding out about her life before stroke, her values and priorities for recovery, and gets to know her as a person. The keyworker documents and feeds this information back to the rest of the rehabilitation team. Members of the interprofessional team begin to set goals for Mrs Wilson to achieve to work towards her aim of returning home. Although returning home is Mrs Wilson's main objective, the rehabilitation team is careful not to make any promises about her recovery, but indicate that they are committed to helping her recover as best she possibly can. Mrs Wilson is still unable to sit on the edge of her bed independently, her left arm is densely hemiplegic, she is incontinent of urine (although this might be partly caused by difficulty with accessing the toilet) and the therapy staff suspect some visual perceptual problems are contributing to her functional deficits. However, Mrs Wilson is fully communicative, has good memory and other cognitive abilities and reports being very determined to work hard at her therapy. She needs a lot of support in her rehabilitation, certainly to begin with, because she is still unable to do very much by herself.

For the purposes of this chapter, early subacute rehabilitation can be considered to start once a person is medically stable and beginning to work towards returning to the community – approximately a week after stroke onset. Depending on how unwell a person is and whether they have significant comorbidities, hospital-based subacute rehabilitation may continue for some weeks to months after the stroke event (Bernhardt et al 2017).

Arguably, in an ideal world (i.e., with unlimited funding) subacute rehabilitation might almost entirely occur in a person's home. The justification for this perspective is that early supported discharge services, which reduce hospital length of stay, appear to result in better functional outcomes and higher patient satisfaction with service delivery than traditional inpatient rehabilitation (Langhorne et al 2017). Although the reasons for these improvements have not been empirically established, it has been suggested that home environments are more enriched and stimulating than hospital environments, which encourages generally greater activity levels, and that training in inpatient rehabilitation has limited transferability to the 'real world' of functioning at home (Indredavik et al 2000).

The primary reason for keeping people in hospital is that stroke rehabilitation is dose dependent, i.e., more intensive rehabilitation is better (Lohse et al 2014), and it is assumed that it is more cost-effective to deliver high-intensity rehabilitation in an institutional environment. Despite best efforts, however, stroke patients often spend most of their day in rehabilitation wards inactive, alone and in their bedrooms (Adey-Wakeling et al 2021, Blennerhassett et al 2018, Jones et al 2021, West & Bernhardt 2012). Many people may well be better served by receiving more of their rehabilitation in the community.

All this means that the main objective (i.e., the main 'goal') of admission to inpatient stroke rehabilitation is often simply discharge – assuming, of course, that rehabilitation can continue in the community. To put it another way, planning for discharge needs to begin on admission to subacute rehabilitation, if not before. This 'goal' is usually repackaged in inpatient stroke rehabilitation to be about a series of achievable, time-bound targets related to a minimum level of functional performance required for community living: walking, talking, eating, toileting, self-cares, arm/hand function and so on. Goals for inpatient rehabilitation can (and should) be individualised to better match the life context and personal values of each person with stroke, but overall the goals of inpatient rehabilitation will necessarily draw on similar activities required for community living. For instance, one person might not particularly care if they can wash independently or have a shower, but all people need be able to deal with hygiene issues one way or another after leaving hospital.

This perspective on inpatient rehabilitation goal planning (i.e., that for all patients the main 'goal' of admission is 'discharge') goes some way to explain why, in observational studies of clinical practice, health professionals still tend to dominate discussion of goal selection (Barnard et al 2010, Levack et al 2011). Inpatient health professionals tend to be oriented towards what needs to be achieved to return someone to the community. Regardless, the subacute stage of rehabilitation is the time when health professionals need to begin relinquishing some control over decision making. From the perspective of a fiduciary model of care, this involves empowering the person with the stroke to take greater control over decisions about their health and recovery once more. Indeed recent studies suggest that it is possible to begin training for self-management after stroke in inpatient subacute rehabilitation (Jones et al 2013) or even in acute stroke units (Mäkelä et al 2014). Central to self-management is the ability and authority to set goals for yourself.

This does not mean that patients should be left entirely to their own devices when it comes to goal setting. Rehabilitation professionals have a role in challenging patients' expectations, encouraging patients to be ambitious when needed and educating them about the consequences of stroke. There are still risks associated with a fully patient-directed approach to goal selection. For instance, in one qualitative study, a stroke patient was found to report regret some months after discharge from hospital because she had not specified a goal to improve her arm function while in inpatient stroke rehabilitation (Brown et al 2014). She stated that, when asked by therapists, she had chosen to prioritise mobility over arm function while in hospital, and believed that the therapists had minimised their attention to her hemiplegic upper limb as a result. Regardless of whether she was right or wrong about the influence of her personal goals on the behaviour of the health professionals, this woman felt at fault for having not prioritised both her upper and lower limb function while in hospital, and thought she had suffered a poorer outcome as a result.

At some point in early subacute rehabilitation, it might become increasingly clear that a patient is not going to achieve their best possible desired outcome. By 2 or 3 months after stroke, a patient's basic motor function will be broadly approaching what they can expect to achieve in the longer term (Meyer et al 2015). At this point, revision of goals is likely to be necessary. A goal for some form of walking with aid might need to be replaced by a goal to achieve mobility by use of transfers and a wheelchair. A goal for independent speech might need to be replaced by communication with the aid of assistive technology. If it appears that a person is going to be completely unable to return home, then the goals of therapy typically move on to maximising functional independence in personally meaningful areas of life in residential care. In this context, opportunities for patients to discuss their disappointment with their recovery ought to be provided and acknowledged. However, patients in this situation also ought to be encouraged to find ways to engage with previously meaningful social roles and occupational pursuits in a modified capacity.

In summary, goal setting in early subacute inpatient rehabilitation needs to primarily provide direction to discharge. Patients need health professionals to provide them with compassion and encouragement, challenging them to be ambitious in terms of their recovery, but updating them about the likely outcomes from their stroke as they progress. Patients also need help to connect the intent of prescribed therapeutic activities and their efforts in inpatient rehabilitation with life outside the hospital after stroke. From the perspective of mood and motivation, patients do also benefit from early experiences of success. This success may be in terms of early goal achievement, but any functional gains can also be used to signal progress.

Community-Based Late Subacute Rehabilitation
Case Description

After 11 weeks in hospital, Mrs Wilson has regained the ability to sit independently on the edge of her bed and can transfer safely by herself from a bed or chair into a wheelchair. She is able to stand up with the aid of a rail for support and take a few shuffling steps, and can even walk short distances with a walking frame plus the assistance of her daughter. Her ongoing problems with balance mean that she is not able to walk safely by herself. She is mostly continent, although now wears pads for extra protection during both night and day. Although her daughter is very concerned about Mrs Wilson's safety and social isolation at home, she is willing to support her mother's strong desire to give home another try rather than move straight into a nursing home. Mrs Wilson is able to self-propel indoors, can get herself on and off the toilet, and can safely make herself a cup of tea and snacks in her kitchen. Although Mrs Wilson wants to continue to work on her physical fitness, her main aim now that she is back at home is to somehow return to a community art group for older adults that she had joined 6 months before her stroke. However, she is really not sure how she is going to be able to manage this. A paid caregiver is visiting her regularly to help with showers, and her daughter, who lives locally, can pop in daily, but otherwise Mrs Wilson is managing alone.

The period shortly after discharge from hospital is one full of new challenges for people with stroke. It is a period that can be characterised by uncertainty and grief as the reality of life after stroke begins to become more apparent (Arntzen et al 2015 Cott 2004, 2007, Timothy et al 2016). While in hospital, people with stroke have a high degree of contact with health professionals and with other people going through similar experiences. Early stroke recovery is also associated with more rapid recovery of functional abilities than later recovery. Although people with stroke may have been told and intellectually understand that their physical recovery is plateauing, these people may not really know what life with physical impairments is actually going to be like until they experience it outside of hospital. Furthermore, once at home, health professional contact reduces to just formally scheduled, less frequent events.

The period after discharge from hospital is also when people begin to reflect on or be troubled by changes to their sense of self after stroke (Arntzen et al 2015, Ellis-Hill et al 2008, Timothy et al 2016). This can include problems with making sense of their experiences of a body that has always been part of them, but now may act, respond and feel subjectively different (Timothy et al 2016). Problems with self-identity can also arise from disruptions of social roles and life goals as a consequence of disability (Ellis-Hill et al 2009, Thomas et al 2015). Timely input from rehabilitation professionals is highly valuable at this stage. In particular, it has been suggested that people do best on return home after a stroke if they are able to maintain a sense of momentum in their recovery, if they feel well supported by health professionals, family and friends and if they feel informed about their recovery and available healthcare services going forwards (Ellis-Hill et al 2009).

Goal setting at this stage helps provide a road map for learning to live with stroke in the community. In early community-based rehabilitation, goal setting should move from a focus on basic functional needs for community living towards being more about personally meaningful occupations and social participation. It is also important to consider goals around holistic well-being (e.g., cardiovascular fitness, eating well) and prevention of secondary problems arising from stroke, such as cardiac or renal disease, fractures from falls and depression (Kumar et al 2010).

Once in the community, rehabilitation professionals have the opportunity to get a lot more creative regarding the goals of therapy. People's lives in the community are far more diverse than they are in the institutional environment of a hospital. Similarly, the selection of goals for therapy can be more diverse, relating to issues such as self-management in the home, hobbies, accessing and making use of community facilities, paid or unpaid work or fulfilling social roles associated with friends and family (e.g., playing with grandchildren). Some people may wish to continue to work on trying to improve their functional abilities in areas such as mobility, upper limb function or speech. Even if physical recovery has plateaued at a biological level, people still have opportunities to learn new ways of being physically active with the function abilities that they have, and health professional input can be highly valuable to guide this learning.

Thus, in community-based rehabilitation, patients should be encouraged to take much more control over the selection of goals and the direction of therapy, with support from their family where needed. In other words, rehabilitation goals should be increasingly patient or family led. The role of health professionals at this point should be to provide targeted therapy or creative solutions to adapt environments or provide aids to achieve these goals. Health professionals may also have a role in helping patients adhere to plans to pursue goals that they have set themselves. McPherson et al (2015) have argued that the theory of intentional action control may be of value in this regard. The theory of intentional action control posits that successful self-regulation of behaviour requires two things: intention and implementation (Achziger et al 2012).

From the perspectives of rehabilitation, goal setting is a process used to identify and articulate a person's (or a team's) *intentions*. However, just having a goal is insufficient to create change. A person (or a team) needs to do something different, and usually keep doing it for a while, to achieve this change. In other words, actions are required to *implement* a plan to achieve a goal. While in hospital, patients have health professionals on hand to help with this implementation. In the community, however, much

of the activity for a patient to achieve a goal needs to be self-directed.

To help patients pursue a goal, McPherson et al (2015) have suggested that a specific type of implementation plan, called *if-then* plans, may be of value. If-then plans are fairly simple, but potentially powerful (Bieleke et al 2021). They involve identifying and documenting what a person will do when certain conditions occur. For instance, '*If* my daughter comes to visit, *then* I will practice getting down onto the floor and back up again three times while she is around'.

This approach also allows the patient and the health professional to consider barriers to implementation of this plan, and to come up with and document alternative strategies if these other conditions occur. These documents, which stay with the patient, then help the patients as reminders or guides for action. For instance, '*If* I'm feeling like I don't want to exercise when my daughter is here, *then* I will remind myself that it is important to stay fit to keep living by myself at home, and that it is much better to practice getting off the floor when she is here than when she isn't'. Alternatively, '*If* my daughter is not able to visit for 3 days, *then* I will ask my caregiver to help me practice getting up off the floor'. Although research into implementation intentions in neurorehabilitation is still developing, a systematic review of clinical trials has shown that implementation intention strategies can result in a modest increase of physical activity levels in populations of adults with general chronic health conditions (da Silva et al 2018).

In summary, once in the community, goal setting should become increasingly patient (or family) led, although health professional involvement may still be important for helping patients identify areas for goal selection. Patients are likely to need support with their transition from hospital to home, and goals around activities or roles in everyday living are likely to be particularly valuable. Patients should be encouraged at this stage to begin to think of themselves as managers of their own recovery, with support from their family. In addition to goal setting, patients may also need help with development of a plan to work towards achieving their goals at times when health professionals are no longer present.

Ongoing Life After Stoke
Case Description

Six months after her stroke, Mrs Wilson is still living independently at home. She had a period of depression that required input from her family physician, but has been feeling a bit better about her life in recent weeks. Mrs Wilson did manage to return to her community art group, which meets fortnightly. Having learnt how to safely transfer by herself from her wheelchair into a car, she is now getting lifts from a friend in the art group. Mrs Wilson was initially embarrassed about being seen in public in a wheelchair but decided that her pride should not stop her getting out and about when opportunities arise. Rather, she has chosen to take pride in her stubbornness. Mrs Wilson is trying to do a little bit of exercise at home – practicing standing and trying to get a little more control and strength in her left arm. She is no longer gaining any more strength in her hemiplegic side but wants to maintain what she has, and it feels good to be doing something for herself. Her last contact with a rehabilitation professional was 2 months ago.

At some point during the recovery process, rehabilitation professionals cease being actively involved, and medical care passes over to the person's general practitioner or family physician. The person with stroke may have largely maximised their physical recovery at this stage, but still has a long way to go in terms of learning to live with a chronic health condition. Opportunities for improving a person's quality of life exist in terms of learning new ways of doing things, starting new occupational activities or returning to old ones, and through positive social connections with others – family, friends or even members of the general public.

People who have survived stroke are no longer 'patients' at this point, having exited the hospital system. Instead, they should be encouraged to think of themselves as their own rehabilitation professionals – experts of their own health condition. If the person with stroke is too impaired to really lead their own recovery, this mantle of 'leader of recovery' can be passed to a close family member or main caregiver. People after stroke still benefit from a rehabilitation approach to recovery at this stage, however, and so can benefit from making use of goal-setting strategies. Rehabilitation goal setting at this stage should be entirely directed by the person with the stroke and/or their family or carers, both in terms of goal selection and development of activities for goal pursuit.

Two examples of using goal setting like this include the Bridges self-management programme in the UK, and the Take Charge intervention that was successfully studied in a clinical trial in New Zealand. Bridges is an individualised, self-management programme with a strong foundation in social cognitive theory and self-efficacy principles (Jones et al 2009, McKenna et al 2015). Bridges involves a training programme for people with stroke and their families to follow, which teaches people to identify their own goals for improving their health and well-being, then to develop their own strategies to pursue these goals. The degree to which people with stroke lead the selection of goals – unrestrained by the priorities, preference or values of health professionals – is one of the key characteristics of the Bridges approach (McKenna et al 2015). Preliminary clinical trials of this programme suggest that it may result in positive

changes in functional activity and social integration after stroke, although designing scientifically robust trials of the programme is challenging because of the highly complex nature of the intervention (Jones et al 2016, McKenna et al 2015).

A similar kind of programme for people with stroke in the community is the Take Charge intervention. Designed as a family-centred approach to community-based stroke rehabilitation, this intervention also involves a focus on helping people pick their own goals for recovery and develop their own strategies to achieve these goals. Two fully powered, randomised controlled trials of this intervention have demonstrated that it results in statistically and clinically significant improvements in quality of life, as well as a reduction of dependency on family carers 1 year after the intervention (Fu et al 2020, Harwood et al 2011).

In summary, goal setting continues to be a potentially useful strategy for people with stroke to use on their own or with their family, long after rehabilitation professionals have otherwise stopped being formally involved. Training for self-management while people are in formal rehabilitation services should include consideration of how they can continue to lead their own recovery after discharge. Further clinical trials of goal-directed, patient- or family-driven self-management programmes are warranted.

KEY POINTS FOR GOAL SETTING IN STROKE REHABILITATION

- Different approaches to goal setting are likely to be needed in different clinical contexts (Levack & Siegert 2015).
- Goal setting needs to be adapted to each stage of the recovery process.
- Goals should progress from a focus on basic functional needs towards meaningful occupation and participation in community living.
- Health professionals can have a tendency to emphasise the importance of setting goals that are realistic, although this may not always be in the best interests of patients (Levack et al 2011).
- Health professionals need to consider the relationship between goals, hope, motivation, expectations and ambitions. Discussion of goals should be separated from the discussion of expectations (Snyder et al 2006).
- Hope is a critical concept in neurological rehabilitation. Goals in the acute stage should focus on the best possible outcomes to instil hope (Bright et al 2011, Snyder et al 2006).

- When in hospital, patients need help to connect the intent of therapy activities and their effects with life outside the hospital (Cott 2007).
- Goal setting requires behaviour changes from both health professionals and patients.
- Having a goal is insufficient to create change; actions are also required. If-then plans may be of value in this regard (McPherson et al 2015).
- Providing training to people with stroke and their family in self-directed goal setting may help them continue to improve their function and well-being long after rehabilitation professionals have stopped being formally involved (Fu et al 2020, Harwood et al 2011, Jones et al 2009, McKenna et al 2015).

GOAL ACHIEVEMENT AS AN OUTCOME MEASURE – CHALLENGING CURRENT ASSUMPTIONS

One attractive idea in goal-setting practice is the notion that individual achievement of a patient's goal (or goals) might be a useful way to evaluate the effectiveness of the rehabilitation services they received. Goal achievement, and in particular Goal Attainment Scaling (GAS), has risen in prominence as a strategy for individualised outcome measurement. In the UK, for instance, reporting on GAS scores is currently a core part of the contracted service specifications for specialised rehabilitation involving patients with highly complex needs and is linked to the benchmarking of performance for those services (NHS England 2013). The question is: Should other countries follow suit? Is individualised goal achievement a good method for judging how successful rehabilitation providers have been in their work or to compare one rehabilitation provider group with another?

The Appeal of Goal Attainment As an Outcome

Goal achievement, and GAS in particular, has gained popularity in neurorehabilitation for a number of reasons. Neurorehabilitation patients often present with a wide variety of problems. One person after a stroke might have difficulty with walking, upper limb function and visual perceptual deficits, but have largely intact memory, communication and cognition. Another person might regain physical functions after stroke fairly quickly and mainly have problems with communication and swallowing. This means that it can be difficult finding a standardised outcome measure that is relevant to all people with neurological illness or injuries, with few redundant items for most

people. It has been argued that individualised goal attainment addresses this problem by converting this heterogeneity in presentation to a common metric: the degree to which a person achieves what they and the rehabilitation team set out to achieve through the provision of targeted therapy (Turner-Stokes 2009).

The individualisation of goals for the purposes of outcome measurement is also attractive because of its potential to address problems around the sensitivity of standardised outcome measures (Turner-Stokes 2009). Because individualised goals can be tailored to reflect relatively small degrees of change in outcome, they can be made to reflect improvements in function that would otherwise be missed by general outcome measures such as the Barthel Index or the Functional Independence Measure.

There is also appeal in the idea of involving patients in the selection of criteria on which to judge the effectiveness of a programme of rehabilitation. A person-centred healthcare service should not only involve patients and family members in setting the direction of therapy, but also involve them in how success in rehabilitation is evaluated and against what criteria. Goal attainment as an outcome appears to support this moral objective.

An Overview of Goal Attainment Scaling

Multiple publications present a GAS approach to outcome measurement in rehabilitation (e.g., Steenbeek et al 2015, Turner-Stokes 2009), so a detailed overview of this method will not be provided here. In summary, however, GAS involves the creation of a multipoint scale, usually with five levels, where each point of the scale represents a different level of achievement or nonachievement of a goal. The midpoint on a GAS scale is established as the *expected* level of achievement and is given a score of 0. This midpoint is operationalised as an objectively described goal for the patient to reach. Then four related outcomes are documented that describe: (1) much worse than expected, (2) a little worse than expected, (3) a little better than expected, and (4) much better than expected levels of achievement related to that goal. They are given the scores −2, −1, +1 and +2, respectively. Often, it is recommended that the patient's current level of performance is set as the description for the −1 score, allowing the −2 score to be used to record deteriorations in outcome if these occur. Turner-Stokes and Williams (2010) have suggested an alternative, which is to add a sixth GAS level to allow for situations where a person might improve somewhat from their baseline performance (i.e., better than the −1 score, as described earlier), but less than the expected level of outcome, suggesting that a score of −0.5 be used to report partial achievement of an expected goal. When an individual person has multiple goals, it is then supposed to be possible to combine the

GAS scores from each of these scales into a single 'T-score' using a prescribed calculation (for more details on calculating T-scores, see Turner-Stokes 2009).

One consideration with using GAS scales in clinical practice is the time it takes to develop them. To make GAS a bit easier for busy rehabilitation teams to use, Ashford and Turner-Stokes (2015) have described a simplified version of the approach, which they call GAS-light. This abbreviated approach to GAS requires health professionals to invest time carefully describing the 0 point on the GAS scale (i.e., the expected outcome), but not the other levels in detail. Then, when a patient's outcome is being evaluated, the +2, +1, −1 and −2 scores are replaced with generic assessments of whether a person has 'greatly exceeded', 'exceeded', 'not quite achieved' or was 'nowhere near' the target goals, respectively. An example of a GAS scale is presented in Table 6.2.

Problems With Goal Attainment As an Outcome

GAS as an outcome measure has a number of criticisms. Grant and Ponsford (2014) have highlighted that setting GAS goals is time consuming, an issue addressed in part by the GAS-light approach described earlier. Grant and Ponsford (2014) have also noted the lack of guidelines for how to interpret T-scores, in particular the range of T-scores that are considered to represent 'acceptable' goal attainment. In addition, they have criticised GAS for its dependence on the user's skill level in setting and documenting GAS scales.

Other authors have criticised the T-score itself. T-scores start with the assumption that GAS produces interval data (i.e., data that are uni-dimensional, ordered, with the same quantity of change between steps on the measure, such as centimetre increments on a ruler). Using Rasch analysis, Tennant (2007) demonstrated that the T-score calculation can manufacture the appearance of clinically important change in 15% of GAS data in situations where no such difference should exist. For this reason, authors such as Steenbeek et al (2015) have argued that T-scores should perhaps be abandoned, and if GAS is to be used, outcome reporting should include only raw GAS data (i.e., the −2 to +2 scores), using nonparametric methods for data analysis (e.g., medians and percentiles rather than means and standard deviations).

There is, however, one more fundamental problem with GAS as an outcome, and indeed with any use of goal attainment to measure success of rehabilitation programmes, which has seldom been raised or discussed. This problem is to do with what measurement construct is actually being evaluated by the attainment of goals. Changes in scores on measures of goal attainment reflect two things: (a) change in a person's health, functioning or well-being from a

baseline state; and (b) the expectations of the person or people setting the goals. In fact, GAS scores are arguably much more of a reflection of a health professional's ability to prognosticate than they are a measure of improvement in a person's health status. It is possible for one person to do

TABLE 6.2 Examples of a Goal Attainment Scaling Scale

Rakesh is a 47-year-old man with secondary progressive multiple sclerosis who lives with his husband in the community. A recent exacerbation of his multiple sclerosis has resulted in Rakesh becoming more ataxic, and he needs help from his husband plus a stick to get up a flight of stairs into their family home. A community physiotherapist visits him to begin work on improving his balance, coordination and muscle strength. The physiotherapist expects that Rakesh should be able to regain the ability to climb stairs independently after 8 weeks of therapy, but anticipates that Rakesh is still likely to need to use a stick for support. This is set as the 0 score for the GAS goal. Rakesh's current performance on stair climbing is set at the −1 score. The following GAS scale is established.

Score	Individual GAS Scale Items	GAS-light Scale Items
+2	Rakesh will walk up and down a flight of 12 steps six times in 2 minutes without use of a stick.	Greatly exceeds expected outcome
+1	Rakesh will walk up a flight of 12 steps without use of stick.	Slightly exceeds expected outcome
0	Rakesh will walk up a flight of 12 steps independently with aid of a stick.	Rakesh will walk up a flight of 12 steps independently with aid of a stick
−1	Rakesh will walk up a flight of 12 steps with assistance of one person and a stick.	Not quite achieving expected outcome
−2	Rakesh will not be able to walk up a flight of 12 steps even with maximal assistance.	Nowhere near the expected outcome

GAS, Goal Attainment Scaling.

worse in terms of their rehabilitation outcomes but score better than another person if the expectation for the first person was initially lower (Fig. 6.2).

Furthermore, if health professionals are 100% accurate with their predictions regarding what outcomes patients will achieve, then all patients should always achieve a GAS score of 0 (the *expected* outcome). Indeed, proponents of

GAS have stated that average GAS scores should always be 0. It has been recommended, for example, that when a clinician or healthcare team consistently scores greater than 0, then this should be taken as evidence that the clinicians lack experience or are attempting to massage the GAS scales to make the outcomes seem more positive, not that the clinician or healthcare team is achieving

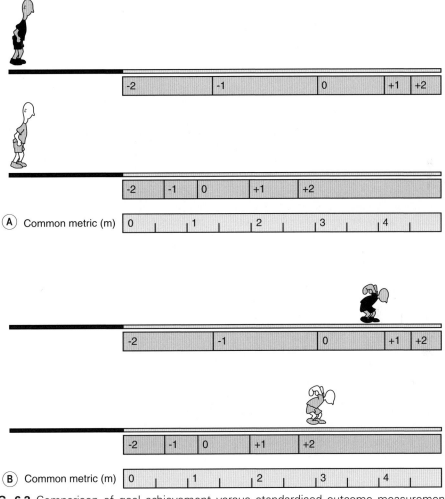

FIG. 6.2 Comparison of goal achievement versus standardised outcome measurement. In this hypothetical scenario, two people undertake a 12-week exercise programme to improve the distance they can jump. Both begin with same jumping ability, but their potential for improvement is thought to differ. Each is set an expected outcome for jumping to be achieved by 12 weeks (the goal), giving this distance a score of 0, with better and worse than expected outcomes being given scores ranging from −2 to +2 (A). At 12 weeks, the person who achieves the best outcome on a common metric (jumping distance) scores worse in terms of goal attainment because the initial expectations for that person were much higher (B).

better-than-average outcomes for their patients (Kiresuk & Sherman 1968, Turner-Stokes 2009). Likewise, it has been recommended that consistently scoring less than 0 is an indication that the clinician or healthcare team has been overly ambitious for their patient population. A third scenario is also possible, however. A rehabilitation team could be both underambitious *and* worse than others at delivering therapy, and thus consistently score 0 as expected on their patients' GAS scales. GAS scores cannot distinguish between substandard therapy oriented towards easily achievable goals and extremely high standard therapy with very ambitious goals.

There are other implications arising from this. For instance, as a rehabilitation team develops in its expertise, so too should its expectations for patient outcomes. As such, even if a rehabilitation team improves the quality of its service delivery, its average GAS score ought to remain at a steady 0. GAS scores therefore cannot be used to meaningfully benchmark performance between two rehabilitation services, nor within one rehabilitation service over time.

This problem is not unique to GAS, however. It is a feature of all types of goal setting where achievement of individualised goals is used to evaluate outcomes. Goal achievement only tells us whether people achieved what they set out to achieve. It cannot tell us if that achievement was better or worse than another person's individual achievement (or nonachievement).

Other approaches to goal setting dodge this particular problem by using a different metric than goal achievement to measure outcomes related to rehabilitation goals. For instance, it is possible to use the Canadian Occupational Performance Measure (COPM) to identify areas of occupation that can be converted into goals for therapy (Phipps & Richardson 2007). The COPM, however, involves measurement of individual people's perception of their current level of performance in these prespecified areas of occupational activity and their current satisfaction with their own performance – both on a 10-point scale (Law et al 2014). Performance and satisfaction with performance can then be measured at the beginning and at the end of a programme of rehabilitation to evaluate change.

Despite the difficulties with interpreting goal attainment scores at the level of a rehabilitation service, there is still value in reflecting on goal attainment at an individual patient level. The degree to which a person achieved or did not achieve a particular goal can provide a useful point for discussion for rehabilitation professionals reflecting on their practice. Talking about goal attainment can also be helpful when reminding patients about how far they have come in their recovery, or as a point of entry into discussions about disappointments regarding poorer than expected outcomes, and what should change as a result.

Furthermore, when a third-party payer, such as an insurance company, is involved in funding an individualised rehabilitation service for a person with a complex presentation, goal attainment can be used as a key performance indicator from a business perspective, as part of an outcome-oriented funding model. In this context, the rehabilitation business makes money only if it achieves its prespecified goals for individual patients. An example of such a model, used successfully in the USA, is the systematic managed care model of insurance for people with complex rehabilitation needs (Sundance et al 2004). Thus, although individual goal achievement can be informative and even drive a healthcare funding model when used at an individual patient level, it is difficult to meaningfully compare goal achievement between patients, between services or within one service over time.

CONCLUSION

Goal setting is an attractive, yet complex and multipurpose tool available for use by rehabilitation providers. Although much of this chapter has focused on goal setting within the context of stroke rehabilitation, the key concepts within it are likely to be relevant to other neurological conditions. For instance, it is increasingly clear that when it comes to goal setting in rehabilitation, one approach is not going to be suitable for all people in all contexts. Rather, approaches to goal setting need to be tailored to the individual disposition of patients, to their clinical context, to their health condition and to their stage of recovery. Open for debate are questions such as how difficult or challenging a goal should be, whether goal achievement actually matters and why, how involved patients or their families should be in the selection of goals at various stages of recovery, what the subject of goals should be and how best to help people work towards their goals. These and other questions are all good targets for future research.

Interestingly, such calls for the development of a more nuanced understanding of goal setting are not limited to rehabilitation research. In a review of goal setting in management literature, Ordóñez et al (2009) commented on how uncritically goal setting has been adopted in business practice. 'Rather than dispensing goal setting as a benign, over-the-counter treatment for motivation', Ordóñez et al (2009) wrote, 'managers and scholars need to conceptualise goal setting as a prescription-strength medication that requires careful dosing, consideration of harmful side effects and close supervision' (p. 14). If this is true for business practice, it must surely be true for rehabilitation.

Ultimately the objective of rehabilitation is not to achieve goals; the main objective of rehabilitation is to help people maximise their opportunities to fulfil their personal preferences, and thus their health, well-being and quality of life. Goal setting is one strategy that can be used to further work towards this objective. Goals and goal achievement should be considered the 'means' not the 'ends' of rehabilitation. Pragmatic approaches to goal setting, such as offered by Randall and McEwen (2000), provide a useful starting point for learning about the application of goal setting to clinical practice. More sophisticated understandings of goal setting are required to maximise the benefits and minimise the possible harms arising from its use in various rehabilitation contexts.

SELF-ASSESSMENT QUESTIONS

1. What strategies can be used to make goal setting more person-centred?
2. What are the advantages and challenges of involving family members in goal setting?
3. Why should health professionals use different approaches to goal setting over the course of recovery after a stroke?
4. What are the limitations of GAS as an outcome measure?

REFERENCES

Achziger, A., Martiny, S.E., Oettingen, G., Gollwitzer, P.M., 2012. Metacognitive processes in the self-regulation of goal pursuit. In: Brinol, P., DeMarree, K.G. (Eds.), Social Metacognition. Psychology Press, New York, pp. 121–139.

Adey-Wakeling, Z., Jolliffe, L., O'Shannessy, E., et al., 2021. Activity, participation, and goal awareness after acquired brain injury: a prospective observational study of inpatient rehabilitation. Ann. Rehabil. Med. 45, 413.

Arntzen, C., Hamran, T., Borg, T., 2015. Body, participation and self transformations during and after in-patient stroke rehabilitation. Scand. J. Disabil. Res. 17, 300–320.

Ashford, S., Turner-Stokes, L., 2015. Goal attainment scaling in adult neurorehabilitation. In: Siegert, R.J., Levack, W.M.M. (Eds.), Rehabilitation Goal Setting: Theory, Practice, and Evidence. CRC Press, Boca Raton, pp. 123–142.

Baird, T., Tempest, S., Warland, A., 2010. Service users' perceptions and experiences of goal setting theory and practice in an inpatient neurorehabilitation unit. Br. J. Occup. Ther. 73, 373–378.

Baker, S.M., Marshak, H.H., Rice, G.T., Zimmerman, G.J., 2001. Patient participation in physical therapy goal setting. Phys. Ther. 81, 1118–1126.

Barnard, R.A., Cruice, M.N., Playford, E.D., 2010. Strategies used in the pursuit of achievability during goal setting in rehabilitation. Qual. Health. Res. 20, 239–250.

Bernhardt, J., Hayward, K.S., Kwakkel, G., et al., 2017. Agreed definitions and a shared vision for new standards in stroke recovery research: the Stroke Recovery and Rehabilitation Roundtable Taskforce. Int. J. Stroke. 12, 444–450.

Bernhardt, J., Langhorne, P., Lindley, R.I., et al., 2015. Efficacy and safety of very early mobilisation within 24 h of stroke onset (AVERT): a randomised controlled trial. Lancet. 386, 46–55.

Bieleke, M., Keller, L., Gollwitzer, P.M., 2021. If-then planning. Eur. Rev. Soc. Psychol. 32, 88–122.

Blackmer, J., 2000. Ethical issues in rehabilitation medicine. Scand. J. Rehabil. Med. 32, 51–55.

Blennerhassett, J.M., Borschmann, K.N., Lipson-Smith, R.A., Bernhardt, J., 2018. Behavioral mapping of patient activity to explore the built environment during rehabilitation. Health. Environ. Res. Des. J. 11, 109–123.

Bovend'Eerdt, T.J.H., Botell, R.E., Wade, D.T., 2009. Writing SMART rehabilitation goals and achieving goal attainment scaling: a practical guide. Clin. Rehabil. 23, 352–361.

Bright, F.A.S., Kayes, N.M., McCann, C.M., McPherson, K.M., 2011. Understanding hope after stroke: a systematic review of the literature using concept analysis. Top. Stroke. Rehabil. 18, 490–508.

Brown, M., Levack, W., McPherson, K.M., et al., 2014. Survival, momentum, and things that make me 'me': patients' perceptions of goal setting after stroke. Disabil. Rehabil. 36, 1020–1026.

Cott, C.A., 2004. Client-centred rehabilitation: client perspectives. Disabil. Rehabil. 26, 1411–1422.

Cott, C.A., 2007. Continuity, transition and participation: preparing clients for life in the community post-stroke. Disabil. Rehabil. 29, 1566–1574.

Culley, C., Evans, J.J., 2010. SMS text messaging as a means of increasing recall of therapy goals in brain injury rehabilitation: a single-blind within-subjects trial. Neuropsychol. Rehabil. 20, 103–119.

da Silva, M.A.V., São-João, T.M., Brizon, V.C., Franco, D.H., Mialhe, F.L., 2018. Impact of implementation intentions on physical activity practice in adults: a systematic review and meta-analysis of randomized clinical trials. PloS One. 13, e0206294.

Doran, G., 1981. There's a S.M.A.R.T way to write management's goals and objectives. Management. Review. 70, 35–36.

Ellis-Hill, C., Payne, S., Ward, C., 2008. Using stroke to explore the Life Thread Model: an alternative approach to understanding rehabilitation following an acquired disability. Disabil. Rehabil. 30, 150–159.

Ellis-Hill, C., Robison, J., Wiles, R., McPherson, K., Hyndman, D., Ashburn, A., 2009. Going home to get on with life: patients and carers experiences of being discharged from hospital following a stroke. Disabil. Rehabil. 31, 61–72.

Foster, A.M., Armstrong, J., Buckley, A., et al., 2012. Encouraging family engagement in the rehabilitation process: a rehabilitation provider's development of support strategies for family members of people with traumatic brain injury. Disabil. Rehabil. 34, 1855–1862.

Fu, V., Weatherall, M., McPherson, K., et al., 2020. Taking Charge after Stroke: a randomized controlled trial of a person-centered, self-directed rehabilitation intervention. Int. J. Stroke. 15, 954–964.

Grant, M., Ponsford, J., 2014. Goal attainment scaling in brain injury rehabilitation: strengths, limitations and recommendations for future applications. Neuropsychol. Rehabil. 24, 661–677.

Hart, T., Hawkey, K., Whyte, J., 2002. Use of a portable voice organizer to remember therapy goals in traumatic brain injury rehabilitation: a within-subjects trial. J. Head. Trauma. Rehabil. 17, 556–570.

Harwood, M., 2010. Rehabilitation and indigenous peoples: the Māori experience. Disabil. Rehabil 32, 972–977.

Harwood, M., Weatherall, M., Talemaitoga, A., 2011. Taking charge after stroke: promoting self-directed rehabilitation to improve quality of life – a randomized controlled trial. Clin. Rehabil. 26, 493–501.

Heidenreich, P.A., 2013. Time for a thorough evaluation of patient-centered care. Circ. Cardiovasc. Qual. Outcomes. 6, 2–4.

Holliday, R.C., Ballinger, C., Playford, E.D., 2007. Goal setting in neurological rehabilitation: patients' perspectives. Disabil. Rehabil. 29, 389–394.

Indredavik, B., Fjaertoft, H., Ekeberg, G., Løge, A.D., Mørch, B., 2000. Benefit of an extended stroke unit service with early supported discharge. Stroke. 31, 2989–2994.

Jones, F., Gage, H., Drummond, A., et al., 2016. Feasibility study of an integrated stroke self-management programme: a cluster-randomised controlled trial. BMJ. Open. 6, e008900.

Jones, F., Gombert, K., Honey, S., et al., 2021. Addressing inactivity after stroke: the Collaborative Rehabilitation in Acute Stroke (CREATE) study. Int. J. Stroke. 16, 669–682.

Jones, F., Livingstone, E., Hawkes, L., 2013. Getting the balance between encouragement and taking over – reflections on using a new stroke self-management programme. Physiother. Res. Int. 18, 91–99.

Jones, F., Mandy, A., Partridge, C., 2009. Changing self-efficacy in individuals following a first time stroke: preliminary study of a novel self-management intervention. Clin. Rehabil. 23, 522–533.

Kiresuk, T., Sherman, R., 1968. Goal Attainment Scaling: a general method for evaluating community health programs. Community. Ment. Health. J. 4, 443–453.

Knutti, K., Björklund Carlstedt, A., Clasen, R., Green, D., 2020. Impacts of goal setting on engagement and rehabilitation outcomes following acquired brain injury: a systematic review of reviews. Disabil. Rehabil. 42, 2581–2590.

Kollen, B., Kwakkel, G., Lindeman, E., 2006. Longitudinal robustness of variables predicting independent gait following severe middle cerebral artery stroke: a prospective cohort study. Clin. Rehabil. 20, 262–268.

Kreutzer, J.S., Marwitz, J.H., Godwin, E.E., Arango-Lasprilla, J.C., 2010. Practical approaches to effective family intervention after brain injury. J. Head. Trauma. Rehabil. 25, 113–120.

Kumar, S., Selim, M.H., Caplan, L.R., 2010. Medical complications after stroke. Lancet. Neurol. 9, 105–118.

Langhorne, P., Baylan, S., 2017. Early supported discharge services for people with acute stroke. Cochrane. Database. Syst. Rev. 7, CD000443.

Law, M., Baptiste, S., Carswell, A., McColl, M.A., Polatajko, H., Pollock, N., 2014. Canadian Occupational Performance Measure, 5th ed. CAOT Publications ACE, Ottawa, Ontario.

Levack, W.M.M., Dean, S.G., McPherson, K.M., Siegert, R.J., 2006a. How clinicians talk about the application of goal planning to rehabilitation for people with brain injury – variable interpretations of value and purpose. Brain. Inj. 20, 1439–1449.

Levack, W.M.M., Dean, S.G., McPherson, K.M., Siegert, R.J., 2015a. Evidence-based goal setting – cultivating the science of rehabilitation. In: Siegert, R.J., Levack, W.M.M. (Eds.), Rehabilitation Goal Setting: Theory, Practice, & Evidence. CRC Press, Boca Raton, pp. 21–44.

Levack, W.M.M., Dean, S., Siegert, R.J., McPherson, K.M., 2006b. Purposes and mechanisms of goal planning in rehabilitation: the need for a critical distinction. Disabil. Rehabil. 28, 741–749.

Levack, W.M.M., Dean, S.G., Siegert, R.J., McPherson, K.M., 2011. Navigating patient-centered goal setting in inpatient stroke rehabilitation: how clinicians control the process to meet perceived professional responsibilities. Patient. Educ. Couns. 85, 206–213.

Levack, W.M.M., Siegert, R.J., 2015. Challenges in theory, practice and evidence. In: Siegert, R.J., Levack, W.M.M. (Eds.), Rehabilitation Goal Setting: Theory, Practice, & Evidence. CRC Press, Boca Raton. pp. 3–20.

Levack, W.M.M., Siegert, R.J., Dean, S.G., McPherson, K.M., 2009. Goal planning for adults with acquired brain injury: how clinicians talk about involving family. Brain. Inj. 23, 192–202.

Levack, W.M.M., Siegert, R.J., Dean, S.G., et al., 2015b. Goal setting and activities to enhance goal pursuit for adults with acquired disabilities participating in rehabilitation. Cochrane. Database. Syst. Rev. 7, CD009727.

Levack, W.M.M., Siegert, R.J., Pickering, N., 2015c. Ethics and goal setting. In: Siegert, R.J., Levack, W.M.M. (Eds.), Rehabilitation Goal Setting: Theory, Practice, & Evidence. CRC Press, Boca Raton, pp. 67–87.

Levack, W.M.M., Taylor, K., Siegert, R.J., et al., 2006c. Is goal planning in rehabilitation effective? A systematic review. Clin. Rehabil. 20, 739–755.

Levack, W., Tomori, K., Takahashi, K., Sherrington, A.J., 2018. Development of an English-language version of a Japanese iPad application to facilitate collaborative goal setting in rehabilitation: a Delphi study and field test. BMJ. Open. 8, e018908.

Lloyd, A., Bannigan, K., Sugavanam, T., Freeman, J., 2018. Experiences of stroke survivors, their families and unpaid carers in goal setting within stroke rehabilitation: a systematic review of qualitative evidence. JBI. Evid. Synth. 16, 1418–1453.

Lloyd, A., Roberts, A., Freeman, J., 2014. 'Finding a balance' in involving patients in goal setting early after stroke: a physiotherapy perspective. Physiother. Res. Int. 19, 147–157.

Locke, E.A., Latham, G.P., 2002. Building a practically useful theory of goal setting and task motivation: a 35-year odyssey. Am. Psychol. 57, 705–717.

Lohse, K.R., Lang, C.E., Boyd, L.A., 2014. Is more better? Using metadata to explore dose–response relationships in stroke rehabilitation. Stroke. 45, 2053–2058.

Maribo, T., Jensen, C.M., Madsen, L.S., Handberg, C., 2020. Experiences with and perspectives on goal setting in spinal cord injury rehabilitation: a systematic review of qualitative studies. Spinal. Cord. 58, 949–958.

Mäkelä, P., Gawned, S., Jones, F., 2014. Starting early: integration of self-management support into an acute stroke service. BMJ. Open. Qual. 3 u202037.w1759.

McClain, C., 2005. Collaborative rehabilitation goal setting. Top. Stroke. Rehabil. 12 (4), 56–60.

McGrath, J.R., Marks, J.A., Davis, A.M., 1995. Towards interdisciplinary rehabilitation: further developments at Rivermead Rehabilitation Centre. Clin. Rehabil. 9, 320–326.

McKenna, S., Jones, F., Glenfield, P., Lennon, S., 2015. Bridges self-management program for people with stroke in the community: a feasibility randomized controlled trial. Int. J. Stroke. 10, 697–704.

McMillan, T.M., Sparkes, C., 1999. Goal planning and neurorehabilitation: the Wolfson Neurorehabilitation Centre approach. Neuropsychol. Rehabil. 9, 241–251.

McPherson, K.M., Kayes, N., Weatherall, M., 2009. A pilot study of self-regulation informed goal setting in people with traumatic brain injury. Clin. Rehabil. 23, 296–309.

McPherson, K.M., Kayes, N.M., Kersten, P., 2015. MEANING as a smarter approach to goals in rehabilitation. In: Siegert, R.J., Levack, W.M.M. (Eds.), Rehabilitation Goal Setting: Theory, Practice, and Evidence. CRC Press, Baton Rouge, pp. 105–119.

Meyer, S., Verheyden, G., Brinkmann, N., et al., 2015. Functional and motor outcome 5 years after stroke is equivalent to outcome at 2 months. Stroke. 46, 1613–1619.

Meyer, T., Pohontsch, N.J., 2015. Goal orientation and goal setting in German medical rehabilitation research. In: Siegert, R.J., Levack, W.M.M. (Eds.), Rehabilitation Goal Setting: Theory, Practice and Evidence. CRC Press, London, pp. 237–250.

Nair, K.P.S., 2003. Life goals: the concept and its relevance to rehabilitation. Clin. Rehabil. 17, 192–202.

NHS England., 2013. NHS standard contract for specialised rehabilitation for patients with highly complex needs (all ages). Available at: http://www.england.nhs.uk/commissioning/wp-content/uploads/sites/12/2014/04/d02-rehab-pat-high-needs-0414.pdf. Accessed 18 June 2023.

Ordóñez, L.D., Schweitzer, M.E., Galinsky, A.D., Bazerman, M.H., 2009. Goals gone wild: the systematic side effects of overprescribing goal setting. Acad. Manag. Perspect. 23, 6–16.

Phipps, S., Richardson, P., 2007. Occupational therapy outcomes for clients with traumatic brain injury and stroke using the Canadian Occupational Performance Measure. Am. J. Occup. Ther. 61, 328–334.

Plant, S.E., Tyson, S.F., Kirk, S., Parsons, J., 2016. What are the barriers and facilitators to goal-setting during rehabilitation for stroke and other acquired brain injuries? A systematic review and meta-synthesis. Clin. Rehabil. 30, 921–930.

Randall, K.E., McEwen, I.R., 2000. Writing patient-centered functional goals. Phys. Ther. 80, 1197–1203.

Rethnam, V., Langhorne, P., Churilov, L., et al., 2022. Early mobilisation post-stroke: a systematic review and meta-analysis of individual participant data. Disabil. Rehabil. 44, 1156–1163.

Rosewilliam, S., Roskell, C.A., Pandyan, A.D., 2011. A systematic review and synthesis of the quantitative and qualitative evidence behind patient-centred goal setting in stroke rehabilitation. Clin. Rehabil. 25, 501–514.

Sherratt, S., Worrall, L., Pearson, C., Howe, T., Hersh, D., Davidson, B., 2011. 'Well it has to be language-related': speech-language pathologists' goals for people with aphasia and their families. Int. J. Speech-Lang. Pathol. 13, 317–328.

Snyder, C.R., Lehman, K.A., Kluck, B., Monsson, Y., 2006. Hope for rehabilitation and vice versa. Rehabil. Psychol. 51, 89–112.

Steenbeek, D., Gorter, J.W., Ketelaar, M., et al., 2015. Goal attainment scaling in paediatric rehabilitation. In: Siegert, R.J., Levack, W.M.M. (Eds.), Rehabilitation Goal Setting: Theory, Practice, and Evidence. CRC Press, Boca Raton, pp. 143–160.

Strubbia, C., Levack, W.M.M., Grainger, R., Takahashi, K., Tomori, K., 2020. Use of technology in supporting goal setting in rehabilitation for adults: a scoping review. BMJ. Open. 10, e041730.

Strubbia, C., Levack, W.M., Grainger, R., Takahashi, K., Tomori, K., 2021. Use of an iPad app (Aid for Decision-making in Occupational Choice) for collaborative goal setting in interprofessional rehabilitation: qualitative descriptive study. JMIR. Rehabil. Assist. Technol. 8, e33027.

Sundance, P., Cope, N., Kirshblum, S., Parsons, S., Apple, S., 2004. Systematic care management: clinical and economic analysis of a national sample of patients with spinal cord injury. Top. Spinal. Cord. Inj. Rehabil. 10, 17–34.

Swann, C., Jackman, P.C., Lawrence, A., et al., 2022. The (over) use of SMART goals for physical activity promotion: a narrative review and critique. Health. Psychol. Rev, 1–16.

Tang Yan, H.S., Clemson, L.M., Jarvis, F., Laver, K., 2014. Goal setting with caregivers of adults in the community: a mixed methods systematic review. Disabil. Rehabil. 36, 1943–1963.

Taylor, W.J., Brown, M., William, L., 2012. A pilot cluster randomised controlled trial of structured goal-setting following stroke. Clin. Rehabil. 26, 327–338.

Tennant, A., 2007. Goal attainment scaling: current methological challenges. Disabil. Rehabil. 29, 1583–1588.

Thomas, E.J., Levack, W.M.M., Taylor, W.J., 2015. Rehabilitation and recovery of self-identity. In: McPherson, K.M., Gibson, B.E., Leplege, A. (Eds.), Rethinking Rehabilitation: Theory & Practice. CRC Press, Boca Raton, pp. 163–189.

Timothy, E.K., Graham, F.P., Levack, W.M., 2016. Transitions in the embodied experience after stroke. A grounded theory study. Phys. Ther. 96, 1565–1575.

Tomori, K., Saito, Y., Nagayama, H., Seshita, Y., Ogahara, K., Nagatani, R., Higashi, T., 2013a. Reliability and validity of individualized satisfaction score in aid for decision-making in occupation choice. Disabil. Rehabil. 35, 113–117.

Tomori, K., Nagayama, H., Saito, Y., Ohno, K., Nagatani, R., Higashi, T., 2013b. Examination of a cut-off score to express the meaningful activity of people with dementia using iPad application (ADOC). Disabil. Rehabil. Assist. Technol. 10, 126–131.

Tomori, K., Uezu, S., Kinjo, S., Ogahara, K., Nagatani, R., Higashi, T., 2012. Utilization of the iPad application: aid for decision-making in occupation choice. Occup. Ther. Int. 19, 88–97.

Turner-Stokes, L., 2009. Goal attainment scaling (GAS) in rehabilitation: a practical guide. Clin. Rehabil. 23, 362–370.

Turner-Stokes, L., Williams, H., 2010. Goal attainment scaling: a direct comparison of alternative rating methods. Clin. Rehabil. 24, 66–73.

Wade, D.T., 1998. Evidence relating to goal planning in rehabilitation. Clin. Rehabil. 12, 273–275.

Wade, D.T., 1999a. Goal planning in stroke rehabilitation: how? Top. Stroke. Rehabil. 6, 16–36.

Wade, D.T., 1999b. Goal planning in stroke rehabilitation: what? Top. Stroke. Rehabil. 6, 8–15.

West, T., Bernhardt, J., 2012. Physical activity in hospitalised stroke patients. Stroke. Res. Treat, 813765.

World Health Organization, 2001. International Classification of Functioning Disability and Health. WHO, Geneva.

Management of Specific Conditions

Stroke

Janne M. Veerbeek and Geert Verheyden

OUTLINE

Introduction, 151
Epidemiology, 152
Pathophysiology, 152
Diagnosis, 152
Medical Management, 152
Setting, 153
Interdisciplinary Team, 153
Clinical Presentation, 153
Assessment, 154
    Hyperacute and Acute Phase, 154
    Subacute Phase, 156
    Chronic Phase, 157
    Prognosis and Time Course of Recovery, 157
Interventions, 159
    General Therapy Principles, 160
Lower Limb and Locomotor Recovery, 163
    Balance Training, 163
    Gait Training, 163

Overground Walking, 163
Speed-Dependent Treadmill Training, 163
Body Weight-Supported Treadmill Training, 164
Robot-Assisted Gait Training, 164
Circuit Class Training, 164
Electrostimulation of the Paretic Lower Limb, 165
Upper Limb Recovery, 165
Constraint-Induced Movement Therapy, 166
Bilateral Arm Training, 167
Virtual Reality, Including Interactive Video Gaming, 167
Electrostimulation of the Paretic Arm and Hand, 168
Robot-Assisted Therapy for the Upper Limb, 168
Therapy Delivery, 168
Conclusion, 169
Case Study, 169

INTRODUCTION

According to the Stroke Association (2017), every 2 seconds, someone in the world has a stroke. One in eight strokes is fatal within the first 30 days, and almost two-thirds of stroke survivors leave hospital with a disability (Stroke Association 2017). Stroke remains the third leading cause of death and disability (expressed as disability-adjusted life-years lost [DALYs]) in the world (Feigin et al 2022) and is therefore a significant cause of people being in need of physical management and rehabilitation.

A stroke or cerebrovascular accident (CVA) is in fact a central nervous system pathology, defined as 'brain, spinal cord or retinal cell death attributable to ischemia, based on: (1) pathological, imaging or other objective evidence of cerebral, spinal cord or retinal focal ischemic injury in a defined vascular distribution; or (2) clinical evidence of cerebral, spinal cord or retinal focal ischemic injury based on symptoms persisting ≥24 hours or until death, and other etiologies excluded' (Sacco et al 2013, p. 2066).

A transient ischaemic attack (TIA) is defined as 'a transient episode of neurological dysfunction caused by focal brain, spinal cord or retinal ischemia, without acute infarction' (Easton et al 2009, p. 2281); it is also called a mini-stroke. Patients present with similar symptoms as a stroke but which last only minutes or hours and are completely resolved within 24 hours.

Because the majority of strokes happen in one of the two brain hemispheres, the typical clinical sign of a person after stroke is a sensorimotor hemiparesis or hemiplegia, contralateral to the side of the lesion in the brain. Hemiparesis is typically defined as weakness on one side of the body, whereas hemiplegia is paralysis of the arm, leg and trunk on one side of the body. Of course this focus on only motor impairment is too limited, as will become clear throughout this chapter. Nevertheless, as this book focuses on physical management, the focus on treatment in this chapter will be on rehabilitation for improving motor function and related activities post-stroke.

EPIDEMIOLOGY

Strokes are classified into two main categories: ischaemic or haemorrhagic (Amarenco et al 2009). An ischaemic stroke is caused by an interruption of the blood supply. A haemorrhagic stroke is caused by a ruptured blood vessel. The majority of strokes are ischaemic accidents (approximately 80%).

In an ischaemic stroke, blood supply to a certain area of the brain is decreased, which causes dysfunction of the brain area supplied by the affected blood vessel.

A haemorrhagic stroke can be an intracerebral or intracranial accident. An intracerebral haemorrhage is a stroke where blood is leaking directly into the brain tissue, building up a haematoma. An intracranial haemorrhage is the buildup of blood anywhere within the skull, typically somewhere between the skull and the meninges surrounding the brain and spinal cord.

PATHOPHYSIOLOGY

The arteries that supply blood to the brain are arranged in a circle called the circle of Willis, after Thomas Willis (1621–1673). All of the principal arteries of the circle of Willis give origin to secondary vessels, which supply blood to the different areas of the brain.

The aetiology of ischemic stroke can be classified according to TOAST (Trial of Org 10172 in Acute Stroke Treatment). This classification differentiates between five subtypes: large-artery atherosclerosis, cardioembolism, small-vessel occlusion, other determined aetiology and undetermined aetiology (Adams Jr. et al 1993). Classifications like TOAST are presented to allow clinical trials to present results according to subtypes. This should then inform clinical practice determining effective medical treatment approaches for different stroke subtypes.

When an ischaemic stroke occurs and part of the brain suffers from lack of blood, the ischaemic cascade starts. Without blood, the brain tissue is no longer supplied with oxygen and after a few hours in this situation, irreversible injury leads to tissue death. Because of the organisation of

the circle of Willis, collateral circulation is possible, so there is a continuum of possible severity. Part of the brain tissue may die immediately, whereas other parts are potentially only injured and could recover. The area of the brain where tissue might recover is called the penumbra. Ischaemia triggers pathophysiological processes, which result in cellular injury and death, such as the release of glutamate or the production of oxygen free radicals.

A haemorrhagic stroke causes tissue injury by diminished (or absent) blood flow to areas in the brain, resulting in lack of oxygen. Additionally, compression of tissue from an expanding haematoma or blood pool can result in subsequent tissue injury; consequently, the increased pressure might lead to a decreased blood supply into the surrounding tissue (and eventually infarction).

DIAGNOSIS

The diagnosis of stroke is based on a clinical assessment and imaging techniques such as computed tomography or magnetic resonance imaging scans.

When a stroke has been diagnosed, determining the underlying aetiology is important with regard to secondary stroke prevention. Common techniques include:
- Ultrasound of the carotid arteries to determine carotid stenosis,
- Electrocardiogram to detect arrhythmias of the heart which may send clots in the heart to the blood vessels of the brain,
- Holter monitor to identify intermittent arrhythmias,
- Angiogram of the blood vessels of the brain to detect possible aneurysms or arteriovenous malformations, and
- Blood test to examine the presence of hypercholesterolemia (high cholesterol).

MEDICAL MANAGEMENT

In the case of an ischaemic stroke, the more rapidly the blood flow is restored to the brain, the fewer brain cells die (Saver 2006). Hyperacute stroke treatment is aimed at breaking down the blood clot by means of medication (thrombolysis) or mechanically removing the blood clot (thrombectomy). Other acute treatments focus on minimizing enlargement of the clot or preventing new clots from forming by means of medication such as aspirin, clopidogrel or dipyridamole. Furthermore, blood sugar levels should be controlled and the patient should be supplied with adequate oxygen and intravenous fluids.

Thrombolysis is performed with a clot-busting drug, for instance, recombinant tissue plasminogen activator. A Cochrane review (Wardlaw et al 2014) including 27 trials with 10,187 patients showed that thrombolytic therapy provided up to 6 hours after stroke significantly reduces the proportion of deaths or dependency. There is an important time window because those treated within the first 3 hours post-stroke demonstrated considerably more benefit compared with later treatment. Thrombolysis is generally provided within a 3- to 4.5-hour post-stroke window, depending on the region of the world. Thrombolytic drugs, however, can cause serious bleeding in the brain. Therefore, patient selection is crucial.

Thrombectomy is another intervention for acute ischaemic stroke and consists of the mechanical removal of the blood clot. This is done by inserting a catheter into the femoral artery, which is then directed into the cerebral circulation next to the thrombus. The clot is then entrapped by the device and withdrawn from the body. A Cochrane review by Roaldsen and colleagues (2021) based on 19 trials including 3,793 patients concluded that there is high-quality evidence that endovascular thrombectomy increases the chance for better functional outcome, without an increased risk for serious side effects such as a bleeding.

In case of a haemorrhagic stroke, being able to stop the bleeding as early as possible is of paramount importance, and patients sometimes do require neurosurgical intervention to achieve this. Therefore, a craniotomy might be indicated, whereby a part of the skull is temporarily removed to decrease elevated intracranial pressure caused by the bleeding.

SETTING

People who have had a stroke are ideally managed in a dedicated acute stroke unit by a specialist multidisciplinary team. There are different types of clinical services, pathways and, indeed, stroke units with varying criteria for admission and discharge. Organised services with specialist interdisciplinary teams have been identified as key to a positive outcome in terms of both mortality and morbidity. Although stroke rehabilitation commences in the hyperacute (0–24 hours) and acute phase (1–7 days) on admission to hospital, active participation in the relearning of mobility and independence broadly takes place during the early (7 days–3 months) and late (3–6 months) subacute phase post-stroke and is sometimes continued into the chronic phase (>6 months), although this is largely dependent on the health service setting (Bernhardt et al 2017).

Post-stroke care comprises a whole continuum, in which patients often progress through different environments. An acute or rehabilitation stroke unit is a dedicated area with specialist staff for managing people with stroke. The length of stay on an acute unit can vary from a few hours to several days; after medical stabilisation, patients are usually referred to a rehabilitation unit for 1 or 2 weeks or several months. Patients may be referred to outpatient rehabilitation services or the domiciliary service when transferred from inpatient care. Some patients may be discharged early from a stroke unit to be cared for in the community through early supported discharge services (Langhorne et al 2017), but patients should be discharged early only if there is specialist stroke rehabilitation in the community. This early supported discharge is most suitable for patients with mild to moderate impairments and with a Barthel Index score of 10 out of 20 points or higher (Royal Dutch Society for Physical Therapy (KNGF) 2014).

Somewhere between 5% and 15% of people with stroke are discharged into residential care or nursing homes. These people with stroke rarely receive any rehabilitation, although stroke remains an indication for continued physical management provision.

INTERDISCIPLINARY TEAM

Specialist stroke services have been shown to be more cost and clinically effective if they are well organised with specialist staff (Stroke Unit Trialists' Collaboration 2013). Healthcare providers with expert knowledge of managing people with stroke are recommended for the interdisciplinary teams. The range of disciplines represented in a team reflects the range of impairments that can emerge after a stroke. People with a suspected stroke should be seen by a specialised physician for diagnosis and be managed by staff with expertise in stroke and rehabilitation. A team typically includes consultant physician(s), nurses, physiotherapists, occupational therapists, speech and language therapists, psychologists, dieticians and social workers. Stroke teams should meet at least once a week to agree on the management of patient problems and documentation of the plan and assessments to be completed. There should be education and specialist training programmes with access to services such as provision of assistive devices. The person with stroke and their carers are also part of the team and should be involved and consulted in the process of identifying and solving problems and setting treatment goals. A recent network meta-analysis based on 29 trials with 5,902 participants showed that there is moderate-quality evidence that stroke patients who are admitted and treated in a stroke unit are more likely to be alive, independent and living at home 1 year after stroke (Langhorne et al 2020).

CLINICAL PRESENTATION

If a stroke occurs in one of the brain arteries, the area normally supplied by the blood will be affected. Ischaemic strokes are commonly further classified according to the

TABLE 7.1   Oxford Community Stroke Project Classification for Ischaemic Strokes

Oxford Community Stroke Project Classification	Deficits
Total anterior circulation infarct (TACI)	All of the following: • Higher dysfunction (e.g., speech or visuospatial impairments) • Visual impairments (homonymous hemianopia) • Severe sensorimotor deficit in face, arm, trunk and leg
Partial anterior circulation infarct (PACI)	Any one of these: • Two out of three as TACI • Higher dysfunction alone • Limited sensorimotor impairments in face, arm, trunk and leg
Lacunar infarct (LACI)	Any one of these: • Pure motor impairments in face, arm, trunk and leg • Pure sensory impairments in face, arm, trunk and leg • Sensorimotor impairments in face, arm, trunk and leg • Ataxic hemiparesis
Posterior circulation infarct (POCI)	Any one of these: • Cranial nerve palsy and sensorimotor impairments • Bilateral sensory or motor impairment • Conjugate eye movement deficit • Isolated cerebellar dysfunction • Isolated homonymous hemianopia

Oxford Community Stroke Project (OCSP) classification, also known as the Oxford or Bamford classification (Bamford et al 1991). The OCSP classification proposes signs and symptoms for the different types of ischaemic accident (Table 7.1).

When evaluating 543 patients with a first-ever cerebral infarct, 17% had a total anterior circulation infarct showing both cortical and subcortical involvement, and consequently high mortality and a poor chance for a good outcome; 34% had a partial anterior circulation infarct with predominantly cortical involvement; 24% had a posterior circulation infarct which showed to be the subtype with the best chance of good functional outcome; and 25% had a lacunar infarct where in spite of the small anatomical size of the infarct, patients remained considerably limited in activities of daily living (ADLs; Bamford et al 1991).

Stroke, whether ischaemic or haemorrhagic, thus leads to a wide diversity of signs and symptoms. Fig. 7.1 provides an overview of the most relevant categories of the *International Classification of Functioning, Disability and Health* (ICF) affected by stroke.

ASSESSMENT

The initial data collection should comprise personal details such as age, contact details, medical history, function and motor ability, sensation, and psychological, social and family status. Descriptions of what happened at the time of stroke and since that period should be recorded. The purpose of the initial assessment is to both identify the level of impairment and individual experiences, and their ability in terms of sensation, posture, movement, function, attention, comprehension and previous skills. Standardised measures of these characteristics are used for the comparative evaluation of recovery over time.

The initial assessment may be performed over more than one session if the person with stroke is tired and unable to complete all the measures. Equally, the therapist may need to observe the impact of the impairments experienced by the individual over several sessions before prioritising a problem and setting a goal for treatment. For example, the therapist may need to decide whether the problem with the sequence of motor control during walking results from a loss of initiation of a component muscle group or as a result of abnormal tone.

Hyperacute and Acute Phase

Patients in the very early phases can be at different levels of consciousness: they may be sedated and intubated, or they may be able to communicate with or without difficulty. It is essential to determine whether the person is medically stable before commencing treatment; talk to

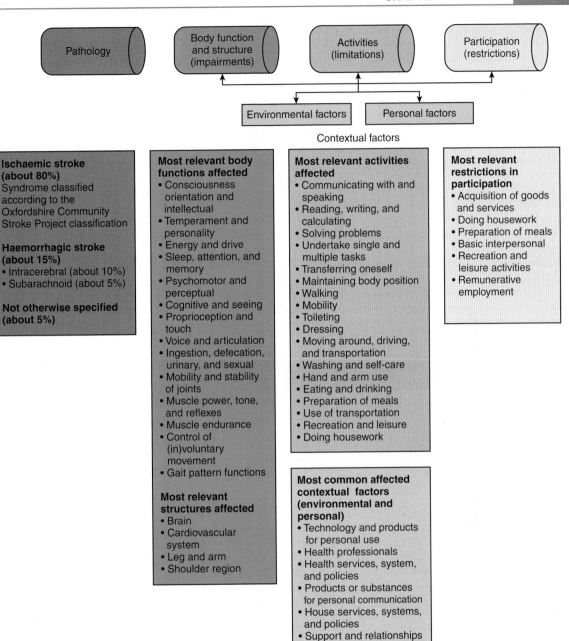

FIG. 7.1 Most relevant *International Classification of Functioning, Disability and Health* (ICF) categories affected after stroke. (Reproduced with permission from Langhorne et al 2011.)

key members of the hospital team and read the medical notes. Find out the age of the patient, the type of stroke, blood pressure, ability to communicate, if an injury occurred at the time of their stroke and information about their medical history, for example, have they experienced a previous stroke or do they have dementia? An outline of their social environment may also provide a guide on cultural issues and language differences. It is important to be informed of those potential risk factors that may influence what a therapist does and the treatment planned. Assume that all patients understand you even though they may not appear to. At a later stage many patients describe conversations overheard between members of staff who were either talking about them or ignoring them in the early period. Remember, a stroke is an event that happens suddenly; the previous day your patient could have been a director of a company, a highly skilled worker or an independent active mother or grandmother. The change in situation can be frightening and a shock. If members of the family are present when you visit, they are also likely to be shocked and confused. Introduce yourself and say what you will be doing. Invite them to ask any questions they have. Most likely they have many questions and not all of them can and should be answered by you. Refer them to the most appropriate member of the healthcare team.

All people with stroke should receive a full interdisciplinary assessment using an agreed procedure as early as possible, with preferable initial contact within the first 24 hours when the medical situation allows this.

EARLY MANAGEMENT AIMS

- Monitoring vital signs for medical stability
- Maintaining respiratory function
- Skin care
- Positioning
- Monitoring muscle length and range of motion
- Early mobilisation

When the medical condition has stabilised, mobilisation should start and the person with stroke should be helped to sit and get out of bed as soon as possible, within 48 hours (e.g., as indicated in the current Stroke Foundation, 2023 guidelines), in close collaboration with nursing staff. In the process of helping a patient to sit or stand up, the therapist needs to assess how much help is required (two people should be available to assist initially), how much the individual can do on their own and whether the patient can follow commands. Remember if two people are assisting a person with a stroke, one therapist must take the lead, explain the task and set the commands. A confused person in the acute stage of a stroke will be more confused during a treatment session if several commands are given (plus feedback) by different people at the same time.

Very early mobilisation (within the first 24 hours) has been investigated after showing promising results in a pilot

(phase II) trial. Cumming and colleagues (2011) showed that starting intensive mobilisation within 24 hours post-stroke resulted in a significantly faster return to walking in comparison with usual case. However, results from the definitive (phase III) trial including 2,104 patients from 56 acute stroke units in five countries could not confirm the initial results. In fact, fewer patients in the very early mobilisation group had a favourable outcome than those in the usual care group (AVERT Trial Collaboration Group 2015). Still, early mobilisation (when medically stable) in terms of bringing people into the upright sitting or standing position should be encouraged, with further analysis of the phase III trial indicating that shorter, more frequent mobilisation sessions are associated with an increased chance of a favourable outcome (Bernhardt et al 2016).

Subacute Phase

People in the subacute phase are generally medically stable, having been assessed in several ways, which may include follow-up evaluation by use of brain scans, level of consciousness, neurological signs, blood pressure, heart rate, respiratory rate, blood gases, swallowing and glucose levels. Intervention at this stage is characterised by programmes of rehabilitation. The emphasis is on determining progress through assessment and active participation in treatments. The first assessment is the baseline against which recovery or deterioration over time can be measured, in the presence or absence of treatment.

The core impairments in body functions include loss or reduction of movement and postural control, altered sensation, abnormalities of tone, fatigue, comprehension, ability to communicate, spatial awareness, visual neglect, visual field impairment, pain and swelling, all contributing to a level of functional dependence and decreased safety. Assessments should identify abilities and potential, as well as impairment and damage. Findings from global assessments of comprehension or communication may indicate where more in-depth assessments from specialist professionals are required, which in turn underlines the importance of team work and multiprofessional staff. The person with stroke and their carers are members of the team. Active participation in physical programmes during and between sessions should be encouraged with practice sessions in hospital, rehabilitation centre or in the community. People with stroke may range from having no activity in their limbs and trunk to advanced movement skills and could experience considerable variability in the degrees of impairment across the body. This variability has consequences for the rehabilitation goals and applied strategies. Rehabilitation objectives should therefore be carefully negotiated with the individual and include consideration of influencing factors such as age. Many young

Diagnostics	Body structure (impairments)	Activity (Disability)	Participation (Handicap)
• CT or MRI scan (with or without contrast) • Doppler • Electrocardiogram **Examinations** • History from patient and family • Clinical examination • Fundoscopic examination • Auscultation • Blood analysis (including pressure)	**Neurological scales** • Glasgow Coma Scale • Mini Mental State Examination • National Institutes of Health Stroke Scale • Scandinavian Stroke Scale • Canadian Neurological Scale **Other scales used by the stroke team** • Cumulative Illness Rating Scale • Bells and Star Cancellation Tests • Western Aphasia Battery • Ontario Society of Occupation Therapists Perceptual Evaluation • Medical Research Council • Motricity Index of Arm and Leg • Fugl-meyer Motor Assessment • Motor Assessment Scale • Fatigue Severity Scale • Hospital Anxiety and Depression Scale • Hamilton Rating Scale for Depression • Cambridge Cognition Examination	**Global ADL-scales** • Barthel Index • Functional Independence Measure • Frenchay Activities Index • (Modified) Rankin Scale **Other scales used by the stroke team** • Trunk Control Test • Timed up-and-go • Berg Balance Scale • Rivermead Mobility Index • 5 or 10 Metre Gait Speed • 2 or 6 Minute Walk Test • Stair Climbing Test • Frenchay Arm Test • Action Research Arm Test • Wolf Motor Function Test • Toronto Bed-side Swallowing Screening Test • American Speech-language-hearing Association Functional Assessment of Communication Skills	• Euroqol-5D • Frenchay activities index • Nottingham extended activities of daily living • Nottingham health profile • General health questionnaire • Stroke impact profile (stroke adapted version) • Medical outcome study short form 36 • Stroke-specific quality of life

Contextual factors
• Caregiver strain index
• Family assessment

Classification of commonly used scales for outcome

FIG. 7.2 Examples of outcome measures to be used with people with stroke, presented according to the *International Classification of Functioning, Disability and Health* (ICF). *ADLs,* Activities of daily living; *CT,* computed tomography; *MRI,* magnetic resonance imaging. (Reproduced with permission from Langhorne et al 2011.)

people with stroke want to return to work and to indulge in leisure activities.

Chronic Phase

Although most recovery takes place in the first few months post-stroke, improvements, adaptation and behavioural changes can continue for many years. The impact of a stroke lasts a lifetime, and most people want to return to their previous roles and to be involved in their community. From a physical management perspective, maintaining an adequate level of physical conditioning and monitoring quality of life are key priorities long term after stroke.

Stroke recovery should be documented by means of standardised outcome measures (Stokes 2009). An increasing number of assessment tools are available. Fig. 7.2 provides examples of stroke-specific and generic clinical measures according to the ICF.

Online summaries of evidence concerning stroke outcome measures and recommendations towards the use of assessment tools in different stages post-stroke are available. As presented in Chapter 4 on outcome measures, knowledge of and understanding psychometric properties are essential for healthcare professionals to decide which outcome measure is best suited to evaluate the patient.

Prognosis and Time Course of Recovery

Fig. 7.3 presents the recovery pattern after stroke (Langhorne et al 2011). There is general agreement across studies that most motor and functional recovery is observed in the first

WEBSITES AND PUBLICATIONS WITH SUMMARY OVERVIEWS ON STROKE OUTCOME MEASURES

- Stroke EDGE documents: http://www.neuropt.org/professional-resources/neurology-section-outcome-measures-recommendations/stroke
- Evidence-based review of stroke rehabilitation – outcome measures in stroke rehabilitation: http://www.ebrsr.com/evidence-review/20-outcome-measures-stroke-rehabilitation
- Rehabilitation measures database – assessments (stroke and nonstroke content): https://www.sralab.org/rehabilitation-measures
- Consensus-based core set of outcome measures for clinical motor rehabilitation after stroke (Pohl et al 2020)

month after stroke. Recovery continues up until 3 months and stagnates between 3 and 6 months after stroke. This recovery seems to be irrespective of impairment assessed. Indeed, Verheyden and colleagues (2008) compared trunk, upper limb, lower limb and basic ADL recovery and found no significant differences in recovery between any of the measures. Long-term recovery post-stroke has been investigated as well, and although between-subjects variation is observed, in a large cohort of European stroke survivors, a 5-year follow-up revealed deterioration in motor and functional outcome, with a return to the motor and functional level at 2 months (Meyer et al 2015).

Predicting stroke outcome has received great attention in the literature, as information concerning prognosis is relevant towards therapy planning, short- and long-term goal setting and discharge destination. For *ADL independence*, a systematic review of 48 studies showed that younger age and less severity of neurological deficits in the early post-stroke phase are associated with better basic ADL outcome at 3 months post-stroke (Veerbeek et al 2011). Further

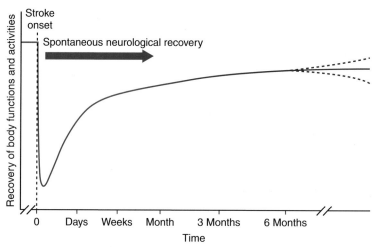

FIG. 7.3 Recovery Pattern post-stroke with therapy intervention goals. (Reproduced with permission from Langhorne et al 2011.)

independent predictive factors for good ADL outcome beyond 6 months, arising from different studies, are better core stability (sitting balance), the absence of urinary incontinence, less severe hemiplegia, limited comorbidity, consciousness at admission, better cognitive status and absence of depression (Kwakkel & Kollen 2013). For regaining *walking ability* at 6 months, information from prospective cohort studies presents the following prognostic factors: younger age, less severe sensory and motor dysfunction of the paretic leg, absence of homonymous hemianopia, no urinary incontinence, adequate sitting balance, better initial ADL function and ambulation, better level of consciousness on admission, no cognitive impairment and no neglect (Kwakkel & Kollen 2013; Preston et al 2021). For regaining *dexterity*, Coupar and colleagues (2012) showed in a review of 58 studies that initial severity of motor impairment and function was found to be the most important predictive factor for upper limb recovery. In addition, Nijland and colleagues (2010) showed that two simple bedside tests, the presence of shoulder abduction and finger extension, measured within 72 hours after stroke onset provide a probability of 0.98 to regain some dexterity at 6 months, as defined by an Action Research Arm Test (ARAT) of 10 points or more out of 57.

Although in general, neuroimaging and neurophysiological measurements have limited added value in prognostic models, research such as the PREP model (Predicting REcovery Potential for the hand and arm) combines clinical with transcranial magnetic stimulation measurements and neuroimaging for predicting upper limb recovery after stroke (Stinear et al 2012). In the updated model (PREP2), these authors presented a revised model without magnetic resonance imaging measurement, with no loss of prediction accuracy (Stinear et al 2017), and further demonstrated that prediction at 3 months was for more than 80% of patients also the correct prediction at 2 years after stroke (Smith et al 2019). Underlying the different elements of these models is the determination of motor pathway (mainly corticomotor) integrity, as patients having this integrity have a much higher chance of achieving good outcome.

Smith and colleagues (2017) have further developed a prediction model for gait. This TWIST algorithm starts from trunk control and hip extension strength evaluation at 1 week and predicts independent gait (short distance, even ground) at 6 or 12 weeks or dependent gait at 12 weeks. The only externally validated model for early prediction of regaining independence is the EPOS model (Early Prediction of Functional Outcome after Stroke) (Veerbeek et al 2011, 2022). Based on assessment of paretic leg strength and sitting balance from day 2 onwards, an accurate prediction of independent gait 6 months after stroke can be made (Veerbeek 2011). External validation

PREDICTORS OF RECOVERY

- For ADL independence:
- Younger age
- Less severe neurological deficits
- Better sitting balance
- Absence of urinary incontinence
- Limited comorbidity
- Consciousness at admission
- Better cognitive status
- Absence of depression
- For walking:
- Younger age
- Less severe sensorimotor dysfunction of the paretic leg
- No cognitive impairment (Preston et al 2021)
- No neglect (Preston et al 2021)
- Absence of homonymous hemianopia
- No urinary incontinence
- Adequate sitting balance
- Better initial ADL function and ambulation
- Better level of consciousness on admission
- For dexterity:
- Initial severity of motor impairment and function, e.g., presence of shoulder abduction and finger extension

showed that the EPOS model is also applicable for predicting independent gait at 3 months (Veerbeek 2022).

It should be clear that assessment of motor and functional performance is a key part of stroke rehabilitation, not just in terms of therapy delivery and outcome, but also in terms of prognosis. Reassessment, at an initial stage with a higher frequency, is needed to improve the accuracy of the prognosis.

INTERVENTIONS

Although this chapter focuses on motor rehabilitation after stroke, there are general management issues and secondary complications after stroke that should be considered during motor rehabilitation. Examples of general management issues are respiratory care, visual impairments, neuropathic pain, fatigue, communication problems and swallowing disorders, cognitive problems, spatial and perceptual problems, dyspraxia, psychosocial issues, bladder and bowel dysfunction and carer support. Soft tissue damage and shoulder subluxation, shoulder pain and falls are examples of secondary complications. However, a detailed description of these issues and complications is outside the scope of this chapter. More information can be found in the national clinical guidelines for all aspects of care that exist in many countries (e.g., see Royal Dutch Society for Physical Therapy (KNGF) 2014, 2021, National Institute for Health and Care Excellence 2008, National Stroke Foundation 2017, Scottish Intercollegiate Guidelines Network 2010, Winstein et al 2016, and more recently Stroke Foundation, 2023). These readily available guidelines guide assessment and treatment, but often lack information regarding which type of patients would benefit from a certain intervention.

After assessment, clinical hypotheses for explaining movement deficits or functional difficulties are stated and used to prioritise goals and planning of treatment. For example, weakness in the trunk or the hip muscles may explain the inability to balance and perform washing and dressing in sitting.

Notably, an informal process of assessment continues throughout the treatment programme. The nature of physiotherapy for people with stroke means that there is a constant monitoring of responses. The treatment plan is dependent on the responsiveness of the individual to intervention and handling. Not only is the physiotherapist aiming to facilitate a change in movement, but they are also teaching the individual to learn how to move and, in so doing, the physiotherapist wants the patient to be able to recognise a poor movement and a good movement. People need to know when they have achieved the movement and task correctly; thus, feedback is crucial. Also, the therapist needs to be certain their patient has remembered to practice the task set. Remembering the task and the importance of practice are positive signs for active participation and potential for improvement.

General Therapy Principles

Characteristics of effective motor rehabilitation interventions after stroke are specificity, intensity including repetition, and the application of motor learning principles.

Specificity of training means that what is trained will improve, whereas a transfer to nontrained tasks has not been clearly demonstrated. Specificity not only accounts for the tasks being practiced but also for the location (i.e., context, environment). However, training of body functions might be a prerequisite before being able to train activities (Royal Dutch Society for Physical Therapy (KNGF) 2014).

Intensity (or dose) of practice can be expressed in many ways, such as time spent in exercise therapy, performed number of repetitions or energy expenditure. In neurorehabilitation, it often refers to the number of hours spent on exercise therapy (Veerbeek et al 2011). People with stroke benefit from more time spent in practice compared with less time spent in practice because this speeds up their recovery in terms of body functions, such as selective movements, walking speed and walking distance (Lohse et al 2014, Veerbeek et al 2014). Positive effects of intensive practice have also been reported on the activities level, such as sitting and standing balance (Lohse et al 2014, Veerbeek et al 2014). For these effects, an additional therapy time of about 17 hours was reported. However, a recent meta-analysis showed no effects on the activities level, although the level of evidence was very low (Clark et al 2021); therefore, it has to be concluded that the optimal dose of therapy is unknown, as well as the long-term effects, and there is no evidence for a ceiling effect (Lohse et al 2014, Veerbeek et al 2014).

Repetition is another often reported measure of intensity of practice in post-stroke rehabilitation. Repetitions are defined as the 'repeated practice of functional tasks' (French et al 2016). There is low- to moderate-quality evidence that the active practice of task-specific motor activities improves upper and lower limb activities, and that these improvements are sustained up to 6 months after termination of the treatment (French et al 2016).

Although the optimal timing of intensive training has not been established, it is generally accepted that rehabilitation should start early after stroke and should be intensified after the first vulnerable days have passed (Bernhardt et al 2016). For clinical practice, it is recommended that patients with limitations in basic ADLs (i.e., <19/20 points on the Barthel Index) should be enabled to exercise for 40–60 minutes a day while at the hospital stroke unit (Royal Dutch Society for Physical Therapy (KNGF) and Dutch Society for Hospital Physical Therapy 2021) and at least 45 minutes a day during inpatient stay (Royal Dutch Society for Physical Therapy (KNGF) 2014). Exercises can be performed in a supervised or nonsupervised manner.

Several general recommendations are assumed to determine the efficacy of motor learning after stroke (Krakauer 2006, Krakauer & Carmichael 2017, Royal Dutch Society for Physical Therapy (KNGF) 2014):

- Exercises should be individually tailored (i.e., relevant and meaningful, on limits of ability).
- Exercises should include repetition, but with variations ('repetition-without-repetition').
- Rest periods between sessions and repetitions are needed.
- Frequent (verbal or nonverbal) feedback on performance and results should be provided.
- For declarative learning (e.g., a complex movement like dressing), feedback (verbal or nonverbal) should be given on performance, with decreasing frequency.
- For procedural learning (e.g., walking), feedback (verbal or nonverbal) should be given on results, with decreasing frequency.

- Patients should be motivated by information about the goal and provision of (positive) feedback.
- Complex movements such as dressing should be fragmented first, whereas automatised movements such as walking should be practiced as a whole.
- Training should be conducted in a meaningful environment.

A large array of therapeutic interventions are available for motor rehabilitation after stroke. Tables 7.2 and 7.3 provide an overview of the interventions for which two or more randomised controlled trials of sufficient quality

are available. The tables include the effects for all of these interventions. Interventions for which the best evidence is available are discussed later. For further details regarding motor rehabilitation interventions, please see, for example, Royal Dutch Society for Physical Therapy (KNGF), 2014, Teasell et al, 2015, Stroke Foundation, 2023, and Wolf et al, 2016. The selection of interventions should be based on the available evidence, as well as the functional prognosis for patients and their preferences.

To date, virtually no differences in intervention effects between the various post-stroke stages have been found.

TABLE 7.2 Interventions for Lower Limb and Locomotor Recovery

	ICF CATEGORY		
Interventions	Body Functions	Activities and Participation	Environmental Factors
Early mobilisation out of bed	~	×	×
Balance training			
Sitting balance, including trunk exercises	✓	✓	?
Standing up and sitting down	~	✓/~	?
Standing balance without visual feedback/virtual reality	✓/~	✓/~	?
Postural control with visual feedback/virtual reality	✓ when combined with standard therapy/~	~	?
Balance during various activities	✓/~	✓/~	?
Gait training			
Overground gait training	✓ in the chronic phase/~	✓ in chronic the chronic phase/~	?
Speed-dependent treadmill training	✓/~ for short-term effects on walking speed and walking endurance for patients who can walk but ~ for long-term effects	~ for walking independence	?
Body weight-supported treadmill training	✓/~	~	?
Robot-assisted gait training	✓ in patients <3 months post-stroke not able to walk independently in combination with regular physical therapy/~	✓ in patients <3 months post-stroke not able to walk independently in combination with regular physical therapy/~	?

(Continued)

TABLE 7.2   Interventions for Lower Limb and Locomotor Recovery—Cont'd

| | ICF CATEGORY | | |
Interventions	Body Functions	Activities and Participation	Environmental Factors
Gait training with external auditory rhythms	✓	✓	?
Gait training in public spaces	~	?	?
Circuit class training	✓ when a large amount of time is spent on a specific function/~ when little time is spent on a specific function	✓ when a large amount of time is spent on a specific activity/~ when little time is spent on a specific activity	?
Exercising with informal caregiver	~	✓ when combined with physical therapy/~	✓ when combined with physical therapy
Muscle strength training	✓/~	✓/~	?
Aerobic training	✓/x	✓/~	?
Muscle strength and aerobic training	✓/~	✓/~	?
Training in water (hydrotherapy)	✓ when combined with physical therapy	✓ when combined with physical therapy/~ when compared with conventional therapy	?
Interventions for somatosensory functions	✓/~	✓/~	?
Electrostimulation combined with physical therapy	✓/~ but to be added to regular therapy	✓/~ but to be added to regular therapy	?
Electromyography biofeedback	✓/~ but to be added to regular therapy	✓/~ but to be added to regular therapy	?
Virtual reality	✓ when additionally provided/~ when compared with conventional therapy	✓ when additionally provided/~ when compared with conventional therapy	?
Mirror therapy for the lower limb	✓ when additionally provided/~	✓ when additionally provided/~	?

?, Unknown effect based on the inability to statistically pool data of randomised controlled trials; ✓, beneficial or likely to be beneficial based on significant positive summary effect sizes; ~, uncertain benefit based on nonsignificant summary effect sizes; x, not beneficial or even harmful based on significant negative summary effect sizes; ✓/~, mixed effects; *ICF*, International Classification of Functioning, Disability and Health.

However, it should be considered that therapy goals might differ between stages. Early after stroke the focus is more on restitution of body functions, whereas later the focus shifts towards optimising activities, preventing learned nonuse, integration in society and secondary prevention (see Fig. 7.3). As a final comment regarding motor rehabilitation interventions after stroke, the long-term effects of motor rehabilitation interventions are generally unknown (Veerbeek et al 2014).

Telerehabilitation As an Alternative Form of Therapy Delivery

Traditionally, therapy is provided during face-to-face contact with the patient. However, in the past 2 decades, more attention has been paid to alternative forms of therapy delivery, such as telerehabilitation (Laver et al 2020). A main driver for other delivery forms was the low-intensity dose provided to patients who were no longer inpatients, and this development was further accelerated by the outbreak of the Covid-19 pandemic in early 2020. With home-based telerehabilitation, patients are enabled to exercise in their home situation by using communication technologies (Cramer et al 2019, Laver et al 2020). Like with regular therapy, the training consists of supervised and nonsupervised training sessions. However, during the supervised training sessions, the patient is remotely instructed and coached by the therapist by using, for example, a videoconferencing application. As telerehabilitation is a new emerging field, high-quality trials are scarce. In a noninferiority randomised controlled trial, it was found that delivery of upper limb rehabilitation for patients living in the community resulted the same upper limb improvements when compared with patients who received the same dose of face-to-face therapy (Cramer et al 2019). A meta-analysis showed that there is low-to-moderate evidence for an equal efficacy of telerehabilitation and face-to-face rehabilitation for ADLs, balance, height-related quality of life and depressive symptoms (Laver et al 2020). The cost-effectiveness of telerehabilitation remains unknown (Laver 2020).

LOWER LIMB AND LOCOMOTOR RECOVERY

Table 7.2 provides an overview of lower limb interventions.

Balance Training

Balance training includes exercises aiming to maintain, achieve or restore a state of balance during any posture (Pollock et al 2014). This training could take place during various activities such as sitting, changing body position (such as a transfer from bed to chair or standing up from a sitting position) or walking (Nindorera et al 2022, Van Duijnhoven et al 2016, Veerbeek et al 2014). Balance cannot only be trained by more conventional exercises such as reaching with the nonparetic upper limb beyond arm length or manipulating objects beyond the supporting surface. Also, the application of technological developments such as force platforms or a (commercially available) virtual reality environment could be considered when training balance.

Training of balance after stroke has postintervention effects on postural stability, balance capacity while sitting and standing and basic ADLs regardless of timing post-stroke (Hugues et al 2019, Van Duijnhoven et al 2016, Veerbeek et al 2014). Therefore, it is recommended to train balance in patients with impaired balance (Royal Dutch Society for Physical Therapy (KNGF) 2014). The training should include various postures and, if possible, walking. Furthermore, variations regarding visual dependence, type of surface, width of the supporting surface, shifting the body's centre of gravity and level of distraction during task performance (i.e., dual tasks) are advised

(Royal Dutch Society for Physical Therapy (KNGF) 2014). Standing balance can also be practiced using a standing frame. However, training postural control while standing on a force platform should only be combined with standard therapy because solely training on this platform has not shown to be beneficial (Royal Dutch Society for Physical Therapy (KNGF) 2014). In the literature, balance training is performed 15–60 minutes per session, 2–7 days a week, for about 4–6 weeks.

Gait Training

For gait training after stroke, several evidence-based interventions are available (Hornby et al 2020, Royal Dutch Society for Physical Therapy (KNGF) 2014, Winstein 2016). The most well-investigated interventions include overground walking, (speed-dependent) treadmill training with or without body weight support and robot-assisted gait training.

Overground Walking

Overground gait training is defined as 'observation and manipulation of the patient's gait over a regular floor surface, and is often accompanied by practice walking overground, and exercises specifically designed to improve gait,' and safety (States et al 2009, p. 3). This kind of gait training can be performed in every setting or place and does not require technological aids.

In stroke patients beyond 6 months with mobility deficits, beneficial effects have been found for walking speed, walking distance, participation and quality of life postintervention (Nindorera et al 2022, States et al 2009). These effects were no longer present at follow-up (States et al 2009, Veerbeek et al 2014). The application of overground walking is recommended in chronic stroke patients with walking deficits. However, keeping in mind the principle of specificity of training, overground training should also be considered in patients who are unable to walk independently or those within the first 6 months post-stroke, when judged feasible. Furthermore, backward walking training can be considered as an additional intervention (Chen et al 2020). In the literature, the mean time per overground walking session varied from 15 to 60 minutes, with a frequency of 1–5 times a week, during 2–6 months (Royal Dutch Society for Physical Therapy (KNGF) 2014).

Speed-Dependent Treadmill Training

With speed-dependent treadmill training (STT), the patient walks on a treadmill and can optionally support with one or both upper limbs on a bar (Hornby 2020, Royal Dutch Society for Physical Therapy (KNGF) 2014, Winstein 2016). A therapist is standing beside or behind the patient to monitor balance and to instruct the patient.

During and over the sessions, the walking speed and walking duration are gradually increased. Advantages of walking on a treadmill are that the walking speed can be more closely controlled, observation of the gait pattern is facilitated and the therapist can more easily give manual support (Royal Dutch Society for Physical Therapy (KNGF) 2014). However, walking on a treadmill induces a different optical flow compared with regular overground walking. In addition, walking speed and stride length are shorter compared with overground walking, with the cadence being higher.

There is evidence that STT has beneficial effects on postintervention gait speed, walking distance and width of the gait pattern compared with overground walking (Mehrholz et al 2014, Veerbeek et al 2014). At follow-up, the effects for walking distance were sustained, but the effects for walking speed were levelled off (Mehrholz et al 2017). There are no beneficial effects on walking independency (Mehrholz et al 2017). For clinical practice, it is recommended to use STT in stroke patients who can walk with or without a walking aid with or without supervision (Functional Ambulation Categories [FAC] score ≥3 out of 5). Walking speed, bouts, total duration and inclination should be progressively increased. In the literature, STT sessions have a duration from 8 to 60 minutes, applied 3–5 days a week, during 2 weeks to 6 months (Royal Dutch Society for Physical Therapy (KNGF) 2014).

Body Weight-Supported Treadmill Training

With body weight-supported treadmill training (BWSTT), the patient walks on a treadmill while the body weight is partially supported by a parachute harness (Royal Dutch Society for Physical Therapy (KNGF) 2014). This enables patients who are unable to support their body weight to walk and put weight on their affected lower limb. The percentage of body weight can be reduced stepwise. This form of gait training allows increasing intensity of practice (i.e., use of the paretic lower limb) in stroke patients who are unable to walk. The application of BWSTT requires most often the presence of two therapists: one for guiding the movements of the paretic leg, and the other one for instruction and monitoring balance. With that, BWSTT has a relatively high burden on personnel resources.

BWSTT has beneficial effects for comfortable walking speed and walking distance directly after termination of the intervention (Mehrholz et al 2017, Veerbeek et al 2014), but BWSTT was found to be no more effective than other interventions for balance outcomes (Veerbeek et al 2014). No evidence was found for effects on independency of walking (Mehrholz et al 2017). The findings were regardless of timing post-stroke. According to the Royal Dutch Society for Physical Therapy (KNGF) (2014), BWSTT is recommended for patients who cannot walk without human support or are physically too weak for 'hands-on' mobilisation. The initial maximum level of support should be 30%–40%, and subsequently be gradually reduced. In the meantime, walking speed and the duration of exercise sessions should be systematically increased, depending on the patient's abilities. In the literature, the duration of treatment sessions varies from 15 to 90 minutes, 3–6 times a week, during 2–6 weeks (Royal Dutch Society for Physical Therapy (KNGF) 2014).

Robot-Assisted Gait Training

Robot-assisted gait training is a form of walking exercise in which the walking cycle is guided by electromechanically controlled footplates ('end-effectors') and/or an orthosis ('exoskeleton'), which control the legs in a preprogrammed walking cycle or parts of the walking cycle. The patient's body weight is partially supported by a harness. This enables patients to engage in high-intensity exercising. Many robots can give support as needed, which allows the patient to be as active as possible. Contrary to BWSTT, only one physiotherapist is needed because the robot moves the legs of the patient. The high costs for buying a robot should also be considered.

The postintervention effects of robot-assisted gait training include walking independence, walking speed, walking distance, heart rate, balance, walking ability and basic ADLs (Mehrholz et al 2020, Veerbeek et al 2014). Virtually all effects were found in patients within 3 months after stroke who are unable to walk independently. Furthermore, the effects in walking speed and distance concerned end-effector devices; the effect in walking independency concerned exoskeleton robots. Robot-assisted gait training in combination with physiotherapy is recommended in patients with a FAC score ≤3 out of 5. In the literature, the duration of a treatment session ranges from 15 to 60 minutes, 3–7 days a week, during 2–10 weeks.

Circuit Class Training

With supervised circuit class training (CCT) for walking and other mobility-related activities, two or more patients practice at the same moment, using workstations that are arranged in a circuit (English & Hillier 2010, Royal Dutch Society for Physical Therapy (KNGF) 2014, Wevers et al 2009). These exercises are individually tailored and progressive in terms of, for example, repetitions or complexity (English & Hillier 2010, Wevers et al 2009). Patients usually spend 5 minutes at each working station. The therapist-to-patient ratio is 1:3, with a total of 12 participants. The intervention has mainly been investigated in stroke patients who are either living in the community or following an inpatient rehabilitation program. Advantages of CCT are the increase in therapy time without an increasing demand on therapists and the peer contact for patients.

CCT has been found to be beneficial for walking speed, walking distance, balance and balance confidence, walking ability and physical activity (English et al 2017, Veerbeek et al 2014). However, to induce effects, the type of practice is important (English et al 2015): patients must spend a considerable amount of time practicing the function or activity that was formulated to be a treatment goal. When only a small amount of additional time is spent in walking, for example, then there are no effects for the distance that the patient can walk within 6 minutes, as assessed with the 6-minute walking test (English et al 2015). This stresses the importance of task-specific training.

The application of CCT is recommended for patients who can at least walk 10 metres with or without supervision (FAC ≥3). However, there are indications that this type of training can also be applied in patients who are unable to walk. The number of working stations should be around 6–10 and can target body functions or activities. In the literature, the duration of a CCT session varied from 30 to 75 minutes, provided 3–5 times a week, during 4–19 weeks (Royal Dutch Society for Physical Therapy (KNGF) 2014).

Electrostimulation of the Paretic Lower Limb

Electrostimulation is frequently added to regular physiotherapy (Stroke Foundation, 2023). Two effective forms of electrostimulation of nerves and muscles of the lower limb with surface electrodes (Pomeroy et al 2006) are neuromuscular electrostimulation (NMS) and electromyography-triggered neuromuscular electrostimulation (EMG-NMS).

Both NMS and EMG-NMS can be applied during performance of a functional task (i.e., functional electrical stimulation [FES]) or when making nonfunctional movements of the lower limb, such as eliciting dorsiflexion of the ankle while sitting.

The application of NMS on the lower limb has postintervention effects on the body function level in terms of motor function, muscle strength and resistance to passive movements postintervention (Veerbeek et al 2014). Evidence for a beneficial effect of EMG-NMS is currently lacking (Veerbeek et al 2014). FES has a positive effect on ADLs when applied within the first 2 months after stroke (Eraifej et al 2017). Long-term effects are unknown.

It is recommended to use electrostimulation of the paretic leg in patients who can stand or walk (with or without support) and have some volitional movement of their paretic leg (Royal Dutch Society for Physical Therapy (KNGF) 2014). Because of large heterogeneity between trials, the optimal settings of the device, as well as the number of repetitions, sessions per week and treatment period duration are to date unknown.

Upper Limb Recovery

Notably, for evidence-based interventions for upper limb recovery as described in Table 7.3 and in the following subsections, it is required that patients have some volitional activity of the paretic upper limb. Currently, there is no evidence-based upper limb rehabilitation intervention for patients with a paralysis of the upper limb.

TABLE 7.3	Interventions for Upper Limb Recovery		
	ICF CATEGORY		
Interventions	**Body Functions**	**Activities and Participation**	**Environmental Factors**
CIMT			
Original CIMT	✓	✗ but ✓ for perceived amount and quality of use	?
Modified CIMT	✓	✗ but ✓ for perceived amount and quality of use	?
Forced use	✗	✗	?
Bilateral arm training	✓ compared with conventional therapy/– compared with unilateral arm training	–	?

(Continued)

TABLE 7.3   Interventions for Upper Limb Recovery—Cont'd

Interventions	ICF CATEGORY		
	Body Functions	Activities and Participation	Environmental Factors
Virtual reality	✓ when additionally provided/x when compared with conventional therapy	✓ when additionally provided/x when compared with conventional therapy	?
Electrostimulation	✓/x but to be added to regular therapy	✓/x but to be added to regular therapy	?
Robot-assisted training	✓§ but to be considered as add-on to exercise therapy	✓§ but to be considered as add-on to exercise therapy	?
Mirror therapy	✓ at least as an adjunct to conventional rehabilitation	✓ at least as an adjunct to conventional rehabilitation	?
Electromyography biofeedback	x	x	?
Muscle strength training	✓/x	?	?
Trunk restraint while training paretic arm	✓ for patients in subacute phase/x for patients in chronic phase	✓ for patients in subacute phase/x for patients in chronic phase	?
Interventions for somatosensory functions	✓ for active somatosensory interventions (effect on motor impairment)/x for active somatosensory interventions (effect on somatosensation) and for passive somatosensory interventions	x for passive and active somatosensory interventions	?
Therapeutic positioning	✓§/x	?	?
Reflex-inhibiting positions and immobilisation techniques	✓§ for positioning orthoses reduced wrist-flexor spasticity when compared with no therapy/x	?	?
Use of air-splints and wrappings	x	?	?
Hemiplegic shoulder pain	✓ for electrical stimulation on pain and external rotation (but high risk of bias) ✓ for kinesio taping on pain, motor function and magnitude of subluxation	✓ for electrical stimulation (but high risk of bias) ✓ for kinesio taping	?

§, Effect not clinically relevant; ?, unknown effect, based on the inability to statistically pool data of randomised controlled trials; ✓, beneficial or likely to be beneficial, based on significant positive summary effect sizes; x, uncertain benefit, based on nonsignificant summary effect sizes; –, not beneficial or likely not to be beneficial, based on significant negative summary effect sizes; ✓/x, mixed effects; –/x, not beneficial; *CIMT*, constraint-induced movement therapy; *ICF*, International Classification of Functioning, Disability and Health.

Constraint-Induced Movement Therapy

Constraint-induced movement therapy (CIMT) was initially developed to promote the use of the paretic upper limb after stroke both in the clinic and in daily life (Morris et al 2006). The original intervention protocol includes three key elements: (1) repetitive, task-oriented training of the more affected upper limb for 6 hours a day with an increasing difficulty; (2) wearing a mitt on the less affected upper limb for 90% of the waking hours to promote the use of the more affected upper limb and (3) the application of a transfer package (Morris et al 2006). This transfer package includes behavioural methods to enhance the transfer of gains made in the clinic to the patients' daily lives. The duration of the original CIMT treatment is each working day for 2 or 3 consecutive weeks (Corbetta et al 2015, Kwakkel et al 2015, Veerbeek et al 2014). A plethora of modified CIMT protocols have been scientifically tested for their efficacy. These modified versions mainly include the first two elements of the original CIMT and are often applied with a lower intensity: the duration of sessions ranges from 30 minutes to 6 hours a day, with number of sessions per week being between 2 and 7, and a treatment period of 2–12 weeks (Kwakkel et al 2015).

The effects of CIMT lie mainly at the activity level of the ICF, such as upper limb activities and patient-reported upper limb use in their home environment, and there is also evidence of effect on patient-reported outcomes of health status (Abdullahi et al 2021, Corbetta et al 2015, Kwakkel et al 2015, Veerbeek et al 2014). Postintervention effects were sustained 20 weeks after termination of the intervention. The size of the effect does not differ between the original form of CIMT and its modified versions, nor is there a difference between the various phases after stroke. The only exception is for motor function of the paretic upper limb, for which only beneficial effects were found when modified CIMT was applied within 3 months after stroke (Kwakkel et al 2015). It should be noted that only wearing a mitt without further training or application of a transfer package (i.e., forced use) has shown not to be beneficial and is therefore not recommended. Finally, it is important to stress that CIMT is a treatment option only for patients who have some volitional movement in their paretic upper limb and especially in the extension direction of one or more fingers and/or thumb.

Bilateral Arm Training

Simultaneous bilateral arm training (BAT) is defined as 'the completion of identical activities with both arms simultaneously', aiming to improve arm function and reduce impairment (Coupar et al 2010, pp. 1–2). This form of training is characterised by a high number of repetitions of the movements. BAT can be applied in functional activities such as grabbing a plate with both hands, or in combination with technological developments such as robotics, EMG-triggered electrostimulation or devices that provide rhythmic auditory cues while training flexion and extension of elbows or wrists (Royal Dutch Society for Physical Therapy (KNGF) 2014). The latter is called BAT with rhythmic auditory cueing.

Currently, the evidence suggests that BAT is not more (or less) effective than unilateral arm training for motor impairment and functional performance (Chen et al 2022). With that, BAT is a treatment option for patients with a paresis of the upper limb. Compared with conventional therapy, BAT demonstrated significant benefit for improving motor impairment but not functional performance. Superior effects appear associated with patients being more mildly impaired in the chronic phase after stroke and receiving a higher dose of the intervention (Chen et al 2022).

Virtual Reality, Including Interactive Video Gaming

Virtual reality is defined as the use of interactive simulations created with computer hardware and software to present users with opportunities to engage in environments that appear and feel similar to real world objects and events (Weiss et al 2006). With sensors placed on the patients' upper limb, a controller for the hand and/or the use of a mouse/keyboard, they can move with their paretic upper limb in a virtually created environment. This virtual environment can either be immersive or nonimmersive. With immersive training, patients wear special glasses and are being 'immersed' in this virtual environment. When with a nonimmersive system, the environment is projected on a TV screen. This is often the case when commercially available video gaming devices are used. Patients training in a virtual environment can receive visual and/or auditory feedback regarding how they move and the results of their movements (Royal Dutch Society for Physical Therapy (KNGF) 2014). Advantages of this kind of training are that it allows a high number of repetitions, motivates and challenges patients and supports training without supervision.

A Cochrane review reports beneficial effects for upper limb function and ADLs when added as an adjunct to regular therapy (to increase overall therapy time), with long-term effects being unclear (Laver et al 2017). However, virtual reality was not more beneficial than conventional therapy in improving upper limb function. One systematic review showed that the application of virtual reality training also induced a higher muscle tone of the paretic upper limb (Veerbeek et al 2014). Large, randomised trials showed no differences in patient outcomes and safety issues when comparing nonimmersive virtual reality training using a Nintendo Wii with the same amount of time spent in recreational training (Saposnik et al 2016), or when specifically designed rehabilitation virtual reality was used in the subacute phase (Brunner et al 2017). For clinical practice, it is recommended to apply virtual reality training as an add-on to regular exercise therapy after stroke. The session duration should amount to 30 minutes, applied 5 days a week for several weeks (Royal Dutch Society for Physical Therapy (KNGF) 2014). Because patients have an increased risk for higher muscle tone in their affected upper limb, the tone should be monitored throughout the treatment period.

Electrostimulation of the Paretic Arm and Hand

Electrostimulation is frequently added to regular physiotherapy. Two effective forms of electrostimulation of nerves and muscles of the upper limb with surface electrodes (Pomeroy et al 2006) are NMS and EMG-NMS. Both NMS and EMG-NMS can be applied during performance of a functional task (i.e., FES) or when making nonfunctional movements of the upper limb, such as extending the wrist without a functional task (Veerbeek et al 2014).

The postintervention effects of electrostimulation of the paretic arm and hand mainly lie on the motor function domain of the paretic upper limb. However, for EMG-NMS, beneficial effects were also found for upper limb activities. How long the effects last after termination of the study remains unclear (Veerbeek et al 2014). Because of large heterogeneity between trials, the optimal settings of the device, as well as the number of repetitions, sessions per week and treatment period duration, are to date unknown. For patients who have some volitional extension function of the paretic wrist and/or fingers, it is recommended to use EMG-NMS and NMS as an add-on therapy (Royal Dutch Society for Physical Therapy (KNGF) 2014). In trials, the stimulation is most often applied in patients who are at least 1 month and more often beyond 6 months after stroke onset (Veerbeek et al 2014). In addition, NMS for the paretic shoulder muscles could be considered for patients less than 3 months after stroke who have a glenohumeral subluxation and hemiplegic shoulder pain (Royal Dutch Society for Physical Therapy (KNGF) 2014).

Robot-Assisted Therapy for the Upper Limb

With robot-assisted therapy for the upper limb (RT-UL), patients train their paretic upper limb by using electronic, computerised control systems to mechanical devices that are designed to assist human functions in rehabilitation. These robotic devices are developed either as an exoskeleton or as an end-effector (Mehrholz et al 2018). Exoskeleton devices are defined as external structural devices with axes aligned with anatomical axes of the human body, providing direct control of individual joints (Chang & Kim 2013). End-effector devices are defined as systems with a single distal attachment point to apply mechanical forces to the distal segment of a limb (Chang & Kim 2013, Loureiro et al 2011). Robotics can also be classified according to the joints they target, with most robots focusing on the shoulder-elbow. Furthermore, they can be classified according to the level of support provided by the robot (e.g., passive, assist-as-needed, resistance) and the type of support (patient or robot in charge while moving) (Veerbeek et al 2017).

The advantage of robotic devices is that they allow patients to increase the number of repetitions of a movement and with that, increase intensity of practice. In addition, they are assumed to increase the patients' motivation and allow semi-independent practice. The application of RT-UL was shown to be safe and well accepted by patients (Veerbeek et al 2017). An updated Cochrane review demonstrates that electromechanical and robot-assisted arm training improves ADLs, arm function and arm muscle strength (Mehrholz et al 2018). However, the effects may not be clinically relevant (Veerbeek et al 2017). Also, with robot-assisted therapy of the upper limb, patients have an increased risk for higher muscle tone in their affected upper limb. When interpreting the findings, one should remark that the studies mainly included patients beyond 3 months after stroke, indicating that to date the effects of RT-UL applied early after stroke remain speculative. Furthermore, a large clinical trial including 770 patients showed that robot-assisted training for 45 minutes, three times per week for 12 weeks did not provide better results for upper limb function and activity compared with usual care or an equally intensive conventional upper limb program (Rodgers et al 2019). Altogether the application of RT-UL could be considered as an add-on to exercise therapy when there are upper limb rehabilitation goals (Royal Dutch Society for Physical Therapy (KNGF) 2014). Nevertheless, its superiority over other interventions for the upper limb has not been proven in a definitive trial, and routine use of these devices to replace therapy is therefore discouraged (Veerbeek et al 2017).

Therapy Delivery

As described earlier, rehabilitation should start as early as possible after stroke onset when the patient is medically stable and should be intensified after the first vulnerable period has passed. For patients discharged home, but for whom there are still treatment goals, various methods of therapy delivery are available. Therapy can be delivered as booster sessions in which patients receive high-frequency therapy bouts alternated with periods without therapy (Hesse et al 2011). An equally effective delivery method is continuous low-frequency therapy in which patients receive therapy over a longer period, but with fewer treatment sessions per week (Hesse et al 2011). Furthermore, patients can be instructed regarding a self-training programme. This self-training programme is usually performed at home and can be extended by telerehabilitation facilitation, such as a video link or telephone (Laver et al 2020). Telerehabilitation often consists of an initial face-to-face instruction session with a therapist after which patients train at home without therapist supervision. Therapist's feedback regarding performance and evaluation of progress is intermittently provided by using information and communication technologies. Patients can also take the initiative to contact their therapist (Royal Dutch Society for Physical Therapy (KNGF) 2014).

Involvement of caregivers could be considered when patients perform exercises without supervision of a therapist. Caregiver-mediated exercises focused on mobility have positive effects on gait and gait-related outcomes, such as balance and walking endurance, without increasing caregiver burden (Vloothuis et al 2016).

CONCLUSION

For the majority of patients, a stroke is a life-changing and chronic condition. Stroke can be caused by a blood clot in or a rupture of an artery in the brain. Symptoms after stroke depend on the localisation of the stroke. With that, symptoms are heterogeneous in terms of modalities affected and severity. Most recovery post-stroke takes place within the first 6 months after stroke onset. Rehabilitation should be started as early as possible and aims to optimise functions, activities and participation of the patients. Knowledge of the functional prognosis is essential to design the rehabilitation of an individual patient. This knowledge is also important for properly informing patients and their carers.

Depending on the rehabilitation goals, the preferences of the patient and the available resources, therapists have various evidence-based rehabilitation interventions to choose from. Some general treatment principles that characterise efficacious motor rehabilitation interventions are intensity, specificity and the application of motor learning principles.

The application of clinimetrics is a prerequisite throughout the rehabilitation period: to determine entry level of the patient, to make a functional prognosis for recovery, to set rehabilitation goals, to evaluate the patient's status over time and to guide therapy content and delivery.

CASE STUDY

David is a 67-year-old retired mathematics teacher who complained of a sudden loss of strength in his right upper and lower limb while attending the school's yearly party. An attentive parent recognised the sudden change in David's condition, noticed also that the right side of his mouth was dropping, and that David's speech and language abruptly became incomprehensible. They immediately called an ambulance (as time is brain!), and David was rushed to Accidents & Emergency (A&E).

At A&E, David was admitted to the acute stroke unit and stroke severity was assessed by means of the National Institute of Health Stroke Scale (NIHSS); he obtained a score of 16 out of 42 (lower is better), indicating a moderate stroke severity. Because he fulfilled the criteria for receiving thrombolysis, he received thrombolysis within the favourable 3-hour window after stroke onset. Back on the acute stroke unit, David's condition was considered medically stable, and therapy was started with short bouts of early mobilisation to bring David up into the sitting and standing position, and to allow him to walk within the room with a walking aid and light physical support of the therapists and nurses.

During the next days, David's condition has improved. He still has upper and lower limb motor deficits, but less pronounced compared with stroke onset. David has good sitting balance, measured by the Trunk Control Test (74/100). Furthermore, he still has language deficits and also swallowing problems for which he receives speech and language therapy. His NIHSS score improved to 6 out of 42 at discharge from the acute stroke unit. When strength of upper and lower limb is measured by means of the Motricity Index, David scores 39 out of 100 for the upper limb and 42 out of 100 for the lower limb, indicating the possibility of volitional activity in the different muscles (including finger extension) tested, but no full range of movement and limited activity against gravity. Furthermore, he can partially extend the fingers of his right hand. Based on these measurements, David has a favourable outcome for functional ability at 6 months. Based on a multidisciplinary approach, key assessment findings are presented in Table 7.4.

After 8 days, David is transferred from the acute stroke unit to an inpatient rehabilitation centre, where he continues to receive interdisciplinary treatment. His main goal is to live at home independently, drive his car again and enjoy life after stroke with his wife, daughter and son-in-law and grandchildren. The therapist's clinical reasoning process is represented in Table 7.5.

Based on the intake assessment showing further progress since his stroke unit assessment, the treatment focus for David was on the following elements:
- Balance activities including transfers to and back up from the floor, addressing the residual balance problem David has and giving him the ability to get back up from the floor should he experience a fall.
- Gait activities including STT (practiced together with the sports therapists), overground walking as part of the physiotherapy sessions which include walking stairs but also walking outdoors over uneven surfaces such as cobblestones, grass and small hills. David is also included in a CCT group focusing on gait and dynamic balance activities.
- For arm activities, David fulfils the criteria for CIMT, and he is entered into a CIMT group for 2 weeks comprising

TABLE 7.4   **David's Key Assessment Body Function Findings From a Multidisciplinary Perspective**

Body Function	Key Findings
Consciousness, orientation and intellectual function	Not affected; David is awake and alert, oriented in space and time without obvious cognitive deficits
Temperament and personality	David appears to be somewhat depressed
Energy and drive	Lack of motivation, David is overwhelmed by the sudden stroke event
Sleep, attention and memory	Attention and memory seem not to be affected, David is not sleeping well
Psychomotor and perceptual ability	Not affected
Cognitive and seeing ability	Not affected
Proprioception and touch	Not affected
Voice and articulation	David has a dysarthria and a mild motor aphasia; he also has swallowing problems
Ingestion, defecation and urinary continence	Not affected
Mobility and stability of joints	Not affected
Muscle strength, tone and reflexes	Reduced muscle strength in both right upper and lower limbs, measured by means of Motricity Index (39/100 for upper limb, 42/100 for lower limb), David has adequate trunk control measured by means of the Trunk Control Test (74/100)
Muscle endurance	Reduced because of reduced muscle power
Control of voluntary movement	Reduced because of reduced muscle power
Gait pattern functions	Asymmetrically because of reduced muscle power in the right side of the body, reduced walking speed (measured by 10-metre walk test: 0.42 m/s with walking aid)

restraining the use of the unaffected left upper limb, intensive therapy for the affected right upper limb and the application of a transfer package, facilitating the use of the affected upper limb during, for example, grooming and washing activities without therapist supervision.

An overview of David's rehabilitation progress is presented in Table 7.6. After 4 months in the rehabilitation centre, David is discharged home with residual deficits. Although he can independently walk outdoors without a walking aid, he still has not regained full dorsiflexion strength in his affected lower limb, which impedes him from making longer walks because of distal motor fatigue (i.e., more pronounced drop-foot when walking longer distances). For that, he will try out a customised ankle-foot orthosis. Furthermore, his dexterity in his affected upper limb is also still limited. Fine motor skills such as zipping up or down his trousers or buttoning his shirt require a lot of attention and effort, which frustrates David. In addition, he has not started yet with car driving lessons. When discharged home, David receives further weekly therapy, which includes a self-exercise programme. He also conducts regular physical activity in line with general recommendations. Together with his medication for high blood pressure and increased cholesterol levels, David is aware that regular physical activity is a factor that he himself can control to prevent a subsequent stroke and, despite his limitations, to enjoy life after stroke with his wife, daughter and son-in-law and grandchildren.

TABLE 7.5   David's Multidisciplinary Problem List, Goals and Treatment Plan, at the Different ICF Levels

Problem list

Body function	• Lack of motivation, although this has improved when attending inpatient rehabilitation, probably also because of improvements observed
Body function and activity	• Speech and language difficulties; David understands everything but sometimes produces slurred speech which frustrates him
Body function and activity	• Reduced muscle power in the right upper and lower limbs, leading to reduced endurance, voluntary movement (distal more than proximal), reduced gait speed and pattern alterations, and balance problems

Goals

Body function and participation	• David is motivated and knows about stroke and life after stroke
Body function and participation	• David feels confident about his speech in everyday conversations
Body function and participation	• To improve muscle strength, walking distance and gait speed. The aim is: (a) to reach 0.80 m/s on the 10-metre walk test (comfortable speed to achieve appropriate gait speed for community ambulation, and (b) to be able to walk independently to the grocery store around the corner and back without a rest (500 m)

Treatment plan

Linked to goal (1)	• Neuropsychological consults including group session to discuss stroke, stroke consequences and possibilities; involve David's hobby as part of the treatment approach
Linked to goals (1) and (3)	• Occupational therapy focusing on facilitating gardening activities as this is one of David's hobbies, as well as linking with grocery store visit
Linked to goal (2)	• Speech and language therapy for slurred speech
Linked to goal (3)	• Physiotherapy and sports therapy with emphasis on improving upper and lower limb proximal and distal muscle power and endurance, gait and balance activities

TABLE 7.6   David's Progress With Physical Rehabilitation

	Status at the End of Inpatient Rehabilitation
Body Function	
Muscle strength	Increased muscle strength in both upper and lower limbs; however, distal function (dorsiflexion of foot and manipulation component of hand and fingers) remains impaired.
	Currently under discussion is the suggestion for David to wear a foot orthosis, which would allow him to walk longer distances.
Muscle endurance	David participated in a 6-minute walking test where he was able to walk 6 minutes but still achieved a lower distance compared with age- and gender-matched controls.
Control of voluntary movement	Improved but distal control in both upper and lower limb shows residual deficits.
Gait pattern and balance	Comfortable gait speed has improved to 0.82 m/s, which is at the lower limit for community ambulation.
	Balance has improved as well; David is confident in walking indoors without walking aid.
Activities and participation	
Functional walking	David can walk to the grocery store and back without needing a break (500 m).
Car driving	Will be assessed and trained in an outpatient situation. David has made contact for a first appointment. The prospect of being able to resume driving motivates David.

SELF-ASSESSMENT QUESTIONS

1. What is a stroke, and which two types of stroke are commonly seen? Explain how for both types the stroke event leads to loss of body functions.
2. Give 10 body functions that can be affected in people after stroke.
3. True or false: 'Based on current literature it is not possible to predict upper limb outcome at 6 months after stroke based on initial assessment within the first days because of the long time period between both assessments.' Explain your answer.
4. Draw the recovery pattern after stroke and provide the corresponding core physical treatment focus according to the following phases: hyperacute, early and late rehabilitation, and chronic phase.
5. What are the evidence-based treatment options for a patient with a paralysis in the upper and lower limbs, respectively?

REFERENCES

Abdullahi, A., Van Criekinge, T., Umar, N.A., Zakari, U.U., Truijen, S., Saeys, W., 2021. Effect of constraint-induced movement therapy on persons-reported outcomes of health status after stroke: a systematic review and meta-analysis. Int. J. Rehabil. Res. 44, 15–23.

Adams Jr., H.P., Bendixen, B.H., Kappelle, L.J., Biller, J., Love, B.B., Gordon, D.L., 1993. Classification of subtype of acute ischemic stroke. Definitions for use in a multicenter clinical trial. Stroke. 24, 35–41.

Amarenco, P., Bogousslavsky, J., Caplan, L.R., Donnan, G.A., Hennerici, M.G., 2009. Classification of stroke subtypes. Cerebrovasc. Dis. 27, 493–501.

AVERT Trial Collaboration Group., 2015. Efficacy and safety of very early mobilisation within 24 h of stroke onset (AVERT): a randomised controlled trial. Lancet. 386, 46–55.

Bamford, J., Sandercock, P., Dennis, M., Burn, J., Wardlow, C., 1991. Classification and natural history of clinically identifiable subtypes of cerebral infarction. Lancet. 337, 1521–1526.

Bernhardt, J., Churilov, L., Ellery, F., AVERT Collaboration Group., 2016. Prespecified dose-response analysis for A Very Early Rehabilitation Trial (AVERT). Neurology. 86, 2138–2145.

Bernhardt, J., Hayward, K.S., Kwakkel, G., et al., 2017. Agreed definitions and a shared vision for new standards in stroke recovery research: The Stroke Recovery and Rehabilitation Roundtable taskforce. Int. J. Stroke. 12, 444–450.

Brunner, I., Skouen, J.S., Hofstad, H., et al., 2017. Virtual Reality Training for Upper Extremity in Subacute Stroke (VIRTUES): a multicenter RCT. Neurology. 89, 2413–2421.

Chang, W.H., Kim, Y.H., 2013. Robot-assisted therapy in stroke rehabilitation. J. Stroke. 15, 174–181.

Chen, S., Qiu, Y., Bassile, C.C., Lee, A., Chen, R., Xu, D., 2022. Effectiveness and success factors of bilateral arm training after stroke: a systematic review and meta-analysis. Front. Aging. Neurosci. 14, 875794.

Chen, Z.H., Ye, X.L., Chen, W.J., et al., 2020. Effectiveness of backward walking for people affected by stroke: a systematic review and meta-analysis of randomized controlled trials. Medicine. 99, e20731.

Clark, B., Whitall, J., Kwakkel, G., Mehrholz, J., Ewings, S., Burridge, J., 2021. The effect of time spent in rehabilitation on activity limitation and impairment after stroke. Cochrane Database Syst. Rev. 10, CD012612.

Corbetta, D., Sirtori, V., Castellini, G., Moja, L., Gatti, R., 2015. Constraint-induced movement therapy for upper extremities in people with stroke. Cochrane Database Syst. Rev. 10, CD004433.

Coupar, F., Pollock, A., van Wijck, F., Morris, J., Langhorne, P., 2010. Simultaneous bilateral training for improving arm function after stroke. Cochrane Database Syst. Rev 4, CD006432.

Coupar, F., Pollock, A., Rowe, P., Weir, C., Langhorne, P., 2012. Predictors of upper limb recovery after stroke: a systematic review and meta-analysis. Clin. Rehabil. 26, 291–313.

Cramer, S.C., Dodakian, L., Le, V., National Institutes of Health StrokeNet Telerehab Investigators., 2019. Efficacy of home-based telerehabilitation vs in-clinic therapy for adults after stroke: a randomized clinical trial. JAMA. Neurol. 76, 1079–1087.

Cumming, T.B., Thrift, A.G., Collier, J.M., Churilov, L., Dewey, H.M., Donnan, G.A., 2011. Very early mobilization after stroke fast-tracks return to walking: further results from the phase II AVERT randomized controlled trial. Stroke. 42, 153–158.

Easton, J.D., Saver, J.L., Albers, G.W., Alberts, M.J., Chaturvedi, S., Feldmann, E., American Heart Association, American Stroke Association Stroke Council, Council on Cardiovascular Surgery and Anaesthesia, Council on Cardiovascular Radiology and Intervention, Council on Cardiovascular Nursing, Interdisciplinary Council on Peripheral Vascular Disease., 2009. Definition and evaluation of transient ischemic attack: a scientific statement for healthcare professionals from the American Heart Association/American Stroke Association Stroke Council; Council on Cardiovascular Surgery and Anaesthesia; Council on Cardiovascular Radiology and Intervention; Council on Cardiovascular Nursing; and the Interdisciplinary Council on Peripheral Vascular Disease. The American Academy of Neurology affirms the value of this statement as an educational tool for neurologists. Stroke. 40, 2276–2293.

English, C., Bernhardt, J., Crotty, M., Esterman, A., Segal, L., Hillier, S., 2015. Circuit class therapy or seven-day week therapy for increasing rehabilitation intensity of therapy after stroke (CIRCIT): a randomized controlled trial. Int. J. Stroke. 10, 594–602.

English, C., Hillier, S.L., 2010. Circuit class therapy for improving mobility after stroke. Cochrane Database Syst. Rev. 7, CD007513.

English, C., Hillier, S.L., Lynch, E.A., 2017. Circuit class therapy for improving mobility after stroke. Cochrane Database Syst. Rev. 6, CD007513.

Eraifej, J., Clark, W., France, B., Desando, S., Moore, D., 2017. Effectiveness of upper limb functional electrical stimulation after stroke for the improvement of activities of daily living and motor function: a systematic review and meta-analysis. Syst. Rev. 6, 40.

Feigin, V.L., Brainin, M., Norrving, B., et al., 2022. World Stroke Organization (WSO): Global Stroke Fact Sheet 2022. Int. J. Stroke. 17, 18–29.

French, B., Thomas, L.H., Coupe, J., McMahon, N.E., Connell, L., Harrison, J., 2016. Repetitive task training for improving functional ability after stroke. Cochrane Database Syst. Rev. 11, CD006073.

Hesse, S., Welz, A., Werner, C., Quentin, B., Wissel, J., 2011. Comparison of an intermittent high-intensity vs continuous low-intensity physiotherapy service over 12 months in community-dwelling people with stroke: a randomized trial. Clin. Rehabil. 25, 146–156.

Hornby, T.G., Reisman, D.S., Ward, I.G., the Locomotor CPG Appraisal Team., 2020. Clinical practice guideline to improve locomotor function following chronic stroke, incomplete spinal cord injury, and brain injury. J. Neurol. Phys. Ther. 44, 49–100.

Hugues, A., Di Marco, J., Ribault, S., et al., 2019. Limited evidence of physical therapy on balance after stroke: a systematic review and meta-analysis. PloS. One. 14, e0221700.

Kwakkel, G., Kollen, B.J., 2013. Predicting activities after stroke: what is clinically relevant? Int. J. Stroke. 8, 25–32.

Kwakkel, G., Veerbeek, J.M., van Wegen, E.E., Wolf, S.L., 2015. Constraint-induced movement therapy after stroke. Lancet. Neurol. 14, 224–234.

Krakauer, J.W., 2006. Motor learning: its relevance to stroke recovery and neurorehabilitation. Curr. Opin. Neurol. 19 (1), 84–90.

Krakauer, J.W., Carmichael, T., 2017. Broken movement: the neurobiology of motor recovery after stroke. MIT Press.

Langhorne, P., Baylan, S., 2017. Early supported discharge trialists. Early supported discharge services for people with acute stroke. Cochrane Database Syst. Rev. 7, CD000443.

Langhorne, P., Bernhardt, J., Kwakkel, G., 2011. Stroke rehabilitation. Lancet. 377, 1693–1702.

Langhorne, P., Ramachandra, S., Stroke Unit Trialists' Collaboration., 2020. Organised inpatient (stroke unit) care for stroke: network meta-analysis. Cochrane Database Syst. Rev. 4, CD000197.

Laver, K.E., Adey-Wakeling, Z., Crotty, M., Lannin, N.A., George, S., Sherrington, C., 2020. Telerehabilitation services for stroke. Cochrane Database Syst. Rev. 1, CD010255.

Laver, K.E., George, S., Thomas, S., Deutsch, J.E., Crotty, M., 2017. Virtual reality for stroke rehabilitation. Cochrane Database Syst. Rev. 11, CD008349.

Lohse, K.R., Lang, C.E., Boyd, L.A., 2014. Is more better? Using metadata to explore dose-response relationships in stroke rehabilitation. Stroke. 45, 2053–2058.

Loureiro, R.C., Harwin, W.S., Nagai, K., Johnson, M., 2011. Advances in upper limb stroke rehabilitation: a technology push. Med. Biol. Eng. Comput. 49, 1103–1118.

Mehrholz, J., Pohl, M., Elsner, B., 2014. Treadmill training and body weight support for walking after stroke. Cochrane Database Syst. Rev. 1, CD002840.

Mehrholz, J., Thomas, S., Elsner, B., 2017. Treadmill training and body weight support for walking after stroke. Cochrane Database Syst. Rev. 1, CD002840.

Mehrholz, J., Pohl, M., Platz, T., Kugler, J., Elsner, B., 2018. Electromechanical and robot-assisted arm training for improving activities of daily living, arm function, and arm muscle strength after stroke. Cochrane Database Syst. Rev. 9, CD006876.

Mehrholz, J., Thomas, S., Kugler, J., Pohl, M., Elsner, B., 2020. Electromechanical-assisted training for walking after stroke. Cochrane Database Syst. Rev. 10, CD006185.

Meyer, S., Verheyden, G., Brinkmann, N., Dejaeger, E., De Weerdt, W., Feys, H., 2015. Functional and motor outcome 5 years after stroke is equivalent to outcome at 2 months: follow-up of the collaborative evaluation of rehabilitation in stroke across Europe. Stroke. 46, 1613–1619.

Morris, D.M., Taub, E., Mark, V.W., 2006. Constraint-induced movement therapy: characterizing the intervention protocol. Eur. Medicophys. 42, 257–268.

National Institute for Health and Care Excellence.,2008. Clinical guideline. Stroke and transient ischaemic attack in over 16s: diagnosis and initial management [CG68]. Available at: www.nice.org.uk. Accessed 9 August 2022.

National Stroke Foundation (NSF).,2017. Clinical guidelines for stroke management. Available at: www.informme.org.au. Accessed 9 August 2022.

Nijland, R.H., van Wegen, E.E., Harmeling-van der Wel, B.C., Kwakkel, G., EPOS Investigators., 2010. Presence of finger extension and shoulder abduction within 72 hours after stroke predicts functional recovery. Early prediction of functional outcome after stroke: the EPOS cohort study. Stroke. 41, 745–750.

Nindorera, F., Nduwimana, I., Thonnard, J.L., Kossi, O., 2022. Effectiveness of walking training on balance, motor functions, activity, participation and quality of life in people with chronic stroke: a systematic review with meta-analysis and meta-regression of recent randomized controlled trials. Disabil. Rehabil. 44, 3760–3771.

Pohl, J., Held, J.P.O., Verheyden, G., et al., 2020. Consensus-based core set of outcome measures for clinical motor rehabilitation after stroke—a Delphi study. Front. Neurol 11, 875. Erratum in: Front. Neurol. 2021; 12, 697935

Pollock, A., Baer, G., Campbell, P., Choo, P.L., Forster, A., Morris, J., 2014. Physical rehabilitation approaches for the recovery of function and mobility following stroke. Cochrane Database Syst. Rev. 4, CD001920.

Pomeroy, V.M., King, L., Pollock, A., Baily-Hallam, A., Langhorne, P., 2006. Electrostimulation for promoting recovery of movement or functional ability after stroke. Cochrane Database Syst. Rev. 2, CD003241.

Preston, E., Ada, L., Stanton, R., Mahendran, N., Dean, C.M., 2021. Prediction of independent walking in people who are nonambulatory early after stroke: a systematic review. Stroke. 52(10), 3217–3224. http://doi:10.1161/STROKEAHA.120.032345.

Roaldsen, M.B., Jusufovic, M., Berge, E., Lindekleiv, H., 2021. Endovascular thrombectomy and intra-arterial interventions for acute ischaemic stroke. Cochrane Database Syst. Rev. 6, CD007574.

Rodgers, H., Bosomworth, H., Krebs, H.I., et al., 2019. Robot assisted training for the upper limb after stroke (RATULS): a multicentre randomised controlled trial. Lancet. 394, 51–62.

Royal Dutch Society for Physical Therapy (KNGF)., 2014. KNGF evidence-based clinical practice guidelines. KNGF-guideline Stroke 2014. Royal Dutch Society for Physical Therapy (Koninklijk Nederlands Genootschap voor Fysiotherapie). Amersfoort, the Netherlands.

Sacco, R.L., Kasner, S.E., Broderick, J.P., American Heart Association Stroke Council, Council on Cardiovascular Surgery and Anesthesia; Council on Cardiovascular Radiology and Intervention; Council on Cardiovascular and Stroke Nursing; Council on Epidemiology and Prevention; Council on Peripheral Vascular Disease; Council on Nutrition, Physical Activity and Metabolism., 2013. An updated definition of stroke for the 21st century: a statement for healthcare professionals from the American Heart Association/American Stroke Association. Stroke. 44, 2064–2089.

Saposnik, G., Cohen, L.G., Mamdani, M., Pooyania, S., Ploughman, M., Cheung, D., Stroke Outcomes Research Canada., 2016. Efficacy and safety of non-immersive virtual reality exercising in stroke rehabilitation (EVREST): a randomised, multicentre, single-blind, controlled trial. Lancet. Neurol. 15, 1019–1027.

Saver, J.L., 2006. Time is brain – quantified. Stroke. 37, 263–266.

Scottish Intercollegiate Guidelines Network (SIGN), 2010. 118. Management of patients with stroke: Rehabilitation, prevention and management of complications, and discharge planning. A national clinical guideline. Available at: www.sign.ac.uk. Accessed 9 August 2022.

Smith, M.C., Ackerley, S.J., Barber, P.A., Byblow, W.D., Stinear, C.M., 2019. PREP2 algorithm predictions are correct at 2 years poststroke for most patients. Neurorehabil. Neural. Repair. 33, 635–642.

Smith, M.C., Barber, P.A., Stinear, C.M., 2017. The TWIST algorithm predicts time to walking independently after stroke. Neurorehabil. Neural. Repair. 31, 955–964.

States, R.A., Pappas, E., Salem, Y., 2009. Overground physical therapy gait training for chronic stroke patients with mobility deficits. Cochrane Database Syst. Rev. 3, CD006075.

Stinear, C.M., Barber, P.A., Petoe, M., Anwar, S., Byblow, W.D., 2012. The PREP algorithm predicts potential for upper limb recovery after stroke. Brain. 135, 2527–2535.

Stinear, C.M., Byblow, W.D., Ackerley, S.J., Smith, M.C., Borges, V.M., Barber, P.A., 2017. PREP2: a biomarker-based algorithm for predicting upper limb function after stroke. Ann. Clin. Transl. Neurol. 4, 811–820.

Stokes, E.K., 2009. Outcome measurement. In: Lennon, S., Stokes, M. (Eds.), Pocketbook of Neurological Physiotherapy. Churchill Livingstone, London, UK, pp. 192–201.

Stroke Association.,January 2017. State of the nation: stroke statistics. Available at: https://www.stroke.org.uk/sites/default/files/state_of_the_nation_2017_final_1.pdf. Accessed 9 August 2022.

Stroke Foundation. Clinical guidelines for stroke management. Available at: https://informme.org.au/guidelines/living-clinical-guidelines-for-stroke-management. Accessed 12 July 2023.

Stroke Unit Trialists' Collaboration., 2013. Organised inpatient (stroke unit) care for stroke. Cochrane Database Syst. Rev. 9, CD000197.

Teasell, R., Foley, N., Hussein, N., Salter, K., Cotoi, A., Richardson, M., 2015. Evidence-based review of stroke rehabilitation. Evidence-based review of stroke rehabilitation, London. Available at: http://www.ebrsr.com. Accessed 9 August 2022.

Van Duijnhoven, H.J., Heeren, A., Peters, M.A., Veerbeek, J.M., Kwakkel, G., Geurts, A.C., 2016. Effects of exercise therapy on balance capacity in chronic stroke: systematic review and meta-analysis. Stroke. 47, 2603–2610.

Veerbeek, J.M., Koolstra, M., Ket, J.C., van Wegen, E.E., Kwakkel, G., 2011. Effects of augmented exercise therapy on outcome of gait and gait-related activities in the first 6 months after stroke. A meta-analysis. Stroke. 42, 3311–3315.

Veerbeek, J.M., Kwakkel, G., Van Wegen, E.E., Ket, J.C., Heymans, M.W., 2011. Early prediction of outcome of activities of daily living after stroke: a systematic review. Stroke. 42 (5), 1482–1488.

Veerbeek, J.M., Langbroek-Amersfoort, A.C., Van Wegen, E.E., Meskers, C.G., Kwakkel, G., 2017. Effects of robot-assisted therapy for the upper limb after stroke. Neurorehabil. Neural. Repair. 31, 107–121.

Veerbeek, J.M., Pohl, J., Held, J.P.O., Luft, A.R., 2022. External validation of the early prediction of functional outcome after stroke prediction model for independent gait at 3 months after stroke. Front. Neurol. 13, 797791.

Veerbeek, J.M., Van Wegen, E.E., Harmeling-Van der Wel, B.C., Kwakkel, G., EPOS Investigators., 2011. Is accurate prediction of gait in nonambulatory stroke patients possible within 72 hours poststroke? The EPOS study. Neurorehabil. Neural. Repair. 25, 268–274.

Veerbeek, J.M., Van Wegen, E., Van Peppen, R., Van der Wees, P.J., Hendriks, E., Rietberg, M., 2014. What is the evidence for physical therapy poststroke? A systematic review and meta-analysis. PLoS. One. 9, e87987.

Verheyden, G., Nieuwboer, A., De Wit, L., Thijs, V., Dobbelaere, J., Devos, H., 2008. Time course of trunk, arm, leg, and functional recovery after ischemic stroke. Neurorehabil. Neural. Repair. 22, 173–179.

Vloothuis, J.D., Mulder, M., Veerbeek, J.M., Konijnenbelt, M., Visser-Meily, J.M., Ket, J.C., 2016. Caregiver-mediated exercises for improving outcomes after stroke. Cochrane Database Syst. Rev. 12, CD011058.

Wardlaw, J.M., Murray, V., Berge, E., del Zoppo, G.J., 2014. Thrombolysis for acute ischaemic stroke. Cochrane Database Syst. Rev. 7, CD000213.

Weiss, P., Kizony, R., Feintuch, U., Katz, N., 2006. Virtual reality in neurorehabilitation. In: Selzer, M., Cohen, L., Gage, F., Clarke, S., Duncan, P. (Eds.), Textbook of Neural Repair and Rehabilitation. Cambridge University Press, Cambridge, UK.

Wevers, L., Van de Port, I., Vermue, M., Mead, G., Kwakkel, G., 2009. Effects of task-oriented circuit class training on walking competency after stroke: a systematic review. Stroke. 40, 2450–2459.

Winstein, C.J., Stein, J., Arena, R., Bates, B., Cherney, L.R., Cramer, S.C., American Heart Association Stroke Council, Council on Cardiovascular and Stroke Nursing, Council on Clinical Cardiology, and Council on Quality of Care and Outcomes Research., 2016. Guidelines for adult stroke rehabilitation and recovery: a guideline for healthcare professionals from the American Heart Association/American Stroke Association. Stroke. 47, e98–e169.

Wolf, S.L., Kwakkel, G., Bayley, M., McDonnell, M.N., Upper Extremity Stroke Algorithm Working Group., 2016. Best practice for arm recovery post stroke: an international application. Physiotherapy. 102, 1–4.

Traumatic Brain Injury

Gavin Williams

OUTLINE

Introduction, 177
Epidemiology, 178
Pathophysiology, 178
    Primary Brain Injury, 178
    Secondary Brain Injury, 179
    Associated Injuries, 179
Diagnosis, 179
    Coma, 180
    Posttraumatic Amnesia, 180
Medical Management, 180
    Intracranial Pressure, 180
    Multidisciplinary Care, 181
Clinical Presentation, 181
Assessment, 182
    Abnormal Tone, 183
    Muscle Paresis, 184
    Disorders of Movement, 184
    Balance and Vestibular Function, 184
    Muscle and Joint Range of Motion, 184

Concurrent Musculoskeletal Injuries, 185
Pain, 185
Function, 185
Summary, 185
Prognosis/Time Course, 185
Interventions, 186
    Hypertonicity and Spasticity, 186
    Muscle Paresis, 187
    Disorders of Movement, 187
    Balance and Vestibular Function, 187
    Muscle and Joint Range of Motion, 188
    Concurrent Musculoskeletal Injuries, 188
    Pain, 188
    Function, 189
Other Considerations, 189
Covid Update, 189
Conclusion, 190
Case Presentation, 190

INTRODUCTION

Traumatic brain injury (TBI) is a particular type of acquired brain injury (ABI) that describes a single-event injury to the brain caused by an external force, whereas ABI is an overarching term applied to describe an injury or pathology to the brain that is not congenital or perinatal in nature. Usually the term ABI is used to describe the outcome of a distinct event, such as a subarachnoid haemorrhage, a hypoxic brain injury or the result of a central nervous system (CNS) tumour. TBI remains the primary cause of death and disability for young adults. The primary causes of TBI are motor vehicle accidents, falls, sporting accidents and assaults. The common theme in the mechanism of injury is a high velocity or high impact blow to the head. This chapter will focus on the epidemiology and pathophysiology of TBI, the common physical sequelae and their management.

This chapter will also discuss physical management after TBI during the acute, rehabilitation and community-based phases, but focuses primarily on the rehabilitation phase. Given the sustained, permanent and life-changing injuries associated with TBI, a multidisciplinary team that includes a range of specialist physicians, nursing staff, therapists, psychologists and social workers is required. Further, an integrated rehabilitation approach also requires the family and wider social networks to be involved. A thorough understanding of the impact and scope of TBI on an individual is essential if the rehabilitation team is to work effectively with patients, families and other healthcare professionals to facilitate community participation.

EPIDEMIOLOGY

TBI is a growing global healthcare burden (Dewan et al 2018). The incidence of TBI affects three distinct age groups. Those most at risk are children younger than 2 years, adolescents and young adults aged 15–45 years, and older adults aged 75 years and older (Harrison-Felix et al 2012, O'Connor 2002). The highest incidence of TBI is in adolescents and younger adults aged 15–45 years, primarily because of road trauma and sport-related concussions. Males are almost three times more likely to be injured and to have more severe injuries (O'Connor & Cripps 1999, Thurman et al 1999). Studies reporting the incidence of TBI in Western countries such as the USA (Thurman et al 1999), Europe (Jennett 1996) and Australia (O'Connor 2002) produce a range of values of around 200–300 new cases presenting for medical evaluation per 100,000 population each year. Sporting-related concussion has received considerable attention in the past decade because of issues related to resumption of activity and the effects of repeat concussion (McCrory et al 2013). Falls and head strikes are a major cause of head trauma in children younger than 2 years and adults older than 75 years. Falls are a major healthcare burden because they are prevalent and associated with high rates of hospitalisation (see Chapter 21 for a detailed discussion of falls management). This chapter will focus on TBI associated with adolescents and younger adults, as it has the highest incidence rate and is the main cause of death and disability in this age group.

In addition to the substantial personal costs, TBI has a major economic impact in industrialised countries. Costs associated with hospitalisation, rehabilitation, equipment and ongoing medical problems run to billions of dollars (Papastrat 1992, Pope & Tarlov 1991). The social and economic costs related to reduced work productivity of the person with TBI, their families and carers are also considerable (Berger et al 1999, Ditunno 1992, Johnston & Hall 1994, Max et al 1991).

Although most cases of severe TBI are caused by road trauma, there is a much higher prevalence of concussion and mild TBI. The terms *concussion* and *mild TBI* are often used interchangeably, but it remains unclear whether these are two distinct neuropathologies (McCrory et al 2017). Full recovery is expected in 80%–90% of cases within 7–10 days (McCrory et al 2013) but may take longer in children and adolescents (McCrory et al 2017). Several key differences exist in the management of concussion/mild TBI compared with more severe classifications of TBI, particularly around assessment tools and 'return-to-play' protocols.

The Sport Concussion Assessment Tool version 5 (SCAT5) is the recommended assessment tool for concussion/mild TBI (Echemendia et al 2017). This field is rapidly evolving because of high public interest, studies that have demonstrated persistent subclinical deficits in balance and motor control, and concerns related to the, as yet, unproven relationship between repeated concussions and chronic traumatic encephalopathy (CTE) (McCrory et al 2013).

PATHOPHYSIOLOGY

Moderate to severe TBI typically occurs as a result of a high-velocity, high-impact blow to the head, most commonly because of road trauma and falls (O'Connor 2002, O'Connor & Cripps 1999). TBI encompasses a wide variety of CNS lesions (Crooks et al 2007). The pathophysiology of TBI is typically classified into primary and secondary injuries. The primary injury relates to the mechanical forces acting on the brain. The secondary injury that occurs in the brain is linked to the primary injury, but relates to the physiological and biomolecular sequelae (see Key Features Associated With Primary and Secondary Brain Injury box).

KEY FEATURES ASSOCIATED WITH PRIMARY AND SECONDARY BRAIN INJURY

Primary Injury	Secondary Injury
• Occurs at the time of injury	• Occurs after the initial impact
• Closed or blunt injury	• Disrupted autoregulation
• Open or penetrating injury	• Compression
• Contrecoup movement	• Reduced blood flow
• Diffuse axonal injury	• Elevated intracranial pressure hypotension
• Haemorrhages (subdural haematoma, extradural haematoma, petechial)	• Hypoxia

---

Primary Brain Injury

The primary injury is associated with the mechanical forces acting on the brain that result in a combination of acceleration, deceleration and rotational forces (Crooks et al 2007). There are two main mechanisms of TBI:
- Closed or blunt injury
- Open or penetrating injuries

When the head strikes an object, such as the windscreen or ground, a TBI may occur without any fracture or significant injury to the skull. This is called a *closed* or *blunt head injury*, as the barrier between the brain and the environment has been maintained. Alternatively, a fracture resulting from a head strike may result in a piece of bone being pushed into brain tissue, or an object such as a bullet may enter the skull. These injuries are termed *open* or *penetrating injuries* and may cause further damage to the brain and thus introduce greater risk of infection.

The mechanism and force both affect the resulting brain injury. In a typical closed TBI, the skull makes contact with an external object leading to an abrupt stop. The area of the brain immediately adjacent to the impact site may sustain a cerebral contusion as the brain collides with the inside of the skull. The brain may then move back and forth within the skull, producing a 'contrecoup' movement and further shearing damage. Brain tissue has little structural support, so it does not tolerate these forces well, and the resulting blood vessel damage may vary from large extradural or subdural bleeds to multiple small petechial haemorrhages (Crooks et al 2007). The neuronal injury associated with contrecoup movement and rotational forces is called diffuse axonal injury (DAI) (Crooks et al 2007). DAI is usually associated with more severe TBI.

After the initial impact and primary brain injury, the injury response leads to oedema, which, in conjunction with contusion, haemotomas and haemorrhage, causes additional compressive forces. These compressive forces can further disturb brain function by distorting brain tissue, elevating intracranial pressure (ICP) or reducing cerebral blood flow. The combination of these factors leads to secondary brain injury.

Secondary Brain Injury

Secondary brain injury relates to the physiological and biomolecular sequelae of the initial trauma. The outcomes of people who survive the initial injury are related to the secondary injury processes. Despite extensive work to reduce the impact of the secondary injury, no trials have demonstrated clinical efficacy to date (Carney et al 2017).

Although there are several mechanisms that protect the brain and maintain constant oxygen and nutritional supplies, these mechanisms may be compromised after TBI. In particular, the blood–brain barrier, which is vital for the autoregulation of cerebral blood flow, is often disrupted. Autoregulation is achieved through control of cerebral vascular resistance, cerebral blood flow and oxygen extraction. The autoregulation mechanisms can compensate for changes to cerebral vascular resistance, cerebral blood flow and oxygen extraction, but compensation has finite limits. Maintenance of autoregulation, whether through the body's own protective mechanisms or medical intervention, is vital because brain tissue is particularly susceptible to ischemia. Hypotension and hypoxia are common after TBI (Carney et al 2017). They are the leading causes of mortality after injury and the reason why trauma centres have been developed that can very quickly receive patients from accident

sites (Jeremitsky et al 2003). Numerous efforts to medically (Nichol et al 2015), surgically (Cooper et al 2011) and pharmacologically (Edwards et al 2005) moderate secondary brain injury are underway; however, initial positive findings in animal models have generally not translated to humans (Stocchetti et al 2015), with some promising studies resulting in sometimes counterintuitive or negative outcomes (Cooper et al 2011).

Associated Injuries

The type of incidents that result in TBI often lead to associated peripheral injuries. Chest, spinal, abdominal and limb injuries are common. Blood loss associated with these injuries further complicates the autoregulation of the secondary physiological response to brain injury. Orthopaedic injuries are common and may involve extensive bony fractures, joint dislocations and ligament ruptures. Bony deformity, leg length discrepancy and pain may all affect gait performance; the impact of orthopaedic lower limb injuries on gait performance has not been investigated in TBI.

DIAGNOSIS

Initial diagnosis is based on factors such as orientation, arousal or conscious state. In many cases, TBI is associated with a period of loss of consciousness. However, this is not necessarily the case with concussion and very mild TBI (McCrory et al 2013). It remains unclear whether concussion and mild TBI are distinct neurological pathophysiologies, whereby mild TBI is associated with less severe diffuse structural changes, whereas concussion is a transient functional disturbance rather than a structural injury (McCrory et al 2017). In addition to initial diagnosis, the severity of TBI is graded and ranges from mild concussion with transient symptoms to very severe injury resulting in death. There are two main areas assessed in relation to severity of TBI: level of consciousness or coma (depth and duration) and posttraumatic amnesia (PTA) (see Table 8.1).

TABLE 8.1 Traumatic Brain Injury Severity: Glasgow Coma Score Depth and Duration (Bond 1986, 1990)

GCS Classification	Depth (Scored in First 24 Hours)	Duration of GCS $\leq$ 8
Mild	13–15	<15 minutes
Moderate	9–12	15 minutes to 6 hours
Severe	3–8	6–48 hours
Very severe		>48 hours

TABLE 8.2 Traumatic Brain Injury: Severity and Duration of Posttraumatic Amnesia (Shores et al 1986)	
Severity of Injury	Duration of Posttraumatic Amnesia
Very mild	<5 min
Mild	5–60 min
Moderate	<24 hours
Severe	1–6 days
Very severe	7–28 days
Extremely severe	>28 days

AIMS OF ACUTE MANAGEMENT

- Stabilise the patient – maintain life
- Prevent further/secondary neurological damage – keep brain oxygenated
- Limit/cease bleeding
- Monitor ICP and conscious state
- Prevent complications – prevent respiratory problems
- Improve level of consciousness
- Manage other chest, abdominal and musculoskeletal injuries

Coma

Coma is defined as 'not obeying commands, not uttering words and not opening eyes' (Teasdale & Jennett, 1974). The Glasgow Coma Scale (GCS) is the most widely used measure of depth and duration of coma (Teasdale & Jennett, 1974). The GCS has three subscales, giving a summated score of 3–15 (see Table 8.1). Higher summed scores represent better performance or less severe injury (see Table 8.1); however, it should be noted that a score of 3 does not discriminate between the most severe grading of TBI and someone who is deceased. Duration of coma may also be used as an indicator of severity, where coma is generally numerically defined as a GCS score ≤8 (Bond 1990).

Posttraumatic Amnesia

PTA is the period from the accident until the person is orientated to their surroundings. It determines the degree to which a person is aware of their surroundings and to some extent determines how responsible they are for their actions. There are a number of measures of length of PTA; the Galveston Orientation and Amnesia Test (GOAT) (Levin et al 1979) and the Westmead PTA scale (Shores et al 1986) are among the most widely used (Table 8.2). Orientation, as quantified by length of PTA, is the preferred method of measuring severity of TBI because it is a better predictor of outcome than the GCS (Shores et al 2008).

MEDICAL MANAGEMENT

The aims of initial emergency and early medical management are to keep the person alive by stabilising the patient, to limit the development of secondary brain damage, and to provide the best conditions for recovery from any reversible damage that has already occurred (see Aims of Acute Management box). Significant improvements in mortality and morbidity have been obtained by early intensive management targeted towards reducing secondary brain damage (Bragge et al 2015). These interventions include immediate resuscitation and early intubation, rapid admission to a dedicated trauma unit, early scanning and evacuation of intracranial haematomas, and monitoring of ICP.

A thorough overview of the medical and surgical management of TBI was published in *Neurosurgery* in 2017 (Carney et al 2017). These guidelines constitute the fourth edition and cover all the evidence for emergency and acute care of TBI. They include 94 new studies published in TBI since the third edition in 2007. Several of the 2007 recommendations have been changed in the 2017 edition. A separate large overview of randomised controlled trials for the acute management of moderate to severe TBI was also published in 2015 (Bragge et al 2015). The guiding principles of the early management of TBI are presented in Table 8.3. A common theme emerging from both of these large bodies of work is the failure to establish effective interventions for the emergency and acute management of moderate to severe TBI.

Patients are often ventilated, sedated, paralysed and intubated during the acute phase. This is done initially to minimise agitation because of the negative cascade of effects of agitation leading to raised blood pressure, raised ICP and reduced brain oxygenation. Intubation and ventilation may be performed if a person is having trouble breathing. Respiratory support (i.e., intubation and ventilation) is usually achieved via an endotracheal tube. A tracheostomy is performed only where facial or spinal fractures preclude endotracheal tube insertion, or when respiratory support is required over a more extended period. Oxygen is usually provided (via nasal prongs or face mask) even when ventilation is not required; oxygen therapy is recommended to help meet the injured brain's increased energy requirements. Respiratory management is covered separately in more depth in Chapter 18.

Intracranial Pressure

The two standard interventions for the treatment of raised ICP are mannitol and hypertonic saline (Bratton et al 2007a). The ultimate goal is to reduce ICP whilst maintaining or improving cerebral perfusion pressure (CPP) and cerebral blood flow. A slightly raised head position (avoiding neck flexion) is usually recommended for raised ICP. Usual

TABLE 8.3 Guiding Principles for Acute Management (Carney et al 2017)

Clinical Problem	Recommended Management
ICP	• Management of severe TBI patients using information from ICP monitoring is recommended (>20 mmHg)
Infection	• Increased risk of infection because of interventions such as ICP monitoring and intubation • Prophylactic antibiotics are no longer recommended for intubation to reduce the risk of pneumonia or external ventricular drains
DVT	• Compression stockings are recommended prophylactically • Blood thinning agents are no longer recommended for prophylactic management of DVT
Metabolism	• Recommendations for timing and method feeding, but not glycemic control or vitamins and supplements
Seizures	• Prophylactic use of antiseizure medication is not recommended for preventing seizures after the first 7 days

DVT, Deep venous thrombosis; *ICP*, intracranial pressure; *TBI*, traumatic brain injury.

paresis, spasticity and hypertonicity mean that the patient is at high risk of developing contractures and pressure areas.

During this early stage of recovery, physiotherapy assessment for respiratory and musculoskeletal health is important, although sessions are typically short and frequent. It is critical to identify any threats to soft tissue extensibility and skin integrity. When a patient has a reduced level of consciousness, with minimal movement and activity to command, physiotherapists use interventions such as positioning, assisted movement, serial splinting or casting, and tilt-tabling in an attempt to maintain range of motion (ROM) and encourage movement. Casting or splinting may need to be used to maintain or prevent the loss of joint ROM and muscle length (Leung et al 2019), but moderate- to long-term benefits remain elusive (Harvey et al 2017). Access to all joints may not be possible because some positions and movements may need to be avoided because of threats to medical status. Frequent repositioning every 2–4 hours may help to prevent musculoskeletal contractures and pressure areas on the skin.

The acute hospital environment is busy and noisy, and often lit throughout the 24-hour period. It may be necessary to *limit* rather than increase sensory stimulation to ensure periods of rest, for example, the use of eye-patching to promote normal diurnal rhythms. It is important for this concept of regulated sensory stimulation to be imparted to friends and family members so they may contribute appropriately to the promotion of recovery.

CLINICAL PRESENTATION

Once a patient has become medically stable, rehabilitative interventions can be commenced. The range and severity of

respiratory care interventions, such as postural drainage or manual hyperinflation, may be contraindicated or used with caution because of the associated rise in ICP (>20 mmHg) (Bratton et al 2007b). Neurosurgery may be required in open or penetrating TBI to remove debris and clean the wound. Decompressive craniectomy, the removal of a bone flap from the skull, is required for some severe cases of raised ICP.

Multidisciplinary Care

Management of these severe trauma cases involves a large team of specialists and is a particularly traumatic time for the patient's family and friends (see Early Team Goals box). Additional injuries associated with the mechanism of injury, such as fractures, dislocations and amputations, also need to be assessed and treated as the medical status of the patient allows. Another important goal at this stage is to prevent or monitor the development of secondary complications. Chest care and prevention of pneumonia have been covered earlier. The combination of a prolonged period of unconsciousness and associated bed rest, fractures, muscle

COMMON TREATMENT GOALS DURING THE ACUTE PHASE

- Ongoing (daily) assessment
- Monitoring of respiratory status
- Prevention of contractures and pressure areas – consider interventions such as positioning and assisted movement, splinting or casting, and tilt-tabling
- Liaising within the multidisciplinary team to ensure a coordinated approach
- Graded sensory stimulation
- Introduction of antigravity activity such as sitting on the edge of the bed, sitting out of bed or standing on a tilt-table
- Provision of information, education and support for family and friends

TABLE 8.4   Disorders of Consciousness

Disorders	Definition/Description
PTA	Not a true disorder of arousal; characterised by disorientation to time, person and place (Shores et al 1986).
Vegetative state or persistent vegetative state	A clinical condition of complete unawareness of the self and the environment, accompanied by sleep–wake cycles with either complete or partial preservation of hypothalamic and brainstem automatic functions (Seel et al 2010). This state is sometimes referred to as unresponsive wakefulness syndrome.
MCS	A condition of severely altered consciousness in which minimal but definite behavioural evidence of self or environmental awareness is demonstrated. (Giacino et al 2002). One or more of four diagnostic criteria confirm MCS and include: (1) following simple commands, (2) yes/no responses, (3) intelligible verbalisation and (4) purposeful behaviour.
'Locked in' syndrome	Normal consciousness and sleep–wake cycle, preserved auditory, visual and emotional function, but limited verbal communication and bodily movement (American Congress of Rehabilitation 1995)
Coma	No verbal response, no obeying commands and the patient does not open the eyes either spontaneously or to any stimulus (Jennett and Teasdale 1977)

MCS, Minimally conscious state; *PTA*, posttraumatic trauma.

the presenting signs and symptoms can be diverse because of the variability in location of focal brain injury and the extent of diffuse and secondary brain injury. The most common and obvious signs and symptoms associated with the more severe TBIs that require rehabilitation relate to the initial altered conscious state, usually referred to as 'disorders of consciousness' such as coma, vegetative state and

the minimally conscious state (MCS) (Table 8.4). This may be short-lived or may extend over weeks or months, and in some cases even years. In recent years, North American (Giacino et al 2018, 2020) and European (Kondziella et al 2020) guidelines for the diagnosis and management of disorders of consciousness have been published. Key recommendations are the importance of imaging and ongoing monitoring of behaviour.

The next section of this chapter is devoted to the physical sequelae of TBI; however, a discussion of the signs and symptoms of TBI is not complete without addressing impairment to the psychosocial, cognitive, behavioural, emotional and sensorimotor domains. Not all impairments are observable immediately after injury, and some may take time to be revealed as a patient's conscious state improves and their environment changes. Chapter 24 on neuropsychology focuses in more depth on cognitive and behavioural impairments.

ASSESSMENT

After the initial life-saving and subsequent brain-saving phase, the next most important phase commences as the patient becomes medically stable. A full physical assessment is required to determine the extent of physical impairment and to develop a prioritised list of goals and treatment plan. It is vital that physiotherapists are involved in developing a physical management plan to guide the management of physical factors over the full 24-hour period, and that this occurs at the earliest possible point after hospital admission.

The range and severity of physical impairments can vary considerably between patients and over time within a patient. Some of the common physical impairments resulting from TBI include:

- Hypertonicity
- Spasticity
- Muscle paresis
- Reduced muscle and joint ROM
- Exaggerated muscle tendon reflexes
- Reduced motor control
- Dyspraxia
- Reduced balance
- Ataxia
- Reduced vestibular function

Given the complex and multifactorial nature of the physical impairments that can result from TBI, the American Physical Therapy Association (APTA) has published recommendations for outcome measures specifically for TBI (McCulloch et al 2016) and more broadly for people with neurological conditions undergoing rehabilitation (Moore et al 2018). Further, at the time of writing, the World Health Organization (WHO) is developing a 'Package of

Interventions for Rehabilitation' for TBI that includes the physical domains to be assessed and, where available, recommended outcome measures.

The list given earlier is by no means extensive. Chapter 3 discusses the management of impairments and their impact on activity. Patients may also have problems with pain, either associated with physical impairments resulting from the TBI or concurrently sustained musculoskeletal injuries. Swallow, cough or gag reflexes may also be affected, which may impact on eating and drinking. Diplopia (double vision) is common after TBI and may resolve over time. A standard early management strategy is the use of an alternating eye patch. Although the positive features of the upper motor neurone (UMN) syndrome are the most common and receive considerable attention after TBI, hypotonicity may also occur and should not be overlooked simply because spasticity is not present, as it too may have a significant impact on a person's mobility.

Because of the initial priorities related to patient survival, some less urgent musculoskeletal injuries may get overlooked. Patients are unable to report pain and discomfort when unconscious, and in the absence of significant bruising, swelling or deformity, musculoskeletal injuries may get missed in the emergency setting because there is no rationale to prescribe a scan or X-ray. In addition to the potential for overlooked musculoskeletal injuries, other conditions such as heterotrophic ossification (HO) may develop weeks or months after the injury. The remainder of this section will deal with assessment and treatment options of the more commonly occurring impairments specific to TBI.

Abnormal Tone

Hypertonicity and spasticity are two of the prevalent positive features of the UMN syndrome after TBI (Brashear & Elovic 2010). Compared with stroke, where there is often a period of low tone before hypertonicity and spasticity may develop, these features can develop very quickly after TBI, particularly in the more severe cases. Hypertonicity and spasticity may be observed as the person begins to emerge from a coma or when sedation is reduced. In severe cases, the arms and legs may be held in a rigid position, making active or passive movement virtually impossible. Although the clinical presentation may be highly variable, two patterns of hypertonicity and spasticity have been described in the more severe cases. They are decerebrate (arms and legs in extension, hands clenched) and decorticate (Fig. 8.1; arms in flexion and legs in extension) posturing (see Abnormal Postures box). Although these patterns have been described, one side of the body may be more affected than the other, or the severity may vary between the arms and legs. Muscle paresis is also usually evident, but easily masked by the hypertonicity and spasticity. Overall, spasticity may lead to significant disability (Brashear & Elovic 2010). Approximately 18%–30% of TBI survivors experience spasticity requiring treatment after their accident (Verplancke et al 2005); however, like hypertonicity, it is more common with the more severe TBIs. This is especially true for those with disorders of consciousness, and regular physical therapy is particularly important to reduce spasticity and the development of contracture (Synnot et al 2017, Thibaut et al 2018).

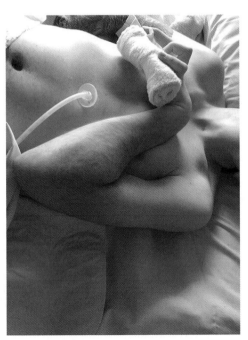

FIG. 8.1 Decorticate posture upper limbs.

ABNORMAL POSTURES	
Decerebrate Posture	**Decorticate Posture**
• Arms and legs are held in extension	• Legs are held in extension
• Hips extended and adducted	• Arms are held in flexion
• Knees extended	• Shoulder flexion, adduction and internal rotation
• Ankles plantarflexed and inverted	• Elbows flexed, forearms pronated
• Shoulders neutral, elbows extended	• Wrists and fingers flexed
• Hands clenched	

Muscle Paresis

Muscle paresis is common after TBI and may originate from several causes. The TBI may lead to focal neurological deficits, and muscle paresis is one of the key negative features associated with the UMN syndrome, along with impaired coordination, motor control and fatigue (Ivanhoe & Reistetter 2004). This may lead to a hemiparetic pattern, but can also present as quadriparesis, and the arms and legs may be differentially affected (Williams 2015). Generalised muscle weakness may also occur as a result of a prolonged period of bed rest or enforced inactivity. Fractures, other musculoskeletal injuries and the associated pain may also lead to focal areas of muscle weakness. It is not uncommon for all of these causes of muscle weakness to be present after severe TBI given the multitrauma mechanism of injury and the subsequent hospitalisation.

Similar to stroke, occasionally a clinical presentation of hemiparesis will be further complicated by nonphysical issues such as neglect or problems with spatial orientation, sometimes referred to as 'pusher syndrome', where a person's orientation to vertical is affected. When either or both of these complications are also present, sometimes a better indication of active movement may be obtained by intermittent observation of spontaneous movement or during basic functional or automatic tasks like clapping or standing.

Disorders of Movement

There are many terms used to describe various disorders of movement that may occur after TBI, such as dyspraxia and dyskinesia (involuntary movements), ataxia or simply reduced motor control. The different disorders of movement usually relate to the mechanism of injury and the resulting location of brain injury. For example, ataxia usually results from a fall or strike to the back of the head and subsequent injury to the cerebellum. Disorders of movement are notoriously difficult to assess and treat.

Balance and Vestibular Function

Balance and vestibular dysfunction are very common after TBI, ranging from those who are unable to sit on the edge of the bed, to those who still display impairment despite having achieved a good recovery from concussion/mild TBI (McFadyen et al 2009). Balance dysfunction is also a leading cause of TBI resulting from a fall in elderly persons (see Chapter 21), contributing to a vicious circle of balance dysfunction leading to TBI that leads to further balance dysfunction. The visual, somatosensory or vestibular systems can all contribute to the patient's balance impairment, and the vestibular disorder could be either central, meaning involvement of the CNS, or peripheral, indicating

TABLE 8.5   Common Assessment Tools in Traumatic Brain Injury

Impairment	Common Assessment Tools
Hypertonicity	• Ashworth scale (Ashworth 1964) • Modified Ashworth scale (Bohannon and Smith 1987)
Spasticity	• Modified Tardieu scale (Haugh et al 2006)
Weakness	• Manual muscle testing (Morris et al 2004) • Hand-held dynamometry (Stark et al 2011)
Reduced voluntary movement	• Stroke Rehabilitation Assessment of Movement (Daley et al 1999)
Balance dysfunction	• Function in Sitting Test (Gorman et al 2010) • Berg Balance Scale (Berg et al 1989)
Loss of range of motion	• Goniometry

pathology associated with the inner ear. Please see Chapter 17 for more detailed information on vestibular assessment and treatment.

Muscle and Joint Range of Motion

Loss of ROM and contractures are also very common after TBI, whether they are primarily caused by hypertonicity and spasticity, a prolonged period of rest in bed, concurrent musculoskeletal injuries or a combination of all or some of these. It is important to thoroughly assess and document ROM, particularly in the more severe cases where the patient's physical status may deteriorate in the early stages, or when other conditions such as HO may develop. Additional care must be taken around areas with musculoskeletal injuries, skin lesions or skin grafts. Further, careful handling is required when assessing patients who are unable to communicate pain, are in an MCS, are paretic and hypotonic, or are restless or agitated. All main joints and all two or multi-joint muscle groups should be assessed. Measurements are usually taken with a goniometer. Often two therapists are required to make accurate assessments, that is, one to handle the patient and one to perform and document the assessment. Some common assessment tools used in TBI are presented in Table 8.5 (McCulloch et al 2016).

Concurrent Musculoskeletal Injuries

Because of the high-velocity/high-impact nature of the injury, it is not uncommon for people who sustain a TBI to have a range of other musculoskeletal, chest and abdominal injuries. Wounds and skin grafts are also common and may affect early assessment and treatment options. Often the need to stretch and maintain ROM because of severe spasticity and hypertonicity is contraindicated by fractures and other musculoskeletal injuries. The trend in recent years to use internal and external fixation, rather than casts, to stabilise fractures has allowed physiotherapists to do a greater amount of early exercise.

Pain

Like so many areas of TBI assessment and management, there are a multitude of potential contributing factors to a patient's pain, and each may differ in their optimal management. Pain may be associated with spasms, spasticity or hypertonicity for some patients who present with these positive features of the UMN syndrome. Injury to the brain itself can also cause pain such as central post-stroke pain syndrome (Flaster et al 2013), usually as a result of injury to the thalamus (also known as thalamic pain syndrome). Alternatively, pain may be associated with any of the musculoskeletal, chest, abdominal or skin injuries that were sustained during the accident. In a subset of these patients, some may develop complex regional pain syndrome (Birklein 2005). Musculoskeletal injuries may also lead to peripheral nerve injuries in the upper and lower limbs, and the resultant nerve pain is often very severe. For a detailed overview of pain in neurological conditions, please refer to Chapter 22.

Function

All the impairments listed here may affect function. In some cases, because of a range of issues related to cognition, behaviour or conscious state, an accurate and thorough physical assessment is not possible. When this occurs, it is still important to assess and document functional status. Assessment of functional status is important for coordinated rehabilitation and nursing care, to determine what help is required and how that help should be provided. For example, one person may require the assistance of two people and a hoist to transfer into a wheelchair, whereas another person may be able to walk independently but require supervision because of confusion. It is important to optimise a patient's engagement in the rehabilitation process, as even those who have some confusion or cognitive impairment may benefit from routine and a consistent approach to their care.

Summary

The clinical presentation after TBI may be severe and complex. Many signs and symptoms can mask the presence of other important injuries or impairments. The clinical presentation may fluctuate from day to day, change over time as things improve (conscious state) or develop (HO) over time. Cognitive and behavioural impairment may also affect the ability to assess and measure physical status, and therefore limit the accuracy and interpretation of the assessment findings. The most important tool at the therapist's disposal is a systematic and thorough assessment process. The assessment process may require several days or more, and repeated checking, to ensure that the findings recorded are representative of the patient's physical status and not an isolated observation.

PROGNOSIS/TIME COURSE

The key initial factor in determining survival is the immediate arrival to a trauma or emergency management unit to limit or reduce the impact of secondary brain injury (Gruen et al 2020, Spaite et al 2019). Once a person has survived their accident, the two main tools used to predict outcome after TBI are measures of the severity of the initial brain injury. These tools are the GCS and length of PTA. The GCS and PTA scores have been used in many TBI outcome studies over recent decades. The length of PTA is marginally better at predicting outcome than GCS (Perrin et al 2015, Shores et al 2008). Other than severity of injury, other factors that may influence outcome after TBI are:

- Age: those who are younger tend to have better outcomes (Perrin et al 2015).
- Cognitive reserve: those who have higher levels of premorbid cognitive function may have greater 'reserve' capacity and therefore may better cope with some levels of cognitive impairment (Schonberger et al 2011).
- Gender: some females may have better outcomes than males (de Guise et al 2014).

Outcome is determined by a range of factors, such as independence in self-care and mobility, ability to work or study, community participation, relationships and quality of life. A number of outcome measures have been specifically developed or adapted for TBI, such as the Glasgow Outcome Scale (Jennett & Bond 1975), Community Integration Questionnaire (Willer et al 1993) and Mayo-Portland Adaptability Inventory (Malec et al 2000). Although these outcome measures vary, they all have common domains that are important for young adults recovering from TBI.

Because of the considerable impact of TBI on cognition, which in turn affects personal, domestic and community activities of daily living, a thorough cognitive or neuropsychological assessment is required (Ponsford et al 2013). A thorough cognitive evaluation can determine relative strengths and weaknesses, and is used to implement compensatory strategies. A key factor that affects TBI outcome is the support of family and friends. Up to 85% of people with moderate to severe TBI do not return to preaccident activities (Ponsford et al 1995), so a strong network of family and friends who are able to assist on a daily basis once they return home tend to have better outcomes, are better integrated into their community and have higher quality of life.

Recovery from TBI is notoriously slow. Ongoing improvement can occur and has been documented for years after TBI, but most recovery occurs by 6 months postinjury (Jennett 1981), with little overall change found when routinely assessed for many years (Ponsford 2014). Even in the less severe injuries, recovery can take many months and people often require a graded return-to-work programme because fatigue has a major impact on day-to-day activity. For the more severe injuries, some people may be in hospital for 6 months or more whilst issues related to future accommodation, modification to existing accommodation, or assessment, supply and fitting of equipment such as wheelchairs is conducted. In contrast with the early medical management of TBI, there are no published peer-reviewed guidelines for the rehabilitation of people with TBI. However, several comprehensive guidelines have been developed by groups in the USA (State of Colorado 2018), UK (Scottish Intercollegiate Guidelines Network 2013), Canada (Bayley et al 2018) and New Zealand (New Zealand Guidelines Group 2006) to provide clinicians with resources, evidence and recommendations for the management of people in the postacute phase of management. Nonetheless, guidelines are important to improve the quality and reduce the variation in healthcare, and specifically in TBI, adherence to guidelines has been shown to improve outcomes (Cnossen et al 2021).

Intensive rehabilitation has been shown to improve people's outcomes after TBI (Turner-Stokes et al 2016), but the nature and method of rehabilitation may vary over time. Typically, intensive inpatient rehabilitation is provided initially as the person becomes medically stable, their conscious state improves and they begin to wake up. Once they are ready or able to return home, a period of outpatient or community-based rehabilitation is often provided. Rehabilitation in a community-based setting is important because it enables a person to learn and practice activities in the environment in which they will be applied, so any barriers to implementation are immediately identified and resolved. Community-based rehabilitation may include programmes directed towards driving, work, study, shopping, banking, parenting or other relationships. Where return to premorbid roles is not possible, rehabilitation may focus on alternative activities.

INTERVENTIONS

Given the extensive range and severity of injuries, and variety of potential impairments, clinicians must be experienced and competent in a considerable range of physical and other interventions. Clinicians also need to know when to advise or refer patients to other members of the multidisciplinary team for related treatments such as botulinum toxin A (BoNT-A) injections, wheelchair seating or a swallowing assessment if it is not within their scope of practice. Further, cognitive (e.g., poor memory, initiation, planning or problem solving) and behavioural (e.g., verbal or physical abuse, disinhibited or inappropriate communication) impairments are common and may influence how physical interventions may be delivered. The management of cognitive and behavioural impairments and the capacity of people with TBI to engage in therapy is a rapidly evolving field. Historically, little therapy was provided during the early PTA phase after TBI. However, emerging evidence in the early rehabilitation stage during PTA has demonstrated that people with TBI may benefit from physical and functional therapies (Spiteri et al 2021, 2022, Trevena-Peters et al 2018). Evidence also suggests that many people are sedated during PTA to assist in managing their agitation and behaviours (Ponsford et al 2021), despite little evidence for the efficacy of sedation during PTA (McKay et al 2021). Once a person has emerged from PTA, the entire multidisciplinary team and family and friends need to implement a consistent behaviour modification management plan to optimise rehabilitative outcomes. The following section touches on some of the many interventions which physiotherapists may need to consider for a person with a TBI.

Hypertonicity and Spasticity

A range of interventions are used to treat and manage hypertonicity and spasticity after TBI. Sometimes these interventions have a focus towards improving function; other times, the primary rationale for treatment is to limit deterioration in secondary musculoskeletal impairments. Interventions targeted towards hypertonicity and spasticity itself include medications such as baclofen, dantrolene sodium, diazepam, tizanidine and BoNT-A. Baclofen is one of the more commonly prescribed systemic medications for hypertonicity and spasticity, and should be considered when hypertonicity and spasticity affect most of the body or the majority of the limbs. In more severe cases, pumps can be inserted to administer baclofen directly to the spinal cord (McCormick et al 2016). The benefit of this application is that it is more effective at reducing hypertonicity and spasticity because the baclofen is being delivered directly to the cerebrospinal fluid, and there are fewer side effects compared with oral administration (McCormick et al 2016). Of the side effects, fatigue is very common, and for some people the impact of baclofen on their fatigue levels negates any reduction in hypertonicity and spasticity they may obtain. The main problem with baclofen pump administration is the complication rate, which is reported to be approximately 40%, with issues related to the surgical procedure, pump problems and catheter malfunctions (Stetkarova et al 2010).

BoNT-A is the most common intervention for focal spasticity. Its use during the past 20 years has greatly reduced the use of phenol nerve blocks. The most recent international consensus statements for use of BoNT-A were published in 2010 (Olver et al 2010, Sheean et al 2010). BoNT-A is injected into the hypertonic or spastic muscle or muscles, usually with some localising technology (e.g., electrical stimulation, ultrasound) to ensure that the correct muscle is targeted (Wissel et al 2009). Guidelines and recommendations have been developed related to patient and muscle selection, dosage and injection site (Olver 2010, Van Campenhout 2011). BoNT-A is very effective at reducing spasticity; however, the impact on function or activity limitations is yet to be established (Olver et al 2010, Sheean et al 2010).

Therapies used to treat hypertonicity and spasticity are rarely used in isolation. Most commonly the medical management of spasticity is supported by a range of interventions provided by physiotherapists, which include stretching, casting, splinting, tilt-tabling, strength training and functional retraining. In cases where hypertonicity and spasticity do not respond to medical and physiotherapy interventions, and secondary musculoskeletal changes such as contractures occur, surgery may be required.

Muscle Paresis

Strength training is a key intervention for muscle paresis associated with the UMN syndrome for many people with a wide variety of neurological conditions. A large number of studies have shown that strength training is safe and effective for improving muscle weakness associated with the UMN syndrome; however, as with the treatment of many physical impairments, the translation of improved muscle strength to improved function is less well established (Taylor et al 2005, Williams et al 2014).

The application of strengthening exercises may range from those with minimal muscle activation to those walking independently in the community. Hydrotherapy may be appropriate for those with considerable muscle paresis, whereas a community-based gym may be more appropriate for those who are stronger and have higher level goals. Strength training should be targeted towards the key muscle groups responsible for improved function to optimise the translation to functional gain (Williams et al 2014). For

example, the hip and knee extensors should be targeted if the goal is to improve standing up, but if the goal is to improve walking, then greater emphasis should be placed on the ankle plantarflexors, and hip flexors and extensors (Neptune et al 2008, Winter 1983).

Disorders of Movement

Task practice is a key intervention in disorders of movement. For example, if a person with ataxia is having difficulty standing up and balancing, then practicing the task of sit to stand is helpful. Disorders of movement often co-occur with other problems, such as weakness, spasticity or reduced ROM. If this occurs, improvement in each of these physical impairments is likely to have a positive effect on the quality of movement. However, conditions such as ataxia may occur in the absence of any other contributing physical impairment. All the key aspects of motor learning or skill acquisition need to be considered (i.e., structured practice, movement specificity, feedback, knowledge of results) to improve performance. The application of these principles may require modification in the presence of cognitive impairment. For example, feedback may need to be simplified and limited to one or two key factors associated with improved performance. In more severe cases, such as the inability to sit independently, physical assistance or facilitation may be required, and this may form part of the feedback on task performance. Disorders of movement are very frustrating for the patient and notoriously difficult to treat.

Balance and Vestibular Function

Findings from the balance and vestibular assessment should direct which types of interventions are used. For example, if a clinical balance assessment indicates a problem with proprioception and a person with TBI was compensating by fixing their gaze, a range of intervention strategies may be implemented. Altering the surface from a firm to a soft surface, or using a foam mat, will require greater proprioceptive demands. Changing the visual input, by asking the person to move their gaze from side to side, or even close their eyes, will restrict the ability to visually compensate and place greater emphasis on the proprioceptive system. The guiding principle in the subacute phase of rehabilitation should be to drive recovery by selection of appropriate interventions, rather than training or consolidation of compensatory patterns.

Vestibular dysfunction (see Chapter 17) requires its own exercises, which are quite distinct from other types of balance exercises. For example, if a person is unsteady on their feet, reports being dizzy, and the clinical assessment indicates benign paroxysmal positional vertigo, the patient is unlikely to benefit from conventional balance exercises. In this case, a repositioning manoeuvre is required to treat the symptoms. The environment in which the person lives and functions is important to assess to ensure potential hazards are identified and removed, and equipment such as rails are put in place, to optimise independence and reduce risk of falling.

Muscle and Joint Range of Motion

A range of physiotherapy interventions are used to maintain or improve ROM, and are frequently used in conjunction with other treatments such as BoNT-A or baclofen. Treatments include serial casting, splinting, stretching or standing on a tilt-table or in a standing frame. Each type of physiotherapeutic intervention has likely advantages and precautions that need to be considered when choosing between potential alternatives.

Serial casting has been used for many years to maintain or improve joint or muscle ROM, and is most commonly applied the distal joints of the arms (elbow, wrists and hands) and legs (knees and ankles) (Singer et al 2003, Verplancke et al 2005). The materials used range from plaster of paris to fibreglass-type products. Once in place, they may be left for 7–10 days until being removed and a new one applied in a better (more stretched) position. An advantage of serial casts is that they provide a prolonged stretch, which is fundamental for improvement. A relative disadvantage is that they cannot be removed daily for exercises or to check the person's skin integrity, particularly if the patient is minimally responsive and is not necessarily able to report discomfort.

Splints are an alternative to serial casts and have similar indications. Splints are generally more expensive than casts, and not all of the materials used to make splints are easily modified to accommodate improvement as the stretching takes effect. Some splints are 'static', that is, they do not move and restrict the person from moving. Other splints are 'dynamic', that is, they allow movement whilst they are in situ. Unlike casts, splints can be removed for showering and dressing, or to perform other exercises during therapy.

Equinovarus is particularly common in severe TBI (Fig. 8.2), and maintenance of plantargrade is an important factor in achieving sitting and standing positions and walking. Considerable time and effort have been devoted over the years to using serial casting and splinting to maintain plantargrade. Alternatives include tilt-tables and standing frames. A tilt-table gives a person with TBI the opportunity for a full body-weight stretch of their calves at a stage in their rehabilitation when they are unlikely to be able to unable to stand independently. An added advantage is that the inclination can be adjusted according to the person's physiological response, particularly when someone has been minimally conscious or rest in bed for a prolonged period.

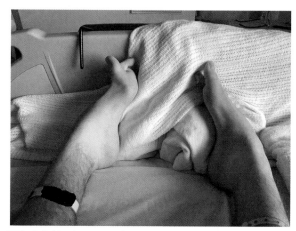

FIG. 8.2 Equinovarus feet.

Concurrent Musculoskeletal Injuries

Musculoskeletal injuries are often sustained concurrently with the TBI. Each of these injuries will come with their own recommended management strategies, contraindications and precautions. The initial management of these injuries may override or take priority over some of the TBI-related interventions. For example, a person with a fractured tibia who is non–weight-bearing is not allowed to stand on a tilt-table even though they may have spastic equinovarus. However, many of the physical treatment priorities for musculoskeletal injuries – i.e., maintain ROM and improve strength and function – overlap with the priorities associated with managing the positive and negative features of the UMN syndrome (Synnot et al 2017).

Pain

Whether it is caused by spasticity and spasms, a central pain syndrome or any of the associated musculoskeletal injuries, many people have significant pain and considerable need for pain relief after TBI. Each different cause of pain may require a different medication, and not all pain requires medication (see Chapter 23). Management of a person's pain is not only important to reduce their discomfort and distress, but also to allow rehabilitative efforts to commence. Pain can be a major barrier to engaging in a range of therapies or exercises. Prescription of medication for pain relief before therapy often allows a patient to better engage in therapy, tolerate stretches or tilt-tabling with more comfort, and provides greater motivation to move. Pain generally subsides over time, but occasionally patients report new or different pain in the subacute phase. If this does occur, the relevant investigations are required because a musculoskeletal injury may have been missed in the acute stage or, alternatively, HO may be developing in the subacute phase.

Function

The overall aim of rehabilitation is to promote independence or function. The previous sections have dealt with interventions aimed at impairments. Functional practice, or task practice, provides the opportunity to 'bring it all together' to improve performance and reduce activity limitations. For example, an activity limitation such as walking may be because of a spastic calf muscle, weak hip muscles, reduced ankle ROM, or pain from toe clawing. Each of these four contributing impairments can be treated and improved. However, task practice – in this case walking – is vital for improved walking performance and to ensure improvements in physical impairments translate into functional gains (Dean et al 2000, Dobkin et al 2010). Improved physical impairments do not necessarily automatically lead to improved participation rates (Sullivan & Cen 2011), and task or functional practice is the vital link in ensuring that rehabilitation outcomes are used in day-to-day life. Adaptive equipment, such as ankle-foot orthoses (AFOs), is commonly prescribed to improve mobility, reduce tripping and falls and enable safe independent walking. Extensive clinical practice guidelines (CPGs) for the use of AFOs have been published (Johnston et al 2021). Although this CPG is focused on stroke, there are no equivalent guidelines in TBI, so the stroke CPG for AFOs may be an adequate interim guide.

Functional retraining also must be context specific. This means that rather than just practicing activities in a clinical setting, it may be more beneficial to the patient for the therapy to be implemented in the community (e.g., the patient's home, workplace or gym). There are many good reasons why therapy implementation may be more effective in a community-based setting. Patients, particularly those with cognitive impairment, do not need to translate task practice from a clinical setting to the home setting, where the setup and layout of the home may be different. Further, family members and friends are more likely to understand and engage in the facilitating rehabilitative interventions that will foster independent practice.

OTHER CONSIDERATIONS

In the presence of severe and complex disability after TBI, simple and general health factors can be easily overlooked. All people, regardless of disability, need to maintain an active lifestyle, with good cardiovascular fitness and body weight. These factors can be very difficult to achieve after TBI, particularly if someone has a dense spastic hemiparesis, which may mean they can only walk indoors with a gait

aid. In such a case, walking does not provide a cardiovascular benefit, running is not possible, and they may not have the ability to balance and ride a bike or the arm and leg function to swim. However, there is a wide range of exercises and adaptive equipment that may be used to facilitate activity levels and cardiovascular fitness. Exercise bikes, recumbent bikes, arm ergometers and other machines can be used to achieve a heart rate in a desired training range to meet guidelines for maintaining general health. The first physical activity guidelines for people living with disability has recently been published (Carty et al 2021). The work by Carty and colleagues (2021) demonstrates that it is safe and effective for people with neurological conditions such as multiple sclerosis, Parkinson's, spinal cord injury and stroke to engage in exercise and physical activity to improve and maintain their cardiovascular health. However, this substantial review did not include TBI. Fewer investigations into cardiovascular fitness have been reported in TBI compared with other adult-onset neurological conditions (Hassett et al 2017).

Cognitive, behavioural and emotional impairments may also have a major impact on how physical interventions are delivered, and independent practice may never be possible for some. However, practice and repetition are vital for improved performance. A person with a TBI may be highly motivated but fail to benefit from their prescribed exercise programme because of poor memory (forgetting to do their exercises unprompted), poor initiation (lack of internal drive), poor self-monitoring (difficulty discriminating between good and poor performance) or fear or anxiety (worried about falling when walking). Each aspect of these related impairments must be addressed to promote independence and optimise outcomes.

COVID UPDATE

The Covid-19 pandemic has had extensive implications for healthcare around the world. There are numerous emerging Covid-19 and 'long' Covid resources, and although they are specific to physical rehabilitation (American Physical Therapy Association 2022a, 2022b), none are specific to TBI. At this stage, it is too early to determine whether Covid-19 has had an impact on TBI outcomes. There is emerging evidence of the impact of societal restrictions on the incidence of TBI (Lester et al 2021). There were initial concerns that some may not seek medical care to avoid Covid-19-overwhelmed hospitals. Road traffic deceased, but there were conflicting reports of associated increases (Prawiroharjo et al 2020) and decreases (Jayakumar et al 2020) in TBI. Government policies and societal restrictions in response to the Covid-19 pandemic have also been reported to have associations with reduced leisure-related TBI (Pinggera et al

2021) yet increases in TBI associated with domestic violence (Toccalino et al 2022). Those that did make it to rehabilitation for TBI during the Covid-19 pandemic found reduced length of stay, shortened session times, restricted services and transition to telehealth-type services (Lester et al 2021). However, in many cases the impact of Covid-19 and the associated societal effects on TBI incidence, healthcare provision and outcomes are yet to be determined.

CONCLUSION

TBI can result in severe and complex injuries. Given the nature of the event that typically causes a TBI, multisystem injuries are often associated with the TBI, which may complicate the early acute and rehabilitation stages of care. Cognitive, behavioural and emotional impairments are likely to be present, but may only become apparent over time as the patient regains consciousness. TBI most commonly occurs in young adults, so survivors are dependent on their rehabilitation outcomes for many decades after their injury. Important physical outcomes can be achieved for many years after TBI. Some people will be unable to return home and require assisted living. Given the complex nature of TBI, a team approach is vital. However, fragmented service delivery is common and leads to suboptimal outcomes, especially once patients return to live in the community. Unlike emergency and acute TBI management, there are no published peer-reviewed consensus guidelines for the provision of rehabilitation after brain injury. Service provision and evaluation of interventions in the rehabilitation phase require much further development so that support for patients and their families become more accessible and available in the longer term.

CASE PRESENTATION

This case study will discuss an 18-year-old young woman, Penny, who sustained a TBI as a passenger in a motor vehicle accident. Her friend died as a result of her injuries sustained in the accident, and two other friends sustained non–life-threatening orthopaedic injuries. Penny's GCS at the scene of the accident was 3. She had also sustained facial fractures and a left humeral fracture and a left femoral fracture. She was stabilised at the scene and air-lifted to a trauma unit. Scans revealed a large left subdural haematoma (SDH), bifrontal contusions, DAI and multiple petechial haemorrhages. A craniectomy was performed to evacuate the SDH the following day; a tracheostomy to assist in maintaining her upper airway and internal fixation of the humeral and femoral fractures were performed 2 days later. Her cervical spine was cleared of injury and the protective hard collar removed. Penny was

---

> **KEY INITIAL ASSESSMENT FINDINGS**
>
> - Extremely severe traumatic brain injury
> - Nonresponsive
> - Non–weight-bearing left upper and lower limbs
> - Decorticate spastic pattern affecting right > left
> - Spontaneous movement left upper limb

in intensive care for 11 days before being transferred to a high-dependency unit (HDU). Whilst she was in the HDU, a percutaneous endoscopic gastrostomy was inserted so the nasogastric feeding tube could be removed. This decision was made because of the likely longer-term requirement of assisted nutrition. The key findings of the physiotherapy assessment are identified in the Key Initial Assessment Findings box.

During her stay in the HDU, Penny's conscious state slowly started to improve, and some spontaneous movement was noticed on the left upper limb. Her sedation was reduced, and her usual resting position was described as decorticate, with the right side more affected than the left. Full passive ROM was restricted on the right during daily stretching, and the left-side ROM was slowly deteriorating as stretching was contraindicated by the fractures. However, in consultation with the orthopaedic surgeon, weight bearing was permitted on the left leg on the tilt-table only, so daily tilt-tabling commenced. Daily tilt-tabling stopped further loss of ROM at her ankles and maintained Penny's loss of dorsiflexion to 10° (i.e., 10° of plantarflexion at best) with inversion. Baclofen was commenced for her spasticity and hypertonicity, the ventilator was weaned and the tracheostomy was extubated a week later. Five weeks after the accident, Penny was transferred to an inpatient rehabilitation facility.

On admission to rehabilitation, Penny was dependent in all areas for self-care and mobility; her conscious state was improving but she remained in PTA. She did not have a reliable yes/no response and was doubly incontinent. After her first week of admission to rehabilitation, an orthopaedic review allowed Penny to commence partial weight bearing on her left upper and lower limbs. Penny displayed some spontaneous active movement in all four limbs, but more so on the left than the right (she was right dominant), and in the upper more so than the lower limbs. Penny received twice-daily physiotherapy on the ward, although the scheduling was challenging given her disrupted sleep–wake cycle. Tilt-tabling continued, sitting out of bed in a supportive tilt-in-space chair commenced with supervision because of restlessness, and a swallowing assessment was performed including videofluoroscopy. All transfers were performed with a hoist. After 6 weeks in rehabilitation, Penny was clear of PTA, for an official duration of 74 days.

Once Penny was out of PTA, physiotherapy commenced in the physiotherapy department. Her equinovarus had not deteriorated or improved, and a higher dose of baclofen was not tolerable because of marked fatigue. BoNT-A was injected into both heads of gastrocnemius, soleus and tibialis posterior on both sides. Serial casting was considered but not implemented because twice-daily tilt-tabling was considered to be more beneficial. However, resting ankle splints were prescribed in an attempt to maintain a plantargrade position overnight. She developed a mild left upper limb tremor that affected eating and drinking because she did not have sufficient active movement in her dominant right upper limb for these activities. Penny was now continent and did not have any substantial pain associated with her musculoskeletal injuries, but was prescribed gabapentin for neuropathic pain in her left arm. She also reported an ache around her left hip. After assessment (about 3 months postinjury), the a problem list, goals and treatment plan were devised (see Table 8.6).

Each day Penny performed stretches, strengthening exercises, transfer training and balance training. Hydrotherapy commenced to improve active movement, strength, balance and commence walking. Eight weeks after the BoNT-A injections, Penny was able to achieve a plantargrade position bilaterally, but only after 10 minutes of stretching on the tilt-table. Walking on land was attempted with a gutter frame and the assistance of three staff, but this exacerbated the spastic equinovarus position and caused foot pain. At this point, as spasticity was considered to be the main barrier to improvement, a decision was made for a baclofen pump trial, which was successful. Two weeks later, Penny had a baclofen pump inserted.

TABLE 8.6 Penny's Problem List, Goals and Treatment Plan

Problem List	Goals	Treatment Plan
Body structure and function		
Severe spasticity affecting lower > upper limbs, right > left side	Reduce the impact of spasticity on function	Baclofen (main side effect is fatigue)
		Botulinum toxin injections for multifocal spasticity
Quadriparesis	Improve strength upper and lower limbs to improve function	Daily physiotherapy targeting strength training using American College of Sports Medicine principles to maximise transfer of muscle strength into function
Loss of ROM, particularly in both ankles, left hip and both shoulders	Maintain current ROM	Daily stretching and standing on a tilt-table
	Improve ROM so that joint and muscle contractures do not affect performance of personal activities of daily living, transfers and mobility	
Left arm pain disrupting sleep	To be able to sleep through the night without being woken by pain	Liaise with medical staff as to likely cause of pain (central, nerve, musculoskeletal) and most appropriate medication
Fatigue limiting therapy time	To last a whole hour in physiotherapy twice daily	Schedule regular breaks within session, and rest breaks after therapy
		Address pain management so Penny gets sufficient rest overnight
Activity limitations		
Dependent on assistance for bed mobility and transfers	Supervised bed mobility (FIM 5)	Daily physiotherapy and occupational therapy to target:
	Assist ×1 for sit to stand and stand transfers (FIM 4)	- Strength training upper and lower limbs
	Independent mobility in a powered wheelchair (FIM 6)	- Balance training
		- Task practice in therapy and on ward (with nursing staff)
	Consider home modifications likely to be required for discharge	- Commence family and carer training for their assistive roles for discharge

(Continued)

TABLE 8.6	Penny's Problem List, Goals and Treatment Plan —Cont'd	
Problem List	**Goals**	**Treatment Plan**
Dependent on assistance for personal activities of daily living and eating and drinking	Set up only required for eating and drinking (FIM 6) Independent upper body washing and dressing with set up (FIM 6) Minimal assistance for lower body washing and dressing (FIM 4) Consider home modifications likely to be required for discharge	Daily physiotherapy and occupational therapy to target: - Task practice in therapy and on ward (with nursing staff) - Commence family and carer training for their assistive roles for discharge

FIM, Functional independence measure; *ROM,* range of motion.

Penny was discharged home 8.5 months after her accident. At this point, she had achieved all the inpatient goals set for her. Penny commenced outpatient physiotherapy three times per week and continued with occupational therapy, speech therapy and psychology. At 6 months post-discharge from inpatient rehabilitation, Penny was independent in transfers, showering, dressing, toileting, eating and drinking. These improvements were largely a result of her ongoing improved physical status, but complemented by several modifications and provision of adaptive equipment. Regular 3-monthly team meetings were held with Penny to review goals and set new ones. Although Penny could walk short distances with a frame and assistance of two physiotherapists, walking remained a physiotherapy exercise and not a functional task.

Although the baclofen pump had allowed several important physical goals to be achieved, walking remained an elusive goal, so an orthopaedic consultation was sought to determine whether correction of her equinovarus could provide an improved level of functional walking. After a thorough assessment process, Penny had a bilateral calf release, bilateral hip adductor releases and a right rectus femoris transfer (where the distal rectus femoris tendon is resected and attached to the semitendinosus tendon so it assists with knee flexion). Six weeks later, Penny commenced walking with 1× assist for balance on a forearm crutch (FAC).

Four years after her accident, Penny was able to walk independently with a four-wheeled frame, independently indoors or with supervision outdoors on 1× FAC (because of anxiety and fear of falling) (Fig. 8.3). Longer distances (> 500 m) were too challenging, and as she was unable to drive a car, Penny used a scooter to access the community and public transport. She worked 3 days/week in an administration role after completing a 12-month course. Penny attended a local gym three times a week to continue

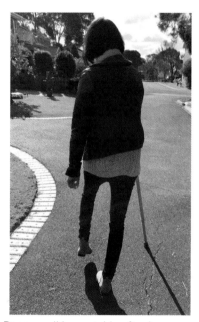

FIG. 8.3 Penny walking outside after her surgery.

to work on her strength, flexibility, balance and cardiovascular fitness. This programme was supervised by a community-based exercise physiologist once a week. She still experienced pain associated with spasticity and spasms. This was managed during attendance at a 3-monthly spasticity clinic by a combination of the baclofen pump and intermittent BoNT-A injections as she had ceased oral medications. Although she lived with her parents, she was able to live independently with some domestic support when they were away on holidays. A summary of Penny's progress is presented in Table 8.7.

TABLE 8.7 Penny's Progress With Rehabilitation	
Time Postinjury (setting)	**Rehabilitation Status**
11 days after TBI (intensive care unit/high dependency unit)	• Comatose (Glasgow Coma Scale = 3) • Postcraniectomy • Internal fixation all fractures • Tracheostomy in situ • Nasogastric feeding • Decorticate posturing • Fully dependent in all areas
5 weeks after TBI (rehabilitation ward)	• Awake but in PTA • Spontaneous breathing • Percutaneous endoscopic gastrostomy feeding • Fully dependent in all areas (transfers by hoist) • Spontaneous movements left upper limb
3 months after TBI (rehabilitation ward)	• Alert, orientated, out of PTA • Self-feeding • Fully dependent in all areas • Spontaneous movements all four limbs • Baclofen pump for spasticity
9 months after TBI (living at home with parents)	• Outpatient rehabilitation • Independent in self-care and transfers • Walking with frame + 2 assist (FIM 1)
4 years after TBI (living at home with parents)	• Orthopedic surgery to improve walking ability • Independently walking with frame (FIM 6) or 1× forearm crutch (FIM 5) • Working 3 days/week • Attending gym

FIM, Functional independence measure; *PTA*, posttraumatic amnesia; *TBI*, traumatic brain injury.

SELF-ASSESSMENT QUESTIONS

1. What does a GCS of 3 indicate?
2. What does a PTA of 74 days indicate?
3. What is the usual predicted outcome for Penny given her GCS and PTA scores?
4. Discuss the relative pros and cons of different strategies for maintaining Penny's ROM in the inpatient phase of rehabilition.
5. What may be the cause of the loss of ROM in her left hip and associated 'ache'?
6. Discuss the changes in roles within the family unit that may occur after significant brain injury and the implications of these changes including carer stress.
7. What are the relevant standardised outcome measures you could use to evaluate the effectiveness of:
   a. Mobility and walking after insertion of the baclofen pump
   b. Mobility and walking after the orthopaedic surgery

REFERENCES

American Congress of Rehabilitation Medicine., 1995. Recommendations for use of uniform nomenclature pertinent to patients with severe alterations in consciousness. Arch. Phys. Med. Rehabil. 76, 205–209.

Ashworth, B., 1964. Preliminary trial of carisoprodol in multiple sclerosis. Practitioner. 192, 540–542.

American Physical Therapy Association., 2022a. Coronavirus (COVID-19) resources for the physical therapy profession. Available at: https://www.apta.org/patient-care/ public-health-population-care/coronavirus. Accessed December 1, 2022.

American Physical Therapy Association., 2022b. COVID-19 core outcome measures. Available at: https://www.apta.org/your-practice/outcomes-measurement/covid-19-core-outcome-measures. Accessed December 1, 2022.

Bayley, M.T., Lamontagne, M.-E., Kua, A., et al., 2018. Unique features of the INESSS-ONF rehabilitation guidelines for moderate to severe traumatic brain injury: responding to users' needs. J. Head. Trauma. Rehabil 33, 296–305.

Berg, K., Wood-Dauphine, S., Williams, J.I., Gayton, D., 1989. Measuring balance in the elderly: preliminary development of an instrument. Physiother. Can. 41, 304–311.

Berger, E., Leven, F., Pirente, N., Bouillon, B., Neugebauer, E., 1999. Quality of life after traumatic brain injury: a systematic review of the literature. Restor. Neurol. Neurosci. 14, 93–102.

Birklein, F., 2005. Complex regional pain syndrome. J. Neurol. 252, 131–138.

Bohannon, R.W., Smith, M.B., 1987. Interrater reliability of a modified Ashworth scale of muscle spasticity. Phys. Ther. 67, 206–207.

Bond, M., 1986. Neurobehavioural sequelae of closed head injury. In: Grant, I., K.M., A. (Ed.), Neuropsychological Assessment of Neuropsychiatric Disorders. Oxford University Press, New York.

Bond, R., 1990. Standardised methods for assessing and predicting outcome. In: Rosenthal, M., Griffith, E., Bond, M., Miller, J. (Eds.), Rehabilitation of the Adult and Child with Traumatic Brain Injury. F.A. Davis, Philadelphia.

Bragge, P., Synnot, A., Maas, A.I., Menon, D.K., Cooper, D.J., Rosenfeld, J.V., Gruen, R.L., 2015. A state-of-the-science overview of randomized controlled trials evaluating acute management of moderate-to-severe traumatic brain injury. J. Neurotrauma. 33, 1461–1478.

Brashear, A., Elovic, E., 2010. Spasticity: Diagnosis and Management. Demos Medical Publishing, New York.

Bratton, S.L., Chestnut, R.M., Ghajar, J., et al., 2007a. Guidelines for the management of severe traumatic brain injury. II. Hyperosmolar therapy. J. Neurotrauma. 24 (Suppl. 1), S14–S20.

Bratton, S.L., Chestnut, R.M., Ghajar, J., et al., 2007b. Guidelines for the management of severe traumatic brain injury. VIII. Intracranial pressure thresholds. J. Neurotrauma. 24 (Suppl. 1), S55–S58.

Carney, N., Totten, A.M., O'Reilly, C., et al., 2017. Guidelines for the Management of Severe Traumatic Brain Injury, 4th ed. Neurosurgery. 80, 6–15.

Carty, C., van der Ploeg, H.P., Biddle, S.J.H., et al., 2021. The first global physical activity and sedentary behavior guidelines for people living with disability. J. Phys. Act. Health, 1–8.

Cnossen, M., Scholten, A., Lingsma, H., et al., 2021. Adherence to guidelines in adult patients with traumatic brain injury: a living systematic review. J. Neurotrauma. 38, 1072–1085.

Cooper, D.J., Rosenfeld, J.V., Murray, L., et al., 2011. Decompressive craniectomy in diffuse traumatic brain injury. N. Engl. J. Med. 364, 1493–1502.

Crooks, C.Y., Zumsteg, J.M., Bell, K.R., 2007. Traumatic brain injury: a review of practice management and recent advances. Phys. Med. Rehabil. Clin. N. Am. 18, 681–710. vi

Daley, K., Mayo, N., Wood-Dauphinee, S., 1999. Reliability of scores on the Stroke Rehabilitation Assessment of Movement (STREAM) measure. Phys. Ther. 79, 8–19. quiz 20–23

De Guise, E., Leblanc, J., Dagher, J., et al., 2014. Outcome in women with traumatic brain injury admitted to a level 1 trauma center. Int. Sch. Res. Notices., 263241.

Dean, C.M., Richards, C.L., Malouin, F., 2000. Task-related circuit training improves performance of locomotor tasks in chronic stroke: a randomized, controlled pilot trial. Arch. Phys. Med. Rehabil. 81, 409–417.

Dewan, M.C., Rattani, A., Gupta, S., et al., 2018. Estimating the global incidence of traumatic brain injury. J Neurosurg, 1–18.

Ditunno Jr., J.F., 1992. Functional assessment measures in CNS trauma. J. Neurotrauma. 9 (Suppl 1), S301–S305.

Dobkin, B.H., Plummer-D'Amato, P., Elashoff, R., Lee, J., 2010. International randomized clinical trial, stroke inpatient rehabilitation with reinforcement of walking speed (SIRROWS), improves outcomes. Neurorehabil. Neural. Repair. 24, 235–242.

Echemendia, R.J., Meeuwisse, W., McCrory, P., et al., 2017. The Sport Concussion Assessment Tool 5th Edition (SCAT5). Br. J. Sports Med. 51, 848–850.

Edwards, P., Arango, M., Balica, L., et al., 2005. Final results of MRC CRASH, a randomised placebo-controlled trial of intravenous corticosteroid in adults with head injury-outcomes at 6 months. Lancet. 365, 1957–1959.

Flaster, M., Meresh, E., Rao, M., Biller, J., 2013. Central poststroke pain: current diagnosis and treatment. Top. Stroke. Rehabil. 20, 116–123.

Giacino, J.T., Ashwal, S., Childs, N., et al., 2002. The minimally conscious state: definition and diagnostic criteria. Neurology. 58, 349–353.

Giacino, J.T., Katz, D.I., Schiff, N.D., et al., 2018. Practice guideline update recommendations summary: disorders of consciousness. Arch. Phys. Med. Rehabil. 99, 1699–1709.

Giacino, J.T., Whyte, J., Nakase-Richardson, R., et al., 2020. Minimum competency recommendations for programs that provide rehabilitation services for persons with disorders of consciousness: a position statement of the American Congress of Rehabilitation Medicine and the National Institute on Disability, independent living and rehabilitation research traumatic brain injury model systems. Arch. Phys. Med. Rehabil. 101, 1072–1089.

Gorman, S.L., Radtka, S., Melnick, M.E., Abrams, G.M., Byl, N.N., 2010. Development and validation of the function in sitting test in adults with acute stroke. J. Neurol. Phys. Ther. 34, 150–160.

Gruen, D.S., Guyette, F.X., Brown, J.B., et al., 2020. Association of prehospital plasma with survival in patients with traumatic brain injury: a secondary analysis of the PAMPer Cluster Randomized Clinical Trial. JAMA. Netw. Open. 3, e2016869.

Harrison-Felix, C., Kolakowsky-Hayner, S.A., Hammond, F.M., et al., 2012. Mortality after surviving traumatic brain injury: risks based on age groups. J. Head. Trauma. Rehabil. 27, E45–E46.

Harvey, L.A., Katalinic, O.M., Herbert, R.D., Moseley, A.M., Lannin, N.A., Schurr, K., 2017. Stretch for the treatment and prevention of contractures: an abridged republication of a Cochrane Systematic Review. J. Physiother. 63, 67–75.

Hassett, L., Moseley, A.M., Harmer, A.R., 2017. Fitness training for cardiorespiratory conditioning after traumatic brain injury. Cochrane. Database. Syst. Rev. 12, CD006123.

Haugh, A.B., Pandyan, A.D., Johnson, G.R., 2006. A systematic review of the Tardieu Scale for the measurement of spasticity. Disabil. Rehabil. 28, 899–907.

Ivanhoe, C.B., Reistetter, T.A., 2004. Spasticity: the misunderstood part of the upper motor neuron syndrome. Am. J. Phys. Med. Rehabil. 83, S3–S9.

Jayakumar, N., Kennion, O., Villabona, A.R., Paranathala, M., Holliman, D., 2020. Neurosurgical referral patterns during the coronavirus disease 2019 pandemic: a United Kingdom experience. World. Neurosurg. 144, e414–e420.

Jennett, B., 1996. Epidemiology of head injury. J. Neurol. Neurosurg. Psychiatr. 60, 362–369.

Jennett, B., Bond, M., 1975. Assessment of outcome after severe brain damage: a practical scale. Lancet. 1, 480–484.

Jennett, B., Teasdale, G., 1977. Aspects of coma after severe head injury. Lancet. 1, 878–881.

Jeremitsky, E., Omert, L., Dunham, C.M., Protetch, J., Rodriguez, A., 2003. Harbingers of poor outcome the day after severe brain injury: hypothermia, hypoxia, and hypoperfusion. J. Trauma. 54, 312–319.

Johnston, M.V., Hall, K.M., 1994. Outcomes evaluation in TBI rehabilitation. Part I: overview and system principles. Arch. Phys. Med. Rehabil. 75, SC1–9.

Johnston, T.E., Keller, S., Denzer-Weiler, C., Brown, L., 2021. A clinical practice guideline for the use of ankle-foot orthoses and functional electrical stimulation post-stroke. J. Neurol. Phys. Ther. 45, 112–196.

Kondziella, D., Bender, A., Diserens, K., et al., 2020. European Academy of Neurology guideline on the diagnosis of coma and other disorders of consciousness. Eur. J. Neurol. 27, 741–756.

Lester, A., Leach, P., Zaben, M., 2021. The impact of the COVID-19 pandemic on traumatic brain injury management: lessons learned over the first year. World. Neurosurg. 156, 28–32.

Leung, J., King, C., Fereday, S., 2019. Effectiveness of a programme comprising serial casting, botulinum toxin, splinting and motor training for contracture management: a randomized controlled trial. Clin. Rehabil. 33, 1035–1044.

Levin, H.S., O'Donnell, V.M., Grossman, R.G., 1979. The Galveston Orientation and Amnesia Test. A practical scale to assess cognition after head injury. J. Nerv. Ment. Dis. 167, 675–684.

Malec, J.F., Moessner, A.M., Kragness, M., Lezak, M.D., 2000. Refining a measure of brain injury sequelae to predict post-acute rehabilitation outcome: rating scale analysis of the Mayo-Portland Adaptability Inventory. J. Head. Trauma. Rehabil. 15, 670–682.

Max, W., Mackenzie, E.J., Rice, D.P., 1991. Head injuries: costs and consequences. J. Head. Trauma. Rehabil. 6, 76–91.

McCormick, Z.L., Chu, S.K., Binler, D., Neudorf, D., Mathur, S.N., Lee, J., Marciniak, C., 2016. Intrathecal versus oral baclofen: a matched cohort study of spasticity, pain, sleep, fatigue, and quality of life. Phys. Med. Rehabil. 8, 553–562.

McCrory, P., Meeuwisse, W.H, Aubry, M., Cantu, B., Dvořák, J., Echemendia, R.J., et al., 2013. Consensus statement on concussion in sport: the 4th International Conference on Concussion in Sport held in Zurich, November 2012. Br. J. Sports. Med. 47, 250–258.

McCrory, P., Meeuwisse, W., Dvorak, J., et al., 2017. Consensus statement on concussion in sport—the 5th international conference on concussion in sport held in Berlin, October 2016. Br. J. Sports. Med. 47, 250–258.

McCulloch, K.L., De Joya, A.L., Hays, K., et al., 2016. Outcome measures for persons with moderate to severe traumatic brain injury: recommendations from the American Physical Therapy Association Academy of Neurologic Physical Therapy TBI EDGE Task Force. J. Neurol. Phys. Ther. 40, 269–280.

McFadyen, B.J., Cantin, J.-F., Swaine, B., Duchesneau, G., Doyon, J., Dumas, D., Fait, P., 2009. Modality-specific, multitask locomotor deficits persist despite good recovery after a traumatic brain injury. Arch. Phys. Med. Rehabil. 90, 1596–1606.

McKay, A., Trevena-Peters, J., Ponsford, J., 2021. The use of atypical antipsychotics for managing agitation after traumatic brain injury. J. Head. Trauma. Rehabil. 36, 149–155.

Moore, J.L., Potter, K., Blankshain, K., Kaplan, S.L., O'Dwyer, L.C., Sullivan, J.E., 2018. A core set of outcome measures for adults with neurologic conditions undergoing rehabilitation: a Clinical Practice Guideline. J. Neurol. Phys. Ther. 42, 174–220.

Morris, S.L., Dodd, K.J., Morris, M.E., 2004. Outcomes of progressive resistance strength training following stroke: a systematic review. Clin. Rehabil. 18, 27–39.

Neptune, R.R., Sasaki, K., Kautz, S.A., 2008. The effect of walking speed on muscle function and mechanical energetics. Gait. Posture. 28, 135–143.

New Zealand Guidelines Group., 2006. Traumatic Brain Injury: Diagnosis, Acute Management and Rehabilitation. Available at: http://www.acc.co.nz/PRD_EXT_CSMP/groups/external_communications/documents/guide/wim2_059414.pdf. Accessed on 14 May 2022.

Nichol, A., Gantner, D., Presneill, J., et al., 2015. Protocol for a multicentre randomised controlled trial of early and sustained prophylactic hypothermia in the management of traumatic brain injury. Crit. Care. Resusc. 17, 92–100.

O'Connor, P., 2002. Hospitalisation due to traumatic brain injury (TBI). Australia 1997–98. Australian Institute of Health and Welfare, Adelaide.

O'Connor, P.J., Cripps, R.A., 1999. Traumatic brain injury (TBI) surveillance issues. AIHW National Injury Surveillance Unit. Flinders University Research Centre for Injury Studies, Adelaide.

Olver, J., Esquenazi, A., Fung, V., Singer, B., Ward, A., 2010. Botulinum toxin assessment, intervention and aftercare for lower limb disorders of movement and muscle tone in adults: international consensus statement. Eur. J. Neurol. 17, 57–73.

Papastrat, L.A., 1992. Outcome and value following TBI: a financial providers perspective. J. Head. Trauma. Rehabil. 7, 11–23.

Perrin, P.B., Niemeier, J.P., Mougeot, J.-L., et al., 2015. Measures of injury severity and prediction of acute traumatic brain injury outcomes. J. Head. Trauma. Rehabil. 30, 136–142.

Pinggera, D., Klein, B., Thomé, C., Grassner, L., 2021. The influence of the COVID-19 pandemic on traumatic brain injuries in Tyrol: experiences from a state under lockdown. Eur. J. Trauma. Emerg. Surg. 47, 653–658.

Ponsford, J., Carrier, S., Hicks, A., McKay, A., 2021. Assessment and management of patients in the acute stages of recovery after traumatic brain injury in adults: a worldwide survey. J. Neurotrauma. 38, 1060–1067.

Ponsford, J., Sloan, S., Snow, P., 2013. Traumatic brain injury: rehabilitation for everyday adaptive living. Psychology Press, East Sussex, UK.

Ponsford, J.L., Olver, J.H., Curran, C., 1995. A profile of outcome: 2 years after traumatic brain injury. Brain. Injury. 9, 1–10.

Pope, A.M., Tarlov, A.R., 1991. Disability in America: toward a national agenda for prevention. National Academy Press, Washington, DC.

Prawiroharjo, P., Pangeran, D., Supriawan, H., et al., 2020. Increasing Traumatic brain injury incidence during COVID-19 pandemic in the emergency department of Cipto Mangunkusumo National General Hospital—a national referral hospital in Indonesia. Neurology. 95 S11–S11

Schonberger, M., Ponsford, J., Olver, J., Ponsford, M., Wirtz, M., 2011. Prediction of functional and employment outcome 1 year after traumatic brain injury: a structural equation modelling approach. J. Neurol. Neurosurg. Psychiatry. 82, 936–941.

Scottish Intercollegiate Guidelines Network (SIGN)., 2013. Brain injury rehabilitation in adults. A national clinical guideline. Scottish Intercollegiate Guidelines Network (SIGN), Edinburgh.

Seel, R.T., Sherer, M., Whyte, J., et al., 2010. Assessment scales for disorders of consciousness: evidence-based recommendations for clinical practice and research. Arch. Phys. Med. Rehabil. 91, 1795–1813.

Sheean, G., Lannin, N., Turner-Stokes, L., Rawicki, B., Snow, B., 2010. Botulinum toxin assessment, intervention and aftercare for upper limb hypertonicity in adults: international consensus statement. Eur. J. Neurol. 17, 74–93.

Shores, E.A., Lammel, A., Hullick, C., Sheedy, J., Flynn, M., Levick, W., Batchelor, J., 2008. The diagnostic accuracy of the Revised Westmead PTA Scale as an adjunct to the Glasgow Coma Scale in the early identification of cognitive impairment in patients with mild traumatic brain injury. J. Neurol. Neurosurg. Psychiatry. 79, 1100–1106.

Shores, E.A., Marosszeky, J.E., Sandanam, J., Batchelor, J., 1986. Preliminary validation of a clinical scale for measuring the duration of post-traumatic amnesia. Med. J. Aust. 144, 569–572.

Singer, B.J., Jegasothy, G.M., Singer, K.P., Allison, G.T., 2003. Evaluation of serial casting to correct equinovarus deformity of the ankle after acquired brain injury in adults. Arch. Phys. Med. Rehabil. 84, 483–491.

Spaite, D.W., Bobrow, B.J., Keim, S.M., et al., 2019. Association of statewide implementation of the prehospital traumatic brain injury treatment guidelines with patient survival following traumatic brain injury: the Excellence in Prehospital Injury Care (EPIC) study. JAMA. Surg. 154, e191152.

Spiteri, C., Ponsford, J., Williams, G., Kahn, M., McKay, A., 2021. Factors affecting participation in physical therapy during posttraumatic amnesia. Arch. Phys. Med. Rehabil. 102, 378–385.

Spiteri, C., Williams, G., Kahn, M., Ponsford, J., McKay, A., 2022. Factors associated with physical therapy engagement during the period of posttraumatic amnesia. J. Neurol. Phys. Ther. 46, 41–49.

Stark, T., Walker, B., Phillips, J.K., Fejer, R., Beck, R., 2011. Hand-held dynamometry correlation with the gold standard isokinetic dynamometry: a systematic review. Phys. Med. Rehabil. 3, 472–479.

State of Colorado., 2018. Traumatic brain injury medical treatment guidelines. In: Department of Labor and Employment, 5th ed. Division of Workers' Compensation, Colorado.

Stetkarova, I., Yablon, S.A., Kofler, M., Stokic, D.S., 2010. Procedure- and device-related complications of intrathecal baclofen administration for management of adult muscle hypertonia: a review. Neurorehabil. Neural. Repair. 24, 609–619.

Stocchetti, N., Taccone, F.S., Citerio, G., et al., 2015. Neuroprotection in acute brain injury: an up-to-date review. Crit. Care. 19, 186.

Sullivan, K.J., Cen, S.Y., 2011. Model of disablement and recovery: knowledge translation in rehabilitation research and practice. Phys. Ther. 91, 1892–1904.

Synnot, A., Chau, M., Pitt, V., et al., 2017. Interventions for managing skeletal muscle spasticity following traumatic brain injury. Cochrane. Database. Syst. Rev. 11, CD008929.

Taylor, N.F., Dodd, K.J., Damiano, D.L., 2005. Progressive resistance exercise in physical therapy: a summary of systematic reviews. Phys. Ther. 85, 1208–1223.

Teasdale, G., Jennett, B., 1974. Assessment of coma and impaired consciousness. A practical scale. Lancet. 2, 81–84.

Thibaut, A., Wannez, S., Deltombe, T., Martens, G., Laureys, S., Chatelle, C., 2018. Physical therapy in patients with disorders of consciousness: impact on spasticity and muscle contracture. NeuroRehabilitation. 42, 199–205.

Thurman, D., Alverson, C., Browne, D., et al., 1999. Traumatic brain injury in the United States: a report to Congress. Centers for Disease Control and Prevention, Atlanta.

Toccalino, D., Haag, H., Estrella, M.J., et al., 2022. Addressing the shadow pandemic: COVID-19 related impacts, barriers, needs, and priorities to healthcare and support for women survivors of intimate partner violence and brain injury. Arch. Phys. Med. Rehabil. 103, 1466–1476.

Trevena-Peters, J., McKay, A., Spitz, G., Suda, R., Renison, B., Ponsford, J., 2018. Efficacy of activities of daily living retraining during posttraumatic amnesia: a randomized controlled trial. Arch. Phys. Med. Rehabil. 99, 329–337.e2.

Turner-Stokes, L.F., Williams, H., Bill, A., Bassett, P., Sephton, K., 2016. Cost-efficiency of in-patient specialist rehabilitation following acquired brain injury: a large multi-centre cohort analysis from the UK. Br. Med. J. Open. 6 (2), e010238.

Verplancke, D., Snape, S., Salisbury, C.F., Jones, P.W., Ward, A.B., 2005. A randomized controlled trial of botulinum toxin on lower limb spasticity following acute acquired severe brain injury. Clin. Rehabil. 19, 117–125.

Willer, B., Rosenthal, M., Kreutzer, J.S., Gordon, W.A., Rempel, R., 1993. Assessment. of community integration following rehabilitation for traumatic brain injury. J. Head. Trauma. Rehabil. 8, 75–87.

Williams, G., Kahn, M., Randall, A., 2014. Strength training for walking in neurologic rehabilitation is not task specific: a focused review. Am. J. Phys. Med. Rehabil. 93, 511–522.

Winter, D.A., 1983. Biomechanical motor patterns in normal walking. J. Mot. Behav. 15, 302–330.

Wissel, J., Ward, A.B., Erztgaard, P., et al., 2009. European consensus table on the use of botulinum toxin type A in adult spasticity. J. Rehabil. Med. 41, 13–25.

Spinal Cord Injury

Sue Paddison and Benita Hexter

OUTLINE

Introduction, 198
Epidemiology, 198
  Incidence Data, 198
Aetiology, 198
Pathophysiology, 199
Diagnosis, 199
Prognosis, 200
Incomplete Syndromes, 200
Early Acute Management, 203
  Discussing Prognosis, 204
  Physical Management, 204
  Facilitation of Range, Muscle Length and Functional
    Movement, 205
  Mobilisation, 207
Respiratory Assessment, 207
Respiratory Treatment, 208
  Weaning From Ventilatory Support, 209
    Respiratory Management and Covid-19, 209
  Long-Term Respiratory Management, 210
Clinical Presentation, 210
  Spinal Shock, 210
  Autonomic Dysreflexia, 210
  Cardiovascular Dysfunction, 210
  Thermoregulation Dysfunction, 211
  Bladder, Bowels and Sexual Dysfunction, 211
  Weakness, 211
  Sensory Changes, 212
  Balance, 212

  Pain, 212
  Spasticity, 212
Assessment, 212
Physical Management, 212
  Strength Training, 214
  Aquatic Therapy, 214
  Facilitation of Movement, 214
  Splinting, 216
  Seating, 216
  Functional Mobility, 217
  Standing, 218
  Gait Training, 218
  Cardiovascular Fitness, 220
  Other Modalities, 220
Special Considerations, 221
  Reduced Bone Density, 221
  Loss of Range of Movement and Postural
    Deformity, 221
  Shoulder Pain, 221
  Tissue Viability, 221
  Heterotropic Ossification, 222
  Syrinx and Syringomyelia, 222
Paediatric Considerations, 222
Discharge Planning and Lifelong Care, 222
Conclusion, 223
Case Study, 223
  Progress With Rehabilitation, 223

INTRODUCTION

Spinal cord injury (SCI) is usually a sudden-onset, life-transforming condition. An SCI denotes disruption of the neural tissue within the spinal canal. It refers to damage to the cord resulting from trauma, disease or degeneration which presents as an upper motor neurone (UMN) lesion with varying loss of sensation, weakness and spasticity. There may also be intracanal damage to the brachial plexus or other peripheral nerves as they make their short journeys from the spinal cord to their foramina.

The term SCI often encompasses damage to the conus medullaris, at the distal end of the spinal cord at around T12/L1 level, and the cauda equina, which is formed by the L1-S5 peripheral nerves as they exit the spinal cord and travel down through the spinal canal before they exit at their neural foramina. Vertebral injury below T12 will often result in cauda equina syndrome as the spinal cord ends at L1 or L2 vertebral level. These injuries result in a lower motor neurone (LMN) lesion, which is characterised by the absence of spasticity.

Paraplegia is used to describe dysfunction of the trunk and lower limbs, arising from damage to the spinal cord below T1.

Tetraplegia refers to loss of function in the upper limbs, trunk and lower limbs caused by injury at cervical spinal levels.

SCI can be classified according to the degree of sparing of movement and sensation below the lesion. Individuals with SCI will need to develop adaptive strategies to return to optimum control of their physical self and instigate their path to reintegration.

In many countries it is recognised as best practice to manage people with SCI in specialist centres. This chapter will focus on the clinical management of SCI initiating at acute phase, through rehabilitation, to restore potential and subsequent interventions to restore function. The Multidisciplinary Association of Spinal Cord Injury Professionals (MASCIP), National Institute for Health and Care Excellence (NICE) 2016 and the International Spinal Cord Injury Society (ISCoS; http://www.elearnsci.org) have developed guidelines and online resources to inform the care and management of SCI including use of the International Classification of Function (Herrmann et al 2011).

EPIDEMIOLOGY

Incidence Data

There are very limited new data available for worldwide incidence because of the Covid-19 pandemic. A literature review of published data between 1993 and 2017 identified a varied worldwide incidence from 13 to 163.4 cases per million population (Kang et al 2018). The ratio of male to female cases varies significantly in the studies reviewed, but the rate of SCI in men is always higher than women. Age at time of injury also differs significantly but is higher in developed countries.

- 12–16 per million population in the UK have SCI per year.
- The international incidence is between 40 and 80 new cases per million of SCI per year (WHO-ISCOS 2013).
- Around 50,000 people in the UK are living with SCI under the care of an SCI centre (www.spinal.co.uk).

AETIOLOGY

SCI can be caused by several mechanisms, with a variety of causes. Traumatic injuries may lead to vascular and compressive damage with bony and/or ligamentous disruption. The main causes of traumatic injury are listed in Table 9.1. The World Health Organization (WHO) reports that 90% of cases are due to traumatic causes, although the proportion of nontraumatic SCIs appears to be growing. In the UK it is estimated that 37% of cases referred to the national SCI centres are because of trauma; this reflects the change to provide specialist rehabilitation funding for nontraumatic SCI.

Nontraumatic aetiology is more common than traumatic and often results from compression caused by degenerative disc disease, spinal canal stenosis, tumours or abscesses (often tuberculous); primary vascular disruption may cause ischaemic damage to the cord after infarct (spinal stroke) and ischaemia following dissecting injury (e.g., ruptured aortic aneurysm or arteriovenous malformation). Viral and bacterial infective diseases can lead to SCI through transverse myelitis and similar pathologies (New & Marshall 2014).

Fig. 9.1 highlights that there are more incomplete than complete lesions with only 1% of admissions achieving a full recovery. There are an increasing number of older people with SCI largely caused by falls, reflecting the increasing ageing of the general population. In addition, there is

TABLE 9.1 **Causes of Traumatic Spinal Cord Injury (New & Marshall 2014)**	
Road traffic accident (RTA)	37.5%
Falls	42.9%
Violence	13.8%
Sports	12%
Other	6.8%

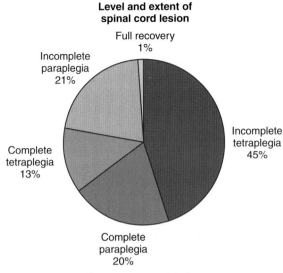

Level and extent of spinal cord lesion

- Full recovery 1%
- Incomplete paraplegia 21%
- Incomplete tetraplegia 45%
- Complete tetraplegia 13%
- Complete paraplegia 20%

FIG. 9.1 Extent of lesions.

TABLE 9.2 Pathological Changes After Spinal Cord Injury (Anscomb 2020)		
Injury Type	**Time Frame**	**Events**
Primary injury	Immediate	Concussion Compression Contusion Laceration/transection
Secondary injury	Minutes to weeks	Cascade of systemic and cellular events Inflammation and vascular damage Apoptosis Ischaemia
Spinal shock	2–6 weeks	Flaccid paralysis
Chronic	12 months	Cyst formation (fluid-filled cavity in the centre of the cord) Glial scar formation

a reduction of mortality and preservation of neurology in new lesions (DiMarco et al 2014, Nakajima et al 2022).

PATHOPHYSIOLOGY

SCI damages the complex neural network involved in transmitting, modifying and coordinating motor, sensory and autonomic control of the organ system, causing variable loss of homeostatic and adaptive mechanisms.

Most traumatic injuries involve contusion or tearing of the underlying cord by displaced bony fragments, disc or ligaments. This results primarily in loss of axons caused by damage of the white matter. Secondary damage, loss of cells in the grey matter, results from a secondary process comprising changes in the cell membrane permeability, leakage of cell contents, release of chemical factors and arrival of blood cells and agents involved in the response to injury and subsequent repair. This process leads to swelling and increasing cord pressure, affecting the venous and arterial supply, and results in ischaemia, lack of necessary proteins and failure to remove the debris of injury. The series of events that take place are outlined in Table 9.2. These inflammatory processes lead to further neurological damage, and hinder recovery and plasticity (Bennett et al 2022).

DIAGNOSIS

Bony injuries are evaluated using X-ray and computed tomography scans. Damage to the cord and ligamentous structures is imaged using magnetic resonance imaging (MRI). Electromyographic testing may be required to assess damage to peripheral nerves.

An internationally accepted assessment nomenclature for SCI is ISNCSCI (International Standard Neurological Classification of Spinal Cord Injury 2019). It was initially called an ASIA examination (American Spinal Injuries Association) and is still commonly referred to as such. Accurate evaluation using this classification allows clear communication between professionals in description of the nature of an SCI.

The assessment is completed with the patient in supine, to enable testing in the acutely unstable injured person. The assessment comprises evaluation of 10 key myotomes and 28 dermatomes (Fig. 9.2). Each dermatome is tested for light touch and pinprick sensation. The full description for these classifications will not be detailed here, but online training is available at http://www.asia-spinalinjury.org/learning.

The ISNCSCI denotes the level of the SCI and the degree of impairment to be found below it. The neurological level of injury may be from C2–S4/5 and represents the highest (most cephalad) myotome and dermatome in which normal function is preserved. The AIS (ASIA Impairment Scale) describes how much function is maintained below the level of injury, ranging from A (no function to S4 and S5) to E (normal function). At S4-5, motor function is examined by assessing voluntary anal contraction and sensory function by the ability to feel deep anal pressure and perineal sensation of light touch and pinprick. This is usually undertaken by medical staff.

PROGNOSIS

From an ISNCSCI assessment, some inferences can be drawn about the likelihood of neurological change and the functional potential of an individual. To embark upon a rehabilitation programme, it is important to have these functional outcomes in mind.

The ISNCSCI result and an evaluation of the likely pattern of injury in the spinal cord can allow some evaluation of the potential for neurological recovery. Functional outcomes after SCI are summarised in Table 9.3. SCI is notoriously heterogenous, and outcomes vary even when ISNCSCI is the same (Table 9.4).

INCOMPLETE SYNDROMES

There are recognised patterns of incomplete cord injury where the signs and symptoms are related to the anatomical areas of the cord affected (Figs. 9.3 and 9.4).

Clinically, patterns of incomplete lesions are referred to as a *syndrome* (Kirshblum et al 2011). The most common ones presented in Table 9.5 are anterior cord syndrome, cauda equina syndrome, Brown–Séquard syndrome and central cord syndrome. Posterior cord syndrome, a rare condition, produces damage to the dorsal columns (sensation of light touch, proprioception and vibration) with preservation of motor function and pain and temperature pathways. However, the patient presents with profound

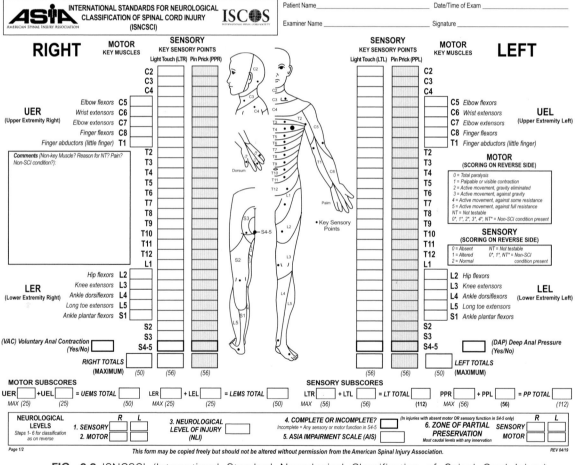

FIG. 9.2 ISNCSCI (International Standard Neurological Classification of Spinal Cord Injury) worksheet. (Reprinted with permission from American Spinal Injury Association. International Standards for Neurological Classification of Spinal Cord Injury, American Spinal Injury Association, Atlanta, GA, Revised 2019.)

Muscle Function Grading

0 = Total paralysis

1 = Palpable or visible contraction

2 = Active movement, full range of motion (ROM) with gravity eliminated

3 = Active movement, full ROM against gravity

4 = Active movement, full ROM against gravity and moderate resistance in a muscle specific position

5 = (Normal) active movement, full ROM against gravity and full resistance in a functional muscle position expected from an otherwise unimpaired person

NT = Not testable (i.e. due to immobilization, severe pain such that the patient cannot be graded, amputation of limb, or contracture of > 50% of the normal ROM)

0*, 1*, 2*, 3*, 4*, NT* = Non-SCI condition present [a]

Sensory Grading

0 = Absent   **1** = Altered, either decreased/impaired sensation or hypersensitivity

2 = Normal   **NT** = Not testable

0*, 1*, NT* = Non-SCI condition present [a]

[a] Note: Abnormal motor and sensory scores should be tagged with a '*' to indicate an impairment due to a non-SCI condition. The non-SCI condition should be explained in the comments box together with information about how the score is rated for classification purposes (at least normal / not normal for classification).

When to Test Non-Key Muscles:

In a patient with an apparent AIS B classification, non-key muscle functions more than 3 levels below the motor level on each side should be tested to most accurately classify the injury (differentiate between AIS B and C).

Movement	Root level
Shoulder: Flexion, extension, abduction, adduction, internal and external rotation **Elbow:** Supination	C5
Elbow: Pronation **Wrist:** Flexion	C6
Finger: Flexion at proximal joint, extension **Thumb:** Flexion, extension and abduction in plane of thumb	C7
Finger: Flexion at MCP joint **Thumb:** Opposition, adduction and abduction perpendicular to palm	C8
Finger: Abduction of the index finger	T1
Hip: Adduction	L2
Hip: External rotation	L3
Hip: Extension, abduction, internal rotation **Knee:** Flexion **Ankle:** Inversion and eversion **Toe:** MP and IP extension	L4
Hallux and Toe: DIP and PIP flexion and abduction	L5
Hallux: Adduction	S1

ASIA Impairment Scale (AIS)

A = Complete. No sensory or motor function is preserved in the sacral segments S4-5.

B = Sensory Incomplete. Sensory but not motor function is preserved below the neurological level and includes the sacral segments S4-5 (light touch or pin prick at S4-5 or deep anal pressure) AND no motor function is preserved more than three levels below the motor level on either side of the body.

C = Motor Incomplete. Motor function is preserved at the most caudal sacral segments for voluntary anal contraction (VAC) OR the patient meets the criteria for sensory incomplete status (sensory function preserved at the most caudal sacral segments S4-5 by LT, PP or DAP), and has some sparing of motor function more than three levels below the ipsilateral motor level on either side of the body. (This includes key or non-key muscle functions to determine motor incomplete status.) For AIS C – less than half of key muscle functions below the single NLI have a muscle grade ≥ 3.

D = Motor Incomplete. Motor incomplete status as defined above, with at least half (half or more) of key muscle functions below the single NLI having a muscle grade ≥ 3.

E = Normal. If sensation and motor function as tested with the ISNCSCI are graded as normal in all segments, and the patient had prior deficits, then the AIS grade is E. Someone without an initial SCI does not receive an AIS grade.

Using ND: To document the sensory, motor and NLI levels, the ASIA Impairment Scale grade, and/or the zone of partial preservation (ZPP) when they are unable to be determined based on the examination results.

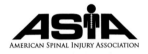

AMERICAN SPINAL INJURY ASSOCIATION

INTERNATIONAL STANDARDS FOR NEUROLOGICAL CLASSIFICATION OF SPINAL CORD INJURY

INTERNATIONAL SPINAL CORD SOCIETY

Page 2/2

Steps in Classification

The following order is recommended for determining the classification of individuals with SCI.

1. Determine sensory levels for right and left sides.
The sensory level is the most caudal, intact dermatome for both pin prick and light touch sensation.

2. Determine motor levels for right and left sides.
Defined by the lowest key muscle function that has a grade of at least 3 (on supine testing), providing the key muscle functions represented by segments above that level are judged to be intact (graded as a 5).
Note: in regions where there is no myotome to test, the motor level is presumed to be the same as the sensory level, if testable motor function above that level is also normal.

3. Determine the neurological level of injury (NLI).
This refers to the most caudal segment of the cord with intact sensation and antigravity (3 or more) muscle function strength, provided that there is normal (intact) sensory and motor function rostrally respectively.
The NLI is the most cephalad of the sensory and motor levels determined in steps 1 and 2.

4. Determine whether the injury is Complete or Incomplete.
(i.e. absence or presence of sacral sparing)
If voluntary anal contraction = **No** AND all S4-5 sensory scores = **0** AND deep anal pressure = **No**, then injury is **Complete**.
Otherwise, injury is **Incomplete**.

5. Determine ASIA Impairment Scale (AIS) Grade.
Is injury <u>Complete</u>?   If YES, AIS=A

NO ↓

Is injury <u>Motor Complete</u>? If YES, AIS=B

NO ↓ (No=voluntary anal contraction OR motor function more than three levels below the <u>motor level</u> on a given side, if the patient has sensory incomplete classification)

Are <u>at least</u> half (half or more) of the key muscles below the <u>neurological level of injury</u> graded 3 or better?

NO ↓   YES ↓
AIS=C   AIS=D

If sensation and motor function is normal in all segments, AIS=E
Note: AIS E is used in follow-up testing when an individual with a documented SCI has recovered normal function. If at initial testing no deficits are found, the individual is neurologically intact and the ASIA Impairment Scale does not apply.

6. Determine the zone of partial preservation (ZPP).
The ZPP is used only in injuries with absent motor (no VAC) OR sensory function (no DAP, no LT and no PP sensation) in the lowest sacral segments S4-5, and refers to those dermatomes and myotomes caudal to the sensory and motor levels that remain partially innervated. With sacral sparing of sensory function, the sensory ZPP is not applicable and therefore "NA" is recorded in the block of the worksheet. Accordingly, if VAC is present, the motor ZPP is not applicable and is noted as "NA".

FIG. 9.2, cont'd

PROGNOSIS

More neurological change is seen in tetraplegia than paraplegia

- 90% of patients with incomplete (AIS C&D) SCI have recovery of a motor level in their upper limbs compared with 70%–85% of the complete injuries (AIS A&B) (Ditunno et al 2000).

Recovery happens over time

- The majority of neurological recovery happens in the first 6–9 months, most in the first 3 months (Kirshblum et al 2021).
- 13.5% of those with a complete presentation (AIS A) went on to become incomplete at a year (Kirshblum et al 2011).

- Pinprick sparing is a good prognostic sign
- Pinprick sparing in a dermatome is an excellent indicator of increased recovery of motor strength (Poynton et al 1997).
- Pinprick preservation below the level of the injury to the sacral dermatomes is the best indicator of useful recovery, with 75% of patients regaining the ability to walk (van Middendorp et al 2011).

Sacral sparing is a good prognostic sign

- 10% of those AIS A and 33% of those AIS B at initial discharge become motor incomplete at year (Kirshblum et al 2016).

TABLE 9.3   Functional Outcomes After Spinal Cord Injury (SCIFERTO Spinal Cord Injury Therapy Leads 2016)

Level of Complete Spinal Cord Injury	Key Movements Added at That Level	Maximal Functional Potential
C0–C4	24 hours ventilated Head and neck flexion and rotation, scapula elevation	Verbally independent in postural adjustment Acceptable posture and seating and skin integrity equipment provided Head/chin-controlled powered wheelchair Potential use of assistive technology for communication and environmental control Verbally independent in directing own care Able to stand using device with assistance
C0–C4	Night ventilated	Inspiratory muscle training programme
C0–C4	Not ventilated	Up in wheelchair for 12 consecutive hours
C5	Biceps Rotator cuff Shoulder abduction	Upper limb–controlled powered mobility Self-propelling wheelchair Assisted same height transfer on and off bed with aids (not including lifting legs) Once set up with adaptive aids, carry out grooming activities in an accessible environment Once set up with adaptive aids, carry out feeding in an accessible environment Once set up with adaptive aids, carry out writing in an accessible environment
C6	Wrist extension	Independent pressure relief Independent positioning in wheelchair Self-propelling on level surfaces Self-propelling on small inclines (1:12) Independent flipping front castors Independent back wheel balance Independent traversing rough terrain in back-wheel balance Independent ascending and descending 7.5-cm kerb Independent rolling in double bed Independent moving between supine lying and long sitting in bed Independent lifting legs on and off the bed Independent same height transfers with TB on and off bed Assisted car transfers with TB Independent lifting lightweight wheelchair in and out of car Independent grooming in an accessible environment Independent writing in an accessible environment Independent feeding in an accessible environment Independent light DADL Independent in upper limb PADL with adaptive aids Independent in lower limb PADL with adaptive aids
C7	Elbow extension	Possibility of supported ambulation options Independent car transfers with TB Independent graduated floor to wheelchair transfer Independent same height transfers on/off bed with no aids Independent stretch programme

TABLE 9.3 Functional Outcomes After Spinal Cord Injury (SCIFERTO Spinal Cord Injury Therapy Leads 2016)—Cont'd

Level of Complete Spinal Cord Injury	Key Movements Added at That Level	Maximal Functional Potential
C8/T1	Finger and thumb movement	Independent in upper limb PADL without aids in an accessible environment
		Independent in lower limb PADL without aids in an accessible environment
		Independent in light DADL without aids in an accessible environment
		Independent in/out standing frame
T2-T6	Increasing trunk stabilisers	Up/downstairs in wheelchair with assistance
		'Bunny hop' in wheelchair
		Independent floor to and from wheelchair transfer
		Independent car transfers with no aids
		Independent in heavy DADL without aids in an accessible environment
T7-T12	Abdominals	Potential for ambulation with knee-ankle-foot-orthosis
L1-L2	Hip flexion	Consideration of functional ambulation
L3	Knee extension	Independent indoor functional ambulation
L4/5	Dorsiflexion	Independent ascend/descend 7.5-cm step/kerb with no rail
S1-5	Plantarflexion	Independent ascend/descend flight of stairs
	Knee flexion	Independent on/off floor
	Hip extension	Independent ascend/descend 1:12 slope
		Independent outdoor functional ambulation

DADL, Domestic activities of daily living; *PADL*, personal activities of daily living; *TB*, transfer board.

TABLE 9.4 Factors That Affect Outcome

Factors	Neurological preservation below the level of injury (Milicevic et al 2014, Ovechkin et al 2013, Scivoletto et al 2014)
	Individual variations in innervation
	Motivation
	Anthropometric considerations
Complications	Heterotopic ossification
	Recurrent infective illness
	Severe spasticity
	Tissue viability problems
	Contracture
Comorbidities	Psychiatric/psychological
	Other fractures/injuries
	Musculoskeletal conditions
	Cardiac/respiratory
	Compromised cognition

ataxia because of loss of proprioception, and there is a poor prognosis for ambulation (Kirshblum & Donovan 2002, cited in Sheerin 2005). Conus medullaris injury presents as a combination of UMN and LMN lesions, with or without the sacral reflexes (anal/bulbocavernous), depending on the injury.

EARLY ACUTE MANAGEMENT

Immediately after injury, maintenance of airway and circulation are primary concerns particularly for those with tetraplegia. This may include intubation and ventilation and circulatory support with fluids and inotropes to maintain a circulation compatible with life in the first instance and secondarily to maximise perfusion to the cord, minimising further avascular damage. Avoidance of further injury is the second priority with a focus on achieving and maintaining spinal alignment to avoid further damage and then acting to reduce compression on the cord (Consortium for Spinal Cord Medicine 2008).

Surgical decompression and stabilisation may be necessary to reinstate a patent spinal canal and maintain it once

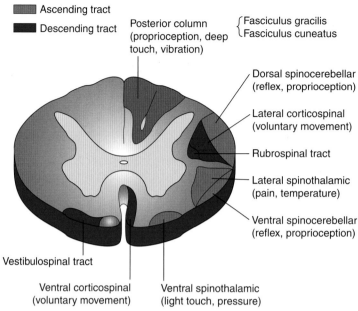

Ascending tract
Descending tract

Posterior column (proprioception, deep touch, vibration)

{ Fasciculus gracilis
  Fasciculus cuneatus

Dorsal spinocerebellar (reflex, proprioception)

Lateral corticospinal (voluntary movement)

Rubrospinal tract

Lateral spinothalamic (pain, temperature)

Ventral spinocerebellar (reflex, proprioception)

Vestibulospinal tract

Ventral corticospinal (voluntary movement)

Ventral spinothalamic (light touch, pressure)

FIG. 9.3 Cross-section of SCI.

NEUROPROTECTION AND FACILITATION OF NEUROLOGICAL RECOVERY

- Preventing immediate adverse reactions to injury such as neuronal death and scar formation
- Minimising inhibitory properties of the central nervous system environment and maximising the growth potential of damaged neurones
- Understanding axonal guidance systems that will be required for directed outgrowth and functional reconnection
- Optimising the function of surviving systems (Ramer et al 2000, Wilson et al 2013)

achieved. Neuroprotection is a key aim. Management aims to minimise neurological deterioration, restore alignment and stabilisation, facilitate early mobilisation, minimise hospital stay and prevent complications (Johnston 2001).

Conservative treatment regimens may be followed with bed rest, careful rolling and positioning, possibly supplemented with traction. While a patient has an unstable spinal column, great care should be taken in rolling and positioning in supine and side lying (MASCIP 2015b). As patients mobilise, orthotic devices may be recommended including collars and braces and cervico- and thoraco-lumbar-sacral orthoses; fabric corsets may also be used. Other restrictions may be imposed by the surgical team.

Discussing Prognosis

SCI is considered one of the most devastating injuries one can experience, often with permanent consequences that affect every aspect of the person's life. An early conversation with clear and sensitive communication is recommended (Kirshblum et al 2016). It is important that all members of the multidisciplinary team (MDT) understand the implications of breaking bad news when undertaking the assessment of a new patient with SCI. Often the physiotherapist is one of the first professionals to compile a thorough physical examination and will be asked for information by the patient. It is an inevitable part of each team member's role to contribute to discussions of prognosis. A planned team approach is the best way to manage such conversations within the context of the process of information giving.

Patients report that a trusted relationship with their MDT is important, and that context, timing and source of information is an essential component of the discussion (Nadeau et al 2021). In this case, any discussion should be based on accurate assessment with evidence-based reasoning where possible. It is unlikely that an exact answer can be given, in which case a positive emphasis on progressive goals will help the patient to focus on each phase of their rehabilitation.

Physical Management

In the early postinjury phase, physical management will involve prevention of respiratory and circulatory

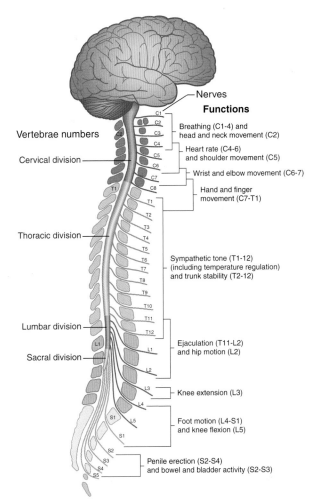

Vertebrae numbers

Cervical division

Thoracic division

Lumbar division

Sacral division

Nerves
Functions

Breathing (C1-4) and
head and neck movement (C2)

Heart rate (C4-6)
and shoulder movement (C5)

Wrist and elbow movement (C6-7)

Hand and finger
movement (C7-T1)

Sympathetic tone (T1-12)
(including temperature regulation)
and trunk stability (T2-12)

Ejaculation (T11-L2)
and hip motion (L2)

Knee extension (L3)

Foot motion (L4-S1)
and knee flexion (L5)

Penile erection (S2-S4)
and bowel and bladder activity (S2-S3)

FIG. 9.4 The spinal cord with functional motor innervations.

complications, maintenance of joint range of movement and preservation of skin integrity. The consequences of weakness and hyperreflexia leading to hypertonus and contracture also require management. The management of emerging spasticity will include pharmacological and physical treatments, although the timing of introduction of antispasmodics is poorly evidenced, as is the use of physiotherapy interventions (Barbosa et al 2021, Theriault et al 2018).

The main objectives in the acute phase are to:
- Institute a prophylactic respiratory regimen and treat any complications.
- Achieve independent respiratory status where possible.
- Maintain full range of motion (ROM) of all joints by managing the effects of spasticity and muscle

imbalances, within the limitations determined by fracture stability.
- Monitor and manage neurological status as appropriate.
- Maintain/strengthen all innervated muscle groups.
- Facilitate functional patterns of movement to assist in restoration of function where possible.
- Support/educate the patient, carers, family and colleagues.

Facilitation of Range, Muscle Length and Functional Movement

During the acute phase, whilst the patient is immobilised in bed, the therapist can assist in exploiting the potential for functional return. Facilitation of meaningful movement should be a priority during the phase of post–spinal shock, when there is an opportunity to optimise recovery of voluntary movement by influencing neuroplasticity (Filipp 2019). Recovery of activity resulting from plasticity of the damaged neurones depends on many factors (Walker & Detloff 2021). The introduction of early therapeutic interventions is essential in restoration of functional activity and focusses on exercise training and preventing secondary complications (Fu 2016, Harvey 2016). Many studies have explored the augmentation of plasticity using transcranial magnetic stimulation, transcutaneous electrical stimulation and implanted stimulators (Gerasimenko et al 2015, Inanici et al 2021, Jo et al 2021).

Splints may be used to provide joint support and maintain joint range of movement and muscle length. Facilitation of movement can be enhanced and promoted by the use of electrical stimulation (Marquez-Chin et al 2020). Movements are monitored and facilitated at least twice a day. Following the precautions defined by the surgeon is essential.

POSSIBLE PRECAUTIONS WITH UNSTABLE SCI

1. Undertake facilitated movements in supine.
2. Unstable paraplegic SCI (T9 and below):
   - Limit hip flexion to 30° (tailor position for knee flexion).
3. Unstable tetraplegic SCI (T4 level and above):
   - Shoulder hold during lower limb movements and upper limb movements above 90°.
4. Severe spasms during limb movements may cause loss of spinal alignment: use shoulder hold if concerned.
5. Respiratory techniques should be applied bilaterally, with a shoulder hold and only when essential.
6. Extreme range of movement must be avoided.

TABLE 9.5　Common Patterns of Incomplete Lesions (McKinley et al 2007)

Syndrome	Frequency (%)	Location	Common Mechanism	Consequences	Prognosis
Anterior cord syndrome	44	Anterior two-thirds of spinal cord or anterior spinal artery	High-velocity hyperflexion	Reduced motor function Reduced sensation to pain and temperature Proprioception preserved	Poor 10%–20% potential of motor recovery (Sheerin 2005)
Cauda equina syndrome	25	Compression of the sacral nerve roots	Intervertebral disc herniation	Flaccid paralysis caused by peripheral nerve damage Flaccid paralysis of bowel and bladder	
Brown–Séquard syndrome	17	Hemisection of spinal cord	Shot or stab wound	Greater ipsilateral proprioceptive and motor loss Contralateral loss of sensitivity to pain and temperature	75%–90% of individuals ambulate after rehabilitation (Johnston 2001)
Central cord syndrome (Avila et al 2021)	10	Occurs in the cervical spinal cord damaging central grey matter, affecting decussating sensory axons and the lateral corticospinal tracts	Low velocity cervical extension compression injury to the spinal cord without fracture or dislocation Often after a fall in the older population with preexisting stenosis	Upper limbs are more affected than the lower limbs Some flaccid weakness of the arms may occur, caused by damage to anterior horn cells at the level of injury Partial bowel and bladder dysfunctions	57%–86% of patients will ambulate, although 97% of patients younger than 50 years ambulate compared with 41% of patients older than 50 years (Foo 1986)

McKinley, W., Santos, K., Meade, M., Brooke, K., 2007. Incidence and outcomes of spinal cord injury clinical syndromes. J. Spinal. Cord. Med. 30, 215–224.

Facilitated movements of weak or paralysed limbs are continued until the patient is mobile and thus capable of ensuring full mobility through their own activities, unless there are complications, such as excessive spasms or stiffness. It has been shown that stretching regimes do not help increase range of movement (Harvey et al 2017). Movements that require special emphasis are identified in the following list. Microtrauma may be a predisposing factor in the formation of heterotropic ossification (HO), which is the formation of normal lamellar bone in the soft tissues around paralysed joints, below the level of the lesion. Insensate and paralysed joints are vulnerable to soft tissue damage. Special emphasis should be placed on the following:

- Stretching the finger flexors with wrist in neutral to preserve tenodesis grip (Bromley 2006);
- Ensuring a full fist can be attained with wrist extension;
- Pronation and supination in elbow flexion and extension;
- Full extension at the elbow (Harvey et al 2016);
- Full elevation and lateral rotation of the shoulder;
- Stretching the long head of the triceps – arm in elevation with elbow flexion;
- Stretching the upper fibres of the trapezius muscle;

- Maintaining plantar grade in extension and flexion of the knee; and
- Avoidance of extreme ROM and aggressive stretching, especially at the hip and knee.

Tenodesis is a functional grip that uses activity in wrist extensors and shortness in hand and forearm flexors to bring about passive opposition of the thumb and finger flexion in level C6-C7 tetraplegia.

Mobilisation

It is common for orthostatic changes in blood pressure to be problematic on initial mobilisation and can remain an ongoing feature for individuals with injuries T6 and above (Claydon et al 2005). Progressive sitting up in bed before getting out is necessary to evaluate a response. Blood pressure should be monitored, with reference to the patient's baseline, which is likely to be lower than those without an SCI. The patient's signs and symptoms are also a guide – colour of the face, dizziness, changes to vision and ringing in the ears being common indicators of low circulation to the head. Spinal shock causes vasodilation of the vascular network and flaccidity of the muscles below the level of the lesion. This is most pronounced in cervical SCI. Careful management of blood pressure is important to avoid fainting and to maintain perfusion to the cord (Alexander et al 2009). It is important that spinal shock is not confused with hypovolaemia. Fluid replacement in the absence of actual blood loss may arise from misinterpretation of clinical signs and may lead to pulmonary oedema (Harrison 2000).

Use of physical compression may limit symptoms (e.g., compression stockings and elastic abdominal binders). Supplementing this with tilting back the chair and putting the feet up may also be necessary for short periods while a patient accommodates. Numerous short-acting medications are also used to successfully manage orthostatic hypotension (www.scireproject.com).

RESPIRATORY ASSESSMENT

SCI affects the active components of inspiration and expiration, the passive resistance of the lungs and chest wall to expansion, and the production of respiratory secretions. Respiratory problems affect 36%–83% of SCI individuals in their acute phase of injury and remain a leading cause of morbidity and mortality (Jaja et al 2019, Steel et al 2018). SCI can result in paralysis of respiratory muscles inspiration (diaphragm-C5 and intercostals-corresponding thoracic level), and muscles of expiration (abdominals: T6-T12) are involved. The patient's cough will be impaired if the level of the lesion is T12 or above.

An unstable spinal column may preclude use of manual techniques or require them to be done in supine with a shoulder hold where necessary. Because of the traumatic nature of many spinal cord injuries, there are often other injuries. In respiratory assessment, particular attention should be paid to rib fractures, pneumothorax and/or haemothorax, and the presence of a chest drain (Table 9.6).

Because of the autonomic changes, there is a high risk for cardiac instability (see later). Bradycardia caused by unopposed vagal stimulation is common and can be exacerbated by tracheal suction. Atropine should be at the bedside in this eventuality. Low blood pressure and heart rate are associated with altered autonomic function.

Because of the changes to bowel function after SCI, constipation is common and paralytic ileus can occur. This can impair respiratory mechanics by upwards pressure from the abdomen affecting expansion of the bases of the lungs. The presence of severe constipation or paralytic ileus is an absolute contraindication to use of manual assisted coughing techniques.

High cervical injury may result in paralysis of the diaphragm necessitating mandatory ventilation via a tracheostomy. As injuries descend, varying degrees of support will be required. Initial endotracheal tube ventilation may

TABLE 9.6 Respiratory Assessment

Subjective Assessment	Objective Assessment
Level of spinal cord injury	Respiratory rate
Spinal precautions	Oxygen saturation (Sa_{O_2})
Other injuries	Fraction of inspired oxygen ($F_{I_{O_2}}$)
Cardiac stability	Heart rate
Medical history – chronic obstructive pulmonary disease, asthma, smoking	Blood pressure
Age	Fluid balance
Cardiovascular fitness	Temperature
Drug history	Auscultation
Steroids	Cough
Anticoagulants	Breathing pattern
Inotropes for cardiac contractility	Abdomen
Bowel management	Forced vital capacity
Ventilation method and history	Cough peak expiratory flow rate
	Chest radiograph
	Arterial blood gases

be converted to a tracheostomy. The use of noninvasive ventilation may avoid both.

Increasing respiratory rate is often the first sign of impending respiratory failure. As the work of breathing (WOB) becomes unsustainable, often 72 hours postinjury, the rate increases in an effort to maintain oxygenation. It is a sign that additional support may be required.

Neural control of mucosal activity is also changed after SCI in lesions of T6 and above. There will be a disproportionate amount of activity of the parasympathetic nervous system, causing hypersecretion and preponderance to infection.

Use of a microspirometer to evaluate forced vital capacity (FVC) gives an indication of the extent to which the respiratory system has been impaired by the restrictive presentation after SCI. A reduction in lung volumes is likely to be observed. If it descends below 500 mL, some invasive or noninvasive ventilator support will be required. The consequences of reduced volumes are increased risk for atelectasis, collapse and consolidation, and a reduced volume of air to cough with.

In a person with an intact neuromuscular system, their WOB will be less in a seated position. In a patient with a complete tetraplegia and above, their WOB will be less in supine because of the upward pressure of the abdominal contents bringing the diaphragm to a more effective position on its length-tension curve, increasing the FVC (Terson de Paleville et al 2014). Assessment of FVC in supine and in sitting will identify how much the change of position is a factor for an individual, and it is particularly useful for those with activity below their level of SCI (Table 9.7).

Assessment of the patient's ability to produce an effective cough is essential. The combination of loss of abdominal-generated active expiration and volume of air reduces the ability to clear secretions, compounding problems of atelectasis, collapse and consolidation. Cough can be objectively evaluated using cough peak expiratory flow (PCF) rate using a peak flow meter and face mask:

- A PCF < 160 L/min is an indicator of an ineffective cough. The patient will require an airway clearance and cough augmentation system such as Nippy Clearway or effective manual assisted cough to clear secretions.

- A PCF < 280 L/min indicates a patient's cough may not be effective.
- Review effectiveness of manual assisted cough, consider lung volume bag (LVB) to increase lung volumes and therefore cough effectiveness, consider need for Clearway.

Breathing patterns should be observed. A paradoxical breathing pattern occurs when the diaphragm is working but the abdominals are flaccid, resulting in the abdomen being pushed out during inspiration as the diaphragm descends. Lack of activity in the intercostals prevents the ribs from elevating during inspiration; instead, they are drawn inwards by negative pressure in the thoracic cavity. Asymmetrical expansion may be observed, possibly associated with the effects of chest trauma or asymmetrical residual innervation of the hemidiaphragms.

Chest X-ray films may show signs of basal collapse and consolidation associated with abdominal distension. Altered heights of hemidiaphragms may be associated with partial de-innervation in high cervical lesions.

RESPIRATORY TREATMENT

The approach to respiratory management is in keeping with the well-established principles. The evidence is set out in SCIRE – Respiratory Management Following Spinal Cord Injury (Steel et al 2018). Principles are based on improving expansion by using active cycle of breathing techniques, postural drainage, effective hydration and humidification, and medical management of hypersecretions, if necessary (see Precautions Box). Please see Chapter 18 for a

---

PRECAUTIONS IN THE USE OF RESPIRATORY TECHNIQUES

Unstable Spinal Column
- Treat in supine
- Bilateral chest techniques with shoulder hold
- Caution with manual assisted cough (MAC) with shoulder hold

MAC
- Contraindicated if there is paralytic ileus, severe constipation or abdominal injuries
- Caution with chest or abdominal injuries and pathologies, clotting disorders, unstable angina and cardiac arrhythmias

Suction
- Undertake suction with care in patients with neurological level of injury T6 or above

---

TABLE 9.7 Forced Vital Capacity Values in Spinal Cord Injury (Linn et al 2001)		
	Complete SCI	**Incomplete SCI**
C3	52	58
C7	67	84
T6	84	99
L1	95	96

comprehensive overview of respiratory management in neurological conditions.

The most dependent patients will require mandatory ventilation. Short-term ventilation is provided via an endotracheal tube, and longer term ventilation requires conversion to a tracheostomy. Long-term mandatory ventilated patients are usually managed with an uncuffed tube. Dependence while sleeping is higher, and many of those who wean to spontaneous ventilation in the day will require support at night. This may be achievable noninvasively.

In general, for patients with lesions of T6 and above there is a reduction in FVC when they sit up. The use of an elastic abdominal binder provides additional abdominal support (Prigent et al 2010), combined with effective wheelchair seating systems.

If FVC decreases to less than 1 L in an average-size adult, positive pressure respiratory support is recommended (Hough 2001, RISCI 2017). Use of devices to deliver higher levels of expansion and encourage deeper active breathing where possible is an important adjunct to acute and chronic management. This may include intermittent positive pressure breathing (IPPB), cough-assisted devices (CADs), manual hyperinflation, lung volume recruitment bag and incentive spirometry. These devices are combined with manual clearance techniques for effective secretion clearance.

The use of inspiratory muscle training to maximise the effectiveness of neurologically preserved muscles should be considered. There is level 1a evidence of positive effect on lung volumes, respiratory muscle strength, reduction in infections and perception of dyspnoea (Mueller et al 2012, 2013, Van Houtte et al 2008). The training can be done with a portable mechanical device.

Reduced lung excursion can lead to the accumulation of secretions. Assistance will often be required to cough and clear secretions. Optimal hydration using humidified O_2 and nebulisers aids in secretion clearance and is combined with good fluid balance. Suction should always be undertaken with care in patients with SCI and is not recommended in the unstable cervical nonintubated patient because the neck cannot be extended to open the airway. Suction causes vagal stimulation via the carotid bodies, which pass impulses to the brain via the glossopharyngeal nerves and are sensitive to lack of oxygen (Karlsson 2006). During suction, the vagus nerve is unopposed, and the patient may become hypotensive and bradycardiac, possibly resulting in cardiac arrest. Endotracheal intubation may produce a similar response. Therefore, it is wise to preoxygenate the patient, monitor heart rate and have atropine on standby.

MACs are a way of producing an effective cough without the use of aids. The aim is to replace the compressive effect of the abdominal musculature using the hands or forearm of an assistant, timed with a deep breath and an active cough. When correct, it should sound like a normal cough. Self-MACs are also possible for those with sufficient arm function. Use of MAC is contraindicated with severe constipation or paralytic ileus and should be approached with caution in the presence of an unstable spine, clotting disorder, chest or abdominal pathologies and injuries, unstable angina and cardiac arrhythmias. The use of a CAD in the hospital and domestic environment can provide deeper breaths and augment cough. The use of electrical stimulation of the expiratory muscles has been found to be beneficial in clearance of secretions (Butler 2011).

Weaning From Ventilatory Support

The recommended algorithm for weaning those with SCI from ventilator support is known as 'ventilator-free breathing' (VFB). It follows training principles to improve the strength and endurance of the respiratory musculature. Prerequisites for initiation of weaning are:

- $FIO_2 < 0.4$;
- Positive end-expiratory pressure (PEEP) preferably around 5 cm H_2O;
- Awake and cooperative, minimal opiates, preferably no delirium;
- No active sepsis; and
- Some evidence of spontaneous respiratory activity.

Based on the patient's vital capacity (VC), all ventilatory support is removed for a specified time. The patient is kept supine during VFB to maximise the efficiency of the diaphragm. Ventilation is then resumed for a rest period of at least 1–2 hours. The patient should not be significantly fatigued. The VC should be retaken after VFB periods. If it is less than 70% of the pre-VFB VC, the rest period should be extended or the duration of VFB reduced. Suggested initial VFB times based on VC are:

- If VC is less than 250 mL, start with 5 minutes of VFB.
- If VC is less than 500 mL, start with 15 minutes of VFB.
- If VC is greater than 750 mL, start with 30 minutes of VFB.

After a day of three or more successful VFB episodes, the next day VFB time can be increased by approximately 20%. The initial aim is for VFB up to 18 hours during daytime, but for ventilation at night, because patients with SCI can have significant hypoventilation during sleep. The assessment of safe VFB overnight requires partial pressure of carbon dioxide ($Paco_2$) or transcutaneous carbon dioxide ($TcCO_2$) monitoring.

Respiratory Management and Covid-19

The Covid-19 pandemic has necessitated a review of the use of personal protective equipment (PPE) when treating respiratory conditions. Cough has been identified as the key aerosol-generating activity, and chest physiotherapy using a MAC technique produces the same aerosol generation as an active cough (Thomas et al 2022). The use of full PPE including FFP3 masks and visors should be used with patients testing positive for Covid-19. Professional and government guidelines are being updated to inform which other procedures are considered to be aerosol generating.

Long-Term Respiratory Management

Ongoing use of incentive spirometry and muscle training devices is potentially beneficial for all those with significant respiratory deficit.

Teaching of self-MACs for those who are able and training care staff in MAC is essential for those with impaired coughs. In the long term, those with a large degree of impairment to coughs may benefit from a domestic CAD. This can be used regularly to deliver good lung expansion and offset the propensity for stiffening of the lungs and chest wall. The cough function can then be used intermittently as required. Patients should be aware of signs of deteriorating respiratory function – reducing volumes on their incentive spirometer, more secretion production and increasing difficulty in clearing, and worsening shortness of breath – and should seek assessment and help early. For some, ongoing use of noninvasive or mandatory ventilation may be required.

Some patients with high cervical injuries may not be able to wean partially or at all. They may be appropriate for consideration of intramuscular diaphragmatic stimulation to produce strengthening of the diaphragm, allowing patients to breathe without the ventilator whilst stimulated (NICE 2017).

CLINICAL PRESENTATION

Acute traumatic management guidelines are well established (NICE 2022). Comprehensive multidisciplinary guidelines in SCI management are also available (ISCoS 2015). The function of all systems below the level of lesion will be changed, causing many and varied physical consequences of SCI.

Spinal Shock

After an insult to the spinal cord, spinal shock occurs to a varying degree depending on the extent of the cord injury itself. It is recognised as the transient suppression and gradual return of reflex activity below the cord lesion (Dittuno et al 2004). Initial paralysis is flaccid; there are no deep tendon reflexes and no reflexic somatic activity. Neural plasticity shaped by experience and activity does occur above and below the level of injury (Dietz 2012). Synapse growth

is likely to be activity dependent and competitive; thus, with good positioning to maintain joint range and muscle length, as well as facilitation of functional movements, a beneficial environment may be maintained for improving outcomes while minimising maladaptive responses. Spinal shock is often associated with hypotension and sometimes bradycardia, and these features are seen more commonly in those with tetraplegia than paraplegia (Ruiz et al 2018).

Autonomic Dysreflexia

Autonomic dysreflexia (AD) is an exaggerated sympathetic nervous system response to a noxious stimulus below the level of SCI. Hypertension 20–40 mmHg above baseline (Krassioukov et al 2021) is the definitive symptom and is often associated with tachycardia and headache with pilo-erection and capillary dilation and sweating above the level of the lesion. Potentially life-threatening AD occurs in those with injuries above T6 (Table 9.8) and is a medical emergency.

First-line treatment is to sit the individual up and seek to find and rectify the cause of the AD. Vascular dilating medication may be required. Unmanaged AD may result in the blood pressure increasing to levels where a stroke or other catastrophic failure may occur. AD affects about 50%–70% of those with cervical injuries (Karlsson 2006).

Cardiovascular Dysfunction

Autonomic dysfunction is often overlooked when considering the impact on neurological control. After SCI, there is altered control of the bowel and bladder, blood vessels, the heart and lungs, and all organs (Tator 1998).

Parasympathetic activity slows the heart rate. Parasympathetic supply to the heart via the vagus nerve is not affected by SCI (Teasell et al 2000). Injury at or above T1-T5 will interrupt sympathetic activity descending from the brain, impairing acceleration of the heart rate and vasoconstriction. The reduction/absence of descending sympathetic output for those with injuries above T6 is partially compensated for in the medium and long term by increasing local sensitivity to adrenaline and noradrenaline by blood vessels.

The unopposed parasympathetic stimulation results in persistent bradycardia. It has been found to peak at day 4 postinjury, resolving in most by day 10 and all by week 6 (Lehmann et al 1987). Asystolic events are managed with pharmacological treatments and perhaps a pacemaker (Alexander et al 2009). The unopposed vagal stimulation elicited by tracheal suction can cause cardiac arrest.

Other problems include hypotension resulting in dizziness and fainting and are significantly correlated with the level of SCI; those with tetraplegia are most affected (Vaccaro et al 2022). Abdominal elasticated binders and

TABLE 9.8	Key Factors in Autonomic Dysreflexia		
Signs and Symptoms	**Potential Causes**	**Responses Required**
• Increased blood pressure (>20% increase in systolic blood pressure above baseline) (Alexander et al 2009) • Rash above level of injury • Pounding headache • Goose bumps above level of spinal cord injury • Bradycardia or tachycardia • Nasal congestion • Vascular constriction below level of injury	• Severe spasticity • Sudden stretch • Fractures • Skin breakdown • Ingrowing toenail • Sepsis (particularly bladder) • Full bladder (blocked catheter) • Constipation	• Sit patient upright • Loosen clothing • Check for and manage any cause of bladder or bowel irritation • Check for and manage other potential triggers • Consider pharmacological management if unable to identify and remove the trigger

compression stockings are routinely used to support blood pressure. Medications to assist in reducing hypotension have been previously identified.

In exercise, the sympathetically mediated increase in venous return, heart rate and myocardial contractility cannot occur in those injured above T6. A degree of responsive tachycardia can occur via reduction in vagal output. Ascending level of spinal injury and reducing levels of activity below the level of lesion restrict maximal heart rate (Eriksson et al 1988).

Thermoregulation Dysfunction

The smooth muscle of the vasculature will also have altered control, and the body's ability to thermoregulate is therefore impaired (Price & Trbovich 2018). This may lead to limbs feeling cold and discolouring. Those with an SCI are unable to use skeletal muscles to shiver in response to cold. Vasodilation cannot occur in response to higher ambient temperatures, and sweating may not be possible below the SCI. This can lead to increased core temperatures in response to ambient temperature of pyrexia. The tendency of those with SCI to adapt to the temperature of their environment is called *poikilothermia*. The degree to which poikilothermia is observed corresponds to the level of SCI, with those with higher levels of lesion having less ability to achieve thermal homoeostasis. In practice, it means environments should avoid extremes of temperature. Clothing should be adjusted accordingly (Handrakis et al 2017).

Bladder, Bowels and Sexual Dysfunction

The impaired coordination of the detrusor muscle and sphincter muscles of the bladder can lead to problems with bladder emptying. Spinal cord damage leads to a neurogenic bladder, with increased contractility of the bladder leading to sudden incontinence and potential reflux of urine into the kidneys. Incomplete emptying may increase risk for

bladder infections and damage the urinary system because of high pressures as urine accumulates. Loss of activity in the skeletal muscle of the pelvic floor may further impair continence. Use of indwelling urethral catheterisation is common in the short term, and self-intermittent catheterisation is encouraged in the longer term. The surgical insertion of suprapubic catheter through the abdomen or use of intermittent self-catheterisation provides longer term management for many with SCI.

Changes in the peristaltic activity of the bowel and paralysis of the anal sphincter results in constipation and continence issues. For most with UMN lesions, training the bowel habit can restore continence with a degree of reliability (MASCIP 2015a). Those with LMN injury and consequent loss of tone in the external anal sphincter will often suffer more significant incontinence. A regular bowel routine will help offset this.

Erectile dysfunction is a common consequence of SCI. Those with UMN lesions often regain capacity for a reflex erection; those with LMN lesions usually experience complete loss of erectile function. Fertility in women is not impaired by SCI. Men often require in vitro fertilisation to become fathers.

Weakness

Loss of muscle power occurs because of disruption of neural control to muscles; some muscles may be completely denervated, whereas others retain partial innervation from above the level of SCI. Sensory changes may reduce the capacity to generate effective contraction even where innervation is preserved. In muscles where the reflex arc is lost through damage to the peripheral nerve or anterior horn cells, flaccid paralysis will be observed. This is seen in the lower spinal injuries of the conus and cauda equina. Weakness is often compounded by disuse atrophy, which quickly sets in while an individual is less active after injury.

Sensory Changes

Changes to sensation after SCI are more complicated than presence or loss of sensation. Additional sensation is common including paraesthesia (commonly pins and needles, tingling, feelings of hot and cold, sensation of running water) and neuropathic pain. These can be very difficult to manage.

Balance

The combination of weakness and loss of sensation impairs balance reactions to perturbation. Changes in postural tone can make it harder to achieve an accurate response to a balance challenge, or sudden spasms can be the cause of a fall. Loss of range of movement can make it harder to achieve a stable alignment. Balance can be affected in the seated position for wheelchair users. It is most affected in the frontal plane and is compensated for by slowing arm movement and using the contralateral arm and trunk to counterbalance when reaching (Peeters et al 2018). Balance in sitting is significantly correlated with functional performance (Abou & Rice 2022).

Pain

Pain is a dominant feature after SCI, related to the neural and musculoskeletal structures. It affects about 40%–50% of patients with SCI (Sidall 2014). A lack of sensation or movement in a part of the body does not mean that pain cannot be experienced there. Neuropathic pain results from sensitisation of input into the dorsal horn (Siddall & Middleton 2015) and to the damaged neural structures.

Spasticity

Spasticity affects about 70% of patients with SCI, with 63% developing signs of spasticity within the first month following injury (Levasseur et al 2021). When the spinal cord is damaged, loss of descending control of reflexes occurs and spasticity results, as in all UMN lesions. If damage within the spinal canal has affected only the cauda equina, there will be no spasticity because these are peripheral nerves rather than spinal cord. It is also possible to get a mixed picture of UMN and LMN disruption after spinal injury. If the conus medullaris has been damaged at the distal end of the spinal cord (varies from T10 down), where it changes from UMNs to LMNs, a mixed presentation may be observed in the legs.

ASSESSMENT

Comprehensive assessment is essential to identify key factors affecting the management starting with the subjective assessment (Table 9.9).

Objectively, it is essential to assess weakness, sensation, spasticity/tone, ROM and the impact of these impairments at the level of activity and participation. Consideration should be given to technique, assistance, aids and appliances in the performance of transfers, bed mobility and ambulation.

The use of ISNCSCI is best practice for motor and sensory assessment (www.asia-spinalinjury.org). This is limited to key and non-key muscles as set out in the assessment and by the strict interpretation of the motor grading scale. Full muscle charting using the modified Oxford Scale and proprioception assessment informs a more comprehensive assessment, particularly where there is preservation of function below their injury.

Use of the Modified Ashworth Scale and the Penn Spasm Frequency Scale allows the capture of the through range resistance to movement and sudden unwanted movements that form the usual presentations of spasticity in SCI. The Tardieu scale can be used for more specific assessment to inform further intervention such as the use of botulinum toxin.

Other common outcome measures used are presented in Table 9.10.

PHYSICAL MANAGEMENT

Physical impairments and their impact on activity and participation in everyday life are addressed by an MDT approach. The aims of rehabilitation are formulated using the *International Classification of Functioning, Disability and Health* (www.who.int). This provides a framework around which the information regarding each individual patient can be organised and assessed to direct rehabilitation outcomes. This involves:

- Establishing an interdisciplinary process which is patient focused, comprehensive and coordinated.
- Addressing physical impairments with early intervention and prophylaxis to prevent further complications.
- Equipping the individual with knowledge to achieve independence, be that physical or verbal.
- Delivering skills and optimising equipment provision to facilitate independence.
- Achieving and maintaining successful reintegration into the community.
- Managing psychological adaptation to the newly acquired physical condition.

Where required, carers are actively involved in the rehabilitation process and are taught how to assist with normal daily activities and to support independent living. Assisted exercises, standing programmes and chest care are taught in addition to moving and handling, whilst paying attention to skin care and their own safety and back care. This

TABLE 9.9 Subjective Assessment

HPC	• Date of SCI • Mode of SCI • Skeletal spinal injury • Other injuries at time of SCI • Spinal surgery	• Other surgery • Inpatient rehabilitation • Outpatient/community rehabilitation • Current International Standard Neurological Classification of Spinal Cord Injury
DH	• Anticoagulants • Steroids • Botulinum toxin	• Antispasmodics • Pain medication
Medical history	• Osteoporosis/osteopenia • Heterotrophic ossification • Rheumatoid arthritis • Fractures (other than at time of SCI) • Musculoskeletal injuries • Hypertension • Cardiovascular disease • Diabetes	• Surgery • Chronic obstructive pulmonary disease • Deep vein thrombosis/pulmonary embolism • Malignancy • Autonomic dysreflexia • Pacemakers/implants • Psychological well-being
SH	• Home • House/flat • Permanent/temporary • Owned/privately rented/HA/council • Steps and stairs inside • Steps and stairs to access • Bedroom	• Bathrooms • Others in residence • Home roles and responsibilities • Work • Driving/transport • Leisure/hobbies/interests • Care
Currently	• Spasticity/spasms • Pain • Skin • Bowel/bladder • Exercise programme • Respiratory • Fitness activities • Standing	• Mobility – indoor, outdoor, important environments • Orthotics • Wheelchair/posture/seating • Activities of daily living/function • Weight • Sleeping • Mood

DH, Drug history; *HPC*, history of present condition; *HA*, social housing; *SCI*, spinal cord injury; *SH*, social history.

TABLE 9.10 Common Outcome Measures in Spinal Cord Injury

Fitness	Borg Perceived Rate of Exertion (Borg 1982)
Gait	Walking Index for Spinal Cord Injury Scale II (Ditunno et al 2008, Ditunno & Ditunno 2001) 10-metre walk (Amatachaya et al 2014) 6-minute walk Berg Balance Scale (Berg 1993) Spinal Cord Injury Functional Ambulation Inventory (Field-Fote et al 2001) Hi-Mat (Williams et al 2006)
Odstock Drop Foot Stimulator	Physiological cost index (MacGregor 1981)
Respiratory	Cough peak expiratory flow rate Forced vital capacity

(Continued)

TABLE 9.10 **Common Outcome Measures in Spinal Cord Injury—Cont'd**	
Spinal cord injury	International Standard Neurological Classification of Spinal Cord Injury
	Spinal Cord Independence Measure III (v6.0 2016 SCIREProject.com)
Spasticity	Modified Ashworth Scale (Bohannon & Smith 1987)
	Penn Spasm Frequency Scale (Penn et al 1989)
	Range of motion
	SCI-SET (Adams et al 2007)
Upper limbs	Wheelchair User's Shoulder Pain Index (Curtis et al 1995)

support is within a holistic educational advocacy provided by case managers during rehabilitation.

It is outside the scope of this chapter to consider all physical interventions used in the rehabilitation phase for SCI; readers are referred to expert reviews and textbooks (Harvey 2007, 2016 and Reznik & Simmons 2020) and comprehensive freely available online materials (http://www.elearnsci.org). Therapists focus on the following interventions during the rehabilitation phase:

- Respiratory care;
- Functional mobility (sitting balance, pressure relief manoeuvres, bed mobility, wheelchair mobility and transfers);
- Strength training;
- Management of range of movement, including standing programmes and spasticity management;
- Cardiovascular fitness training;
- Upper limb management and shoulder protection; and
- Gait training

It must be acknowledged that there is limited evidence to demonstrate the effectiveness of commonly used physical interventions. Most controlled trials have focused on demonstrating the effectiveness of high-technology, high-cost interventions such as treadmill training with body weight support and robotics (Harvey 2016).

Strength Training

Strengthening can be achieved through prescription of exercises, ranging from facilitated, gravity eliminated, gravity opposed to resisted exercises, as indicated by the assessment. Augmenting the exercise programme into functionally specific activity-based patterns of movement, as soon as possible, will maximise efficacy. Progressive resisted exercise is effective for grade 3 and 4 muscles that require hypertrophy to enable the patient to be as functionally independent as possible (Bye et al 2017). Activity-based rehabilitation (ABR) focusses on producing activation of the neuromuscular system to restore activity below the lesion through neuroplasticity (Sadowsky et al 2009). Studies of movement relearning and strengthening enhanced by electrical stimulation have

---

STRENGTH TRAINING PRINCIPLES IN SCI (GINIS ET AL 2018)

The scientific exercise guidelines for adults with SCI:
- Exercise moderately to vigorously, twice a week for 20 minutes, to develop fitness.
- In addition, the recommendation is for three sets of moderate to vigorous strength training, twice a week.
- For improved metabolic health, it is advised to exercise for 30 minutes, three times a week.

For partially innervated muscles:
- Neuromuscular electrical stimulation (NMES) in UMN lesion (with an intact peripheral nerve supply)
- Direct muscle stimulation in LMN injury

---

demonstrated positive results (Martin et al 2012, van der Scheer 2021).

Aquatic Therapy

Aquatic therapy/hydrotherapy is used for strengthening and as preparation for swimming (Fig. 9.5). Patients are taught how to roll in the water and to swim. If the patient is wearing a brace, this will limit activities in the water. Careful consideration is given to individuals with an FVC of less than 1 L before shoulder-deep water immersion, although there is some evidence that shoulder-deep immersion can improve pulmonary function for tetraplegic individuals during the immersion (Thomaz et al 2005). There is no evidence for longer term effects.

Facilitation of Movement

The effectiveness of stretch and passive movements is controversial, with some authors refuting its efficacy as a therapeutic intervention (Harvey et al 2017). The use of facilitated movements, encouraging participation where possible for the purpose of movement reeducation and avoidance of loss of range, remains part of clinical practice, and the ongoing provision of range of movement exercises as part of a care programme to ameliorate loss of range of movement has not been researched.

Maintaining range of movement requires early institution of a facilitated range of movement programme, taking joints and muscles through their full available range on a daily basis. Positioning to avoid adoption of potentially problematic postures can provide the sustained stretch that is likely to best avoid loss of range and can address the early onset of stiffness. Care must be taken with:

- Maintaining alignment and spinal stability;
- Movements to end of range when joints may be vulnerable;
- Planes of movement across joints left unprotected by paralysed muscles – avoid torsional forces and valgus/varus strains; and
- The effects on neural dynamics when moving a traumatised neural system.

People with cervical SCI from a functional perspective have impaired ability to actively extend their elbow during transfers (level C5-C6) and inability to grasp (level C5-C7). These movements can be retrained in a different way using substitute movements (Mateo et al 2015). Tenodesis is a functional grip that uses activity in wrist extensors and shortness in hand and forearm flexors to bring about passive opposition of the thumb and finger flexion. Moving the wrist in extension or flexion then causes the fingers to grip when the wrist is extended and to release when the wrist is flexed. It provides a functional grasp for C6/C7 injuries. In those with partially preserved active hand function, a full assessment of all motor and sensory activity should be undertaken to decide whether to pursue a tenodesis grip or work for active flexion. When facilitating a tenodesis grip, passive movements in wrist neutral should include wrist extension with finger flexion and wrist flexion with finger extension (also see Fig. 9.6).

In SCI, loss of agonist/antagonist pairs of muscle groups across a joint can exacerbate problems. For example, at the elbow, with a C5 SCI, biceps activity will be retained, and triceps activity lost. The elbow will be held in a flexed position, particularly when in bed where gravity does not deliver extension. Loss of range of extension quickly ensues. This scenario can be catastrophic for function if the individual later needs full elbow extension to achieve an activity, for example, transfers.

Where there is the potential for recovering activity, augmentation techniques, for example, proprioceptive neuromuscular facilitation (PNF), functional electrical stimulation (FES), and deweighting, should be considered (Fig. 9.7). The use of ABR programmes has been developed to facilitate restoration of activity, although further evidence to support the variety of programmes is required (Mehrholz et al 2015).

Range of movement can change very quickly, and careful monitoring, particularly in the early stages, is important. Early intervention is more likely to be successful, and quick escalation of treatment is necessary to avoid the development of contractures if changes are detected. In the

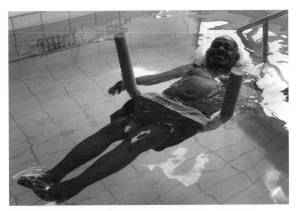

FIG. 9.5 Aquatic therapy.

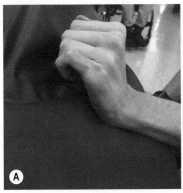
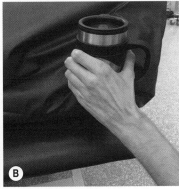

FIG. 9.6. Tenodesis series (A) and (B).

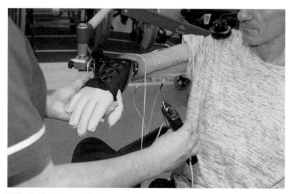

FIG. 9.7 Upper limb deweighted with functional electrical stimulation.

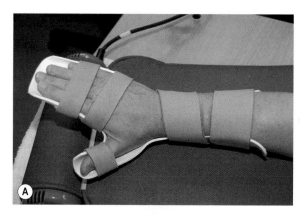

longer term, for those with the physical ability, often completion of functional tasks in the daily routine is enough to maintain range of movement. Others might have some specific stretches that they are able to complete independently. Where necessary to maintain range of movement, carers can be trained to undertake daily facilitated movements, and this should be encompassed in care packages. The requirements for maintaining range should be assessed with recommendations made on an individual basis. Patients can also be taught passive movements and stretching to perform independently as a home programme (see http://www.physiotherapyexercises.com).

Splinting

Splinting in the upper limbs may be necessary to maintain range of movement, particularly when unopposed activity and significant spasticity are present (see Fig. 9.8A; Association of Chartered Physiotherapists in Neurology [ACPIN] 2014). Dynamic splinting systems, FES, and botulinum toxin are of great value in restoration of functional movement. In the lower limbs, soft splints may be required to maintain dorsiflexion at the ankles. This can also be accomplished using pillows and the end of the bed. Caution when restraining movement must be exercised because of the increased risk for tissue viability problems associated with SCI. The use of compression garments can also increase stability and proprioception (Ghai et al 2017).

Several routine positions may be considered to minimise contractures or mild loss of range of movement through prolonged stretch.

Seating

When sitting, great care in achieving and maintaining a good postural alignment is the most effective way of distributing loading equally, preventing excess pressure on any one point (Table 9.11). This requires careful choice

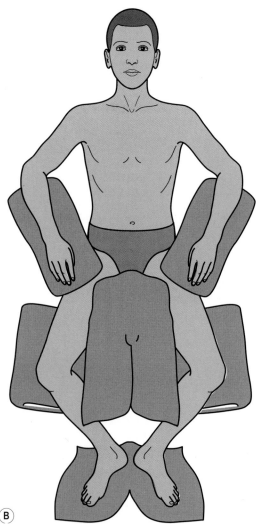

FIG. 9.8 (A) Custom-made thermoplastic resting splint. (B) "Frogged" position.

REASONS TO CONSIDER SPLINTING AND POSITIONING (ACPIN 2014)

- Reduce oedema;
- Maintain soft tissue length;
- Prevent overstretching;
- Support anatomical alignment;
- Prevent contractures and deformity with prolonged stretch;
- Manage spasticity;
- Promote function; and
- Replace function.

Positioning

Some patterns of contracture are characteristic and more predictable because of unopposed pull of innervated muscles. According to Ghai et al (2013), risk factors for development of contractures are:

- Higher level of spinal cord injury;
- High levels of spasticity;
- Long periods of bed rest;
- Low levels of mobility;
- Dependence on others for changing position;
- Unopposed muscle activity across a joint; and
- Underlying joint problems.

RECOMMENDATIONS FOR POSITIONING IN BED

- Cervical spine in neutral (avoidance of prolonged flexion)
- Elbow extension in pronation and supination
- Shoulder abduction and external rotation
- Prone lying
- Alternating between hip and knee flexion and extension
- Dorsiflexion
- 'Frogged' position – supine with hips flexed and externally rotated, knees flexed (see Fig. 9.8b)

TABLE 9.11 Checklist for Good Seated Posture

Body Segment	Optimal Position
Trunk	• Adequate lumbar lordosis supported by a back rest • Buttocks back in the chair
Pelvis	• Neutral position • Avoid posterior tilt • Neutral lateral alignment (indicated by level anterior superior iliac spine [ASIS])
Arms	• Arms should rest without scapula elevation but high enough to reduce any glenohumeral subluxation • Able to reach, when possible, without stabilising with other arm or falling forward
Thighs	• Thighs supported on cushion, which should finish 2–3 cm behind the knees • Hips in neutral rotation, using inserts if required
Knees	• 90° flexion and aligned over ankles
Ankle	• Plantargrade, with soles of feet well supported

of cushion, back rest and wheelchair frame, as well as adequate setup. Those who can adjust their own posture should be taught to do so. Those who cannot should be able to instruct those assisting them. Patients should be able to lift their arms to table height without losing their postural alignment.

Specialised pressure-relieving cushions help to maintain even pressure over seated surfaces. Hourly forwards-leaning pressure relief, chest on lap, arms forwards, for 2 consecutive minutes has been found to be the optimum for allowing capillary reperfusion. Tetraplegic individuals will require assistance of one or two people initially, but paraplegic patients should manage this technique independently. Sideways leaning produces lateral pressure relief and is also effective but less favourable because of the change in postural alignment that occurs. It also takes twice as long because each side must be relieved for 2 minutes. For some patients, this may be necessary because of pain and musculoskeletal issues causing stiffness and loss of joint range.

Functional Mobility

Initial rehabilitation focuses on restoration of functional independence and utilisation of functional activity. Rolling from side to side is taught first, then lying to sitting, and sitting to lying. Function is dependent on the level of the lesion and whether there is spared activity below the level of the lesion.

Sitting supported in the wheelchair is progressed to a plinth supported, then unsupported. Static and dynamic balance are practiced in short and long sitting to aid independence in activities of daily living. Lifting in preparation for transfer begins on the plinth. Long sitting is more stable, with knees flexed to accommodate range in hamstrings. Hand blocks may be used initially, and most will progress to no longer need them. Females often find achieving an effective lift more difficult because of body shape and arm length.

Depending on the level of the lesion and functional ability, a transfer board may be used for legs-up and legs-down transfers onto the bed. Progression to managing without a board is achieved where possible. More challenging transfers require practice in lifting from various levels for functional activities: between two plinths, floor to plinth, floor to chair and chair to car, bath and easy chair.

Assessment using a variety of wheelchairs is helpful when a patient is developing their confidence in wheelchair mobility. Essential principles of safety and wheelchair skills are taught. As patients progress, they should be given the opportunity to develop advanced skills, such as varied height kerbs, slopes, uneven terrain, tight corners, and, if possible, stairs and escalator techniques. A wheelchair skills training programme available at https://wheelchair-skillsprogram.ca/en/ is freely available.

Power-assisted wheeling systems provide the wheelchair user with the ability to push over difficult terrain, uphill and for longer distances. Numerous additions are available to attach to a manual wheelchair such as power trikes, third wheels and hand cycle systems. Skills in powered chairs are based around safe use of the chair functions, manoeuvring and experience of outdoor terrain. These chairs may have kerb-climbing functions and standing systems.

Standing

The use of devices to support a standing position remains prevalent in the management of SCIs (Figs. 9.9 and 9.10). The ability to achieve this is recommended for everyone after an SCI (MASCIP 2019). Carers are trained to assist where necessary. Standing two to three times per week for up to an hour is recommended. Standing offers the opportunity for a sustained stretch in a position of dorsiflexion, hip, knee and trunk extension. Loss of joint range is a common sequela of SCI, and standing can be part of a strategy to maintain range of movement. It is assumed clinically that weight bearing by approximating joint surfaces and stimulating normal activity with the consequent 'normal' sensory response can reduce spasticity, but there is limited evidence for this assumption to date (Newman & Barker 2012). Practically, passive standing is often initiated using a tilt-table where gradual increase in tilt allows careful monitoring for signs and symptoms of orthostatic hypotension, and descent can be achieved swiftly when required. Many will progress from tilt-table to less supportive devices.

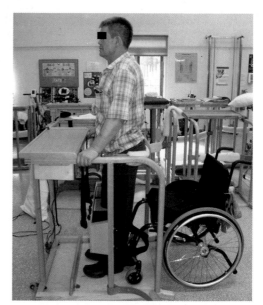

FIG. 9.9 Oswestry standing frame.

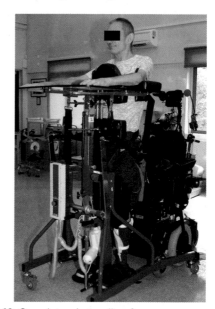

FIG. 9.10 Grandstand standing frame.

Gait Training

Despite the availability of new technologies, their cost is prohibitive to nearly all. Walking orthoses may still be the only option available. The ability to walk with callipers and the degree of support required depends on the functional level of injury. In principle, the energy expenditure, wear and tear on the upper limbs and the functional constraints of using the upper limbs in walking aids make ambulating using orthoses with L3 or above something some consider for very specific purposes.

The benefits of orthoses are outlined in the following list. Examples of orthoses used for different levels of injury are:

- C7-L1: hip guidance orthosis, advanced reciprocal gait orthosis, reciprocal gait orthosis, walkabout
- T6-T12: calliper walk/walkabout with rollator; progress to crutches depends on patient's function
- T9-L3: calliper walk with comfortable handle crutches
- L3 and below: appropriate orthoses or walking aid

BENEFITS OF ORTHOSES AND EXOSKELETONS

- Reduction in spasms and pain
- Enhancement or improvement in functional muscle activity
- Restoration of activities and hobbies that cannot be achieved independently when seated in a wheelchair
- Sense of well-being in returning to participation in pre-injury activities

Techniques used for gait training are discussed in detail by Bromley (2006). Initial training can be undertaken using a temporary calliper or a fibreglass backslab. Criteria to consider before calliper training include:

- Appropriate risk assessment;
- Sufficient upper limb strength to lift body weight;
- No upper limb injuries;
- Full ROM of hips, knees and ankles;
- Cardiovascular (CV) fitness sufficient to sustain walking activity;
- Assessment of spinal deformity (e.g., scoliosis) that may hinder standing balance;
- Motivation of the patient; and
- Assessment of spasticity that may make walking unsafe.

Those individuals with activity in their lower limbs should be rehabilitated using the usual principles in the presence of a UMN lesion. Those with LMN lesions benefit from appropriate orthosis and aids, strength, fitness and balance training and assistance in gaining the skills to achieve gait with their neurological presentation.

Technological advances in SCI such as treadmill training with body weight support, robotics, exoskeletons (Fig. 9.11) and neural prostheses hold great promise for the future, but it is challenging to implement the use of these technologies outside the research arena because of high costs and accessibility for most people with SCI (Reznik 2020).

Exoskeletons and lightweight orthotics are becoming more available to support rehabilitation. Some exoskeletons

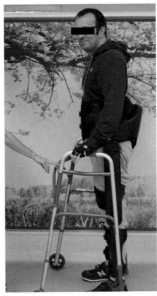

FIG. 9.11 'Indego' Exoskeleton worn by T4 paraplegic.

provide fully supportive walking and can even be used to climb stairs. Other devices can provide graduated support to the user allowing them to access their own active movement. Latest models include electrical stimulation to augment activity and produce muscle function (del-Ama et al 2014). The benefits of the hybrid exoskeletons include reduction of spasticity, maintained/improved bone density, circulatory improvement, improved bladder drainage, improved muscle bulk and protection of bony prominences, maintenance of joint range of movement, CV fitness and sense of psychological well-being.

The benefits of these technologies are clear, but the costs remain very high. It must also be borne in mind that some individuals would prefer not to use these systems because they may require assistance to use them and most require upper limb support using walking aids. For both reasons, the systems can limit function as well as enhance it.

The use of body weight support to facilitate gait has been extensively investigated. A treadmill is used to create the movement necessary of the deweighted lower limbs to activate the central pattern generators (CPGs; Fig. 9.12).

There is evidence that neural networks exist in isolation in the spinal cord. They generate outputs of rhythmic motor bursts reciprocally organised between agonist and antagonist muscle groups. The CPGs activate in the absence of efferent descending control and all movement-related afferent sources (Grillner & Wallen 1985, Kandel et al 2012, Polese et al 2013). The afferent activation originates at spinal and supraspinal levels, then will feedback to the CPGs. Complex patterns of movement can be generated by

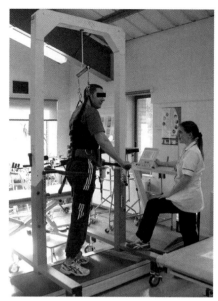

FIG. 9.12 Treadmill deweighting gantry.

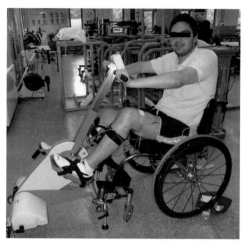

FIG. 9.13 Functional electrical stimulation (FES) lower limb ergometer.

the central nervous system without specific input from the limbs (Dietz et al 2002).

Some other systems such as the Lokomat can provide robotic-assisted gait combined with body weight–supported treadmill training. Research identifies that limb loading and hip afferent input are essential in effecting change in locomotion (Dietz et al 2002).

Cardiovascular Fitness

Improving CV fitness of an individual after SCI is an important element of rehabilitation. There are evidence-based guidelines that recommend for cardiorespiratory fitness and muscle strength benefits, adults with an SCI should engage in at least 20 minutes of moderate to vigorous intensity aerobic exercise two times per week and three sets of strength exercises for each major functioning muscle group, at a moderate to vigorous intensity, two times per week (strong recommendation). For cardiometabolic health benefits, adults with an SCI are suggested to engage in at least 30 minutes of moderate to vigorous intensity aerobic exercise three times per week (conditional recommendation) (Hoekstra et al 2020, Ginis et al 2018). Group exercise and participation in sports and circuit training activities are encouraged during rehabilitation. Wheeling, using a hand cycle or static upper limb ergometry, can provide cardiovascular exercise.

The use of FES ergometry has become a well-accepted modality to improve CV fitness. Most of the studies suggested that FES lower limb cycling used for periods of

12 weeks or up to 6 months produced CV and muscle strength benefits (van der Scheer 2021).

Other Modalities

New developments also include the use of virtual reality (VR) in movement reeducation. This technology proposes that the motivation and fun components of using VR can enhance the potential neuroplastic benefits of movement retraining (Tamar Weiss et al 2014).

FES is an effective adjunct to movement reeducation and to maintain range of movement The use of electrical stimulation is well documented in enhancing movement and has been demonstrated to be most effective when used in functional task-specific activities (Patil et al 2014, Santos et al 2006). There is some preliminary evidence that it can also inhibit spasticity (van der Salm et al 2006). FES has previously been found to have a therapeutic or 'carryover' effect in gait reeducation and lower limb strengthening in studies on both stroke and SCI patients (Barbeau et al 2002, Duffel et al 2019, Field-Fote 2001, Postans et al 2004). It can be used as an alternative to orthotics to assist movement, such as reach and grasp or stepping and foot clearance.

FES motor-assisted ergometers have been devised to provide stimulated cycling of the upper and lower limbs producing movement assisted by the user's own stimulated muscles (Fig. 9.13).

Now many studies demonstrate benefits to individuals with SCI although intensity, duration and frequency of these interventions all vary in the studies (van der Scheer 2021). The gains in muscle mass can help to protect vulnerable skin areas over bony prominences, as well as producing an improved cosmetic appearance of the lower limbs.

Evidence suggests that FES cycling can produce benefits in improving CV fitness when combined with resisted upper limb exercise (Backus et al 2009). Other studies demonstrate improvements in bone density, mainly showing gains in areas around the lower femur and upper tibia. These benefits are maintained only whilst the equipment is regularly used.

The muscles of an individual with an LMN lesion cannot be stimulated using the same form of electrical stimulation; however, alternative stimulation can be used providing direct muscle stimulation (Kern et al 2010).

SPECIAL CONSIDERATIONS

Reduced Bone Density

After SCI, because of the reduced demands on the bony skeleton, a rapid loss of bone density is observed. After SCI, there is an increased risk for fractures associated with osteopaenia and osteoporosis. These are often observed in the bones of the lower limbs and require careful management to prevent long-term postural deformity. There is some evidence to suggest a passive standing programme, and FES ergometry can reduce bone demineralisation in some bones. There are also pharmacological interventions that can prove effective (Soleyman-Jahi et al 2018).

Loss of Range of Movement and Postural Deformity

Loss of muscle power and reduced levels of mobility can quickly lead to a range of consequences outlined in the Consequences of Loss of Range box. Unchecked, the progression to contracture can be rapid. Once loss of range of movement has occurred, short-duration stretches quickly become ineffective. More sustained stretching with positioning and splinting may have some impact. Depending on the analysis of risk and benefit, the use of botulinum toxin (if there is a muscular component), manipulation under anaesthetic, tenotomies and serial casting may be considered.

CONSEQUENCES OF LOSS OF RANGE

- Undesired aesthetics
- Increased spasticity
- Pain
- Impaired hygiene of closely approximated tissue
- Reduced active range of movement
- Impaired function
- Postural deformity
- Increased risk for tissue viability failure

Shoulder Pain

Of those with SCI, 39% will report shoulder pain within the last week (Bossuyt et al 2017). Shoulder pain is associated with less effective transfers and an increase fear of falling (Rice et al 2022). Careful positioning in the acute phase can reduce early problems from developing. This may include avoidance of lying on the point of the shoulder by bringing the shoulder girdle through when in side lying, use of a hip twist when in side lying when spinal stability allows, and positioning in abduction and external rotation for a period each day to offer a capsular stretch. Loss of range of movement during the acute phase is a significant predictor of high levels of pain at 5 years (Eriks-Hoogland et al 2014).

Additional support from Lycra garments across the shoulder may provide relief for those with limited arm function. Enhancing stability through adequate seating and other means allows the muscles across the shoulder girdle to pattern most effectively, which may help avoid impingement.

Specific exercises to address muscle imbalance and maintenance of full range have been shown to reduce incidence of pain, including posterior strengthening and anterior stretching exercises (Curtis et al 1999, van Straaten et al 2017). Activity modification is a significant contributor. Options for reducing strain on the upper limbs should be considered, such as good transfer technique, adapted environments, minimising the need for overhead reaching and the use of power-assisted wheelchair options being a starting point.

Tissue Viability

After an SCI, independently adjusting position is likely to be more difficult. Tissues are less able to tolerate compression and heal less efficiently because of reductions in affective circulation associated with reduced muscle activity and less responsive vasculature. Muscle mass is often reduced, leaving bony prominences more exposed. Sensation is impaired, reducing awareness of impending problems.

Pressure ulcers are a significant cause of morbidity after SCI; in the USA, 15.2% of those with SCI will experience pressure ulcer in their first year of injury, with the incidence increasing year on year with 40.6% of those with tetraplegia developing an ulcer in the 20 years after their injury (McKinley et al 1999). In a Swiss study, 51% of patients were found to have developed a pressure ulcer during their first episode of rehabilitation (Najmanova et al 2022). A categorisation system is used to assess pressure ulcers (National Pressure Ulcer Advisory Panel 2019).

A regular turning regimen is developed to reduce pressure over bony prominences and forms part of a 24-hour positioning plan. In all activities and use of splints and orthosis, skin vulnerability is a main consideration and steps are taken to ensure it is carefully monitored. Successful management of oedema can contribute to avoidance.

Good seating posture supplemented with an appropriately pressure-relieving cushion in the wheelchair and regular pressure relief are essential. Pressure relief should take place for 2 consecutive minutes in every hour (Coggrave & Rose 2003). This can be effectively achieved for most in a forward lean position, deweighting the sacrum and ischial tuberosities. Care may be required to maintain forward stability. An effective transfer technique will prevent scuffing the skin during a transfer.

To achieve effective self-management, patients need a working knowledge of pressure ulcer risk factors; they should be able to check their skin or instruct others to do so and be aware of what to do initially and how to contact their general practitioner and SCI centre for further advice.

Heterotropic Ossification

HO is the formation of normal lamellar bone in the soft tissues around paralysed joints, below the level of the lesion. Clinically, it has been found to be present in around 4%–20% of patients with SCI (Teasell et al 2010). The most common locations are around the hip joints. Stretch of the affected muscle and use of electrical stimulation in the area should be avoided during the active phase of HO, when there is evidence of an inflammatory process. Pharmacological treatment is with etidronate and nonsteroidal antiinflammatory medications to help to slow the development. Surgical resection may be required, but it is complicated because of the invasion of the bone into the soft tissue and vascular structures. HO has been found to significant impair function in continence management, self-care and mobility (Franz et al 2022).

Syrinx and Syringomyelia

After a traumatic injury to the spinal cord, there may be formation of a posttraumatic syrinx, a cavity filled with cerebrospinal fluid. It is often a late complication of SCI and presents with symptoms of pain, deteriorating neurology and changes in spasticity. A syrinx is most likely to occur in the cervical and thoracic spine, is likely to manifest more quickly in older people and is associated with more severe, complete injuries (Krebs et al 2016). The clinical incidence of posttraumatic syringomyelia in SCI has been estimated to be 0.3%–3.2% (Umbach & Heilporn 1991), although MRI reports greater incidence rates of 12%–22% (Vannemreddy et al 2002). Most syrinx do not require surgical management, but where symptoms are problematic it may be necessary to introduce a shunt to drain the fluid.

PAEDIATRIC CONSIDERATIONS

SCI in children and adolescents is rare and mostly results from trauma. Throughout Europe, the average cumulative incidence of traumatic and acquired non-traumatic SCI in children is from 0.9 to 27 per million per annum (Smith et al 2017).

Special considerations for children with SCI extracted from the NHS England Service Standards for Children and Young People (0–19 years) Requiring Spinal Cord Injury Care (NHS England Service Specifications 2014) and the MASCIP Guidance for Paediatric Physiotherapists Managing Childhood Onset Spinal Cord Injuries (2017) document entitled 'Children Requiring Domiciliary/Long Term Ventilation' (available at https://www.mascip.co.uk/wp-content/uploads/2016/10/Approved-vent-paeds-appendix.pdf) are:

- Children are very sensitive to hypotension, autonomic dysfunction and thermoregulatory dysfunction. There is potential for damage of the immature brain from chronic hypotension when first mobilising.
- Children have a high metabolism and therefore have high calorific needs for healing and recovery.
- Paralytic ileus is a very common problem in cervical and thoracic lesions.
- Standing is a priority in rehabilitating children. It is important for social skills and development of curiosity, is essential in preventing osteoporosis and facilitates the development of the epiphyseal growth plates.
- There is a greater potential for plasticity in children and may lead to quicker recovery.
- The child must be closely monitored during growth spurts for the development of spinal deformity (e.g., scoliosis).
- Support and education of the parents about the implications of the SCI will enable them to educate their child and family and monitor the child for any complications.
- Transitioning of adolescents into adult services requires a greater amount of support and planning from the professionals involved in the individual's care.

DISCHARGE PLANNING AND LIFELONG CARE

The process of rehabilitation and reintegration is complex, involving many agencies and resources. The development of the case management process has helped to coordinate the complex process of discharge into the community. A home visit is made by the community team and members of the inpatient team as required. This may include school or workplace. If home adaptations or rehousing are not completed but the patient is ready for discharge, transfer to an interim placement may be necessary.

On discharge all patients will require further close follow-up and reassessment, usually involving community teams. Ideally, there will be a multidisciplinary review to maintain continued support, monitor physical well-being and facilitate reintegration. During rehabilitation, patients are introduced to groups and organisations, such as the Spinal Injuries Association, ASPIRE and Back Up, who can offer social and peer support and leisure activities, whilst also providing advisory role, to assist in the reintegration process.

Lifelong care is provided in many countries by national spinal cord injury centres, offering follow-up, further restorative surgery, further rehabilitation and intervention for new problems as required (www.scireproject.com/community/) (Reznik et al 2020).

CONCLUSION

The management of SCI is complex. Although the most obvious impairments of SCI are paralysis and sensory loss, SCI affects many other body functions, including CV, bowel and bladder, respiratory, gastrointestinal and sexual function. There are many factors, physical and psychological, complications and comorbidities that will affect the likely ultimate outcome after SCI. In the early postinjury phase, physical management will mainly involve prevention of respiratory and circulatory complications, and care of pressure areas with attention directed to the consequences of weakness. Prophylaxis to prevent further complications is critical. In the rehabilitation phase, therapists focus on respiratory care, functional mobility, strength training, implementing a daily standing programme, gait training with orthotics, fitness training and upper limb management. A functional, goal-oriented, interdisciplinary rehabilitation programme should enable the patient with SCI to live as full and independent a life as possible. Evidence-based interventions are continuing to emerge, but it must be acknowledged that there is limited evidence to demonstrate the effectiveness of commonly used physical interventions; therefore, more research into these interventions is required. Medical developments, technology and pharmacology offer exciting prospects for the future management of SCI.

CASE STUDY

This highly complex case of paediatric incomplete SCI with high cervical pathology AIS D demonstrates the integration of all aspects of SCI management and coordination of the whole MDT. This 4-year-old female was diagnosed in February 2016 with rhombencephalitis (Campos et al 2016). This is a brainstem encephalitis or acute descending encephalomyelitis, a rare autoimmune inflammatory demyelinating condition affecting the white matter of the brain and spinal cord. There is complete recovery in 50%–70% of cases and partial recovery in 70%–90%, with a mortality rate of 5%. There is a poorer prognosis when there is severe neurological deficit and no response to steroid treatment.

The patient presented at the emergency department in February with paralysis of all limbs, neck and facial muscles, and was transferred to the SCI centre in March. At that time, she was medically unstable, experiencing AD and associated autonomic dysfunction leading to fits. The initial management plan is presented in Table 9.12. Communication was very limited because of a tracheostomy; therefore, the team was unable to fully assess using INSCSCI. MDT liaison to provide advice, education and support to the family was critical.

Progress With Rehabilitation

The management plan during the rehabilitation phase is presented in Table 9.13. Fig. 9.14 through Fig. 9.19 illustrate sitting and standing postures achieved. Sufficient progress was made to stabilise her respiratory function and to educate family members in how to assist in ongoing rehabilitation. The patient was able to independently drive her wheelchair using good distal right-hand control.

Trials of FES to improve muscle strength were not well tolerated because of hypersensitivity. Her motor recovery continued, and she regained weak proximal control of her left shoulder and some functional distal activity. Her right upper limb remained flaccid with flickers of finger movements. Both her legs regained antigravity power in most major muscle groups with the left slightly stronger than the right.

MDT discharge liaison meetings involved community paediatric services, as the initial plan was for discharge to a paediatric hospice because of the complexities of the carer training and risk assessment. The MDT prepared a carer training booklet for discharge and handover to family and care team at the hospice. This involved the assessments of hoist and slings to enable safe transfer with assistance of two people. Seating and orthotic postural bracing ensured optimum stability and alignment was achieved. However, it remained unsafe to return the patient to her home, and the complexity of her management necessitated a return to the spinal injuries centre for 4 weeks for further carer training.

Funding was obtained for domiciliary respiratory management. The patient was discharged home after 11 months of inpatient rehabilitation. Clear monitoring plans were established to maintain good spinal alignment with regular monitoring every 6 months as she grows. Lower limb power improvement continues to date, and she has achieved walking 50 metres with two assisting.

TABLE 9.12   Initial Management Plan

Body Structure and Function Impairments	Problem List	Treatment Goal	Treatment
Impaired respiratory function resulting from brain and cervical spinal white matter inflammation	• Intubated and ventilated • Left lower lobe collapse • Right mid and lower lobe consolidation • Increased secretions	• Clear secretions • Strengthen active respiratory function • Initiate weaning from ventilator	• Trial of ventilator-free breathing – no diaphragmatic activity identified • Establish cough assist programme using the Clearway Cough Assist Device • Vest therapy (high-frequency chest wall oscillation) setup • Progress deflated cuff for speaking
Diffuse weakness with developing increased tone/ankle clonus	• Flaccid trunk • Poor head control • Flickers of distal activity of right upper limb • No activity of left upper limb • Flickers in lower limbs • Orthostatic hypotension	• Manage increased tone • Provide postural stability • Maintain range of movement in all joints • Strengthen/facilitate active movements	• Ankle splinting (initially hindered by Venflons [intravenous cannula] in situ) • 24-hour positioning plan • Resting splints for upper limbs • Passive and active facilitated movements • Strengthening facilitated by functional electrical stimulation • Liaison with orthotics team to develop thoraco-lumbo-sacral orthosis and collar • Medication to support low blood pressure, compression stockings and abdominal binder to facilitate sitting and standing
Neuropathic pain in left upper limb	• Pain affects activity and facilitated movements	• Assist in holistic pain management	• Refer to pain team • Focus treatment on desensitisation
Activity Limitations			
Inability to breathe independently	• Respiratory muscles remain weak	• Facilitate independence and mobility	• Use of adapted power wheelchair to enable mobilisation whilst on domiciliary ventilator
Loss of postural stability	• Unable to sit or stand • Loss of proximal stability for upper and lower limb function	• Establish strategies of postural support	• Identify medication to reduce hypotension to support upright posture • Support posture using orthotics as activity returns
Loss of independent personal activities and functional activities	• Loss of bilateral hand function due to diffuse weakness	• Establish strategies to compensate for hand function	• Use of custom splints and arm supports to utilise any available activity in assisted functional movements

TABLE 9.13 Updated Problem List, Goals and Treatment Plan During Rehabilitation Phase

Body Structure and Function Impairments	Problem List	Goals	Treatment Plan
Impaired respiratory function	• Ongoing ventilatory support	• Maintain clear airways • Strengthen improving abdominal activity to assist cough • Review speech and swallow	• Monitor respiratory function for recovering activity • Secretion clearance as required • Use of spirometry to assess forced vital capacity • Liaise with speech and language therapist
Diffuse muscle weakness	• Loss of independent movement	• Strengthen all active movements of limbs	• Functional electrical stimulation/deweighting upper limb to triceps, deltoid and wrist extensors of right upper limb • Active leg bike for strengthening and endurance in activity • Plinth work for trunk facilitation, rolling and sitting balance
Loss of postural stability in sitting and standing	• Unable to sit or stand • Loss of proximal stability for upper and lower limb function	• Strengthen trunk stability • Maintain postural alignment and review orthoses • Develop standing endurance • Increase active standing with assistance	• Standing with a tilt-table progressing to specific paediatric standing equipment • Custom-made trunk orthosis including cervical component • Serial casting ankles to improve range of movement • AFOs used for standing • Left upper limb support created to support arm when sitting and standing
Neuropathic pain in left upper limb with variable loss of sensation in all limbs	• Impaired control of movement • Hypersensitivity in left upper limb • Inhibition of facilitated movement	• Support pain management	• Team management of pain including pressure garments to reduce hypersensitivity
Spasticity developing with underlying diffuse weakness in all limbs and trunk	• Loss of selective movement • Risk of loss of muscle length and development of contractures	• Maintain range of lower limb joints • Manage soft tissue mobility and pain • Promote active recovery	• Regular standing programme • Facilitated weight bearing through legs during transfers • Facilitate active movement including leg bike • Stepping with adapted rollator and assistance using AFOs

(Continued)

TABLE 9.13   Updated Problem List, Goals and Treatment Plan During Rehabilitation Phase—Cont'd

Body Structure and Function Impairments	Problem List	Goals	Treatment Plan
Activity Limitations			
Unable to sit or stand unaided	• Limited participation in personal and functional activities of daily living	• Establish strategies to compensate for weakness and sensory impairments	• Use of orthotics and equipment to facilitate independent sitting and to assist in standing/stepping
Participation Limitations			
Loss of ability to participate in academic and social activities	• Inaccessible environments to wheelchair users • Environments not adapted for activities performed from a wheelchair • Unable to participate in educational activities due to upper limb weakness	• Facilitate participation in school and play	• Timetable coordinated with play therapist and on-site school involvement • Trial of aquatic therapy with long ventilator tube, monitored and supported by anaesthetist • Trained ability to drive power chair via right hand on joystick with supervision • Use of technologies to access education
Altered family dynamics and support systems	• Prolonged hospitalisation • Anxiety caused by complexity of needs • Risk of respiratory and cardiac event	• Support and educate family in understanding of sudden cardiac injury and respiratory complications	• Psychosocial team involvement with close liaison with community teams for discharge
Environmental Limitations			
Difficulties in accessing school building and in the use of facilities within school	• School not accessible to power chair	• Provide appropriate adaptations to enable access to education, utilising technologies to enable participation	• Coordination with local services and education authorities to facilitate access
Limitations in accessing home environment and buildings to participate in social situations	• Family home not accessible to a power chair • Family car inappropriate • Difficult to access family and peer leisure activities	• To provide access to an appropriate home environment • Assist in providing contacts to source a wheelchair-accessible vehicle • Identify options for accessible leisure activities	• Utilisation of specialist equipment to facilitate access • Coordinate with local services to facilitate a safe discharge • Identify appropriate organisations and charities

AFO, Ankle–foot orthosis.

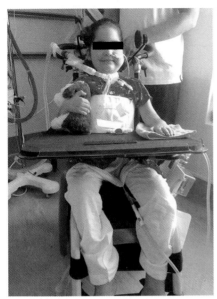

FIG. 9.14 Case study: seated in manual wheelchair with corset, left arm support and head supports.

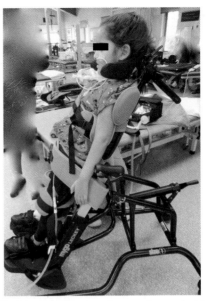

FIG. 9.16 Case study: standing system providing postural support.

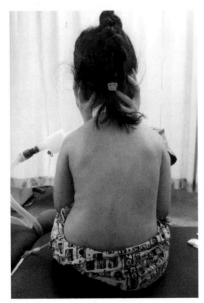

FIG. 9.15 Case study: posture with only head supported showing postural scoliosis.

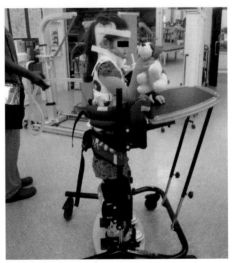

FIG. 9.17 Case study: improved standing in cervico-thoraco-lumbo-sacral orthosis (CTLSO).

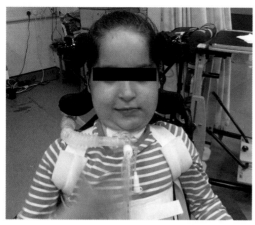

FIG. 9.18 Case study: modular head control system.

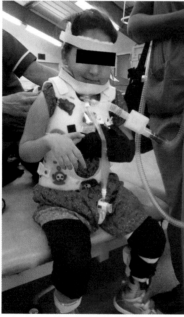

FIG. 9.19 Case study: independent sitting balance achieved wearing bilateral ankle–foot orthoses, cervico and thoraco-lumbar-sacral orthoses and left arm support.

SELF-ASSESSMENT QUESTIONS

1. What tool do you use to assess impairment in a patient with SCI?
2. How can you quickly assess respiratory function in a patient with SCI?
3. At what level of SCI would you expect a patient to present with impaired ability to cough and clear chest secretions?
4. Which body systems are affected by SCI?
5. Do patients with SCI experience pain below their level of SCI?
6. What factors should you consider when assessing a person with SCI for an appropriate wheelchair?

REFERENCES

Abou, L., Rice, L.A., 2022. The associations of functional independence and quality of life with sitting balance and wheelchair skills among wheelchair users with spinal cord injury. J Spinal. Cord. Med. 7, 1–8.

Adams, M.M., Ginis, K.A., Hicks, A.L., 2007. The spinal cord injury spasticity evaluation tool: development and evaluation. Arch. Phys. Med. Rehabil. 88, 1185–1192.

Alexander, M.S., Biering-Sorensen, F., Bodner, D., et al., 2009. International standards to document remaining autonomic function after spinal cord injury. Spinal. Cord. 47, 36–43.

Amatachaya, S., Naewla, S., Srisim, K., Arrayawichanon, P., Siriratatiwat, W., 2014. Concurrent validity of the 10-meter walk test as compared with the 6-minute walk test in patients with spinal cord injury at various levels of ability. Spinal. Cord. 52, 333–336.

Anscomb, H., 2020. Introduction to *spinal cord injury*. In: Reznik, J.E., Simmons, J. (Eds.), *Rehabilitation* in *Spinal Cord Injuries*. Elsevier Press, Australia.

Association of Chartered Physiotherapists in Neurology (ACPIN), 2015. Splinting for the prevention and correction of contractures in adults with neurological dysfunction. Available at: https://www.acpin.net/pdfs/Splinting_Guidelines.pdf. Accessed on 13 July 2023.

Barbeau, H., Ladouceur, M., Moirbagheri, M.M., Kearney, R.E., 2002. The effect of locomotor training combined with functional electrical stimulation in chronic spinal cord injured subjects: walking and reflex studies. Brain. Res. Rev. 40, 274–291.

Barbosa, P.H., Glinsky, J.V., Fachin-Martins, E., 2021. Physiotherapy interventions for the treatment of spasticity in people with spinal cord injury: a systematic review. Spinal. Cord. 59, 236–247.

Berg, K., 1993. Measuring Balance in the Elderly: Validation of an Instrument (PhD Thesis). McGill University, Montreal.

Bennett, J., Das, J.M., Emmady, P.D., 2022. Spinal Cord Injuries. StatsPearls Publishing, Tampa, FL.

BOAST 8., 2014. The management of traumatic spinal cord injury. Available at: http://boa.ac.uk. Accessed on 13 July 2023.

Bohannon, R.W., Smith, M.B., 1987. Interrater reliability of modified Ashworth scale of muscle spasticity. Phys. Ther. 67, 206–207.

Borg, G.A., 1982. Psychophysical bases of perceived exertion. Med. Sci. Sport. Exerc. 14, 377–381.

Bossuyt, F.M., Arnet, U., Brinkhof, M.W.G., et al., 2017. Shoulder pain in the Swiss spinal cord injury community: prevalence and associated factors. Disabil. Rehabil. 13, 1–11.

Bromley, I., 2006. Tetraplegia and Paraplegia, sixth ed. Churchill Livingstone, London.

Butler, J.E., Lim, J., Gorman, R.B., Boswell-Ruys, C., Saboisky, J.P., Lee, B.B., Gandevia, S.C., 2011. Posterolateral surface electrical stimulation of abdominal expiratory muscles to enhance cough in spinal cord injury. Neurorehabil. Neural. Repair. 25, 158–167.

Bye, E.A., Harvey, L.A., Gambhir, A., et al., 2017. Strength training for partially paralysed muscles in people with recent spinal cord injury: a within-participant randomized controlled trial. Spinal. Cord. 55, 460–465.

Cameron, T., Broton, J.G., Needham-Shropshire, B., Klose, K.J., 1998. J Spinal Cord Med. 21, 1–6.

Campos, L.G., Régis, A.R.T., Faistauer, A., et al., 2016. Rhombencephalitis: pictorial essay. Radiol. Bras. 49, 329–336.

Calydon, V.E., Steeves, J.D., Krassioukov, A., 2005. Orthostatic hypotension following spinal cord injury: understanding clinical pathophysiology. Spinal. Cord. 44, 341–351.

Coggrave, M.J., Rose, L.S., 2003. A specialist seating assessment clinic: changing pressure relief practice. Spinal. Cord. 41, 692–695.

Consortium for Spinal Cord Medicine., 2008. Early acute management in adults with spinal cord injury: a clinical practice guideline for health-care professionals. J. Spinal. Cord. Med. 31, 403–479.

Curtis, K.A., Drysdale, G.A., Lanza, R.D., et al., 1999. Shoulder pain in wheelchair users with tetraplegia and paraplegia. Arch. Phys. Med. Rehabil. 80, 453–457.

Curtis, K.A., Roach, K.E., Apllegate, E.B., et al., 1995. Development of the Wheelchair User's Shoulder Pain Index (WUSPI). Paraplegia 33, 290–293.

del-Ama, A.J., Gil-Agudo, A., Pons, J.L., Moreno, J.C., 2014. Hybrid gait training with an overground robot for people with incomplete spinal cord injury: a pilot study. Front. Hum. Neurosci. 8, 298.

Dietz, V., 2012. Neuronal plasticity after a human spinal cord injury: positive and negative effects. Exp. Neurol. 235, 110–115.

Dietz, V., Müller, R., Colombo, G., 2002. Locomotor activity in spinal man: significance of afferent input from joint and load receptors. Brain 125, 2626–2634.

DiMarco, A.F., Dawson, N.V., 2014. Risk factors for mortality in spinal cord injury. J Spinal. Cord. Med. 37, 670–671.

Ditunno Jr., J.F., Cohen, M.E., Hauck, W.W., Jackson, A.B., Sipski, M.L., 2000. Recovery of upper extremity strength in complete and incomplete tetraplegia: a multicenter study. Arch. Phys. Med. Rehabil. 81, 389–393.

Ditunno, J.F., Little, J.W., Tessler, A., Burns, A.S., 2004. Spinal shock revisited: a four-phase model. Spinal. Cord. 42, 383–395.

Ditunno Jr., J.F., Scivoletto, G., Patrick, M., et al., 2008. Validation of the walking index for spinal cord injury in a US and European clinical population. Spinal. Cord. 46, 181–188.

Ditunno, P.L., Ditunno, J.F., 2001. Walking index for spinal cord injury (WISCI II): scale revision. Spinal. Cord. 39, 654–656.

Duffell, L.D., Paddison, S., Alahmary, A.F., Donaldson, N., Burridge, J., 2019. The effects of FES cycling combined with virtual reality racing biofeedback on voluntary function after incomplete SCI: a pilot study. J. Neuroeng. Rehabil. 16, 149.

Eriks-Hoogland, I.E., Hoekstra, T., de Groot, S., Stucki, G., Post, M.W., van der Woude, L.H., 2014. Trajectories of musculoskeletal shoulder pain after spinal cord injury: Identification and predictors. J. Spinal. Cord. Med. 37, 288–298.

Eriksson, P., Lofstrom, L., Ekblom, B., 1988. Aerobic power during maximal exercise in untrained and well-trained persons with quadriplegia and paraplegia. Scand. J. Rehabil. Med. 20, 141–147.

Field-Fote, E.C., 2001. Combined use of body weight support, functional electric stimulation, and treadmill training to improve walking ability in individuals with chronic incomplete spinal cord injury. Arch. Phys. Med. Rehabil. 82, 818–824.

Field-Fote, E., Fluet, G., Schafer, S., et al., 2001. The Spinal Cord Injury Functional Ambulation Inventory (SCI-FAI). J. Rehabil. Med. 33, 177–181.

Filipp, M.E., Travis, B.J., Henry, S.S., et al., 2019. Differences in neuroplasticity after spinal cord injury in varying animal models and humans. Neural. Regen. Res. 14, 7–19.

Foo, D., 1986. Spinal cord injury in forty-four patients with cervical spondylosis. Paraplegia 24, 301–306.

Franz, S., Rust, L., Heutehaus, L., Rupp, R., Schuld, C., Weidner, N., 2022. Impact of heterotopic ossification on functional recovery in acute spinal cord injury. Front. Cell. Neurosci. 16, 842090.

Fu, J., Wang, H., Deng, L., Li, J., 2016. Exercise training promotes functional recovery after spinal cord injury. Neural. Plast. 2016, 4039580.

Gerasimenko, Y., Gorodnichev, R., Moshonkina, T., et al., 2015. Transcutaneous electrical spinal-cord stimulation in humans. Ann. Phys. Rehabil. Med. 58, 225–231.

Ghai, A., Nidhi, G., Sarla, H., et al., 2013. Spasticity pathogenesis, prevention and treatment strategies. Saudi. J. Anaesth. 7, 453–460.

Ghai, S., Driller, M., Ghai, I., 2017. Effects of joint stabilizers on proprioception and stability: a systematic review and meta-analysis. Phys. Ther. Sport. 25, 65–75.

Ginis, M., van der Scheer, J.W., Latimer-Cheung, A.E., et al., 2018. Scientific exercise guidelines for adults with spinal cord injury. Spinal. Cord. 56, 308–321.

Grillner, S., Wallen, P., 1985. Central pattern generators for locomotion, with special reference to vertebrates. Ann. Rev. Neurosci. 8, 233–261.

Handrakis, J.P., Trbovich, M., Hagen, E.M., Price, M., 2017. Thermodysregulation in persons with spinal cord injury: case series on use of the autonomic standards. Spinal. Cord. Ser. Cases. 3, 1–8.

Harvey, L., 2016. Physiotherapy rehabilitation for people with spinal cord injuries. J. Physiother. 62, 4–11.

Harvey, L.A., 2007. Management of Spinal Cord Injuries. Elsevier, London.

Harvey, L.A., Glinsky, J.V., Bowden, J.L., 2016. The effectiveness of 22 commonly administered physiotherapy interventions for people with spinal cord injury: a systematic review. Spinal. Cord. 54, 914–923.

Harvey, L.A., Katalinic, O.M., Herbert, R.D., et al., 2017. Stretch for the treatment and prevention of contracture: an abridged republication of a Cochrane Systematic Review. J. Physiother. 63, 67–75.

Harrison, P., 2000. HDU/ICU Managing Spinal Injury: Critical Care. Spinal Injuries Association, London.

Herrmann, K.H., Kirchberger, I., Stucki, G., Cieza, A., 2011. The comprehensive ICF core sets for spinal cord injury from the perspective of physical therapists: a worldwide validation study using the Delphi technique. Spinal. Cord. 49, 502–514.

Hoekstra, F., McBride, C.B., Borisoff, J., et al., 2020. Translating the international scientific spinal cord injury exercise guidelines into community and clinical practice guidelines: a Canadian evidence-informed resource. Spinal. Cord. 58, 647–657.

Hough, A., 2001. Physiotherapy in Respiratory Care: An Evidence Based Approach to Respiratory Management and Cardiac Conditions, 3rd ed. Nelson Thornes Ltd, Cheltenham.

Inanici, F., Brighton, L.N., Samejima, S., et al., 2021. Transcutaneous spinal cord stimulation restores hand and arm function after spinal cord injury. IEEE. Trans. Neural. Syst. Rehabil. Eng. 29, 310–319.

International Spinal Cord Injury Society (ISCoS)., 2015. In: Chhabra, H.S. (Ed.), Textbook on Comprehensive Management of Spinal Cord Injuries. Lippincott Williams & Wilkins, Philadelphia.

ISCOS-WHO International Perspectives on Spinal Cord Injury., 2013. Available at www. https://www.iscos.org.uk/international-perspectives-on-spinal-cord-injury. Accessed on 13 July 2023.

Jaja, B.N.R., Jiang, F., Badhiwala, J.H., et al., 2019. Association of pneumonia, wound infection, and sepsis with clinical outcomes after acute traumatic spinal cord injury. J. Neurotrauma. 36, 3044–3050.

Jo, H.J., Richardson, M.S.A., Oudegan, M., et al., 2021. Paired corticospinal-motoneuronal stimulation and exercise after spinal cord injury. J. Spinal. Cord. Med. 44 (Suppl. 1), S23–S27.

Johnston, L., 2001. Human spinal cord injury: new and emerging approaches to treatment. Spinal. Cord. 39, 609–613.

Kang, Y., Ding, H., Wei, Z.J., et al., 2018. Epidemiology of worldwide spinal cord injury: a literature review. J. Neurorestoratol. 6, 1–9.

Kandel, E.R., Schwartz, J.H., Jessell, T.M., Siegelbaum, S.A., Hudspeth, A.J., 2012. Principles of Neural Science, 5th ed. McGraw-Hill, New York City.

Karlsson, A.-K., 2006. Autonomic dysfunction in spinal cord injury: clinical presentation of symptoms and signs. Prog. Brain. Res. 152, 1–8.

Kern, H., Carraro, U., Adami, N., et al., 2010. Home-based functional electrical stimulation rescues permanently denervated muscles in paraplegic patients with complete lower motor neuron lesion. Neurorehabil. Neural. Repair. 24, 709–721.

Kirshblum, S., Burns, S.P., Biering-Sorensen, F., et al., 2011. International Standards for Neurological Classification of Spinal Cord Injury. J. Spinal. Cord. Med. 34, 535–546.

Kirshblum, S., Botticello, A., Lammertse, D.P., Marino, R.J., Chiodo, A.E., Jha, A., 2016. Patterns of sacral sparing components on neurologic recovery in newly injured persons with traumatic spinal cord injury. Arch. Phys. Med. Rehabil. 97, 1647–1655.

Kirshblum, S.C., Botticello, A.L., Benaquista, G., et al., 2016. Breaking the news: a pilot study on patient perspectives of discussing prognosis after traumatic spinal cord injury. J. Spinal. Cord. Med. 39, 155–161.

Kirshblum, S., Snider, B., Eren, F., Guest, J., 2021. Characterising natural recovery after traumatic SCI. J. Neurotrauma. 38, 1267–1284.

Krassioukov, A., Linsenmeyer, T.A., Beck, L.A., Elliott, S., Gorman, P., Kirshblum, S., Clay, S., 2021. Evaluation and management of autonomic dysreflexia and other autonomic dysfunctions: preventing the highs and lows: management of blood pressure, sweating, and temperature dysfunction. Top. Spinal. Cord. Inj. Rehabil. 27, 225–290.

Krebs, J., Koch, H., Hartmann, K., Frotzler, A., 2016. The characteristics of posttraumatic syringomyelia. Spinal. Cord. 54, 463–466.

Lehmann, K.G., Lane, J.G., Piepmeier, J.M., Batsford, W.P., 1987. Cardiovascular abnormalities accompanying acute spinal cord injuries in humans: incidence, time course and severity. J. Am. Coll. Cardiol. 10, 46–52.

Levasseur, A., Mac-Thiong, J.-M., Richard-Denis, A., 2021. Are early clinical manifestations of spasticity associated with long-term functional outcome following spinal cord injury? A retrospective study. Spinal. Cord. 59, 910–916.

Linn, W.S., Spungen, A.M., Gong Jr., H., Adkins, R.H., Bauman, W.A., Waters, R.L., 2001. Forced vital capacity in two large outpatient populations with chronic spinal cord injury. Spinal. Cord. 39, 263–268.

Marquez-Chin, C., Popovic, M.R., 2020. Functional electrical stimulation therapy for restoration of motor function after spinal cord injury and stroke: a review. Biomed. Eng. Online. 19, 34.

Martin, R., Sadowsky, C., Obst, K., et al., 2012. Functional electrical stimulation in spinal cord injury: theory to practice. Top. Spinal. Cord. Rehabil. 18, 28–33.

Mateo, S., Roby-Brami, A., Reilly, K.T., et al., 2015. Upper limb kinematics after cervical spinal cord injury: a review. J. Neuroeng. Rehabil. 12, 9–12.

MacGregor, J., 1981. The evaluation of patient performance using long-term ambulatory monitoring technique in the domicillary environment. Physiotherapy. 67, 30–33.

McKinley, W.O., Jackson, A.B., Cardenas, D.D., DeVivo, M.J., 1999. Long term medical complications after a traumatic spinal cord injury: a regional model systems analysis. Arch. Phys. Med. Rehabil. 80, 1402–1410.

McKinley, W., Santos, K., Meade, M., Brooke, K., 2007. Incidence and outcomes of spinal cord injury clinical syndromes. J. Spinal. Cord. Med. 30, 215–224.

Mehrholz, J., Pohl, M., Platz, T., Kugler, J., Elsner, B., 2015. Electromechanical and robot-assisted arm training for improving activities of daily living, arm function, and arm muscle strength after stroke. Cochrane. Database. Syst. Rev. 7, CD006876.

Milicevic, S., Piscevic, V., Bukumiric, Z., et al., 2014. Analysis of the factors influencing outcomes in patients with spinal cord injury. J. Phys. Ther. Sci. 26.

Mueller, G., Hopman, M.T.E., Perret, C., 2013. Comparison of respiratory muscle training methods in individuals with motor and sensory complete tetraplegia: a randomized controlled trial. J. Rehabil. Med. 45, 248–253.

Multidisciplinary Association of Spinal Cord Injury Professionals (MASCIP)., 2017. Guidance for Paediatric Physiotherapists Managing Childhood Onset Spinal Cord Injuries. Available at: https://www.mascip.co.uk/wp-content/uploads/2017/11/guidance_for_paediatric_physiotherapists_managing_childhood_onset_spinal_cord_injuries_2017.pdf.

Multidisciplinary Association of Spinal Cord Injury Professionals (MASCIP), 2015a. MASCIP Bowel Guidelines. Available at: https://www.mascip.co.uk/wp-content/uploads/2015/02/CV653N-Neurogenic-Guidelines-Sept-2012.pdf.

Multidisciplinary Association of Spinal Cord Injury Professionals (MASCIP), 2019. Clinical guideline for standing adults following spinal cord injury. Spinal Cord Injury Centre Physiotherapy Lead Clinicians. Available at: https://www.mascip.co.uk/wp-content/uploads/2015/05/Clinical-Guidelines-for-Standing-Adults-Following-Spinal-Cord-Injury.pdf.

Multidisciplinary Association of Spinal Cord Injury Professionals (MASCIP), 2015b. The patient is for turning: the role and use of mechanical turning beds for patients with spinal cord injury, associated major trauma and complex care scenarios. Available at: https://www.mascip.co.uk/wp-content/uploads/2015/02/The-Patient-is-for-Turning-MASCIP-final-290813.pdf.

Nadeau, M., Singh, S., Bélanger, L., et al., 2021. Patient perspective: diagnosis and prognosis of acute spinal cord injuries. Spinal. Cord. 59, 865–873.

Najmanova, K., Neuhauser, C., Krebs, J., et al., 2022. Risk factors for hospital acquired pressure injury in patients with spinal cord injury during first rehabilitation: prospective cohort study. Spinal. Cord. 60, 45–52.

Nakajima, H., Yokogawa, N.M., Sasagawa, T., et al., 2022. The prognostic factors for cervical spinal cord without major bone injury in elderly patients. J. Neurotrauma. 39, 658–666.

National Institute for Health and Care Excellence (NICE)., 2016. Guideline 41: Spinal Injury: Assessment and Initial Management. National Clinical Guideline Centre, London. Available at: https://www.nice.org.uk/guidance/ng41. Accessed on 13 July 2023.

National Institute for Health and Care Excellence (NICE)., 2017. Interventional Procedure overview of intramuscular diaphragm stimulation for ventilator-dependent chronic respiratory failure caused by high spinal cord injuries. Interventional procedures guidance IPG594.

National Institute for Health and Care Excellence (NICE)., 2022 Rehabilitation after traumatic injury (NG211).

National Pressure Ulcer Advisory Panel (NPUAP)., 2019. Prevention and treatment of pressure ulcers: clinical practice guideline. Available at: https://internationalguideline.com/2019.

New, P.W., Marshall, R., 2014. International spinal cord injury data sets for non-traumatic spinal cord injury. Spinal. Cord. 52, 123–132.

Newman, M., Barker, K., 2012. The effect of supported standing in adults with upper motor neurone disorders: a systematic review. Clin. Rehabil. 26, 1059–1077.

NHS England Service., 2013. Standards for children and young people (<19 yrs) requiring spinal cord injury care. Available at: https://www.england.nhs.uk/commissioning/wp-content/uploads/sites/12/2014/04/d13-spinal-cord-0414.pdf. Accessed on 13 July 2023.

Ovechkin, A.V., Vitaz, T.W., Terson de Paleville, D.G., et al., 2013. Quality of residual neuromuscular control and functional deficits in patients with spinal cord injury. Front. Neurosci. 4, 174.

Patil, S., Raza, W.A., Jamil, F., et al., 2014. Functional electrical stimulation for the upper limb in tetraplegic spinal cord injury: a systematic review. J. Med. Eng. Technol. 39, 419–423.

Peeters, L.H.C., de Groot, I.J.M., Geurts, A.C.H., 2018. Trunk involvement in performing upper extremity activities while seated in neurological patients with a flaccid trunk – A review. Gait Posture. 62, 46–55.

Penn, R.D., Savoy, S.M., Corcos, D., et al., 1989. Intrathecal baclofen for severe spinal spasticity. N. Engl. J. Med. 320, 1517–1521.

Polese, J.C., Ada, L., Dean, C.M., Nascimento, L., Teixeira-Salmela, L., 2013. Treadmill training is effective for ambulatory adults with stroke: a systematic review. J. Physiother. 59, 73–80.

Postans, N.J., Hasler, J.P., Granat, M.H., et al., 2004. Functional electric stimulation to augment partial weight-bearing supported treadmill training for patients with acute incomplete spinal cord injury: a pilot study. Arch. Phys. Med. Rehabil. 85, 604–610.

Poynton, A.R., O'Farrel, D.A., Shannon, F., et al., 1997. Sparing of sensation to pinprick predicts motor recovery of a motor segment after injury to the spinal cord. J. Bone. Joint. Surg. 79, 952–954.

Price, M., Trbovich, M., 2018. Thermoregulation following spinal cord injury. Handbook. Clin. Neurol. 157, 799–820.

Prigent, H., Roche, N., Laffont, I., et al., 2010. Relation between corset use and lung function postural variation in spinal cord injury. Eur. Respir. J. 35, 1126–1129.

Ramer, M.S., Harper, G.P., Bradbury, E.J., 2000. Progress in spinal cord research. A refined strategy for the International Spinal Research Trust. Spinal. Cord. 38, 449–472.

Reznik, J., Simmons, J., 2020. Rehabilitation in Spinal Cord Injuries. Elsevier, Sydney Australia.

Rice, L.A., Peters, J., Fliflet, A., Sung, J., Rice, I.M., 2022. The influence of shoulder pain and fear of falling on level and non-level transfer technique. J. Spinal. Cord. Med. 45, 364–372.

RISCI, 2017. Weaning guidelines for spinal cord injured patients in critical care units. Available at: http://risci.org.uk/weaning-guidelines-for-spinal-cord-injured-patients-in-critical-care-units. Accessed on 13 July 2023.

Ruiz, I.A., Squiar, J.W., Phillips, A.A., et al., 2018. Incidence and natural progression of neurogenic shock after traumatic spinal cord injury. J. Neurotrauma. 35, 461–466.

Sadowsky, C.L., McDonald, J., 2009. Activity-based restorative therapies: concepts and applications in spinal cord injury-related neurorehabilitation. Dev. Disabil. Res. Rev. 15, 112–116.

Santos, M., Zahner, L.H., McKiernan, B.J., Mahnken, J.D., Quaney, B., 2006. Neuromuscular electrical stimulation improves severe hand dysfunction for individuals with chronic stroke: a pilot study. J. Neurol. Phys. Ther. 30, 175–183.

SCIFERTO Spinal Cord Injury Therapy Leads., 2016. Available at: mascip.co.uk. Accessed on 13 July 2023.

Scivoletto, G., Tamburella, F., Laurenza, L., Torre, M., Molinari, M., 2014. Who is going to walk? A review of the factors influencing walking recovery after spinal cord injury. Front. Hum. Neurosci. 8, 141.

Sheerin, F., 2005. Spinal cord injury: causation and pathophysiology. Emerg. Nurse. 12, 29–38.

Siddall, P., McCabe, R., 2014. The Spinal Cord Injury Pain Book. Hammond Care Media, Australia.

Siddall, P., Middleton, J.W., 2015. Spinal cord injury-induced pain: mechanisms and treatments. Pain. Manag. 5, 493–507.

Smith, E., Finn, S., Fitzpatrick, P., 2017. Epidemiology of pediatric traumatic and acquired nontraumatic spinal cord injury in Ireland. Top. Spinal. Cord. Inj. Rehabil. 23, 279–284.

Soleyman-Jahi, S., Yousefian, A., Maheronnaghsh, R., et al., 2018. Evidence-based prevention and treatment of osteoporosis after spinal cord injury: a systematic review. Eur. Spine. J. 27, 1798–1814.

Steel, A.W., Welch, J.F., Townson, A., 2018. Respiratory management following spinal cord injury. Available at: https://scireproject.com/wp-content/uploads/FINAL-Resp-V6-Chapter-May-30-2018.pdf. Accessed on 13 July 2023.

Tamar Weiss, P.L., Keshner, E.A., Levin, M.F., 2014. Virtual Reality for Physical and Motor Rehabilitation. Springer-Verlag, New York.

Tator, C.H., 1998. Biology of neurological recovery and functional restoration after spinal cord injury. Neurosurgery. 42, 696–707.

Teasell, R.W., Arnold, J.M., Krassioukov, A., Delaney, G.A., 2000. Cardiovascular consequences of loss of supraspinal control of the sympathetic nervous system after spinal cord injury. Arch. Phys. Med. Rehabil. 81, 506–516.

Teasell, R.W., Mehta, S., Aubut, J.L., 2010. A systematic review of the therapeutic interventions for heterotopic ossification after spinal cord injury. Spinal. Cord. 48, 512–521.

Terson de Paleville, D.G., Sayenko, D.G., Aslan, S.C., et al., 2014. Respiratory motor function in seated and supine positions in individuals with chronic spinal cord injury. Resp. Physiol. Neurobiol. 203, 9–14.

Theriault, E.R., Huang, V., Whiteneck, G., et al., 2018. Antispasmodic medications may be associated with reduced recovery during inpatient rehabilitation after traumatic spinal cord injury. J. Spinal. Cord. Med. 41, 63–71.

Thomas, P., Baldwin, C., Beach, L., et al., 2022. Physiotherapy management for Covid-19 in the acute hospital setting and beyond: an update to clinical practice recommendations. J. Physiother. 68, 8–26.

Thomaz, S., Beraldo, P., Mateus, S., Horan, T., Leal, J.C., 2005. Effects of partial isothermic immersion on the spirometry parameters of tetraplegic patients. Chest 128, 184–189.

Umbach, I., Heilporn, A., 1991. Review article: post-spinal cord injury syringomyelia. Paraplegia. 29, 219–221.

Vaccaro, D.H., Weir, J.P., Noonavath, M., et al., 2022. Orthostatic systemic and cerebral hemodynamics in newly injured patients with spinal cord injury. Autonom. Neurosci. 240, 102973.

Van Houtte, S., Vanlandewijck, Y., Kiekens, C., Spengler, C.M., Gosselink, R., 2008. Patients with acute spinal cord injury benefit from normocapnic hyperpnoea training. J. Rehabil. Med. 40, 119–125.

van der Salm, A., Veltink, P.H., Maarten, J., et al., 2006. Comparison of electric stimulation methods for reduction of triceps surae spasticity in spinal cord injury. Arch. Phys. Med. Rehabil. 87, 222–228.

Van der Scheer, J.W., Goosey-Tolfrey, V., Valention, S.E., et al., 2021. Functional electrical stimulation cycling exercise after spinal cord injury: systematic review of health and fitness – related outcomes. J. Neuroeng. Rehabil. 18, 99.

van Middendorp, J.J., Hosman, A.J., Donders, A.R., et al., 2011. A clinical prediction rule for ambulation outcomes after traumatic spinal cord injury: a longitudinal cohort study. Lancet. 377, 1004–1010.

van Straaten, M.G., Cloud, B.A., Zhao, K.D., Fortune, E., Morrow, M.M.B., 2017. Maintaining shoulder health after spinal cord injury: a guide to understanding treatments for shoulder pain. Arch. Phys. Med. Rehabil. 98, 1061–1063.

Vannemreddy, S.S., Rowed, D.W., Bharatwal, N., 2002. Posttraumatic syringomyelia: predisposing factors. Br. J. Neurosurg. 16, 276–286.

Walker, J.R., Detloff, M.R., 2021. Plasticity in cervical motor circuits following spinal cord injury and rehabilitation. Biology. 10, 976.

Wilson, J.R., Forgione, N., Fehlings, M.G., 2013. Emerging therapies for acute traumatic spinal cord injury. Can. Med. J. 185, 485–492.

Williams, G.P., Greenwood, K.M., et al., 2006. High-Level Mobility Assessment Tool (HiMAT): interrater reliability, retest reliability, and internal consistency. Phys. Ther. 86, 395–400.

USEFUL WEBSITES

American Spinal Injury Association (ASIA): http://www.asia-spinalinjury.org/learning

British Orthopaedic Association: http://Boa.ac.uk

elearnSCI.org: http://www.elearnsci.org

International Spinal Cord Society: http://www.iscos.org.uk

University of Louisville: http://louisville.edu/medicine/news/spinal-cord-injury-research-bonus-benefit-to-activity-based-training

Multidisciplinary Association for Spinal Cord Injury Professionals: http://www.mascip.co.uk

National Spinal Cord Injury Statistical Center—University of Alabama: https://www.nscisc.uab.edu

Neuro Orthopaedic Institute: http://www.noigroup.com

http://www.nscisc.edu

PhysioTherapy eXercises: http://www.physiotherapyexercises.com

http://www.rehabmeasure.com

National Spinal Cord Injury Database: http://www.spinalcordinjury.nhs.uk

Spinal Cord Injury Research Evidence: http://www.scireproject.com

World Health Organization: http://www.WHO.int

10

Multiple Sclerosis

Jennifer A. Freeman and Hilary Gunn

OUTLINE

Introduction, 235
　Epidemiology, 235
Pathophysiology, 236
Clinical Presentation, 237
Diagnosis, 237
Classification, 238
Medical Management, 239
　Disease-Modifying Therapies in Active Disease, 239
　Challenges Associated With Disease-Modifying
　　Therapies, 239
　Prognosis, 239
　Sign and Symptoms, 240
　The Health and Social Care Team, 240
　Physiotherapy Assessment, 241
　Time Course and Corresponding Management, 242
　Health Promotion, Lifestyle Modifications and
　　Comorbidities, 243
　Restorative Rehabilitation, 243
　Maintenance Rehabilitation, 243
　Service Delivery, 244
Interventions, 244
　Impaired Mobility, Balance and Falls, 244
　Sedentary Behaviour, Weakness and Deconditioning, 246

　Upper Limb Impairment, 247
　Ataxia, 247
　Spasticity, 247
　Fatigue, 248
　Pain, 250
　Vestibulopathy, 250
　Respiratory Dysfunction, 251
　Heat Sensitivity, 251
　Bladder and Bowel, 251
　Cognitive Impairment, 252
　Anxiety and Depression, 252
Secondary Complications, 252
　Contractures, 252
　Pressure Ulcers, 252
Conclusion, 253
Case Study, 253
　History of Presenting Complaint, 253
　Medication: Vitamin D, Amantandine for Fatigue, 254
　Key Assessment Findings, 254
　Treatment Plan, 254
　Progress Review at 3 Months, 255

INTRODUCTION

Multiple sclerosis (MS) is a progressive long-term neurological disorder of the central nervous system (CNS) that directly affects the lives of individuals with the condition, their family and friends. The physical, cognitive and psychosocial consequences of MS are often wide-ranging, variable and complex. Because the disease progresses at differing rates over several decades, the needs of the individual change over time, sometimes suddenly and unexpectedly.

Effective management therefore requires a long-term and proactive rehabilitation approach, with a multidisciplinary team working in partnership with the person with MS and their family. Ideally this begins from the point of diagnosis and evolves as the disease progresses.

Epidemiology

MS is the most common cause of nontraumatic neurological disability in young adults, affecting approximately 2.8

million individuals worldwide (Walton 2020). Its documented prevalence generally rises with increasing distance from the equator, although there are exceptions to this pattern (Leray et al 2016). Whilst most people are diagnosed with MS in young adulthood, there are at least 30,000 people under the age of 18 living with MS worldwide (Walton 2020). The incidence of MS declines in those older than 50 years of age (Kamm et al 2014), and most people presenting in later life (over the age of 60 years) have a progressive course from the start (McGinley et al 2021). The ratio of females to males diagnosed with MS is around 3:1; however, a higher predominance of males are diagnosed with primary progressive MS (Lassmann 2019).

The cause of MS is uncertain, although epidemiological evidence suggests involvement of environmental, genetic and epigenetic factors. Environmental (low vitamin D levels, infection with Epstein–Barr virus) and lifestyle factors (diet, cigarette smoking and obesity) are now thought to play a bigger part in susceptibility than genetic factors (Thompson et al 2018a). This is important because some of these risk factors are modifiable (Olsson et al 2017). Although MS is not considered a hereditary disease, multiple gene involvement has been demonstrated. It remains unknown how these factors interact in the development of the disease, but the current consensus is that environmental factors trigger an autoimmune reaction against CNS myelin in genetically susceptible individuals (Dobson & Giovannoni 2019).

PATHOPHYSIOLOGY

MS is a chronic disease of the CNS, whereby autoimmune-mediated inflammatory processes lead to primary demyelination and later degeneration in the white and grey matter of the brain and spinal cord. Such responses might be initiated intrinsically (i.e., from within the CNS) or extrinsically (e.g., an abnormal autoimmune response following systemic infection or exposure to other trigger factors) (Thompson 2018a). Inflammatory demyelination interrupts saltatory conduction, typically leading to the acute onset of symptoms, which gradually reduce over time as the inflammatory cycle resolves (Thompson 2018a). Diffuse inflammation and neurodegeneration throughout the brain leading to more progressive symptoms is also a feature. This is more pronounced later in the disease course, but imaging evidence suggests that these processes may also be present at an early stage. Neurodegeneration is thought to be associated with loss of neural reserve and the gradual accumulation of disability over time (Lassman 2019) (Fig. 10.1).

Research suggests that the pathological processes in MS include two distinct types of inflammatory response. The first is an acute inflammatory response, where an autoimmune cascade leads to changes to the blood–brain barrier

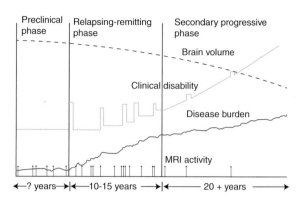

FIG. 10.1 Typical clinical and MRI activity of MS. MRI measuring inflammatory activity (vertical arrows), total volume of MRI lesions (purple), clinical disability (grey) and brain volume (dotted line). (Adapted from Fox & Cohen 2001 with permission).

that enable migration of T and B lymphocytes into the CNS, and activation of proinflammatory macrophage and microglial cells within the CNS. These processes typically lead to acute episodes of neurological deficits known as relapses, which are characterized by the development of focal areas of demyelination with variable axonal injury, which are commonly called lesions or plaques. Symptoms depend on the size and location of the lesions, which may manifest at any point throughout the brain and spinal cord (McGinley et al 2021). In contrast, chronic inflammatory processes are associated with minimal invasion of the blood–brain barrier and are more frequently seen within the meninges and periventricular areas of the brain (Lassmann 2019). Features of the innate immune response such as microglial activation and diffuse lymphocytic and monocytic infiltration are characteristic (Ponath 2018). The resultant inflammatory damage is associated with slow expansion of existing focal lesions, subpial cortical demyelination and widespread damage within cortical white and grey matter (Lassmann 2019).

Alongside the inflammatory mechanisms summarised above, other neurodegenerative processes are likely to contribute to the gradual accumulation of disability over time, which is characteristic of progressive forms of MS. These processes include degeneration of chronically demyelinated axons, which may be associated with mitochondrial dysfunction and/or loss of myelin trophic support (Mahad et al 2015). In addition, damage to or dysfunction of glial cells including astrocytes may affect neuronal homeostasis via a range of mechanisms, including disrupted glutamate handling and impaired redox homeostasis (Ponath 2018).

Neurodegeneration can be demonstrated on magnetic resonance imaging (MRI) scans as loss of brain white matter, ventricular dilation and degeneration of the long ascending and descending tracts of the brainstem and spinal cord. This element of MS pathology is considered a key component of the accelerated rates of brain atrophy that are seen in people with MS when compared with people of a similar age. It is critically important because of its significant contribution to the development of irreversible disability (Mahad et al 2015).

Despite the significant inflammatory and degenerative CNS changes associated with MS, many people experience symptomatic improvements after relapses. Again, there are several contributory mechanisms. During acute episodes, myelin debris is absorbed as part of the cascade of inflammation and repair, and lesions eventually reach a burned-out stage consisting of demyelinated axons surrounded by glial scar tissue. In the earlier stages of MS, there is evidence of limited, although incomplete, remyelination. Oligodendroglial progenitor cells, which can mature into oligodendrocytes, infiltrate the demyelinated area and provide partial remyelination of axons (Thompson 2018a). In addition to myelin repair, the recovery of clinical symptoms could also be secondary to cortical plasticity, which is associated with reorganisation of the functional activation of cortical regions to maintain clinical function (Prosperini 2019). In later stages of the disease, several processes may interact, meaning that recovery typically becomes more limited. Firstly, the repaired myelin sheath typically has a reduced density and quality compared with unaffected myelin, which may eventually affect neuronal function. Secondly, oligodendrocyte function is affected by recurrent inflammatory attacks, and repeated gliosis creates physical barriers between the oligodendrocytes and their axonal targets. Finally, gradual loss of neural reserve associated with repeated inflammatory episodes and ongoing neurodegeneration means that the capacity for neuroplasticity becomes increasingly limited over time. Thus, early intervention, through targeted disease-modifying treatments to reduce the frequency and severity of inflammatory activity, is a clinical priority (Cerqueira et al 2018).

CLINICAL PRESENTATION

Early MS is usually characterised by an acute relapsing presentation. Presenting symptoms depend on both the area of the CNS affected by the acute inflammatory demyelinating lesions and the extent of the inflammatory process (Thompson 2018a). Initial symptoms are highly variable but commonly include sensory disturbance, pain, fatigue and visual problems (McGinley et al 2021). For approximately 20% of patients, optic neuritis, which is characterised by visual impairment and pain on eye movements, is the first symptom of MS, as demyelination affects the optic

nerves as they pass through the cerebral cortex. Other visual symptoms may include blurred or double vision, altered colour vision, partial or complete visual loss, usually in one eye at a time. Sudden-onset visual symptoms will often resolve spontaneously; however, ongoing visual problems can be an issue for some people as their MS course progresses (van der Feen 2022).

Not all episodes of inflammation lead to clinically apparent symptoms, and people often report experiencing several 'low level' symptoms before the onset of those which are significant enough to lead them to seek medical input. MRI evidence often indicates the presence of lesions that have developed in the absence of any obvious signs (known as 'silent' lesions). This is likely because of early lesions being small and relatively isolated, along with the significant reserve capacity within many areas of the human CNS. The mismatch between frequency of inflammatory episodes and the appearance of clinical symptoms tends to continue throughout the disease course, although the incidence of inflammatory episodes usually decreases over time as the degenerative aspects of the disease become more significant.

As the clinical course continues, people will often develop multiple primary symptoms, related to specific lesions, which may be interrelated. For example, there can be a combination of motor, sensory, visual and vestibular impairments, fatigue, and cognitive and emotional factors. Many of these issues are described later in the section on symptomatic management. In addition, secondary problems, which develop over time, may compound the clinical situation. For example, age-related neurological changes alongside the accumulation of comorbidities are now recognised as significantly affecting recovery from relapses and contributing to the gradual accumulation of disability over time (Inojosa 2021).

DIAGNOSIS

The diagnosis of MS is based on the integration of clinical, imaging and laboratory findings. It uses specific evidence-based criteria known as the McDonald Criteria (Thompson 2018b). These criteria are regularly updated and are widely used in research and clinical practice. Cardinal signs include evidence of multiple episodes of demyelination that are separated in both time and lesion location within the CNS. The use of MRI to supplement clinical findings is central to the diagnostic process, as scanning techniques can enable the identification of both clinical and subclinical (silent) lesions. MRI can also provide supportive evidence of lesion separation over time, using contrast methods to distinguish active from burned-out lesions.

There is no definitive test for MS, and people will typically undergo a range of investigations and a period of uncertainty before a diagnosis is confirmed. Tests that are commonly used alongside MRI scanning and clinical examination include examination of cerebrospinal fluid samples (obtained via a lumbar puncture) to test for the presence of oligoclonal bands. These bands are indicative of inflammatory processes within the CNS; however, this does not exclude inflammation from other causes, for example, infection or other neurological disease.

Neurophysiological assessment of the integrity of the neuronal pathways may also be undertaken by testing evoked potentials. These tests measure the electrical activity of the brain in response to stimulation of specific sensory nerve pathways. They can detect the slowing of electrical conduction caused by demyelination along these pathways even when the change is too subtle to be observed clinically. Evoked potential testing can evaluate any sensory pathway, but current diagnostic criteria only incorporate the findings of visual-evoked potential testing because these tests are considered the most reliable (Thompson 2018b).

CLASSIFICATION

Whilst there are defined clinical subtypes of MS, it is important to recognise that the presentation and course for each person will be variable and unpredictable. The main differentiation is between relapsing and progressive presentations, which broadly correspond to acute inflammatory and degenerative processes described above. However, it is important to remember that this is a generalisation, and the presence of both pathological elements is noted at all stages. Current thinking is that all types of MS are likely to form part of the same disease continuum, where different pathological processes predominate at different stages (Inojosa 2021).

The three main clinical subtypes of MS are relapsing remitting, secondary progressive and primary progressive (Fig. 10.2). Most people initially present with a relapsing-remitting MS (RRMS) course. This is established if they present with at least two clearly defined acute episodes of neurological deficits (relapses). Symptoms of a clinical relapse typically arise over hours to days, worsen over several weeks, and then gradually subside over several weeks or months. Residual enduring neurological symptoms are common. On average, after 10–15 years the disease in most patients converts into a course of slow progression (secondary progressive MS [SPMS]), where disability gradually accumulates over time, although fluctuations in symptoms (as against distinct relapses) can be

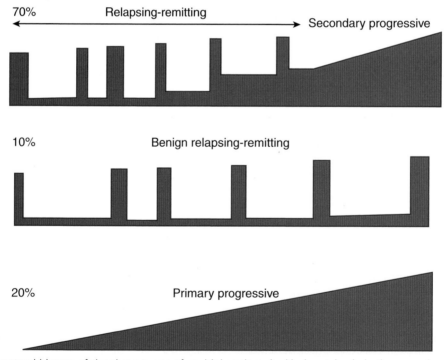

FIG. 10.2 The natural history of the three types of multiple sclerosis. Horizontal axis is time passing, vertical axis is 'disability'. (Reproduced from Coles A. Multiple sclerosis. Pract. Neurol. 2009;9:118–26.).

experienced (Lublin 2014). The transition from relapsing to SPMS is clinically, psychologically and therapeutically significant, particularly because there are limited disease-modifying therapies (DMTs) available to people with progressive forms of MS (Bogosian 2019). However, defining the point at which people enter this progressive phase is not straightforward because some of the symptoms and deterioration in function can occur as a result of the concurrent impacts of ageing and comorbidities (Marrie 2017).

An estimated 15% of people show progression in disability from the outset in the absence of previous relapses, known as primary progressive MS (PPMS) disease. Whilst the pathological processes are similar, lesions in PPMS tend to be more diffuse, less inflammatory and less likely to remyelinate than those occurring in RRMS and SPMS; there are also fewer focal lesions in the brain and proportionately more spinal cord involvement (Tsagkas 2019). Disease onset in this group of patients is typically later than in those with RRMS, usually after the age of 40 years (Harding et al 2015).

In approximately 10% of cases, individuals remain fully functional with little or no disability for a prolonged period following diagnosis (Tallantyre et al 2019). Despite this initial course, some individuals will go on to develop more progressive symptoms, although there is conflicting evidence as to the frequency of this progression (McFaul et al 2021, Schaefer et al 2019).

MEDICAL MANAGEMENT

The medical management of MS is, like the condition itself, complex. There are currently three main pharmacological approaches to management:

- Disease Modifying Therapies (DMTs): Treatments that aim to alter the disease course itself. These include injectable, oral and infusion therapies. The majority of DMTs treat the relapsing-remitting types of MS. As the disease progresses, when neurodegenerative mechanisms predominate, response to DMT typically declines. However, options for people with progressive MS are rapidly evolving and hold considerable promise for the future.
- Treatments to manage relapses: Short courses of oral or intravenous corticosteroids are used to shorten the length of relapses and may improve long-term outcomes.
- Treatments to help manage the symptoms associated with MS: Identification and treatment of symptoms should be considered throughout the disease course. These are discussed in the following section, which describes key symptoms and associated management strategies.

Disease-Modifying Therapies in Active Disease

Currently available DMTs act in a variety of ways to improve the course of MS, primarily through reductions in inflammatory activity leading to improved MRI outcomes, such as reduced number and volume of lesions. For people with RRMS, the use of DMTs is associated with a lower risk of disability accumulation and may delay the onset of secondary progression (Inojosa 2021), although measures of long-term disability, patient satisfaction and quality of life remain underresearched (Rae-Grant et al 2018).

People with PPMS and SPMS may also be eligible for DMT when there is evidence of active (inflammatory) disease, with evidence to suggest reductions in disability progression and measures of brain atrophy. However, these changes may be relatively modest, and when neurodegenerative mechanisms predominate, the response to DMT typically declines. Developing effective therapies for people with MS remains a priority (Faissner & Gold 2019).

Challenges Associated With Disease-Modifying Therapies

Early treatment with DMTs in active MS is now widely recommended with the aim of reducing clinical and subclinical inflammatory disease activity. However, evidence has identified that some of these treatments can also carry significant risks. Current guidelines encourage the development of 'personalised' strategies, which balance the potential implications of ongoing disease activity against possible risks of treatments. Meaningful discussions between neurologists/specialist MS nurses and patients are essential to achieve this balance. The main MS charities (e.g., MS Society [UK], MS Trust [UK], National MS Society [USA]) provide excellent, user-friendly guides to the DMTs that are currently available and are recommended as up-to-date sources for reference purposes. Whatever the approach, regular reviews to assess tolerability, adherence, side effects and the potential benefit of DMTs, and adjust dosage accordingly, are essential (Wingerchuck & Weinshenker 2016).

The Covid-19 pandemic, in situ since 2020, has led to a period of uncertainty for many because of the impact of DMTs on the immune system and the potential for increased risk of contracting or experiencing complications of Covid-19 infection. However, evidence suggests the risks for people with MS are generally moderate, and that the potential benefits of therapy outweigh any risks, provided appropriate monitoring and support is available (Giovannoni 2020).

Prognosis

Advances in healthcare mean that people with MS are living longer, with estimates suggesting that, on average, people with MS live approximately six years less than the general population (Kaufman 2014). The variability of the disease means that prognosis is difficult to predict. It is likely that both disease and person-specific factors are important, with current theories proposing five key factors associated with clinical outcome: localisation and number of lesions (as characterised by a high radiological lesion density), frequency, severity and recovery of relapses, and brain volume at baseline and subsequent atrophy (Inojosa 2021). However, for people affected by MS, prognostic features that are suggestive of developing progression/conversion to a secondary progressive course may be more clinically meaningful. These include multifocal disease manifestation at onset, presence of spinal cord lesions in the first 3 years, an initial presentation that includes balance and walking problems, and the presence of cerebellar and pyramidal symptoms (Degenhardt et al 2009).

Alongside disease-specific factors that influence prognosis, increased life expectancy has highlighted the important potential interaction between processes associated with 'normal' ageing and MS pathology. In particular, the reduction in neurological compensatory mechanisms (which are to a great extent age-related) over time may be key to worsening clinical manifestations of disease as people with MS get older (Cree et al 2019).

Sign and Symptoms

The nature of MS means that a wide range of clinical signs and symptoms may be experienced by each person (Fig. 10.3). For many people, most of their MS symptoms may be relatively 'invisible' to others, whilst still negatively affecting their emotional and social well-being (Parker et al 2021).

Many primary symptoms (those which are caused directly by the neuropathological processes of MS) directly relate to the anatomical area of the CNS region affected, with symptoms developing as lesions appear in different areas of the cerebral hemispheres, cerebellum, brainstem and the spinal cord (see Table 10.1 for examples).

Other symptoms, such as fatigue and pain, appear to be more global in their origin. In addition, demyelinated axons can become hyperexcitable and spontaneously generate impulses that can be distressing for individuals, such as the perception of flashing light upon eye movements or sudden shooting pain in a limb.

The Health and Social Care Team

Physiotherapists are important members of the multidisciplinary team (MDT) involved in the management of people with MS. Given the wide range of symptoms associated with MS, issues around progressive physical and cognitive disability, psychosocial adaptation, and limitations in activity and participation levels will occur over long periods. A collaborative and coordinated multidisciplinary teamwork approach (including health and social care and third sector organisations) is essential to ensure access to the right professional at the right time and in the right place (Amatya et al 2019).

Clinical guidelines (NICE 2022) advocate comprehensive, flexible and responsive review and reassessment systems to ensure ongoing support is available for people with MS and their carers. The traditional approach to review, where set reassessments are scheduled, regardless of any changes in the person's clinical or personal situation, is unlikely to meet this need. Flexible systems (e.g., self-referral, telephone support and web-based resources) that allow individuals to access services when their needs change may be more effective to help people to self-manage their condition. The increased use of remote delivery of services accelerated by the Covid-19 pandemic has highlighted some of the opportunities and challenges that telerehabilitation may present (Portaccio et al 2022). Regardless of the means of communication, to work successfully, people

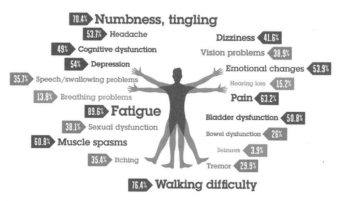

FIG. 10.3 The range of MS symptoms (Reproduced with permission from MS Wellington).

TABLE 10.1 Examples of MS Symptoms and Possible Lesion Locations[a]

CNS Location	Possible Symptoms
Cerebral cortex	Cognitive issues, motor problems (including weakness and spasticity), sensory dysfunction, visual deficits, dysarthria and dysphagia
Optic tracts[b]	Visual deficits
Cerebellum	Ataxia (including speech issues) and tremor
Brainstem	Vestibular and balance issues (including dizziness and vertigo), autonomic problems, dysarthria and dysphagia
Spinal cord	Weakness, sensory dysfunction, bladder and bowel issues, sexual dysfunction, spasticity/spasms

[a]This list is not exhaustive. Remember that each individual will present with different problems, and that lesion location/size is not always directly associated with symptom severity.
[b]Although the optic nerves are part of the peripheral nervous system, they are myelinated by oligodendrocytes and are therefore often affected in MS.

with MS and their families need to know how, why and when they should make contact. Mechanisms should be provided to support people with marked cognitive impairment, emotional issues or those who may struggle to identify when professional input may be of value. Importantly, the need to manage disability and deficits over time should be anticipated, systems to support functional independence provided and 'crisis management' avoided where possible.

Physiotherapy Assessment

The unpredictable and fluctuating nature of MS means that physiotherapy assessment cannot be a one-off process, even during a single episode of care. The presence of MS-related fatigue and cognitive impairments emphasises the need for assessments to be adapted to individual circumstances, with therapists working flexibly and sensitively, prioritising where necessary. Where appropriate, support and advice should be sought from other members of the MDT to ensure that assessments are appropriately tailored.

Each assessment will draw on a variety of skills from across the spectrum of clinical practice to evaluate the range of factors that are contributing to the person's problems. Central to this is the need to use the same principles of best practice that underpin all physiotherapy assessments:

good communication, patient-centredness and a holistic, problem-solving approach.

Building an in-depth understanding of the individual's problems and the impact of these issues at an activity and participation level is a priority. People with long-term conditions, such as MS, constantly make adaptations to their daily lifestyle and functional activities as symptoms develop and change over time; therefore, they may not spontaneously identify problems that have gradually evolved. In addition, the invisibility of many symptoms, as well as people's wish not to 'give in', can mean that problems are minimised or not disclosed on initial discussion (Parker et al 2021). Therefore, guidelines (NICE 2022) recommend that assessments include a comprehensive annual review of a person's activities and participations alongside specific questions about common MS symptoms to aid the identification of problems that may not otherwise be mentioned by the patient (Table 10.2). Including significant others in this discussion may also be valuable, especially when the person with MS has cognitive impairments. However, care should be taken to maintain the person with MS at the centre of the discussion to ensure the problem list accurately reflects their circumstances and priorities.

Effective assessment enables the therapist and the person with MS to develop a working hypothesis about the key issues contributing to their problems. Subsequently, they need to work together to agree the desired outcome(s) of therapy and to develop a feasible and achievable plan. It is essential that this process involves a meaningful dialogue between the patient and therapist, where the patient is supported to identify their desired course of action. As with all shared goal-setting processes, the role of the therapist is to provide appropriate support, guidance and information to enable the person to reach an informed decision and comprehensive action plan, having identified the potential risks and benefits of the available options (Kang et al 2022). Types of information that may be presented include:

- General and MS-specific health education advice;
- Management options for specific symptoms;
- Implications/avoidance/management of secondary complications; and
- Resources required (including time, energy, finance and logistics).

Guidelines highlight the importance of including appropriate outcome measures within assessment practice (NICE 2022). The range of issues experienced by people with MS, and their varying levels of functional ability, mean that no single measure will be suitable for all patients and circumstances. It is essential that clinicians consider the characteristics and performance of outcome measures before use to ensure suitability because effective targeting of intervention, evaluation of progress and demonstration

---

TABLE 10.2   Checklist of Issues to Explore as Part of the Comprehensive Assessment Process (reproduced from Petty & Davies 2008 with permission)

This is not a list of questions to be asked of every person with MS on every occasion. It is a list to remind clinicians of the wide range of potential problems that people with MS may face, and which should be actively considered. A positive answer should lead to a more detailed assessment and management.

Initial question
It is best to start by asking an open-ended question, such as 'Since you were last seen or assessed, has any activity you used to undertake been limited, stopped or affected?'

Activity domains
Then, especially if nothing has been identified, it is worth asking questions directly, choosing those appropriate to the situation based on your knowledge of the person with MS:
'Are you still able to undertake, as far as you wish:

- vocational activities (work, education, other occupations)?
- leisure activities?

- family roles?

- shopping and other community activities?
- household and domestic activities?

- washing, dressing, using the toilet?

- getting about (either by walking or in other ways) and getting in and out of your house?
- controlling your environment (opening doors, switching things on and off, using the phone)?'

If restrictions are identified, the reasons for these should be identified as far as possible considering impairments (see later), and social and physical factors (contexts).

Common impairments
It is worth asking about specific impairments from the subsequent list, again adapting to the situation and what you already know.
'Since you were last seen have you developed any new problems with:

- fatigue, endurance, being overtired
- speech and communication
- balance and falling
- chewing and swallowing food and drink
- unintended change in weight
- pain or painful abnormal sensations
- control over your bladder or bowels

- control over your movement
- vision and your eyes
- thinking, remembering
- your mood
- your sexual function or partnership relations
- how you get on in social situations?'

Final question
It is always worth finishing off with a further open-ended question: 'Are there any other new problems that you think might be caused by MS that concern you?'

---

of the value and impact of therapy depend on the use of appropriate outcome measures. The ability of a measure to reflect progress towards the agreed aims of therapy is particularly important, especially given that for many people with MS, maintenance or slowing of deterioration may be considered positive outcomes.

See Academy of Neurologic Physical Therapy Outcome Measures Recommendations (EDGE) (2012) for further information and associated references.

Time Course and Corresponding Management

To ensure management is successful, there should be good communication and timely referral between professionals to meet an individual's needs. The physiotherapist's role focuses on physical management, although consideration of cognitive and emotional issues is fundamental to this.

The approach to management can be viewed in three ways. Whilst each has a varying emphasis, together they provide a continuum of care across the disease course.

MS-SPECIFIC OUTCOME MEASURES

- 12-item Multiple Sclerosis Walking Scale Version 2.0 (Hobart et al 2003)
- Multiple Sclerosis Impact Scale-29 Version 2.0 (Hobart et al 2001)
- Fatigue Scale for Motor and Cognitive Functions (Penner et al 2009)
- Brief International Cognitive Assessment for Multiple Sclerosis (Langdon 2012) (cognition)

Other Relevant Measures
- 9-Hole Peg Test (upper limb function)

- 2-Minute Walk Test (gait)
- Timed 25-Foot/10-Metre Walk Test (gait)
- 6-Minute Walk Test (endurance)
- Functional Reach Test (balance)
- MiniBEST (balance)
- ABC Balance Confidence
- 4 Square Step Test
- Minimum Inspiratory/Expiratory Pressures (respiratory function)

Health Promotion, Lifestyle Modifications and Comorbidities

There is evidence to suggest a role for behavioural and lifestyle modification in the medical management of MS. Although more research is required, some studies suggest that vitamin D supplementation and cessation of tobacco smoking could enhance the benefits of DMTs. The promotion of a 'brain-healthy' lifestyle to optimise brain volume and cognitive reserve is also now being emphasised as a priority. The brain health approach emphasises the maintenance of neural reserve to help mitigate the negative impact of neurodegenerative changes (Giovannoni et al 2017), thus minimising the effects of MS pathology (Brandstadter et al 2019). This includes avoidance of smoking and excessive alcohol consumption, promoting participation in aerobic exercise and weight loss, as evidence suggests these changes can positively affect MS outcomes (Giovannoni et al 2016).

Health promotion is also an increasing focus, as evidence emerges that rates of diabetes, hypertension and hyperlipidaemia are greater amongst people with MS than the general population (Marrie 2017). It is essential that these are identified and managed appropriately because they may directly increase disability, reduce quality of life and life expectancy and affect DMT selection and treatment concordance. There is a key role for physiotherapists in facilitating behaviour change, particularly with regard to physical activity and exercise, as well as working with MDT members to ensure a full range of healthy lifestyle changes are embedded and supported.

Restorative Rehabilitation

Clinical guidelines recommend early referral for rehabilitation with the aim of restoring recent functional deterioration and helping people to maintain their usual roles (NICE 2022). The approaches used are based on a comprehensive assessment of the unique needs of the individual. Modifiable impairments (such as weakness, spasticity, pain

and emotional distress) may be the focus where these are identified as the primary contributors to functional limitations. However, where changes are not possible/limited, then improvements can often still be achieved through the acquisition of new skills. For those with complex disability, this may require provision of adaptive equipment and modifications to the environment.

There is also a growing evidence base for many of the other rehabilitation interventions used for people with MS; this evidence is presented later in this chapter. However, the nature of MS means that the benefits gained will often reduce over time. Therefore, rehabilitation cannot be viewed as a 'one-off' intervention, and targeted rereferral will usually be required at various time points throughout the disease course.

Maintenance Rehabilitation

The personal and economic costs of worsening disability over many years may be significant (Ernstsson et al 2016). People with severe disabilities may endure complications such as aspiration pneumonia, urinary tract infections, falls and fractures, and sepsis secondary to pressure ulcers over many years (Higginson et al 2006). All these issues are major causes of morbidity and mortality; therefore, timely support from health and social care professionals is essential to aid management.

Much of the physical and emotional burden of caring for a person with severe disability falls on family members, many of whom become lifelong caregivers. The physical tasks of caring can be daunting and exhausting; however, carers describe adjusting to and managing the cognitive impairments associated with MS as being particularly difficult (Borreani et al 2014). Feelings of loneliness and isolation are also significant, not only for the person with MS, but also for their family and caregivers (Freeman et al 2020).

Caregiver support needs are often overlooked (Maguire 2020), and this can be compounded by the fact that carers themselves may reject offers of support (Davies et al 2015).

Provision of respite, community and/or long-term care, and support to address complex mobility issues may all be valuable options. For example, educating carers about how they can best help the person with MS to move and to achieve a comfortable position in bed and in the wheelchair can go some way to help to reduce the burden of care. Key too is the provision of equipment such as hoists, transfer aids, specialist beds, mattresses and seating to assist carers and to ensure care can be provided safely and effectively.

In the latter stages of the disease, there is an increasing overlap between neurorehabilitation and neuropalliative care. Unlike other palliative contexts, coping with disability rather than end of life is reported to be the major concern of people with MS and their carers. There is increasing evidence supporting the effectiveness of palliative care in improving symptoms and the quality of life of patients with MS and their families (Solari et al 2020).

Service Delivery

Alongside the range of management approaches, there is increasing variety in the methods by which physiotherapy may be accessed and delivered. Traditionally, most contacts were face to face, delivered in a variety of contexts. Whilst most physiotherapy contacts remain outpatient and community based, there is evidence that specialist inpatient rehabilitation for people with neurological problems (including MS) can be highly cost-efficient, yielding significant savings in ongoing care costs, especially in those with more complex disability (Turner-Stokes et al 2016, Zuber et al 2020).

More recently (partly driven by the Covid-19 pandemic), there has been an increase in telerehabilitation, where rehabilitation services are provided remotely through telephone, video calls, software applications (apps) and online platforms (Yeroushalmi et al 2022) (Fig. 10.4). These methods offer advantages in terms of accessibility when there are barriers such as geographical remoteness, economic constraints or physical disabilities with some preliminary evidence to support the benefits gained using this method of delivery (Karakas 2021). The increasing use of technology such as apps and online platforms may also offer benefits in terms of providing ongoing information, supporting people to self-manage or as a supplementary resource for rehabilitation. However, issues such as digital exclusion must not be ignored, and feedback from therapists and people with MS highlights limitations to the potential loss of face-to-face contact. Together, this suggests that in the long term telerehabilitation is likely to become part of the range of approaches rather than a replacement for other contact methods (Buckingham et al 2022).

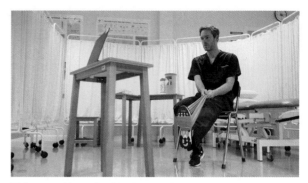

FIG. 10.4 Use of telerehabilitation.

INTERVENTIONS

Impaired Mobility, Balance and Falls

People with MS consistently rate mobility as one of their most important yet challenging daily functions (Heesen 2018). Moreover, gait and balance issues are among the most frequently reported symptoms, with an estimated 93% of people experiencing walking difficulties 10 years after diagnosis (Soler et al 2020). Mobility impairments frequently restrict participation in work, family, social, vocational and leisure activities. Therefore, maintaining walking ability for as long as possible is a key priority for people with MS, and hence should be an important focus of therapy throughout the disease course.

Studies show that even in the early stages of the disease course, changes occur in the speed and pattern of walking (Brandstadter et al 2020). Typical spatiotemporal and kinematic factors affected include slower speed, shorter strides, lengthened double limb support, increased step width, reduced heel strike and push-off, reduced knee range of motion and increased variability of movements – all indicative of reduced balance when walking (Chee 2021). Although these deficits can initially be subtle, they can significantly affect the levels of concentration and mental and physical effort that are required when undertaking everyday activities. Particularly affected are dual task activities (e.g., carrying a drink whilst walking) and those requiring higher levels of dynamic balance (e.g., playing sport) or endurance (e.g., walking outdoors).

When disability is mild to moderate, assistive devices such as orthotics (e.g., ankle–foot orthoses, foot-up splints) can be effective at minimising the impact of foot drop, which is a common problem. Another evidence-based alternative is functional electrical stimulation wherein the peroneal nerve is stimulated to activate the dorsiflexors to assist foot clearance and improve foot placement during gait (Miller 2017). Exercise interventions (aerobic, resistance and combined), undertaken regularly and at a moderate to high intensity, can significantly improve walking capacity (Pearson et al 2015) and should be encouraged and supported from the outset. Pharmacological treatments such as fampridine, or those targeting symptoms such as spasticity (e.g., baclofen, gabapentin), are also commonly used to optimise mobility (Soler et al 2020, Valet 2019).

For most people, mobility difficulties gradually increase over time, with accelerated trajectories of impaired walking capacity as people age (Hvid et al 2020). As difficulties progress, the therapist's role in mobility management moves towards the assessment and provision of standing and mobility aids, which includes the use of supported standing frames (Dennett 2020, Freeman et al 2019), manual and powered wheelchairs and scooters (van der Feen 2020) (Fig. 10.5). This is important because an estimated 25% of people eventually rely almost exclusively on a wheelchair (Noseworthy 2000).

Impaired balance is an important contributor to mobility difficulties and falls. Falls are common in MS, with more than half of people falling regularly (Nilsagard 2015). Falls occur across the spectrum of disability, with falls risk relating to an interaction between both physiological and psychological factors (Gunn et al 2018). Whilst the highest rate of recurrent falls occurs in those who do not yet use a

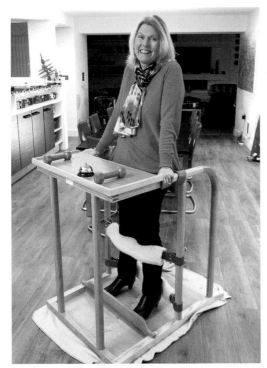

FIG. 10.5 Client in standing frame.

mobility device, the risk of falls is doubled in people with progressive MS, with an estimated 75% of wheelchair or scooter users falling (Coote 2020). Crucially, falling and a fear of falling means that people lose confidence in their walking. In response to this, they may markedly restrict their activities, which can lead to a downward spiral of immobility, deconditioning and accumulation of disability. Physiotherapists play a key role in optimising safe mobility, maintaining physical activity and preventing falls. It is important to ask about falls at all stages of the condition and provide appropriate interventions in a timely manner. The complex nature of falls means that targeted multifactorial interventions examining physiological (e.g., balance impairments, cognitive dysfunction), behavioural (e.g., fear of falling) and environmental (e.g., use of mobility aids) risk are required. This may need input from a variety of MDT members. From a physiotherapy perspective, a range of strategies can be helpful, including balance training and dual task activities, strength training, task-specific training (including overground walking, treadmill walking, body weight-supported treadmill training and robot-assisted gait training), functional electrical stimulation, exercise and gaming technology (Calafiore et al 2021, Karakas 2021, Soler 2020). Systematic reviews of exercise-based interventions suggest that physiotherapy has some beneficial effects on mobility and balance in people with mild to moderate disability (Campbell 2016) but that there is currently insufficient evidence to conclude that this results in a reduction of falls (O'Malley 2021). Although less research has been undertaken in people with more severe disability, there are encouraging data from studies evaluating body weight-supported treadmill training and robot-assisted ambulatory training to indicate that functional gains in mobility and balance can be made in these individuals (Calabro et al 2021). However, it is probable that there is a point at which neural reserve becomes so low that balance and gait impairments do not respond to training.

A wide range of assistive devices can be provided to support safe and effective mobility. The therapist's role is to ensure that these devices are used to their best effect. This includes appropriate assessment, provision and monitoring, as well as education about their use. Over time, the progressive and variable nature of MS means that people with MS may accumulate and use multiple walking devices, choosing to use them according to their current circumstances. For example, they may 'furniture walk' in their own home, use a single stick 'on a good day' or when out with friends, but have a pair of crutches or a wheelchair available to manage longer distances or outdoor terrain. Whilst many people report increased feelings of competence, adaptability and self-esteem through the use of this equipment (Cohen et al 2021), it is not uncommon for them to express reluctance when initially offered these devices because they can be viewed as a symbol of loss of function and a major life transition. The therapist's role is to sensitively support rather than impose the appropriate choice of device, and to educate the individual about their potential benefits, which may include improvements in safety and autonomy, reduced fatigue by energy conservation, reduced risk of falls and increased occupational performance (Rice et al 2021, Stevens 2013).

Sedentary Behaviour, Weakness and Deconditioning

MS has shown to be associated with reduced physical activity levels at all stages of the disease (Backus 2016). Supporting people to be less sedentary and to undertake regular physical activity (including exercise) is important, particularly given the evidence, which suggests that secondary deconditioning contributes to at least some of this disability. There is strong evidence from systematic reviews and meta-analyses demonstrating that both aerobic and resistance training is safe and feasible, offering benefits in improving aerobic capacity, muscle strength, mobility, fatigue, balance, depression and quality of life in people with mild to moderate disability (Andreu-Caravaca et al 2021, Motl et al 2017, Razazian et al 2020). There is also some evidence to support this in those who are more severely disabled (Edwards and Pilutti 2017). In addition, there is some evidence that exercise may improve pain (Demaneuf et al 2019) with variable evidence regarding its impact on cognition (Gharakhanlou et al 2020). Encouragingly, physiological studies suggest that exercise may also have a neuroprotective role (Dalgas 2019), although further research is needed to draw firm conclusions (Sandroff et al 2020).

Exercise and lifestyle physical activity recommendations for people with MS throughout the disease course are available to guide clinicians and people with MS (Kalb et al 2020). These guidelines recommend that people should be encouraged to undertake ≥150 min/week of exercise and/or ≥150 min/week of lifestyle physical activity. Progress toward these targets should be gradual and based on the person's abilities, preferences and safety. More specifically, evidence-based guidelines recommend that people with mild to moderate disability undertake 30 minutes of moderate intensity aerobic exercise (e.g., stationary bicycle, treadmill or rowing machine) and 30 minutes of moderate intensity strength training for major muscle groups twice a week (Latimer-Cheung 2013). This may not be achievable for everyone, and it should be noted that these recommendations are based predominately on studies undertaken with people with RRMS with mild to moderate levels of disability (Feinstein 2015). People with higher levels of disability may have difficulty in tolerating high-intensity training because of motor fatigue and reduced neural reserve and may therefore benefit from longer training duration at low intensity. They may require the use of more sophisticated equipment (such as total body recumbent steppers, body weight-supported treadmill training and robot-assisted training) and/or the support of a trained assistant to achieve these training intensities. Further research is required to provide evidence to further inform exercise prescription in this group, both within supervised and unsupervised environments (Ghahfarrokhi et al 2021).

Supporting people to incorporate physical activity (including exercise) into their lifestyle is key to sustaining benefits over the longer term. This is important because studies repeatedly show that benefits gained are not maintained when exercise is stopped. Ensuring people have the confidence, knowledge, skills, resources and strategies (such as identifying barriers and problem solving) to optimise successful long-term engagement in physical activity/exercise is essential (Silveira et al 2021). Therefore, the use of personally relevant behaviour change techniques alongside exercise interventions is recommended (Plow & Finlayson 2019). Staying active can be challenging at all stages of the disease. Early on, irregular and unpredictable relapses may occur that make planning and adjusting to symptoms difficult. As the disease progresses, physical activity/exercise is often further complicated by the interaction of multiple symptoms that are the hallmark of MS. To navigate these challenges, people may need access to guidance and support from health professionals, sports instructors and voluntary organisations working in partnership, to adapt programmes as circumstances change and to support them to remain physically active and exercise effectively within the limits of their disability (Fig. 10.6).

Upper Limb Impairment

Up to 75% of people with MS experience difficulties with upper limb function, and this is even more common for people in the progressive phase (Lamers 2016). Weakness, ataxia, sensory impairment and fatigue can all contribute to these difficulties. Reduced manual dexterity has found to be a key predictor of activity and participation (Cattaneo 2017). Therefore, it is important that management of the upper limb is incorporated within physiotherapy treatment.

As has shown to be the case for other neurological conditions such as stroke, high-intensity, repetitive, task-specific training is important to achieve successful outcomes. A

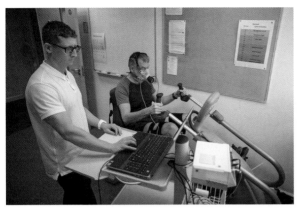

FIG. 10.6 Supervised practice for intensity.

range of interventions can be used, which include task-oriented upper limb training, constraint-induced therapy, strengthening and sensory reeducation training (Lamers 2016, Ortiz et al 2016). New technologies such as active console games and virtual reality are increasingly being incorporated into physical therapy programmes and can transfer well into the home environment (Webster 2021). Robot-based training is a fast-growing field that shows promise, but as is the case for all of these technology-based interventions, its superiority compared with conventional treatment programs as yet remains unclear (Karakas 2021, Lamers 2018).

Ataxia

Approximately 80% of people with MS experience ataxia, which is a lack of voluntary coordination of movements. Ataxia can be the result of damage to the cerebellum (cerebellar ataxia), the posterior columns of the spinal cord (sensory ataxia) or dysfunction of the vestibular system (vestibular ataxia). This can be seen as clumsiness, imbalance, unsteady gait, impaired limb coordination and accuracy of movement, limb and body tremor, dysarthria and oculomotor abnormalities. Ataxia is very challenging to manage, and none of the available treatments are particularly effective (Marquer et al 2014).

Drug treatments include isoniazid, pyridoxine and cannabis; however, these tend to have minimal impact (Zesiewicz 2018). They are often used in conjunction with rehabilitation interventions, which can be either compensatory or restorative in their approach, but evidence to support the use of these interventions is limited. Restorative strategies, such as intensive balance and coordination exercises (Vergaro 2010), gait training using the treadmill (Zesiewicz 2018) or balance and ocular exercises, aim at treating the underlying coordination

impairment. As disability levels increase, compensatory strategies typically become the main approach. Breaking movement patterns into simpler single joint movements, using visual and verbal cues when walking and loading the limbs or trunk with weights to dampen the tremor all demonstrate variable success (Marsden 2011). Walking aids can help improve posture, balance and mobility when used effectively; wheeled frames are usually preferable to sticks/crutches because they are easier for people to coordinate. Occupational therapists can provide adaptive appliances to improve independence in functional tasks such as eating and drinking (e.g., neater eaters which dampen tremor), use of computers (e.g., voice recognition software), household activities (e.g., kettle tippers) (Fonteyn et al 2014) and use of sensory dynamic orthoses have begun to be explored for upper limb tremor (Miller 2016). Another potential avenue of treatment is the use of repetitive transcranial magnetic stimulation. Whilst this shows some promise, studies to date indicate that benefits gained appear transient (Leon Ruiz 2022). When ataxia is severe, stereotactic neurosurgery such as thalamotomy or deep brain stimulation can be used with good outcomes for some individuals (Roy et al 2020).

Spasticity

Spasticity, which can be either focal or generalised, has reported to be experienced by up to 90% of people with MS during the disease course (Milinis et al 2016). It is often associated with pain, spasms, soft tissue stiffness, contractures and pressure areas. For many people, spasticity can contribute to disability and lead to a restriction in social participations; it can dramatically affect quality of life (Milinis et al 2016). However, for some, particularly in those with weak lower limbs, it can help to maintain lower limb function for activities such as transfers, standing and walking. Therefore, it is important to undertake a careful assessment and clearly determine the goals of treatment, particularly before antispasticity pharmacological interventions are initiated. Physiotherapists, working alongside other members of the MDT, play an important role in this assessment.

Identifying and alleviating factors that may trigger or worsen spasticity is an important first step in the assessment and treatment plan. Triggers may include pain (e.g., from ingrown toenails, tight fitting orthoses or pressure sores), constipation, infection (e.g., urinary or respiratory infections) and poor posture or movement patterns (e.g., pulling up strongly with arms into standing). Physical management approaches are typically multifactorial in their approach, involving a variety of individually tailored interventions. As a result, single intervention studies tend to lack face validity, and systematic reviews are often inconclusive (Etoom et al 2018). Buchanan and Hourihan (2016) provide a practical and evidence-based overview of spasticity management strategies, which include education of the individual about avoiding trigger factors and minimising effort during mobility/functional tasks, stretching regimes, orthotics and lower limb splints, functional electrical stimulation, active exercises and strengthening, reeducation of posture and movement, standing programmes and optimising seating and positioning through the use of equipment. Fig. 10.7 provides a helpful algorithm for selecting appropriate physical modalities to help manage a person's spasticity.

Pharmacological treatment should be undertaken only if spasticity is negatively affecting function or associated symptoms such as pain, and once trigger factors have been alleviated and physical approaches have demonstrated to be inadequate in managing the problem (Stevenson 2016). Although there is no agreed evidence-based model for pharmacological management, clinical guidelines (NICE 2022) and consensus reviews (Gold et al 2013, Otero-Romero 2016) are available to inform practice. Whilst some physiotherapists will have trained as supplementary or full prescribers, it is the role of all physiotherapists to monitor the effect of pharmacological interventions in relation to agreed goals, and communicate closely with the neurologist, MS nurse specialist and GP to optimise outcomes.

Importantly, treatment options will vary significantly dependent on the goal of intervention; for example, the approach taken to maintain or optimise walking will be very different from those for an immobile patient where improvement of sitting and lying posture, hygiene and comfort may be the priority.

Medications can be administered via different routes, dependent on the severity of the spasticity and whether it is focal or generalised (Stevenson 2016):

1. Oral medications: With generalised spasticity, commonly prescribed medications include baclofen, tizanidine, diazepam and clonazepam, all of which work at CNS level. Gabapentin and pregabalin (antiepileptic drugs) can also help reduce spasticity and spasms and can be particularly beneficial when the person is experiencing both pain and spasticity. Dantrolene is also used as an antispasmodic drug, but this works peripherally, acting directly on the muscles.
2. Intramuscular botulinum toxin: When spasticity is focal, for example, in the adductors of the lower limbs, it can be used in conjunction with therapy to minimise the effects of troublesome spasticity (e.g., when hygiene is difficult because of adductor spasms). These injections need to be repeated approximately every 3 months as the effect reduces over time.

3. Intrathecal baclofen: When high doses of oral baclofen are needed to manage generalised spasticity, then people can often experience disabling side effects, such as drowsiness and loss of concentration. Intrathecal baclofen delivers the drug directly to the nerve cells in the spinal cord, and so allows high doses to be tolerated with fewer side effects. This requires a baclofen pump to be surgically placed in the abdomen, whereby a catheter delivers the baclofen into the intrathecal space in the spinal cord (Abbatemarco 2021, Sammaraiee et al 2019).

Finally, neurosurgical procedures or more destructive techniques such as intrathecal phenol are available when spasticity is not manageable with these approaches; however, these are rarely used (Anwar et al 2019).

Fatigue

MS-related fatigue has been defined as 'a decrease in physical and/or mental performance that results from changes in central, psychological and/or peripheral factors' (Rudroff 2016). Fatigue is common in MS, and two-thirds of people report this as one of their most troubling symptoms (Rommer et al 2019). Fatigue can have significant consequences on functional performance, societal participation, economic burden and quality of life (Oliva Ramirez et al 2021). Despite this, it is typically undertreated, with a large UK-based survey indicating that less than one-third of people experiencing fatigue had been offered a fatigue treatment (Picariello et al 2022).

As the definition suggests, the concept of 'fatigue' in MS is multidimensional. 'Perceived fatigue' is characterised by a lack of energy or overwhelming sense of physical and/or mental tiredness with no obvious cause and out of proportion to the activity undertaken. In contrast, 'performance fatigability' refers to the objectively measurable use-dependent declines in capacity, such as an observable decrease in performance during a cognitive or motor task because of fatigue (Zijdewind et al 2016). This differentiation is important to guide both assessment choices (e.g., patient-reported outcome versus objective measure) and management approaches.

Many factors contribute to fatigue. These can be categorised as either:

1. Primary factors: nervous system damage leading to increased energy exertion, altered brain metabolism, altered regulation of the immune system and endocrine system; or
2. Secondary factors: interrupted sleep, side effects of medicines, psychological factors such as anxiety, depression and stress, comorbidities or reduced physical activity.

It has also been postulated that fatigue is perpetuated by certain cognitions and beliefs (Enoka et al 2021, Manjaly et al 2019, Wendebourg et al 2017).

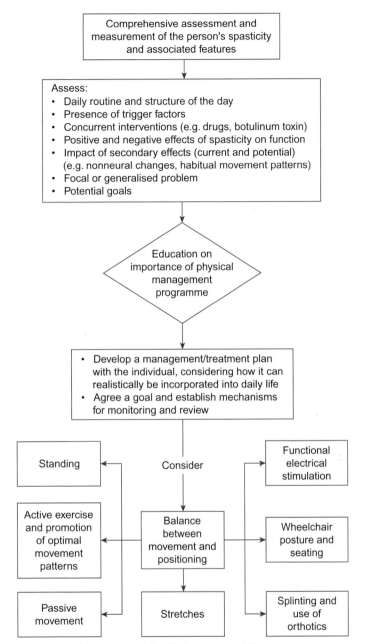

FIG. 10.7 Selecting modalities for managing spasticity (Stevenson 2016).

In recognition of the multifactorial nature of fatigue, medication is often used in conjunction with rehabilitation strategies. The most commonly used drug treatments are amantadine, modafinil and pemoline, but there is no convincing evidence to support their effectiveness (Bourdette 2021, Miller & Soundy 2017). In contrast, there is evidence to demonstrate that significant benefits can be gained from nonpharmacological rehabilitation interventions (Asano et al 2014, Harrison et al 2021). These include aerobic, resistance and balance exercises (including yoga and Pilates), vestibular rehabilitation and personalised advice on healthy living (nutritious diet, regular sleeping patterns). Also effective is the use of cognitive behavioural therapy (CBT) where the individual is guided to identify factors that perpetuate their fatigue and then techniques for managing these behavioural, cognitive, emotional and external factors. This CBT approach appears to be superior to energy conservation interventions, which focus on modifying activity to reduce energy expenditure, for example, through prioritising activities and taking rest breaks (Harrison et al 2021). Such interventions can be successfully provided face to face (Moss-Morris 2021), via self-guided online programmes (Pottgen et al 2018) or telephone (Plow et al 2019).

Pain

Chronic pain is one of the most prevalent, disabling and persistent symptoms associated with MS and is experienced by an estimated 60% of people (Foley 2013). Pain prevalence, intensity and interference with quality of life and everyday activities appear to be similar across MS types (Knowles et al 2021). Pain can occur for a variety of reasons, which may include central neuropathic pain caused by lesions of the ascending somatosensory pathways or nociceptive pain caused by spasticity, muscle tightness, prolonged sitting or abnormal gait and posture. It is now also recognised as being part of a complex interplay between other common symptoms or comorbidities, such as fatigue, anxiety and depression, or caused by other comorbid conditions (Wright 2012). Therefore, the first step in managing pain is to investigate and establish the cause, through detailed history taking and a physical examination, to ensure it is managed correctly.

Neuropathic pain is a commonly reported type of pain in MS. It includes unpleasant dysesthesia and paraesthesias, typically described as burning, tingling, jabbing, electrical and itching sensations (Harrison et al 2015a). Other types of pain include eye pain and photophobia from optic neuritis, restless legs, migraines, painful spasms and trigeminal neuralgia. Pharmacological treatments used for pain relief include analgesics, antiepileptics, antidepressants, cannabinoids, spasmolytics and muscle relaxants, although their efficacy is limited (Yilmazer et al 2022), so their use should be regularly reviewed. Psychosocial factors (e.g., pain beliefs, coping behaviours, depression and anxiety) have been shown to be strongly associated with pain intensity and associated distress (Harrison et al 2015b). Therefore, behavioural techniques such as CBT, relaxation, meditation, imagery and mindfulness training can be beneficial for many people (Yilmazer et al 2022). There is also some evidence that other nonpharmacological interventions such as exercise (Demaneuf et al 2019), transcutaneous electrical nerve stimulation, reflexology and transcranial stimulation may be beneficial to pain management (Amatya et al 2018).

Nociceptive pain is also common in people with MS. For example, an estimated 50% of people with MS experience low back pain (Massot 2021). This is frequently underdiagnosed because it is assumed that the pain is caused by MS nerve damage. This is concerning because musculoskeletal pain can improve with physical activity and therapy (Knowles et al 2021). Musculoskeletal pain often occurs secondary to problems with weakness, immobility, postural malalignment, inactivity and fall-related injuries. For example, people can experience back or extremity pain because of prolonged sitting or excessive strain on joints (e.g., hyperextended knees when standing and walking). A comprehensive assessment of the cause of pain is important to offer relevant patient education and targeted treatment, using a similar approach to people who do not have MS (NICE 2020, 2021); physiotherapists have an important role to play in this. Referral to chronic pain programmes should be considered if pain remains inadequately controlled.

Vestibulopathy

Vestibular system dysfunction is common in people with MS, with an estimated 50% experiencing symptoms that may include vertigo, dizziness, abnormalities in the control of eye movements, balance and mobility impairment (Cochrane et al 2021). These symptoms affect a wide range of everyday functional activities and contribute to falls. As a consequence, they can markedly affect people's quality of life, work and social participation (Marrie et al 2013).

The vestibular system consists of a peripheral pathway (the inner ear and vestibular nerve) and central pathways in the brain (e.g., the vestibular nuclei and cerebellum) that process vestibular signals. In MS, symptoms that arise can be caused by either, or both, of these pathways. Differentiation of the cause of the vestibular symptoms is important in targeting vestibular rehabilitation/physical treatment, which is the recommended treatment rather than the use of antivertigo drugs (van Vugt et al 2017). For example, in those with benign paroxysmal positional vertigo, affecting the inner ear, bedside physical manoeuvres such as Epley or Semont can be effective in reducing symptoms of vertigo in a single treatment by moving dislodged otoconia crystals back into the otoliths (Chen et al 2018), although recurrence can occur over time.

Vestibular symptoms of central origin may be treated with a graded programme of exercises involving varied eye, head and body movements in different positions (sitting, standing and walking). The aim of these exercises is to stimulate the vestibular system to optimise adaptive changes in the brain, called vestibular compensation. Although there is good evidence from clinical trials regarding the effectiveness of vestibular rehabilitation, there remains uncertainty as to the most effective approach (Synnott et al 2020). For example, some programmes are supervised in the clinic, whereas others are unsupervised home-based programmes;

some use generic exercises and others are customised. So too are there marked variations in programmes regarding intensity (variations from twice daily to once weekly) and duration (variations from 4 to 14 weeks) (Garcia-Munoz et al 2020, Synnott et al 2020). Therefore, further evidence-based guidance is needed to inform best practice.

Several factors have shown to influence the effectiveness of vestibular rehabilitation and therefore should be carefully considered during the planning of treatment. For example, long-term use of antivertigo medication, fatigue, depression, anxiety, loss of confidence, immobility and restricted neck movement all need to be addressed to optimise outcomes. See also Chapter 17 on vestibular disorders.

Respiratory Dysfunction

Respiratory impairment occurs in people with MS even at the early stages of the disease. It is typically not recognized by clinicians until later in the disease course when problems become more apparent (Dereli 2022). Impairments include respiratory muscle weakness and fatigue, deterioration in diffusion capacity and ventilation–perfusion ratio, change in pulmonary volumes and inefficiency of cough (Levy 2018). Abnormalities of breathing control can also occur, which include sleep disordered breathing, central sleep apnoea and central respiratory dysregulation (Tzelepis & McCool 2015). Although the primary cause of respiratory impairment is CNS demyelination, secondary contributory factors include medication (e.g., steroids), fatigue, malnutrition, sedentary lifestyle and deconditioning. It is important to consider these factors in overall management because these secondary factors are amenable to change.

Impairment in respiration can interfere with the process of speech and voice production, making it more difficult and tiring for people to speak loudly or carry on a conversation. Difficulty in clearing secretions and reduced lung volumes are associated with a higher risk of infections and pneumonia, and at the end stage of MS, respiratory failure and infection is a common cause of death (Harding 2020). Therefore, systematic evaluation of respiratory status, from an early stage, regardless of disease severity, is recommended to enable early detection and prevention (Muhtaroglu et al 2020). This is important because there is evidence that rehabilitation strategies such as respiratory muscle training, Pilates, yoga and continuous positive airway pressure treatment can be effective in improving inspiratory and expiratory muscle strength, fatigue, cough efficiency and dyspnoea in people with MS from across the disease spectrum (Dereli 2022).

Heat Sensitivity

An estimated 60%–80% of people with MS show sensitivity to increases in temperature where they experience a temporary exacerbation of symptoms, such as blurred vision, sensory disturbance, cognitive problems, weakness and fatigue (Davis et al 2018). This heat sensitivity is thought to primarily be driven by temperature-dependent slowing or blocking of neural conduction within the CNS because of changes in a combination of internal (core) and external (skin) temperature (Christogianni et al 2018). Importantly, exercise can generate internal heat that temporarily exacerbates symptoms. Although in approximately 85% of individuals these symptoms resolve/return to normal within 30–60 minutes of stopping the exercise, or more rapidly with body cooling (Smith et al 2006), they can nevertheless cause distress to individuals and lead them to avoid activities that have triggered the symptoms to occur. Practical strategies can help to minimise the impact of heat, including drinking ice slush drinks, fans/air conditioners to cool the environment, cooling garments, precooling with cold showers and baths, and ice packs (Kaltsatou & Flouris 2019). More advanced cooling garment technology and body immersion in cold water have been investigated, showing some benefits, but can raise practical issues when incorporating into daily life (Meyer-Heim et al 2007, White et al 2000).

Bladder and Bowel

Bladder and bowel symptoms are common in MS, with estimates suggesting up to 80% of people experience problems at some time (Medeiros 2020). These symptoms can be present regardless of disease duration, type or level of disability. They markedly affect a person's quality of life and social interactions. Urinary problems experienced may include incontinence, urgency, frequency and infections. Such infections are a major cause of hospitalization and mortality (Harding 2020). As with many MS symptoms, bladder problems vary from person to person; therefore, referral to specialist nurses and urologists who specialise in this area is important to ensure appropriate assessment and targeting of interventions. There are a range of management options available, depending on the type of problem and the person's level of disability. These include monitoring and regulation of fluid intake, pelvic floor reeducation and ensuring that toilets are accessible and transfers are safe. Oral medication, botulinum toxin A injections, intermittent self-catheterisation or long-term catheterisation may be required to optimise management (Medeiros 2020).

The causes of bowel symptoms in MS are less well understood than bladder issues; however, it is likely that a combination of reduced peristalsis speed, sensory loss and weakness or lack of coordination around the anal sphincters and pelvic floor muscles may be significant. Polypharmacy, behavioural elements and ability to access the toilet are also contributory factors (Preziosi et al 2018).

The most common complaint is constipation, but the most distressing is faecal incontinence. Appropriate intake of dietary fibre and fluids, together with establishment of a bowel regime, are important general management strategies. Medication and management approaches such as abdominal massage and biofeedback can help where problems persist. Exercise can also be beneficial; this can include general physical activity, standing and walking as appropriate to the person's level of disability (Preziosi 2018).

Cognitive Impairment

A significant factor that can contribute to the complexity of managing disability is the presence of cognitive impairments. Prevalence varies across the lifespan, with estimates of cognitive impairment ranging between 34% and 65% (Benedict et al 2020). The domains most frequently involved are information processing speed, memory (visual and verbal) and learning, although a wide range of other cognitive problems can be seen (Brochet 2021). These deficits can influence almost every aspect of daily living and have shown to negatively influence rehabilitation outcomes. Therefore, it is important to take cognitive impairments into consideration with rehabilitation intervention, for example, by tailoring the speed and complexity of information delivery, providing written information to support verbal advice and encouraging involvement and support from family members and friends. Targeted neuropsychological rehabilitation using both restorative (e.g., memory rehabilitation, computerised training programmes) and compensatory approaches (e.g., using aids such as diaries or calendars and counselling in how to cope better with cognitive problems) has shown to be beneficial (Goverover 2018, Taylor et al 2021). There is also some preliminary evidence that exercise may improve deficits such as processing speed (Rademacher 2021), although its impact on global cognitive performance remains uncertain (Gharakhanlou et al 2020).

Anxiety and Depression

Approximately 30%–50% of people with MS will develop major depression or anxiety at some point in their life (Boeschoten et al 2017). The causes can be both biological (site of lesions) and psychological (e.g., dealing with the uncertainties of an unpredictable disease course, significant life changes and an unknown prognosis) (Hanna & Strober 2020). Regardless of cause, these symptoms significantly affect the quality of peoples' lives and their ability to engage in rehabilitation (Feinstein 2014) and social participation (Freeman et al 2020). Antidepressant medications (such as paroxetine, desipramine and sertraline) may provide some benefit, but can have significant side effects. CBT, psychotherapy (Sesel et al 2018) and psychological interventions (such as mindfulness) aimed at reducing stress and enhancing self-efficacy and self-esteem can be beneficial (Carletto et al 2020, Fiest 2016).

Alongside this specialist intervention, it is important for professionals to develop a positive relationship with the person affected by MS and their family, whether an individual is diagnosed with anxiety and/or depression. For instance, it is important to provide reassurance that rehabilitation interventions/symptomatic treatments are available to help manage physical, cognitive and emotional problems as they arise so that people do not feel that they will be left alone to manage their disability by themselves. By providing honest explanations in a sensitive manner, professionals can give people confidence that they will form part of a supportive network for the future (Davies et al 2015).

SECONDARY COMPLICATIONS

Contractures

Joint contractures (limited passive range of joint motion) are prevalent among people with MS, with evidence to demonstrate that almost 60% have contracture in at least one joint, most commonly in the ankle joint (Hoang 2014). Contractures are more common in people with progressive disease and those who are more severely disabled (Hoang 2014), but they are evident at all stages of the disease.

Joint contracture can affect standing and walking balance, walking pattern by limiting heel-to-toe progression during weight transfer (Psarakis et al 2017) and risk of falls, even at relatively low levels of disability. They can also affect postural alignment in a range of different positions. For example, tight calf muscles can prevent the foot from resting in a plantargrade position on the footplate/floor when seated and can result in compensatory knee hyperextension when standing and walking (Schmid et al 2013). Regular assessment and (self/carer) monitoring is important to detect and minimise loss of range at an early stage. Although the most effective ways to maintain soft tissue and joint range have yet to be determined, those commonly used include stretching regimes, splinting, functional electrical stimulation, active exercises, and standing programmes (Buchanan & Hourihan 2016, Freeman 2019, Psarakis 2021).

Pressure Ulcers

Pressure ulcers are a secondary complication, with estimates that approximately 15% of people with MS will develop a pressure ulcer at some point in the disease course (Cramp 2004). They may develop when the skin breaks down from constant pressure, typically in sitting or lying, or from friction to the skin (called shear). Pressure ulcers are associated with increased morbidity, mortality and costs of healthcare, and have been recognised as both a Patient Safety and Quality of Care Indicator for patients in hospital and community care settings (NICE 2022). Pressure ulcers have a significant impact on people's lives, affecting it physically, psychologically and socially (McGinnis 2015). It is the responsibility of all health and social professionals to minimise their development, and the assessment of areas at risk of pressure ulcers should be integral to the formal review process (NICE 2014, 2022).

People with impaired mobility, spasticity, decreased sensation, bladder/bowel incontinence, malnutrition and cognitive impairment are at higher risk of pressure ulcers; thus, assessment and monitoring are particularly important in these people as disability progresses (Jaul et al 2019). For example, regular inspection of the toes and feet in ambulant individuals and the sacrum and bottom for those restricted to a wheelchair/bed is important to detect areas of redness/skin abrasions and prevent them from developing into pressure ulcers. Education and advice to enable self/carer monitoring of this is essential. Nutritional advice is also important (Stratton 2005).The provision of equipment such as pressure-relieving cushions (for chairs/wheelchairs) and mattresses (for people who spend large amounts of time in bed), specialist seating, standing frames and simple devices such as T-rolls, wedges and resting splints can help to prevent development of pressure ulcers. Physiotherapists have an important role to play in educating other professionals, people with MS and carers about effective moving and handling procedures to minimise trauma through shear of tissues, which can occur, for example, when sliding across a bed or wheelchair seat. This is particularly important when the person is unable to reposition themselves.

CONCLUSION

MS presents significant challenges to those living with the condition and those involved in their care. The use of DMTs is an integral part of management for people in the relapsing remitting phase. However, despite recent advances, this is not currently the case in progressive MS, where rehabilitation strategies and symptomatic therapy are the mainstay of clinical practice. Person-centred management, based on assessment of the individual's needs and provided in a timely and coordinated manner, is essential. The evidence base for physiotherapy in this area continues to advance, and this, together with an improved understanding of brain health and neuroprotection is informing the development of new and potentially effective approaches.

CASE STUDY

History of Presenting Complaint

Mrs A is 54 years old and was diagnosed with RRMS 16 years ago, having had variable sensory symptoms and weakness over 3 years. Her diagnosis was confirmed by MRI, lumbar puncture and evoked potentials. She was commenced on a DMT, with relative stability of her disease for a number of years. In the past year, Mrs A reports that her walking is more difficult, and at the last review appointment with her neurologist she was told she is now in the secondary progressive phase. She says she was worried that this would be the case, but that she is 'slowly beginning to come to terms with it'.

Mrs A said that her mobility and balance is very variable, with some 'good and bad days', although she feels 'the bad days are more often now'. A key issue is that her walking distance has gradually reduced over the past year or so, and that she must constantly concentrate whilst walking in order to keep her balance; she finds this very tiring. At home she feels more confident because she can steady herself on furniture and the walls. When outside, she uses either a stick or a crutch (which she bought via the internet) depending on how well she feels, but still 'doesn't feel safe' when walking. She finds that her left leg is stiff and weak, and her foot frequently scuffs the floor when she walks, which can cause her to trip or slip. Although she can save herself on most occasions, she has had a couple of falls recently, which have resulted in bruises and scrapes. Mrs A lives in a two-storey house, and whilst she can manage the stairs, she is finding these increasingly difficult and is reliant on the bannister for support. On her 'bad days' she moves up and down the stairs on her bottom. She reports being unable to walk up or down stairs where no rail is available, for example, in cinemas. She feels very anxious if this situation arises and has started to curtail activities to avoid this.

Mrs A reports long-standing problems with urinary frequency and urgency and has had several urinary tract infections (UTIs) in the past 2 months. Recently, she has had a few episodes of urinary incontinence, which she finds very embarrassing, and she has cancelled a few social activities as a result. Fatigue has also been worse over the past few months, which Mrs A partly attributes to needing to get up several times in the middle of the night to go to the toilet. This is frustrating for her husband because she needs to turn on the light each time she gets up, as her balance is much worse in the dark. Her sleep is also interrupted by the nighttime spasms, which have been worse over the past few months.

Mrs A continues to work 2 days a week as a school teaching assistant, and although she enjoys her work, she is finding this increasingly difficult to manage. She lacks confidence to walk through the busy, noisy corridors from the classroom to the staffroom at break times because she is concerned about falling. She frequently stays in the classroom to avoid this. She also reports feeling exhausted by the time she gets home and is getting worried about the drive to work because her legs are stiffer and weaker, which makes it harder to work the brake. Her lack of energy also means that she is not currently undertaking any regular exercise. She would like to try to do more because she is aware how important this is.

Medication: Vitamin D, Amantadine for Fatigue

Mrs A attended the clinic with her husband, and it was apparent that they had a very supportive relationship. They were keen to work as a team, together with professionals, to best manage her condition. It became clear that Mrs A's mood had been particularly low since being told that she had SPMS. Qualitative research highlights that this is a common reaction because this is a time when the person is having to come to terms with the uncertainties related to having a progressive disease in which they face declining mobility, physical and cognitive function, and where disease-modifying drug treatments are more limited. Therefore, emotional support and information provision is particularly important at this time.

Key Assessment Findings

This case illustrates how several factors can interact to contribute to impaired mobility and falls. Here, weakness, fatigability, increased tone and loss of range, combined with cognitive issues and poor selection and use of walking aids, have resulted in balance and mobility problems

and increased risk of falling. Key findings are presented in Table 10.3.

Treatment Plan

The therapist's clinical reasoning to identify an *International Classification of Functioning, Disability and Health*-based problem list, goals and plan is highlighted in Table 10.4.

The initial physiotherapy session focused on gait reeducation, stair practice, a discussion about functional electrical stimulation for footdrop and a home programme including stretching (see Outpatient Physiotherapy box). This type of initial session is typical given the range of problems Mrs A is experiencing. However, the inclusion of so many elements could be overwhelming; therefore, it is essential to discuss carefully with the patient and to be prepared to prioritise when necessary. Writing down a summary of what has been covered in the session, any exercises that may have been given and physiotherapy contact details should any queries arise, is important. Some people may need only a few sessions to adequately cover their issues and enable them to integrate this advice and activities into their self-management plan. Others may require more supervised sessions and/or extra support to enable effective management. Different options exist for providing this intervention: face to face, videoconferencing (telerehabilitation) or a hybrid approach. Key is that the person with MS feels that they can incorporate these activities

TABLE 10.3	Key Assessment Findings
Tone	• Increased in the left leg; deep tendon reflexes brisk
Gait	• Heavily dependent on walking stick in right hand (stick too short)
	• Pattern poor: continued catching/scuffing of left foot because of foot drop/tight and stiff calf muscles; tendency to circumduct left leg and to walk on flexed right knee and hip, which further aggravates the difficulty in clearing the left leg; walks in a forwards flexed position at the trunk
	• Able to safely walk up and down stairs using alternate steps when holding on to one or two rails; however, when no rail available, unsteady and clearly very anxious
Muscle strength	• Bilateral lower limb weakness, right greater than left, generally grade 3 throughout (although effortful)
	• All lower limb muscle groups fatigable with repetition
	• Upper limb muscle strength grade 4 throughout
Range of movement	• Calf muscles both tight, barely able to achieve plantargrade position on left calf
Coordination	• Upper limbs no abnormality detected
	• Reduced coordination in both lower limbs – probably because of weakness
Balance	• Impaired in standing: Romberg's positive, able to maintain stride stance independently but significantly worse with dual tasks (both cognitive and motor); unable to tandem stance or to stand on a single leg
	• Unsteady when reaching in all directions and with height changes
	• Stepping reactions delayed when displaced, but able to regain balance with several steps

TABLE 10.4 Problem List, Goals and Plan

Problem List	Goals	Plan
Impairments: • Poor gait pattern, with lower limb weakness, increased tone and impaired balance • Reduced level of fitness and a lack of energy • Recent increase in severity of longstanding bladder problems, including urinary tract infections and incontinence **Activity limitations** • Reduced walking distance and occasional falls • Loss of confidence with outdoor mobility and climbing stairs **Participation restrictions** • Increasing difficulties engaging in work and social activities	• To walk safely and confidently around the school during the course of her workday • To be able to safely climb up and down the entrance stairs at the local cinema	• Provision of exercises to increase strength of lower limbs and to continue stretching and gait reeducation work • Education and advice regarding minimising spasticity and avoiding triggers of spasms (e.g., sleeping position at night), and managing clonus should it occur • Referral to local continence team • Discussion of physical activity recommendations and options for increasing physical activity • Follow-up discussion about walking aid preference

INITIAL OUTPATIENT PHYSIOTHERAPY SESSION

1. Gait reeducation within session: Advice given to more fully extend knee and hip during stance phase on the right leg, provision of a drop foot ankle–foot orthosis (AFO) on left leg and raising of stick by one notch – noticeable improvement in gait pattern noted with these changes. Mrs A observed walking with a rollator (provided at physiotherapy clinic) with a very significant improvement in walking pattern, level of effort and confidence. A discussion was held with Mrs A as to whether she might consider using this walking aid at work/within the community.

2. Education regarding managing stairs using slow, careful step-by-step approach when only one rail or no rails. Advised to practice this at home with a small step and a rail nearby (to build confidence and ensure safety), with the aim of achieving her goal of being able to negotiate stairs at the cinema. Advised that, whenever possible, it was preferable to take someone's arms to negotiate step if no rail available, to ensure safety.

3. Functional electrical stimulation (FES) discussed as an option with Mrs A to assist with her foot drop. She expressed a preference to trial the AFO in the first instance, but to consider FES as an alternative option at a later stage. AFO provided for left foot. Instructions were provided regarding wearing time, sensation and checking skin integrity.

4. Taught stretches of calf muscles to undertake daily; written instructions were provided.

Plan for Subsequent Sessions

1. Provision of progressive resistance exercise programme to increase strength of lower limbs, balance activities, revisit stretching and gait reeducation work undertaken at first visit.

2. Education and advice regarding minimising spasticity and avoiding triggers of spasms (e.g., sleeping position at night), and managing clonus should it occur.

3. Referral to MS specialist nurse/local continence team (depending on local services) for management of bladder.

4. Discussion of physical activity/exercise recommendations and options for increasing this, such as use of web-based exercise programmes (e.g., Simple exercises for MS, Multiple Sclerosis Society UK (mssociety.org.uk, https://www.mssociety.org.uk/care-and-support/everyday-living/staying-active/simple-exercises-for-ms) and community-based activities (e.g., local leisure centre, yoga, Pilates, tai chi and community-based MS groups).

5. Follow-up discussion about walking aid preference.

within their daily life so that the benefits can be sustained in the longer term. Provision of a contact name and number is helpful to reassure people that they can ask questions if they arise, rather than feeling that they have 'been left to get on with it'.

Progress Review at 3 Months

At Mrs A's request, this review session was undertaken via videoconferencing. Mrs A reported feeling more positive since her last review and feels she has made some progress.

KEY NEEDS AND INTERVENTIONS AT DIFFERENT STAGES OF MULTIPLE SCLEROSIS (ADAPTED FROM **FREEMAN ET AL 2003**)

Stage of Multiple Sclerosis	Key Needs	Focus of Intervention by the MDT
Diagnosis	• Certain clear diagnosis • Appropriate support • Access to information • Continuing education • Disease-modifying drugs	• Emphasis is on *health promotion* to maintain current levels of activities and participations by management of fatigue, regular exercise and a healthy lifestyle • Team working with the neurologist and nurse specialist to provide support, advice and information, either on an individual or group basis • Provision of physiotherapy on an outpatient basis as required
Minimal impairment	• Advice, support and information • Self-management options • Treatment of relapses • Disease-modifying drugs • Management of symptoms	• *Guided self-management and health promotion* to facilitate regular exercise, maintain usual activities and prevent complications • Symptomatic management by MDT • Relapse management alongside steroid treatment to improve residual deficits • Physiotherapy on an outpatient basis or in a hospital setting during relapse • Liaison with specialist professionals (e.g., continence advisors, employment advisors)
Moderate disability	• Rehabilitation and symptomatic management • Easy access to well-coordinated services • Clear and consistent communication	• *Restorative rehabilitation* and symptomatic management to optimise activities and participations; often achieved through comprehensive MDT rehabilitation programme • Liaison with specialist services, such as posture and seating clinics • Assess carer's needs, and provide education and support • Implement/reinforce links with community care
Severe disability	• Access to information and expertise • Good communication and coordinated care within the community • Respite care • Palliative care	• *Maintenance rehabilitation* usually within the community, aimed at maintaining autonomy wherever possible • Management by all involved in care and throughout 24 hours of the day, rather than intensive 'hands-on' physiotherapy • Emphasis on preventing or improving secondary complications such as pressure areas and contractures • Provision of appropriate equipment, environmental controls, wheelchairs, home adaptations and community mobility; joint working between healthcare and social care • Supportive care to increase comfort

MDT, Multidisciplinary team; *NICE,* National Institute for Health and Care Excellence.

She saw the local continence team and was assessed, including a postmicturition ultrasound for volume, which showed incomplete emptying. The continence team recommended strategies to improve bladder emptying and reduce bladder sensitivity, which Mrs A has found helpful; she is now less anxious about this at work and when out socially, and feels this has helped her confidence and mood.

Mrs A found her course of physiotherapy helpful, and she felt that the exercises she did during the sessions and worked on at home improved her walking and balance. Since finishing her course of physiotherapy, Mrs A feels she has regressed somewhat and feels this is primarily because of stopping doing much of the home programme she was given. She has been using the stick and AFO consistently but has not used the rollator outside. In discussion, Mrs A says the main reason is 'vanity'. After a long discussion regarding advantages and disadvantages of the rollator (e.g., fear of looking 'disabled' versus the potential to reduce the embarrassment of falls and to walk for longer distances with less effort), Mrs A decided this was a positive way forward.

After this review, the therapist contacted Mrs A's general practitioner to request a referral to the local community exercise prescription service. She also gave Mrs A the contact details of the local MS society coordinator to investigate the availability of exercise groups.

This case highlights the need for ongoing support to maintain motivation and engagement with exercise and physical activity. It illustrates the need to engage with the community sector, such as voluntary organisations and leisure centres, to help people sustain physical activity (including exercise) over the longer term.

SELF-ASSESSMENT QUESTIONS

1. Can you describe the underlying pathophysiology of MS?
2. Who might be involved in the management of people with MS, and what are their roles? What are the different types of MS? How might your management approach differ at different stages of the disease?
3. How might you evaluate the effectiveness of your input, and what are some commonly used outcome measures?
4. What approaches are available to help manage ataxia in MS?
5. How might cognitive problems affect your physiotherapy intervention? What strategies could be used to help deal with this?
6. What advice would you give a person with MS about maintaining a healthy lifestyle and physical fitness, both in the early and latter stages of the disease?
7. What are the common comorbidities experienced in MS? And what are the potential impacts of these comorbidities?
8. What are the different factors that can contribute to the development of fatigue in someone with MS? What treatment options are available to help them manage their fatigue?
9. What advice could you give a person with MS and their carers to help them gauge when they might need to request a physiotherapy review?
10. What are the different ways you can maintain contact/undertake reviews with your patient, and what are the pros and cons of each approach?
11. What guidance and support might you provide people to ensure they can access relevant and high-quality digital resources?

REFERENCES

Abbatemarco, J.R., Griffin, A., Jones, N.G., et al., 2021. Long-term outcomes of intrathecal baclofen in ambulatory multiple sclerosis patients: a single-center experience. Mult. Scler. 27, 933–941.

Amatya, B., Khan, F., Galea, M., 2019. Rehabilitation for people with multiple sclerosis: an overview of Cochrane Reviews. Cochrane. Database. Syst. Rev. 1, Cd012732.

Amatya, B., Young, J., Khan, F., 2018. Non-pharmacological interventions for chronic pain in multiple sclerosis. Cochrane. Database. Syst. Rev 12, Cd012622.

Andreu-Caravaca, L., Ramos-Campo, D.J., Chung, L.H., Rubio-Arias, J., 2021. Dosage and effectiveness of aerobic training on cardiorespiratory fitness, functional capacity, balance, and fatigue in people with multiple sclerosis: a systematic review and meta-analysis. Arch. Phys. Med. Rehabil. 102, 1826–1839.

Anwar, F., Antiga, S., Mee, H., Al Khayer, A., 2019. Management of spasticity with intrathecal phenol injections: the past and the present. J. Int. Soc. Phys. Rehabil. Med 2, 94–99.

Asano, M., Finlayson, M.L., 2014. Meta-analysis of three different types of fatigue management interventions for people with multiple sclerosis: exercise, education, and medication. Mult. Scler. Int. 2014, 798285.

Backus, D., 2016. Increasing physical activity and participation in people with multiple sclerosis: a review. Arch. Phys. Med. Rehabil. 97 (9 Suppl.), S210–217.

Benedict, R.H.B., Amato, M.P., DeLuca, J., Geurts, J.J.G., 2020. Cognitive impairment in multiple sclerosis: clinical management, MRI, and therapeutic avenues. Lancet. Neurol. 19, 860–871.

Boeschoten, R.E, Braamse, A.M.J., Beekman, A.T.F., et al, 2017. Prevalence of depression and anxiety in Multiple Sclerosis: A systematic review and meta-analysis. J Neurological Sciences. 372, 331–341.

Bogosian, A., Morgan, M., Moss-Morris, R., 2019. Multiple challenges for people after transitioning to secondary progressive multiple sclerosis: a qualitative study. BMJ. Open. 9, e026421.

Borreani, C., Bianchi, E., Pietrolongo, E., Rossi, I., Cilia, S., et al., 2014. Unmet needs of people with severe multiple sclerosis and their carers: qualitative findings for a home-based intervention. PLoS One. 9, e109679.

Bourdette, D., 2021. Are drugs for multiple sclerosis fatigue just placebos? Lancet. Neurol. 20, 20–21.

Brandstadter, R., Sand, Katz, I., Sumowski, J.F., 2019. Beyond rehabilitation: a prevention model of reserve and brain maintenance in multiple sclerosis. Mult. Scler. 25, 1372–1378.

Brandstadter, R., Ayeni, O., Krieger, S.C., et al., 2020. Detection of subtle gait disturbance and future fall risk in early multiple sclerosis. Neurology. 94, e1395–e1406.

Brochet, B., 2021. Cognitive rehabilitation in multiple sclerosis in the period from 2013 and 2021: a narrative review. Brain. Sci. 12, 55.

Buchanan, K., Hourihan, S., 2016. Physical and postural management of spasticity. In: Stevenson, V.L., Jarrett, L. (Eds.), Spasticity Management: A Practical Multidisciplinary Guide. CRC Press, London.

Buckingham, S.A., Anil, K., Demian, S., et al., 2022. Telerehabilitation for people with physical disabilities and movement impairment: a survey of United Kingdom Practitioners. JMIRx Med 3, e30516.

Calabrò, R.S., Cassio, A., Mazzoli, D., et al., 2021. What does evidence tell us about the use of gait robotic devices in patients with multiple sclerosis? A comprehensive systematic review on functional outcomes and clinical recommendations. Eur. J. Phys. Rehabil. Med. 57, 841–849.

Calafiore, D., Invernizzi, M., Ammendolia, A., et al., 2021. Efficacy of virtual reality and exergaming in improving balance in patients with multiple sclerosis: a systematic review and meta-analysis. Front. Neurol. 12, 773459.

Campbell, E., Coulter, E.H., Mattison, P.G., Miller, L., McFadyen, A., Paul, L., 2016. Physiotherapy rehabilitation for people with progressive multiple sclerosis: a systematic review. Arch. Phys. Med. Rehabil. 97, 141–151.

Carletto, S., Cavalera, C., Sadowski, I., et al., 2020. Mindfulness-based interventions for the improvement of well-being in people with multiple sclerosis: a systematic review and meta-analysis. Psychosom. Med. 82, 600–613.

Cattaneo, D., Lamers, I., Bertoni, R., Feys, P., Jonsdottir, J., 2017. Participation restriction in people with multiple sclerosis: prevalence and correlations with cognitive, walking, balance, and upper limb impairments. Arch. Phys. Med. Rehabil. 98, 1308–1315.

Cerqueira, J.J., Compston, D.A.S., Geraldes, R., et al., 2018. Time matters in multiple sclerosis: can early treatment and long-term follow-up ensure everyone benefits from the latest advances in multiple sclerosis? J. Neurol. Neurosurg. Psychiatry. 89, 844–850.

Chee, J.N., Ye, B., Gregor, S., Berbrayer, D., Mihailidis, A., Patterson, K.K., 2021. Influence of multiple sclerosis on spatiotemporal gait parameters: a systematic review and meta-regression. Arch. Phys. Med. Rehabil. 102, 1801–1815.

Chen, C.-C., Cho, H.-S., Lee, H.-H., Hu, C.-J., 2018. Efficacy of repositioning therapy in patients with benign paroxysmal positional vertigo and pre-existing central neurologic disorders. Front. Neurol. 9, 486.

Christogianni, A., Bibb, R., Davis, S.L., Jay, O., Barnett, M., Evangelou, N., Filingeri, D., 2018. Temperature sensitivity in multiple sclerosis: An overview of its impact on sensory and cognitive symptoms. Temperature. 5, 208–223.

Cochrane, G.D., Christy, J.B., Motl, R.W., 2021. Comprehensive clinical assessment of vestibular function in multiple sclerosis. J. Neurol. Phys. Ther 45, 228–234.

Cohen, E.T., Huser, S., Barone, K., Barone, D.A., 2021. Trekking poles to aid multiple sclerosis walking impairment: an exploratory comparison of the effects of assistive devices on psychosocial impact and walking. Int. J. MS. Care. 23, 135–141.

Coote, S., Comber, L., Quinn, G., Santoyo-Medina, C., Kalron, A., Gunn, H., 2020. Falls in people with multiple sclerosis: risk identification, intervention, and future directions. Int. J. MS. Care. 22, 247–255.

Cramp, A.F.L., Warke, K., Lowe-Strong, A.S., 2004. The incidence of pressure ulcers in people with multiple sclerosis and persons responsible for their management. Int. J. MS. Care. 6, 52–54.

Cree, B.A.C., Hollenbach, J.A., Bove, R., et al., 2019. Silent progression in disease activity-free relapsing multiple sclerosis. Ann. Neurol. 285, 653–666.

Dalgas, U., Langeskov-Christensen, M., Stenager, E., Riemenschneider, M., Hvid, L.G., 2019. Exercise as medicine in multiple sclerosis – time for a paradigm shift: preventive, symptomatic, and disease-modifying aspects and perspectives. Curr. Neurol. Neurosci. Rep. 19, 88.

Davies, F., Edwards, A., Brain, K., et al., 2015. 'You are just left to get on with it', qualitative study of patient and carer experiences of the transition to secondary progressive multiple sclerosis. BMJ. Open. 5, e007674.

Davis, S.L., Jay, O., Wilson, T.E., 2018. Thermoregulatory dysfunction in multiple sclerosis. Handbook Clin. Neurol. 157, 701–714.

Degenhardt, A., Ramagopalan, S.V., Scalfari, A., Ebers, G.C., 2009. Clinical prognostic factors in multiple sclerosis: a natural history review. Nat. Rev. Neurol. 5, 672–682.

Demaneuf, T., Aitken, Z., Karahalios, A., et al., 2019. Effectiveness of exercise interventions for pain reduction in people with multiple sclerosis: a systematic review and meta-analysis of randomized controlled trials. Arch. Phys. Med. Rehabil. 100, 128–139.

Dennett, R., Hendrie, W., Jarrett, L., et al., 2020. "I'm in a very good frame of mind": a qualitative exploration of the experience of standing frame use in people with progressive multiple sclerosis. BMJ. Open. 10, e037680.

Dereli, M., Kahraman, Ozcan, Kahraman, T., B., 2022. A narrative review of respiratory impairment, assessment, and rehabilitation in multiple sclerosis. Dubai Med. J. 5, 78–88.

Dobson, R., Giovannoni, G., 2019. Multiple sclerosis – a review. Eur. J. Neurol. 26, 27–40.

Edwards, T., Pilutti, L.A., 2017. The effect of exercise training in adults with multiple sclerosis with severe mobility disability: a systematic review and future research directions. Mult. Scler. Relat. Disord. 16, 31–39.

Enoka, R.M., Almuklass, A.M., Alenazy, M., Alvarez, E., Duchateau, J., 2021. Distinguishing between fatigue and fatigability in multiple sclerosis. Neurorehabil. Neural. Rep. 15459683211046257.

Ernstsson, O., Gyllensten, H., Alexanderson, K., Tinghög, P., Friberg, E., Norlund, A., 2016. Cost of illness of multiple sclerosis – a systematic review. PloS One. 11, e0159129.

Etoom, M., Khraiwesh, Y., Lena, F., et al., 2018. Effectiveness of physiotherapy interventions on spasticity in people with multiple sclerosis: a systematic review and meta-analysis. Am. J. Phys. Med. Rehabil. 97, 793–807.

Faissner, S., Gold, R., 2019. Progressive multiple sclerosis: latest therapeutic developments and future directions. Ther. Adv. Neurol. Disord. 12, 175628641987832 (e-collection).

Feinstein, A., Freeman, J., Lo, A.C., 2015. Treatment of progressive multiple sclerosis: what works, what does not, and what is needed. Lancet Neurol. 14, 194–207.

Feinstein, A., Magalhaes, S., Richard, J.-F., Audet, B., Moore, C., 2014. The link between multiple sclerosis and depression. Nat. Rev. Neurol. 10, 507–517.

Fiest, K.M., Walker, J.R., Bernstein, C.N., et al., 2016. Systematic review and meta-analysis of interventions for depression and anxiety in persons with multiple sclerosis. Mult. Scler. Relat. Disord. 5, 12–26.

Foley, P.L., Vesterinen, H.M., Laird, B.J., et al., 2013. Prevalence and natural history of pain in adults with multiple sclerosis: systematic review and meta-analysis. Pain. 154, 632–642.

Fonteyn, E.M., Keus, S.H., Verstappen, C.C., Schols, L., de Groot, I.J., van de Warrenburg, B.P., 2014. The effectiveness of allied health care in patients with ataxia: a systematic review. J. Neurol. 261, 251–258.

Fox, R.J., Cohen, J.A., 2001. Multiple sclerosis: the importance of early recognition and treatment. Cleveland Clin. J. Med. 68, 157–171.

Freeman, J.A., Ford, H., Mattison, P., et al., 2003. Developing multiple sclerosis healthcare standards: evidence based recommendations for service providers. Multiple Sclerosis Society of Great Britain and Northern Ireland.

Freeman, J., Gorst, T., Gunn, H., Robens, S., 2020. "A non-person to the rest of the world", experiences of social isolation amongst severely impaired people with multiple sclerosis. Disabil. Rehabil. 42, 2295–2303.

Freeman, J., Hendrie, W., Jarrett, L., et al., 2019. Assessment of a home-based standing frame programme in people with progressive multiple sclerosis (SUMS): a pragmatic, multi-centre, randomised, controlled trial and cost-effectiveness analysis. Lancet Neurol. 18, 736–747.

Garcia-Munoz, C., Cortes-Vega, M.D., Heredia-Rizo, A.M., Martin-Valero, R., Garcia-Bernal, M.I., Casuso-Holgado, M.J., 2020. Effectiveness of vestibular training for balance and dizziness rehabilitation in people with multiple sclerosis: a systematic review and meta-analysis. J. Clin. Med. 9, 590.

Ghahfarrokhi, M.M., Banitalebi, E., Negaresh, R., Motl, R.W., 2021. Home-based exercise training in multiple sclerosis: a systematic review with implications for future research. Mult. Scler. Relat. Disord. 55, 103177.

Gharakhanlou, R., Wesselmann, L., Rademacher, A., et al., 2020. Exercise training and cognitive performance in persons with multiple sclerosis: a systematic review and multilevel meta-analysis of clinical trials. Mult. Scler. 27, 1977–1993.

Giovannoni, G., Butzkueven, Helmut, H., et al., 2017. Brain Health: Time Matters in Multiple Sclerosis. Available at: www.msbrainhealth.org. Accessed 2 June 2023.

Giovannoni, G., Hawkes, C., Lechner-Scott, J., Levy, M., Waubant, E., Gold, J., 2020. 'The COVID-19 pandemic and the use of MS disease-modifying therapies'. Mult. Scler. Relat. Disord. 39, 102073.

Gold, R., Oreja-Guevara, C., 2013. Advances in the management of multiple sclerosis spasticity: multiple sclerosis spasticity guidelines. Expert. Rev. Neurother. 13 (12 Suppl.), 55–59.

Goverover, Y., Chiaravalloti, N.D., O'Brien, A.R., DeLuca, J., 2018. Evidenced-based cognitive rehabilitation. for persons with multiple sclerosis: an updated review of the literature from 2007 to 2016. Arch. Phys. Med. Rehabil. 99, 390–407.

Gunn, H., Cameron, M., Hoang, P., Lord, S., Shaw, S., Freeman, J., 2018. The relationship between physiological and perceived fall risk in people with multiple sclerosis: implications for assessment and management. Arch. Phys. Med. Rehabil. 99, 2022–2029.

Hanna, M., Strober, L.B., 2020. Anxiety and depression in multiple sclerosis (MS): antecedents, consequences, and differential impact on well-being and quality of life. Mult. Scler. Relat. Disord. 44, 102261.

Harding, K., Zhu, F., Alotaibi, M., Duggan, T., Tremlett, H., Kingwell, E., 2020. Multiple cause of death analysis in multiple sclerosis. Neurology. 94, e820.

Harding, K.E., Wardle, M., Moore, P., et al., 2015. Modelling the natural history of primary progressive multiple sclerosis. J. Neurol. Neurosurg. Psychiatry. 86, 13–19.

Harrison, A.M., Bogosian, A., Silber, E., et al., 2015a. 'It feels like someone is hammering my feet': Understanding pain and its management from the perspective of people with multiple sclerosis. Mult. Scler. 21, 466–476.

Harrison, A.M., Safari, R., Mercer, T., et al., 2021. Which exercise and behavioural interventions show most promise for treating fatigue in multiple sclerosis? A network meta-analysis. Mult. Scler. 27, 1657–1678.

Harrison, A.M., Silber, E., McCracken, L.M., et al., 2015b. Beyond a physical symptom: the importance of psycho-social factors in multiple sclerosis pain. Eur. J. Neurol. 22, 1443–1452.

Heesen, C., Haase, R., Melzig, S., et al., 2018. Perceptions on the value of bodily functions in multiple sclerosis. Acta. Neurol. Scand. 137, 356–362.

Higginson, I., Hart, S., Silber, E., Burman, R., Edmonds, P., 2006. Symptom prevalence and severity in people severely affected by multiple sclerosis. J. Palliat. Care. 22, 158–165.

Hoang, P.D., Gandevia, S.C., Herbert, R.D., 2014. Prevalence of joint contractures and muscle weakness in people with multiple sclerosis. Disabil. Rehabil. 36, 1588–1593.

Hobart, J., Lamping, D., Fitzpatrick, R., Riazi, A., Thompson, A., 2001. The Multiple Sclerosis Impact Scale (MSIS-29): a new patient-based outcome measure. Brain. 124, 962–973.

Hobart, J.C.J., Riazi, A., Lamping, D.L.D., Fitzpatrick, R., Thompson, A.J.A., 2003. Measuring the impact of MS on walking ability – the 12-Item MS Walking Scale (MSWS-12). Neurology. 60, 31–36.

Hvid, L.G., Feys, P., Baert, I., Kalron, A., Dalgas, U., 2020. Accelerated trajectories of walking capacity across the adult life span in persons with multiple sclerosis: an underrecognized challenge. Neurorehabil. Neural. Rep. 34, 360–369.

Inojosa, H., Proschmann, U., Akgün, K., Ziemssen, T., 2021. Should we use clinical tools to identify disease progression? Front. Neurol. 11, 628542.

Jaul, E., Factor, H., Karni, S., Schiffmiller, T., Meiron, O., 2019. Spasticity and dementia increase the risk of pressure ulcers. Int. Wound J. 16, 847–851.

Kalb, R., Brown, T.R., Coote, S., et al., 2020. Exercise and lifestyle physical activity recommendations for people with multiple sclerosis throughout the disease course. Mult. Scler. J 26, 1459–1469.

Kaltsatou, A., Flouris, A.D., 2019. Impact of pre-cooling therapy on the physical performance and functional capacity of multiple sclerosis patients: a systematic review. Mult. Scler. Relat. Disord. 27, 419–423.

Kamm, C.P., Uitdehaag, B.M., Polman, C.H., 2014. Multiple sclerosis: current knowledge and future outlook. Eur. Neurol. 72, 132–141.

Kang, E., Kim, M.Y., Lipsey, K.L., Foster, E.R., 2022. Person-centered goal setting: a systematic review of intervention components and level of active engagement in rehabilitation goal-setting interventions. Arch. Phys. Med. Rehabil. 103, 121–130.e3.

Karakas, H., Seebacher, B., Kahraman, T., 2021. Technology-based rehabilitation in people with multiple sclerosis: a narrative review. J. Mult. Scler. Res. 1, 54–68.

Kaufman, D.W., Reshef, S., Golub, H.L., et al., 2014. Survival in commercially insured multiple sclerosis patients and comparator subjects in the U.S. Mult. Scler. Relat. Disord. 3, 364–371.

Knowles, L.M., Phillips, K.M., Herring, T.E., et al., 2021. Pain intensity and pain interference in people with progressive multiple sclerosis compared with people with relapsing-remitting multiple sclerosis. Arch. Phys. Med. Rehabil. 102, 1959–1964.

Lamers, I., Feys, P., Swinnen, E., 2018. Robot-supported rehabilitation in persons with multiple sclerosis. In: Colombo, R., Sanguineti, V. (Eds.), Rehabilitation Robotics. Academic Press. https://www.elsevier.com/books/rehabilitation-robotics/colombo/978-0-12-811995-2. Accessed 2 June 2023.

Lamers, I., Maris, A., Severijns, D., et al., 2016. Upper limb rehabilitation in people with multiple sclerosis: a systematic review. Neurorehabil. Neural. Repair. 30, 773–793.

Langdon, D.W., Amato, M.P., Boringa, J., et al., 2012. Recommendations for a Brief International Cognitive Assessment for Multiple Sclerosis (BICAMS). Mult. Scler. J. 18, 891–898.

Lassmann, H., 2019. Pathogenic mechanisms associated with different clinical courses of multiple sclerosis. Front. Immunol. 9, 3116.

Latimer-Cheung, A.E., Pilutti, L.A., Hicks, A.L., et al., 2013. Effects of exercise training on fitness, mobility, fatigue, and health-related quality of life among adults with multiple sclerosis: a systematic review to inform guideline development. Arch. Phys. Med. Rehabil. 94, 1800–1828.e3.

León Ruiz, M., Sospedra, M., Arce Arce, S., Tejeiro-Martínez, J., Benito-León, J., 2022. Current evidence on the potential therapeutic applications of transcranial magnetic stimulation in multiple sclerosis: a systematic review of the literature. Neurología. 37, 199–215.

Leray, E., Moreau, T., Fromont, A., Edan, G., 2016. Epidemiology of multiple sclerosis. Rev. Neurol. 172, 3–13.

Levy, J., Prigent, H., Bensmail, D., 2018. Respiratory rehabilitation in multiple sclerosis: a narrative review of rehabilitation techniques. Ann. Phys. Rehabil. Med. 61, 38–45.

Lublin, F.D., Reingold, S.C., Cohen, J.A., et al., 2014. Defining the clinical course of multiple sclerosis: the 2013 revisions. Neurology. 83, 278–286.

Maguire, R., Maguire, P., 2020. Caregiver burden in multiple sclerosis: recent trends and future directions. Curr. Neurol. Neurosci. Rep. 20, 18.

Mahad, D.H., Trapp, B.D., Lassmann, H., 2015. Pathological mechanisms in progressive multiple sclerosis. Lancet Neurol. 14, 183–193.

Manjaly, Z.-M., Harrison, N.A., Critchley, H.D., et al., 2019. Pathophysiological and cognitive mechanisms of fatigue in multiple sclerosis. J. Neurol. Neurosurg. Psychiatry. 90, 642.

Marquer, A., Barbieri, G., Perennou, D., 2014. The assessment and treatment of postural disorders in cerebellar ataxia: a systematic review. Ann. Phys. Rehabil. Med. 57, 67–78.

Marrie, R.A., 2017. Comorbidity in multiple sclerosis: implications for patient care. Nat. Rev. Neurol. 13, 375–382.

Marrie, R.A., Cutter, G.R., Tyry, T., 2013. Substantial burden of dizziness in multiple sclerosis. Mult. Scler. Relat. Disord. 2, 21–28.

Marsden, J., Harris, C., 2011. Cerebellar ataxia: pathophysiology and rehabilitation. Clin. Rehabil. 25, 195–216.

Massot, C., Donze, C., Guyot, M.A., Leteneur, S., 2021. Low back pain in patients with multiple sclerosis: a systematic review and the prevalence in a French multiple sclerosis population. Rev. Neurol. 177, 349–358.

McFaul, D., Hakopian, N.N., Smith, J.B., Nielsen, A.S., Langer-Gould, A., 2021. Defining benign/burnt-out MS and discontinuing disease-modifying therapies. Neurol. Neuroimmunol. Neuroinflamm. 8 (2). Available at: https://nn.neurology.org/content/8/2/. Accessed 2 June 2023.

McGinley, M.P., Goldschmidt, C.H., Rae-Grant, A.D., 2021. Diagnosis and treatment of multiple sclerosis: a review. JAMA. 325, 765–779.

McGinnis, E., Nelson, A.E., Gorecki, C., Nixon, J., 2015. What is different for people with MS who have pressure ulcers: a reflective study of the impact upon people's quality of life? J. Tissue. Viability. 24, 83–90.

Medeiros Jr., W.L.G., Demore, C.C., Mazaro, L.P., et al., 2020. Urinary tract infection in patients with multiple sclerosis: an overview. Mult. Scler. Relat. Disord. 46, 102462.

Meyer-Heim, A., Rothmaier, M., Weder, M., et al, 2007. Advanced lightweight cooling-garment technology: functional improvements in thermosensitive patients with multiple sclerosis. Multiple Sclerosis J. 13, 232–237.

Miller, L., McFadyen, A., Lord, A.C., et al., 2017. Functional electrical stimulation for foot drop in multiple sclerosis: a systematic review and meta-analysis of the impact on gait speed. Arch. Phys. Med. Rehabil. 98, 1435–1452.

Miller, L., van Wijck, F., Lamont, L., Preston, J., Hair, M., 2016. Sensory dynamic orthoses in mild to moderate upper limb tremor in multiple sclerosis: a mixed methods feasibility study. Clin. Rehabil. 30, 1060–1073.

Miller, P., Soundy, A., 2017. The pharmacological and non-pharmacological interventions for the management of fatigue related multiple sclerosis. J. Neurol. Sci. 381, 41–54.

Milinis, K., Tennant, A., Young, C.A., 2016. Spasticity in multiple sclerosis: associations with impairments and overall quality of life. Mult. Scler. Relat. Disord. 5, 34–39.

Moss-Morris, R., Harrison, A.M., Safari, R., et al., 2021. Which behavioural and exercise interventions targeting fatigue show the most promise in multiple sclerosis? A systematic review with narrative synthesis and meta-analysis. Behav. Res. Ther. 137, 103464.

Motl, R.W., Sandroff, B.M., Kwakkel, G., et al., 2017. Exercise in patients with multiple sclerosis. Lancet. Neurol. 16, 848–856.

Muhtaroglu, M., Mut, Ertugrul, Selcuk, S., Malkoc, M., F., 2020. Evaluation of respiratory functions and quality of life in multiple sclerosis patients. Acta. Neurol/ Belg. 120, 1107–1113.

National Institute for Clinical Excellence (NICE)., 2022. Multiple sclerosis in adults: management. NICE guideline (NG220)., Available at: https://www.nice.org.uk/guidance/ng220. Accessed 2 June 2023.

National Institute for Clinical Excellence (NICE)., 2020. Low back pain and sciatica in over 16s: assessment and management. NICE guideline [NG59]. Available at: https://www.nice.org.uk/guidance/ng59. Accessed April 26, 2022.

National Institute for Clinical Excellence (NICE)., 2021. Chronic pain (primary and secondary) in over 16s: assessment of all chronic pain and management of chronic primary pain. NICE guideline [NG193]. https://www.nice.org.uk/guidance/ng193. Accessed April 26, 2022.

National Institute for Health and Care Excellence (NICE)., 2014. RCN RCoN. Pressure ulcers: prevention and management of pressure ulcers. NICE Guideline CG 1792014. Available at: https://www.nice.org.uk/Guidance/CG179. Accessed April 26, 2022.

Nilsagård, Y., Gunn, H., Freeman, J., et al., 2015. Falls in people with MS: an individual data meta-analysis from studies from Australia, Sweden, United Kingdom and the United States. Mult. Scler. 21, 92–100.

Noseworthy, J.H., Lucchinetti, C., Rodriguez, M., Weinshenker, B.G., 2000. Multiple sclerosis. N. Engl. J. Med. 343, 938–952.

Oliva Ramirez, A., Keenan, A., Kalau, O., Worthington, E., Cohen, L., Singh, S., 2021. Prevalence and burden of multiple sclerosis-related fatigue: a systematic literature review. BMC. Neurol. 21, 468.

Olsson, T., Barcellos, L.F., Alfredsson, L., 2017. Interactions between genetic, lifestyle and environmental risk factors for multiple sclerosis. Nat. Rev. Neurol. 13, 25–36.

O'Malley, N., Clifford, A.M., Conneely, M., Casey, B., Coote, S., 2021. Effectiveness of interventions to prevent falls for people with multiple sclerosis, Parkinson's disease and stroke: an umbrella review. BMC. Neurol. 21, 378.

Ortiz-Rubio, A., Cabrera-Martos, I., Rodriguez-Torres, J., Fajardo-Contreras, W., Diaz-Pelegrina, A., Valenza, M.C., 2016. Effects of a home-based upper limb training program in patients with multiple sclerosis: a randomized controlled trial. Arch. Phys. Med. Rehabil. 97, 2027–2033.

Otero-Romero, S., Sastre-Garriga, J., Comi, G., et al., 2016. Pharmacological management of spasticity in multiple sclerosis: systematic review and consensus paper. Mult. Scler. 22, 1386–1396.

Parker, L.-S., Topcu, G., De Boos, D., das Nair, R., 2021. The notion of "invisibility" in people's experiences of the symptoms of multiple sclerosis: a systematic meta-synthesis. Disabil. Rehabil. 43, 3276–3290.

Pearson, M., Dieberg, G., Smart, N., 2015. Exercise as a therapy for improvement of walking ability in adults with multiple sclerosis: a meta-analysis. Arch. Phys. Med. Rehabil. 96, 1339–1348.e7.

Penner, I.K., Raselli, C., Stöcklin, M., Opwis, K., Kappos, L., Calabrese, P., 2009. The Fatigue Scale for Motor and Cognitive Functions (FSMC): validation of a new instrument to assess multiple sclerosis-related fatigue. Mult. Scler. J. 15, 1509–1517.

Petty, J., Davies, A., 2008. Translating the NICE and NSF guidance into practice: A guide for physiotherapists. Multiple Sclerosis Society (UK), London.

Picariello, F., Freeman, J., Moss-Morris, R., 2022. Defining routine fatigue care in multiple sclerosis in the United Kingdom: what treatments are offered and who gets them? Mult. Scler. J. 8, 20552173211072274.

Ponath, G., Park, C., Pitt, D., 2018. The role of astrocytes in multiple sclerosis. Front. Immunol. 9, 217.

Plow, M., Finlayson, M., 2019. Beyond supervised therapy: promoting behavioral changes in people with MS. Mult. Scler. 25, 1379–1386.

Plow, M.P., Finlayson, M.P., Liu, J.M.S., Motl, R.W.P., Bethoux, F.M.D., Sattar, A.P., 2019. Randomized controlled trial of a telephone-delivered physical activity and fatigue self-management interventions in adults with multiple sclerosis. Arch. Phys. Med. Rehabil. 100, 2006–2014.

Portaccio, E., Fonderico, M., Hemmer, B., et al., 2022. Impact of COVID-19 on multiple sclerosis care and management: Results from the European Committee for Treatment and Research in Multiple Sclerosis survey. Mult. Scler. J 28, 132–138.

Pöttgen, J., Moss-Morris, R., Wendebourg, J.M., et al., 2018. Randomised controlled trial of a self-guided online fatigue intervention in multiple sclerosis. J. Neurol. Neurosurg. Psychiatry 89, 970–976.

Preziosi, G., Gordon-Dixon, A., Emmanuel, A., 2018. Neurogenic bowel dysfunction in patients with multiple sclerosis: prevalence, impact, and management strategies. Degen. Neurol. Neuromusc. Dis. 8, 79–90.

Prosperini, L., Filippo, M., Di, 2019. Beyond clinical changes: rehabilitation-induced neuroplasticity in MS. Mult. Scler. 25, 1348–1362.

Psarakis, M., Greene, D., Moresi, M., et al., 2017. Impaired heel to toe progression during gait is related to reduced ankle range of motion in people with multiple sclerosis. Clin. Biomech. 49, 96–100.

Psarakis, M., Lord, S.R., Hoang, P.D., 2021. Safety, feasibility, and efficacy of eccentric exercise intervention in people with multiple sclerosis with ankle contractures. Int. J. MS Care. 23, 31–36.

Rademacher, A., Joisten, N., Proschinger, S., et al., 2021. Cognitive impairment impacts exercise effects on cognition in multiple sclerosis. Front. Neurol. 11, 619500.

Rae-Grant, A., Day, G.S., Marrie, R.A., et al., 2018. Practice guideline recommendations summary: disease-modifying therapies for adults with multiple sclerosis: report of the Guideline Development, Dissemination, and Implementation Subcommittee of the American Academy of Neurology. Neurology. 90, 777–788.

Razazian, N., Kazeminia, M., Moayedi, H., et al., 2020. The impact of physical exercise on the fatigue symptoms in patients with multiple sclerosis: a systematic review and meta-analysis. BMC. Neurol. 20, 93.

Rice, L.A., Yarnot, R., Peterson, E.W., Backus, D., Sosnoff, J., 2021. Fall prevention for people with multiple sclerosis who use wheelchairs and scooters. Arch. Phys. Med. Rehabil. 102, 801–804.

Rommer, P.S., Eichstädt, K., Ellenberger, D., et al., 2019. Symptomatology and symptomatic treatment in multiple sclerosis: results from a nationwide MS registry. Mult. Scler. 25, 1641–1652.

Roy, H., Aziz, T., 2020. Indications and approaches for functional neurosurgery in multiple sclerosis, including the role for lesional surgery and deep brain stimulation. Med. Res. Arch. 8, 1–14.

Rudroff, T., Kindred, J.H., Ketelhut, N.B., 2016. Fatigue in multiple sclerosis: misconceptions and future research directions. Front. Neurol. 7, 122.

Sammaraiee, Y., Yardley, M., Keenan, L., Buchanan, K., Stevenson, V., Farrell, R., 2019. Intrathecal baclofen for multiple sclerosis related spasticity: a twenty-year experience. Mult. Scler. Relat. Disord. 27, 95–100.

Sandroff, B.M., Jones, C.D., Baird, J.F., Motl, R.W., 2020. Systematic review on exercise training as a neuroplasticity-inducing behavior in multiple sclerosis. Neurorehabil. Neural. Rep. 34, 575–588.

Schaefer, L.M., Poettgen, J., Fischer, A., Gold, S., Stellmann, J.-P., Heesen, C., 2019. Impairment and restrictions in possibly benign multiple sclerosis. Brain. Behav. 9, e01259.

Schmid, S., Schweizer, K., Romkes, J., Lorenzetti, S., Brunner, R., 2013. Secondary gait deviations in patients with and without neurological involvement: a systematic review. Gait. Posture. 37, 480–493.

Sesel, A.L., Sharpe, L., Naismith, S.L., 2018. Efficacy of psychosocial interventions for people with multiple sclerosis: a meta-analysis of specific treatment effects. Psychother. Psychosom. 87, 105–111.

Silveira, S.L., Huynh, T., Kidwell, A., Sadeghi-Bahmani, D., Motl, R.W., 2021. Behavior change techniques in physical activity interventions for multiple sclerosis. Arch. Phys. Med. Rehabil. 102, 1788–1800.

Smith, R.M., Adeney-Steel, M., Fulcher, G., Longley, W.A., 2006. Symptom change with exercise is a temporary phenomenon for people with multiple sclerosis. Arch. Phys. Med. Rehabil. 87, 723–727.

Solari, A., Giordano, A., Sastre-Garriga, J., et al., 2020. EAN guideline on palliative care of people with severe, progressive multiple sclerosis. Eur. J. Neurol. 27, 1510–1529.

Soler, B., Ramari, C., Valet, M., Dalgas, U., Feys, P., 2020. Clinical assessment, management, and rehabilitation of walking impairment in MS: an expert review. Exp. Rev. Neurother., 1–12.

Stevens, V., Goodman, K., Rough, K., Kraft, G.H., 2013. Gait impairment and optimizing mobility in multiple sclerosis. Phys. Med. Rehabil. Clin. N. Am. 24, 573–592.

Stevenson, V., 2016. Oral medication. In: Stevenson, V.L., Jarrett, L. (Eds.), Spasticity Management: A Practical Multidisciplinary Guide. CRC Press, London.

Stratton, R.J., Ek, A.-C., Engfer, M., et al., 2005. Enteral nutritional support in prevention and treatment of pressure ulcers: a systematic review and meta-analysis. Ageing Res. Rev. 4, 422–450.

Synnott, E., Baker, K., 2020. The effectiveness of vestibular rehabilitation on balance related impairments among multiple sclerosis patients: a systematic review. J. Mult. Scler. 7, 1–8.

Tallantyre, E.C., Major, P.C., Atherton, M.J., et al., 2019. How common is truly benign MS in a UK population? J. Neurol. Neurosurg. Psychiatry. 90, 522–528.

Taylor, L.A., Mhizha-Murira, J.R., Smith, L., et al., 2021. Memory rehabilitation for people with multiple sclerosis. Cochrane. Database. Syst. Rev. 10, Cd008754.

Thompson, A.J., Baranzini, S.E., Geurts, J., Hemmer, B., Ciccarelli, O., 2018a. Multiple sclerosis. Lancet. 391, 1622–1636.

Thompson, A.J., Banwell, B.L., Barkhof, F., et al., 2018b. Diagnosis of multiple sclerosis: 2017 revisions of the McDonald criteria. Lancet. Neurol. 17, 162–173.

Tsagkas, C., Magon, S., Gaetano, L., et al., 2019. Preferential spinal cord volume loss in primary progressive multiple sclerosis. Mult. Scler. J. 25, 947–957.

Turner-Stokes, L., Williams, H., Bill, A., Bassett, P., Sephton, K., 2016. Cost-efficiency of specialist inpatient rehabilitation for working-aged adults with complex neurological disabilities: a multicentre cohort analysis of a national clinical data set. BMJ. Open. 6, e010238.

Tzelepis, G.E., McCool, F.D., 2015. Respiratory dysfunction in multiple sclerosis. Respir. Med. 109, 671–679.

Valet, M., Quoilin, M., Lejeune, T., et al., 2019. Effects of fampridine in people with multiple sclerosis: a systematic review and meta-analysis. CNS. Drugs. 33, 1087–1099.

van der Feen, F.E., de Haan, G.A., van der Lijn, I., Heersema, D.J., Meilof, J.F., Heutink, J., 2020. Independent outdoor mobility of persons with multiple sclerosis – a systematic review. Mult. Scler. Relat. Disord. 37, 101463.

van der Feen, F.E., de Haan, G.A., van der Lijn, I., et al., 2022. Recognizing visual complaints in people with multiple sclerosis: Prevalence, nature and associations with key characteristics of MS. Mult. Scler. Relat. Disord. 57, 103429.

van Vugt, V.A., van der Horst, H.E., Payne, R.A., Maarsingh, O.R., 2017. Chronic vertigo: treat with exercise, not drugs. BMJ. 358, j3727.

Vergaro, E., Squeri, V., Brichetto, G., et al., 2010. Adaptive robot training for the treatment of incoordination in multiple sclerosis. J. Neuroeng. Rehabil. 7, 37.

Walton, C., King, R., Rechtman, L., et al., 2020. Rising prevalence of multiple sclerosis worldwide: insights from the Atlas of MS, 3rd edition. Mult. Scler. 26, 1816–1821.

Webster, A., Poyade, M., Rooney, S., Paul, L., 2021. Upper limb rehabilitation interventions using virtual reality for people with multiple sclerosis: a systematic review. Mult. Scler. Relat. Disord. 47, 102610.

Wendebourg, M.J., Heesen, C., Finlayson, M., Meyer, B., Pöttgen, J., Köpke, S., 2017. Patient education for people with multiple sclerosis-associated fatigue: a systematic review. PLoS One. 12, e0173025.

White, A.T., Wilson, T.E., Davis, S.L., et al, 2000. Effect of precooling on physical performance in multiple sclerosis. Multiple Sclerosis J. 6, 176–180.

Wingerchuk, D.M., Weinshenker, B.G., 2016. Disease modifying therapies for relapsing multiple sclerosis. BMJ. i3518.

Wright, L.J., 2012. Identifying and treating pain caused by MS. J. Clin. Psych. 73, e23.

Yeroushalmi, S., Maloni, H., Costello, K., Wallin, M.T., 2022. Telemedicine and multiple sclerosis: a comprehensive literature review. J. Telemed. Telecare. 26, 400–413.

Yilmazer, C., Lamers, I., Solaro, C., Feys, P., 2022. Clinical perspective on pain in multiple sclerosis. Mult. Scler. J. 28, 502–511.

Zesiewicz, T.A., Wilmot, G., Kuo, S.H., et al., 2018. Comprehensive systematic review summary: treatment of cerebellar motor dysfunction and ataxia: Report of the Guideline Development, Dissemination, and Implementation Subcommittee of the American Academy of Neurology. Neurology. 90, 464–471.

Zijdewind, I., Prak, R.F., Wolkorte, R., 2016. Fatigue and fatigability in persons with multiple sclerosis. Exer. Sport. Sci. Rev. 44, 123–128.

Zuber, P., Tsagkas, C., Papadopoulou, A., et al., 2020. Efficacy of inpatient personalized multidisciplinary rehabilitation in multiple sclerosis: behavioural and functional imaging results. J. Neurol. 267, 1744–1753.

Parkinson's

Bhanu Ramaswamy and Mariella Graziano

OUTLINE

Introduction, 265
Epidemiology and Aetiology, 266
Pathophysiology, 267
Neuroanatomy, 267
Medical Management, 268
   Diagnosis and Clinical Presentation, 268
   Pharmacological Management, 270
   Surgical Management, 270
   Research into Newer Technologies, 271
Team Management, 271
   Time Course From Diagnosis of Parkinson's, and Communication, 272

Physiotherapy Management, 274
   Referral to Physiotherapy, 274
   Physiotherapy History Taking, 275
   Physical Assessment, 276
   Goal Setting and Choosing Treatments, 276
      Exercise, 279
      Practice, 281
      Movement Strategies Training, 282
Conclusion, 284

INTRODUCTION

Parkinson's is the fastest growing neurodegenerative disorder in the world, with no known cure. It is not infectious, yet the figures projected of nearly 13 million people diagnosed with Parkinson's across the globe by 2040 are requiring the condition be considered in pandemic terms (Dorsey et al 2018).

Parkinson's progressive nature, plus range and variability of motor and nonmotor symptoms affect function, mobility and life quality of people with the condition. Progress is less predictable now that increased treatments are available; therefore, an individually tailored approach is required to inform and intervene appropriately both for those diagnosed with Parkinson's and close family members.

The Covid-19 pandemic highlighted how the breakdown of support mechanisms can adversely affect the health and activity of people with Parkinson's (Simpson et al 2020), with an enforced change in routine negatively affecting psychological and physical health, plus reducing important social contact (Brown et al 2020, Helmich & Bloem 2020).

Physiotherapy forms an important part of the shared management of the condition, and can have a positive effect on the lifestyle and quality of life for people with Parkinson's, with a greater emphasis on early referral, and for the use of exercise from diagnosis onward to minimise progression of both the pathological processes directly related to Parkinson's, as well as to counter the effects of secondary complications (Keus et al 2014, National Institute of health and Clinical Excellence [NICE] 2017, Osborne et al 2022, Rafferty et al 2017).

The effective practice of physiotherapists working alongside people diagnosed with Parkinson's requires an ability to apply knowledge and skills about this pathology appropriately. Despite diagnosis being based on physical presentations, the impact on the individual with Parkinson's is seldom experienced in isolation, but as physical, psychological and sociocultural contexts requiring the support of family, friends, neighbours and work colleagues. The effects of ageing and secondary pathological processes often compound the progression of the condition.

Therefore, the recommended intervention for people with the condition is through multi- or interdisciplinary management (Lindop & Skelly 2021). Where such as service is unavailable, the physiotherapist should know when and where to act as a referral point to other services. This includes provision through the voluntary or private sectors.

Because this chapter has been written to assist the development of therapy practice, although demography, pathology and multidisciplinary intervention is considered in the first part of the chapter, there is greater focus on the practical aspects of assessment and management to help practitioners form appropriate clinical judgements to plan and share management of the condition effectively with those affected by Parkinson's.

EPIDEMIOLOGY AND AETIOLOGY

The global incidence of Parkinson's is rising (Dorsey et al 2018). It affects an estimated 10 million people (Bridgeman & Arsham 2017, p. 47), although numbers are inconsistently recorded because of differing administrative processes, countries where communities may not seek medical care and people awaiting diagnosis (Hirsch et al 2016).

Across the UK, there are 145,000 people living with Parkinson's. The average incidence is 286 cases per 100,000 population and around 17,000 new diagnoses per year (Parkinson's UK 2018), although this varies in incidence by age, gender, social deprivation score and urban/rural status (Horsfall et al 2013).

With regards to aetiology, although the condition was first described 200 years ago by Dr James Parkinson in his essay *The Shaking Palsy*, its cause remains largely unknown. Hence, the common form is referred to as 'idiopathic Parkinson's', 'idiopathic Parkinson's disease' or 'IPD', which accounts for 70% of people with 'Parkinsonism'. Multicausal possibilities include interaction between infective or toxic environmental factors from increasing industrialisation within our societies, for example, air pollution, pesticide use, solvent or heavy metal exposure (Dorsey et al 2018). These affect mitochondrial function on dopamine-producing neurones (Subramaniam & Chesselet 2013) or cause genetic mutations in Parkinson's-related proteins, such as misfolding, aggregation, inflammatory and immunological processes leading to cell death (Blesa et al 2015).

Parkinson's is largely considered a sporadic disease (i.e., not inherited but arising from a mutation), despite a few clear cases of familial genetic forms of Parkinson's (Goedert et al 2017). More is being discovered about the pathology and treatments available for people with Parkinson's and the atypical Parkinson's conditions, that is, those with similar characteristics to be grouped within this neurological umbrella (Goedert et al 2017).

Parkinson's is most commonly diagnosed in the older generation, accounting for about 1% of adults 65 years or older. Increasing numbers are being identified in younger people too, including those younger than 40 years (Bridgeman & Arsham 2017, p. 51, Parkinson's UK 2018). The gender difference is typically 1.5:1 male to female, but because women live longer, numbers even out over time (Hirsch et al 2016, Parkinson's UK 2018).

Studies of mortality in Parkinson's are limited by the accuracy of death certification and diagnostic confusion between other neurodegenerative conditions, but they suggest that life expectancy is reduced because of Parkinson's (Okunoye et al 2021), with the increased risk of respiratory complications as the highest cause of mortality (Pennington et al 2010). Age of onset and chronological age at diagnosis, motor severity, cognitive impairment plus dementia, and psychotic symptoms independently predict an increased mortality risk (Aarsland 2008, Forsaa et al 2010).

Health and social care, plus societal costs, increase as the condition progresses. People with Parkinson's have a higher risk of hospital and (subsequent) care home admission (Klaptocz et al 2019, Low et al 2015, Osborne et al 2022). In-patient stay from nonelective causes such as pneumonia, Parkinson's management review, urinary infections and hip fractures are longer than for people without the condition (Low et al 2015), with an increased likelihood of extended stay from the development of secondary complications (e.g., infection) (Low et al 2015) and recovery below their preadmission ability (Shahgholi et al 2017).

Parkinson's also generates indirect and hidden costs by affecting employment status through loss of productivity and reduced personal financial circumstances from early retirement, reduction in working hours or altered work roles to better manage the symptoms, or from stress on carers (Gumber et al 2016).

KEY POINTS

Parkinson's is the second most common neurodegenerative disorder in the world, with no known cure, likely caused by an interaction between infective or toxic environmental factors and genetic mutations.

It is most common in the older population, although increasing numbers of individuals are being diagnosed younger, and initially diagnosed more in males.

Parkinson's results in direct health and social care costs, as well as indirect costs from affected employment, use of personal finances and intangible psychosocial costs, such as stress, all experienced over the course of the condition.

PATHOPHYSIOLOGY

The prion hypothesis was initially suggested as the pathophysiology behind Parkinson's, whereby the prion (an infectious agent made solely of misfolded protein) spreads from cell to cell. In neurodegenerative conditions, such as Parkinson's, Lewy body dementia (LBD) and multiple system atrophy (MSA), misfolded and aggregated proteins called alpha-synuclein (α-syn) have been found inside nerve cells (Chu & Kordower 2015).

The pathophysiology of Parkinson's is complex, with interactions between the damaged α-syn inside the nerve cells, mitochondrial dysfunction, vesicle or synaptic transport system malfunction and neuroinflammation (Kalia & Lang 2015). Each system has a part to play in accelerating neuronal death within nervous system pathways, particularly in the dopaminergic neurones affecting the body's movement control (Dorsey et al 2018).

Also, it is thought that 10% of Parkinson's diagnoses result from a genetic cause (Dorsey et al 2018). The younger the person at age of onset, the more likely genetic factors play a role in the aetiology (Crosiers et al 2011). Although only a small proportion of the people living with Parkinson's are linked with genetic causation, their pathology offers a valuable window into the mechanism of the disease process by highlighting specific molecular pathways and their effects at the cellular level (Vázquez-Vélez & Zoghbi 2021).

The role of gut microbiota is increasingly under investigation since histological studies of the brains of people with Parkinson's postmortem led Braak et al (2003) to conceive a staging model emphasising sequential development of increasing degrees of Lewy pathology in anatomically interconnected regions, starting in the bowel with a 'slow virus' entering the central nervous system after passing through the intestinal mucosa (Braak & del Tredici 2017). The interactions between the enteric nervous system, the parasympathetic nerves frequently affected by α-syn pathology and the intestinal microbiota provide a possible cause of the spread of disease to the brain via the vagus nerve (with preganglionic neurons that innervate the distal oesophagus and stomach (Braak & del Tredici 2017, Scheperjans et al 2015a), and other nonnigral regions like the locus coeruleus, pedunculopontine nucleus and Meynert's nucleus in the basal forebrain. Possible neuroprotective effects to a Parkinson's risk from intake of high doses of nicotine and caffeine are also under investigation (Scheperjans et al 2015b).

Much less is known about the atypical parkinsonism conditions, including progressive supranuclear palsy (PSP), MSA, corticobasal disease (CBD) and LBD, than of idiopathic Parkinson's. New insights into the overlaps and differences between the Parkinson's-like conditions complicates diagnosis in the absence of a reliable, disease-specific biomarker (Aerts et al 2012).

NEUROANATOMY

Understanding the neuroanatomical changes during the disease process provides a physiotherapist insight into the complexity of Parkinson's, and why individual makeup, lifestyle choices and their environment make it so variable between individuals.

Motor symptom pathology in Parkinson's is linked primarily to grey matter structures in the subcortical region of the cerebrum and ventral midbrain, the basal ganglia, through interrelationships with neighbouring areas (Lanciego et al 2010). The deep nuclei comprise the striatum (caudate and putamen) and globus pallidus (internus and externus), with related structures including the subthalamic nucleus (STN) (diencephalon), mesencephalon's substantia nigra (pars compacta and reticulata) and pedunculopontine nucleus (pons). Neurodegeneration occurs mostly in the pars compacta, an area rich in neuromelanin-containing cells, giving the region a pigmented appearance (Lanciego et al 2010).

The role of the basal ganglia and related nuclei are broadly threefold. The caudate, putamen and accumbens nucleus (part of a dopaminergic pathway stimulated during rewarding experiences) act as input nuclei to receive information (mainly cortical, thalamic and nigral in origin); the internal globus pallidus (GPi) segment and substantia nigra pars reticulata act as output nuclei, sending information to the thalamus; and the external segment of the globus pallidus (GPe), the STN and substantia nigra pars compacta form the intrinsic nuclei relay of information between the other two structures (Lanciego et al 2010). Functionally, the basal ganglia and related nuclei form part of a series of parallel loops linking with the thalamus and cerebral cortex (particularly the motor cortex and frontal lobe). The basal ganglia are thought to work through direct or indirect pathways, each with an opposing excitatory or inhibitory effect on basal ganglia output according to the motor task required.

It is proposed in Parkinson's that apoptosis as opposed to necrosis (programmed versus accidental cell death) results in the destruction of more than 70% of the neuromelanin-containing neurones, with an effect of depleting the neurotransmitter dopamine in the substantia nigra. As dopamine levels fall, compensatory changes occur in the basal ganglia circuitry, responsible for parkinsonian features. For example, increases in the inhibitory output to the thalamus cause onward circuitry paths to the cortex to suppress movement, resulting in bradykinesia. Being a modulatory neurotransmitter, dopamine deficiency affects background tone, resulting in rigidity and releasing the inhibition of tremor (Lanciego et al 2010), plus it affects the three parallel corticostriatal loops (i.e., the motor, associative and limbic loops. The effect on the associative loop (includes the caudate nucleus and prefrontal cortex) is linked with working memory, apathy and depression (Hirano et al 2012).

Investigations into other neurotransmitters reveal their roles in clinical manifestation. For example, gait and postural instability problems in sporadic Parkinson's have been related to cholinergic and glutaminergic rather than dopaminergic nerve cell and neurotransmitter loss (Karachi et al 2010, Pahapill & Lozano 2000), whilst dopaminergic and cholinergic-mediated systems are considered critical in cognition (Hirano et al 2012).

As knowledge of nondopaminergic-cell dysfunction evolves, more is understood about the development of nonmotor symptoms. Sleep, for example, may be affected by abnormalities in the sleep–wake cycle pathways mediating thalamocortical arousal, including brainstem nuclei such as the raphe nucleus (serotonin), the locus coeruleus (norepinephrine) and pedunculopontine nucleus – all areas related to visual hallucinations and rapid eye movement (REM) sleep behavioural disorder (RBD) in Parkinson's (Chaudhuri & Schapira 2009).

Exploration into where sporadic Parkinson's begins, and whether other (nonnigral) regions of the human anatomy are vulnerable to the degenerative processes and spread underlying Parkinson's pathology, continues. Increasing emphasis is being placed on the development of biomarkers to detect changes early in the disease course and monitor this over time through imaging, permitting in vivo monitoring of progression (Ryman & Poston 2020).

The staging hypothesis mapping the neuropathology of LBD from the brainstem, advancing via midbrain nuclear grey regions into the neocortex (Braak & del Tredici 2017), alongside the prion hypothesis linking gut pathology to Parkinson's, explains the prodromal features of slow transition (autonomic dysregulation, e.g., leading to constipation), hyposmia (loss of smell from olfactory bulb involvement), sleep disorders and mood and cognitive changes (extranigral pathology from involvement at the limbic system level and cortices) (Pagán 2012).

However, Parkinson's rarely presents as a single condition, particularly as pathogenesis parallels natural ageing changes in our nervous and musculoskeletal systems. For example, cognitive impairment worsens, and cardiac disease or metabolic syndromes such as type 2 diabetes develop secondary to increased sedentary behaviour. The consequence of falling may be physical injury to soft tissue or bone fracture and psychological fear slowing movement

> **KEY POINTS**
>
> The motor symptoms of Parkinson's (for which the condition is best known) are primarily associated with deep subcortical nuclei, the basal ganglia and their relationships with neighbouring lobes.
>
> The basal ganglia work through direct and indirect pathways, modulated by varied neurotransmitters, but mainly dopamine, to excite or inhibit output for a required motor task.
>
> The diverse pathology on neuroanatomy from Parkinson's, however, produces varied subjective experiences and symptomatic presentation, including nonmotor symptoms affecting sleep, gut motility, mood and smell.

and increasing disability, both independent risk factors of morbidity. Links of anecdotal reports of the longer-term effects of Covid-19 affecting Parkinson's risk are under investigation.

Therapists require the knowledge and skills to deal with multiple and complex interactions of the conditions.

MEDICAL MANAGEMENT

Diagnosis and Clinical Presentation

James Parkinson (1817) described movement qualities (motor symptoms) still recognised today as major clinical features of the condition.

Research and investigative advances into Parkinson's, new pathological insights and increasing recognition of nonmotor symptoms manifesting prodromally (before motor symptoms) provide the accepted diagnostic criteria for Parkinson's (Bloem et al 2021, Chaudhuri et al 2006a, Postuma et al 2015, 2016).

Diagnosis allows for the presence of dementia but remains based on expert history taking and neurological examination. No single reliable diagnostic test exists to definitively confirm the diagnosis during life. Where uncertainty exists, monitoring symptoms over subsequent consultations improves diagnostic accuracy.

Parkinson's is divided into three stages:

1. A preclinical stage where neurodegeneration is present (detected by molecular biomarkers and imaging) but asymptomatic.
2. Prodromal Parkinson's where motor or nonmotor symptoms are present but clinical Parkinson's criteria have not yet been met. Some symptoms may be experienced 20 years before the observation of a motor symptom. The most widely experienced changes (some noted in other neurological conditions) are:

- Hyposmia – reduced or loss of smell
- Constipation
- RBD
- Low mood and fatigue

3. Clinical Parkinson's with motor parkinsonism: This remains defined by dopamine-responsive motor features of bradykinesia (must be present) plus rigidity or rest tremor or both, which are initially unilateral. Postural instability has been removed as a core feature of Parkinson's; if present early in the condition, it indicates investigation into other neuropathology.

The International Movement Disorder Society (MDS) diagnostic criteria (Postuma et al 2015), the European Physiotherapy Guideline for Parkinson's disease (henceforth referred to as the European Guideline) (Keus et al 2014) and the MDS-sponsored revision of the Unified Parkinson's Rating Scale (MDS-UPDRS) updated examination (Goetz et al 2008) describe the clinical features of Parkinson's in the following way:

Bradykinesia is defined both by slowness (possibly at initiation and movement quality) and by hypokinesia (decreased speed and movement amplitude) of repetitive actions. This is observed in writing, slowness and lack of spontaneous facial expression, and reduced arm swing during walking. Bradykinesia is tested by observing the performance of repetitive opposition with the thumb and each of the other fingers in turn. The expectation is of this sign showing the greatest improvement with medication.

Rigidity is judged by slowness to passive movement of major joints when the patient is relaxed but the assessor is manipulating their limbs and neck. It has a lead-pipe nature of resistance that is velocity independent to the movement direction, usually tested by flexing and extending the wrist or elbow. 'Cogwheeling' describes the rigidity felt in the presence of an underlying tremor, usually at the wrist or ankle.

Tremor is observed in 70% of individuals, primarily as a rest tremor of 4–6 Hz (a slower frequency than an action tremor) and should be inhibited on initiating movement. There are different types of tremors; however, a rest tremor must be observed when the limb is fully relaxed. It is most noticeable in the upper limb as a reciprocal movement of the thumb and forefinger, named for its resemblance of a 'pill-rolling' motion. Resting tremor may be observed during the interview and examination of an individual. Over time, the quality of the tremor may change or disappear.

Later features of Parkinson's include *postural instability*, the most common physical reason being from a flexed posture with weakness in antigravity musculature and tonal changes affecting the ability to support postural adjustments for upright balance. Individuals are tested for their response to counter the loss of balance from a pull backwards (retropulsion) or push forwards (propulsion) test.

Commonly assessed alterations to walking include a shuffling gait (short-stepped, poor foot clearance) as joint range reduces in response to tonal changes. The centre of mass falls relatively forwards to the base of support, resulting in a poorly controlled pattern with increased step frequency but reduced amplitude (festination) or difficulty maintaining the amplitude of pelvic motion during leg loading causing freezing (experienced as problems of movement initiation and the inability to sustain movement when attention is compromised). Freezing and festination can occur together, making activities such as turning and moving in narrow spaces a challenge. These sorts of intrinsic mechanisms affect balance more than extrinsic (environmental) mechanisms and are a main reason for falls.

Overlap in symptomatic experience occurs with individuals (especially with ageing and other pathology); however, certain physical red flags should cause the therapist to question the accuracy of diagnosis of Parkinson's and consider an atypical parkinsonism. For example, falls early in diagnosis (from postural instability), bilateral presentation of increased tone (more pronounced in MSA and CBD) and lower body symptoms only are more indicative of vascular causes of parkinsonism, especially if changes occur in a more definite stepwise manner; more axial presentation (especially back and neck) is more likely to be PSP (Abdo et al 2010, Aerts et al 2012).

The 55 acknowledged nonmotor symptoms can be divided into the following categories:

- Neuropsychiatric: depression, anxiety, apathy, cognitive changes, hallucinations and delusions
- Sleep: restless legs, RBD and loss of atonia during REM sleep, insomnia and daytime sleepiness
- Autonomic: bladder disturbance, excessive sweating, orthostatic hypotension and sexual dysfunction
- Gastrointestinal: dribbling (saliva), choking or dysphagia, nausea and constipation
- Sensory: presenting as pain, paraesthesia and olfaction disturbance
- Other symptoms: fatigue, visual changes, weight loss and weight gain (related to certain medications)

Those experienced may manifest through the course of the condition affecting quality of life (Chaudhuri et al 2006a, 2007, Schrag et al 2014). A few are responsive to dopaminergic treatment (Chaudhuri & Schapira 2009). They can be identified with a simple nonmotor symptom questionnaire (Chaudhuri et al 2006a, 2006b), but ensure people understand they will not experience all the symptoms over the course of the condition.

Imaging is currently not used routinely for diagnosis but is assistive through the varied technology available. In terms of detecting and monitoring Parkinson's progression, magnetic resonance imaging (MRI), positron emission tomography (PET), single-photon emission computed tomography (SPECT) and proton magnetic resonance spectroscopy (MRS) may be used to diagnose and differentiate between the atypical parkinsonisms (NICE 2017).

Pharmacological Management

Parkinson's medication is prescribed to manage symptoms, particularly the motor systems for improved movement ability (NICE 2017).

A discovery in the 1960's linking Parkinson's pathology to a reduction of striatal dopamine in patients with extrapyramidal features (Ehringer & Hornykiewicz 1960) and understanding that the amino acid L-3,4-dihydroxyphenylalanine (L-DOPA) could increase the levels of dopamine in the brain revolutionised treatment, and L-DOPA became the gold standard drug for Parkinson's treatment (Hornykiewicz 2017).

Uncomplicated, idiopathic Parkinson's should respond well to dopaminergic therapy at diagnosis, with a return to a normal or near-normal level of function for the first few years of therapy. The dopaminergic drugs available work by increasing the amount of dopamine in the brain, by stimulating the parts of the brain where dopamine acts or by blocking the action of other factors (enzymes) that break down dopamine (NICE 2017).

A pragmatic, 7-year UK-based trial of long-term medication prescribing practice found slightly greater benefit for patient-rated mobility scores using levodopa as initial treatment compared with levodopa-sparing therapy; the latter drugs demonstrated equivalence in effect when chosen as the initial medication (PD MED Collaborative Group 2014).

In addition to the dopaminergic medications, anticholinergic therapy is also used with a rationale of restoring impaired acetylcholine neurotransmission and striatal dopamine balance, hence reducing the tremor. Symptoms such as dystonia, a cramping and often painful involuntary response seen in Parkinson's, may respond positively to dopaminergic drugs; however, some people will benefit from medications that affect a different neurotransmitter to dopamine or a drug that blocks the action of a nerve on muscle so it cannot contract, for example, botulinum toxin injection.

Although current medications assist in the management of Parkinson's symptoms, there are none that can cure, slow, stop or reverse the progression of the condition. Therefore, Parkinson's is treated symptomatically, increasing doses and mixes of available drugs to control the presenting symptoms. Where symptoms are mild, people might discuss with their specialist postponing drug treatment until their symptoms increase (NICE 2017).

In countries like the UK, varied health professionals, including physiotherapists, prescribe medicines according to their professional role and competence. The priority for Parkinson's medication choice is placed on symptomatic improvement and the prevention or reduction of side effects, motor complications (off periods, where medication is ineffective) and psychiatric complications that occur over the course of Parkinson's.

The most common general effect on starting replacement medications is nausea and/or vomiting. Longer-term use of levodopa therapy can result in the development of abnormal involuntary movements (dyskinesias) and fluctuations in motor control, known as 'on' and 'off' periods, and orthostasis. The effect of dopamine-sparing therapy does not depend on the metabolism of dopamine, so motor complications are seen less frequently with these types of drugs compared with levodopa, suggesting that longer-term symptomatic control could be better with these classes of drugs. Nonmotor side effects such as nausea, hallucinations, oedema, and sleep disturbance are more frequent with the dopamine agonists, as are impulsive and compulsive behaviours. These symptoms can be of greater impact for individuals with Parkinson's and their families than the motor complications (Kincses & Vecesi 2011, PD MED Collaborative Group 2014).

Not all Parkinson's symptoms are related to movement, with careful treatment needed for people who develop neuropsychiatric nonmotor symptoms (e.g., psychosis, hallucinations or dementia) (NICE 2017). In addition to these, treatments are required to manage symptoms of anxiety, pain and constipation, to name but a few, that are not specific to only people with Parkinson's.

To counter some side effects and minimise the numbers of daily tablets prescribed (poor concordance with medications has adverse health and cost implications) (Malek & Grosset 2015), different modes of administering the medications have been manufactured. Drugs are available as skin patches, inhalers, slow-release and once-daily versions, plus invasive delivery through subcutaneous infusions, and a gel directly infused through the duodenum.

Investigation is ongoing into the repurposing drugs for Parkinson's use, that is, use of approved and available drugs for other conditions such as type 2 diabetes (possible neuroprotective role) or nonsteroidal medication (possible anti-inflammatory effects on the oxidative stress processes) (Athauda & Foltynie 2018).

Surgical Management

The commonly described surgical methods for treating people with Parkinson's include stimulation of dopaminergic pathways through deep brain (high frequency) stimulation (DBS), insertion of new cells which either deliver genes so new dopamine cells might form or might repair damaged dopaminergic neurones (still experimental), surgery to destroy parts of the brain and abdominal surgery that includes the insertion of a system to directly infuse levodopa through the duodenum to achieve a stable plasma levodopa concentration (Dorsey et al 2018). All surgery carries a high risk of complications.

The mainstay of surgery is through DBS (NICE 2017) for people with Parkinson's who:

- Have motor complications refractory to best medical treatment;
- Are biologically fit with no clinically significant active comorbidity;
- Are levodopa responsive; or
- Have no clinically significant active mental health problems, for example, depression or dementia.

Although not everyone with Parkinson's is suitable for surgery (Hariz 2017), as technology enhances surgical accuracy and inclusion criteria for the procedures improve, large randomised trials show surgery to be of more benefit into the longer term to the people with advanced Parkinson's than for those only taking medication (Rizzone et al 2014, Williams et al 2010). Self-reported quality of life improves in those who have undergone the procedures through the control of motor symptoms and related complications, although people continue to demonstrate a decline in activities of daily living consistent with the progression of Parkinson's (Deuschl et al 2006, Rizzone et al 2014, Schuenbach et al 2013, Williams et al 2010).

Research Into Newer Technologies

As technology advances, newer less invasive treatments are being investigated to reduce involuntary movement when medication is less effective, for example, MRI-guided focused ultrasound, a treatment that uses ultrasonic energy to target tissue deep in the body.

TEAM MANAGEMENT

The overall goal of management is around enabling people to live life fully by remaining active, engaged, and participating in activities, whilst considering issues affecting their personal and environmental factors. The focus on symptomatic control uses pharmacological, surgical and exercise means to maintain activity and is delivered by experts in Parkinson's collaborating via multidisciplinary teams (MDTs) from diagnosis to the end of life (Lindop & Skelly 2021, Osborne et al 2022, Post et al 2011).

Research advances, developments in technology, escalating healthcare costs and people with Parkinson's demanding a more active role in the shared management of their condition are revolutionising the management of

---

KEY POINTS

The diagnosis of Parkinson's is based on expert clinical observation and assessment using agreed criteria (allowing for the presence of dementia), dividing Parkinson's into three stages: an asymptomatic preclinical stage, a prodromal Parkinson's of emergent motor or nonmotor symptoms and clinical Parkinson's.

Motor symptoms are defined by dopamine-responsive features (initially unilateral) of bradykinesia (slowness and reduced amplitude), rigidity (stiffness) or rest tremor, whereas nonmotor features are numerous and include neuropsychiatric, autonomic and gastrointestinal symptoms; sleep disorders; sensory impairment and other symptoms such as fatigue

Medical management primarily uses drugs to manage motor symptoms, but side effects worsen over time. The 'on' and 'off' phases induced by long-term medication use influence how the person with Parkinson's moved and feels, and therefore affects physiotherapy intervention.

Neurosurgical intervention is mainly through DBS.

Advances in technology are permitting the investigation into the use of less invasive techniques to aid movement quality.

---

chronic neurological conditions, like Parkinson's (Dorsey et al 2018, NICE 2017).

The European Parkinson's Disease Association (EPDA) in conjunction with the World Health Organization (WHO) launched a Charter for People with Parkinson's in 1997, delineating their rights to certain standards of care. These include referral to a doctor with a special interest in Parkinson's to receive an accurate diagnosis, have access to support services, receive continuous care and take part in managing their condition (Bloem & Stocchi 2012). The role of the person with Parkinson's central to their own condition management is increasingly evolving. To date more than 25 professional disciplines can offer benefits for people with Parkinson's throughout the course of their condition, with anecdotal reports of a positive professional intervention impact on life quality for people affected by Parkinson's (Dorsey et al 2018). Fig. 11.1 illustrates the recommended (in green) team members and professionals for referral to if suggested criteria are met (in red) (Keus et al 2014, Appendix 11).

Many centres around the world offer MDT care for people affected by Parkinson's; however, diversity of healthcare systems, educational standards and defined roles of MDT members vary according to resources, professional regulation and expectation (Nijkrake et al 2009).

Rehabilitation medicine[1] or elderly care physician[2] always involved in case of complex motor and non-motor impairments deals with:
- interdisciplinary analyses of limitations and restrictions
- day hospital referral or continuous interdisciplinary care
- support in employment[1]
- assessment of (e.g. walking) aids & home adjustments[1]
- palliative care[2]

Pharmacist deals with:
- provision of medication, including verification and interaction / side effects
- treatment adherence

Psychiatrist deals with:
- energy and drive impairments, e.g. reduced motivation and impulse control
- emotional impairments, e.g. anxiety
- temperament & personality impairments, e.g. mood
- depression
- impairments in perceptual functions, e.g. hallucinations
- sleep impairments
- dementia

Speech therapist deals with:
- reduced voice pitch &loudness
- impaired articulation (e.g. dysarthria)
- impaired swallowing (including drooling)
- reduced speech fluency

Clinical geriatrician deals with:
- frail elderly with complex problems, not well managed with medicines & psychiatry
- comorbidity, falls and polypharmacy

National Parkinson's Society
- advice & support from fellow members and health professionals
- representation of interests

Sexologist deals with:
- impaired sexual functions, e.g. altered performance or interest
- changed sexual perception
- information, e.g. sexual aids
- restrictions in intimate and sexual relationships

Supraregional Parkinson centre of excellence
- to provide multidisciplinairy diagnostics and resultant treatment plan)
- provide specialised treatment (e.g. DBS)

Neurosurgeon deals with:
- severe, unpredictable response fluctuations or dyskinesias
- resistant tremor

Social worker deals with:
- psychosocial problems, e.g. coping
- carer burden (mental and financial)
- limitations & restrictions in interpersonal relationships, e.g. with carer
- loss of meaningful daytime activities
- information & support (financial) benefits

Occupational therapist deals with:
- home l.ife, work, leisure time related limitations & restrictions (incl. cognitive problems, need for assistive devices & home adjustments)
- carer experienced limitations in providing support or care

Physical therapist deals with:
- (risk of) reduced physical capacity & performance
- gait limitations (e.g. freezing)
- limitations in transfers
- limitations in manual activities
- reduced balance; falls
- pain experience & perception

Neuropsychologist deals with:
- patient/carer stress
- complex psychosocial limitations & restrictions
- limitations in acceptance & coping
- limitations in interpersonal relationships, e.g. with carer
- impairments in temperament, in personality and in fear, with or without medication
- cognitive impairments

Dietician deals with:
- weight loss; risk: >5% in 1 month or >10% in 6 months
- reduced quality or quantity of nutritional intake
- medication related nutritional advice (e.g. peri operative)
- constipation

Home care services deals with:
- restrictions in self- care, e.g. dressing
- restrictions in domestic life, e.g. housework

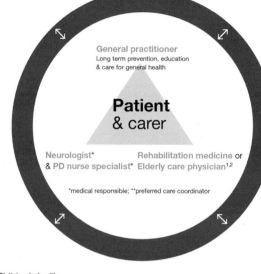

General practitioner
Long term prevention, education & care for general health

Patient & carer

Neurologist*
& PD nurse specialist*

Rehabilitation medicine or Elderly care physician[1,2]

*medical responsible; **preferred care coordinator

FIG. 11.1 Model for collaborative Parkinson's care: health professionals and referral criteria. [Intellectual property of KNGF/ParkinsonNet and reproduced with permission (Keus et al 2014).]

The innovative patient-centred community of ParkinsonNet in the Netherlands in 2004 demonstrated that an MDT approach of healthcare training and delivery for people affected by Parkinson's improved access and care quality whilst reducing healthcare costs for Parkinson's (Keus et al 2012, Nijkrake et al 2010). The ParkinsonNet regional networks of specially trained health professionals link together through a shared online platform to which patients also have access, providing publicly available comments, have been replicated elsewhere with professionals working according to evidence-based guidelines to provide decision support for everyday clinical practice (Bloem & Munneke 2014). This success has inspired other countries to adapt this community, evidence-informed model to their own healthcare systems requirements. The Parkinson's UK (2015a) strategy, for example, has responded to consultation with its wider membership through the voluntary sector to collaborate with National Health Service (NHS) professionals (public sector) through the Parkinson's Excellence Network.

Such services can improve availability of provision for people with Parkinson's in a timely manner and, more importantly, provide access to health professionals with interest and expertise in this condition (Bloem & Munneke 2014, Osborne et al 2022, Post et al 2011).

Time Course From Diagnosis of Parkinson's, and Communication

The impact of diagnosis of a degenerative condition requires communication and education through honest, yet affirmative language. Although the pathological process of Parkinson's is known to be degenerative and incurable, information should be presented in ways that enable people to positively manage the condition (NICE 2017).

Health professionals categorise Parkinson's through motor-defined stages (e.g., a disease stage rating scale from 1 to 5) (Hoehn & Yahr 1967) (Table 11.1) as used in the Clinical Practice Guideline from the American Physical Therapy Association (henceforth referred to as the American Guideline) (Osborne et al 2022), the European

TABLE 11.1 The Modified Hoehn and Yahr Scale

Stage	Scale Descriptors	Disease Phase
1	Unilateral involvement only	Early
1.5	Unilateral and axial involvement	Early
2	Bilateral involvement without impairment of balance	Early
2.5	Mild bilateral disease and recovery on pull test	Early
3	Mild to moderate bilateral disease, some postural instability, physically independent	Complicated/middle
4	Severe disability, still able to walk or stand unassisted	Complicated/middle
5	Wheelchair bound or bedridden unless aided	Late

Guideline (Keus et al 2014) clinical phases (MacMahon & Thomas 1998) and subtypes (Dorsey et al 2018) to identify condition progression. This is useful for research purposes, for charting effective management (particularly of drug therapy and exercise) and considering the point at which to increase support networks to facilitate best care.

These professional-perspective models emphasise difficulties people will experience over the course of Parkinson's, adding to issues of poor acceptance and shock at the diagnosis in people with Parkinson's (Bramley & Eatough 2005, Stanley-Hermanns & Engebretson 2010). They request timely education and availability of support networks, which include experience sharing with others, enable them to live more normally, improving their understanding and management of Parkinson's throughout its course (Bloem & Munneke 2014, Ramaswamy 2016, Wensing et al 2011).

A UK model of the way people with Parkinson's describe their journey not as a linear view of their rate of decline with defined time periods but as a model of shared experience and enriching relationships (Fig. 11.2). The interdependent social model acknowledges that people affected by Parkinson's are aware of the impending decline and the impact poor communication can have on their outlook, but seek activities with others to provide, then maintain, a positive attitude, enabling better coping with the impact of Parkinson's and other comorbidities (Ramaswamy 2016, Webster 2014). It fits observed clinical practice whereby people can show improvements over a 2- to 3-year period after the introduction of a new intervention of interest to them, for example, singing (Elefant et al 2012) or exercise (Combs et al 2014, McConaghy 2014), at whatever stage of their condition.

At 'prediagnosis', people are seeking information to maintain normality in life at a time of minimal motor disturbance. As health consultations are few at this stage, input may come from social groups (often run through the voluntary sector) and self-management groups.

People with Parkinson's consider their journey over the 'elapsing' years as meandering rather than the straight decline seen in the medical models, and it requires relevant support for both the people with Parkinson's and their carers.

The future is seen as requiring positivity: 'holding onto hope', awaiting the cure promised by research while understanding that taking part in activity (attitude, behaviour) slows decline and improves coping despite increases in the experience of apathy and depression.

The model of interdependence promotes empowerment by recognising the evolution of people's individual needs and a way to harness our daily practice through a more positive lens. In addition to shared management, individuals are ultimately supported to engage education and management of others with Parkinson's, as well as in research, and physiotherapists are reminded to consider the importance of quality of life in our clinical dialogue and decisions.

KEY POINTS

People with Parkinson's should be encouraged to participate in activities that enhance life quality.

This is best managed by professionals with expertise in Parkinson's collaborating via multidisciplinary team and the voluntary sector to provide shared management of the condition.

Health professionals categorise Parkinson's through stages that clarify expected condition progression to provide effective management and support.

People with Parkinson's want professionals to nurture interactive relationships and provide education through language that emphasises positive options for management so they can better accept the decline of the condition and share experiences with others.

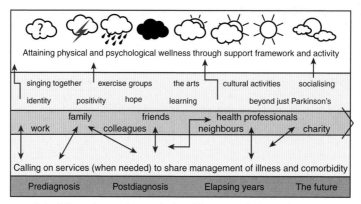

FIG. 11.2 New model of interdependent relationships: needs based as experienced by people affected by Parkinson's. [Model of interdependent relationships produced with permission of Bhanu Ramaswamy, Pamela Goff, Janice Forder and Denise Webster (2014). © B.Ramaswamy]

PHYSIOTHERAPY MANAGEMENT

World Physiotherapy (WP) (the global body for 125 worldwide physiotherapy organisations; https://world.physio/) acknowledges the responsibility of individual national physical therapy associations to support and recognise the distinctive and autonomous nature of physical therapy practice. They advocate for dynamic and responsive practice to the needs of the client, as well as to societal health needs using evidence-informed knowledge and technological advances.

The European Guideline (Keus et al 2014) was a unique initiative of a clinical interest group, the Association of Physiotherapists in Parkinson's Disease Europe (APPDE) (now evolved into the wider global arena of the WP's neurology subgroup). The collaborative project involved 20 European physiotherapy associations plus the EPDA, an organisation with membership of individual country associations concerned with the health and welfare of people living with Parkinson's, their families and carers (https://www.epda.eu.com/), ensuring contribution with people affected by the condition throughout its development.

It uses the *International Classification of Functioning, Disability and Health* (ICF) (World Health Organization [WHO] 2001) domains to describe the health condition (dividing this into body structure and function, the activity and the participation domains), and contextual factors include consideration of environmental and personal issues.

The subsequent American Guideline (Osborne et al 2022) was also developed through wide collaboration of various representative academic and neurological bodies plus the American Parkinson's Disease Association.

Both provide frameworks for physiotherapy intervention using internationally recommended models, plus service user and research-based literature to inform practice. The evidenced reference list is comprehensive, so readers of this chapter will be directed to sources other than in the two guidelines only if there is a specific issue of note that requires an individual reference.

Referral to Physiotherapy

Referral to physiotherapy can come from many sources and at any stage of the condition. It is recommended that an appointment be made soon after diagnosis (NICE 2017) with recommendations for referral criteria tabulated in Table 11.2.

In the past, benefits of early physiotherapy intervention for people with Parkinson's have been poorly represented (Clarke et al 2016), inappropriately provided by therapists with insufficient or no expertise (Nijkrake et al 2009) or service access is inadequate or nonexistent (Parkinson's UK 2015b). Referral to therapy usually occurs in the mid to later stages when the risk of falling and injury increases (particularly if the person is hospitalised) or where impairment to cognition deteriorates, affecting mobility and daily task management (Keus et al 2014). Evidence is building, however, demonstrating that physiotherapy or professional-led exercise interventions in early-stage Parkinson's (some with self-referral criteria) show both the maintenance of function and wellness traits through social interaction with others affected by Parkinson's, as well as health professionals (Combs et al 2014, Keus et al 2014, McConaghy 2014).

TABLE 11.2 Recommended Referral Criteria for People With Parkinson's to Physiotherapy

Based on:[a]	Description
Stage: early	Soon after the diagnosis of Parkinson's disease for: Self-management advice, education and coaching, including support to stay physical active; and If required, tailored intervention to prevent limitations in functional mobility through motor learning, to reduce fear of falling and to improve physical capacity.

Specific impairments or limitations in activities	Presence of:
	• Reduced physical capacity;
	• Functional mobility limitations regarding:
	  • Transfers, such as rising from a chair or rolling in bed,
	  • Gait including freezing,
	  • Balance including falls, and
	  • Manual activities (including upper limb freezing[b])
	• Pain, nonrelated to medication; and
	• Breathing dysfunction.[b]

Context: hospital or nursing home	If admitted to a hospital for any cause or to a nursing home, aim to educate and, if necessary, train people with Parkinson's and health professionals to improve physical capacity or limitations in functional mobility, or to support prevention of falls (e.g., using walking aids) and pressure sores.

[a]Physiotherapists in the UK with a nonmedical prescribing qualification can prescribe, as well as supply and administer, medicines to individually named patients (CSP 2011). The terms by which this process occurs are legislated and monitored under strict guidance.
[b]Added by chapter authors.
[Intellectual property of KNGF/ParkinsonNet and reproduced with permission (Keus et al 2014).]

KEY POINTS

People with Parkinson's should be referred soon after to diagnosis for therapy assessment.
A framework for physiotherapy assists therapists in recognising the impact of pathology, the medication, reduced activity, comorbidity, environmental and personal contextual factors when considering intervention.

Physiotherapy History Taking

As with any intervention, the physiotherapist should incorporate their knowledge with the perspective of the individual seeking treatment. An understanding of the presenting problems, goals, expectations and priorities opens dialogue towards a shared action plan that is realistic, although sometimes requires compromise on both parts.

A 'Preassessment Information Form' (PIF) is available in the Appendices in the European Guideline, recommended to be sent before the first appointment. It assists in the process of building an interdependent relationship by asking questions about previous treatment and expectations (checking what problems the individual would like to tackle first, and in what way they have tried themselves; if they have consulted other professionals, the PIF asks about the effectiveness of prior interventions).

Individuals are prompted to consider more widely the impact of having Parkinson's, their current management, and also relevant information about the role of close family and friends in supporting any needs (Keus et al 2014). The PIF questions lead to personalised treatment suggestions and identify any 'tricks', mentioned in the history taking, that the person may use to overcome the problem. This helps the physiotherapist understand the possible application of compensation strategies, which include cueing for and other strategies to break down and aid complex movements.

The actual history should consider challenges faced around movement-related functional problems, including of the hand, because hand and upper limb function are increasingly affected by freezing, as are gait and speech (Capato et al 2019). Some movement challenges are related to environmental factors, but also personal anxiety-producing factors such as the effect of medication, financial worries, stigma, mood affecting participation in activities and the person's level of coping (Jenkinson et al 1995, 1997, Keus et al 2014) (Fig. 11.3).

Although research trials attempt to eliminate people with other conditions so as not to affect the outcome of an intervention on the Parkinson's element, in clinical practice many of the individuals will have comorbidities such as hypertension, constipation, coronary heart disease and metabolic disorders, as well as Parkinson's, as they fall into the older population (McLean et al 2017, Santos Garcias et al 2017). These added conditions have an impact on history and physical assessment, and their prevalence increases as the person ages or the longer they have had Parkinson's (Santos Garcias et al 2017). The impact of the Covid-19 crisis on the lives of people with Parkinson's in terms of the disease, the deconditioning from lockdown and increased vulnerability to mental health involvement from the isolation (Helmich & Bloem 2020, Simpson et al 2020) must be considered, as should specific questioning about work-related or family issues that might be affecting a person with younger-onset Parkinson's (Gumber et al 2016).

Where mobility of an individual has been affected for a while, they will have often developed compensatory methods to overcome the problem, sometimes subconsciously avoiding a task that takes too long to complete, that fatigues them or that has become difficult, for example, using self-adhesive fastening rather than buttons where dexterity is affected, or simple strategies to initiate movement. The latter are worth noting and checking during the physical assessment as adequate and safe for the person's current needs.

The interview period provides opportunities to observe the person, for example, signs of stress like an exaggerated tremor, limited concentration and engagement with the questioning, affected posture and reduced use of the Parkinson's side, to gain a complete picture of presentation. The presence of a family member or carer alters the dynamics of the session but add richness to the understanding of the social support network and insight into their attitude to the diagnosis.

Physical Assessment

The physical assessment permits a linking of information gathered during the history taking and observations of movement quality to be able to match intervention with expectation(s) of the person with Parkinson's (Fig. 11.3). The physiotherapist must use their knowledge to differentiate between the effects of different pathologies during the assessment to judge which can be treated and which are not amenable to intervention.

It is worthwhile looking at the European Guideline divisions of the assessment section into five areas for which there is evidence available on the effectiveness of physiotherapy (Fig. 11.4): physical capacity, transfers, manual activities, balance and gait. Respiratory function (a morbidity risk

factor) and pain management are also part of therapy care, with chronic pain experienced in 50%–85% of people with Parkinson's, affecting identity and body image (Fil et al 2013, Keus et al 2014, Marques & Brefel-Courbon 2021).

Each section contains triggers for further investigation, or which might limit performance, but are not limited solely to that column. For example, in the Physical Capacity column (see Fig. 11.4), the physiotherapist is guided to check muscle power of hip, knee and ankle (especially extensors known to be weak in people with Parkinson's), with suggested tools useful to measure the ability and possibly monitor change after physical therapy. Weakness in turn affects the transfer of sit to stand when rising from a chair (Inkster et al 2003, Pääsuke et al 2004), recorded in the Transfers column, but also is a known risk factor in walking (causes a reduction in speed) and is a falls risk (Allen et al 2010), and hence recorded in both the Balance and the Gait columns. Tonal differences in those with younger-onset Parkinson's (more dystonic issues) will also alter movement quality and appear as if the muscle is weak (Post et al 2020), or reduction in movement range will affect recruitment of muscle fibres to generate sufficient movement force (Zijlstra et al 2012).

The measurement tools in European Guideline have been chosen on the basis that they had been validated and are reliable for use with a Parkinson's population, are capable of being completed in time-limited clinical appointments and have clear relationships to the ICF framework domains (Keus et al 2014). Be aware that some suggested tools are valid as assessment instruments but not sensitive or designed to measure the outcome of intervention.

Goal Setting and Choosing Treatments

Physiotherapy intervention aims to optimise levels of function and independence to improve a person's quality of life for as long as possible. In neurodegenerative processes, however, it is important to discuss openly that the longer-term aims alter from expecting improvement to maintenance and eventually towards managing physical and mental decline.

Where intervention is indicated, the therapist and person with Parkinson's negotiate and agree to goals of treatment including the time, plus number of sessions it should take to achieve short-term and long-term goals. Goals will address both Parkinson's-specific needs plus relate to the prevention of secondary complications. Engagement of the person with Parkinson's and someone close to them in a supportive role is essential to maintain motivation to achieve set goals into the longer term.

People with Parkinson's may have cognitive impairment even at the point of diagnosis (Litvan et al 2012), affecting memory, visuospatial and attention/executive abilities

European Physiotherapy Guideline for Parkinson's disease

Quick Reference Card 1. History taking

Interest		Supportive	Paying attention to
Perceived problems		PIF 5As model	• The pwp most important problems: support the pwp to prioritise problems • Carer involvement
Medical information		Preferably upon referral from physician	• Parkinson: diagnosis; year of diagnosis; disease stage# • Motor complications: motor fluctuations, unpredictable on and off states*, dyskinesias* and off state dystonia* (if severe, advise pwp to anticipate medical consultation) • Mental complications: executive dysfunction such as in concentration, holding and using information, decision-making, planning, shifting attention from one to another stimulus and dual task performance; anxiety; apathy; depression*; illusions*; hallucinations*; impulse control disorders (e.g. repetitive activities)* • Pain: time of the day, location (e.g. specific or general), quality (e.g. cramping, tingling, shooting), severity* • Comorbidity: heart failure; osteoporosis; COPD; arthritis; diabetes; pressure sores • Current (non)medical treatment: type, intensity and adverse events possibly influencing physiotherapy options • Earlier treatment for problem referred for: type and outcome
Participation			Problems with relationships; profession and work; social life, including leisure activities
Functions & activities	Transfers	PIF	Getting in and out of bed; rolling over; rising from a chair or toilet seat and sitting down; getting into and out of a car; getting up from the floor (after a fall)
	Balance and falls	PIF History of falling ABC or FES-I Falls Diary	While standing, bending forward, reaching, making transfers, walking (backward), turning or dual tasking In pwp reporting on the PIF: • a (near) fall, use the History of Falling for insight in frequency and circumstances (e.g. orthostatic hypotension and difficulty dual tasking) • a (near) fall or fear of falling, use the ABC or (for less ambulant pwp) the FES-I for insight in activities related balance confidence Provide a Falls Diary to all pwp who have fallen for insight in fall frequency and circumstances
	Manual dexterity	PIF	Reaching, grasping and moving objects in household activities, such as small repairs, cleaning, cooking, slicing food and holding a glass or cup without spilling; or in personel care, such as bathing and getting (un)dressed
	Gait	PIF FOG video New FOGQ	• Upon step initiation, while walking (backward), turning or dual tasking; freezing of gait; gait speed and safety; location and circumstances when limitations arise • Use of aids; walking short and long distances; relation to falls • In pwp reporting freezing of gait on the PIF: use the New FOGQ for insight in frequency and duration of freezing related to step initiation and turning
	Physical capacity	PIF	• Exercise tolerance, including feeling easily out of breath, rapid onset of fatigue* and general tiredness; joint mobility; muscle tone, power and endurance • Physical activity levels compared to WHO recommendation: 75 min/wk vigorous exercise or 150 min/wk moderate intensity
Tips & tricks			Tips & tricks the pwp uses to reduce or compensate for the problems: are these adequate?
External factors	Personal		Age and gender; insight into the disease; coping; experiences; preferences; motivation; coping skills; feeling isolated and lonely; being tearful; anger; concern for the future; awareness (to change); motivation (to adhere to a specific intervention)
	Environmental		Drugs (see Medical information); assistive devices; financial assets; attitudes of and support from carer, family or friends, the primary care physician and the employer; accommodation (interior, kind of home); work (content, circumstances and conditions); transportation
Expectations pwp			With regard to: • general prognosis • physiotherapy treatment: contents, frequency and outcome • self-management: need for information, advice and coaching

#such as using the Hoehn and Yahr classification; *items included in the (MDS-)UPDRS

© ParkinsonNet | KNGF 2014

188

FIG. 11.3 Quick reference card 1: History taking. [Intellectual property of KNGF/ParkinsonNet and reproduced with permission (Keus et al 2014).]

European Physiotherapy Guideline for Parkinson's disease

Quick Reference Card 2. Physical examination

	Physical capacity and pain	Transfers	Manual dexterity	Balance	Gait
Tick list Observe the pwp well when rising from the waiting room chair, walking into your clinic, closing the door and taking of a coat. Include any reported or detected sensory alterations plus description	Muscle power ○ hip extensors ○ knee extensors ○ ankle flexors ○ other, namely: Muscle tone ○ hamstrings ○ calf muscles ○ other, namely: Joint mobility ○ cervical spine ○ thoracic spine ○ other, namely: Exercise tolerance ○ exertion ○ respiration control Pain ○ musculoskeletal ○ neuropathic ○ other, namely:	○ sitting down on chair/sofa ○ rising from chair/sofa ○ getting up from the floor ○ getting in bed ○ getting out of bed ○ rolling over in bed ○ sitting down on toilet seat ○ rising from toilet seat ○ getting in car ○ getting out of car ○ other, namely: Safety ○ a fall ○ a near fall ○ other, namely:	○ reaching ○ grasping ○ moving objects Limited activities:	○ while standing ○ while rising from a chair ○ during forward walking ○ during backward walking ○ when turning ○ when freezing ○ when bending forward ○ when reaching and grasping ○ when dual tasking, to know: Safety ○ a fall ○ a near fall ○ other, namely:	Gait pattern impairments ○ decreased walking speed ○ decreased trunk rotation ○ decreased arm swing ○ shortened stride length ○ variable stride length Festination or freezing: ○ upon step initiation ○ upon turning ○ when avoiding obstacles ○ when passing doorways ○ during forward walking ○ during backward walking ○ when dual tasking, to know: Safety ○ a fall ○ a near fall ○ other, namely:
Supportive tools * can also be used for evaluative purposes	○ 6MW & Borg 6-20 ○ 5STS	Bed: ○ M-PAS Bed Chair: ○ M-PAS Chair ○ TUG* ○ 5STS	-	General: ○ Push and Release test Transfers: ○ M-PAS Chair ○ 5STS Gait: ○ M-PAS Gait ○ TUG* ○ DGI* / ○ FGA / ○ Mini-BESTest ○ Rapid Turns Stationary: ○ BBS*	○ M-PAS Gait ○ TUG* ○ 10MWT* ○ 6MW* ○ Rapid Turns
In all pwp	3-step Falls Prediction Model: to identify pwp requiring interdisciplinary falls assessment, individualised physiotherapy or general exercising Goal Attainment Scaling (GAS): to describe and evaluate a SMART treatment goal				

© ParkinsonNet | KNGF 2014

189

FIG. 11.4 Quick reference card 2: Physical assessment. [Intellectual property of KNGF/ParkinsonNet and reproduced with permission (Keus et al 2014).]

(Aarsland et al 2010). The younger person will also have very different expectations to their life course than someone older (Post et al 2020). The therapist must take such issues into account when discussing treatment and goal selection, including the use of appropriate measurement tools. They should ensure the process is apparent to the person with Parkinson's and document input appropriately.

The treatment choice will depend on decisions related to location (space, travel, equipment availability) of intervention, whether to have 1:1 or group input, or both, plus regularity of attendance and duration.

A person with Parkinson's may experience several symptoms at once or certain ones creating challenges at different times of the day; correct history taking and physical assessment elicit the issue(s) to prioritise in the management strategy. For example, at night when the body has reduced activity and medication levels are low, the individual with Parkinson's will find it difficult to turn in bed because movement ability is reduced (Mirelman et al 2020).

Although physiotherapy treatment concentrates on physical manifestations of a disorder targeting identified impairments and activity limitations, attention should be paid to how other symptoms affect the person's lifestyle and participation. Using the example above, the inability to get comfortable can adversely affect sleep, concentration and energy levels to engage in normal activities, with a negative effect on family relationships and employment (Hodgson et al 2004, Mirelman et al 2020), as well as an impact on morbidity (Kim et al 2018).

The European Guideline appraised research literature from key clinical questions asked of physiotherapists, developing interventions into three modalities: exercise (related to conditioning), practice (related to motor learning and performance) and movement strategy training (Fig. 11.5). The evidence has subsequently been updated through a meta-analysis of effective treatment modalities (Osborne et al 2022, Pang 2021), but the framework and message remain the same, even for interventions where more research is indicated (Pang 2021, Radder et al 2020).

Each intervention is supported by appropriate information and education provided to the people affected by Parkinson's (Pang 2021, Radder et al 2020, Rochester et al 2011), with the American Guideline considering the importance of ensuring the use of behaviour change approaches (Osborne et al 2022). The rationale for all recommendations still depends ultimately on the treatment goal, type of intervention, person's character traits and their response to treatment.

For example, when promoting self-management, it would be best to increase the number of unsupervised sessions over time, whilst delivering clear instructions and continuous feedback on performance and goal assessment. These strategies support the individual's control, which in turn leads to increased motivation and treatment adherence (Chiviacowsky et al 2012). For many, whether they have mental health issues or not, the prospect of 'self'-managing a long-term condition over the years can be daunting, and they would rather the use of a shared-care model (Coulter & Collins 2011). Working together with people they trust because of an established relationship enables the individual to clarify treatment aims and to support goal achievement, sharing information about options and preferred outcomes with the aim of reaching mutual agreement on the best course of action. The opportunity to receive information and education should be from the point of diagnosis at a pace the person can take in, so they best manage changes in impairments, activity limitations and restrictions in participation.

Exercise

Healthy lifestyle choices, amongst other bio-psycho-social factors, include eating a balanced diet, taking sufficient exercise and breaking sedentary behaviour (Urtamo et al 2019). Exercise is strongly advocated for anyone with a long-term condition to remain physically active, reduce discomfort from conditions affecting mobility and to continue living a chosen lifestyle for as long as possible. It is suggested that exercise protects and preserves function, can modify progression of symptoms and possibly restore brain function, but the dosage – especially intensity at which to exercise – remains unanswered (Rodríguez et al 2020).

For the disease process of Parkinson's, exercise has demonstrated widespread neuromolecular changes, including improved vascularisation and angiogenesis (new blood vessel growth), levels of proteins associated with

European Physiotherapy Guideline for Parkinson's disease

Quick Reference Card 3. Treatment goals

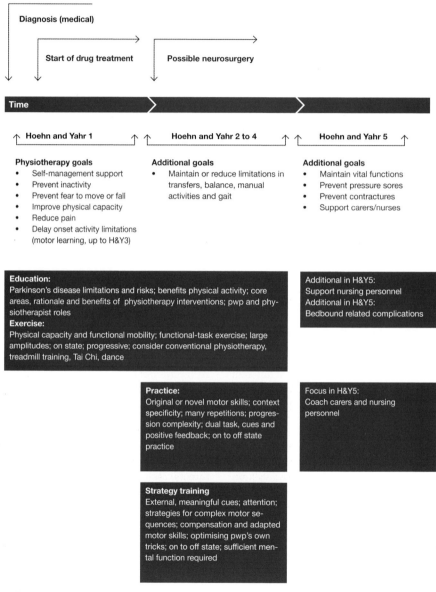

FIG. 11.5 Quick reference card 3: Treatment goals. [Intellectual property of KNGF/ParkinsonNet and reproduced with permission (Keus et al 2014).]

promotion of dopaminergic neurone survival (e.g., brain- or glial-derived neurotropic factors) and transmission through synaptogenesis (strengthening of neuronal health) (Lindop & Skelly 2021). The consequent reduction in neuroinflammatory mechanisms preserves the condition of the Parkinson's-diseased brain and use of dopamine (Ellis & Rochester 2018). Exercise also benefits management of nonmotor symptoms and mental health of people with Parkinson's (Cusso et al 2016).

For those with Parkinson's with compromised physiological systems, exercise has even been suggested to enhance protection against the Covid-19 infection through the building of immune factors (Hall & Church 2020).

People with Parkinson's, however, are generally less active than the general public, particularly women over 70 (Lord et al 2013, Mantri et al 2018), so it is vital to introduce exercise or ensure those already exercising are doing the correct exercise for their needs, and 'prescribe' it to be taken daily as one would take medications – working towards a minimal goal of 2.5 hours of exercise a week (NICE 2017, Rafferty et al 2017). No exercise done correctly has been demonstrated as harmful, and when done properly, it can help recalibrate slow and small movement (motor symptoms) associated with Parkinson's, preventing secondary complications, reducing pain and preventing the fear of moving and falling. The converse appears that a lack of sufficient physical activity and dosage has been associated with higher rates of all-cause mortality (Yoon et al 2021). Given the detrimental effects of bradykinesia and rigidity on lung function (dos Santos et al 2019), the usefulness of respiratory exercise needs to be considered as part of the wider exercise prescription (van de Wetering-van Dongen et al 2020).

The challenges people with Parkinson's face when considering uptake of exercise relate to the complexity of their motor and nonmotor symptoms. The Parkinson's UK exercise framework (Parkinson's UK 2017) divides exercise into three sections incorporating research evidence into the benefits of progressive resistance strength training, cardiovascular training, specific interventions such as Nordic walking and also higher level balance challenge training (Fig. 11.6), alongside the dosage shown to be effective in different trials in both the European and American guidelines, plus the subsequent meta-analysis of effective interventions (Keus et al 2014, Pang 2021, Radder et al 2020).

The first section of the exercise framework advocates that people invest in exercise from the point of diagnosis and develop an exercise-focused lifestyle. Activity counteracts inactivity and complications of sedentary behaviour; using this early period to optimise physical fitness and slow the progression of the Parkinson's should be encouraged. Introducing body conditioning maximises specific components of fitness whilst targeting the conventional areas of physiotherapy

intervention to use exercise for gait, balance, transfers or physical capacity (Radder et al 2020). Motor-cognitive exercise is advocated (e.g., dual tasking and exergaming) and measured through their effect on returning or preserving activities of daily living like writing, buttoning clothes or shrugging shoulders to getting a coat on properly. The Covid-19 pandemic has seen the increased use of technology, with people being educated about physical activity early in the diagnosis period (Quinn et al 2020) or accepting to partake in exercise from diagnosis onwards (Ramaswamy et al 2021).

The second section suggests that people stay active by increasing the focus on Parkinson's-specific issues, including nonmotor symptoms like maintaining cognitive function and dealing with mood and sleep. Motivation and planning are vital because Parkinson's has a profile of higher levels of depression and apathy, so finding different means of keeping up the activity is paramount, such as monitored home exercise programmes (van der Kolk et al 2019).

The third section advises the use of exercise to manage physical challenges of this progressive condition, preserving fitness and functional daily activities where possible, and managing the discomfort from likely postural changes. The variability in motor and nonmotor presentation necessitates an increased focus on supporting others to assist the person with Parkinson's with exercise, particularly for transfers and gait-related activities (Rukavina et al 2021). Although this variability negates the inclusion of people in the later stages from most exercise intervention research, the longer someone with Parkinson's is supported to exercise, the better their future physical ability (Hunter et al 2019, Mak et al 2017).

Exercise can be performed throughout most of the condition by the individual alone or in a group, increasing the positive qualities of socialisation, and can be supervised or unsupervised. A belief in the benefit of exercise, and a competitive and supportive streak when exercising in company will sustain motivation to exercise.

The use of technology can enhance exercise performance. For example, fitness levels can be monitored through apps and wrist monitors, exercise might use game technology (e.g., Kinect or Wii Fit components) and people can access exercise examples through the Internet, DVDs or digital platforms to act as 'rainy day' alternatives to going out for exercise (see Table 11.3).

Practice

Practice refers to improvement of motor skill performance, and its use is no different than any other condition a physiotherapist will encounter.

The issues to bear in mind with someone who has Parkinson's is that the ability to continue learning and upkeeping practice later in the condition will depend on their cognitive ability. For some, it is better to first watch

Parkinson's Exercise Framework (for exercise professionals and health professionals)
Key messages for professionals to give the people they support and examples of exercise styles to focus on

	Investing in exercise from diagnosis onwards	Staying active	Managing complex (physical) challenges
Focus	**Emerging evidence suggests that increasing exercise to 2.5 hours a week can slow the progression of Parkinson's symptoms, so:** • seek referral to an informed professional to discuss exercise and its benefits, the individual's physical state and motivation • exposure to an exercise-focused lifestyle (that is sociable and fun), using family, friends or Parkinson's networks, supports regular exercise behaviour • if symptoms are mild, this is the optimal time to improve physical condition to remain well, prevent inactivity and the complications of sedentary behaviour (weight gain, heart disease and metabolic disorders such as diabetes and osteoporosis)	**Keeping moving is important for people with Parkinson's, so:** • stay as (or more) active than at diagnosis and increase exercise targeting Parkinson's-specific issues such as balance and doing two things at once (dual tasking) • continue to keep the progression of symptoms to a minimum by exercising both the body and the mind (especially for memory, attention, and learning) • use the positive effects of exercise to better manage non-motor symptoms such as mood and sleep	**Movement, ability and motivation change over time, so:** • pay attention to specific physical functions that focus on daily activities such as getting up out of a chair, turning or walking safely • continue to maintain general fitness for physical wellbeing, finding ways to make sure this is kept up • prevent discomfort related to postural changes
Exercise style (bearing in mind fitness and any barriers to exercise such as travel or fatigue)	**Target postural control, balance, large movement (including twisting) and coordination through:** • moderate and vigorous intensity exercise to get the best performance from the body. Best done 5 x week in 30 minute bouts (can be built over time) • progressive resistance exercise to build muscle strength and power. Best results if done 2 x week • Parkinson's-specific exercise prescribed by health professionals such as dual-tasking and stretching for flexibility. Best results if done 2 x week • (Evidence from animal models that vigorous intensity exercise may have neuroprotective effects is in its infancy with humans, so more research is needed.)	**Target flexibility (dynamic stretching), plus slower exercise to control postural muscles for balance through:** • maintaining effortful exercise that pushes people according to their fitness levels • continuing resistance exercises • increasing balance exercises • increasing postural exercises • Parkinson's-specific review by health professionals	**Target better movement through:** • functional exercise (chair-based with the use of resistance bands) • supervised classes with a professional reviewing safety to perform exercise • home programmes to stay moving, avoid sedentary behaviour, reduce flexed position and the secondary effects of being less mobile
Examples	• Sport: racket sport, cycling, jogging, running and swimming • Leisure centre and other classes: aerobics, vigorous intensity training (such as boot camps with high level balance work), Nordic walking • Home DVDs or high intensity exergaming • Parkinson's-specific exercise such as PD Warrior, boxing training classes, the Parkinson's Wellness Recovery (PWR!) programme, some exercise classes run by the Parkinson's UK network	• Golf, bowling, (paired) dance, health walks, swimming • Flexibility with strength: tai chi, Pilates and yoga • Specific classes for people with Parkinson's such as LSVT BIG and balance and walking classes (run by the Parkinson's UK network)	• Specific classes for people with mobility and balance challenges, especially dance • Pedal exerciser • Resistance band workouts • Supervised balance and mobility challenge tasks • Seated exercise groups (some run by the Parkinson's UK network)

Registered charity in England and Wales (258197) and Scotland (SC037554). © Parkinson's UK 09/17 (CS2783)

PARKINSON'S^UK CHANGE ATTITUDES. FIND A CURE. JOIN US.

FIG. 11.6 Parkinson's UK exercise framework for professionals. (Reproduced in concise form with permission of Parkinson's UK.)

the task done by the therapist, then use sensory input and integrate this with mental imagery.

Intervention includes motor-cognitive work to preserve the person's ability to dual- and multi-task for as long as it is safe to do and consider the effectiveness of practice when someone is less medicated (off) compared with during optimal medication effect (on).

Parkinson's pathology results in automaticity deficits with the loss of habitual movement, so practice aims to achieve a level of automaticity. This can be checked in the following ways:

1. If testing for automatisation, look for the individual's response to dual task and how much one task interferes with the other (this can be done with the Timed Up and Go test, using a second motor task or a cognitive task).
2. If testing for transfer of motor learning, observe the ability to carry out an untrained task with a similar context.
3. If testing for retention, determine whether the individual can automatically retrieve their ability after a period of time has lapsed.

Movement Strategies Training

Movement strategy training is based around an expectation to compensate for automatic behaviour affected by cognitive impairment even early on around diagnosis. Strategies include the use of cues, attention, and strategies for complex motor sequences, but to be shown as effective, they must be tailored to the individual and specific to the context in which the strategy needs application (Osborne et al 2022, Tosserams et al 2021). The use of the PIF before a consultation will identify if the individual has already worked out their own little trick to aid movement in different circumstances.

Strategies used to improve functional (meaningful) activities induce motor learning, with commands kept short and simple. For example, to improve the efficiency of the

TABLE 11.3 Summary of Recommendations

Intervention	Quality of Evidence	Strength of Recommendation	Recommendation
Aerobic exercise	High	◆◆◆◆	Physical therapists should implement moderate- to high-intensity aerobic exercise to improve VO$_2$, reduce motor disease severity and improve functional outcomes in individuals with Parkinson disease
Resistance training	High	◆◆◆◆	Physical therapists should implement resistance training to reduce motor disease severity and improve strength, power, nonmotor symptoms, functional outcomes, and quality of life in individuals with Parkinson disease
Balance training	High	◆◆◆◆	Physical therapists should implement balance training intervention programs to reduce postural control impairments and improve balance and gait outcomes, mobility, balance confidence, and quality of life in individuals with Parkinson disease
Flexibility exercises	Low	◆◆◇◇	Physical therapists may implement flexibility exercises to improve ROM in individuals with Parkinson disease
External cueing	High	◆◆◆◆	Physical therapists should implement external cueing to reduce motor disease severity and freezing of gait and to improve gait outcomes in individuals with Parkinson disease
Community-based exercise	High	◆◆◆◆	Physical therapists should recommend community-based exercise to reduce motor disease severity and improve nonmotor symptoms, functional outcomes, and quality of life in individuals with Parkinson disease
Gait training	High	◆◆◆◆	Physical therapists should implement gait training to reduce motor disease severity and improve stride length, gait speed, mobility, and balance in individuals with Parkinson disease
Task-specific training	High	◆◆◆◆	Physical therapists should implement task-specific training to improve task-specific impairment levels and functional outcomes for individuals with Parkinson disease
Behavior-change approach	High	◆◆◆◇	Physical therapists should implement behavior-change approaches to improve physical activity and quality of life in individuals with Parkinson disease
Integrated care	High	◆◆◆◆	Physical therapist services should be delivered within an integrated care approach to reduce motor disease severity and improve quality of life in individuals with Parkinson disease
Telerehabilitation	Moderate	◆◆◇◇	Physical therapist services may be delivered via telerehabilitation to improve balance in individuals with Parkinson disease

ROM, range of motion; VO$_2$, oxygen consumption.
(Reproduced with permission from Osborne et al 2022.)

compensatory mechanisms to aid transfers, a physiotherapist might combine a cue to stand with attention paid to the task using a sequencing strategy, such as 'feet back, body forward, now stand'. We recommend you refer to the Resources section to access links to video clips of examples of different strategies.

Regarding the use of dual-task training to improve gait, particularly speed without adding to falls risk, both consecutive and integrated dual-task training demonstrated similar and sustained improvements, thus supporting their use in clinical practice (Strouwen et al 2017, Tosserams et al 2021).

CONCLUSION

Parkinson's is the second most common global neurodegenerative disorder in older adults. It is currently incurable and caused by varied factors, some of which remain unknown, with a higher likelihood of a genetic link where the person is diagnosed when young. There are similar conditions to this idiopathic form but with different causes and prognoses, called the atypical parkinsonism conditions.

Parkinson's is recognised by the presence of motor symptoms, mostly resulting from progressive destruction of neuronal pathways in the substantia nigra of the basal ganglia, reducing the availability of the neurotransmitter dopamine. Dopamine modulates basal ganglia pathways, with other neurotransmitters, thus interacting with neighbouring areas of the brain both directly and indirectly to enable movement. The complexity of the neurodegenerative processes is responsible for diverse nonmotor symptoms experienced by people with Parkinson's (e.g., sleep disturbance or cognitive impairments), all of which affect social participation and quality of life of the person with Parkinson's and their families. In addition to these symptoms, people with Parkinson's can be prone to secondary comorbidity, especially from reduced activity.

The diagnosis of Parkinson's is primarily based on expert clinical observation and assessment of motor and nonmotor symptoms that emerge several years after the onset of the condition starts. Motor symptoms (initially dopamine responsive and unilateral) include bradykinesia (slowness and reduced amplitude), rigidity (stiffness) or rest tremor. Other involuntary movement can be present, such as dystonia and dyskinesia, that may be debilitating or perceived as stigmatising. Nonmotor features are numerous and include neuropsychiatric, autonomic and gastrointestinal symptoms; sleep disorders; sensory impairment and other symptoms such as fatigue.

Parkinson's is best managed through multidisciplinary intervention to effect symptomatic control (e.g., through medication prescription), encouraging physical activity and social participation, optimising the person's potential from the moment of diagnosis, throughout the condition course, until the end of life. People affected by Parkinson's hope to work with professionals to nurture interactive relationships with positive options for management so they may better accept the diagnosis and regression of the condition.

With regards to physiotherapy, people with Parkinson's should be referred for assessment soon after diagnosis to a therapist with experience in Parkinson's. The goal of therapy is to optimise function and independence to improve quality of life, particularly through the promotion of an active lifestyle. In Parkinson's, the longer-term aim alters towards managing physical decline.

Guidance is provided through the European Guideline framework, assisting therapists' history taking (with questions informed by people with Parkinson's) and physical assessment. Evidence exists for effective physiotherapy for improving physical capacity, transfers, manual activities, balance, gait, respiratory function and pain management, approached through the combined knowledge of the therapist and perspective of the individual seeking treatment.

A realistic and shared action plan of intervention should be supported where able using a PIF before the first appointment to develop dialogue towards goal planning and help keep the individual motivated to achieve their goals, especially where cognitive impairment affects memory, planning and attention.

Physiotherapy can have a positive effect on the lifestyle and quality for people with Parkinson's using evidence-informed interventions of exercise (related to conditioning), practice (related to motor learning and performance) and movement strategy training.

CASE STUDY: USE OF EXERCISE THROUGH THE THREE STAGES OF PARKINSON'S

The case study below uses the WHO model from the European Guideline for Parkinson's Disease Appendices 9 and 10 (Keus et al 2014, pp. 155–156) for ICD-10: G20 (Parkinson's Disease), and the UK Parkinson's Exercise Framework for professionals (Parkinson's UK 2017) as a model to present the case of someone with Parkinson's over a 12-year period. It is written from the perspective of neurologically specialised physiotherapists who have worked across the public, the private and voluntary sectors.

About the Person: Conventional Subdivisions of Parkinson's

Jennifer (Jenny) was a 75-year-old woman when she self-referred for information about the benefits of higher (vigorous) intensity exercise programmes for active people newly diagnosed with Parkinson's. She was active, a widow of 4 years, a busy grandmother, socialite and wished to remain so.

At her self-referral, Jenny would be considered as having early Parkinson's (Hoehn & Yahr stages 1–2/2.5) with main symptom of a stiff right shoulder. Her activity levels meant she was not offered public sector physiotherapy services, but the specialist nurse gave her information about exercise classes run locally through the Parkinson's UK voluntary group.

Around 5 years after diagnosis, Jenny noted a decline in her mobility (her balance and endurance) and less effectiveness in her medications. Although she was keeping active, she was aware that she was the slowest member in her walking group, and that she occasionally requested they have a break in places they would not have previously had to stop. She found it hard, however, to know what were normal changes now that she had entered her 80's, and what was Parkinson's.

A little after her 87th birthday, Jenny was forced into isolation in her house because of the restrictions of the Covid-19 pandemic. The effect of deconditioning brought on both a physical and mental decline affecting Jenny's daily life routines, and she had a fall and fractured a vertebra. In hospital, Jenny was told that her memory problems meant they would send her for cognitive testing to consider whether there was an onset of dementia, and that in healthcare terms, she was considered as having late-stage Parkinson's (Hoehn & Yahr stage 5). It was at this point that an NHS therapy service was offered.

Special test results: No specific investigations were done at Jenny's initial specialist appointment; her diagnosis of Parkinson's was based on clinical presentation and examination.

Other MDT involved: Parkinson's consultant and specialist nurse at the point of diagnosis, therapy services (short term) following her more recent fall 12 years into diagnosis and a referral to the social services to consider her living situation.

About the Person: Assessment Aspects of Note From History Taking Providing an Understanding of Environmental and Personal Factors

PMH: Apart from a frozen shoulder Jenny had in her 50's, she occasionally experienced what she called a 'grumbling right knee and low back' from what her general practitioner had described as arthritic changes. She had received no investigations or bone density scans despite her age. She had a bowel resection for cancer 20 years previously but managed the regularity of bowel movement with exercise and a good diet.

FH: Jenny's grandfather had Parkinson's.

DH: Dopamine replacement therapy (Sinemet) for Parkinson's 3 x daily, with doses increased over the years. During the Covid-19 pandemic, this was increased to 4 x day, plus she was started on low-dose monoamine oxidase-B inhibitor (Rasagiline); she took the occasional over-the-counter pain killer if her knee or back were troublesome and kept a supply of senokot tablets in case she felt constipated.

SH: Jenny is a retired teacher and lives alone in a house. At diagnosis, she was able to drive or catch the train across country to visit friends and family, but as the condition progressed, her family and friends either met her halfway or came to visit her. She has three children with eight grandchildren who she saw regularly and, up until the pandemic, would accompany them abroad for holidays. Jenny was still able to see to personal care independently of help and, until the fall, was shopping for herself, although she described experiencing slowness completing tasks as her balance was affected by freezing episodes when walking and multitasking.

Agreed Goals According to Stage of Disease

In the early disease stage (Hoehn & Yahr stages 1–2/2.5) Jenny wanted to know more about how exercise would help her stay active into the longer term, and the 'best' exercise for her.

As she entered the middle stage (Hoehn & Yahr 3–4) and the changes to her mobility became more debilitating, Jenny requested additional emphasis on helping her keep safe on her feet, as she had witnessed some class participants falling over time.

As Jenny approached the later stage (Hoehn & Yahr 5), setting goals became harder because she had not anticipated such a catastrophic event, making even the most basic functional task painful or hard to achieve. Low mood set in and ways to keep Jenny motivated were needed.

(Continued)

Summary of Physiotherapy Assessment (using European Guidelines Quick Reference Cards for guidance)

This section will follow the guidance in the Quick Reference Cards of History Taking (Fig. 11.3), Physical Assessment (Fig. 11.4) and Treatment Goals (Fig. 11.5). Because the focus of this case study is on the use of exercise, we have emphasised the changes to components of fitness and function Jenny was experiencing over time. There were other factors considered and reflected on to provide a full picture of aspects for Jenny that required additional interventions over the years, i.e., education, clinic treatment techniques, assistive devices and referral onwards to other professionals.

History Taking (Fig. 11.3)

Early stage: There was nothing particular to note from the PIF from Jenny's past. She had been an independent and fit woman, had not long been diagnosed, so had no experience of physiotherapy for any ailment before. She was still self-sufficient and had not noticed developing tricks to compensate for altered movement whether in her house or when out with friends and family.	**Mid stage:** At about 5 years into diagnosis, we reviewed Jenny's balance, strength and gait. She had been attending varied exercise classes run either by a physiotherapist or exercise professional, but not returned for a physiotherapy assessment. At the review, although Jenny had not had a fall, she noted changes to her confidence when out, describing short-duration episodes of freezing of gait when in crowded or stressful situations and was needing to use her hands to push up from a seat. She also admitted to being a little 'lazy' with her exercise routine if tired.	**Later stage:** On returning from hospital, Jenny required a full assessment at home to consider the adaptations and assistance required for safe mobility in the house, as well as equipment with which to do exercise. The period of lockdown before hospitalisation had left her deconditioned (poor balance, less safe with transfers and walking) and dispirited (low confidence and motivation to be active). Her inability to access classes she attended before was experienced as a loss of a support system that motivated her to attend exercise. She was keen to regain some of her previous activity but found it hard to remember what to do.

Physical Assessment (Fig. 11.4)

Physical capacity: 6-minute walk distance: Jenny did 610 m (>400 m expected of someone with Parkinson's and within the lower range of a community-dwelling person who does not have the diagnosis, i.e., >600 m)	A repeat of fitness components: **Physical capacity:** 6-minute walk distance: Jenny did 490 m (still >400 m for someone with Parkinson's but <600 m community-dwelling adult mark)	All aspects of Jenny's fitness were affected by recent events: **Physical capacity:** She was unable to do a 6-minute walk. In a 2-minute march holding the back of a high sturdy chair, she completed 30 right knee-to-hip-height marches.
Leg strength: 5 times sit to stand: Jenny managed well within the 16-second cutoff time	**Leg strength:** 5 times sit to stand: Jenny just managed the 16-second cutoff time	**Leg strength:** 5 times sit to stand: Jenny did 3 stands, each using her hands and demonstrated reluctance to let go of the chair when she stood
Leg power: Jenny did not have the explosive power to coordinate five consecutive jumping jacks	**Leg power:** Jenny could do five consecutive jumping jacks, but slow with little height	**Leg power:** Not attempted as Jenny was still recovering from vertebral fracture after her fall
Hand grip strength: Although a weaker right hand, both were within the range for her age and gender (between 15 and 25 kg)	**Hand grip strength:** Jenny's right hand had weakened further but was still within the range for her age and gender	**Hand grip strength:** Jenny was too weak to squeeze either hand to get a recording within the range for her age and gender

Balance: MiniBEST (Balance Evaluation Systems Test) – full marks for the anticipatory, reactive and sensory sections, but was slow on a couple of the dynamic gait sections. Still .19/20 (cutoff score for people with Parkinson's with a risk of falling)	**Balance:** MiniBEST – all sections (anticipatory, reactive, sensory and dynamic gait) had components Jenny scored lower on sections. She scored overall 18/28, the changes now identifying her at risk of falling	**Balance:** MiniBEST not tested because Jenny was too unsteady. She was unable to attempt a timed unsup-ported static stand without reaching for support
Flexibility: Back scratch test >12.5 cm distance with right arm (stiff from old frozen shoulder and Parkinson's), but within range for age and gender on left	**Flexibility:** Back scratch test – neither left or right achieved the measure to be within range for age and gender. Jenny's overall posture was noted as becoming more flexed at hips and stooping at her shoulders and neck	**Flexibility**: Back scratch test – neither left or right achieved the measure to be within range for age and gender. Jenny's posture was now fixed in forward flexion, resting onto a walking frame because of her back pain
Gait: Tested with the MiniBEST dynamic gait components and the Timed Up and Go (TUG) – both within cutoff times, no balance losses or episodes of gait freezing	**Gait:** Tested with the MiniBEST dynamic gait components and the TUG – both tests revealed changes in balance For the TUG, Jenny was slower when asked to do a dual cognitive task, demonstrating interference between cognitive and motor tasks	**Gait:** TUG – took over 45 seconds to complete the test, freezing on initiation and using her wheeled walker as an assistive device
Exercise-Related Treatment Goals (Fig. 11.5)		
Discussion revolved around setting realistic levels of exercise given Jenny's age and current busy lifestyle. 'Best' exercise, as per her wishes, were agreed as building muscular power whilst maintaining her strength and balance. A programme was set using an exercise wheel of ideal exercise (see Resources), made easier because Jenny had use of a set of dumbbells and kettle bells her grandson had left in his room when he moved to university. She was also introduced to the local charity support group who ran varied classes so she could also meet others with the condition.	There were global changes noted in Jenny's fitness scores. Even in those which were still within normal ranges, the decline over a 5-year period was clear. Although Jenny's goals were to continue with the walking group and the classes she attended (one for dance and one for general fitness), we discussed the possibility of using a personal trainer for one-to-one sessions. Jenny did not wish to attend a gym – something she had no experience of. She also did not have much money as a widow, so did not feel able to pay for weekly sessions. She agreed to try certain chosen videos found online and see a trainer once a month to monitor her fitness.	Jenny's pain levels severely affected her motivation. Her lack of sleep and energy affected her concentration. It was organised that as Jenny would have carers for personal care needs and cooking, they would encourage Jenny to incorporate sit-to-stand and walking speed/posture during her movement around the house as she become less stiff and painful. The family organised a rota for someone to visit daily, and a small chair-based exercise programme using dumbbells and a resistance band was demonstrated and left for them to do on 5 of 7 days. Zoom calls were arranged with old classmates for a social chat.

SELF-ASSESSMENT QUESTIONS

1. How would you discuss Parkinson's with an individual in terms of what it is, what causes it and an expected prognosis?
2. What are the main motor symptoms doctors use as diagnostic criteria, and how is the diagnosis currently arrived at these days? See if you can name the three stages that can lead to a diagnosis, and at which stage a clinical diagnosis is given.
3. How is Parkinson's best managed?
4. At what point should people with Parkinson's be referred to therapy, and to whom?
5. Thinking of physiotherapy assessment for people with Parkinson's, what areas do we have expertise in assessing that responds to physiotherapy intervention?
6. What are the main evidence-informed physiotherapy interventions?

REFERENCES

Aarsland, D., Bronnick, K., Williams-Gray, C., et al., 2010. Mild cognitive impairment in Parkinson disease: a multicenter pooled analysis. Neurology. 75, 1062–1069.

Aarsland, D., Beye, M.E., Kreuz, M.W., 2008. Dementia in Parkinson's disease. Curr. Opin. Neurol. 21, 676–682.

Abdo, W., van der Warrenburg, B., Burn, D., et al., 2010. The clinical approach to movement disorders. Nat. Rev. Neurol. 6, 29–37.

Aerts, M., Esselink, R., Post, B., et al., 2012. Improving the diagnostic accuracy in parkinsonism: a three-pronged approach. Pract. Neurol. 12, 77–87.

Allen, N., Sherribngton, C., Canning, C., et al., 2010. Reduced muscle power is associated with slower walking velocity and falls in people with Parkinson's disease. Parkinsonism. Relat. Disord. 16, 261–264.

Athauda, D., Foltynie, T., 2018. Drug repurposing in Parkinson's disease. CNS Drugs. 32, 747–761.

Blesa, J., Trigo-Damas, I., Quiroga-Varela, A., et al., 2015. Oxidative stress and Parkinson's disease. Front. Neuroanat. 9, 91.

Bloem, B., Munneke, M., 2014. Revolutionising management of chronic disease: the ParkinsonNet approach. BMJ. 348, g1838.

Bloem, B.R., Okun, M.S., Klein, C., 2021. Parkinson's disease. Lancet. 397, 2284–2303.

Bloem, B.R., Stocchi, F., 2012. Move for change part I: a European survey evaluating the impact of the EPDA Charter for people with Parkinson's disease. Eur. J. Neurol. 19, 402–410.

Braak, H., del Tredici, K., 2017. Neuropathological staging of brain pathology in sporadic Parkinson's disease: separating the wheat from the chaff. J. Parkinson. Dis. 7, S71–S85.

Braak, H., Del Tredici, K., Rüb, U., et al., 2003. Staging of brain pathology related to sporadic Parkinson's disease. Neurobiol. Aging. 24, 197–211.

Bramley, N., Eatough, V., 2005. The experience of living with Parkinson's disease: an interpretative phenomenological analysis case study. Psychol. Health. 20, 223–235.

Bridgeman, K., Arsham, T., 2017. The Comprehensive Guide to Parkinson's Disease. Viartis, London.

Brown, E., Chahine, L., Goldman, S., et al., 2020. The effect of the Covid-19 pandemic on people with Parkinson's. disease. J. Parkinson. Dis. 10, 1365–1377.

Capato, T.T.C., Nonnekes, J., Barbosa, E.R., Bloem, B.R., 2019. Internal and external compensation strategies to alleviate upper limb freezing in Parkinson's disease. Parkinsonism. Relat. Disord. 64, 335–336.

Chartered Society of Physiotherapy., 2011. Practice Guidance for Physiotherapy Supplementary Prescribers. PD026 ed. London, CSP.

Chaudhuri, K.R., Martinez-Martin, P., Brown, R.G., et al., 2007. The metric properties of a novel non-motor symptoms scale for Parkinson's disease: results from an international pilot study. Mov. Disord. 22, 1901–1911.

Chaudhuri, K.R., Martinez-Martin, P., Schapira, A.H., et al., 2006b. International multicenter pilot study of the first comprehensive self-completed nonmotor symptoms questionnaire for Parkinson's disease: the NMSQuest study. Mov. Disord. 21, 916–923.

Chaudhuri, R., Healy, D., Schapira, A., 2006a. Non-motor symptoms of Parkinson's disease: diagnosis and management. Lancet. Neurol. 5, 235–245.

Chaudhuri, R., Schapira, A., 2009. Non-motor symptoms of Parkinson's disease: dopaminergic pathophysiology and treatment. Lancet. Neurol. 8, 464–474.

Chiviacowsky, S., Wulf, G., Lewthwaite, R., et al., 2012. Motor learning benefits of self-controlled practice in persons with Parkinson's disease. Gait. Posture. 35, 601–605.

Chu, Y., Kordower, J.H., 2015. The prion-hypothesis of Parkinson's disease. Curr. Neurol. Neurosci. Rep. 15, 28.

Clarke, C., Patel, S., Ives, N., et al., 2016. Physiotherapy and occupational therapy vs no therapy in mild to moderate Parkinson disease. A randomized clinical trial. JAMA Neurol. 73, 291–299.

Combs, S., Diehl, D., Chrzastowski, C., 2014. Community-based group exercise for persons with Parkinson disease: a randomized controlled trial. NeuroRehabilitation. 32, 117–124.

Coulter, A., Collins, A., 2011. Making Shared Decision-Making a Reality: No Decision About Me, Without Me. The King's Fund, London.

Crosiers, D., Theuns, J., Cras, P., et al., 2011. Parkinson's disease: insights in clinical, genetic and pathological features of monogenic disease subtypes. J. Chem. Neuroanat. 42, 131–141.

Cusso, M.E., Donald, K.J., Khoo, T.K., 2016. the impact of physical activity on non-motor symptoms in Parkinson's disease: a systematic review. Front. Med. 3, 35.

Deuschl, G., Schade-Brittinger, C., Krack, P., et al., 2006. A randomized trial of deep-brain stimulation for Parkinson's disease. N. Engl. J. Med. 355, 896–908.

Dorsey, E.R., Sherer, T., Okun, M., Bloem, B.R., 2018. The emerging evidence of the Parkinson pandemic. J. Parkinson. Dis. 8, S3–S8.

Dos Santos, R.B., Fraga, A.S., de Sales Corioilano, M., et al., 2019. Respiratory muscle strength and lung function in the stages of Parkinson's disease. J. Bras. Pneumonol. 45, e20180148.

Ehringer, H., Hornykiewicz, O., 1960. Distribution of noradrenaline and dopamine (3-hydroxytyramine) in the human brain and their behavior in diseases of the extrapyramidal system. Klin. Wochenschr. 38, 1236–1239.

Elefant, C., Baker, F., Lotan, M., et al., 2012. The effect of group music therapy on mood, speech, and singing in individuals with Parkinson's disease—a feasibility study. J. Music. Ther. 49, 278–302.

Ellis, T., Rochester, L., 2018. Mobilizing Parkinson's disease: the future of exercise. J. Parkinson. Dis. 8, S95–S100.

Fil, A., Cano-de-la-Cuerdaa, R., Munoz-Hellin, E., et al., 2013. Pain in Parkinson's disease: a review of the literature. Parkinsonism. Relat. Disord. 19, 285–294.

Forsaa, E.B., Larsen, J.P., Wentzel-Larsen, T., et al., 2010. What predicts mortality in Parkinson disease? A prospective population-based long-term study. Neurology. 75, 1270–1276.

Goedert, M., Jakes, R., Spillantini, M.G., 2017. The synucleinopathies: twenty years on. J. Parkinson. Dis. 7, S51–S69.

Goetz, C.G., Tilley, B.C., Shaftman, S.R., et al., 2008. Movement Disorder Society-sponsored revision of the Unified Parkinson's Disease Rating Scale (MDS-UPDRS): scale presentation and clinimetric testing results. Mov. Disord. 23, 2129–2170.

Gumber, A., Ramaswamy, B., Ibbotson, R., et al., 2016. Economic, Financial and Social Cost of Parkinson's on Individuals, Their Carers and Families in the UK: Final Report. Sheffield Hallam University, Sheffield.

Hall, M.-F.E., Church, F.C., 2020. Exercise for older adults improves the quality of life in Parkinson's disease and potentially enhances the immune response to COVID-19. Brain. Sci. 10, 612.

Hariz, M., 2017. My 25 stimulating years with DBS in Parkinson's disease. J. Parkinson. Dis. 7, S33–S41.

Helmich, R.C., Bloem, B.R., 2020. The impact of the COVID-19 pandemic on Parkinson's disease: hidden sorrows and emerging opportunities. J. Parkinson. Dis. 10, 351–354.

Hirano, S., Shinotoh, H., Eidelberg, D., 2012. Functional brain imaging of cognitive dysfunction in Parkinson's disease. J. Neurol. Neurosurg. Psychiatry. 83, 963–969.

Hirsch, L., Jette, N., Frolkis, A., et al., 2016. The incidence of Parkinson's disease: a systematic review and meta-analysis. Neuroepidemiology. 46, 292–300.

Hodgson, J.H., Garcia, K., Tyndall, L., 2004. Parkinson's disease and the couple relationship: a qualitative analysis. Fam. Syst. Health. 22, 101.

Hoehn, M.M., Yahr, M.D., 1967. Parkinsonism: onset, progression and mortality. Neurology. 17, 427–442.

Hornykiewicz, O., 2017. L-DOPA. J. Parkinson. Dis. 7, S3–S10.

Horsfall, L., Petersen, I., Walters, K., et al., 2013. Time trends in incidence of Parkinson's disease diagnosis in UK primary care. J. Neurol. 260, 1351–1357.

Hunter, H., Lovegrove, C., Haas, B., Freeman, J., Gunn, H., 2019. Experiences of people with Parkinson's disease and their views on physical activity interventions: a qualitative

systematic review. JBI Database. Syst. Rev. Implement. Rep. 17, 548–613.

Inkster, L., Eng, J., MacIntyre, D., et al., 2003. Leg muscle strength is reduced in Parkinson's disease and relates to the ability to rise from a chair. Mov. Disord. 18, 157–162.

Jenkinson, C., Fitzpatrick, R., Peto, V., et al., 1997. The Parkinson's Disease Questionnaire (PDQ-39): development and validation of a Parkinson's disease summary index score. Age. Ageing. 26, 353–357.

Jenkinson, C., Peto, V., Fitzpatrick, R., et al., 1995. Self-reported functioning and wellbeing in patients with Parkinson's disease: comparison of the Short Form Health Survey (SF-36) and the Parkinson's Disease Questionnaire (PDQ-39). Age. Ageing. 22, 505–509.

Kalia, L.V., Lang, A.E., 2015. Parkinson's disease. Lancet. 386, 896–912.

Karachi, C., Grabli, D., Bernard, F.A., et al., 2010. Cholinergic mesencephalic neurons are involved in gait and postural disorders in Parkinson disease. J. Clin. Invest. 120, 2745–2754.

Keus, S.H.J., Munneke, M., Graziano, M., et al., 2014. European Physiotherapy Guideline for Parkinson's Disease. KNGF/ParkinsonNet, The Netherlands.

Keus, S.H.J., Nijhuis, O., Nijkrake, M.J., et al., 2012. Improving community healthcare for patients with Parkinson's disease: the Dutch model. Parkinson. Dis. 543426, 1–7.

Kim, Y., Kim, Y.E., Park, E.O., Shin, C.W., Kim, H.-J., Jeon, B., 2018. REM sleep behavior disorder portends poor prognosis in Parkinson's disease: a systematic review. J. Clin. Neurosci. 47, 6–13.

Kincses, Z.T., Vecesi, L., 2011. Pharmacological therapy in Parkinson's disease: focus on neuroprotection. CNS Neurosci. Ther. 17, 345–367.

Klaptocz, J., Gray, W., Marwood, S., et al., 2019. The pattern of hospital admissions prior to care home placement for people with Parkinson's disease: evidence of a period of crisis for patients and carers. J. Aging. Health. 31, 1616–1630.

Lanciego, J., Luquin, N., Obeso, J., 2010. Functional neuroanatomy of the basal ganglia. Cold. Spring. Harb. Perspect. Med. 2, a009621.

Lindop, F., Skelly, R., 2021. Parkinson's disease: a multidisciplinary guide to management. Elsevier, Amsterdam.

Litvan, I., Goldman, J.G., Tröster, A.I., et al., 2012. Diagnostic criteria for mild cognitive impairment in Parkinson's disease: Movement Disorder Society Task Force guidelines. Mov. Disord. 27, 349–356.

Lord, S., Godfrey, A., Galna, B., et al., 2013. Ambulatory activity in incident Parkinson's: more than meets the eye? J. Neurol. 260, 2964–2972.

Low, V., Ben-Shlomo, Y., Coward, E., et al., 2015. Measuring the burden and mortality of hospitalisation in Parkinson's disease: a cross-sectional analysis of the English Hospital Episodes Statistics database 2009–2013. Parkinsonism. Relat. Disord. 21, 449–454.

MacMahon, D., Thomas, S., 1998. Practical approach to quality of life in Parkinson's disease: the nurse's role. J. Neurol. 245 (Suppl 1), S19–S22.

Mak, M., Wong-Yu, I., Shen, X., Chung, C.L., 2017. Long-term effects of exercise and physical therapy in people with Parkinson disease. Nat. Rev. Neurol. 13, 689–703.

Malek, N., Grosset, D., 2015. Medication adherence in patients with Parkinson's disease. CNS Drugs. 29, 47–53.

Mantri, S., Fullard, M., Duda, J., Morley, J., 2018. Physical activity in early Parkinson's disease. J. Parkinson. Dis. 8, 107–111.

Marques, A., Brefel-Courbon, C., 2021. Chronic pain in Parkinson's disease: clinical and pathophysiological aspects. Rev. Neurol. 177, 394–399.

McConaghy, M., 2014. The New Parkinson's Treatment: Exercise Is Medicine. New South Wales, Australia, Publish-Me.

McLean, G., Hindle, J.V., Guthrie, B., Mercer, S.W., 2017. Co-morbidity and polypharmacy in Parkinson's disease: Insights from a large Scottish primary care database. BMC. Neurol. 17, 126.

Mirelman, A., Hillel, I., Rochester, L., et al., 2020. Tossing and turning in bed: nocturnal movements in Parkinson's disease. Mov. Disord. 35, 959–968.

National Institute of Health and Care Excellence., 2017. Parkinson's Disease in Adults. NG71. London, NICE.

Nijkrake, M.J., Keus, S.H.J., Oostendorp, R.A.B., et al., 2009. Allied health care in Parkinson's disease: referral, consultation, and professional expertise. Mov. Disord. 24, 282–286.

Nijkrake, M.J., Keus, S.H.J., Overeem, S., et al., 2010. The ParkinsonNet concept: development, implementation and initial experience. Mov. Disord. 25, 823–829.

Okunoye, O., Horsfal, L., Marston, L., Walters, K., Schrag, A., 2021. Mortality of people with Parkinson's disease in a large UK-based cohort study: time trends and relationships to disease duration. Mov. Disord. 36, 2811–2820.

Osborne, J.A., Botkin, R., Colon-Semenza, C., et al., 2022. Physical therapist management of Parkinson disease: a clinical practice guideline from the American Physical Therapy Association. Phys. Ther. 102, pzab302.

Pääsuke, M., Erelinem, J., Gapeyeva, H., et al., 2004. Leg-extension strength and chair-rise performance in elderly women with Parkinson's disease. J. Aging. Phys. Act. 12, 511–524.

Pagán, F., 2012. Improving outcomes through early diagnosis of Parkinson's disease. Am. J. Manag. Care. 18, S176–S182.

Pahapill, P.A., Lozano, A.M., 2000. The pedunculopontine nucleus and Parkinson's disease. Brain. 123, 1767–1783.

Pang, M.Y.C., 2021. Physiotherapy management of Parkinson's disease. J. Physiother 67, 163–176.

Parkinson's, U.K., 2017. Exercise Framework for Parkinson's. Available at: https://www.parkinsons.org.uk/information-and-support/parkinsons-exercise-framework. Accessed 14 June 2023.

Parkinson's, U.K., 2018. The incidence and prevalence of Parkinson's in the UK. Results from the Clinical Practice Research Datalink. Parkinson's UK, London.

Parkinson's, U.K., 2015a. The strategy for 2015–2019: bringing forward the day when no one fears Parkinson's. Parkinson's UK, London.

Parkinson's, U.K., 2015b. Your Parkinson's services 2015. Parkinson's UK, London.

Parkinson, J., 1817. An Essay on Shaking Palsy. London, Whitington and Rowland for Sherwood, Neely and Jones.

PD MED Collaborative Group, 2014. Long-term effectiveness of dopamine agonists and monoamine oxidase B inhibitors compared with levodopa as initial treatment for Parkinson's disease (PD MED): a large, open-label, pragmatic randomised trial. Lancet. 384, 1196–1205.

Pennington, S., Snell, K., Lee, M., et al., 2010. The cause of death in idiopathic Parkinson's disease. Parkinsonism. Relat. Disord. 16, 434–437.

Post, B., van der Eijk, M., Munneke, M., et al., 2011. Multi-disciplinary care for Parkinson's disease: not if, but how! Practical Neurol. 11, 58–61.

Post, B., van den Heuvel, L., van Prooije, T., van Ruissen, X., van de Warrenburg, B., Nonnekes, J., 2020. Young onset Parkinson's disease: a modern and tailored approach. J. Parkinson. Dis. 10 (Suppl 1), S29–S36.

Postuma, R., Berg, D., Adler, C., et al., 2016. The new definition and diagnostic criteria of Parkinson's disease. Lancet. Neurol. 15, 546–548.

Postuma, R., Berg, D., Stern, M., et al., 2015. MDS clinical diagnostic criteria for Parkinson's disease. Mov. Disord. 30, 1591–1601.

Quinn, L., MacPherson, C., Long, K., Shah, H., 2020. Promoting physical activity via telehealth in people with Parkinson disease: the path forward after the Covid-19 pandemic? Phys. Ther. Rehabil. J. 100, 1730–1736.

Radder, D.L.M., Lígia Silva de Lima, A., Domingos, J., Keus, S.H.J., van Nimwegen, M., Bloem, B.R., 2020. Physiotherapy in Parkinson's disease: a meta-analysis of present treatment modalities. Neurorehabil. Neural. Rep. 34, 871–880.

Rafferty, M.R., Schmidt, P., Sheng, L., et al., 2017. Regular exercise, quality of life, and mobility in Parkinson's disease: a longitudinal analysis of National Parkinson Foundation quality improvement initiative data. J. Parkinson. Dis. 7, 193–202.

Ramaswamy, B., 2016. Reconceptualising Parkinson's from illness to wellness: advancing physiotherapy practice through action research (Doctoral thesis). Accessed from Sheffield Hallam University Research Archive http://shura.shu.ac.uk/15257/.

Ramaswamy, B., Haddad, El, Schoch, L., L., 2021. Investigation into the suitability and acceptance of online-delivered exercise classes for people with Parkinson's. Synapse. 13–19.

Rizzone, M.G., Fasano, A., Daniele, A., et al., 2014. Long-term outcome of subthalamic nucleus DBS in Parkinson's disease: from the advanced phase towards the late stage of the disease? Parkinsonism. Relat. Disord. 20, 376–381.

Rochester, L., Nieuwboer, A., Lord, S., 2011. Physiotherapy for Parkinson's disease: defining evidence within a framework for intervention. Neurodegen. Dis. Manag. 1, 57–65.

Rodriguez, M.A., Albillos-Almarez, L., Lopez-Aguado, I., Crespo, I., del Valle, M., Olmedillas, H., 2020. Vigorous aerobic exercise in the management of Parkinson's disease: a systematic review. PM&R. 13, 890–900.

Ryman, S.G., Poston, K.L., 2020. MRI biomarkers of motor and non-motor symptoms in Parkinson's disease. Parkinsonism. Relat. Disord. 73, 85–93.

Rukavina, K., Batzu, L., Boogers, A., Abundes-Corona, A., Bruno, V., Chaudhuri, R.K., 2021. Non-motor complications in late stage Parkinson's disease: recognition, management and unmet needs. Exp. Rev. Neurother. 21, 335–352.

Santos Garcia, D., Suárez Castro, E., Expósito, I., et al., 2017. Comorbid conditions associated with Parkinson's disease: a longitudinal and comparative study with Alzheimer disease and control subjects. J. Neurol. Sci. 373, 210–215.

Scheperjans, F., Aho, V., Pereira, P., et al., 2015a. Gut microbiota are related to Parkinson's disease and clinical phenotype. Mov. Disord. 30, 350–358.

Scheperjans, F., Pekkonen, E., Kaakkola, S., Auvinen, P., 2015b. Linking smoking, coffee, urate, and Parkinson's disease – a role for gut microbiota? J. Parkinson. Dis. 5, 255–262.

Schrag, A., Horsfall, L., Walters, K., et al., 2014. Prediagnostic presentations of Parkinson's disease in primary care: a case-control study. Lancet. Neurol. 14, 57–64.

Schuepbach, W.M., Rau, J., Knudsen, K., et al., 2013. Neurostimulation for Parkinson's disease with early motor complications. N. Engl. J. Med. 368, 610–622.

Shahgholi, L., De Jesus, S., Wu, S.S., et al., 2017. Hospitalization and rehospitalization in Parkinson disease patients: data from the National Parkinson Foundation centers of excellence. PLoS One. 12, e0180425.

Simpson, J., Eccles, F., Doyle, C., 2020. The Impact of Coronavirus Restrictions on People Affected by Parkinson's: The Findings From a Survey by Parkinson's UK. Lancaster University and Parkinson's UK.

Stanley-Hermanns, M., Engebretson, J., 2010. Sailing stormy seas: the illness experience of persons with Parkinson's disease. Qual. Rep. 15, 340–369.

Strouwen, C., Molenaar, E., Munks, L., et al., 2017. Training dual tasks together or apart in Parkinson's disease: results from the DUALITY trial. Mov. Disord. 32, 1201–1210.

Subramaniam, S., Chesselet, M.-F., 2013. Mitochondrial dysfunction and oxidative stress in Parkinson's disease. Progr. Neurobiol. 106-107, 17–32.

Tosserams, A., Wit, L., Sturkenboom, I.H.W.M., Nijkrake, M., Bloem, B.R., Nonnekes, K., 2021. Perception and use of compensation strategies for gait impairment by persons with Parkinson disease. Neurology. 97, e1404–e1412.

Urtamo, A., Jyväkorpi, S.K., Strandberg, T.E., 2019. Definitions of successful ageing: a brief review of a multidimensional concept. Acta. Biomed. 90, 359–363.

van der Kolk, N.M., de Vries, N.M., Kessels, R.P.C., et al., 2019. Effectiveness of home-based and remotely supervised aerobic exercise in Parkinson's disease: a double-blind, randomised controlled trial. Lancet. Neurol. 18, 998–1008.

van de Wetering-van Dongen, V.A., Kalf, J.G., van der Wees, P.J., Bloem, B.R., Nijkrake, M.J., 2020. The effects of respiratory training in Parkinson's disease: a systematic review. J. Parkinson. Dis. 104, 1315–1333.

Vázquez-Vélez, G.E., Zoghbi, H.Y., 2021. Parkinson's disease genetics and pathophysiology. Annu. Rev. Neurosci. 44, 87–108.

Webster, D., 2014. My Parkinson's journey. Picture produced for MontyZoomer project in Ramaswamy B (2016). Reconceptualising Parkinson's from illness to wellness: Advancing Physiotherapy practice through Action Research (Doctoral thesis). Accessed from Sheffield Hallam University Research Archive at: http://shura.shu.ac.uk/15257/.

Wensing, M., Van der, E.M., Koetsenruijter, J., et al., 2011. Connectedness and healthcare professionals involved in the treatment of patients with Parkinson's disease: a social networks study. Implement. Sci. 6, 67.

Williams, A., Gill, S., Varma, T., et al., 2010. Deep brain stimulation plus best medical therapy versus best medical therapy alone for advanced Parkinson's disease (PD SURG trial): a randomised, open-label trial. Lancet. Neurol. 9, 581–591.

World Health Organization., 2001. International Classification of Functioning, Disability and Health: ICF. WHO, Geneva.

Yoon, S.Y., Suh, J.H., Yang, 2021. Association of physical activity, including amount and maintenance, with all-cause mortality in Parkinson's disease. JAMA Neurol. 78, 1446–1453.

Zijlstra, A., Mancicn, M., Lindemann, U., Chiari, L., Zijlstra, W., 2012. Sit-stand and stand-sit transitions in older adults and patients with Parkinson's disease: event detection based on motion sensors versus force plates. J Neuroeng. Rehabil. 9, 75.

RESOURCES

The European Physiotherapy Guideline for Parkinson's Disease (European Guideline) is available at: https://www.parkinsonnet.com/discipline/physiotherapy/

The guideline is available in English, German, Portuguese, Czech and Finnish.

Also available to download at the same site are the accompanying:

- Guideline information for people with Parkinson's;
- Guideline information for clinicians, and
- Development and scientific justification.

The American Physical Therapy Association's Clinical Practice Guideline for the Physical Therapist Management of Parkinson's DISEASE is available at: https://academic.oup.com/ptj/article/102/4/pzab302/6485202?login=false.

It is also available in Spanish.

Resources in the form of podcasts, apps, books and DVDs can be found on the following sites, either driven by or codeveloped alongside people with Parkinson's:

European Parkinson's Disease Association: https://www.epda.eu.com/

Parkinson's Life: https://parkinsonslife.eu/

Parkinson's UK tab for professionals: https://www.parkinsons.org.uk/professionals/uk-parkinsons-excellence-network with links to the Exercise Framework and a selection of videos for people to do at home.

ParkinsonNet Luxemburg Multidisciplinary videos available in English, French and German: https://www.parkinsonnet.lu/en/living-parkinsons/videos

There are educational associations to join, such as the International Parkinson and Movement Disorder Society, with a dedicated health professionals (nonphysician) special interest group, accessed through: https://www.movementdisorders.org/

The special interest group or physiotherapy body professional network with a neurological interest of World Physiotherapy association, the International Neurological Physical Therapy Association: https://www.inpaneuropt.org/.

In the UK, the CSP professional networks of physiotherapists in neurology, ACPIN, can be joined at: https://www.acpin.net and of physiotherapists working with the older person, AGILE, joined at: https://agile.csp.org.uk.

ACKNOWLEDGEMENT

Adam Poulter is a specialist neurophysiotherapist, for support with the Case Study.

Inherited Neurological Conditions

*Monica Busse, Jonathan Marsden,
Noit Inbar, and Lori Quinn*

OUTLINE

Introduction, 294
Huntington's Disease, 294
 Epidemiology, 294
 Genetics, 294
 Anatomy and Pathophysiology, 295
 Clinical Presentation, 295
 Medical Management, 296
  *A Standard of Care for Huntington's
   Disease, 297*
  Physiotherapy Assessment and Prognosis, 297
  *Time Course and Corresponding Physiotherapy
   Management, 298*
 Treatment Selection and Secondary Complications/
  Special Problems, 300
Hereditary Ataxias, 303
 Epidemiology and Genetics, 303
 Autosomal Dominant Cerebellar Ataxias, 303
 Autosomal Recessive Ataxias, 303
 Anatomy, Pathophysiology and Clinical
  Presentation, 303
  Autosomal Dominant Cerebellar Ataxias, 303
  Friedreich's Ataxia, 305
 Diagnosis and Genetic Testing, 305
 Medical Management, 305
  Symptomatic Treatments of Nonataxic Signs, 305
  Spasticity and Dystonia, 305
  Scoliosis and Orthotic Management, 305
  Cardiac Symptoms, 306
  *Pharmacological and Surgical Management of
   Ataxia, 306*
  *Pharmacological Management of Friedreich's
   Ataxia, 306*

 Physiotherapy Assessment, 307
  Disease-Specific Scales, 307
 Time Course and Corresponding
  Management, 308
 Treatment Selection and Secondary
  Complications/Special Problems, 308
  Upper Limb Function, 308
  Balance, Walking and Mobility, 309
Hereditary Spastic Paresis, 309
 Epidemiology and Genetics, 309
 Anatomy, Pathophysiology and Clinical
  Presentation, 310
 Diagnosis, 311
 Medical Management, 311
  Antispasticity Medication, 311
 Physiotherapy Assessment, 311
  Disease-Specific Scales, 312
  *Time Course and Corresponding
   Management, 312*
 Treatment Selection, Secondary Complications
  and Special Problems, 312
Summary, 313
Case Study, 314
 Condition Overview, 314
 Classification, 316
 Examination, 316
  History, 316
  Body Structures and Function, 317
  Activities, 318
 Prognosis, 318
 Intervention, 318
 Outcomes (8 months), 318

293

INTRODUCTION

This chapter outlines the presentation of three inherited, neurodegenerative conditions: Huntington's disease (HD), the hereditary ataxias (spinocerebellar ataxias [SCAs], Friedreich's ataxia [FRDA]) and hereditary spastic paraparesis (HSP). The conditions predominantly affect different systems (the basal ganglia, the cerebellum and the pyramidal system, respectively), but all primarily result in disorders of movement. In manifest HD, chorea and dystonia predominate, whilst in HSP, spasticity will be a primary problem, and in the hereditary ataxias, the movement disorder is usually related to incoordination. Despite these relative differences in movement disorders, impairments in motor control, gait and balance are common across the conditions. These common impairments lead to activity limitations and participation restrictions and may reflect the greater levels of sedentary behaviour often seen in individuals living with these diseases. Thus secondary prevention physical activity strategies within a condition-informed framework are important components of physiotherapy interventions (Busse & Ramdharry 2020).

Although age of onset of these conditions can vary widely between and even within conditions, from childhood to adulthood, the inherited nature of the diseases means that many people may know they have the condition before symptom onset (Hagen 2018). In addition, people will ultimately be confronted with a progression of symptoms, potentially over many decades, and will have become highly aware of the need to develop strategies to manage these symptoms and the functional sequelae of their disease.

Inherited neurological conditions such as HD, SCA and HSP have relatively low prevalence and are typically understudied. A rare disease is defined as one that affects fewer than 5 people in 10,000 of the general population. When considered cumulatively, however, it is likely that many individuals are significantly affected by the 6000–8000 currently known types of rare diseases. More than 50% of known rare diseases are adult onset, and many are neurodegenerative; at least 700 known conditions result in a movement disorder, ataxia or gait disturbance that results in loss of independence in activities of daily living and detrimentally affect quality of life. Clearly the complexity and resultant cumulative burden and cost of these rare, inherited neurodegenerative diseases represent a significant public health challenge from a medical, care and societal perspective.

In this chapter, we provide a clinical overview of HD, SCA and HSP. In each condition we prioritise a top-down, participation-based approach, which focuses on understanding the personal factors contributing to an individual's health condition and promoting health and wellness throughout the life span. We conclude with a review of ethical considerations.

HUNTINGTON'S DISEASE

Epidemiology

HD is a neurodegenerative condition for which there are no disease-modifying treatments and only limited symptomatic treatments (Dash & Mestre 2020, Ferreira et al 2022, McColgan & Tabrizi 2018). HD is the most frequent autosomal dominant neurodegenerative disease and may affect between 10.6 and 13.7 individuals per 100,000 persons (McColgan & Tabrizi 2018). On average, the condition will develop in half of the offspring of an affected person, with both males and females being affected. Although considered a rare disease, recent figures report up to 12 per 100,000 people affected by the condition across the UK (Evans et al 2013, Pringsheim et al 2012). However, this is likely to be an underestimate because many families with HD either choose not to, or are not able to, access services (Baig et al 2016, Jones et al 2016a).

Genetics

Because HD is a dominant disorder, each cell contains one normal copy and one abnormal copy of the gene. The gene for HD was discovered in 1993 (Huntington Study Group 1993), and the protein for which it codes was named huntingtin. The first part of the HD gene has a sequence CAGCAGCAG, which is repeated several times. CAG codes for the amino acid glutamine so that the huntingtin protein (Htt) contains a sequence called a polyglutamine repeat. Htt is expressed ubiquitously (Walker 2007), and although the precise function is yet to be fully elucidated, it has important roles in axonal trafficking and mitochondrial dysfunction, regulation of gene transcription and cell survival (Schulte & Littleton 2011, Sharma et al 2021). The mutation causing HD (mHtt) is an expansion of the number of CAG repeats in the gene and, consequently, the polyglutamine repeat in the protein that leads to a toxic gain-of-function phenotype (Kshirsagar et al 2021, Schulte & Littleton 2011, Walker 2007).

The normal Htt allele contains a sequence of between 6 and 35 CAG triplet repeats. A CAG triplet expansion of 40 repeats or greater is called a full penetrance gene, meaning that the person will definitely experience development of HD in their life, as long as they do not die prematurely of another cause. The CAG repeat number in Htt plays a dominant role in HD phenotype. Generally, the CAG repeat number in the expanded allele is critical to age of onset and contributes to approximately 70% of the variation of age of onset (Sun et al 2017).

Although there is a correlation between the average age of onset and the CAG repeat length, it is not possible to unequivocally predict the age of onset for an individual from the CAG repeat size (Penney Jr et al 1997, Podvin et al 2019, Rosenblatt et al 2006). It is important for physiotherapists to be aware of the contribution of environment and lifestyle factors that are associated with age of onset of symptoms (Garcia-Gorro et al 2019, Lopez-Sendon et al 2011, Mees 2019, Trembath et al 2010, Wexler et al 2004).

An asymptomatic individual with an affected parent has a prior probability of 50% of inheriting the HD gene, and at this stage could choose to have a genetic test to confirm the number of CAG repeats. This is called a predictive test. Because there is no effective treatment to alter the natural history of HD, such tests are used with caution in conjunction with counselling and according to international guidelines originally published in 1994 and recently updated by the European Huntington Disease Network 'Genetic Testing Counselling' Working Group (MacLeod et al 2013). The relatively recent option of preimplantation genetic diagnosis (PGD) (Bouchghoul et al 2016, van Rij et al 2012) has introduced new options for people at risk for HD who wish to have children, and the importance of skilled counselling cannot be overemphasised.

Before PGD, the options for at-risk individuals were remaining childless, prenatal diagnosis, gamete donation or adoption. If couples decide to go through PGD, they will have to undergo in vitro fertilisation (IVF) procedures, even if they are fertile, to produce embryos for biopsy and testing. Only embryos found to be unaffected by the family's inherited condition are transferred to the uterus. For some, PGD is a safe alternative which decreases the possible risks and the emotional burden of postnatal depression (Ben-Nagi et al 2016, Blancato et al. 2017). It is critical that regardless of the choices, health professionals should have an understanding of some of the dilemmas faced by these families and be able to accommodate this within their professional boundaries (Genoff Garzon 2018, Piña-Aguilar, 2019, Stark et al 2016).

Anatomy and Pathophysiology

In HD, the most abundant cells in the striatum, namely the medium spiny projection neurones, are particularly sensitive to mHtt toxic accumulation (Raymond et al 2011). This leads to selective neuropathological changes and prominent cell loss and atrophy in the caudate and putamen of the striatum. Projections to the external globus pallidus are more involved than neurones that project to the internal globus pallidus, and the dominant feature of chorea early in the course of HD is suggested to be caused by this preferential involvement of the indirect pathway of basal ganglia–thalamocortical circuitry (Walker 2007). As the disease progresses, neurodegeneration is also seen in deep layers of the cerebral cortex, the globus pallidus, thalamus, subthalamic nucleus, substantia nigra and cerebellum (Hadzi et al 2012). This widespread neurodegeneration eventually leads to a triad of symptoms encompassing motor, cognitive and behavioural impairments (Walker 2007). Peripheral organ dysfunction including severe metabolic phenotype, weight loss, HD-related cardiomyopathy and skeletal muscle wasting is also considered to be part of the HD phenotype given the ubiquitous presence of the Htt protein (Zielonka et al 2014).

Clinical Presentation

HD can develop at almost any age from younger than 20 years (and occasionally <10 years) to older than 75 years, but the condition develops in most people between the ages of 35 and 55 years, which is after the usual years of reproduction (Harper 1992). The mean age of symptom onset is 35–44 years, and the median survival time is 15–18 years after onset (Caron et al 2020).

Approximately 5% of individuals will present with a juvenile form of HD and an age of onset of younger than 20 years (Quarrell et al 2012). Young people with juvenile HD may experience problems with speech earlier in the course of the illness, and rigidity and seizures occur more commonly (Quigley 2017).

Diagnosis of HD is typically based on a clinical assessment when an individual shows signs of an involuntary movement disorder, that is, becomes 'motor manifest'. It is now well established, however, that cognitive and behavioural abnormalities can be present 15–20 years before motor symptoms appear, and this time period is termed *presymptomatic HD* (Harrington et al 2015) (Fig. 12.1). Although impaired oculomotor function is an early and established feature of HD (Avanzini et al 1979, Leigh et al 1983), chorea is the most common motor impairment in people with HD (Albin et al 1989, Joel 2001). The movement disorder will typically begin in the distal extremities such as the fingers and in small facial muscles (Roos 2010). As the disease progresses, these involuntary movements increase in severity and begin to affect other muscle groups. With disease progression, chorea will often become less obvious and dystonia, defined by abnormal postures and involuntary twisting in the trunk and limbs, will usually become more established (de Zande et al 2016, Louis et al 1999). In the later stages of the disease, bradykinesia and rigidity become more evident (Fenney et al 2008). Altogether this complex movement disorder leads to balance and gait impairments, falls and loss of independence in functional skills (Busse et al

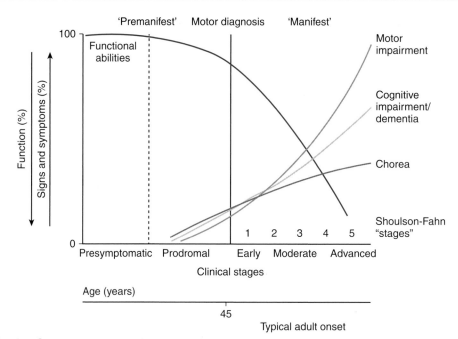

FIG. 12.1 Symptom progression across the Huntington's disease life cycle. Motor diagnosis is made based on the observable presence of movement disorder (usually chorea). Cognitive impairment will, however, be present years before the motor diagnosis and will gradually increase over time. As the disease progresses, motor impairment (bradykinesia and dystonia) will increase with associated dementia and loss of function. (Reproduced with permission. Nature Reviews Neurology from Huntington disease: natural history, biomarkers and prospects for therapeutics. Nature Reviews Neurology. License number 4056010016080.)

2009). Respiratory failure is also integral to the disease process (Alves et al 2016, Jones et al 2016b), and early efforts are required to minimise the effect of respiratory muscle weakness and swallow impairments given the main cause of death is aspiration pneumonia (Heemskerk & Roos 2012).

Cognitive deficits in HD are generally associated with executive function abnormalities, an umbrella term for processes such as task switching, motor planning and sequencing of tasks (Elliott 2003, Menon et al 2000). These cognitive problems may be reflected clinically as impairments in dual tasking ability (Reyes et al 2021).

Core neuropsychiatric symptoms in HD include apathy, a deficit in goal-directed behaviour associated with impaired instrumental learning (McLauchlan et al 2019), irritability (lower threshold for loss of temper) and depressed mood (van Duijn et al 2014). Apathy typically progresses throughout the course of the disease (Thompson et al 2012) and is thus thought to be inherent to the evolution and progression of HD. Indeed, Thompson et al (2012) reported that more than 95% of patients at

some point in the disease process reported reduced activity/energy and more than 90% reported lack of initiative. In contrast, irritability initially progresses before remitting in the mid stages, and depression occurs in a random pattern throughout the course of the illness (Thompson et al 2012).

Regardless of age of onset, managing the symptoms of HD often requires extensive engagement with healthcare and social care services. For this reason, HD is often described as a 'two-person disease' because of the burden it places on families and carers. Families face challenges with caring for affected loved ones because of the debilitating nature of the disease with varied, and somewhat misunderstood, cognitive, motor and behavioural symptoms (Simpson et al 2016). There may also be intergenerational caring requirements and progressive escalation of healthcare costs over time (Jones et al 2016a).

Medical Management

No current treatments will prevent, delay or slow the progressive neurodegeneration, although there are ongoing international efforts to identify potential candidates (Filipe & Wild 2020, Ross et al 2014, Ross & Tabrizi 2011, Tabrizi et al 2019). A small number of treatments are available to alleviate the chorea with variable success (Reilmann 2013), but no pharmacological treatments have been demonstrated to reduce the effect of other movement deficits, including gait impairments and altered postural control (Ferreira et al 2022). Several nonpharmacological approaches are also being explored in various international efforts. There is now preliminary evidence of safety and chorea reduction as a result of deep brain stimulation (DBS) in HD (Wojtecki et al 2016). Other therapies such as primary-foetal neural transplantation and more recently stem cell replacement therapies also have potential, although clinical trials are still in the early stages of development (Bachoud-Lévi 2017, Barker et al 2013, Dunnett & Rosser 2011, Rosser & Svendsen 2014, Wijeyekoon & Barker 2011). Compounds aiming to reduce mHtt expression through ribonucleic acid interference or antisense oligonucleotides are also an important focus of therapeutic development (Filipe & Wild 2020, Wild et al 2014). Given the established role of environmental enrichment in animal models of HD (Harrison et al 2013, Hockly et al 2002, Mo et al 2015, Nithianantharajah & Hannan 2006, van Dellen et al 2000, 2008), it is highly likely that approaches that focus on enhancing general physical activity and promoting engaging in aerobic exercise will be complementary to these novel pharmacological and surgical interventions with the ultimate aim of disease modification. Until such time as a treatment becomes available, end-of-life planning and care is an important consideration for the entire care team (Dellefield & Ferrini 2011, Klager et al 2008, Simpson 2007).

A Standard of Care for Huntington's Disease

HD is a complex disease and there is global agreement that comprehensive, multidisciplinary care involving a range of services is required across the disease stages (Frich et al 2016, Nance 2007, van Walsem et al 2015, Veenhuizen & Tibben 2009, Veenhuizen et al 2011). Critically, family caregivers should be acknowledged across the disease continuum and should be involved as contributors in partnerships with healthcare professionals (Frich et al 2014, Røthing et al 2015).

International consensus guidelines for the treatment of HD (Bachoud-Levi et al 2019) provide evidence-based recommendations for everyday clinical practice with the intention of standardising pharmacological, surgical and nonpharmacological treatment approaches to improve care and quality of life of patients. This follows from the European Huntington's Disease Network (EHDN) published standards of care for healthcare professionals focusing on occupational therapy, speech therapy, nutrition, oral health and physiotherapy (Cook et al 2012, Manley et al 2012, Quinn & Busse 2012). Updated clinical recommendations to guide physiotherapy practice were published in 2020 (Quinn et al 2020). These specifically recommend aerobic exercise, alone or in combination with resistance training, to improve fitness and motor function, and supervised gait training to improve spatiotemporal features of gait. They also recommend training of transfers including getting up from the floor, and in the later stages of HD, the use of positioning devices, seating adaptations and caregiver training.

Physiotherapy Assessment and Prognosis

Although the primary focus for physiotherapy assessment in HD should be on activities and their effect on quality of life and participation, it is also important that the physiotherapy assessment takes the broader HD-specific impairments into consideration. Although this may extend to evaluation of the hallmark voluntary and involuntary movement disorder using the gold standard Unified Huntington's Disease Rating Scale (Huntington Study Group 1996) Total Motor Score, additional performance-based outcome measures will be essential to evaluate any physiotherapy intervention outcomes. Assessment of balance and falls risks (Busse et al 2009, Grimbergen et al 2008), mobility in and outside of the home, and exercise capacity and/or respiratory function should always be included in an in-depth physiotherapy assessment.

Since 2008, there has been a concerted effort in the physiotherapy literature to validate performance-based measures of gait and balance for people with HD. A systematic review of functional outcome measures for HD (Mestre 2018) recommended the Tinetti Mobility Test for the purpose of screening for gait and balance problems in HD, and the Berg Balance Scale for balance assessment. The 6-minute walk test was found to be useful as a measure of walking endurance in ambulatory patients with HD. The 10-metre walk test, the Four-Square Step Test, the Mini Balance Evaluation Systems Test, the Physical Performance Test, the six-condition Romberg test and the Timed Up and Go test were also found to be reliable and valid for use in HD (Jacobs et al 2015, Kloos et al 2014, Quinn et al 2013, Rao et al 2009). Development of a clinical disease-specific measure of balance is needed in HD, as current assessments do not fully capture the range of balance impairments seen in HD. Recent studies also support the use of wearable monitors (e.g., inertial measurement units) to provide quantitative measures of balance and gait, including measures related to postural sway in sitting and standing, as well as measures of gait quality and quantity, as potential clinical endpoints (Desai et al 2021, Keren et al 2021, Muratori et al 2021, Porciuncula et al 2020). Additionally, dual-task function is becoming established as an important domain to consider, particularly in the earlier stages of disease (Fritz et al 2016, Tommaso et al 2017). Individuals with HD have complex cognitive and motor impairments, and research has shown that cognitive interference increases with task complexity during walking, with greater cognitive interference while turning and then walking in a straight path (Purcell et al 2020). The Timed Up and Go Cognitive test has been shown to be a sensitive measure of walking dual-task performance in people with HD (Muratori et al 2021).

Recognising the relative scarcity of specialist HD physiotherapists, members of the EHDN physiotherapy working group have developed a physiotherapy screening tool (Table 12.1) (Inbar et al 2016). The screening tool provides a structure to guide the assessment process that specifically covers issues (e.g., apathy and cognitive and behavioural function) that most commonly affect people with HD and are relevant to the physiotherapy clinical reasoning process. It is the intention that such a screening tool can guide a participation-based approach to HD physiotherapy, where initial assessment first and foremost considers the participation needs of the individual. The HD physiotherapy screening tool is intended to be used to provide initial guidance in intervention planning according to stage of disease (i.e., premanifest, early, early to mid and late stage) and functional level.

Other aspects covered by the screening tool include consideration of cognitive ability and behavioural impairment, which may affect intervention planning and implementation. Critically at each stage of the assessment process and indeed at any reassessment, it is important to consider potential comorbidities that may be unrelated to impairments that are typically seen in HD (Clenaghan et al 2016). The physiotherapist should always treat signs and symptoms that could be indicative of other neurological or peripheral illness as such and manage accordingly. This process of assessment, goal setting, treatment planning and evaluation is reflected in the iterative approach to patient or client management for individuals with HD as set out in the 2020 clinical practice recommendations (Quinn et al 2020) (Fig. 12.2).

Time Course and Corresponding Physiotherapy Management

HD is a progressive disease, which results in a range of motor, cognitive and behavioural impairments that affect daily physical functioning. Although primary prevention (i.e., prevention of the onset of the disease) is not possible, secondary and tertiary prevention strategies can be used.

The goal of secondary prevention is to slow the progress of a disease in its earliest stages to minimise long-term disability (Quinn & Morgan 2017, Quinn et al 2020). In HD, this may involve intervention at the premanifest stages of the disease, when clinical signs and symptoms are not evident but degenerative changes in the brain are occurring (Ross & Tabrizi 2011, Scheller et al 2013). Tertiary prevention focuses on the management of long-term conditions, with the goal to minimise the effect of physical impairments and maximise quality of life.

Therapists who are working with people with HD should incorporate shared goal setting and importantly consider ways in which the caregiver can contribute to the goal setting process so as to facilitate independent mobility for as long as is reasonably possible. Goals should typically be focused around specific functional problems or participation restrictions that are amenable to physiotherapy intervention (Quinn et al 2014). Goals to decrease chorea or dystonia are not realistic. Importantly, alleviation of any particular impairment in HD may not translate into functional improvements; therefore, therapists should focus on functional gains while attempting to ascertain the influence of various impairments on activity limitations. Exercise, including strengthening and cardiovascular conditioning, is recommended for people who are in the premanifest, early and middle stages of the disease (Quinn et al 2020). A recent study found that individuals with early- to mid-stage HD who engaged in a 12-week aerobic and strengthening exercise programme demonstrated improved fitness and disease-specific motor function compared with a control group (Quinn et al 2016). Exercise and physical activity engagement may be helpful in minimising any neuromuscular or musculoskeletal effects that come with disease progression. It is particularly important for therapists to provide behavioural interventions to physical activity uptake. A 14-week physical activity coaching programme was found to improve levels of physical activity in individuals with mid-stage HD (Busse et al 2017), and simple tools to support conversations about incorporating physical activity in daily life are also now available (Jones et al 2021). It is likely that exercise interventions have the potential to be most effective in either delaying disease onset or slowing disease progression when implemented at the earliest stages of the disease; however, this concept still needs empirical testing.

As the disease progresses and specific problems become evident, therapists must begin to ascertain those impairments that may be contributing to specific activity limitations or participation restrictions. For example, involuntary movements (e.g., chorea and dystonia) could contribute to balance problems, but inactivity may also be a contributing factor. Impairments that may affect

TABLE 12.1 Physiotherapy Screening for Huntington's Disease

#				
1	Highlights of issues or concerns: impairments of body functions: • observed and/or concerns raised by the patient or caregiver	Cognitive function Cardiovascular and respiratory functions Involuntary movements (dystonia, chorea) Muscle strength and muscle tone	Sensory function and pain Skin Coordination Balance	Speech, voice, swallow Posture Slowness Slips, trips, falls (see row 6)	
2	Issues described by the patient in their own words.				
3	Does the patients have any symptoms which might not be related to HD? **YES** Details (including referral if needed):		**NO**		
4	**Activity limitations and participation restrictions**	**Learning and applying knowledge** (reading, writing, etc.) **Self-care** (washing, dressing, eating, etc.)	**General tasks and demands** (undertaking single/multiple tasks) **Domestic life** (housework, preparation of meals, etc.)	**Communication** (conversation, speaking, nonverbal messages) **Interpersonal interactions and relationships** (social, family)	**Mobility** (lifting, fine motor control, using transportation) **Community, social and civic life** (leisure, etc.)
5	**Disease stage**	**Presymptomatic/early stage**	**Early-mid stage**	**Mid-late stage**	**Late stage**
6	If falls were mentioned (see row 1): How many falls occurred in the past 6 months? Where was the fall? How did the patient manage to get up from the floor?				
7	Is the patient engaged in regular physical activity? (structured or self-managed) **YES** What kind? How often?	**NO** Why not?			
8	In a usual weekday (morning till night, how much time (%) does the patient spend sitting?				
9	**Gait** Qualitative comments (gait analysis):				
10	Assistive devices (any in use, any required)				
11	**10-Step tandem walk**	Normal	1–3 Deviations from straight line	>3 Deviations from straight line	Cannot complete tandem walk	Cannot attempt tandem walk
12	Quick screening of respiratory function	(a) When asked to cough, is the patient able to self-clear any secretions? **YES NO** (b) Note: NO = In your opinion, is the patient at risk for aspiration? **YES NO**			

HD, Huntington's disease.

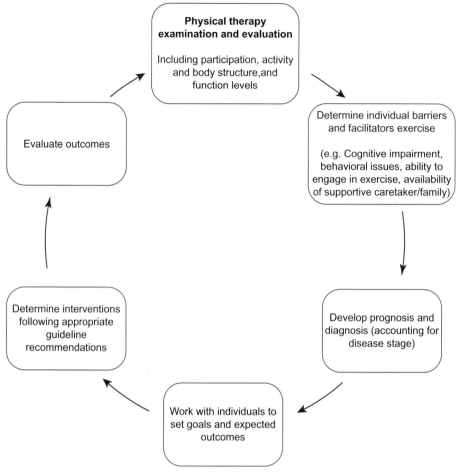

FIG. 12.2 The iterative approach to patient or client management for individuals with Huntington's disease as set out in the 2020 clinical practice guidelines (Reproduced with permission. Neurology. Clinical recommendations to guide physical therapy practice for Huntington disease. License number 5233121289470.)

function include dystonia, bradykinesia, chorea, rigidity, impaired respiratory function and fatigue (Busse et al 2008). It is important to manage the secondary effects of such impairments. For example, for patients with chorea, protective equipment (e.g., helmets, shin guards) can be provided, and for patients with dystonia, loss of range of motion and muscle imbalance should be prevented through stretching and positioning programmes. Functional problems that may occur include impaired fine motor skills and manual dexterity; impaired sitting posture and sitting ability; impaired mobility, transfers and gait; impaired balance and risk for falls; and reduced cardiovascular fitness. The potential effect of psychiatric impairments and a patient's cognitive status cannot be

overlooked. Therapists should consider whether a patient has memory loss, depression, aggression, obsessive-compulsive tendencies or anxiety, to name a few, and these impairments must be considered in development of a physiotherapy programme.

Treatment Selection and Secondary Complications/Special Problems

One of the difficulties in providing guidance for physiotherapy in HD is the heterogeneity of clinical signs and symptoms. Although staging of the disease process (e.g., early, middle, late) can provide a general framework for intervention, within each stage there is a wide range of potential impairments that can affect an individual's level of functional activity and life participation. Through a process of consensus and review of published literature, treatment-based classifications were developed as part of the initial consensus guideline development with a view to guiding clinical decision making across the life course of the disease (Quinn & Busse 2012) (Table 12.2). These classifications can be used by physiotherapists after assessment and decision making as to which classification may be most important to consider in the treatment planning process. The classifications were revised in the 2020 clinical

TABLE 12.2 Summary of Modified Treatment-Based Classifications for Huntington's Disease (Quinn 2020)

Category	Description of Primary Movement Impairments	Clinical Recommendations
Exercise capacity and/or physical activity	Absence of or limited motor impairment or specific limitations in functional activities	Primary interventions: Aerobic exercise (55%–90% age-predicted heart rate maximum) and resistance exercise (upper and lower body, core) 3–4 times per week (minimum of 12 weeks for fitness and motor function benefits); home-based exercise and walking programmes Setting: Home, outpatient Primary outcomes: Motor function (UHDRS total motor or modified motor), fitness (VO_2 max) Secondary outcomes: Physical performance test, 6-minute walk test, Lorig Self-Efficacy for Exercise, physical activity (measured by pedometers or IPAQ), cognitive battery (e.g., Symbol Digit Modality Test), quality of life (SF-36), gait speed (10-metre walk test), Berg Balance Scale
Mobility and function	Impairments in strength or fatigue resulting in mobility limitations; slow gait	Primary interventions: Task-specific training of walking and transfers; multidisciplinary rehabilitation Setting: Inpatient, outpatient, home, supervised at gym Primary outcomes: Gait speed, TUG, spatiotemporal measures of gait, 10-metre walk test Secondary outcomes: Balance (Romberg, Berg Balance Scale, Functional Reach Test, Pastor Test, Four Square Step Test), balance confidence (ABC Scale)
Balance and falls risk	Impairments in balance; increased falls risk	Primary interventions: Task-specific training of balance; multidisciplinary rehabilitation Setting: Outpatient clinic, inpatient rehabilitation hospital, community, and home settings Primary outcomes: None Secondary outcomes: Balance (Romberg, Berg Balance Scale, Functional Reach Test, Pastor Test, Four Square Step Test), balance confidence (ABC Scale); goal attainment scaling
Respiratory function	Impaired respiratory function and capacity, limited endurance, limited airway clearance, resulting in restrictions in functional activities and risk for infection	Primary interventions: Inspiratory and expiratory training, with and without resistance Setting: Home Primary outcomes: Respiratory muscle strength, cough effectiveness Secondary outcomes: Swallowing, breathlessness, exercise capacity/endurance

(Continued)

TABLE 12.2 Summary of Modified Treatment-Based Classifications for Huntington's Disease (Quinn 2020)—Cont'd

Category	Description of Primary Movement Impairments	Clinical Recommendations
Secondary musculoskeletal and postural changes	Musculoskeletal and/or respiratory changes resulting in physical deconditioning and subsequent decreased participation in daily living activities or social/work environments. Altered alignment in sitting or standing because of secondary adaptive changes, involuntary movements, muscle weakness, and incoordination resulting in limitations in functional activities in sitting or standing	Primary interventions: Transfer training, postural stability training. Setting: Outpatient, inpatient rehabilitation. Primary outcomes: Gait (double support %, stride length, gait speed), Force Plate (length, speed of center of mass projection), Physical Performance Test, and Tinetti. Secondary outcomes: Berg Balance Scale, TUG Barthel Index and UHDRS TFC score
End stage	Active or passive ROM limitations and poor active movement control resulting in inability to ambulate; dependent for most ADLs; difficulty maintaining upright sitting posture	Primary interventions: Multisensory stimulation, hydrotherapy, video-based exercise. Setting: Home, specialized unit for late-stage HD. Primary outcomes: Behavior Mood Disturbance Scale, quality of life measures. Secondary outcomes: Blood pressure, heart rate and respiratory rate

ADLs, Activities of daily living; *HD*, Huntington's disease; *IPAQ*, International Physical Activity Questionnaire; *ROM*, range of motion; *SF-36*, 36-Item Short-Form Survey; *TUG*, Timed Up and Go Test; *UHDRS*, Unified Huntington's Disease Rating Scale.

practice recommendations to include exercise capacity and/or physical activity, mobility and function, balance and falls risk, respiratory function, secondary musculoskeletal and postural changes, and end-stage care. For each of the classifications, aims and intervention strategies are proposed (Quinn et al 2020).

Since the initial classification development, there has been a significant increase in the number and quality of physiotherapy and exercise studies in HD (Fritz et al 2017b) that provides validation of the treatment-based classification approach clustered around exercise capacity and performance, balance and mobility, and falls risk. Short- and long-term exercise and physical activity programmes (Busse et al 2013, 2017, Khalil et al 2013, Quinn et al 2016, Thompson et al 2013) and videogame and task-specific training home interventions (Kloos et al 2013, Quinn et al 2014) have been shown to be feasible and beneficial in improving motor function, mobility, self-efficacy and patient-specific goals. A recently completed 1-year physiotherapy-led physical activity intervention was also shown to be feasible, with effect estimates showing improvements in fitness, endurance and self-reported physical activity

for the intervention group compared with a control group (Quinn et al 2022).

Intensive inpatient multidisciplinary rehabilitation programmes (Ciancarelli et al 2013, 2015, Piira et al 2013, Zinzi et al 2007) have also been found to help people with HD maintain functional independence. Studies have shown preliminary evidence that multidisciplinary rehabilitation can improve cognitive functioning, with supportive neuroimaging findings (Cruikshank et al 2015). Published case studies have shown that people with mid- to late-stage HD are able to achieve meaningful functional improvements related to physical therapy interventions in relation to balance, mobility and falls risk (Fritz et al 2017a). There are also emerging data to suggest that respiratory failure in HD is not necessarily the consequence of immobility and postural impairment but could be part of the disease process (Jones et al 2016b). Regular breathing exercises may therefore be an important intervention that can lead to increased respiratory muscle capacity, and home-based respiratory muscle training programmes have been found to have beneficial effects on pulmonary function but little impact on swallowing ability and dyspnoea (Reyes et al 2015).

All studies on physiotherapy and exercise, to date, have been feasibility, pilot or otherwise limited sample size studies without adequate comparator groups, and larger scale studies are needed to provide definitive guidance.

HEREDITARY ATAXIAS

Epidemiology and Genetics

The hereditary ataxias are a large group of neurodegenerative disorders that vary in terms of the clinical signs and symptoms (phenotype) and their underlying genetic deficits (genotype). The hereditary ataxias are mainly inherited in an autosomal dominant or autosomal recessive manner, although rare X-linked ataxias do exist (e.g., fragile X syndrome).

Autosomal Dominant Cerebellar Ataxias

Autosomal dominant cerebellar ataxias (ADCAs) present with slowly progressive cerebellar signs of dysmetria and dyssynergia affecting the limbs, dysarthria, oculomotor signs and disorders of balance and gait. ADCAs with a known genetic locus are referred to as spinocerebellar ataxias (SCAs) and are numbered (e.g., SCA1, SCA3) according to the time they were discovered. There are currently 48 known genetic causes of autosomal dominant ataxias, with more being discovered every year (Scott et al 2020). The prevalence of the ADCAs varies from 2 to 5.6 per 100,000 (Sun et al 2016). ADCAs tend to have an onset in adulthood with a mean age of onset of 35 years (±11 years) (Rossi et al 2014). Seven of the 48 SCAs are caused by CAG repeat expansion, a similar mutation to that seen in HD but occurring at different genetic locus. In these conditions, the age of onset is inversely proportional to the length of the CAG repeat (Scott et al 2020). Episodic ataxias are rare, mainly autosomal dominant ataxias affecting less than 1 per 100,000. They are types of channelopathies that affect ion channels within the neurone membrane. They are characterised by minutes to hours of ataxia involving unsteady gait often associated with nystagmus or dysarthria. Episodes can be triggered by environmental factors such as emotional stress, caffeine, alcohol, certain medications, physical activity and illness. Permanent ataxia may result late in the disease course (Choi & Choi 2016).

Autosomal Recessive Ataxias

Most autosomal recessive ataxias have symptoms of limb ataxia and impaired balance and walking. Additional signs include vertigo, dysphagia and diplopia (Fogel & Perlman 2007). People often have associated neuropathy resulting in loss of proprioception and vibration sense (Fogel & Perlman 2007) that contributes to the ataxia. FRDA is the most common autosomal recessive ataxia, affecting Whites with a prevalence of 2–5 per 100,000. In ~98% of cases, it is caused by a GAA repeat expansion on the Frataxin gene on chromosome 9q13. The age of symptom onset is between 5 and 15 years with earlier onset age being seen in people with larger GAA repeat size in the affected gene (Fogel & Perlman 2007, Parkinson et al 2013a).

Anatomy, Pathophysiology and Clinical Presentation

Autosomal Dominant Cerebellar Ataxias

Clinically, the ADCAs were broadly classified into types I to III (Harding 1983):

Type I: Cerebellar ataxia with additional signs such as ophthalmoplegia, spasticity, extrapyramidal signs, peripheral neuropathy and dementia. The most common SCA is SCA3, which is also known as *Machado-Joseph disease*. Depending on ethnicity, SCA3 accounts for between 21% and 56% of SCA cases (Subramony & Paraminder 2002). It is a polyglutamate (polyQ) disease caused by a CAG repeated expansion of a gene on chromosome 14q. The age of onset varies from childhood to late adult life, and there is an inverse correlation between the number of CAG repeats and the age of onset and disease severity (Watanabe et al 1996). SCA3 is an example of a type I presentation with people showing symptoms of progressive ataxia and a variable combination of other symptoms including pyramidal signs, extrapyramidal signs that can resemble Parkinson's, peripheral amyotrophy and ophthalmoplegia. In addition, in this and other SCAs, people can have nonmotor disorders such as sleep disorders, attention and executive disorders (Matos et al 2019, Maas et al 2021).

Type II: Cerebellar ataxia with pigmentary macular degeneration – this is rare and caused by a CAG expansion on chromosome 3 and is referred to as SCA7.

Type III: This presents with a relatively pure presentation of cerebellar ataxia. SCA6 is an example of a type III presentation. The prevalence of SAC6 varies across the world, being more common in Korean, Japanese and German populations (up to 23%) compared with the UK (5%) (Sun et al 2016).

The Type I–III classification has been largely superseded by the classification based on genetic diagnosis.

Progressive ataxia is seen in all SCAs; cerebellar signs include:
- Limb dyssynergia and dysmetria;
- Tremor (postural and action);
- Oculomotor deficit ('saccadic' smooth pursuit, dysmetric saccades, nystagmus [e.g., gaze evoked, downbeat]);
- Impaired balance and gait; and
- Dysarthria and dysphagia.

The most frequent symptoms at onset in the ADCAs is gait ataxia (observed in 68%) (Luo et al 2017). Loss of walking occurs approximately 15 years after symptom onset. Tremor is more frequently seen in the severe stages of the disease (Lai et al 2019).

Additional nonataxia symptoms are seen in 50% of cases, and these can be the presenting symptoms (e.g., retinal degeneration in SCA7). Nonmotor symptoms in the SCAs include poor executive function (e.g., reduced verbal fluency and working memory), impaired spatial cognition (e.g., poor visuospatial memory) and linguistic difficulties (e.g., dysprosody and agrammatism) (Moriarty et al 2016, Schmahmann & Sherman 1998). Together these are referred to as a cerebellar cognitive affective syndrome and reflect damage to the interconnections between the cerebellum and frontoparietal, superior temporal and paralimbic circuits (Maas et al 2021). Other nonmotor disorders such

as fatigue, sleep disorders (such as restless legs syndrome), depression and anxiety are also common in the SCAs and significantly affect quality of life (Moro et al 2019). Because of the complexity of symptoms in SCA, mild lower urinary tract symptoms such as urinary urgency or frequency are often overlooked and untreated pharmacologically despite being common (e.g., 86.3% in one cohort study) and having a significant impact on quality of life (Afonso Ribeiro et al 2021). The interrelationship of the main nonataxic symptoms in SCA and the genetic diagnosis is summarised in Fig. 12.3.

The affected genes causing the ADCAs tend to be highly expressed in the output neurones of the cerebellar cortex (the Purkinje cells). The affected genes encode a variety of proteins including ion channels, proteins that can phosphorylate or dephosphorylate cellular targets (an essential part of intracellular signalling) termed *kinases* and

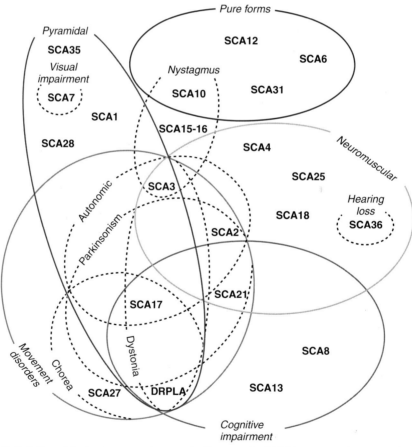

FIG. 12.3 Relationship between spinocerebellar ataxia (SCA) type and presenting symptoms. (Reproduced with permission. Rossi, M., et al., 2014. Autosomal dominant cerebellar ataxias: a systematic review of clinical features. Eur. J. Neurol. 21, 607–615.)

phosphatases and proteins of unknown function (Meera et al 2016). Purkinje cells are normally very active and play an integral role in synaptic changes that underlie motor learning and adaptation (Tada et al 2015). Disease models of the ADCAs highlight that early in the disease there is a reduction in the regular firing of the Purkinje cells. This may affect the normal function of the cell and therefore the function of the circuits which the cerebellum is part of, such as those linking the cerebellum with cerebral cortical areas and the brainstem. Disease models of the ataxias also show that a type of glutamate receptor present in Purkinje cells, the metabotropic receptor, alters its signalling leading to excessive calcium influx. This can in turn activate more metabotropic receptors causing further calcium influx, a type of positive feedback. Because calcium activates a number of enzymes within the cell that in turn can damage components of the cells (e.g., DNA, cell membrane and cytoskeleton), this ultimately leads to degeneration of the Purkinje cell, a type of excitotoxicity (Huang & Verbeek 2019).

Friedreich's Ataxia

In FRDA, there is degeneration of the dorsal columns, spinocerebellar tracts and dentate nucleus (the deep cerebellar nucleus that connects the cerebellar hemispheres to the cerebral cortex via the thalamus). It is characterised by progressive ataxia (affecting balance, walking limbs and speech) and sensory signs. Axonal sensory neuropathy results in areflexia and a loss of proprioception and vibration sense. Corticospinal tract involvement leads to paresis and extensor plantar responses. Nonneurological involvement includes cardiomyopathy in ~50% and diabetes mellitus in ~10%. With disease progression, symptoms of kyphoscoliosis and pes cavus/equinovarus occur that affect respiratory function and walking, respectively (Pandolofo 2002).

Variations of the typical FRDA presentation exist in the 10% of cases having a positive molecular test for FRDA. People can show FRDA with retained reflexes and also late-onset FRDA (LOFA) or very late-onset FRDA, where symptom onset occurs after 25 and 40 years, respectively (Parkinson et al 2013b). Unlike typical FRDA, people with LOFA show signs of spasticity (40% of cases) and have retained reflexes (46% of cases) (Bhidayasiri et al 2005, Gates et al 1998). Nonneurological symptoms such as cardiomyopathy, sphincter disturbances, scoliosis and pes cavus are less frequent in atypical FRDA (Bhidayasiri et al 2005). Oculomotor abnormalities may be absent in atypical FRDA. People with LOFA have a slower progression.

In FRDA, the frataxin gene is affected. Frataxin encodes for a protein that localises to the mitochondria and is associated with iron metabolism and homoeostasis (Parkinson et al 2013b). A deficiency in Frataxin causes mitochondrial iron accumulation, oxidative stress and impaired adenosine triphosphate production. Oxidative stress in turn can damage mitochondrial DNA, resulting in further mitochondrial dysfunction leading to neuronal degeneration.

Diagnosis and Genetic Testing

The hereditary ataxias tend to have a slow onset of symptoms unlike the acute onset seen with a cerebellar stroke. Autosomal recessive disorders have an earlier onset than autosomal dominant ataxias. Family history aided by molecular and genetic tests can confirm the diagnosis. The diagnosis of hereditary ataxias requires the exclusion of other conditions such as multiple sclerosis, posterior fossa tumours, alcoholic cerebellar ataxia or nonmetastatic manifestations of malignancy. Further information on common diagnostic investigations required to rule out other pathology is provided in the Ataxia UK Medical Guidelines (de Silva et al 2019).

Before genetic testing, experts in genetic counselling (e.g., neurologists/geneticists) should discuss the implications of the test with the patient. Tests are available via the UK genetic testing network for many of the hereditary ataxias (de Silva et al 2019). Genetic counselling should also be considered for people who are planning a family.

Medical Management
Symptomatic Treatments of Nonataxic Signs
Nonataxic signs seen in the ADCAs and FRDA frequently may require symptomatic treatment. More commonly encountered symptoms are highlighted later.

Spasticity and Dystonia
Recommendations for the pharmacological symptomatic treatment of spasticity, parkinsonism, dystonia and cramps have been outlined and include benzodiazepines, baclofen and carbamazepine (Bettencourt & Lima 2011, Ogawa 2004). Some people with SCA3 (Machado-Joseph disease) can show levodopa-responsive dystonia; therefore patients should undergo a levodopa trial if dystonia is present (Bettencourt & Lima 2011, Ogawa 2004).

Scoliosis and Orthotic Management
Children with FRDA can present with a variety of curves, including a long, thoracolumbar curve and pelvic obliquity, double lumbar and thoracic curves, or hyperkyphosis. The curves tend to progress even after reaching skeletal maturity (Cady & Bobechko 1984). Children between ages 10 and 16 years and with curves between 20° and 40° should be monitored yearly (Corben et al 2014). Orthotic bracing may slow curve progression, but surgical correction with

a posterior spinal fusion may be required for curves >40° (Corben et al 2014, Tsirikos & Smith 2012).

Cardiac Symptoms

Cardiac manifestations of FRDA include cardiomyopathy, dilated cardiomyopathy and electrophysiological disturbances. They are caused by the mitochondrial dysfunction that also affects the nervous system. Heart failure and arrhythmias account for approximately 60% of the mortality in FRDA. Electrocardiogram (ECG), ambulatory ECG (Holter) and an echocardiogram are recommended at the time of diagnosis. If the ECG is abnormal (e.g., left ventricular hypertrophy), then yearly checks are recommended (Sommerville et al 2017). A cardiologist opinion should be sought before commencing hydrotherapy or surgery (e.g., for scoliosis). Exercise including a structured aerobic programme and light weights is recommended as good clinical practice, but there are no trials to date to support their effect. Angiotensin-converting enzyme inhibitors for heart failure, diuretics for fluid overload and β-blockers for the prevention of atrial arrhythmias are recommended (Corben et al 2014). Drugs that have negative inotropic effects (i.e., reduce force of muscle contraction) should be avoided (Corben et al 2014). Cardiac transplant may be considered for severe heart failure. Idebenone may improve cardiac function (see later).

Pharmacological and Surgical Management of Ataxia

Generally, the pharmacological management of hereditary ataxias is limited (Ilg et al 2014, Perlman 2000). One exception is the episodic ataxias. In about two-thirds of people with episodic ataxia type II (a type of channelopathy) the number of attacks and quality of life can be improved with aminopyridines, a blocker of voltage-gated potassium channels (Strupp et al 2017). These are believed to increase the excitability of the inhibitory cerebellar cortex output neurones (the Purkinje cells) and increase the threshold for the episodic attacks (Strupp et al 2017).

The low prevalence of SCA and diversity in both the underlying genetics and clinical presentation are significant challenges requiring a multinational consortium approach to ascertain natural disease progression via cohort studies and undertake randomised clinical trials (RCTs) (Brooker et al 2021, Ilg et al 2014).

Ataxia UK guidelines suggest initially trying propranolol (a β-blocker) for the treatment of cerebellar tremor. If there is no effect, then primidone (a barbiturate derivative) should be tried in isolation and then in combination with propranolol (Bonney et al 2016). Downbeat nystagmus is a symptom associated with postural ataxia, oscillopsia and reduced visual acuity. The nonselective potassium channel blockers 3,4-Diaminopyridine (3,4-DAP) and

4-Aminopyridine (4-AP) reduce downbeat nystagmus in people with cerebellar atrophy and SCA6, and are associated with improvements in visual acuity. Postural symptoms may also improve, but this finding is not consistent (Ilg et al 2014, Strupp et al 2003, Tsunemi et al 2010). Pharmacological treatments for SCAs tend to focus on regulating cerebellar neurone firing rate (e.g., riluzole), modulating function by affecting nicotinic acetylcholinergic receptors and reducing glutamate-mediated excitotoxicity (e.g., with N-methyl-D-aspartate antagonists).

With severe cerebellar tremor, DBS of the ventral intermediate nucleus of the thalamus (the thalamic relay in humans) may be considered. Reductions in cerebellar tremor in cohorts of people with multiple sclerosis (Berk et al 2002, Torres et al 2010) and in isolated cases of people with ADCA (Herzog et al 2007, Pirker et al 2003, Shimojima et al 2005) have been reported. Functional benefits with DBS may be seen, although these tend to be variable and short-lived in people with multiple sclerosis as the disease progresses (Hooper et al 2002), and this may also be the case in ADCA. Greater benefits of surgery are seen in people with isolated tremor (i.e., oscillatory movement around one frequency) compared with people with combined tremor and dysmetria/dyssynergia (Berk et al 2002, Liu et al 2000).

Preliminary studies of direct stimulation of the cerebellum using transcranial magnetic stimulation or direct current stimulation suggest that certain stimulation paradigms (e.g., inhibitory stimuli using repetitive 1-Hz stimulation) are safe and associated with clinical improvements in symptoms of cerebellar disease such as tremor (Manor et al 2019, Shiga et al 2002). Initial trials in cohorts with ataxic symptoms that included SCA as well as other degenerative conditions such as multisystem atrophy further suggest improvements in ataxia rating scales with repetitive 1-Hz stimulation (França et al 2020) or cerebellospinal transcranial direct current stimulation (Benussi et al 2021). The significant association between changes in clinical ratings of ataxia and cognitive scores with changes in physiological measures of cerebellar-cortical interactions (termed cerebellar inhibition) suggests changes in cerebellar functional connectivity occur after stimulation (Benussi et al 2021).

Pharmacological Management of Friedreich's Ataxia

Coenzyme Q10 is a mitochondrial molecule that is part of the electron transfer chain. It is a potent antioxidant and can maintain other antioxidants such as vitamin E. Idebenone is a structural analogue of coenzyme Q10, but it is more water soluble and has a lower molecular weight and may thus show greater bioavailability (Parkinson et al 2013b). However, systematic reviews suggest there is no improvement with idebenone in ataxia rating scales

(Delatycki & Bidichandani 2019, Kearney et al 2016). There is some evidence from RCTs in the USA and Europe to suggest improved cardiac function and maintenance/ improvements in fine motor skills after idebenone (Ilg et al 2014, Parkinson et al 2013b). However, this seems to be dependent on the prescribed dose and baseline disease severity. Improvements may be more marked in ambulant, less severely affected children. The effect on neurological signs and in particular functional ability and quality of life is unclear (Parkinson et al 2013b), and trials of other antioxidants are ongoing (Delatycki & Bidichandani 2019, Ilg et al 2014).

More recently animal models suggest that inflammation may play a role in the pathogenesis of FRDA, a finding supported by improvements in a 1-minute timed walk following methylprednisolone administration in a 26-week open-labelled trial (Delatycki & Bidichandani 2019).

Physiotherapy Assessment

Deficits in gait and balance are the most common presenting symptom, and falls are frequent (Luo et al 2017). Therefore subjective and objective assessment should enquire about difficulties in these areas, in particular ascertaining frequency, circumstances and causes of falls (e.g., intrinsic or extrinsic/environmental).

Increases in postural sway and deficits in reactive balance and anticipatory responses accompanying voluntary movements have been reported in cerebellar disease and should be assessed (Marsden & Harris 2011), for example, using the BEST or brief-BESTest (Kondo et al 2020, Lo et al 2022). Often preparatory muscle activity is ill-timed or absent, resulting in imbalance and falls. People with ataxia are often worse when faced with moving visual stimuli (Bunn et al 2015b). Therefore people may experience particular difficulties when walking in crowds, down shopping aisles or when having to move their head while walking or may avoid these situations. Assessment should therefore examine balance under different sensory conditions.

An ataxic gait may be caused by difficulties with balance, but also inaccurate foot placement associated with limb dyssynergia (Morton & Bastain 2004). Assessments should therefore assess limb dyssynergia (e.g., with heel shin test) while the person is fully supported (e.g., in supine) to ascertain the importance of this component. Joint movements and interjoint coordination and temporospatial parameters of walking are more variable in people with SCA (Ilg et al 2007). Wearable inertial sensors provide the future possibility of measuring these aspects more easily outside of the laboratory setting (Shah et al 2021).

Balance, gait and upper limb deficits can be further affected by inaccuracies in oculomotor control. Therefore nystagmus in primary position and on looking to the side

(gaze-evoked nystagmus), saccades, smooth pursuit and vestibulo-ocular reflex suppression should be also assessed (Marsden & Harris 2011).

Vertigo often accompanies cerebellar ataxia because of the intimate interconnections between the cerebellar and vestibular systems. As with many neurological conditions, people report difficulties having to attend to another task when walking, so undertaking dual tasks can be associated with a worsening of balance (Ilg & Timmann 2013). Performance can also be affected by fatigue (Fruhmann Berger et al 2006). Upper limb and head/truncal ataxia can affect activities of daily living such as eating, drinking and dressing, occupation and leisure activities. Further, ataxia can affect communication and swallowing. Therefore an assessment should occur as part of a multidisciplinary team including speech and language therapists and occupational therapists.

Disease-Specific Scales

Several scales share common features, evaluating symptoms such as tremor or dysmetria on standard tests using an ordinal scale. Because 50% of people with hereditary ataxia have additional nonataxic signs, it is also important to undertake a holistic assessment with the aim of ascertaining the cause of a person's functional limitations (Perez-Lloret et al. 2021). The scales described measure impairment and may not therefore always relate to people's perceived difficulties with activities of daily living (ADL) (Maas & van de Warrenburg 2021).

Examples of ataxia-specific scales include the scale for the assessment and rating of ataxia (SARA), the International Classification of Ataxia Rating Scale (ICARS) and the Brief Ataxia Rating Scale (BARS) (Storey et al 2004, Yabe et al 2008). The SARA has eight items: gait, stance, sitting, speech, finger chase, nose-to-finger, fast alternating hand movements and heel-shin test. There is an additional inventory of nonataxia symptoms (Jacobi et al 2013). The ICARS has four subscales: (1) postural and gait disturbances, (2) limb movement disturbances, (3) speech disturbances and (4) oculomotor disturbances. The BARS consist of five tests from the ICARS: gait and posture, kinetic function–arm, kinetic function–leg, speech and oculomotor function. The BARS has higher intrarater and interrater reliability compared with the ICARS (Schmahmann et al 2009). The ICARS takes three times longer to complete compared with the SARA, and the BARS takes only 3–5 minutes to complete (Storey et al 2004, Trouillas et al 1997, Weyer et al 2007). Clinically, the ICARS is believed to be sensitive in describing mild cerebellar dysfunction and if an oculomotor assessment is required, whereas the SARA may be more suited in assessing people with pure cerebellar disease (Timmann et al 2009). A video-based version of the SARA that can be performed at home and correlates with the conventional SARA score has been developed but shows high interindividual variation when tested in people with SCA (Grobe-Einsler et al 2021). In conditions such as SCA3 (Machado-Joseph disease), where there is a significant extrapyramidal component, other scales such as the unified multiple system atrophy rating scale are valid (D'Abreu et al 2007).

The Friedreich's Ataxia Rating Scale combines timed measures of performance, a functional disability stage and patient-reported outcomes. It correlates with other scales (e.g., the ICARS and the Functional Independence measure) and can show a change over 1 year. Other performance-based measures (e.g., nine-hole peg test, 10-metre walking test) can also be used to monitor disease progression and the effects of treatment in FRDA (Fahey et al 2007, Lynch et al 2006).

Time Course and Corresponding Management

Over time, symptoms, as measured by clinical rating scales, progress with a yearly change in the SARA score of 0.8 to 2.1 (out of a maximum of 40) depending on SCA subtype. Nonataxic symptoms also develop, and these have a faster progression in type I presentations compared with type III such as SCA6. People also frequently experience cognitive deficits, in particular in the areas of executive functions, speed, attention and visual memory, but the extent varies across SCA subtype (Moriarty et al 2016).

In FRDA, scores on clinical rating scales (Friedreich's Ataxia Rating Scale) and performance measures predict functional ability, activities of daily living and disease duration (Croarkin et al 2009, Lynch et al 2006). Clinical severity is predicted by age and the size of the GAA genetic repeat. In FRDA, ~60% of people die of heart failure with associated symptoms of shortness of breath at rest or with minimal exertion (Corben et al 2014).

Initially management should aim to maintain occupation and leisure activities. As outlined later, clinical trials suggest that intensive exercise can be effective in SCAs at least for balance and walking. People with ataxia should be encouraged to try activities that are enjoyable, meaningful, satisfying and appropriately challenging to maximise long-term engagement (Cassidy et al 2018). Improvements in balance with horse riding, climbing, swimming and yoga, for example, have been reported in case reports (Bonney et al 2016).

With time, the maintenance of function requires the use of aids and adaptations. These can further reduce fatigue. Motor learning and adaptation is affected in people with cerebellar disease, so it may be useful to introduce these earlier in the disease course to allow people to learn to use any adaption that is/may be required (Bastian 2008).

With disease progression, increasing dysarthria can make communication difficult. Early input of speech and language therapists to explore different techniques is required. Speech and language therapists can also aid with swallowing difficulties that may develop (Bonney et al 2016). These can lead to aspiration pneumonias and breathlessness. In light of the potential communication difficulties, people should be made aware of advanced care planning options in ample time. In the later stages of the disease, they should receive access to specialist palliative care services with aftercare for bereaved families and carers (Bonney et al 2016, Perlman 2000, 2004).

Treatment Selection and Secondary Complications/Special Problems
Upper Limb Function

Maintenance of upper limb function should be explored in collaboration with occupational therapists. Addressing trunk and postural control, either through retraining or adaptations, should theoretically aid proximal arm control and function, although the evidence base for this remains poor. Distal hand ataxia can be difficult to improve and may require early use of aids and adaptations (Bonney et al 2016).

In the early stages, different pens and postural support of the head, trunk and forearm may help with writing. Computer use can be improved by strategies such as slowing the movement of the mouse either directly or through external resistance (e.g., tracker ball). Referral to IT solutions experts (e.g., AbilityNet) is recommended in cases where computer use is affected. Other adaptations could be explored with occupational therapists, including larger buttons on phones, nonslip mats (e.g., Dycem) to limit movements of plates or cups, plate guards, weighted cutlery and lidded or insulated cups, and the use of straws to help maintain or improve independence within the home (Bonney et al 2016).

Upper limb function may be improved with the use of weights to dampen tremor. This does not produce any lasting effect on tremor, and it may in fact lead to a temporary increase after the initial removal of tremor (Manto et al 1994). Therefore, weights need to be used to address specific functional goals. Increasing the viscous resistance of the arm experimentally can also reduce tremor and incoordination (Marsden & Harris 2011). This may be exploited clinically by using Lycra garments, although there have been no trials to date showing their effect on cerebellar ataxia. Devices that provide external damping such as the 'neater eater' (http://www.neater.co.uk) can also help with eating for people with more severe cerebellar disease.

Balance, Walking and Mobility

There is increasing evidence from animal models (Chuang et al 2019) and clinical trials that intensive rehabilitation of balance and walking leads to clinical improvements in SCAs (Ilg & Timmann 2013, Lanza et al 2020). In children with hereditary ataxias, high exercise intensity and compliance have been achieved by using exergaming to aid motivation (Synofzik et al 2013). In adults, intensive progressive balance exercises combined with strengthening exercises can achieve similar effects in isolation or when combined with occupational therapy (Ilg et al 2014, Miyai et al 2012, Synofzik & Ilg 2014, Velázquez-Pérez et al 2019). The exercises used in these trials have factors in common such as an emphasis on static and dynamic balance often under different sensory conditions, whole-body movements, strategies to prevent falling and movements to treat or prevent contracture. Training is progressive, challenging and intensive (between 1 and 11 hours per week for 4–8 weeks). Improvements have been observed in fundamental deficits, such as interjoint coordination while walking (Ilg et al 2007), suggesting that these changes may reflect real improvements in how the cerebellum is controlling movement, rather than the development of a compensatory strategy. Noncontrolled trials and case studies suggest that exoskeletons may also provide a high intensity practice of walking that could lead to improvements in spatiotemporal gait parameters and clinical rating scales (Kim et al 2021, Matsushima et al 2021).

Deficits are seen in the sensory control of balance with cerebellar disease. In people with SCA6, balance was particularly worse when viewing moving visual stimuli (Bunn et al 2015b). Improvements in balance have been found with home-based exercises that retrained standing balance in the presence of moving visual stimuli (Bunn et al 2015a). Given the high incidence of falls with the hereditary ataxias (Fonteyn et al 2010, 2013), it is also important to address intrinsic and extrinsic factors that may contribute to falling.

With disease progression, compensation may be required to maintain mobility. Initially light touch support may be sufficient, for example, using Nordic walking poles. Walking frames, with or without additional weighting, may prove useful (Bonney et al 2016, Marsden & Harris 2011). With disease progression, mobility may be maintained with the use of a wheelchair. In people with gross truncal and upper limb ataxia exacerbated by head titubation, specialised seating may be required. Specialist seating improves posture and support (Clark et al 2004). The aim of improved postural control may be to also improve upper limb function, respiratory function and dysarthria, although this was not observed in a case series of people with FRDA (Clark et al 2004).

Consideration needs to be given to psychological and cognitive issues. The incoordination and dysarthria associated with cerebellar disease can be mistaken for the person being drunk with alcohol. Being accused or assumed to be drunk is a common report in people with ataxia and can greatly stigmatise people and limit their participation in the community (Cassidy et al 2011, 2018). This may limit people's desire to access public places (e.g., gyms). Damage to the cerebellum may also result in a cerebellar cognitive affective syndrome. Cognitive issues such as poor visuospatial memory, working memory and executive dysfunction may influence factors such as the ability to plan and instigate new strategies (e.g., fatigue management) or remember instructions (Moriarty et al 2016, Schmahmann & Sherman 1998).

Rehabilitation studies of balance and walking to date suggest that improvements are seen with intensive treatments of at least 3–12 hours per week for 4 weeks (Ilg et al 2014). Lower intensities of training (e.g., six sessions) do not seem to be effective (Daker-White et al 2013). It is suggested that continuous therapy is required; effects of training are lost within 6 months of nonactivity (Miyai et al 2012). One hour per day of home-based therapy seems to result in a partial slowing down of clinical progression (Ilg et al 2010). Recently, case studies ($n = 4$) suggest that focused episodes of therapy can have similar effects to an initial burst of treatment, and recommendations of one to two 'bursts' per year may be helpful (Ilg et al 2014) (Fig. 12.4). The importance of exercise intensity and regularity clearly highlights the need for people with hereditary ataxias to adopt changes in behaviour and ideally make exercise and physical activity a habit which is part of everyday living. This requires people with hereditary ataxias working with therapists and exercise professionals to learn about and explore appropriate physical activities and understand people's attitudes to and expectations of physical activity and associated social and environmental factors that may limit participation and long-term adoption of physical activity programmes (Daker-White et al 2013). The aim is to work in partnership to develop patient-centred, personalised self-managed programmes that may require intermittent review and bursts of more intensive training (Martin et al 2010).

HEREDITARY SPASTIC PARESIS

Epidemiology and Genetics

HSP has a prevalence of 4–6 per 100,000 (Salinas et al 2008). The age of onset can vary from childhood to late adult life (up to 70 years) (Noreau et al 2014). It is a heterogeneous genetic condition with autosomal dominant (70% of cases), autosomal recessive, X-linked and maternal mitochondrial

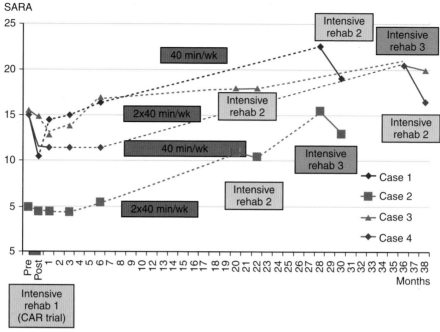

FIG. 12.4 Effect of bursts of treatment on disease progression as measured by the scale for the assessment and rating of ataxia (SARA) in four cases. The first intervention resulted in a 2.5-point improvement on the SARA on average. After an average of 26 weeks, the SARA worsened by 7.6 points and a burst of therapy resulted in a 2.0-point improvement. Solid lines represent intervention periods of intensive rehabilitation. Dotted lines represent follow-up periods with home-based rehabilitation of 40–80 minutes per week. Note the progression of symptoms during the home therapy periods. (Reproduced with permission. Ilg, W. et al. 2014. Consensus paper: management of degenerative cerebellar disorders. Cerebellum. 13, 248–268.)

inheritance described. The most common type, SPAST (SPG4 gene that codes for the spastin protein) is autosomal dominant and occurs in 40%–45% of cases. Spontaneous mutations are common (Brugman et al 2005, McMonagle et al 2002). In SPG4, for example, spontaneous mutations can be seen in 13% of cases, meaning these people will not have a family history of the condition. Although there are many gene loci that can result in HSP (>50), not all are routinely tested, resulting in between 45% and 82% of people having no specific genetic diagnosis even after systematic testing (Ruano et al 2014).

Anatomy, Pathophysiology and Clinical Presentation

There are two main presentations of HSP (Harding 1983): type I and type II. The type I or 'uncomplicated' presentation is seen in most cases of autosomal dominant HSP. It is characterised by lower limb spasticity, hyperreflexia, paresis and a positive (upgoing) Babinski response often with

additional symptoms of urinary urgency and impaired vibration thresholds. Pes cavus is also clinically described. The type II, or 'complicated', presentation features are often seen with autosomal recessive cases. It is characterised by the signs seen in type I with the addition of other signs, such as (Salinas et al 2008):

- Cerebellar ataxia and signs;
- Dementia and cognitive deficits (associated with thinning of the corpus callosum);
- Amyotrophy;
- Peripheral neuropathy;
- Cataracts or pigmentary retinopathy; and
- Dry, itchy skin (ichthyosis).

HSP is caused by a dying-back axonal degeneration; the longer tracts that supply the lower limbs are affected first, with shorter tracts supplying arms being affected later (DeLuca et al 2004). The earlier onset of symptoms in the feet may explain why, like FRDA, pes cavus is often described. The cause of the axonal degeneration varies depending on the gene affected and type of HSP. Many causes of HSP affect axonal transport within the neurone (Noreau et al 2014). Axonal transport is responsible for the movement of organelles and substances such as mitochondria, lipids and synaptic proteins to and from the cell body. Axonal transport occurs along microtubule 'tracts' within the neurone. Motor proteins attach to these tracts to move substances up and down the neurone. HSP can, for example, affect the motor proteins and microtubule processing (Noreau et al 2014), altering axonal transport leading to neuronal degeneration.

The neuronal tracts affected in HSP include the corticospinal tracts. Structural magnetic resonance imaging is usually normal, although thinning of the spinal cord at the cervical and thoracic level has been reported (Duning et al 2010). White matter changes affecting the internal capsule are evident on diffusor tensor imaging scans, and these predict disease duration and severity (Lindig et al 2015). The responses to transcranial magnetic stimulation of the leg area of the motor cortex are reduced and/or prolonged with preserved responses to stimulation of the arm area (Cruz Martinez & Tejada 1999, Ginanneschi et al 2014, Schady et al 1991, Sue et al 1997). Degeneration of the fasciculus gracilis of the dorsal columns carrying somatosensory information from the lower limbs and the spinocerebellar tracts can also occur (Sartucci et al 2007, Scuderi et al 2009). Vibration sense is affected in ~40%–60% of patients (Bruyn et al 1994).

Diagnosis

The diagnosis of HSP requires the detection of clinical symptoms of progressive lower limb weakness and spasticity affecting walking often with urinary symptoms and impaired vibration sense (Fink 2000, 2003, 2013). A family history can be present but, because of the large number of spontaneous mutations, this is not always the case. Further, genetic tests are not always positive (Ruano et al 2014). It is therefore important to exclude other conditions that may have a similar presentation. Differential diagnoses by neurologists include structural abnormalities (e.g., spinal cord compression), other myelopathies (e.g., amyotrophic lateral sclerosis), leukodystrophies (e.g., multiple sclerosis), SCAs (e.g., SCA3), infection (e.g., tropical spastic paraplegia), early-onset dementia, dopa-responsive dystonia and metabolic disorders (e.g., phenylketonuria) (Fink 2000).

Medical Management
Antispasticity Medication

Uncontrolled studies of botulinum toxin injections into proximal and distal lower limb muscles result in a reduction in muscle tone. Changes in function are more variable.

Changes in walking velocity have been seen, but minimal or no global subjective effect has been reported in ~30% and increased weakness noted in ~15% (Geva-Dayan et al 2010, Hecht et al 2008, Rousseaux et al 2007). Obturator nerve blocks have also been used to decrease adductor tone and scissoring of the legs while walking. Although assessed in other conditions (e.g., stroke or cerebral palsy) (Viel et al 2002), the effects have not been formally evaluated in people with HSP. Clinically adductor tone can decrease after an obturator nerve block, but some people may find activities such as lifting the legs to climb the stairs more difficult because the secondary role of the hip adductors in flexing the hip is affected.

There have been no trials of oral baclofen (a Gamma aminobutyric acid [GABA] agonist) and tizanidine in HSP, although clinical opinion suggests that they can be associated with widespread fatigue and improve spasticity and function in only a limited number of people (Hecht et al 2008, Rousseaux et al 2007). A crossover trial of gabapentin (a GABA agonist) showed no effect on tone or walking (Scheuer et al 2007).

Intrathecal baclofen (ITB) has the advantage of reducing side effects such as weakness and fatigue. It has been implanted in children and adults with HSP (Pointon et al 2022, Pucks-Faes et al 2019). ITB given as a bolus (as part of the trial for ITB) or continuous infusion has led to improvements in walking speed and kinematics, although the studies lacked a control group. Satisfaction with the effects of ITB is higher in people in whom the implant occurs while they are still ambulant (Dan & Cheron 2000, Dan et al 2000, Klebe et al 2005, Meythaler et al 1992, Molteni et al 2005). A retrospective review of ITB suggests that spasticity improves for 2–3 years postimplantation followed by a 4- to 5-year stable phase. However, functional improvements in walking and ADLs are less marked (Pointon et al 2022, Pucks-Faes et al 2019). Bladder function has also been reported to improve with ITB (Saltuari et al 1992).

Physiotherapy Assessment

People with HSP will often have increased tone. Experimental studies suggest that this can be caused by changes in passive stiffness, possibly caused by changes in the amount of connective tissue and/or shortening of muscle fibres, as well as enhanced spasticity (enhanced stretch reflexes) (Marsden et al 2012). Increased tone is accompanied by muscle weakness that in particular affects the ankle dorsiflexors and hip abductors (Klebe et al 2004). The increased passive stiffness and weakness can contribute to changes in walking kinematics, such as a stiff knee gait, ankle equinus, a trendelenburg gait or excessive lateral trunk flexion (Bickley et al 2021, van Vugt et al 2019). It should therefore not be assumed that spasticity is the main cause of walking deficits. Hyperextension of the knee when walking, for example, may be associated with spasticity in the ankle plantarflexors and an increase in plantarflexion/knee extension coupling, but also with weakness in the knee extensors (Cimolin et al 2007, Piccinini et al 2011). The finding that walking can deteriorate after pharmacological treatment of spasticity suggests that it may in some cases aid with standing stability (Marsden & Stevenson 2013). Muscle contracture affecting the two joint muscles of the leg but particularly the hip flexors and ankle plantarflexors is observed clinically. Muscle weakness and hip flexor contracture can lead to an increased lumbar lordosis in standing and when walking. Walking is often associated with low back pain. This may reflect the increased lordosis and the increased trunk and pelvic movement that are associated with walking because people compensate proximally for weak and stiff legs to maintain progression and balance (Serrao et al 2016). Falls rates are high with 61.3% of cases reporting a fall in the previous 3 months in a retrospective survey (Chapman & Marsden, unpublished observations). Falls frequently result in people being unable to get up from the floor independently, and the causes of falls such as trips or loss of balance should be explored in more detail.

In the complicated presentations people will have additional symptoms that can affect function and thus the management approach. Cerebellar dysfunction may be seen (e.g., in SPG7) that clinically can affect balance and is potentially amenable to balance retraining. Peripheral neuropathy may limit the effect of adjuncts to therapy such as functional electrical stimulation. Mild cognitive decline and dementia can also affect the ability to remember information, and people may require more time to properly encode information.

Disease-Specific Scales

The Spastic Paraplegia Rating Scale (SPRS) is a 13-item scale that measures symptoms (spasticity, weakness) seen in type I HSP. There is an inventory to record the presence of additional symptoms seen in complicated, type II presentations (Schule et al 2006). It takes less than 15 minutes to complete and is reliable. Disease severity predicts the effect on quality of life measures, and lower quality of life is seen in people with type II, complicated presentations (Klimpe et al 2012).

Time Course and Corresponding Management

Prospective cohort studies monitoring disease progression over time using the SPRS suggest that earlier onset of the disease is associated with less severe progression. Later onset, type II complicated presentation and the SPG11 genotype are associated with more severe disease progression. People are able to walk for a median of 22 years after

symptom onset (Schule et al 2016). Earlier onset presentations are less likely to become wheelchair dependent, reflecting differences in disease progression rate with age of symptom onset.

Treatment approaches may vary over the time course of the disease. Initially emphasis should be on maintaining mobility, balance and aerobic capacity. With disease progression, management of symptoms such as spasticity, urinary dysfunction and impaired balance may need to be addressed alongside falls prevention strategies. Although self-management should be encouraged, professional input may be required at times of transition, for example, ongoing from paediatric into adult services, or after an illness or reduction in mobility. People with HSP report that it can be difficult to regain fitness lost during these periods.

As mobility decreases, consideration of ways of maintaining mobility and participation is required. Elbow crutches with flexible ferrules can aid balance. With time, increased fatigue and effort of walking requires increased use of wheelchairs and/or mobility scooters. By reducing fatigue and improving mobility, these can directly lead to better participation. Therefore these can be used alongside walking aids as a means of fatigue management. Consideration also needs to be given to partners and family members throughout the disease course. Increased time needed to prepare to go out, as well as reduced mobility, can directly affect the partner's participation and quality of life. Low back pain and reductions in fitness have been reported by partners/family members of people with HSP (Grose et al 2014).

Treatment Selection, Secondary Complications and Special Problems

Management should be goal oriented and encourage increased participation. Focus groups with people with HSP highlight that people find benefit with programmes that encourage increased activity (Grose et al 2014), although there are no current trials to support this. People have reported benefit with exercises that incorporate progressive lower limb stretches, strengthening exercise and aerobic activity (Richardson & Thompson 1999). Initially in-shoe orthotics may accommodate pes cavus, but with time, these may need to be combined with heel raises as the ankle plantarflexor muscles become contracted. Bilateral functional electrical stimulation of the common peroneal nerve to address foot drop may improve walking speed and subjectively reduces tripping (Marsden et al 2013). Other stimulation parameters, such as targeting proximal muscles (hip abductors and trunk side flexors) to reduce trunk motion while walking, have been described (Marsden et al 2013). However, issues such as prolonged time to don and doff the device should be considered, and some people prefer more rigid ankle foot orthoses, especially as the disease progresses. In cases where there is knee hyperextension during stance phase of gait, an assessment needs to be made whether this is associated with plantarflexor hypertonia or knee extensor weakness. In the latter case, rigid ankle–foot orthoses could worsen knee stability (Cimolin et al 2007, Piccinini et al 2011).

The management of fatigue is an important consideration. Walking is described as effortful and attention demanding with cognitive fatigue potentially affecting walking ability as much as physical fatigue. Therefore consideration needs to be made of fatigue management principles of pacing and planning the day. People with HSP report that their legs feel stiffer and that their walking is slower in cold weather. Directly cooling the legs increases spasticity and reduces nerve conduction velocity, muscle strength and power (Denton et al 2016). The reverse is seen when warming the legs. This suggests that insulation in cold weather may be useful.

HSP, along with the other conditions described in this chapter, are rarely experienced, and knowledge of the condition with general practitioners and allied health professionals can frequently be limited (Fjermestad et al 2020). This often leads to delays in diagnosis and results in people with the condition travelling long distances to seek specialist help from regional centres, which can be tiring and expensive (Grose et al 2014). In the future, uptake of telehealth may minimise the burden, especially for people in more remote communities. People with HSP benefit from the support and understanding offered by support group meetings, and therapists should direct people to these wherever possible (Grose et al 2014).

SUMMARY

Inherited, progressive central neurological conditions present with particular challenges. The conditions are rare and so can be infrequently seen by clinicians. They are often heterogeneous in their presentation even for people with the sample general disease classification (e.g., SCA) or having the same genetic deficit (e.g., HD). Because they are progressive, the symptoms seen vary across the disease course, and this in turn affects the management strategy. Because of the availability of genetic testing, there may be a period when the genetic mutation is known but there are no overt symptoms. Importantly, healthcare professionals who are involved in diagnosis, treatment, research and long-term follow-up of families of individuals living with inherited neurological conditions may encounter a wide range of ethical dilemmas. Sincere efforts must be made to implement principles of bioethics – respect for autonomy, beneficence, non-maleficence and justice – into the professional relationship.

Ethical considerations may extend to discussions surrounding genetic testing (e.g., diagnostic, carrier, predictive/presymptomatic, prenatal, preimplantation) and confidentiality and truth telling (Baum & Domaradzki 2018, Pierron et al 2021).

Understanding the ramifications of knowledge of gene status is a delicate process and should be supported by an expert multidisciplinary team, striving to eliminate any judgmental views (McCusker & Loy 2017). For those who take the leap into genetic testing, expert teams should have an in-depth understanding of the moral dilemmas faced by carriers and by noncarriers (Eno et al 2020, Erez et al 2010, Hakimian 2000, Keenan et al 2009, Winnberg et al 2018). Healthcare professionals may also be asked prognostic questions such as: Will I be disabled? Will I lose my cognitive abilities? How long will I be able to work? Alongside questions such as: Will my children be affected? Are there new medications or research trials aiming to prevent the disease? From an ethical point of view, those who ask questions are aware, curious and knowledgeable or would like to be informed. In these cases, healthcare providers should carefully word the answers whilst ensuring that they are delivering accurate information (Anestis et al 2021). Other patients or family members might wish to avoid information being provided to them, in the form of denial, minimisation, reluctance, repression or withdrawal (Mahmood et al 2022). From the perspective of person-centred care, tailored support should be crafted to enhance beneficence by meeting needs, discussing viewpoints and promoting wellness. Because there is a thin and fragile line between truth telling, preservation of hope and false hope, healthcare teams should expand their knowledge of the ethical and legal aspects in providing ongoing information about the relevant inherited condition. Health professionals should strive to expand their understanding of ethical issues and cultivate ethical sensitivity (e.g., the ability to identify ethical dilemmas) to ensure that they are able to implement ethical reasoning into daily professional decision making (de Snoo-Trimp et al 2020, Jones-Bonofiglio 2020, Koskenvuori et al 2019). It is also important to acknowledge the important role of family, friends and carers in these long-term conditions and the effect that this may also have on their health and well-being.

Although there are clear overarching commonalities across inherited progressive neurological conditions, there are also differences. The promotion of self-management approaches is a cornerstone across all conditions. The therapist should understand the factors that may affect the development and engagement in a self-management programme including an understanding of the rationale for interventions, people's attitudes and expectations of an intervention and limiting social and environmental factors. To support this, interventions should be goal directed and personalised. Interventions should be appropriate for the point on the disease course trajectory, at first concentrating on prevention of functional decline. Later, maintenance of function using compensatory strategies, aids and adaptations is indicated before entering into an end-of-life and palliative care stage. The similarities and differences as well as potential treatment approaches are summarised in Tables 12.3 and Table 12.4.

CASE STUDY

Condition Overview

This case discusses an individual in the late stage of HD. Patients in this stage show minimal volitional control of limbs and often present with a predominance of rigidity rather than chorea. Passive range of motion is limited, and contractures may be present. Ambulation is limited or even

TABLE 12.3   Summary of the Main Inherited Neurological Conditions Covered in this Chapter

Condition	Cause and Main Locus of Pathology	Prevalence/ Age of Onset	Presentation	Medical Management
Huntington's disease	AD Neurodegeneration in the striatum (caudate and putamen) with additional pathology in cerebral cortex	Prevalence: 12/100,000 Onset: 20–75 years, commonly 35–55 years	Motor: chorea and later dystonia, bradykinesia and rigidity, oculomotor dysfunction leading to deficits in upper limb control, balance, gait, falls and respiratory failure Cognitive: executive dysfunction Behavioural: apathy, irritability, depression	Genetic counselling Symptomatic medical management of chorea (Tetrabenazine, Olanzapine, risperidone, Tiapride, Pimozide, Sulpiride and Aripiprazole); Botulinum toxin in presence of focal dystonias; Levodopa for partial and temporary relief of the akinetic–rigid symptoms of HD (especially in juvenile forms); antidepressants; SSRIs for irritability, aggression and anxiety; Neuroleptics for hallucinations.
Hereditary spastic paraparesis	Heterogeneous: can be AD, AR, X-linked or mitochondrial; many gene loci; 40%–45% AD Type I: mainly dying-back axonal degeneration of the corticospinal tract Type II: additional pathology such as cerebellar degeneration, myopathy, neuropathy can be seen	Prevalence: 4–6 per 100,000 Onset: childhood to 70 years	Motor: mainly affects legs; spasticity, paresis, extensor plantar response, 60% reduced vibration sensation, contracture and changes in passive stiffness Additional signs in type II presentation (e.g., weakness, sensory loss caused by myopathy/ neuropathy and cerebellar signs)	Genetic counselling Symptomatic management of spasticity (e.g., oral and intrathecal antispasticity medication, focal botulinum toxin injections)

TABLE 12.3 Summary of the Main Inherited Neurological Conditions Covered in this Chapter — Cont'd

Condition	Cause and Main Locus of Pathology	Prevalence/ Age of Onset	Presentation	Medical Management
Friedreich's ataxia	AR: chromosome 9q13 Degeneration of the dorsal columns, spinocerebellar tracts, dentate nucleus (cerebellum), corticospinal tract	Prevalence: 2–5 per 100,000 Onset: 5–15 years	Motor: distal sensory loss (vibration sense, proprioception); paresis, extensor plantar responses Kyphoscoliosis Pes cavus/equinovarus Cardiomyopathy	Genetic counselling Coenzyme Q and idebenone Orthotic bracing and surgical bracing (>40° curves) Electrocardiogram monitoring if left ventricular hypertrophy (angiotensin-converting enzyme inhibitors; diuretics and β-blockers for atrial arrhythmias)
SCA	AD many gene loci Type I: cerebellar degeneration with additional signs (e.g., extrapyramidal) Type II: cerebellar ataxia with pigmentary macular degeneration Type III: relatively pure cerebellar degeneration	Prevalence: 2–5.6/100,000 Onset: mean 35 years (±11)	Motor: cerebellar signs: limb dyssynergia, dysmetria, tremor (postural and action), oculomotor deficits, impaired balance and gait, dysarthria and dysphagia Cognitive affective cerebellar syndrome Nonataxia symptoms seen in 50% of cases	Genetic counselling Symptomatic management of non-ataxia signs (e.g., rigidity, spasticity) Limited pharmacological management (e.g., β-blockers for tremor; potassium channel blockers in SCA6)

AD, Autosomal dominant; *AR*, autosomal recessive; *HD*, Huntington's disease; *SCA*, spinocerebellar ataxia.

TABLE 12.4 Summary of Nonpharmacological Treatment Approaches and Considerations for the Main Inherited Neurological Conditions Covered in this Chapter

Condition	Treatment Approaches	Considerations
Generally	Aerobic training Balance and mobility reeducation, balance and reduction of falls risk Maintain joint range of movement with disease progression Mobility aids and use of wheelchair to help with fatigue management and mobility Upper limb aids and adaptations to maintain function	Patient goals and incorporating self-management into everyday life Link into support groups Carer support and management of associated musculoskeletal problems Treatment emphasis varies with stage of disease

(Continued)

TABLE 12.4   Summary of Nonpharmacological Treatment Approaches and Considerations for the Main Inherited Neurological Conditions Covered in this Chapter —Cont'd

Condition	Treatment Approaches	Considerations
Huntington's disease	Aerobic training (e.g., increasing walking distance) Balance and mobility reeducation, balance and reduction of falls risk Breathing exercise	Effect of cognitive and behavioural symptoms Develop individualised patient-centred goals to improve ability to perform functional tasks, maximise safety and aid with sequencing difficulties
Hereditary spastic paraparesis	Progressive resisted exercises Stretches FES for foot drop Mobility aids and wheelchair provision	Effect of antispasticity medication of walking and balance in the presence of paresis Effect of additional symptoms (e.g., cerebellar dysfunction or neuropathy if trialling FES) Associated musculoskeletal problems (e.g., low-back pain)
Ataxia (FRDA and spinocerebellar)	Balance and mobility retraining including varying the sensory inputs available (e.g., moving visual stimuli) Aerobic training Stretches Bracing for kyphoscoliosis in FRDA Orthoses for pes cavus in FRDA Mobility aids and postural support Weights and viscous resistance (e.g., Lycra garments) to reduce tremor Computer modifications Adaptations to aid upper limb function (e.g., dressing)	Cardiomyopathy symptoms in FRDA to commencing hydrotherapy and aerobic exercise Effect of additional cognitive and affective signs with cerebellar degeneration Training intensity and use of exergaming to aid motivation Fatigue management Psychological effect of disease presentation Rate of improvement with cerebellar disease may be slower than in other conditions because of its role in motor learning and recovery

FES, Functional electrical stimulation; *FRDA,* Friedreich's ataxia.

impossible, and maintaining a sitting position is often difficult. As a result, there is a considerable risk for aspiration or respiratory infections, pressure sores, and/or contractures. Patients may exhibit difficulty with communication or may be unable to vocalise at all.

The general aim in this stage is to maintain the patient's quality of life. This includes minimising the risks for aspiration, bed sores and contractures; facilitating an upright sitting position; maintaining overall range of motion; and promoting participation in activities of daily living as much as the patient is able. Because patients are often dependent on caregivers or nursing staff, it is of utmost importance to maintain regular support and to closely coordinate care.

Because the possibilities to walk, stand and sit decrease during this stage, it is important to customise walking aids, wheelchairs, mattresses and cushioning on a regular basis. Normally patients are dependent on a high amount of medication to reduce pain, rigidity, spasticity and/or infections. Table 12.5 provides a summary of the problems, specific physiotherapy goals and treatment plan.

Classification

Dr H is a 74-year-old man with HD diagnosed 18 years ago. Over time there has been a slow but steady deterioration of his general condition.

Examination

History

The patient lives in a two-storey home with his wife, who is his primary caregiver. She is worried about the deterioration of his range of motion and ability to ambulate, as well as how she can maintain his remaining activities of daily life at home. He is fully dependent on his wife for all daily care needs. A chair lift was installed in their house for mobility between the first and second floors. There are no stairs to enter the house. She regularly takes him to meetings with his former colleagues, as he had to quit his job as a surgeon when he was diagnosed.

Dr H's medical history is insignificant, except for regular injections of Botox every 3–4 months in bilateral biceps brachii, hamstrings and hip adductor muscles.

TABLE 12.5 Problem List, Goals and Treatment Plan for the Case Study

Problem List	Goals	Plan
Reduced sitting and standing balance	To independently sit for approximately 1 minute, so his wife has her hands free for a short time To stand with moderate assistance for 30 seconds	Task-specific training in sitting Sit to stand practice Progressive standing training
Severe rigidity in limbs leading to limitations in ROM	To maintain/improve passive and active ROM: hands, extension of the elbow joint, extension of the hip and knee joints	Passive and active ROM: hands, extension of the elbow joint, extension of the hip and knee joints Close collaboration with the neurologist regarding the injections of Botox and subsequent management plan Focused on positioning and ROM
Requires moderate assistance for bed mobility Requires maximal assistance for transfers Requires moderate assistance for walking 10 m	To perform bed mobility with minimal assistance to decrease caregiver burden To perform transfers with moderate assistance and verbal cues	Bed mobility and transfer training for Dr H and his wife to focus on incorporating his available active movements
Limited diaphragmatic breathing resulting in several respiratory infections	To improve diaphragmatic breathing and productive cough for airway clearance	Practice diaphragmatic breathing exercises Posture management in sitting and in bed to promote effective cough techniques
Minor red spots on buttocks; intact skin but at risk for development of pressure sores	To minimise risk for pressure sores on buttocks	Positioning schedule for bed and upright positioning to minimise risk for pressure sores Refer for seating assessment (review current wheelchair and pressure-relieving provision)

ROM, Range of motion.

Body Structures and Function

Details relating to impairment of body structures and function of relevance are described below.

Balance: Dr H is unable to walk, stand or sit without support. The patient is able to sit with the help of his wife. (See later for level of assistance for functional activities.)

Posture: He only stands when pulled forwards, but otherwise shows strong retropulsion. He only walks when pulled forwards, supported by verbal cues. The physiotherapist observes severe bradykinesia and rigidity.

Respiratory function: Dr H's diaphragmatic breathing is very limited; upper chest breathing is noted. Several respiratory infections over the past year were reported by his wife.

Skin integrity: Per wife, he has minor red spots and pressure sores on his buttocks; skin is intact.

Pain: Dr H shows pain when his left hand is moved into wrist flexion or extension. Although he cannot articulate the pain, he moans or screams.

Sensation: Sensation is not testable.

Reflexes: Negative for ankle clonus. Reflexes not testable.

Range of motion: The patient shows no chorea, but exhibits spasticity, rigidity and beginning contractures in every joint. Dr H has severe limitations of both shoulders, elbows, wrists and finger joints. His hands are clenched into fists, except when sleeping. He also has severe limitations on both lower extremities, especially in his hip and knee joints.

Involuntary movement: The physiotherapist notes strong dystonia in the face and strongly limited mouth opening.

Cognition: Dr H seems to understand and react to simple commands. He can perform transfers with minimal help but is still unable to move voluntarily without cue. He remembers his family members and friends, as evidenced by his facial expressions.

Activities

The Extended Barthel Index score is 16/64. Dr H can walk 10 m with moderate support by one person. He is unable to sit unsupported, as he frequently slides down in his chair, requiring repositioning. He sits with support but maintains a forwards flexed position. The patient requires moderate assistance for bed mobility and maximal assistance for transfers with verbal cueing. He has used a manual wheelchair (pushed by wife) with pressure-relieving cushion for primary means of mobility over the past 4 years. Dr H can still chew and swallow, but his wife has to feed him.

Prognosis

Dr H is in the late stage of HD and even though his wife assists him in moving quite regularly, he presents with a high risk for contractures, pressure sores and aspiration because of his decreased postural stability and decreased ability to chew properly. Frequent examination of range of motion, trunk control and ability to stand is necessary, as is referral to a speech therapist. Physiotherapist palliative care intervention can help to mitigate the risk for falls, respiratory infections and contractures through education and training.

Intervention

Dr H attended 45-minute physiotherapy sessions once per week to maintain current abilities and prevent further loss of range of motion and mobility. The physiotherapist instructed his wife on how to achieve or improve his mobility at home. Regular meetings and discussions with his wife were conducted, as well as close collaboration with the neurologist regarding the injections of Botox. The physiotherapist actively involved the patient in treatment (e.g., by moving active-assistive activities in sitting, practicing the sit-to-stand transition).

The intervention included the following mutually agreed goals:

- Bed mobility and transfer training for Dr H and his wife to focus on incorporating his available active movements;
- Passive and active range of motion: hands, extension of the elbow joint, extension of the hip and knee joints;
- Improve the ability to sit: allowing independent sitting for approximately 1 minute, so his wife has her hands free for a short time; and
- Standing and walking training: 10 m walking with support daily; instructing wife in proper guarding and assistance techniques.

Outcomes (8 months)

Dr H's mobility and walking capability stayed consistent. He experienced no falls, respiratory infections, or contractures.

The patient demonstrated improved transfer capability:

- Sit-to-stand transition (including wheelchair to bed and reverse): Dr H can transition with moderate assistance of one person. With a minimal assist, the patient lowers his feet independently; with verbal cueing, he brings the upper body forwards independently; he attempts to rise to stand but still falls backwards.
- Sitting position to supine in bed: self-initiated movement but cannot control movement to supine because of absent trunk control.
- Bed mobility: Dr H turns right and left with minimal assistance and tactile inputs.

During therapy, the left hand can be opened without signs of pain. He can sit for 10 minutes with slight tactile inputs. Dr H can stand for 15 minutes with minimal assistance of one person or at a standing table.

This case study was reprinted from PTNow (http://www.ptnow.org), with permission of the American Physical Therapy Association. © 2016 American Physical Therapy Association.

SELF-ASSESSMENT QUESTIONS

Huntington's Disease

1. HD is an autosomal dominant disease which leads to a triad of symptoms. Aside from the most usual feature of an involuntary movement disorder, describe the impact that the other impairments may have on treatment planning and implementation.
2. People with HD are at risk for falling. Given the nature of the disease and the risks of inactivity, consider appropriate physiotherapy strategies and implications of this for the wider care team.
3. What is the role of the physiotherapist in people with premanifest HD, or in the very early stages of manifest HD?
4. Summarise the evidence in support of exercise as a physiotherapy intervention in people with HD.
5. Cognitive and behavioural impairments are common in people with HD. Describe three common impairments and discuss how a physiotherapist might consider these when planning an intervention.

Hereditary Ataxia

1. Describe the symptoms seen in a cognitive affective syndrome? How may these symptoms influence physiotherapy management?

2. Describe the evidence base for the management of balance in people with adult- and child-onset hereditary ataxia. What are the potential advantages of exergaming-based therapies?

3. Describe the oculomotor impairments seen in hereditary cerebellar ataxias and how these affect upper and lower limb functional movements.

4. Describe three strategies that could aid computer use and writing in people with hereditary ataxia.

5. How may the symptoms of cardiomyopathy in FRDA modify your treatment approach?

Hereditary Spastic Paraparesis

1. What are the key determinants of walking ability in people with type I, uncomplicated HSP?

2. Name three additional symptoms that may be seen in type II, complicated presentations.

3. How may functional electrical stimulation be used to aid walking ability in people with HSP? How may additional symptoms seen in complicated forms of HSP affect symptom management?

4. What service delivery issues may people with rare hereditary neurological conditions encounter? How may this vary geographically?

ACKNOWLEDGEMENT

We would like to acknowledge the European Huntington's Disease Network, the Huntington Study Group and Griffin Foundation for their support of the new clinical recommendations to guide physical therapy practice for Huntington's disease endorsed by the American Academy of Neurology and published in *Neurology* in 2020.

REFERENCES

Afonso Ribeiro, J., Simeoni, S., De Min, L., et al., 2021. Lower urinary tract and bowel dysfunction in spinocerebellar ataxias. Ann. Clin. Transl. Neurol. 8, 321–331.

Albin, R.L., Young, A.B., Penney, J.B., 1989. The functional anatomy of basal ganglia disorders. Trends. Neurosci. 12, 366–376.

Anestis, E., Eccles, F.J., Fletcher, I., Triliva, S., Simpson, J., 2021. Healthcare professionals' involvement in breaking bad news to newly diagnosed patients with motor neurodegenerative conditions: a qualitative study. Disabil. Rehabil. 1–14.

Alves, T.C., et al., 2016. Swallowing endoscopy findings in Huntington's disease: a case report. CoDAS 28, 486–488.

Avanzini, G., et al., 1979. Oculomotor disorders in Huntington's chorea. J. Neurol. Neurosurg. Psychiatry. 42, 581–589.

Bachoud-Lévi, A.-C., 2017. Neural grafts in Huntington's disease: viability after 10 years. Lancet. Neurol. 8, 979–981.

Bachoud-Levi, A., Ferreira, J., Massart, R., et al., 2019. International guidelines for the treatment of Huntington's disease. Front. Neurol. 10, 710.

Baig, S.S., Strong, M., Quarrell, O.W., 2016. The global prevalence of Huntington's disease: a systematic review and discussion. Neurodegen. Dis. Manag. 6, 331–343.

Barker, R.A., et al., 2013. The long-term safety and efficacy of bilateral transplantation of human fetal striatal tissue in patients with mild to moderate Huntington's disease. J. Neurol. Neurosurg. Psychiatry. 84, 657–665.

Bastian, A.J., 2008. Understanding sensorimotor adaptation and learning for rehabilitation. Curr. Opin. Neurol. 21, 628–633.

Baum, E., Domaradzki, J., 2018. Chapter 13: Geneticization and bioethics: ethical dilemmas in genetic counselling. In: Soniewicka, M. (Ed.). In: The Ethics of Reproductive Genetics. Philosophy and Medicine, vol 128. Springer, Cham.

Ben-Nagi, J., et al., 2016. Preimplantation genetic diagnosis: an overview and recent advances. Obstet. Gynaecol. 18, 99–106.

Benussi, A., Cantoni, V., Manes, M., et al., 2021. Motor and cognitive outcomes of cerebello-spinal stimulation in neurodegenerative ataxia. Brain 144, 2310–2321.

Berk, C., et al., 2002. Thalamic deep brain stimulation for the treatment of tremor due to multiple sclerosis: a prospective study of tremor and quality of life. J. Neurosurg. 97, 815–820.

Bettencourt, C., Lima, M., 2011. Machado-Joseph disease: from first descriptions to new perspectives. Orphanet. J. Rare. Dis. 6, 35.

Bhidayasiri, R., et al., 2005. Late-onset Friedreich ataxia: phenotypic analysis, magnetic resonance imaging. Arch. Neurol. 62, 1865–1869.

Bickley, C., Mitchell, K., Scott, A., Bury, M., Oyelami, M., 2021. Familiarity with hereditary spastic paraplegia (HSP) and differentiation of upper body gait characteristics between children with HSP and spastic diplegic cerebral palsy. Phys. Occup. Ther. Pediatr. 41, 99–113.

Blancato, J.K., Wolfe, E., Sacks, P.C., 2017. Preimplantation genetics and other reproductive options in Huntington disease. Handbook. Clin. Neurol. 144, 107–111.

Bonney, H., et al., 2016. Management of the ataxias towards best clinical practice, 3rd ed. Available at: https://pure.strath.ac.uk/ws/portalfiles/portal/54224679/Ataxia_UK_2016_Management_of_the_ataxias_towards_best_clinical.pdf. Accessed 5 June 2023.

Bouchghoul, H., et al., 2016. Prenatal testing in Huntington disease: after the test, choices recommence. Eur. J. Hum. Genet. 24, 1535–1540.

Brooker, S.M., Edamakanti, C.R., Akasha, S.M., Kuo, S.H., Opal, P., 2021. Spinocerebellar ataxia clinical trials: opportunities and challenges. Ann. Clin. Transl. Neurol. 8, 1543–1556.

Brugman, F., et al., 2005. Spastin mutations in sporadic adult-onset upper motor neuron syndromes. Ann. Neurol. 58, 865–869.

Bruyn, R.P.M., et al., 1994. Clinically silent dysfunction of dorsal columns and dorsal spinocerebellar tracts in hereditary spastic paraparesis. J. Neurol. Sci. 125, 206–211.

Bunn, L.M., Marsden, J.F., Giunti, P., et al., 2015a. Training balance with opto-kinetic stimuli in the home: a randomized controlled feasibility study in people with pure cerebellar disease. Clin. Rehabil. 29, 143–153.

Bunn, L.M., Marsden, J.F., Voyce, D.C., et al., 2015b. Sensorimotor processing for balance in spinocerebellar ataxia type 6. Mov. Disord. 30, 1259–1266.

Busse, M., et al., 2013. A randomized feasibility study of a 12-week community-based exercise program for people with Huntington's disease. J. Neurol. Phys. Ther. 37, 149–158.

Busse, M., et al., 2017. Physical activity self-management and coaching compared to social interaction in Huntington's disease: results from the ENGAGE-HD randomized, controlled, pilot feasibility trial. Phys. Ther. 97, 625–639.

Busse, M., Ramdharry, G., 2020. Targeting sedentary behaviour in neurological disease. Pract. Neurol. 20, 187–188.

Busse, M.E., et al., 2008. Physical therapy intervention for people with Huntington disease. Phys. Ther. 88, 820–831.

Busse, M.E., Wiles, C.M., Rosser, A.E., 2009. Mobility and falls in people with Huntington's disease. J. Neurol. Neurosurg. Psychiatry. 80, 88–90.

Cady, R.B., Bobechko, W.P., 1984. Incidence, natural history, and treatment of scoliosis in Friedreich's ataxia. J. Pediatr. Orthopaed. 4, 673–676.

Caron, N.S., Wright, G.E.B., Hayden, M.R., 2020. Huntington disease. In: Adam, M.P. (Ed.), GeneReviews. [Internet]. University of Washington, Seattle, Seattle (WA), pp. 1993–2022. Available from: https://www.ncbi.nlm.nih.gov/books/NBK1305/

Cassidy, E., et al., 2011. Using interpretative phenomenological analysis to inform physiotherapy practice: an introduction with reference to the lived experience of cerebellar ataxia. Physiother. Theory. Pract. 27, 263–277.

Cassidy, E., Naylor, S., Reynolds, F., 2018. The meanings of physiotherapy and exercise for people living with progressive cerebellar ataxia: an interpretative phenomenological analysis. Disabil. Rehabil. 40, 894–904.

Choi, K.D., Choi, J.H., 2016. Episodic ataxias: clinical and genetic features. J. Mov. Disord. 9, 129–135.

Chuang, C.S., Chang, J.C., Soong, B.W., et al., 2019. Treadmill training increases the motor activity and neuron survival of the cerebellum in a mouse model of spinocerebellar ataxia type 1. Kaohsiung. J. Med. Sci. 35, 679–685.

Ciancarelli, I., Ciancarelli, Tozzi, Carolei, A., M.G., 2013. Effectiveness of intensive neurorehabilitation in patients with Huntington's disease. Eur. J. Physiol. Rehabil. Med. 49, 189–195.

Ciancarelli, I., et al., 2015. Influence of intensive multifunctional neurorehabilitation on neuronal oxidative damage in patients with Huntington's disease. Funct. Neurol. 30, 47–52.

Cimolin, V., et al., 2007. Are patients with hereditary spastic paraplegia different from patients with spastic diplegia during walking? Gait evaluation using 3D gait analysis. Funct. Neurol. 22, 23–28.

Clark, J., Morrow, M., Michael, S., 2004. Wheelchair postural support for young people with progressive neuromuscular disorders. Int. J. Rehabil. Ther. 11, 365–373.

Clenaghan, C., et al., 2016. Recognising serious comorbidities in Huntington's disease. J. Neurol. Neurosurg. Psychiatry. 87 (Suppl 1), A75.

Cook, C., et al., 2012. Development of guidelines for occupational therapy in Huntington's disease. Neurodegener. Dis. Manag. 2, 79–87.

Corben, L.A., et al., 2014. Consensus clinical management guidelines for Friedreich ataxia. Orphanet. J. Rare. Dis. 9, 184.

Croarkin, E., et al., 2009. Characterizing gait, locomotor status, and disease severity in children and adolescents with Friedreich ataxia. J. Neurol. Phys. Ther. 33, 144–149.

Cruikshank, T.M., et al., 2015. The effect of multidisciplinary rehabilitation on brain structure and cognition in Huntington's disease: an exploratory study. Brain. Behav. 5, e00312.

Cruz Martinez, A., Tejada, J., 1999. Central motor conduction in hereditary motor and sensory neuropathy and hereditary spastic paraplegia. Electromyogr. Clin. Neurophysiol. 39, 331–335.

D'Abreu, A., et al., 2007. The international cooperative ataxia rating scale in Machado-Joseph disease. Comparison with the unified multiple system atrophy rating scale. Mov. Disord. 22, 1976–1979.

Daker-White, G., Greenfield, J., Ealing, J., 2013. "Six sessions is a drop in the ocean": an exploratory study of neurological physiotherapy in idiopathic and inherited ataxias. Physiotherapy. 99, 335–340.

Dan, B., Cheron, G., 2000. Intrathecal baclofen normalizes motor strategy for squatting in familial spastic paraplegia: a case study. Neurophysiol. Clin. 30, 43–48.

Dan, B., et al., 2000. Effect of intrathecal baclofen on gait control in human hereditary spastic. Neurosci. Lett. 280, 175–178.

Dash, D., Mestre, T.A., 2020. Therapeutic update on Huntington's disease: symptomatic treatments and emerging disease-modifying therapies. Neurotherapeutics. 17, 1645–1659.

Delatycki, M.B., Bidichandani, S.I., 2019. Friedreich ataxia – pathogenesis and implications for therapies. Neurobiol. Dis. 132, 104606.

Dellefield, M.E., Ferrini, R., 2011. Promoting excellence in end-of-life care. J. Neurosci. Nursing. 43, 186–192.

DeLuca, G.C., Ebers, G.C., Esir, M.M., 2004. The extent of axonal loss in the long tracts in hereditary spastic paraplegia. Neuropathol. Appl. Neurobiol. 30, 576–584.

Denton, A., Bunn, L., Hough, A., et al., 2016. Superficial warming and cooling of the leg affects walking speed and neuromuscular impairments in people with spastic paraparesis. Ann. Phys. Rehabil. Med. 59, 326–332.

Desai, R., et al., 2021. Evaluation of gait initiation parameters using inertial sensors in Huntington's disease: insights into anticipatory postural adjustments and cognitive interference. Gait. Posture. 87, 117–122.

de Silva, R., Greenfield, J., Cook, A., et al., 2019. Guidelines on the diagnosis and management of the progressive ataxias. Orphanet. J. Rare. Dis. 14, 51.

de Snoo-Trimp, J.C., De Vet, H.C.W., Widdershoven, G.A.M., Molewijk, A.C., Svantesson, M., 2020. Moral competence, moral teamwork and moral action – the European Moral

Case Deliberation Outcomes (Euro-MCD) Instrument 2.0 and its revision process. BMC Med. Ethics. 21, 1–18.

Duning, T., et al., 2010. Specific pattern of early white-matter changes in pure hereditary spastic paraplegia. Mov. Disord. 25, 1986–1992.

Dunnett, S.B., Rosser, A.E., 2011. Clinical translation of cell transplantation in the brain. Curr. Opin. Transplant. 16, 632–639.

Elliott, R., et al., 2003. Executive functions and their disorders: imaging in clinical neuroscience. Br. Med. Bull. 65, 49–59.

Eno, C.C., Barton, S.K., Dorrani, N., Cederbaum, S.D., Deignan, J.L., Grody, W.W., 2020. Confidential genetic testing and electronic health records: a survey of current practices among Huntington disease testing centers. Mol. Genet. Genom. Med. 8, e1026.

Erez, A., Plunkett, K., Sutton, V.R., McGuire, A.L., 2010. The right to ignore genetic status of late onset genetic disease in the genomic era: prenatal testing for Huntington disease as a paradigm. Am. J. Med. Genet. 152, 1774–1780.

Evans, S.J.W., et al., 2013. Prevalence of adult Huntington's disease in the UK based on diagnoses recorded in general practice records. J. Neurol. Neurosurg. Psychiatry. 84, 1156–1160.

Fahey, M.C., et al., 2007. How is disease progress in Friedreich's ataxia best measured? A study of four. J. Neurol. Neurosurg. Psychiatry. 78, 411–413.

Fenney, A., Jog, M.S., Duval, C., 2008. Bradykinesia is not a "systematic" feature of adult-onset Huntington's disease; implications for basal ganglia pathophysiology. Brain. Res. 1193, 67–75.

Ferreira, J.J., et al., 2022. An MDS evidenced based review on treatments for Huntington's disease. Mov. Disord. 37, 25–35.

Filipe, R.B., Wild, E.J., 2020. Clinical trials corner. J. Huntington. Dis. 9, 185–197.

Fink, J.K., 2000. Hereditary Spastic Paraplegia Overview. In: Adam, M.P., Ardinger, H.H., Pagon, R.A., et al. (Eds.), GeneReviews.

Fink, J.K., 2003. Advances in the hereditary spastic paraplegias. Exp. Neurol. 184, S106–S110.

Fink, J.K., 2013. Hereditary spastic paraplegia: clinico-pathologic features and emerging molecular. Acta. Neuropathol. 126, 307–328.

Fjermestad, K.W., Kanavin, Ø., Nyhus, L., Hoxmark, L.B., 2020. Health service experiences among adults with hereditary spastic paraparesis or neurofibromatosis type 1. Mol. Genet. Genom. Med. 8, e1399.

Fogel, B.L., Perlman, S., 2007. Clinical features and molecular genetics of autosomal recessive cerebellar. Lancet. Neurol. 6, 245–257.

Fonteyn, E.M., et al., 2010. Falls in spinocerebellar ataxias: results of the EuroSCA Fall Study. Cerebellum 9, 232–239.

Fonteyn, E.M., et al., 2013. Prospective analysis of falls in dominant ataxias. Eur. Neurol. 69, 53–57.

França, C., de Andrade, D.C., Silva, V., et al., 2020. Effects of cerebellar transcranial magnetic stimulation on ataxias: a randomized trial. Parkinsonism. Relat. Disord. 80, 1–6.

Frich, J.C., Røthing, M., Berge, A.R., 2014. Participants', caregivers', and professionals' experiences with a group-based rehabilitation program for Huntington's disease: a qualitative study. BMC Health. Serv. Res. 14, 395.

Frich, J.C., et al., 2016. Health care delivery practices in Huntington's disease specialty clinics: an international survey. J. Huntington. Dis 5, 207–213.

Fritz, N.E., et al., 2016. Motor-cognitive dual-task deficits in individuals with early-mid stage Huntington disease. Gait. Posture. 49, 283–289.

Fritz, N.E., Busse, M., Jones, K., Khalil, H., Quinn, L., Members of the Physiotherapy Working Group of the European Huntington's Disease Network, 2017a. A classification system to guide physical therapy management in Huntington's disease: a case series. J. Neurol. Phys. Ther. 41, 156–163.

Fritz, N.E., Rao, A.K., Kegelmeyer, D., et al., 2017b. Physical therapy and exercise interventions in Huntington's disease: a mixed methods systematic review. J. Huntington. Dis. 6, 217–235.

Fruhmann Berger, M., et al., 2006. Deviation of eyes and head in acute cerebral stroke. BMC Neurol. 26, 23.

Garcia-Gorro, C., Garau-Rolandi, M., Escrichs, A., et al., 2019. An active cognitive lifestyle as a potential neuroprotective factor in Huntington's disease. Neuropsychologia. 122, 116–124.

Gates, P.C., et al., 1998. Friedreich's ataxia presenting as adult-onset spastic paraparesis. Neurogenetics. 1, 297–299.

Genoff Garzon, M.C., Rubin, L.R., Lobel, M., Stelling, J., Pastore, L.M., 2018. Review of patient decision-making factors and attitudes regarding preimplantation genetic diagnosis. Clin. Genet. 94, 22–42.

Geva-Dayan, K., et al., 2010. Botulinum toxin injections for pediatric patients with hereditary spastic paraparesis. J. Child. Neurol. 25, 969–975.

Ginanneschi, F., et al., 2014. Hand muscles corticomotor excitability in hereditary spastic paraparesis type 4. Neurol. Sci. 35, 1287–1291.

Grimbergen, Y.A., et al., 2008. Falls and gait disturbances in Huntington's disease. Mov. Disord. 23, 970–976.

Grobe-Einsler, M., Taheri Amin, A., Faber, J., et al., 2021. Development of SARA(home), a new video-based tool for the assessment of ataxia at home. Mov. Disord. 36, 1242–1246.

Grose, J., Freeman, J., Marsden, J., 2014. Service delivery for people with hereditary spastic paraparesis living in the South West of England. Disabil. Rehabil. 36, 907–913.

Hadzi, T.C., et al., 2012. Assessment of cortical and striatal involvement in 523 Huntington disease brains. Neurology. 79, 1708–1715.

Hagen, N., 2018. The lived experience of Huntington's disease: a phenomenological perspective on genes, the body and the lived experience of a genetic disease. Health (London). 22, 72–86.

Hakimian, R., 2000. Disclosure of Huntington's disease to family members: the dilemma of known but unknowing parties. Genet. Test. 4, 359–364.

Harding, A.E., 1983. Classification of the hereditary ataxias and paraplegias. Lancet. 1, 115–1151.

Harper, P., 1992. The epidemiology of Huntington's disease. Hum. Genet. 89, 365–376.

Harrington, D.L., et al., 2015. Network topology and functional connectivity disturbances precede the onset of Huntington's disease. Brain 138, 2332–2346.

Harrison, D.J., et al., 2013. Exercise attenuates neuropathology and has greater benefit on cognitive than motor deficits in the R6/1 Huntington's disease mouse model. Exp. Neurol. 248, 457–469.

Hecht, M.J., et al., 2008. Botulinum neurotoxin type A injections reduce spasticity in mild to moderate. Mov. Disord. 23, 228–233.

Heemskerk, A.-W., Roos, R.A.C., 2012. Aspiration pneumonia and death in Huntington's disease. PLoS Curr. 4 RRN1293

Herzog, J., et al., 2007. Kinematic analysis of thalamic versus sub-thalamic neurostimulation in postural and intention tremor. Brain. 130, 1608–1625.

Hockly, E., et al., 2002. Environmental enrichment slows disease progression in R6/2 Huntington's disease mice. Ann. Neurol. 51 (2), 235–242.

Hooper, J., et al., 2002. A prospective study of thalamic deep brain stimulation for the treatment of movement disorders in multiple sclerosis. Br. J. Neurosurg. 16, 102–109.

Huang, M., Verbeek, D.S., 2019. Why do so many genetic insults lead to Purkinje cell degeneration and spinocerebellar ataxia? Neurosci. Lett. 688, 49–57.

Huntington Study Group, 1996. Unified Huntington's Disease Rating Scale: reliability and consistency. Mov. Disord. 11, 136–142.

Ilg, W., Bastian, A.J., Boesch, S., et al., 2014. Consensus paper: management of degenerative cerebellar disorders. Cerebellum. 13, 248–268.

Ilg, W., Golla, H., Thier, P., Giese, M.A., 2007. Specific influences of cerebellar dysfunctions on gait. Brain. 130, 786–798.

Ilg, W., et al., 2010. Long-term effects of coordinative training in degenerative cerebellar disease. Mov. Disord. 25, 2239–2246.

Ilg, W., Timmann, D., 2013. Gait ataxia – specific cerebellar influences and their rehabilitation. Mov. Disord. 28, 1566–1575.

Inbar, N., et al., 2016. Functional screening for Huntington's disease: a phased approach. J. Neurol. Neurosurg. Psychiatry. 87 (Suppl 1), A74.

Jacobi, H., et al., 2013. Inventory of non-ataxia signs (INAS): validation of a new clinical assessment. Cerebellum. 12, 418–428.

Jacobs, J.V., et al., 2015. Domains and correlates of clinical balance impairment associated with Huntington's disease. Gait. Posture. 41, 867–870.

Joel, D., 2001. Open interconnected model of basal ganglia-thalamocortical circuitry and its relevance to the clinical syndrome of Huntington's disease. Mov. Disord. 16, 407–423.

Jones-Bonofiglio, K., 2020. Health Care Ethics Through the Lens of Moral Distress. Springer, Cham.

Jones, C., et al., 2016a. The societal cost of Huntington's disease: are we underestimating the burden? Eur. J. Neurol. 23, 1588–1590.

Jones, U., et al., 2016b. Respiratory decline is integral to disease progression in Huntington's disease. Eur. Resp. J. 48, 585–588.

Jones, U., Hamana, K., O'Hara, F., Busse, M., 2021. The development of PAT-HD: a co-designed tool to promote physical activity in people with Huntington's disease. Health. Expect. 24, 638–647.

Keren, K., et al., 2021. Towards the quantification of daily-living gait quantity and quality in people with Huntington's disease: preliminary results based on a wrist-worn accelerometer. Front. Neurol. 12, 719442.

Kearney, M., Orrell, R.W., Fahey, M., Brassington, R., Pandolfo, M., 2016. Pharmacological treatments for Friedreich ataxia. Cochrane. Database. Syst. Rev. 8 CD007791

Keenan, K.F., van Teijlingen, E., McKee, L., Miedzybrodzka, Z., Simpson, S.A., 2009. How young people find out about their family history of Huntington's disease. Soc. Sci. Med. 68, 1892–1900.

Khalil, H., et al., 2013. What effect does a structured home-based exercise programme have on people with Huntington's disease? A randomized, controlled pilot study. Clin. Rehabil. 27, 646–658.

Kim, S.H., Han, J.Y., Song, M.K., Choi, I.S., Park, H.K., 2021. Effectiveness of robotic exoskeleton-assisted gait training in spinocerebellar ataxia: a case report. Sensors (Basel) 21, 4874.

Klager, J., et al., 2008. Huntington's disease: a caring approach to the end of life. Care. Manag. J. 9, 75–81.

Klebe, S., et al., 2004. Gait analysis of sporadic and hereditary spastic paraplegia. J. Neurol. 251, 571–578.

Klebe, S., et al., 2005. Objective assessment of gait after intrathecal baclofen in hereditary spastic paraplegia. J. Neurol. 252, 991–993.

Klimpe, S., et al., 2012. Disease severity affects quality of life of hereditary spastic paraplegia. Eur. J. Neurol. 19, 71–168.

Kloos, A.D., et al., 2013. Video game play (Dance Dance Revolution) as a potential exercise therapy in Huntington's disease: a controlled clinical trial. Clin. Rehabil. 27, 972–982.

Kloos, A.D., et al., 2014. Clinimetric properties of the Tinetti Mobility Test, Four Square Step Test, Activities-specific Balance Confidence Scale, and spatiotemporal gait measures in individuals with Huntington's disease. Gait. Posture. 40, 647–651.

Kondo, Y., Bando, K., Ariake, Y., et al., 2020. Test-retest reliability and minimal detectable change of the Balance Evaluation Systems Test and its two abbreviated versions in persons with mild to moderate spinocerebellar ataxia: a pilot study. NeuroRehabilitation. 47, 479–486.

Koskenvuori, J., Stolt, M., Suhonen, R., Leino-Kilpi, H., 2019. Healthcare professionals' ethical competence: a scoping review. Nursing. Open. 6, 5–17.

Kshirsagar, P.B., Kanhere, H.S., Bansinge, P.C., Sawan, K., Khandare, V.S., Das, R.K., 2021. Huntington's disease: pathophysiology and therapeutic intervention. GSC Biol. Pharmaceut. Sci. 15, 171–184.

Lai, R.Y., Tomishon, D.K., Figueroa, P., et al., 2019. Tremor in the degenerative cerebellum: towards the understanding of brain circuitry for tremor. Cerebellum. 18, 519–526.

Lanza, G., Casabona, J.A., Bellomo, M., et al., 2020. Update on intensive motor training in spinocerebellar ataxia: time to move a step forward? J. Int. Med. Res. 48 300060519854626

Leigh, R.J., et al., 1983. Abnormal ocular motor control in Huntington's disease. Neurology. 33, 1268–1275.

Lindig, T., et al., 2015. Gray and white matter alterations in hereditary spastic paraplegia type SPG4 and clinical correlations. J. Neurol. 262, 1961–1971.

Liu, X., et al., 2000. Frequency analysis of involuntary movements during wrist tracking: a way to identify MS patients with tremor who benefit from thalamotomy. Stereotactic. Funct. Neurosurg. 74, 53–62.

Lo, C.W.T., et al., 2022. Psychometric properties of brief-balance evaluation systems test among multiple populations: a systematic review and meta-analysis. Arch. Phys. Med. Rehabil. 103, 155–175.

Lopez-Sendon, J.L., et al., 2011. What is the impact of education on Huntington's disease? Mov. Disord. 26, 1489–1495.

Louis, E.D., et al., 1999. Dystonia in Huntington's disease: prevalence and clinical characteristics. Mov. Disord. 14, 95–101.

Luo, L., et al., 2017. The initial symptom and motor progression in spinocerebellar ataxias. Cerebellum. 16, 615–622.

Lynch, D.R., et al., 2006. Measuring Friedreich ataxia: complementary features of examination and performance measures. Neurology. 66, 1711–1716.

Maas, R., Killaars, S., van de Warrenburg, B.P.C., Schutter, D., 2021. The cerebellar cognitive affective syndrome scale reveals early neuropsychological deficits in SCA3 patients. J. Neurol. 268, 3456–3466.

Maas, R., van de Warrenburg, B.P.C., 2021. Exploring the clinical meaningfulness of the Scale for the Assessment and Rating of Ataxia: a comparison of patient and physician perspectives at the item level. Parkinsonism. Relat. Disord. 91, 37–41.

MacLeod, R., et al., 2013. Recommendations for the predictive genetic test in Huntington's disease. Clin. Genet. 83, 221–231.

Mahmood, S., Law, S., Bombard, Y., 2022. "I have to start learning how to live with becoming sick": a scoping review of the lived experiences of people with Huntington's disease. Clin. Genet. 101, 3–19.

Manley, G., et al., 2012. Guideline for oral healthcare of adults with Huntington's disease. Neurodegener. Dis. Manag. 2, 55–65.

Manor, B., Greenstein, P.E., Davila-Perez, P., Wakefield, S., Zhou, J., Pascual-Leone, A., 2019. Repetitive transcranial magnetic stimulation in spinocerebellar ataxia: a pilot randomized controlled trial. Front. Neurol. 10, 73.

Manto, M., Godaux, E., Jacquy, J., 1994. Cerebellar hypermetria is larger when the inertial load is artificially increased. Ann. Neurol. 35, 45–52.

Marsden, J., Harris, C., 2011. Cerebellar ataxia: pathophysiology and rehabilitation. Clin. Rehabil. 25, 195–216.

Marsden, J., Stevenson, V., 2013. Balance dysfunction in hereditary and spontaneous spastic paraparesis. Gait. Posture. 38, 1048–1050.

Marsden, J., et al., 2012. Muscle paresis and passive stiffness: key determinants in limiting function in hereditary and sporadic spastic paraparesis. Gait. Posture. 35, 266–271.

Marsden, J., et al., 2013. The effects of functional electrical stimulation on walking in hereditary and spontaneous spastic paraparesis. Neuromodulation. 16, 256–260.

Martin, L.R., Haskard-Zolnierek, K.B., DiMatteo, M.R., 2010. Health Behaviour Change and Treatment Adherence: Evidence Based Guidelines for Improving Healthcare. Oxford University Press, Oxford.

Matos, C.A., de Almeida, L.P., Nóbrega, C., 2019. Machado-Joseph disease/spinocerebellar ataxia type 3: lessons from disease pathogenesis and clues into therapy. J. Neurochem. 148, 8–28.

Matsushima, A., Maruyama, Y., Mizukami, N., Tetsuya, M., Hashimoto, M., Yoshida, K., 2021. Gait training with a wearable curara® robot for cerebellar ataxia: a single-arm study. Biomed. Eng. Online. 20, 90.

McColgan, P., Tabrizi, S.J., 2018. Huntington's disease: a clinical review. Eur. J. Neurol. 25, 24–34.

McCusker, E.A., Loy, C.T., 2017. Huntington disease: the complexities of making and disclosing a clinical diagnosis after premanifest genetic testing. Tremor. Other. Hyperkinet. Mov. 7, 467.

McLauchlan, D.J., Lancaster, T., Craufurd, D., Linden, D., Rosser, A.E., 2019. Insensitivity to loss predicts apathy in Huntington's disease. Mov. Dis. 34, 1381–1391.

McMonagle, P., Webb, S., Hutchinson, M., 2002. The prevalence of 'pure' autosomal dominant hereditary spastic paraparesis in the island of Ireland. J. Neurol. Neurosurg. Psychiatry. 72, 43–46.

Mees, I., Tran, H., Renoir, T., Hannan, A.J., 2019. Experience-dependent modulation of neurodegenerative disorders: Huntington's disease as an exemplar. In: Degenerative Disorders of the Brain. Routledge, 116–142.

Meera, P., Pulst, S.M., Otis, T.S., 2016. Cellular and circuit mechanisms underlying spinocerebellar ataxias. J. Physiol. 594, 4653–4660.

Menon, V., et al., 2000. Basal ganglia involvement in memory-guided movement sequencing. Neuroreport. 11, 3641–3645.

Mestre, T.A., 2018. Rating scales for function in Huntington's disease. Mov. Dis. Clin. Pract. 5, 111–117.

Meythaler, J.M., et al., 1992. Intrathecal baclofen in hereditary spastic paraparesis. Arch. Phys. Med. Rehabil. 73, 794–797.

Miyai, I., et al., 2012. Cerebellar ataxia rehabilitation trial in degenerative cerebellar diseases. Neurorehabil. Neural. Repair. 26, 515–522.

Mo, C., Hannan, A.J., Renoir, T., 2015. Environmental factors as modulators of neurodegeneration: insights from gene-environment interactions in Huntington's disease. Neurosci. Behav. Rev. 52, 178–192.

Molteni, F., et al., 2005. Instrumental evaluation of gait modifications before and during intrathecal baclofen therapy: a 2-year follow-up case study. Arch. Phys. Med. Rehabil. 84, 303–306.

Moriarty, A., et al., 2016. A longitudinal investigation into cognition and disease progression in spinocerebellar ataxia types 1, 2, 3, 6, and 7. Orphanet. J. Rare. Dis. 11, 82.

Moro, A., Moscovich, M., Farah, M., Camargo, C.H.F., Teive, H.A.G., Munhoz, R.P., 2019. Nonmotor symptoms in spinocerebellar ataxias (SCAs). Cerebellum. Ataxias. 6, 12.

Morton, S.M., Bastain, A.J., 2004. Cerebellar control of balance and locomotion. Neuroscientist 10, 247–259.

Muratori, L., et al., 2021. Measures of postural control and mobility during dual-tasking as candidate markers of instability in Huntington's disease. Hum. Mov. Sci. 80, 102881.

Nance, M.A., 2007. Comprehensive care in Huntington's disease: a physician's perspective. Brain. Res. Bull. 72, 175–178.

Nithianantharajah, J., Hannan, A.J., 2006. Enriched environments, experience-dependent plasticity and disorders of the nervous system. Nat. Rev. Neurosci. 7, 697–709.

Noreau, A., Dion, P.A., Rouleau, G.A., 2014. Molecular aspects of hereditary spastic paraplegia. Exp. Cell. Res. 325, 18–26.

Ogawa, M., 2004. Pharmacological treatments of cerebellar ataxia. Cerebellum. 3, 107–111.

Pandolofo, M., 2002. Friedreich's ataxia. In: Manto, M.U., Pandolfo, M. (Eds.), The Cerebellum and Its Disorders. Cambridge University Press, Cambridge.

Parkinson, M.H., Boesch, S., et al., 2013a. Clinical features of Friedreich's ataxia: classical and atypical phenotypes. J. Neurochem. 126 (Suppl), 17–103.

Parkinson, M.H., Schulz, J., Giunti, P., 2013b. Co-enzyme Q10 and idebenone use in Friedreich's ataxia. J. Neurochem. 126 (Suppl), 41–125.

Penney Jr., J.B., et al., 1997. CAG repeat number governs the development rate of pathology in Huntington's disease. Ann. Neurol. 41, 689–692.

Perez-Lloret, S., van de Warrenburg, B., Rossi, M., et al., 2021. Assessment of Ataxia Rating Scales and Cerebellar Functional Tests: Critique and Recommendations. Mov. Disord. 36, 283–297.

Perlman, S.L., 2000. Cerebellar ataxia. Curr. Treat. Options. Neurol. 2, 215–224.

Perlman, S.L., 2004. Symptomatic and disease-modifying therapy for the progressive ataxias. Neurologist. 10, 275–289.

Piccinini, L., et al., 2011. 3D gait analysis in patients with hereditary spastic paraparesis and spastic diplegia: a kinematic, kinetic and EMG comparison. Eur. J. Paed. Neurol. 15, 138–145.

Pierron, L., Hennessy, J., du Montcel, S.T., et al., 2021. Informing about genetic risk in families with Huntington disease: comparison of attitudes across two decades. Eur. J. Hum. Genet. 29, 672–679.

Piña-Aguilar, R.E., Simpson, S.A., Alshatti, A., Clarke, A., Craufurd, D., Dorkins, H., Miedzybrodzka, Z., 2019. 27 years of prenatal diagnosis for Huntington disease in the United Kingdom. Genet. Med. 21, 1639–1643.

Piira, A., et al., 2013. Effects of a one year intensive multidisciplinary rehabilitation program for patients with Huntington's disease: a prospective intervention study. PLoS Curr., 5.

Pirker, W., et al., 2003. Chronic thalamic stimulation in a patient with spinocerebellar ataxia type 2. Mov. Disord. 18, 222–225.

Podvin, S., Reardon, H.T., Yin, K., Mosier, C., Hook, V., 2019. Multiple clinical features of Huntington's disease correlate with mutant HTT gene CAG repeat lengths and neurodegeneration. J. Neurol. 266, 551–564.

Pointon, R., Whelan, H., Raza, R., et al., 2022. The use of intrathecal baclofen for management of spasticity in hereditary spastic paraparesis: a case series. Eur. J. Paediatr. Neurol. 36, 14–18.

Porciuncula, F., Wasserman, P., Marder, K.S., Rao, A.K., 2020. Quantifying postural control in premanifest and manifest Huntington's disease using wearable sensors. Neurorehabil. Neural. Repair. 34, 771–783.

Pringsheim, T., et al., 2012. The incidence and prevalence of Huntington's disease: a systematic review and meta-analysis. Mov. Disord. 27, 1083–1091.

Pucks-Faes, E., Dobesberger, J., Hitzenberger, G., et al., 2019. Intrathecal baclofen in hereditary spastic paraparesis. Front. Neurol. 10, 901.

Purcell, N.L., Goldman, J.G., Ouyang, B., et al., 2020. The effects of dual-task cognitive interference on gait and turning in Huntington's disease. PLoS ONE. 15, e0226827.

Quarrell, O., et al., 2012. The prevalence of juvenile Huntington's disease: a review of the literature and meta-analysis. PLoS Curr. 4, e4f8606b742ef3

Quigley, J., 2017. Juvenile Huntington's disease: diagnostic and treatment considerations for the psychiatrist. Curr. Psychiatry. Rep. 19, 9.

Quinn, L., Busse, M., 2012. Development of physiotherapy guidance and treatment-based classifications for people with Huntington's disease. Neurodegener. Dis. Manag. 2, 11–19.

Quinn, L., Kegelmeyer, D., Kloos, A., Rao, A.K., Busse, M., Fritz, N.E., 2020. Clinical recommendations to guide physical therapy practice for Huntington disease. Neurology. 94, 217–228.

Quinn, L., Morgan, D., 2017. From disease to health: physical therapy health promotion practices for secondary prevention in adult and pediatric neurologic populations. J. Neurol. Phys. Ther. 41 (Suppl. 3), S46–S54.

Quinn, L., et al., 2013. Reliability and minimal detectable change of physical performance measures in individuals with premanifest and manifest Huntington disease. Phys. Ther. 93, 942–956.

Quinn, L., et al., 2014. Task-specific training in Huntington disease: a randomized controlled feasibility trial. Phys. Ther. 94, 1555–1568.

Quinn, L., et al., 2016. A randomized, controlled trial of a multi-modal exercise intervention in Huntington's disease. Parkinsonism. Relat. Dis. 31, 46–52.

Quinn, L., et al., 2022. Physical activity and exercise outcomes in Huntington's disease (PACE-HD): results of a 12-month trial-within-cohort feasibility study of a physical activity intervention in people with Huntington's disease. Parkinsonism. Relat. Dis. 101, 75–89.

Rao, A.K., et al., 2009. Clinical measurement of mobility and balance impairments in Huntington's disease: validity and responsiveness. Gait. Posture. 29, 433–436.

Raymond, L.A., et al., 2011. Pathophysiology of Huntington's disease: time-dependent alterations in synaptic and receptor function. Neuroscience. 198, 252–273.

Reilmann, R., 2013. Pharmacological treatment of chorea in Huntington's disease – good clinical practice versus evidence-based guideline. Mov. Disord. 28, 1030–1033.

Reyes, A., et al., 2015. Respiratory muscle training on pulmonary and swallowing function in patients with Huntington's disease: a pilot randomised controlled trial. Clin. Rehabil. 29, 961–973.

Reyes, A., et al., 2021. Clinical determinants of dual tasking in people with premanifest Huntington disease. Phys. Ther. 101 pzab016

Richardson, D.F., Thompson, A.J., 1999. Management of spasticity in hereditary spastic paraplegia. Physiother. Res. Int. 4, 68–76.

Roos, R.A.C., 2010. Huntington's disease: a clinical review. Orphanet. J. Rare. Dis. 5, 40.

Rosenblatt, A., et al., 2006. The association of CAG repeat length with clinical progression in Huntington disease. Neurology. 66, 1016–1020.

Ross, C., et al., 2014. Huntington disease: natural history, biomarkers and prospects for therapeutics. Nat. Rev. Neurol. 10, 204–216.

Ross, C.A., Tabrizi, S.J., 2011. Huntington's disease: from molecular pathogenesis to clinical treatment. Lancet. Neurol. 10, 83–98.

Rosser, A., Svendsen, C.N., 2014. Stem cells for cell replacement therapy: a therapeutic strategy for HD? Mov. Disord. 29, 1446–1454.

Rossi, M., et al., 2014. Autosomal dominant cerebellar ataxias: a systematic review of clinical features. Eur. J. Neurol. 21, 607–615.

Røthing, M., Malterud, K., Frich, J.C., 2015. Family caregivers' views on coordination of care in Huntington's disease: a qualitative study. Scand. J. Caring. Sci. 29, 803–809.

Rousseaux, M., et al., 2007. Botulinum toxin injection in patients with hereditary spastic paraparesis. Eur. J. Neurol. 14, 206–212.

Ruano, L., et al., 2014. The global epidemiology of hereditary ataxia and spastic paraplegia: a systematic review of prevalence studies. Neuroepidemiology. 42, 174–183.

Salinas, S., et al., 2008. Hereditary spastic paraplegia: clinical features and pathogenetic mechanisms. Lancet. Neurol. 7, 1127–1138.

Saltuari, L., et al., 1992. Long-term intrathecal baclofen treatment in supraspinal spasticity. Acta. Neurol. (Napoli) 14, 195–207.

Sartucci, F., et al., 2007. Motor and somatosensory evoked potentials in autosomal dominant hereditary spastic paraparesis (ADHSP) linked to chromosome 2p, SPG4. Brain Res. Bull. 74, 243–249.

Schady, W., et al., 1991. Central motor conduction studies in hereditary spastic paraplegia. J. Neurol. Neurosurg. Psychiatry. 54, 775–779.

Scheller, E., et al., 2013. Interregional compensatory mechanisms of motor functioning in progressing preclinical neurodegeneration. NeuroImage. 75, 146–154.

Scheuer, K.H., et al., 2007. Double-blind crossover trial of gabapentin in SPG4-linked hereditary spastic. Eur. J. Neurol. 14, 663–666.

Schmahmann, J.D., Sherman, J.C., 1998. The cerebellar cognitive affective syndrome. Brain. 121, 561–579.

Schmahmann, J.D., et al., 2009. Development of a brief ataxia rating scale (BARS) based on a modified form of the ICARS. Mov. Disord. 24, 1820–1828.

Schule, R., et al., 2006. The Spastic Paraplegia Rating Scale (SPRS): a reliable and valid measure of disease severity. Neurology. 67, 430–434.

Schule, R., et al., 2016. Hereditary spastic paraplegia: clinicogenetic lessons from 608 patients. Ann. Neurol. 79, 646–658.

Schulte, J., Littleton, J.T., 2011. The biological function of the Huntingtin protein and its relevance to Huntington's disease pathology. Curr. Trends. Neurol. 5, 65–78.

Scott, S.S.O., Pedroso, J.L., Barsottini, O.G.P., França-Junior, M.C., Braga-Neto, P., 2020. Natural history and epidemiology of the spinocerebellar ataxias: insights from the first description to nowadays. J. Neurol. Sci. 417, 117082.

Scuderi, C., et al., 2009. Posterior fossa abnormalities in hereditary spastic paraparesis with spastin mutations. J. Neurol. Neurosurg. Psychiatry. 80, 440–443.

Serrao, M., et al., 2016. Gait patterns in patients with hereditary spastic paraparesis. PLoS One. 11, e0164623.

Sharma, A., Behl, T., Sharma, L., Aelya, L., Bungau, S., 2021. Mitochondrial dysfunction in Huntington's disease: pathogenesis and therapeutic opportunities. Curr. Drug. Targets. 22, 1637–1667.

Shah, V.V., Rodriguez-Labrada, R., Horak, F.B., et al., 2021. Gait variability in spinocerebellar ataxia assessed using wearable inertial sensors. Mov. Disord. 36, 2922–2931.

Shiga, Y., et al., 2002. Transcranial magnetic stimulation alleviates truncal ataxia in spinocerebellar degeneration. J. Neurol. Neurosurg. Psychiatry. 72, 124–126.

Shimojima, Y., et al., 2005. Thalamic stimulation for disabling tremor in a patient with spinocerebellar degeneration. Stereotact. Funct. Neurosurg. 83, 131–134.

Simpson, J.A., et al., 2016. Survey of the Huntington's disease patient and caregiver community reveals most impactful symptoms and treatment needs. J. Huntington. Dis. 5, 395–403.

Simpson, S.A., 2007. Late stage care in Huntington's disease. Brain. Res. Bull. 72, 179–181.

Sommerville, R.B., et al., 2017. Diagnosis and management of adult hereditary cardio-neuromuscular disorders: a model for the multidisciplinary care of complex genetic disorders. Trends. Cardiovasc. Med. 27, 51–58.

Stark, Z., et al., 2016. Predictive genetic testing for neurodegenerative conditions: how should conflicting interests within families be managed? J. Med. Ethics. 42, 640–642.

Storey, E., et al., 2004. Inter-rater reliability of the International Cooperative Ataxia Rating Scale (ICARS). Mov. Disord. 19, 190–192.

Strupp, M., et al., 2003. Treatment of downbeat nystagmus with 3,4-diaminopyridine: a placebo-controlled study. Neurology. 61, 165–170.

Strupp, M., et al., 2017. Aminopyridines for the treatment of neurologic disorders. Neurol. Clin. Pract. 7, 65–76.

Subramony, S.H., Paraminder, J.S.V., 2002. Spinocerebellar ataxia type 3. In: Manto, M.U., Pandolofo, M. (Eds.), The Cerebellum and Its Disorders. Cambridge University Press, Cambridge.

Sue, C.M., et al., 1997. Transcranial cortical stimulation in disorders of the central motor pathways. J. Clin. Neurosci. 4, 19–25.

Sun, Y.M., Lu, C., Wu, Z.Y., 2016. Spinocerebellar ataxia: relationship between phenotype and genotype – a review. Clin. Genet. 90, 305–314.

Sun, Y.-M., Zhang, Y.-B., Wu, Z.-Y., 2017. Huntington's disease: relationship between phenotype and genotype. Mol. Neurobiol. 54, 342–348.

Synofzik, M., Ilg, W., 2014. Motor training in degenerative spinocerebellar disease: ataxia-specific improvements by intensive physiotherapy. Biomed. Res. Int. 2014, 583507.

Synofzik, M., et al., 2013. Videogame-based coordinative training can improve advanced, multisystemic early-onset ataxia. J. Neurol. 260, 2656–2658.

Tabrizi, S.J., et al., 2019. Targeting Huntingtin expression in patients with Huntington's disease. N. Engl. J. Med. 380, 2307–2316.

Tada, M., Nishizawa, M., Onodera, O., 2015. Redefining cerebellar ataxia in degenerative ataxias: lessons from recent research on cerebellar systems. J. Neurol. Neurosurg. Psychiatry. 86, 922–928.

The Huntington's Disease Collaborative Research Group, 1993. A novel gene containing a trinucleotide repeat that is expanded and unstable on Huntington's disease chromosomes. Cell. 72, 971–983.

Thompson, J.A., et al., 2013. The effects of multidisciplinary rehabilitation in patients with early-to-middle-stage Huntington's disease: a pilot study. Eur. J. Neurol. 20, 1325–1329.

Thompson, J.C., et al., 2012. Longitudinal evaluation of neuropsychiatric symptoms in Huntington's disease. J. Neuropsychiatry. Clin. Neurosci. 24, 53–60.

Timmann, D., et al., 2009. Current advances in lesion-symptom mapping of the human cerebellum. Neuroscience. 162, 836–851.

Tommaso, M., et al., 2017. Walking-related dual-task interference in early-to-middle-stage Huntington's disease: an auditory event related potential study. Front. Psychol. 8, 1292.

Torres, C.V., et al., 2010. Deep brain stimulation of the ventral intermediate nucleus of the thalamus for tremor in patients with multiple sclerosis. Neurosurgery. 67, 646–651. discussion 651.

Trembath, M.K., et al., 2010. A retrospective study of the impact of lifestyle on age at onset of Huntington disease. Mov. Disord. 25, 1444–1450.

Trouillas, P., et al., 1997. International Cooperative Ataxia Rating Scale for pharmacological assessment of the cerebellar syndrome. The Ataxia Neuropharmacology Committee of the World Federation of Neurology. J. Neurol. Sci. 145, 205–211.

Tsirikos, A.I., Smith, G., 2012. Scoliosis in patients with Friedreich's ataxia. J. Bone. Joint. Surg. Br. 94, 684–689.

Tsunemi, T., et al., 2010. The effect of 3,4-diaminopyridine on the patients with hereditary pure cerebellar ataxia. J. Neurol. Sci. 292, 81–84.

van de Zande, N.A., Massey, T.H., McLauchlan, D., et al., 2016. Clinical characterisation of dystonia in patients with Huntington's disease. J. Neurol. Neurosurg. Psychiatry. 87 (Suppl 1), A46–A47.

van Dellen, A., et al., 2000. Delaying the onset of Huntington's in mice. Nature. 404, 721–722.

van Dellen, A., et al., 2008. Wheel running from a juvenile age delays onset of specific motor deficits but does not alter protein aggregate density in a mouse model of Huntington's disease. BMC Neurosci. 9, 34.

van Duijn, E., et al., 2014. Neuropsychiatric symptoms in a European Huntington's disease cohort (REGISTRY). J. Neurol. Neurosurg. Psychiatry. 85, 1411–1418.

van Rij, M.C., et al., 2012. Preimplantation genetic diagnosis (PGD) for Huntington's disease: the experience of three European centres. Eur. J. Hum. Genet. 20, 368–375.

van Vugt, Y., Stinear, J., Claire Davies, T., Zhang, Y., 2019. Postural stability during gait for adults with hereditary spastic paraparesis. J. Biomech. 88, 12–17.

van Walsem, M.R., et al., 2015. Unmet needs for healthcare and social support services in patients with Huntington's disease: a cross-sectional population-based study. Orphanet. J. Rare. Dis. 10, 124.

Veenhuizen, R.B., et al., 2011. Coordinated multidisciplinary care for ambulatory Huntington's disease patients. Evaluation of 18 months of implementation. Orphanet. J. Rare. Dis. 6, 77.

Veenhuizen, R.B., Tibben, A., 2009. Coordinated multidisciplinary care for Huntington's disease. An outpatient department. Brain. Res. Bull. 80, 192–195.

Velázquez-Pérez, L., Rodríguez-Diaz, J.C., Rodríguez-Labrada, R., et al., 2019. Neurorehabilitation improves the motor features in prodromal SCA2: a randomized, controlled trial. Mov. Disord. 34, 1060–1068.

Viel, E.J., et al., 2002. Neurolytic blockade of the obturator nerve for intractable spasticity of adductor thigh muscles. Eur. J. Pain. 6, 97–104.

Walker, F.O., 2007. Huntington's disease. Lancet 369, 218–228.

Watanabe, M., et al., 1996. Analysis of CAG trinucleotide expansion associated with Machado-Joseph disease. J. Neurol. Sci. 136, 101–107.

Wexler, N.S., et al., 2004. Venezuelan kindreds reveal that genetic and environmental factors modulate Huntington's disease age of onset. Proc. Nat. Acad. Sci. U S A. 101, 3498–3503.

Weyer, A., et al., 2007. Reliability and validity of the scale for the assessment and rating of ataxia: a study in 64 ataxia patients. Mov. Disord. 22, 1633–1637.

Wijeyekoon, R., Barker, R.A., 2011. The current status of neural grafting in the treatment of Huntington's disease. A review. Front. Integr. Neurosci. 5, 78.

Wild, E.J., et al., 2014. Targets for future clinical trials in Huntington's disease: what's in the pipeline? Mov. Disord. 29, 1434–1445.

Winnberg, E., Winnberg, U., Pohlkamp, L., Hagberg, A., 2018. What to do with a second chance in life? Long-term experiences of non-carriers of Huntington's disease. J. Genet. Counsel. 27, 1438–1446.

Wojtecki, L., et al., 2016. Deep brain stimulation in Huntington's disease-preliminary evidence on pathophysiology, efficacy and safety. Brain. Sci. 6, E38.

Yabe, I., et al., 2008. Usefulness of the scale for assessment and rating of ataxia (SARA). J. Neurol. Sci. 266, 164–166.

Zielonka, D., et al., 2014. Skeletal muscle pathology in Huntington's disease. Front. Physiol. 5, 380.

Zinzi, P., et al., 2007. Effects of an intensive rehabilitation programme on patients with Huntington's disease: a pilot study. Clin. Rehabil. 21, 603–613.

Motor Neurone Disease

Caroline Brown and Vanina Dal Bello-Haas

OUTLINE

Introduction, 327
Epidemiology, 327
Anatomy and Pathophysiology, 328
Genetic Factors, 328
Geographical and Environmental Factors, 329
Clinical Phenotypes, 329
Diagnosis, 329
(Early) Medical Management, 330
Signs, Symptoms and Clinical Presentation, 333
Assessment and Prognosis, 334
    Disease-Specific Measures, 336
    Prognosis, 337

Time Course and Corresponding Management, 338
Treatment Selection and Secondary Complications and
    Special Problems, 339
    Assistive Devices and Orthoses, 341
    Exercise in Motor Neurone Disease, 341
        Overwork Damage Versus Disuse Atrophy, 341
    Types of Exercise, 342
    Evolving Wheelchair Needs, 343
    Respiratory Issues, 344
Conclusion, 347
Case Study, 348

INTRODUCTION

Motor neurone disease (MND) is the term given to a group of chronic neurodegenerative diseases that selectively affect motor neurones, leading to progressive muscle loss and dysfunction. In the UK, MND is synonymous with amyotrophic lateral sclerosis (ALS), a term more commonly used in Canada and the USA. ALS is the most common MND (Leighton et al 2019); many studies have explored its incidence, finding it makes up between 67% and 95% of MND cases (Burchardt et al 2022). This interchangeable use of terms when talking about the same disease can be a source of much confusion, particularly for patients, although neurologists generally agree that they are referring to the same pathology. MND is known as ALS when both upper and lower motor neurones are affected; over time other forms of MND can progress to become ALS (Hardiman et al 2017).

MND is a progressive and inevitably fatal disease associated with destruction of both lower motor neurones (LMNs) arising from the spinal cord and brainstem, and upper motor neurones (UMNs) from the cerebral cortex. The aetiology of MND is often unknown; there is no cure and median life expectancy after diagnosis is 2–4 years (Park et al 2022). Supportive measures can be tailored to meet a person's needs when delivered by a multidisciplinary team (MDT), with a focus on alleviating symptoms and maintaining functional ability, enabling people with MND to live as full a life as possible. In this regard, a knowledgeable and suitability skilled physiotherapist is considered a core member of the MDT. The aim of this chapter is to outline the physiotherapist's role in the MND MDT and provide the theory and evidence to equip the physiotherapist to address the individual needs of patients.

EPIDEMIOLOGY

The crude incidence rate of MND is estimated to be 1.59–1.75 cases per 100,000 worldwide with deaths resulting from MND said to be 12.39%. A lower frequency (<1 per 100,000) has been demonstrated in the South and East Asian community with 2.35 cases reported per 100,000 in Western Europe (Burchardt et al 2022). MND is a relatively rare disease primarily affecting adults, with neurologists estimating that the incidence of MND in England ranges from 1.06 to 2.98 per 100,000 (Opie-Martin et al 2021). A large study (Burchardt et al 2022) analysing the incidence of MND in England based on the records of 16.8 million patients drawn from national general practitioner (GP) records, hospital episode statistics and death certificates suggests an increased incidence of 5.75 per 100,000. This study which aligns with other studies (Longinetti & Fang 2019, Park et al 2022) found MND to be more common in men, with a ratio of 2:1. Median age of diagnosis is 72 years with incidence rates peaking in the 80- to 84-year age group for men and the 75- to 79-year age group for women. Age-standardised incidence for MND was similar in Bangladeshi, Caribbean, Indian, other Asian, Pakistani and White people and relatively lower in Black African and Chinese people.

A person's lifetime risk for development of MND is up to 1 in 300. Based on mostly UK population studies, 1–2 cases per 100,000 people are diagnosed with MND each year, which represents an estimated 6 cases diagnosed per day (Brown & Al-Chalabi 2017). As the progression of MND can be rapid, fewer people are living with this disease than one might expect with a 1 in 300 risk. Median survival is 24–50 months (Park et al 2022), meaning that approximately 5000 individuals have MND at any given time (which is why MND is not seen as a common disease). The global prevalence and impact of MND is continuously increasing as life expectancy increases, especially in middle- and high-income areas. Modelling has predicted a 30% increase in UK cases between 2016 and 2040, based on detailed survival estimates (by age group and by sex) (Gowland et al 2019).

ANATOMY AND PATHOPHYSIOLOGY

Jean-Martin Charcot first described the clinical features of MND in a series of lectures in the 1860's and 1870's. Although his description of the clinical and pathological features of MND remains relevant, the pace of recent research discoveries has significantly advanced the understanding of disease triggers and mechanisms. Arora and Khan (2022) notes that although the exact cause of MND remains unknown, it is thought to be initiated by a complex interaction between several underlying contributory factors which include genetic, environmental and lifestyle influences. These factors must all coincide to trigger the disease process and, once the disease begins, several processes occur in both neurones and glial cells, although

how these mechanisms transpire is another area of active research. Almost all knowledge regarding the pathophysiology of motor neurone degeneration in MND is derived from inferences drawn from cellular changes postmortem or from the SOD1 mouse model (a genetically modified mouse that presents with ALS symptoms). There are several shared themes between MND and other neurodegenerative diseases put forwards as potential cellular mechanisms contributing to degeneration after disease onset (Sweeney et al 2017). Some of the suggested mechanisms are:

- Protein misfolding (aggregation): The aggregation of misfolded protein in degenerating neurones may influence wild protein and disrupt their normal function, which explains how a disease that begins in one area can be widely transmitted in the brain.
- Defects in ribonucleic acid (RNA) processing: Evidence increasingly points to abnormal RNA processing and metabolism underlying the disease, which may occur by local spread, through neuronal networks or through effecting populations of cells made vulnerable by developmental errors.
- Other cellular mechanisms implicated as a primary mechanism of motor neurone death (Morrice et al 2017) include mitochondrial dysfunction, oxidative stress, disrupted axonal transport, glutamate-induced excitotoxicity, inflammation and apoptosis.

GENETIC FACTORS

Emerging evidence of the complex interaction between the molecular and genetic pathways underlying the development of MND has dramatically advanced the understanding of familial forms of MND (fMND), with several abnormal genes identified. Of all MND cases, 10%–15% can be attributed to pathological variants in a single identifiable gene. The two most common forms of fMND are related to mutations on the *SOD 1* gene (20%) and *C90FR72* gene (40%). VariantsFUS and TARDBP account for less than 5% each, and variants in more than 20 other genes each account for less than 1% (Dharmadasa et al 2022).

The *C90RF72* mutations are most common in those with European ancestry, associated with a specific type of MND, characterised by earlier onset, a more aggressive course of the disease, bulbar onset and the occurrence of cognitive and behavioural deficits (Burrell et al 2016). Hence the *C9ORF72* mutation has a high association with disability and death (Park et al 2022). About 35% of people will demonstrate signs of mild cognitive change, affecting their ability to make decisions and plan ahead, whereas 10%–15% of people will show signs of frontotemporal dementia (FTD), which causes cognitive dysfunction, behavioural changes and issues with decision making (Dharmadasa et al 2022).

GEOGRAPHICAL AND ENVIRONMENTAL FACTORS

Approximately 5%–10% of MND cases are fMND, with the rest attributed to sporadic MND (sMND). The cause of sMND is not known, although several geographical and environmental risk factors are suspected. Attention has been focused more recently on repetitive head trauma and a link to chronic traumatic encephalopathy, but no consistent causal factor has been identified. Other factors commonly mentioned in studies include physical athleticism, military service, maternal age, pesticide or heavy metal exposure, statins, cigarette smoking and infectious causes, but there is little evidence to support any of these reasons (Chen et al 2022). It seems likely that there are some relevant environmental exposure factors that have yet to be discovered.

FURTHERING KNOWLEDGE COMMENT

The relationship between MND and physical activity, especially contact sports, is an active area for research following the diagnosis of several high-profile professional athletes. Former Leeds Rhinos scrum-half and MND Association Patron Rob Burrow MBE is the most high profile in the UK because of his campaign to raise awareness of MND. He was diagnosed with MND in December 2019, 2 years after retiring, after captaining Leeds to a record-extending eighth Super League Grand Final. The documentary Rob Burrow: My Year with MND shared Rob's journey since his diagnosis, allowing the world to see how MND affects thousands of families in the UK every day. It is available via this link: https://www.youtube.com/watch?v=y-y014GAhKo.

A cohort study of Italian professional football players demonstrated a severe increase in the incidence of ALS. The study by Chio et al (2005) showed a correlation between head injuries in football players and an increased risk for ALS. Trauma to other parts of the body was not associated with increased risk. A small, updated study suggested a twofold risk of ALS for professional football players and a 20-year earlier disease onset (Pupillo et al 2020) with similar findings echoing this outcome in a Scottish cohort of players (Mackay et al 2019). A study by Chen et al (2022) supports findings that exposure to repeated head injury with concussion as a result of physical activity (especially from heading the ball in football) could be associated with an increased risk of MND. They also extended this finding to potentially include individuals with head injuries that occurred secondary to trauma such as domestic violence or a road traffic collision.

CLINICAL PHENOTYPES

MND can be classed into four main phenotypes depending on the site of origin and severity of neurological involvement (Arora & Khan 2022, Oliver 2016):

1. ALS: Accounts for 60%–80% of all cases of MND, patients present with combined UMN and LMN involvement. Average survival is 2–5 years; incidence is greater in men and peaks around 75–79 years of age.

2. Bulbar-onset ALS: Accounts for 20% of all cases of MND and is the term to describe MND selectively affecting the bulbar muscles, causing dysarthria and dysphasia, although most patients have some limb involvement. Bulbar-onset ALS, which is well known for its poor prognosis compared with limb-onset ALS, is more common in regions of European ancestry than in Asia.

3. Progressive muscular atrophy: Accounts for 5%–10% of cases and is the term describing the LMN-only form of MND, although some patients experience UMN signs later. It is more common in men than women (5:1) and is associated with slower disease progression, with patients typically living 12 months longer than individuals with ALS.

4. Primary lateral sclerosis: Is less common, accounting for 0.5% of cases, and is the term used to describe pure UMN involvement, although 50% of cases progress to the ALS phenotype. Disease progression is slower; therefore patients have a better prognosis.

DIAGNOSIS

Early diagnosis of MND is vital in ensuring an individual receives early access to appropriate multidisciplinary care to optimise their quality of life and survival. People with MND experience a diagnostic delay of 10–16 months from symptom onset (Richards et al 2020), although studies indicate this period has significantly increased because of the Covid-19 pandemic lockdown periods. Pre-Covid data note a median time to diagnosis of 399 days with 5.2% of MND patients presenting as undiagnosed emergencies. Post-Covid diagnostic delays of between 558 and 915 days have been described with emergency presentations ranging from 15% to 45% depending on the demand on primary and secondary care (Burchill et al 2023).

For people living with MND any delay results in diagnosis occurring at a later stage of disease progression. The impact of these delays on those living with and affected by MND should be considered in pandemic recovery planning. Receiving a diagnosis of a terminal condition in later-stage disease progression results in reduced time to process the implications of the diagnosis for both the patient and their loved ones. Practically it limits the opportunity for access to supportive measures offered by MDTs to people living with MND. This includes voice banking, respiratory and nutritional support in addition to advanced care planning, all of which are important factors in securing improved quality of life and survival.

The increase in emergency and late-stage presentations reflects this reduced access to complex but time-sensitive conversations and decision-making on gastrostomy tube placement and noninvasive respiratory support. Late diagnosis restricts this opportunity, potentially resulting in people with MND experiencing rapid escalation to palliative care and respiratory care services.

Before the pandemic the recognised lag in symptom onset to diagnosis of MND led to the UK implementation of the Red Flags checklist in 2014 which was updated in 2022 (MNDA & Royal College of General Practitioners 2022). The MNDA's red flag diagnosis tool for GPs, produced in partnership with the Royal College of General Practitioners (MNDA & Royal College of General Practitioners 2022), aims to prompt GPs to look for additional symptoms, consider the possibility of a neurodegenerative condition, improve timely referrals to neurology, and therefore speed up the time to accurate diagnosis (Fig. 13.1).

FURTHERING KNOWLEDGE LINK

MNDA's red flag diagnosis tool: https://www.mndassociation.org/app/uploads/2013/10/red-flags-final-2.pdf

Because of a lack of definitive diagnostic tests or biological markers, MND diagnosis can be made by clinical findings of a progressive course of weakness, with both UMN and LMN findings in four anatomically defined regions of the body: brainstem (bulbar), cervical, thoracic and lumbosacral. Differential medical diagnosis includes exclusion of other musculoskeletal, neurological or systemic conditions. The El Escorial World Federation of Neurology criteria for the diagnosis of ALS (possible, probable and definite) have been widely accepted since 1994 (Arora & Khan 2022) as a means to include or exclude patients from clinical trials and research, and they were revised in 2000. These criteria are considered too rigorous for application in clinical practice and do not improve accuracy of diagnosis over that of an experienced neurologist and potentially could contribute to diagnostic delays. Therefore diagnosis remains clinical, using investigations to exclude other causes.

Electrophysiological, muscle biopsy and neuroimaging studies can be used to support the diagnosis of MND and to rule out other diagnoses. Nerve conduction studies of peripheral sensory and motor neurones are usually normal or near normal in MND, whereas electromyographic

(EMG) studies typically reveal signs of active denervation. Muscle biopsy studies corroborate EMG findings, showing signs of denervation (i.e., atrophied muscle fibres) and reinnervation (i.e., fibre type grouping). Degeneration of corticospinal tracts and altered cortical activation during motor tasks have been detected in patients with MND using conventional magnetic resonance imaging (MRI), transcranial magnetic stimulation, proton magnetic resonance spectroscopy, functional MRI (fMRI) and diffusion tensor MRI. Blood tests exclude hypothyroidism, hyperparathyroidism, HIV and Lyme disease. Lumbar puncture is considered in atypical presentations of the condition to exclude infiltrative or inflammatory disease. Genetic testing may be considered in individuals with relevant clinical characteristics such as young onset or a family history of neurodegenerative disorders. Genetic counselling may also be important to complement genetic testing given the potential impact of the diagnosis of the family.

Ideally the diagnosis, prognosis and information regarding the subsequent management of MND should be sensitively delivered by a consultant neurologist who has up-to-date knowledge and experience of treating people with MND. The NICE guidelines for the assessment and management of MND (NICE 2016) recommend that a neurologist takes the time to discuss an individual's (and their family's) concerns and questions, if the patient wishes to discuss them at the time of diagnosis. An emphasis on the treatment and support available including the role of the MDT should be explained with the patient given a single point of contact for access to the MND MDT. Because people with MND can experience problems communicating, it is important that individuals are offered a range of different contact options including text or e-mail to access support. Early and continuing follow-up is advised, with guidelines suggesting that an initial follow-up should be arranged 4 weeks after diagnosis (NICE 2016, Shoesmith et al 2020).

FURTHERING KNOWLEDGE LINK

NICE guideline for MND: https://www.nice.org.uk/guidance/ng42/resources/motor-neurone-disease-assessment-and-management-pdf-1837449470149

(EARLY) MEDICAL MANAGEMENT

Although there is no cure for MND, clinical trials to evaluate medications for reducing mortality and treating symptoms are ongoing. At present, riluzole (Rilutek®) is the only medication approved to treat MND in the UK. The drug, a glutamate inhibitor, delays disease progression modestly, extending survival for approximately 3 months (Rafiq

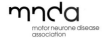

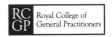

Painless, progressive weakness – Could this be Motor Neurone Disease?

1. Does the patient have one or more of these symptoms?

Bulbar features

- Dysarthria
  - Slurred or quiet speech often when tired
- Dysphagia
  - Liquids and/or solids
  - Excessive saliva
  - Choking sensation especially when lying flat
- Tongue fasciculations

Limb features

- Focal weakness
- Falls/trips – from foot drop
- Loss of dexterity
- Muscle wasting
- Muscle twitching/ fasciculations
- Cramps
- No sensory features

Respiratory features

- Hard to explain respiratory symptoms
- Shortness of breath on exertion
- Excessive daytime sleepiness
- Fatigue
- Early morning headache
- Orthopnoea

Cognitive features (rare)

- Behavioural change
- Emotional lability
  (not related to dementia)
- Fronto-temporal dementia

2. Is there progression?

Supporting factors

- Asymmetrical features
- Age – MND can present at any age
- Positive family history of MND or other neurodegenerative disease

Factors NOT supportive of MND diagnosis

- Bladder / bowel involvement
- Prominent sensory symptoms
- Double vision / Ptosis
- Improving symptoms

If yes to 1 and 2 query MND and refer to Neurology

If you think it might be MND please state explicitly in the referral letter.
Common causes of delay are initial referral to ENT or Orthopaedic services.

Additional resources:

MND Association downloads and publications at www.mndassociation.org/gp

FIG. 13.1 Motor Neurone Disease Association's Red Flag Diagnosis Tool for Motor Neurone Disease. *MND*, Motor neurone disease. (From https://www.mndassociation.org/app/uploads/2013/10/red-flags-final-2.pdf.)

Bulbar features

25% of patients present with bulbar symptoms

- Dysarthria
  - Quiet, hoarse or altered speech
  - Slurring of speech often when tired
- Dysphagia – more often liquids first and later solids. Initially can be sensation of catching in throat or choking when drinking quickly.
- Excessive saliva
- Choking sensation when lying flat
- Weak cough – often not noticed by the patient

Painless progressive dysarthria – consider neurological referral rather than ENT.

Limb features

70% of patients present with limb symptoms

- Focal weakness – painless with preserved sensation
- Distal weakness
  - Falls/trips – from foot drop
  - Loss of dexterity eg problems with zips or buttons
- Muscle wasting – hands and shoulders. Typically asymmetrical
- Muscle twitching/fasciculations
- Cramps

Respiratory features

Respiratory problems are often a late feature of MND and an unusual presenting feature. Patients present with features of neuromuscular respiratory failure

- Shortness of breath on exertion
- Excessive daytime sleepiness
- Fatigue
- Early morning headache. Patients often describe a 'muzziness' in the morning, being slow to get going or as if hung over
- Un-refreshing sleep
- Orthopnoea
- Frequent unexplained chest infections
- Weak cough and sniff
- Nocturnal restlessness and/or sweating

Consider MND if investigations for breathlessness do not support a pulmonary or cardiac cause.

Cognitive features

Frank dementia at presentation is rare. Cognitive dysfunction is increasingly recognised, as evidenced by:

- Behavioural change such as apathy or lack of motivation
- Difficulty with complex tasks
- Lack of concentration
- Emotional lability (not related to dementia)

Ask specifically about a family history of these features.

Development group for this resource:

RCGP (L Davies, R Pizzaro-Duhart, I Rafi) MND Association (J Bedford, H Fairfield)
Neurology (P Callagher, C McDermott, K Morrison, R Orrell, A Radunovic, S Weatherby, A Wills) Palliative Medicine (I Baker)

FIG. 13.1, cont'd

2018). The drug is usually well tolerated, but adverse effects do occur and include asthenia, nausea, vomiting, dizziness, liver toxicity and neutropaenia (Arora & Khan 2022). Regular blood testing every month for the first 3 months, followed by every 3 months for 9 months and then yearly, is recommended.

A new medicine called edaravone for use in selected patients with ALS has been approved for use in Canada and the USA. The Food and Drug Administration (FDA) approved an oral form of edaravone known as Radicava ORS. Radicava ORS is an orally administered version of Radicava, which was approved by the FDA in 2017 as an intravenous infusion. Radicava ORS can be self-administered at home and has been shown to impede disease progression in patients with early-onset disease and rapid disease progression (Takei et al 2017). The drug acts as an antioxidant, which has been shown to prevent the nitration of tyrosine residues in experimental animal models.

FURTHERING KNOWLEDGE LINK

European Clinical Trial of Edaravone: Radicava (edaravone) is currently not approved for use in the UK for people living with MND. A new trial, called ADORE, which is investigating an oral form of edaravone (FAB122) recently started recruiting in Europe. Trial sites in the UK are currently 'in preparation'. The trial is randomised, double-blind and placebo controlled and aims to recruit 300 participants (ClinicalTrials.gov Identifier: NCT05178810).

SIGNS, SYMPTOMS AND CLINICAL PRESENTATION

Muscle weakness is considered the cardinal sign of MND and may be caused by LMN or UMN loss, but LMN loss weakness causes much more significant dysfunction than the UMN loss weakness. The 'classic' presentation of MND is slowly progressive asymmetric muscular weakness and atrophy indicative of LMN involvement along with UMN signs of hyperreflexia.

In 70%–80% of patients, symptoms begin in the extremities (i.e., limb-onset MND), whereas 20%–30% of patients present with bulbar symptoms (i.e., bulbar-onset MND) (Connolly et al 2020). Patients with early lower extremity (LE) involvement may notice tripping, stumbling or awkwardness when walking or running. For example, an individual may notice the foot 'slaps' when walking or increased frequency of tripping. Those with upper extremity (UE) involvement may notice difficulties with fine motor tasks, such as picking up small objects or buttoning shirts.

Bulbar-onset MND occurs more frequently in middle-aged women, and initial symptoms may include changes in voice quality, difficulty moving the tongue, decreased ability to move the lips or open or close the mouth, and difficulty chewing, swallowing and speaking (Connolly et al 2020). As MND progresses, the number of muscles that are weak and the extent of muscle weakness increases.

In addition to limb and bulbar weakness, individuals with MND also experience cervical and thoracic extensor muscle weakness. Early symptoms may include neck stiffness, heaviness and fatigue with holding up the head (e.g., with reading or writing), or difficulties in keeping the head upright with unexpected movements, such as in an accelerating car. With more severe weakness, the head may fall forwards and may become completely flexed causing cervical pain, because of overstretching of the posterior musculature and soft tissues, and patients may experience problems with swallowing and ambulation. Truncal weakness results in poor sitting postures, with patients slouching in attempts to keep their gaze horizontal. During walking some patients will attempt to compensate for the forwards flexed head posture with excessive lumbar lordosis, as they attempt to maintain their posture during ambulation.

As the muscle fibres progressively denervate, muscle fibre volume decreases, resulting in atrophy. Fasciculations are common in individuals with MND, although they are rarely an initial symptom (Rafiq 2018). Other LMN signs include hyporeflexia, decreased or absent reflexes, decreased muscle tone or flaccidity, and muscle cramps, which are also very common. In individuals with MND, muscle cramps may occur in uncommon sites such as the tongue, jaw, neck, abdomen, arms and hands, in addition to more common sites such as the calf or thigh.

UMN degeneration causes impaired activation of motor neurones (reduced central motor drive) and results in decreased firing rates, motor unit recruitment and diminished muscle activation. UMN pathology is characterised by spasticity, hypertonicity, hyperreflexia, clonus and pathological reflexes such as a Babinski or Hoffmann sign. Although UMN loss may also cause muscle weakness, the extent of muscle weakness is overshadowed by the muscle weakness caused by LMN loss. Spasticity can cause contractures and deformities, as well as dyssynergic movement patterns, abnormal timing, loss of dexterity and fatigue, all which affect motor control and function. For example, distal spasticity can cause difficulties with the swing phase of ambulation, and generalised spasticity may cause balance problems.

Approximately one-third of individuals with MND may have clinically significant cognitive impairments (Connolly et al 2020). MND-associated FTD is characterised by cognitive decline; executive functioning impairments; difficulties with planning, organisation and concept abstraction; and personality and behavioural changes. Individuals with MND, without FTD, have been reported to have a variety of cognitive impairments, such as generalised impairments in intellectual function, as well as difficulties with verbal fluency, language comprehension, memory and abstract reasoning. Individuals with bulbar-onset MND are more likely to have cognitive impairments than those with limb-onset disease. Physiotherapists will need to consider that some patients with MND will lack capacity, and therefore any interventions they provide should be provided in line with the Mental Capacity Act (Department of Health 2005). Pseudobulbar affect is a term used to describe emotional incontinence or emotional lability. Although pseudobulbar affect is commonly treated with antidepressants, it is not a mood disorder. Mood incongruence or uncontrolled, spontaneous crying or laughter occurs without the necessary emotional triggers, or emotional responses are exaggerated. Pseudobulbar affect occurs in as many as 50% of individuals with MND and is more common in individuals with spastic bulbar palsy.

Clinical features that are not typical of MND include sensory dysfunction, sphincter impairment, autonomic dysfunction, abnormalities of eye movements, movement disorders and cognitive dysfunction. Sensory pathways for the most part are spared in MND, although studies have reported pathological findings in peripheral sensory neurones, Clarke's neurones and the spinocerebellar tracts, and the dorsal columns. Some individuals with MND may describe vague, ill-defined sensory symptoms of paraesthesia or focal pain. Motor neurones in the Onufrowicz nucleus (Onuf's nucleus) at the second sacral level in the spinal cord that control the anal and external urethral sphincter muscles and muscles of the pelvic floor are also generally spared. However, some individuals do experience urinary symptoms, such as urgency, obstructive micturition, or both, suggesting that supranuclear control over sympathetic, parasympathetic and somatic neurones may be abnormal in MND (Arora & Khan 2022). The oculomotor, trochlear and abducens nerves that control external ocular muscles are typically spared until late stages of the disease. Individuals who are maintained on long-term ventilation may experience development of ophthalmoplegia, a complete ocular paralysis and inability to tightly close the eyes because of degeneration of these nerves.

ASSESSMENT AND PROGNOSIS

Because of the variety and various combinations of regions affected in MND, therapists must conduct a careful and comprehensive examination of each patient to determine the extent of their primary, secondary and composite impairments, and how those impairments are related to their activity limitations and participation restrictions. Reexamination at regular intervals using standard outcome measures is necessary to determine the extent and rate of progression of the disease, and to ensure that therapeutic interventions are administered in a timely manner (e.g., percutaneous endoscopic gastrostomy [PEG] placement before a patient's forced vital capacity [FVC] is <50% of predicted vital capacity [VC]) (NICE 2016, Walsh et al 2021). The extent and timing of reexaminations may depend on whether the therapist is part of an MND MDT or an independent, clinic-based therapist and the severity of the patient's disease. Therapists who are working as team members may have a more circumscribed role related to assessment of gross motor function and activities of daily living (ADLs), whereas clinic-based therapists may need to carry out more comprehensive assessments that also examine bulbar and respiratory function, environmental barriers to independence and caregiver demands. The NICE (2016) MND guidelines suggest carrying out coordinated assessments in the MDT team clinic, every 2–3 months, to assess patients' symptoms and needs, although the frequency should be tailored to a person's individual requirements. Therapists must consider whether the benefits of repeated testing of patients who are in a weakened and debilitated state, particularly during the late-middle and late stages of the disease, outweigh the potential negative psychological impact on the patient.

The Covid-19 pandemic necessitated major changes to the delivery of multidisciplinary care across all neurological services with face-to-face appointments postponed or cancelled, causing significant delays and disruptions to MND specialist care. Furthermore, MND-specific services such as provision of gastrostomy, respiratory function testing and noninvasive ventilation (NIV) have been reported to be adversely affected (Glasmacher et al 2021). Healthcare provision for people with MND has had to adapt new delivery models, with increased use of telehealth and remote monitoring.

Although telephone appointments were generally regarded positively, concerns were raised by people with MND and healthcare professionals (HCPs) about the suitability of these for patients with bulbar dysfunction or communication difficulties, and a fear of missing MND-related symptoms requiring urgent treatment (Musson et al 2022). A balance was required between the provision of remote (telephone or video call) appointments to keep people safe and being able to adequately assess and monitor symptoms. Musson et al (2022) recommends that HCPs advocate patient choice regarding the type of consultation they receive, particularly for patients with dysarthria or when patients require initiation of NIV, with the option of home visits offered when feasible. Drive-through testing was recommended (e.g., phlebotomy and respiratory blood gases) to avoid patients coming into hospital for these tests. To ensure a multidisciplinary approach to MND care continues, it is recommended that HCPs hold regular virtual MDT meetings and provide e-mail, telephone or virtual support to other services to maintain access to coordinated multidisciplinary care.

A regular thorough holistic assessment of the patient should be conducted including assessment of cognition, psychosocial function, pain, range of motion (ROM), muscle length and performance, UE and LE motor function, reflex and cranial nerve integrity, the sensory system, the respiratory system, fatigue, the integumentary system, balance, gait, functional performance posture, body mechanics and ergonomics. Few tests and measures specifically validated in MND are available at the impairment and activity levels (Table 13.1). It is important to include participation tests and measures because they may be more positively affected by physical therapy interventions than impairment and activity level measures because of the progressive nature of the disease. Environmental barriers to ADLs and quality of life should also be assessed. The need to self-isolate during the pandemic resulted in individuals with MND describing increased feelings of loneliness, anxiety and depression, with the need for additional contact and reassurance from HCPs (Cabona et al 2021, Consonni et al 2021).

The types of pain in ALS patients have not been well described, but pain is a common (prevalence 15%–85%) (Chio et al 2017, Kwak 2022) and significant symptom of MND which is deserving of more consideration by HCPs. A recent review outlines how primary pain in patients with MND includes neuropathic pain and pain from spasticity or cramps. Secondary pain is mainly nociceptive, occurring with the progression of muscle weakness and atrophy, prolonged immobility causing degenerative changes in joints and connective tissue, and long-term home mechanical ventilation (HMV) either noninvasively by mask interface or invasively by tracheostomy (Kwak 2022). Pain should be assessed subjectively and objectively during the course of the disease, possibly using a numerical rating scale (0 = no pain to 10 = the worst pain imaginable) or the Visual Analogue Scale (VAS) to detect individual fluctuations of pain (Akerblom et al 2021). Whilst the use of standardised procedures for pain assessment is uncommon, the Brief Pain Inventory is a validated tool for people with MND that uses both open questions and VAS (Keller et al 2004).

ROM, muscle length, muscle performance and sensory integrity should be assessed using standard assessment methods, and initiation, modification and control of movement patterns and voluntary postures can be assessed

TABLE 13.1 Outcome Measures for Use With People With Motor Neurone Disease

Motor Neurone Disease Specific

Disease Specific
- Amyotrophic Lateral Sclerosis Functional Rating Scale
- LSFRS-Revised
- Appel ALS Scale
- ALS Severity Scale
- Norris Scale

Cognition and Behaviour
- ALS Cognitive Behavioral Screen
- Edinburgh Cognitive and Behavioural ALS Screen

Psychosocial Function
- ALS Depression Inventory 12

Quality of Life
- ALS Assessment Questionnaire 40
- ALS Assessment Questionnaire 5
- ALS-Specific Quality of Life Instrument

Other

Psychosocial Function
- Spielberger State-Trait Anxiety Inventory
- Pain
- Visual Analogue Scale

Postural Control and Balance
- Tinetti Performance Oriented Mobility Assessment
- Timed Up and Go

Fatigue
- Fatigue Severity Scale
- Multidimensional Fatigue Inventory

Function
- Functional Independence Measure

ALS, Amyotrophic lateral sclerosis; *ALSFRS,* Amyotrophic Lateral Sclerosis Functional Rating Scale.

through observations. Deep tendon reflexes, pathological reflexes (e.g., Babinski or Hoffman sign) and muscle tone using the Modified Ashworth Scale should be assessed to determine UMN versus LMN involvement. Evaluation of bulbar function includes testing of cranial nerves III, IV, V, VI, VII, IX, X, and XII. Oral motor function, phonation and speech production can be assessed through the interview and observation. Referral to a nutritionist and speech language pathologist for consultation is recommended.

Because respiratory failure is the major cause of death in MND, respiratory status and function should be closely monitored. Regular assessment (every 2–3 months) of

TABLE 13.2 Respiratory Function Test Results Indicating Need for Noninvasive Ventilation (NICE MND Guidelines 2016)

FVC or VC	SNIP and/or MIP (if both tests are performed, base the assessment on the better respiratory function reading)
VC or VC <50% of predicted value	SNIP or MIP <40 cm H_2O
FVC or VC <80% of predicted value plus any symptoms or signs of respiratory impairment (see Table 13.4), particularly orthopnoea	SNIP or MIP <65 cm H_2O for men or 55 cm H_2O for women plus any symptoms or signs of respiratory impairment (see Table 13.4), particularly orthopnoea
	Repeated regular tests show a rate of decrease of SNIP or MIP of >10 cm H_2O per 3 months

FVC, Forced vital capacity; *MIP,* maximal inspiratory pressure; *SNIP,* sniff nasal inspiratory pressure; *VC,* vital capacity.

respiratory function includes the patient's report of respiratory symptoms and inspection of the patient's respiratory rate, rhythm, depth, chest expansion, work of breathing, auscultation of breath sounds, cough, sniff effectiveness, oxygen saturations and VC or FVC testing using a handheld spirometer (Table 13.2). Aerobic capacity and endurance may be assessed in earlier stages of MND using standardised exercise test protocols to evaluate and monitor responses to aerobic conditioning and should be assessed during functional activities.

No MND-specific measures for fatigue exist; however, the (Krupp) Fatigue Severity Scale, Edmonton Symptom Assessment Scale (a generic tool which documents changes in patient-reported symptoms) and VAS to document patient-reported symptoms have been used in clinical studies (Beswick et al 2022). Skin integrity is usually not compromised in MND, even in the late stage, because sensation is normally preserved. Skin inspection at contact points between the body and assistive, adaptive, orthotic, protective and supportive devices, mobility devices and the sleeping surface should be performed regularly, especially when the patient becomes immobile. Swelling of the distal limbs because of a lack of muscle pumping action from weakened limbs should also be evaluated. HCPs are encouraged to consider venous thromboembolism (VTE) as a potential root cause for new leg swelling or pain because there appears to be an increased risk of VTE in MND

patients with leg onset and in patients with poor mobility (Shoesmith et al 2020).

No MND-specific balance test or measure exists; balance tests that have been used in other neuromuscular patient populations include the Tinetti Performance Oriented Mobility Assessment (Tinetti 1986), the Timed Up and Go (TUG) (Podsiadlo & Richardson 1991) test, Berg Balance Scale (Berg et al 1992) and the Functional Reach Test (Duncan et al 1990). Low total Tinetti Balance Test scores, indicating impaired balance, were found to be moderately to strongly related to LE muscle weakness and activity limitations in individuals with MND (Kloos et al 2004) and have been found to be a reliable measure for individuals in the early or early to middle stages of MND (Kloos et al 2004). A recent study found that TUG times increased linearly over 6 months, were negatively correlated with manual muscle testing scores and functional measures and predicted falls using a cutoff of 14 seconds in 31 patients with MND (Montes et al 2007, Sukockienė et al 2021).

Gait stability, efficiency, safety and endurance with or without the use of orthotic and assistive devices should be assessed regularly. Timed 15-foot walk tests have been used to assess gait in clinical trials. Functional mobility skills, safety and energy expenditure should be assessed. The Functional Independence Measure has been used to document functional status in clinical trials. Basic and instrumental ADLs and the need for adaptive equipment may also be assessed by an occupational therapist. Static and dynamic postural alignment and position, ergonomics and body mechanics during self-care, home management, work, community or leisure activities should be assessed. Caregivers should also be assessed in these areas when the patient requires physical assistance from them.

Disease-Specific Measures

The ALS Functional Rating Scale (ALSFRS) (ALS CNTF Treatment Study Phase I-II Study Group 1996) and the revised version, which includes additional respiratory items (ALSFRS-R) (Cederbaum et al 1999), are used to measure functional status and change in patients with MND. The individual is asked to rate their function for the 10–12 items on a scale from 4 (normal function) to 0 (unable to attempt the task). Both scales have been found to be valid and reliable for measuring the decline in function that results from loss of muscular strength when administered in the clinic and via telephone interview, and to predict 9-month survival in individuals with ALS. The NICE (2016) MND guidelines recommend considering a lower ALSFRS-R score as a prognostic factor when planning care, which could be associated with shorter survival if present at diagnosis. Other disease-specific scales include the Appel ALS Scale, ALS Severity Scale and Norris Scale. ALSFRS-R is the primary outcome measure used in clinical trials and research in ALS but is limited by floor and ceiling effects, meaning clinically meaningful changes for individuals can be missed (Hayden et al 2022). Research has begun to focus on the development of assessment devices that adequately address the current limitations of measurement instruments such as the ALSFRS-R in a reproducible, user-friendly and inexpensive manner. Although no currently available device has met all the necessary criteria to ensure universal acceptance in clinical practice, there is clearly a demand for use of technological innovation that is easy to set up, user suitable and which can be used remotely.

There are several tools available to assess cognitive or behavioural impairment, but no standard tool is currently in use. ALS-specific neuropsychological screening instruments have been developed that consider people with MND motor and communication difficulties.

The ALS Cognitive Behavioural Screen (ALS-CBS), an executive function screen, assesses two components: (1) cognitive function, including attention, concentration, working memory, fluency and tracking; and (2) behavioural function via 15 questions completed by the caregiver. The Edinburgh Cognitive and Behavioural ALS Screen (ECAS) assesses executive functions, memory, language, visuospatial skills and social cognition with the patient, and also includes a brief behavioural and psychosis interview with family or caregivers. The ALS-CBS and ECAS appear to be the most suitable tools to evaluate cognitive and behavioural changes in patients with MND (Gosselt et al 2020). If cognitive screens are abnormal, referral for a neuropsychological evaluation may be indicated.

The ALS Depression Inventory 12 is an MND-specific screening instrument for depression that excludes statements addressing activities that depend on an intact motor system. Patients with MND who test positive on depression or anxiety screens (i.e., Spielberger State-Trait Anxiety Inventory has been used in clinical trials) may need to be referred to a psychologist or psychiatrist for further evaluation.

Quality of life (QOL) has become a key outcome measure to be assessed, alongside functional status, because of the longer survival times of people with MND. MND-specific QOL measures include the ALS Assessment Questionnaire 40 (ALSAQ-40) (Jenkinson & Fitzpatrick 2001) and the ALS-specific QOL instrument (ALSSQOL). The ALSAQ-40 contains 40 items that assess five distinct areas of health: mobility (10 items), ADLs (10 items), eating and drinking (3 items), communication (7 items) and emotional functioning (10 items). The ALSAQ-40 was shortened to five items (ALSAQ-5) and was found to be valid and reliable (Jenkinson et al 2007) in instances when

a brief evaluation of health status is required clinically. The ALSSQOL was recently developed and contains 59 items that assess psychological, support, existential and spiritual domains, in addition to a physical domain (Simmons et al 2006). The shortened ALSSQOL-20 disease-specific measure of QOL is considered more suitable for use in clinical practice given the reduced administration time required to complete it (Hartmaier et al 2022).

Prognosis

Validated tools for predicting survival include the ALS Prognostic Index; however, the underpinning research was subjective and considered to be of poor quality (NICE 2016). The NICE (2016) guidelines suggested several key prognostic factors in people with MND including:

- Bulbar presentation;
- Weight loss;
- Poor respiratory function;
- Older age; and
- Shorter time from first symptoms to diagnosis.

One of the strongest predictors of prolonged survival is age (Chiò et al 2009). A longer symptom onset to diagnosis interval (ODI) predicted a better prognosis; patients who had an ODI >12 months were eight times more likely to have a prolonged survival than those with an ODI ≤12 months (Su et al 2021). Other factors that have been associated with a better prognosis include less severe involvement at onset, limb symptoms at onset versus bulbar onset, predominance of UMN signs, psychological well-being and maintenance of adequate nutrition (Su et al 2021).

Studies have examined the prognostic value for respiratory function measures and the use of ventilatory assistance for survival in patients with MND. Baseline measures of FVC or sniff nasal inspiratory pressure (SNIP) (i.e., a short, sharp, voluntary inspiratory manoeuvre used to assess inspiratory muscle strength) are early predictors of survival (Prigent et al 2004). SNIP can be performed more easily than spirometry and in patients with advanced disease, and is a reliable predictor of mortality and a better indicator of early respiratory muscle dysfunction than FVC because its measurement does not require a tight mouth seal which may not be possible for many patients with bulbar-onset MND (Polkey et al 2017, Walsh et al 2021).

Several studies have reported prolonged survival times from initiation of NIV ranging from 7 to 18 months in patients with MND with respiratory compromise or moderately impaired bulbar function who used NIV compared with those who did not. Among patients who used NIV, those who used it more than 4 hours per day survived an average of 7 months longer than those who used it less frequently. Early use of NIV (i.e., before FVC was ≤65% predicted) prolonged life by 329 days (11 months) compared with patients who started when their FVC was less than 65% (O'Brien et al 2019). Survival rates after initiation of NIV were reported to be 18% and 20% at 2 years and 5% at 5 years, whereas survival rates after initiation of tracheostomy invasive ventilation were 69% at 2 years and 33% at 5 years. The clinical management of patients with MND is complex and requires a comprehensive and multidisciplinary approach (Table 13.3). Specialist centres are considered the most advantageous and cost-effective healthcare setting for the management of individuals with MND in terms of survival time, fewer hospital admissions, increased use of adaptive equipment and enhanced quality of life more for patients than those not followed in a multidisciplinary clinic (de Almeida et al 2021). Two studies compared a cohort of patients attending a multidisciplinary clinic versus those attending a general neurology clinic and found that the median survival of the MND clinic cohort was 7.5 and 10.2 months longer than for patients in the general neurology cohort, and the prognosis of bulbar-onset patients was extended by 9.6 months (Aridegbe et al 2013, Rooney et al 2015). This suggests that more active and aggressive MDT management prolongs survival through increased use of NIV, attention to nutrition and earlier referral to palliative care services (Shoesmith et al 2020).

TABLE 13.3 Core Motor Neurone Disease Multidisciplinary Team Members and Extended Team Members

Core Multidisciplinary Team Members (Suggested)	Extended Team Members and Services for People With MND
Neurologist	Clinical psychology/ neuropsychology
Specialist MND nurse	Social care
Physiotherapist	Counselling
Occupational therapist	Respiratory and ventilation services
Respiratory healthcare professional	Gastroenterology
Speech and language therapist	Orthotics
Palliative care expertise	Wheelchair services
Dietitian	Alternative and augmentative technology services
	Community neurology teams
	Specialist palliative care

MND, Motor neurone disease.

TIME COURSE AND CORRESPONDING MANAGEMENT

MND is a steadily progressive disease and does not usually have periods of remission so stable plateaus are rare. The rate of progression is usually consistent for each patient but varies widely between individuals, with disease durations ranging from a few months to 20 years. Population-based studies have reported median survival times from symptom onset ranging between 23 and 52 months and median survival times from diagnosis between 12 and 31 months. Three- and 5-year survival rates after diagnosis have been found to range from 25% to 44% and 4% to 27%, respectively (Huisman et al 2011). Death occurs on average 3–5 years from the time of diagnosis, primarily from respiratory failure (Westeneng et al 2018). Other frequent causes of death are aspiration pneumonia and malnutrition (Chiò et al 2009).

Longitudinal studies of the natural history of MND have revealed several patterns in the progression of signs and symptoms. Loss of strength was found to progress more rapidly in the UEs than LEs. Symptoms progressed in a contiguous manner, meaning that they spread from one focal region to an anatomically adjacent area. For example, symptoms that started in one arm spread the fastest to the opposite arm, then to the ipsilateral leg, contralateral leg and brainstem in that order. Thus patients with initial unilateral arm or leg involvement had symptoms in spinal cord levels before they experienced bulbar symptoms. Bulbar symptoms developed sooner in patients with initial arm involvement than in those with leg involvement. Symptoms also appeared to spread faster in a caudal-to-rostral direction within the spinal cord and from the cervical regions to the bulbar region than in a rostral-to-caudal direction within the spinal cord. Bulbar involvement occurred much faster in female patients than males with initial limb symptoms, whereas limb involvement was more aggressive in male patients with bulbar onset (Fujimura-Kiyono et al 2011, Gargiulo-Monachelli et al 2012, Körner et al 2011).

Dal Bello-Haas (2002) proposed a three-stage model for the progression of MND as a framework for clinical management. In the early stage, individuals are independent with mobility, ADLs and speech despite mild to moderate weakness in specific muscle groups. The person may experience some difficulty with mobility and ADLs towards the end of the stage. During the middle stage, the person with MND has severe muscle weakness in some groups and mild to moderate weakness in others. There is a progressive decline in mobility and ADLs, along with increasing fatigue and pain that results in some compensation or dependence on others. In the late stage, the person is totally dependent with mobility and ADLs because of severe weakness of axial and extremity muscles. Dysarthria, dysphagia, respiratory compromise and pain are all common features of this stage.

It is important to note that the presentation and progression of MND are variable across patients. For example, some individuals present with UE weakness followed by LE weakness, and others present with LE weakness followed by trunk weakness. Some individuals present with speech and swallowing problems initially, whereas others experience development of these problems in the late stages of the disease. Some individuals with MND have a rapidly progressive disease course, dying a few months after their first symptoms, whereas others have very slowly progressive disease and remain ambulatory years after their diagnosis. This variability should be considered in all decision making and when planning interventions.

TREATMENT SELECTION AND SECONDARY COMPLICATIONS AND SPECIAL PROBLEMS

Muscle weakness leads to decreased ROM, and decreased ROM can result in joint subluxation (e.g., shoulder joint), tendon shortening (e.g., Achilles), joint contractures (e.g., claw-hand deformity) and adhesive capsulitis. A weak and dependent-positioned extremity can experience oedema distally because of the decrease or failure of the muscle-pump action.

Although MND does not primarily involve the pain pathways, secondary musculoskeletal impairments and immobility can cause pain. Pain may develop in or around joints because of decreased joint mobility or decreased support from the supporting structures because of muscle weakness. Pain may be directly caused by muscle strains, joint sprains or an acute injury, such as a fall. As described previously, neck and trunk muscle weakness leads to poor spinal support, and individuals with MND may experience neck or back pain. In addition, spasticity, especially if severe, and preexisting conditions can contribute to pain. Shoulder pain is common in people with MND for a variety of reasons: abnormal scapulohumeral rhythm secondary to spasticity or weakness, causing imbalance and leading to impingement; overuse of strong muscles; muscle strain; poor resting position; glenohumeral subluxation secondary to weakness; or a fall. In addition, individuals may also present with capsular patterns of restriction or a frozen shoulder. Adhesive capsulitis has been found to occur in up to 20% of individuals with MND (Ingels et al 2001).

It is important to regularly assess for pain because pain may exacerbate depression and fatigue, both of which have been associated with decreased QOL in people with MND. Edge et al (2020) highlight how pain influences physical QOL more than psychological QOL, whereas depression has a significant influence on both physical and psychological QOL. Anxiety is highly correlated with psychological QOL but only mildly correlated with physical QOL. Repeated assessments of pain, depression and anxiety emerge as valuable additions to comprehensive care provision because these are common and treatable symptoms which affect the QOL of those living with MND. Depending on the cause of physical pain, interventions may include modalities, ROM exercises, passive stretching, joint mobilisations and education about proper joint support and protection.

Respiratory impairments in MND are related to the loss of respiratory muscle strength. Early signs and symptoms of respiratory muscle weakness (RMW) may include fatigue, shortness of breath, orthopnoea, disturbed sleep, poor concentration, confusion, daytime sleepiness and morning headaches (Table 13.4). In addition, weak expiratory muscles result in a decreased ability to cough and clear secretions, increasing the risk for both aspiration and pneumonia. Often individuals will not initially report respiratory symptoms because they tend to decrease their overall level of physical activity because of extremity muscle weakness. Although the decline of respiratory muscle strength differs among individuals, for the most part it tends to progress at a linear rate (Czaplinski et al 2006, de Carvalho et al 2019). As weakness progresses, truncated speech, orthopnoea, shortness of breath at rest, paradoxical breathing and accessory muscle use develop. A decrease in FVC or VC of 50% of predicted is associated with the onset of respiratory symptoms, and a VC or an FVC of less than 25%–30% of predicted is indicative of a significant risk of impending respiratory failure or death. If an individual does not receive ventilatory support, eventual CO_2 retention will lead to acidosis, coma and respiratory failure.

Weakness of the tongue, lip and jaw muscles, larynx and pharynx causes dysarthria, secondary to UMN or LMN bulbar degeneration. Initial symptoms may include the inability to project the voice (e.g., shouting, singing) and problems with enunciation. With spastic dysarthria, the voice sounds forced because more effort is needed to move air through the upper airway, whereas with flaccid dysarthria, the voice sounds hoarse or breathy. With pharyngeal weakness, air in the mouth leaks into the nose during enunciation, resulting in a nasal tone. As MND progresses, speech becomes more difficult and unintelligible, and eventually the individual becomes completely unable to speak (Arora & Khan 2022, Shoesmith et al 2020). During all therapy interventions, the physiotherapist should consider the communication needs of the individual. Communication aids may include both low-level technology such as alphabet, word or picture boards, or high-level technology such

TABLE 13.4   Symptoms and Signs of Potential Respiratory Impairment (NICE MND Guidelines 2016)

Symptoms of Respiratory Impairment	Signs of Respiratory Impairment
Breathlessness	Increased respiratory rate
Orthopnoea	Shallow breathing
Recurrent chest infections	Weak cough
Disturbed sleep	Weak sniff
Nonrefreshing sleep	Abdominal paradox (inwards movement of the abdomen during inspiration)
Nightmares	Use of accessory muscles of respiration
Daytime sleepiness	Reduced chest expansion on maximal inspiration
Poor concentration and/or memory	
Confusion	
Hallucinations	
Morning headaches	
Fatigue	
Poor appetite	

A weak cough can be assessed by measuring peak cough flow.

as iPad- or tablet-based voice output communication aids. Physiotherapists may also need to liaise with occupational therapy or speech and language therapy colleagues when providing equipment, aids and adaptation to ensure aids will anticipate the changing need of patients and their relatives and carers, and that all equipment can be integrated (e.g., the patient's wheelchair can be integrated with their communication and environmental control systems) to maintain QOL and ease of use. Because the disease is progressive it is important that patients are not discharged from these services to guarantee continuity of care and regular reassessment to ensure that any equipment provided continues to meet patient's needs, helps maintain QOL and reduces the risk for adverse events (i.e., falls).

Impaired chewing or swallowing, dysphagia, also occurs secondary to UMN or LMN bulbar degeneration. Manipulating food inside the mouth or moving food into the oesophagus is difficult, and swallowing is impaired. In individuals with flaccid dysphagia, liquids may regurgitate into the nose because of pharyngeal weakness, and the cough reflex may be weak or absent, greatly increasing the risk for aspiration. Individuals with spastic dysphagia will have uncoordinated closure of the epiglottis, which may allow liquids or solids to pass to the larynx, causing aspiration. Because individuals experience dysphagia, choking and slowed eating, they are less likely to take in optimal fluid and caloric needs, which results in constipation and weight loss. Weight loss, choking episodes, aspiration and tiring at mealtimes may indicate the need for supplementary feeding. The option for PEG insertion should be discussed early because research suggests that the best outcome is achieved if the procedure occurs before major loss in body weight and a significant decline in respiratory function (Brotman et al 2022).

An absence of automatic, spontaneous swallowing response causes difficulties with clearing excessive saliva. Lower facial muscle weakness results in muscles that are too weak to close the lips tightly to prevent saliva leakage. Thus individuals with MND frequently experience sialorrhea, excessive saliva and drooling (Banfi et al 2015, Brotman et al 2022). Individuals with bulbar onset will experience sialorrhea relatively early and may notice the pillow is wet in the morning (e.g., drooling at night). As muscle weakness progresses, the individual may require the repeated use of a tissue to wipe away the saliva. Sialorrhea affects up to 50% of people with MND and is often poorly controlled. Antimuscarinics are used as a first line of treatment, but there is no evidence to inform which antimuscarinic or at what dose. Botulinum is used as either the second- or third-line option, although there is little evidence to guide botulinum choice, which salivary gland to inject or at what dose.

Fatigue in MND is thought to be related to a variety of factors. As motor neurones die, remaining neurones or sprouted neurones are overburdened. Weak muscles work at a higher percentage of their maximal strength to perform the same activity as someone without weakness. This hastens the time of muscle to fatigue. Sleep disturbances, respiratory impairments, hypoxia and depression are common in people with MND and may also contribute to fatigue (Abraham & Drory 2012, Lou 2008). It has been suggested that muscle fatigue in patients with MND may be caused in part by impaired contraction activation rather than dysfunction at the neuromuscular junction or within the muscle membrane (Sharma et al 1995). In addition, central factors may contribute to muscle fatigue in moderately impaired individuals with MND (Abraham & Drory 2012).

Because of the typically rapid, progressive and deteriorating nature of MND, physiotherapists are constantly challenged to determine the interrelationships among impairments, activity limitations, and participation restrictions and the best course of action. Physiotherapists must have a solid understanding of the nature and course of MND to effectively make decisions about which of the individual's problems can be restored, which require compensatory strategies and which cannot be affected by physical therapy interventions at all. Future functional losses, in addition to current status, need to be considered, and management needs to be planned accordingly.

Determining whether compensation or restoration interventions should be implemented is predicated on numerous factors that the therapist needs to consider. In people with MND, it may be useful to think about which stage of MND the person is in (early, middle, late) as an initial guide to focusing decision making. During therapy discussions regarding a person's needs, the therapists should consider the individual's cognitive status, communication ability and mental capacity alongside the needs of the carer or relatives.

Assistive Devices and Orthoses

Determining which type of assistive ambulation device to prescribe for a person with MND is dependent on the degree of proximal muscle strength or instability, the extent of UE muscle weakness, the pattern, extent and rate of progression of MND, acceptance of the patient and economic constraints. The weight of the device is an important overall factor to consider in decision making, while also considering which device will ensure optimal function and safety. Walking sticks are prescribed for individuals with mild LE weakness or balance problems, typically individuals with early-stage MND. Rollator frames, which do not require the patient to lift the device, are usually recommended over a Zimmer frame. In general, crutches are rarely prescribed for individuals with MND, but if they are, elbow crutches are preferred.

Orthoses are prescribed for a variety of reasons: to improve function by offering support to weakened muscles and the joints they surround, to decrease the stress on remaining functioning or compensatory muscles, to conserve energy or to minimise local or general muscle fatigue. Deciding between a premanufactured versus custom orthosis is certainly dependent on financial resources; however, the rate of disease progression should also be considered. For example, a premanufactured orthosis may suffice for an individual with rapidly progressive MND and who is likely to use the orthosis for limited time.

Solid ankle–foot orthoses (AFOs) are a good choice for patients who have mediolateral instability of the ankle with quadriceps weakness; however, the fixed ankle position, combined with the quadriceps weakness, may make it difficult for sit-to-stand transfers, stairs and climbing inclines. Hinged AFOs allow dorsiflexion and may be appropriate for the patient with adequate knee extensor strength with

mild ankle strength loss. Posterior leaf spring AFOs may be prescribed for individuals with mild spasticity and a slight foot drop, and for people with severe spasticity, antispasticity features can be built into the AFO (Lin et al 2000). Controlling knee instability can often be achieved through stabilising the ankle with an AFO, and so this should be considered first.

Again it is important to consider the weight of the orthosis because individuals with MND will have energy expenditure issues, and it may be more fatiguing for the patient to ambulate with a heavy orthosis than to ambulate without the impairment being corrected. For this reason, a knee-AFO or metal uprights are not recommended.

Because muscle weakness is one of the key features of MND, head drop can result from weakness in the neck, shoulder girdle and long back extensor muscles. For mild to moderate weakness, a soft foam collar may be recommended and may be worn during specific activities. Soft collars are comfortable and usually well tolerated. However, compressibility is an issue, and thus the time span for use is limited. For moderate to severe weakness, a semirigid or rigid collar is prescribed. These are usually made of padded rigid plastic or leather and provide very firm support. Patients may find them very warm; may experience discomfort at points of body contact, such as the chin, mandible, sternum or over clavicles; and may feel confined. Some models put pressure on the trachea. Some individuals with combined cervical and upper thoracic weakness may benefit from a cervical-thoracic orthosis or a sterno-occipital mandibular immobiliser. These devices provide maximum support but are more expensive, heavy and may be difficult to don and doff. For patients with severe or intractable neck weakness, referral to an orthotist or biomedical engineers for a custom-made device may be necessary.

Exercise in Motor Neurone Disease

The effects of exercise in the MND population are not well understood, and the role of resistance and aerobic exercise and fitness in the pathogenesis and management of people with MND has been controversial. Despite the lack of research evidence, some clinicians discourage any formal exercise programmes because of fear of overuse weakness and recommend no exercise other than everyday activities. Exercise, when prescribed appropriately, may be physiologically and psychologically beneficial for patients with MND, especially when implemented in the early (and possibly middle) stages of the disease.

Overwork Damage Versus Disuse Atrophy

The possibility of inducing overwork damage in individuals with MND through excessive exercise (resistance or aerobic) is a concern and stems from early research (e.g., people with denervated muscles resulting from post-polio syndrome). Some epidemiological studies have suggested a higher incidence of MND in people performing intense physical activity at work or for leisure before disease onset (e.g., Chio et al 2005, Harwood et al 2016, Okamoto et al 2009, Sutedja et al 2009). More recently a positive causal relationship between ALS and physical exercise has been shown and with certain risk genotypes (e.g., C9ORF72) (Julian et al 2021). Some evidence from people with other neuromuscular disorders suggests 'supramaximal' exercise (e.g., highly repetitive or heavy resistance or eccentric exercise) may induce damage and inflammation and failure of skeletal muscle to repair itself, causing prolonged loss of muscle strength (Kostek & Gordon 2018).

The safe range for therapeutic exercise for people with MND may be narrowed, and the range continues to narrow as the disease progresses. The degree to which the range narrows is dependent on the extent of disease involvement, the rate of disease progression and individual variability. In people with MND up to one-half of the motor neurones innervating a muscle may be lost before clinical signs of weakness or atrophy are present. A weak or denervated muscle may be more susceptible to overwork damage because it is already functioning closer to its maximal limits. ADLs alone may cause impaired muscles to act as though in training, and exercise that would improve normal muscles may cause overwork damage in impaired muscles. The remaining motor units will respond to training, and these motor units must work harder to handle a given amount of exercise stress. Thus special attention

needs to be paid when prescribing an exercise programme (Table 13.5 and Fig. 13.2).

In contrast, a marked reduction in activity levels secondary to MND can lead to decreased endurance and disuse weakness, superimposed on the muscle weakness caused by the disease itself. Reduced physical activity, particularly if prolonged, produces muscle atrophy, reduced strength of tendons and ligaments and osteoporosis. Strength loss through inactivity and disuse may significantly debilitate individuals with MND, making them susceptible to deconditioning and muscle and joint tightness, which lead to contractures and pain. Interestingly, studies of individuals with other neuromuscular diseases have found that exercise programmes are beneficial and did not produce overuse weakness (Stefanetti et al 2020, Voet et al 2019).

Types of Exercise

ROM and stretching exercises are typically accepted modes of exercise for people with MND. Resistance exercises of unaffected muscles (and possibly affected muscles with strength at least grade ≥3) using a low to moderate load and intensity, and aerobic activities, such as swimming, walking and bicycling, at submaximal levels (between 50% and 65% of heart rate reserve or intermittent exercise with repetitive exercise–rest periods tend to be safer) may also play an important role in achieving an individual's goals or overall therapeutic goals (Dal Bello-Haas & Krivickas 2008). Aerobic and resistance exercises should be prescribed as soon as possible after diagnosis and are more appropriate for individuals in the early or early-middle stage of MND and those with more slowly progressive disease. When designing any exercise programme for a person

TABLE 13.5	Prescribing Exercise for People With Motor Neurone Disease (From Dal Bello-Haas & Krivickas 2008)		
	Goals	Suggested Exercise Parameters	Special Considerations
Resistance exercise	• Maximise strength of unaffected or mildly affected muscles. • Prevent disuse. • Attempt to delay time to when function is impaired.	• Resistance exercises for muscles > grade 3 strength only • Low to moderate intensity • Low to moderate load • 1–2 sets of 8–12 repetitions	• Reduce resistance and repetitions as weakness progresses. • Monitor for overuse.
Aerobic exercise	• Increase or maximise work capacity and endurance. • Prevent disuse. • May have beneficial effects on mood, psychological well-being, appetite and sleep.	• 50%–80% peak heart rate, 11–13 rate of perceived exertion scale • 3 times per week, nonresistance exercise days • As tolerated, without excessive fatigue	• Mode is determined by safety considerations. • Monitor for overwork.

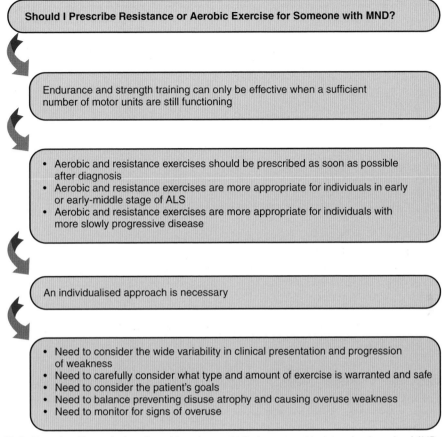

FIG. 13.2 Exercise Prescription Considerations. *ALS,* Amyotrophic lateral sclerosis; *MND,* motor neurone disease.

with ALS, physiotherapists must continuously balance underwork and overwork, and adjust based on the individual's response to exercise and other disease-specific factors. The type and intensity of the exercise programme should be carefully monitored and adjusted by the physiotherapists to prevent excessive fatigue and potential overwork damage, while at the same time promoting optimal use of intact muscle groups. Individuals should be advised not to carry out any activities to the point of extreme fatigue and should keep track of symptoms of overuse, including the inability to perform daily activities after exercise because of exhaustion or pain, a reduction in maximum muscle force that gradually recovers or increased excessive muscle cramping, soreness, fatigue or fasciculations. Individuals should be educated regarding self-monitoring and should use an exercise log the physiotherapists can review. In particular the exercise programme needs to be recorded and any adverse signs and symptoms noted. Last, individuals

may also be advised to exercise for several brief periods throughout the day with sufficient rest in between. If signs of overuse occur, exercises should be stopped until symptoms resolve and the physiotherapists should reevaluate.

Evolving Wheelchair Needs

At some time point as the disease progresses, the extent of muscle weakness or the energy requirements for ambulation will necessitate that a patient use a wheelchair for mobility.

In the early or early-middle stage of MND, a manual wheelchair, preferably lightweight or ultra-lightweight, may be used for traveling long distances to conserve energy. As the condition progresses, it has been estimated that about 80% of people with MND will need to use a wheelchair (MNDA 2015). It is important that a person with MND has access to an appropriate posture and mobility assessment as early as possible to identify their individual requirements and determine the type of wheelchair that will best suit the changing needs of someone with the condition.

Because MND is a rapidly progressive condition and the waiting times for the provision of a wheelchair through wheelchair services can be lengthy, an anticipatory and timely referral to this service is critical. Someone with MND should be referred to the local wheelchair services when they are starting to experience mobility problems and are ready to accept the need for a wheelchair. Once someone has been referred to this service, the request will be triaged to determine the priority for an assessment. The assessment will cover the person's postural and mobility needs and consider their home and the local environment where the wheelchair is to be used.

Powered wheelchair systems have become smaller and lighter and can be folded to fit inside the trunk of a car or the back of a van. The optimum wheelchair that should be provided (1) has a high back and adequate head and neck support to support weakened trunk muscles; (2) has a reclining or tilt-in-space seat that facilitates postural changes for resting and pain and pressure relief; and (3) can be modified to add a ventilator tray or communication device. The assessment should also consider how the wheelchair will be transported and anticipate how the user's needs may change in the future.

Respiratory Issues

As the disease progresses, almost all individuals with MND will eventually require some form of respiratory intervention to alleviate respiratory symptoms. One of the most common and distressing symptoms faced by people with MND with RMW (diaphragmatic and intercostal) is the inability to cough effectively and clear secretions from the airway (de Carvalho et al 2019), reducing quality of life and further impairing respiratory function (Shoesmith et al 2020). An effective cough is a necessary protective mechanism to guard against respiratory tract infections (RTIs). In patients with MND, RTIs are one of the most common causes of acute hospital admissions (Chatwin et al 2018). An RTI may lead to acute or acute-on-chronic respiratory failure, which remains one of the most common causes of death in patients with MND (Sancho et al 2019).

There are three main components of an effective cough: the inspiratory phase, the compressive stage and the expulsive phase. In those with MND, inspiratory muscle weakness limits inspiratory airflow, which in an effective cough would be up to 85%–90% of total lung capacity (Anderson et al 2005). Bulbar involvement impairs glottis closure, the buildup of pressure within the lungs and rapid opening of the glottis. Expiratory muscle weakness alters expiratory airflow leading to a decrease in cough efficacy and secretion clearance. A simple, easily

reproducible measure of cough effectiveness is to assess a patient's peak cough flow (PCF). Bott et al (2009) defined this as the peak flow an individual can generate with a cough through a peak flow meter (a paediatric peak flow meter will enable a more sensitive measurement in a patient with RMW). PCF can be measured with other devices including portable spirometers or calibrated pneumotachographs. Pneumotachographs have been suggested to be preferable because of their greater accuracy, although portable spirometers may provide satisfactory measurements at flows >270 L/min. PCF measurements from modern mechanical insufflation-exsufflation (MI-E) devices should be taken only as a trend because their measurements are not calibrated (Chatwin et al 2018).

Although the PCF is not specific enough to evaluate the separate components of cough limitation, it does provide a global measure of cough strength. Research indicates that a PCF of 160 L/min is required to clear secretions from the airway (Bach & Saporito 1996). Respiratory muscle strength is further compromised during an RTI by secretion retention, fatigue and worsening dysfunction of RMW (Poponick et al 1997, Rafiq et al 2016a, 2016b, Toussaint et al 2018). Therefore a PCF of 270 L/min when a person with MND is well is considered the threshold level for the introduction of techniques to enhance cough effectiveness (Toussaint et al 2009) and secretion clearance.

Conventional physiotherapy techniques to aid secretion clearance (e.g., active cycle of breathing technique [ACBT]) may be impractical and ineffective with patients who have advanced RMW (Rafiq et al 2016a, 2016b). The techniques are tiring for patients and if vigorous can precipitate episodes of desaturation (Chatwin et al 2003, Vianello et al 2005), so suction has often been used in combination with these techniques. Patients with MND are often awake and alert, so they are not ideal candidates for suction; therefore those who do not tolerate it well may decline this type of physiotherapy intervention. Alternative techniques have been explored which compensate for RMW, enhance cough effectiveness and are better tolerated by people with MND.

Cough augmentation techniques is an umbrella term encompassing inspiratory, expiratory and combined inspiratory/expiratory muscle aids (Fig. 13.3). The use of these techniques has grown significantly since the early 1990's and has added further noninvasive secretion management options, commonly used with patients with neuromuscular diseases, to the physiotherapists' toolbox (see Fig. 13.3). Despite a plethora of research in relation to these techniques, there is an absence of randomised control trials supporting the use of cough augmentation techniques in patients with MND. Mixed population, cohort studies or case studies provide evidence to suggest that these aids can increase secretion clearance (Anderson et al 2005, Cleary

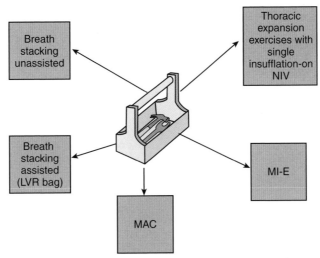

FIG. 13.3 Summary of Cough Augmentation Techniques. *LVR*, Lung-volume recruitment; *MAC*, manual assisted coughing; *MI-E*, mechanical insufflation/exsufflation; *NIV*, noninvasive ventilation.

et al 2013, Rafiq et al 2016a, Rafiq et al 2016b, Shoesmith et al 2020), decrease hospitalisation rates (Tzeng & Bach 2000), prevent or delay the need for tracheostomy (Bach 1995) and prolong survival when used in conjunction with NIV (Gomez-Merino & Bach 2002). Inspiratory aids improve PCF by enabling patients to achieve a precough inhalation to their maximal insufflation capacity (MIC). MIC is defined as the maximum volume of air you can hold with a closed glottis and accounts for 44% of variance in PCF effectiveness (Trebbia et al 2005) as lung expansion to MIC optimises lung recoil pressure to drive the cough manoeuvre. Physiotherapy adjuncts used to facilitate MIC include a modified ACBT using an NIV (Chatwin & Simmonds 2009), intermittent positive-pressure breathing (IPPB), unassisted breath stacking, assisted breath stacking using a lung volume recruitment (LVR) bag or MI-E. A study by Mellies and Goebel (2014) where they assisted precough inhalations below MIC using IPPB still demonstrated an increase in VC and PCF in a cohort group that included NIV-dependent patients. As their insufflations were significantly below MIC, the authors concluded that a submaximal insufflation can still generate an effective PCF, even in patients with severely reduced respiratory system compliance.

Unassisted breath stacking to MIC can be achieved by stacking consecutive inhalation breaths on top of one another, closing the glottis after each one until the patient reaches the maximum volume they can inspire before coughing. The assisted breath stacking technique most commonly uses an LVR bag, which is an Ambu-Bag with a one-way valve acting as the glottis to enable the patient to take successive assisted breaths to their MIC before coughing. Studies suggest that regular breath stacking to MIC may be beneficial as an ROM exercise in patients who have early restrictive respiratory defects but who do not require NIV (Toussaint et al 2018).

Manual assisted coughing (MAC) is used to enhance the expiratory component of the cough manoeuvre by increasing expiratory airflow by compression of the chest wall or abdomen, or both, timed as the glottis opens in synchrony with the patient's own cough effort. The greatest improvements in PCF can be achieved by combining inspiratory and expiratory aids. When using both techniques, patients and their carers often report more confidence when managing secretions, and patients themselves report that their cough is stronger.

MI-E (also known as Cough Assist®) is a combined inspiratory/expiratory aid and is considered of benefit when MAC or breath stacking is no longer effective or because of RMW and fatigue, especially during episodes of acute deterioration and hospitalisation (Shoesmith et al 2020). The MI-E device provides positive inspiratory pressure with a rapid switch to negative pressure and generates high expiratory airflows, mimicking a cough. The greatest improvements in PCF are generated by combining MI-E and MAC (Sheers et al 2019, Toussaint et al 2018). The use of the MI-E with patients who have bulbar muscle involvement remains an area of some debate (Rafiq et al 2015) because of the increased risk for upper airway collapse. Hypopharyngeal constriction during exsufflation is most prominently observed in patients with ALS and bulbar symptoms, reducing airflow and treatment efficacy.

Andersen et al (2017) suggested that individually customised settings can improve the use of MI-E in patients with bulbar involvement by preventing airway obstruction. Settings proposed (see algorithm in Fig. 13.4) are triggered insufflation, decreasing the inspiratory flow and pressures and allowing a longer insufflation time to allow equilibrium of pressure from the device to the lung. Recent MI-E devices now provide the option to add high-frequency oscillations (HFOs) during insufflation, exsufflation or both. HFO added to insufflation, exsufflation and in combination has not been proved to have any effect on PCF in medically stable subjects with ALS (Sancho et al 2019). Chatwin and Simonds (2020) advise that it is difficult to have a protocol that dictates one MI-E setting for all MND patients, advocating for individually prescribed settings. Further studies are required to fully evaluate the impact of manipulating the various parameter options open to HCPs by the MI-E device setting options. Effective secretion clearance plans also require co-optimisation of mucolytics, nebulisers, mouth care, positioning and feeding/hydration regimes.

Both clinical and research interest in cough augmentation techniques have developed considerably since the early 1990's. The techniques are considered to have contributed to the success of NIV with neuromuscular patients. Respiratory failure in patients with MND is a real possibility, especially in the late stages of the disease when global and RMW occurs. Research indicates that NIV significantly prolongs survival and improves QOL in patients with MND (Baxter 2019, Bourke et al 2006, O'Brien et al 2019). The survival benefit is considered to be greater in those patients without bulbar involvement. Patients with MND with cognitive change or FTD may have considerable difficulty in coping with the equipment and the restrictions that come with NIV. In patients with severe bulbar dysfunction, the survival benefit is limited, but hypoventilation symptom-related QOL has been shown to improve (e.g., sleep disruption or severe orthopnoea). Those with more severe bulbar impairment were considered to be at an increased risk of poor adherence with NIV. Although it can potentially be more complex to treat hypoventilation in patients with bulbar dysfunction, initiating NIV via an MDT approach through strategies aimed at promoting its effective use suggests that they may gain both symptom and survival benefit that could be at least equal to that of patients without bulbar dysfunction (O'Brien et al 2019). Such strategies include interface optimisation, adequate initial acclimatisation and ongoing active management with vigilant monitoring and regular adjustments.

NICE (2016) recommends that respiratory function tests should be carried out at diagnosis of MND or soon after and patients monitored for signs and symptoms of

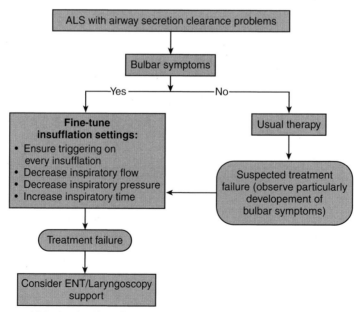

FIG. 13.4 Proposed Mechanical Insufflation/Exsufflation Algorithm for Patients With Bulbar Motor Neurone Disease (Andersen et al 2017). *ALS*, Amyotrophic lateral sclerosis; *ENT*, ear, nose and throat.

potential respiratory impairment every 2–3 months. NIV will be offered if a person's signs and symptoms (see Table 13.4) and the results of the respiratory function tests indicate that a person is likely to benefit from this treatment (see Table 13.2). Clinical practice guidelines recommend that physicians sensitively discuss the use of NIV with a person with MND and at an appropriate time. This discussion should be appropriate to the stage of the person's disease process and may take place soon after diagnosis, when monitoring respiratory function, if a person asks for information or when their respiratory function declines. It should include information on the different ways people can manage their breathless symptoms and include:

- NIV and its advantages and disadvantages, that is, the use of NIV is to relieve symptoms and prolong life but not to halt disease progression;
- Role of medication for breathing problems (e.g., benzodiazepines for anxiety-related shortness of breath);
- Options for treating infections;
- Possibility of becoming dependent on NIV; and
- Means of support and information on how to recognise and cope with distressing situations.

Throughout the disease stages the physiotherapist's roles as part of the MDT may include education regarding shortness of breath management techniques, such as breathing control, positions of ease, pacing and energy conservation techniques. Individuals and caregivers should also be educated about signs and symptoms of aspiration, positioning to avoid aspiration such as upper cervical spine flexion during feeding, causes and signs of respiratory infection and strategies for managing oral secretions or choking episodes.

Before starting NIV, it is recommended that the MDT, together with the respiratory ventilation service, should prepare a comprehensive care plan, in discussion with the patient and their relatives. When initiating NIV, the patient will usually begin using NIV overnight whilst they are sleeping after an initial period of acclimatisation, when they build up their hours of use. The most frequently used method of delivering NIV is bilevel positive-pressure ventilation in which different levels are delivered on inspiration and expiration. As the disease progresses, the amount of time the person will use NIV increases during the daytime up to 24-hour use. It is important that the individual with MND knows that they can stop NIV at any time and can ask for help and advice if they need it, particularly if they are dependent on the device 24 hours a day or become distressed when they try to stop it.

Permanent ventilatory support (via tracheostomy) is an option for some individuals wishing to prolong survival. The rate of tracheostomy in MND is rare, about 2%–3%, although higher in some countries such as Italy (10%) and Japan (30%) (Oliver 2019). There is no evidence to suggest that the use of tracheostomies has increased as a result of greater access to NIV. It is suggested that this more controlled route and less crisis-driven approach to the management of respiratory failure in MND patients may have led to a reduction in tracheostomy ventilation because of early discussion and documentation around the patient's end-of-life choice. People with MND may wish to discuss end-of-life issues and may make advanced directives at any time during disease progression. It is suggested that these conversations take place at clinic reviews or trigger points. A patient with MND may need extra support at certain times during disease progression, such as at diagnosis when they face an unknown disease, when mobility is affected, when gastrostomy is discussed, when respiratory function is declining and NIV is discussed and towards the end of life (Breen et al 2018). It is also important that these conversations take place early, before the patient experiences communication or cognitive problems, when feasible.

A person's decision to accept invasive ventilation has numerous ramifications for the patient and family, and needs to be made after thorough discussion with the physician and family–caregiver unit. It is an expensive option and may be emotionally and socially taxing for those with MND and their caregivers, as well as members of the MDT. People with MND and their physicians often consider NIV more desirable than invasive ventilatory support with tracheostomy. Most individuals with MND in North America and the UK do not choose invasive mechanical ventilation, and client satisfaction has been reported to be higher with NIV compared with invasive ventilation. Invasive ventilation may increase survival more effectively but with a greater financial and caregiver burden (de Wit et al 2018).

A critical issue with NIV and invasive ventilation for patients with MND is the consideration of the withdrawal of ventilatory support. A cognitively competent, informed person has the legal and ethical right to refuse or to discontinue any treatment, including life support and mechanical ventilation, and HCPs are required to respect the patient's decision. As MND progresses, the person becomes completely dependent on ventilatory support and may eventually become unable to communicate. Therefore it is essential that the individual, family–caregiver unit and physician agree, before this point, which circumstances will trigger withdrawal of the ventilator.

CONCLUSION

The care of patients with MND is becoming more complex and challenging as research continues to better our understanding of the disease, its symptoms and progression. Supportive interventions can improve survival time and QOL for patients with MND. Clarity in relation to the individualised pathway of care for both the patients and their families and the MDT is essential to ensure cost-effective, timely and appropriate symptom management that is responsive to the changing needs and wishes of the individual with MND. The physiotherapist plays a core role in working with their MDT colleagues, patients and relatives to ensure regular assessment and anticipatory intervention to manage symptoms, maintain function and improve the QOL for people living with MND as this ultimately fatal condition progresses.

CASE STUDY

David is a 59-year-old married man with three children aged 22 and 24 years who live locally. He took early retirement from his job as an industrial engineer with Jaguar Land Rover 12 months ago. He had smoked in his early twenties but gave up when his children were born. He first noticed symptoms 18 months ago, including diminished grip strength (objects would slip out of his hand and he struggled buttoning his shirts), prone to tripping, fatigue, cramps and muscle spasms in his lower limbs (which he initially dismissed as being related to his hobbies). David liked to take part in triathlons and played football until his mid-thirties. His wife prompted him to go and see his GP after he complained to her that his legs felt tired after limited exertion and he'd had a couple of falls when walking the dog. His GP noted distal leg weakness and a positive Babinski sign and thus referred him to a neurologist for further investigations (blood tests, MRI, EMG and nerve conduction studies). David was diagnosed 6 months later once other causes of symptoms had been ruled out and progression was in keeping with MND; his care was transferred to the MND MDT, and he was started on medication. David, who had been planning to travel in his retirement and devote more time to his hobbies and family, felt his dream had come crashing down and was initially devastated. The MND MDT and the people he met at the local MNDA support group were a good source of support to him postdiagnosis, especially because David wanted answers to lots of questions regarding his condition and its management. He also joined the MNDA Online Forum where he and his wife met a wide range of people, offering first-hand experience of MND who could provide medical, emotional and practical support as well as a sense of community. He wanted to keep exercising for as long as possible, and guided by the MND physiotherapist, he initially continued to attend regular personal training sessions. He hoped that this would help him psychologically and maintain his function and independence for as long as possible, which would maintain his QOL.

Twelve months later, David's mobility had declined; the physiotherapist noted wasting of leg and thigh muscles,

some active movement of lower limbs (proximal > distal), but that he was unable to walk or stand unaided. He had some active movement of his upper limbs and was able to assist with eating and drinking using adapted utensils, as well as assist with dressing, but is limited by bilateral shoulder weakness. David's wife helped him when he went for a shower and to put on his clothes. David was unable to stand by himself, so she had to guide him to the shower and assist with his transfers. David could easily move around the downstairs of the house with an electric wheelchair enabling him to watch television with his grandchildren. He could no longer negotiate stairs, so the occupational therapist suggested a bed downstairs. A ramp was laid to the property so David and his wife could still maintain their social independence.

Six months later, David began to have difficulty speaking. His voice quality was quieter, and he began having trouble holding a conversation. David felt more fatigued but put this down to nightmares that affected his quality of sleep, and he reported shortness of breath when lying flat. David thought that this might be related to recent chest infections he had had. David also reported morning headaches, which prompted an early clinic review for respiratory function tests. During his clinic review, it was noted that David had an FVC of less than 50% predicted and had lost 20% of his body weight; his PCF was 240 L/min.

The treatment options of feeding tubes and ventilation were discussed with David and his wife, Sue. The advantages of tube feeding (possibility of prolonging life, improved nutrition and a reduced time for his wife to spend feeding him) were discussed. Risks of a PEG tube, such as local infection and complications related to insertion, were also discussed. It was explained to David that he would need to be admitted to local hospital to have the tube inserted, and at the same time NIV could be initiated. David understood the potential benefits such as improved QOL, better sleep (including possibly for his wife because he would be more settled) and possibility of prolonging life, as this had been discussed with him at every clinic visit. He was concerned that this may increase his need for care and the carer burden on his wife whilst prolonging his life but not adding any quality. David did understand that if ventilation was commenced he needed to make an advanced decision for the future regarding ceasing ventilation.

His son was due to get married in 6 months' time, so David decided that he would like to live long enough to be part of this important event. He believed that he would then be ready to accept death. He decided to be admitted to hospital for a feeding tube and to initiate NIV. Whilst in the hospital, a physiotherapist taught David how to breath stack using an LVR bag and his wife how to perform a MAC to help him cough and clear secretion more effectively. David believed he would cease life-prolonging treatment at a point in the future if his care needs became too much of a burden on his wife. He also requested that when he was close to death, he be transferred to a hospice close to his home. He believed dying at home would not be in the best interests of his wife because he did not want her to remember him dying in the home they had shared. Six months later David was admitted to a hospice and died, 2 and a half years after he had been diagnosed with MND.

Refer to Table 13.6 for a summary of David's physiotherapy problems, goals and treatment plans.

TABLE 13.6 Case Study: Physiotherapy Problems List, Goals and Plans		
Problems List	**Goals**	**Plan**
Evidence of limb-onset MND evidenced by history of trips, falls and reduced fine movements, e.g., dropping objects and difficulty buttoning shifts	Maintain and optimise functional independence with activities, mobility and (personal) ADLs.	After an initial assessment (including muscle strength, balance, mobility, function) as part of the MND MDT clinic, ensure regular coordinated monitoring and reviews.
Reduced exercise tolerance, ability to continue hobbies and fatigue	Develop an individualised resistance and moderate-intensity aerobic exercise prescription for David.	Therapist to liaise with patient, carer, and personal trainer to ensure programme performed at an intensity that maintains a balance between intensity of activity and fatigue management in the short term. Review longer-term goals and intervene as David's condition progresses.
Difficulty accepting his diagnosis and anxiety regarding the condition, its long-term impact upon his independence and its prognosis	Assist David's understanding of MND and how it affects daily living, and discuss concerns he may have in relation to accepting and coping with the diagnosis and adjusting to the changes it has on his life and his plans. Consider how David's difficulty accepting his condition may affect his ability to accept aids and adaption or the provisions of care.	Discuss the psychological and emotional impact of MND with David and ask if he requires any psychological or care support needs. Offer information about sources of emotional and psychological support including support groups and online forums, and if needed refer on to counselling or psychological services. Consider the impact on David's family members and carers, and their ability and willingness to provide personal care or use equipment.
Muscle wasting, decreased mobility and functional ability, i.e., requires assistance with his (personal) ADLs	Continue to maintain functional mobility and quality of life through: • maintenance of range of movement • prevention of contractures • managing muscle tone • managing pain • monitoring for symptoms of respiratory compromise • education on good posture/ positioning and manual handling	Timely provision and regular review of aids and adaptations, and close liaison with occupational therapist, orthotics, SALT, social care team required. Complete a manual handling risk assessment and provide training to David's carer on manual handling technique, shoulder care and stretching/range of motion exercises for any joints David cannot move himself. Refer to wheelchair services in liaison with the MND MDT.

(Continued)

Problems List	Goals	Plan
Reduced voice quality and weight loss, signs and symptoms of respiratory failure and reduced cough efficacy	Monitor for and address any signs or symptoms of respiratory insufficiency. Regularly monitor David's PCF and instigate cough augmentation techniques should PCF fall below the threshold level for cough efficacy.	Once signs and symptoms of respiratory compromise identified, refer to respiratory ventilation team in conjunction with the MND MDT for review. Consider David's communication needs and liaise with SALT as required. Facilitate cough augmentation techniques to assist in secretion management and to maintain chest wall mobility and lung compliance. Be prepared to discuss end-of-life issues whenever David wishes to and be aware of any advance care plans.

TABLE 13.6   Case Study: Physiotherapy Problems List, Goals and Plans—Cont'd

ADLs, Activities of daily living; MDT, multidisciplinary team; MND, motor neurone disease; PCF, peak cough flow; SALT, speech and language therapy.

SELF-ASSESSMENT QUESTIONS

1. What is the most common MND that affects the bulbar, limb, and respiratory muscles?
   a. progressive bulbar palsy
   b. ALS
   c. Guillain-Barré syndrome
   d. polymyositis
2. Which medication would David have been prescribed to help slow the progressive damage to the motor neurone cells and increase his survival time?
   a. riluzole
   b. quinine
   c. baclofen
   d. gabapentin
3. Which of the following is NOT usually true in MND?
   a. commonly affects men more than women
   b. affects the bladder and bowel in the early stage of the condition
   c. may lead to early-morning headache as the condition progresses
   d. brisk reflexes
4. Which diagnostic limb features for MND did David have that would have prompted his GP to refer him to the neurologist? (more than one response may be selected)
   a. distal limb weakness
   b. history of trips and falls
   c. behavioural changes
   d. tongue fasciculations

5. Despite the lack of research evidence to support, which of the exogenous factors mentioned in David's history have been considered potential triggers for the disease? (more than one response may be selected)
   a. hobbies: physical activity/football
   b. age
   c. gender
   d. occupational history: industrial engineer
6. Which gene is considered to be the most common gene mutation associated with familial MND?
   a. NEK1
   b. SOD1
   c. C9ORF72
   d. TDP-43
7. What aspects might the physiotherapist include when advising David on continuing physical activity post-diagnosis? (more than one response may be selected)
   a. education on preventing the cycle of deconditioning
   b. considering and managing fatigue
   c. advice on suitable aerobic and resistance exercise programmes
   d. balancing the intensity and type of exercise
   e. ceasing all physical activity immediately to prevent overuse injury
8. Which of the following are considered prognostic factors in MND?
   a. bulbar presentation
   b. age of onset
   c. weight loss
   d. impaired respiratory function
   e. all of the above

9. Which of the following would NOT form part of the routine assessment process completed by all Wheelchair Services before provision of a wheelchair?
   a. postural needs
   b. person's home environment
   c. local environment in which the chair will be used
   d. eye test
   e. how the wheelchair will be transported
   f. anticipating the person's future needs as the condition progresses

10. What measurement of PCF is considered the minimal level to facilitate an effective cough and to clear secretions from the airway?
    a. 160 L/min
    b. 470 L/min
    c. 270 L/min
    d. 180 L/min

11. Which sign and symptom of respiratory impairment did David NOT display?
    a. orthopnoea
    b. nightmares
    c. confusion
    d. morning headaches
    e. recurrent chest infections

REFERENCES

Abraham, A., Drory, V.E., 2012. Fatigue in motor neuron diseases. Neuromuscul. Disord. 22, S198–S202.

Åkerblom, Y., Zetterberg, L., Larsson, B.J., et al., 2021. Pain, disease severity and associations with individual quality of life in patients with motor neuron diseases. BMC. Palliat. Care. 20, 154.

ALS CNTF Treatment Study (ACTS) Phase I–II Study Group, 1996. The amyotrophic sclerosis functional rating scale: assessment of daily living in patients with amyotrophic lateral sclerosis. Arch. Neurol. 53, 141–147.

Andersen, T., Sandnes, A., Brekka, A.K., et al., 2017. Laryngeal response patterns influence the efficacy of mechanical assisted cough in amyotrophic lateral sclerosis. Thorax. 72, 221–229.

Anderson, J.L., Hasney, K.M., Beaumont, N.E., 2005. Systematic review of techniques to enhance peak cough flow and maintain vital capacity in neuromuscular disease: the case for mechanical insufflation–exsufflation. Phys. Ther. Rev. 10, 25–33.

Aridegbe, T., et al., 2013. The natural history of motor neuron disease: assessing the impact of specialist care. Amyotroph. Lateral Scler. Frontotemporal Degener. 14, 13–19.

Arora, R.D., Khan, Y.S., 2022. Motor Neuron Disease. StatPearls Publishing, Treasure Island, Florida, Available at: https://www.ncbi.nlm.nih.gov/books/NBK560774/. Accessed 29 April 2022.

Bach, J.R., 1995. Respiratory muscle aids for the presenting of pulmonary morbidity and mortality. Semin. Neurol. 15, 72–83.

Bach, J.R., Saporito, L.R., 1996. Criteria for extubation and tracheostomy tube removal for patients with ventilatory failure. A different approach to weaning. Chest. 110, 1566–1571.

Banfi, P., et al., 2015. A review of options for treating sialorrhea in amyotrophic lateral sclerosis. Respir. Care. 60, 446–454.

Baxter, S.K., Johnson, M., Clowes, M., et al., 2019. Optimizing the noninvasive ventilation pathway for patients with amyotrophic lateral sclerosis/motor neuron disease: a systematic review. Amyotroph. Lateral Scler. Frontotemporal Degener. 20, 461–472.

Berg, K.O., et al., 1992. Measuring balance in the elderly: validation of an instrument. Can. J. Public. Health. 83 (Suppl. 2), S7–S11.

Beswick, E., Forbes, D., Hassan, Z., et al., 2022. A systematic review of non-motor symptom evaluation in clinical trials for amyotrophic lateral sclerosis. J. Neurol. 269, 411–426.

Bott, J., et al., 2009. Guidelines for the physiotherapy management of the adult, medical, spontaneously breathing patient. Thorax. 64 (Suppl. 1), 11–52.

Bourke, S.C., et al., 2006. Effects of non-invasive ventilation on survival and quality of life in patients with amyotrophic lateral sclerosis: a randomised controlled trial. Lancet Neurol. 5, 140–147.

Breen, L.J., Aoun, S.M., O'Connor, M., 2018. Family caregivers' preparations for death: a qualitative analysis. J. Pain Symptom Manage. 55, 1473–1479.

Brotman, R.G., Moreno-Escobar, M.C., Joseph, J., et al., 2022. Amyotrophic Lateral Sclerosis. StatPearls Publishing, Treasure Island, Florida. Available at: https://www.ncbi.nlm.nih.gov/books/NBK556151. Accessed 28 April 2022.

Brown, R.H., Al-Chalabi, A., 2017. Amyotrophic lateral sclerosis. N. Engl. J. Med. 277, 167–172.

Burchardt, J., Mei, X., Ranger, T., et al., 2022. Analysis of incidence of motor neuron disease in England 1998–2019: use of three linked datasets. Amyotroph. Lateral Scler. Frontotemporal Degener. 23, 363–371.

Burchill, E., Rawji, V., Styles, K., et al., 2023. When months matter; modelling the impact of the COVID-19 pandemic on the diagnostic pathway of Motor Neurone Disease (MND). PLoS One. 18, e0259487.

Burrell, J.R., et al., 2016. The frontotemporal dementia-motor neurone disease continuum. Lancet. 338, 919–931.

Cabona, C., Ferraro, P.M., Meo, G., et al., 2021. Predictors of self-perceived health worsening over COVID-19 emergency in ALS. Neurol. Sci. 42, 1231–1236.

Carleton, M., Brown, W.F., 1979. Changes in motor unit populations in motor neuron disease. J. Neurol. Neurosurg. Psychiatry. 42, 42–51.

Cedarbaum, J.M., et al., 1999. The ALSFRS-R: a revised ALS functional rating scale that incorporates assessments of respiratory function. J. Neurol. Sci. 169, 13–21.

Chatwin, M., et al., 2003. Cough augmentation with mechanical insufflation–exsufflation in patients with neuromuscular weakness. Eur. Respir. J. 21, 502–508.

Chatwin, M., Simonds, A.K., 2009. The addition of mechanical insufflation/exsufflation shortens airway-clearance sessions in neuromuscular patients with chest infection. Respir. Care. 54, 1473–1479.

Chatwin, M., Simonds, A.K., 2020. Long-term mechanical insufflation-exsufflation cough assistance in neuromuscular disease: patterns of use and lessons for application. Respir. Care. 65, 135–143.

Chatwin, M., Toussaint, M., Gonçalves, M.R., et al., 2018. Airway clearance techniques in neuromuscular disorders: a state of the art review. Respir. Med. 136, 98–110.

Chen, G.X., Douwes, J., van den Berg, L.H., et al., 2022. Sports and trauma as risk factors for Motor Neurone Disease: New Zealand case–control study. Acta Neurol. Scand. 145, 770–785.

Chio, A., et al., 2005. Severely increased risk of amyotrophic lateral sclerosis among Italian professional football players. Brain. 128, 472–476.

Chiò, A., Hammond, E.R., Mora, G., et al., 2015. Development and evaluation of a clinical staging system for amyotrophic lateral sclerosis. J. Neurol. Neurosurg. Psychiatry. 86, 38–44.

Chiò, A., Logroseine, G., Hardiman, O., et al., 2009. Prognostic factors in ALS: a critical review. Amyotroph. Lateral Scler. 10, 310–323.

Chiò, A., Mora, G., Lauria, G., 2017. Pain in amyotrophic lateral sclerosis. Lancet Neurol. 16, 144–157.

Chiò, A., Mora, G., Moglia, C., et al., 2017. Piemonte and Valle d'Aosta Register for ALS (PARALS). Secular trends of amyotrophic lateral sclerosis: the Piemonte and Valle d'Aosta Register. JAMA Neurol. 74, 1097–1104.

Cleary, S., et al., 2013. The effects of lung volume recruitment on coughing and pulmonary function in patients with ALS. Amyotroph. Lateral Scler. Frontotemporal Degener. 14, 111–115.

Connolly, O., Le Gall, L., McCluskey, G., et al., 2020. A systematic review of genotype–phenotype correlation across cohorts having causal mutations of different genes in ALS. J. Pers. Med. 10, 58.

Consonni, M., Telesca, A., Dalla Bella, E., et al., 2021. Amyotrophic lateral sclerosis patients' and caregivers' distress and loneliness during COVID-19 lockdown. J. Neurol. 268, 420–423.

Czaplinski, A., Yen, A.A., Appel, S.H., 2006. Forced vital capacity (FVC) as an indicator of survival and disease progression in an ALS clinic population. J. Neurol. Neurosurg. Psychiatry. 77, 390–392.

Dal Bello-Haas, V., 2002. A framework for rehabilitation in degenerative diseases: planning care and maximizing quality of life. Neurol. Rep 26, 115–129. (now Journal of Neurologic Physical Therapy)

Dal Bello-Haas, V., Krivickas, L., 2008. Amyotrophic lateral sclerosis. In: Durstine, J.L., Moore, G.E., Painter, P.L. (Eds.), ACSM's Exercise Management for Persons with Chronic Diseases and Disabilities, 3rd ed. Human Kinetics, Champaign, Illinois, pp. 336–341.

de Almeida, F.E.O., Santana, do Carmo, A.K., de Carvalho, F.O., 2021. Multidisciplinary care in amyotrophic lateral sclerosis: a systematic review and meta-analysis. Neurol. Sci. 42, 911–923.

de Carvalho, M., Swash, M., Pinto, S., 2019. Diaphragmatic neurophysiology and respiratory markers in ALS. Front. Neurol. 10, 143.

de Wit, J., Bakker, L.A., van Groenestijn, A.C., et al., 2018. Caregiver burden in amyotrophic lateral sclerosis: a systematic review. Palliat. Med. 32, 231–245.

Department of Health, 2005. Mental Capacity Act: Code of Practice. HMSO, Office of the Public Guardian, London.

Dharmadasa, T., Scaber, J., Edmond, E., et al., 2022. Genetic testing in motor neurone disease. Pract. Neurol. 22, 107–116.

Duncan, P.W., et al., 1990. Functional reach: a new clinical measure of balance. J. Gerontol. 45, M192–M197.

Edge, R., Mills, R., Tennant, A., et al.; TONiC Study Group., 2020. Do pain, anxiety and depression influence quality of life for people with amyotrophic lateral sclerosis/motor neuron disease? A national study reconciling previous conflicting literature. J. Neurol. 267, 607–615. Erratum in: J. Neurol. 2020; 267, 616–617.

Fujimura-Kiyono, C., et al., 2011. Onset and spreading patterns of lower motor neuron involvements predict survival in sporadic amyotrophic lateral sclerosis. J. Neurol. Neurosurg. Psychiatry. 82, 1244–1249.

Gargiulo-Monachelli, G.M., et al., 2012. Regional spread pattern predicts survival in patients with sporadic amyotrophic lateral sclerosis. Eur. J. Neurol. 19, 834–841.

Glasmacher, S.A., Larraz, J., Mehta, A.R., et al., 2021. The immediate impact of the COVID-19 pandemic on motor neuron disease services and mortality in Scotland. J. Neurol. 268, 2038–2040.

Gomez-Merino, E., Bach, J.R., 2002. Duchenne muscular dystrophy: prolongation of life by noninvasive ventilation and mechanically assisted coughing. Am. J. Phys. Med. Rehabil. 81, 411–415.

Gosselt, I.K., Nijboer, T.C.W., Van, Es, M.A., 2020. An overview of screening instruments for cognition and behavior in patients with ALS: selecting the appropriate tool for clinical practice. Amyotroph. Lateral Scler. Frontotemporal Degener. 21, 324–336.

Gowland, A., Opie-Martin, S., Scott, K.M., et al., 2019. Predicting the future of ALS: the impact of demographic change and potential new treatments on the prevalence of ALS in the United Kingdom, 2020–2116. Amyotroph. Lateral Scler. Frontotemporal Degener. 20, 264–274.

Hadjikoutis, S., Wiles, C.M., Eccles, R., 1999. Cough in motor neuron disease: a review of mechanisms. Q. J. Med. 92 (9), 487–494.

Hardiman, O., Al-Chalabi, A., Chio, A., et al., 2017. Amyotrophic lateral sclerosis. Nat. Rev. Dis. Primers. 3, 17071.

Hartmaier, S.L., Rhodes, T., Cook, S.F., et al., 2022. Qualitative measures that assess functional disability and quality of life in ALS. Health Qual. Life Outcomes. 20, 12.

Harwood, C.A., Westgate, K., Gunstone, S., et al., 2016. Long-term physical activity: an exogenous risk factor for sporadic amyotrophic lateral sclerosis. Amyotroph. Lateral Scler. Frontotemporal Degener. 17, 377–384.

Hayden, C.D., Murphy, B.P., Hardiman, O., et al., 2022. Measurement of upper limb function in ALS: a structure review of current methods and future directions. J. Neurol. 269, 4089–4101.

Huisman, M.H.B., et al., 2011. Population based epidemiology of amyotrophic lateral sclerosis using capture-recapture methodology. J. Neurol. Neurosurg. Psychiatry. 82, 1165–1170.

Ingels, P.L., et al., 2001. Adhesive capsulitis: a common occurrence in patients with ALS. Amyotroph. Lateral Scler. Mot. Neuron Disord. 2 (S2), 60.

Jenkinson, C., Fitzpatrick, R., 2001. Reduced item set for the amyotrophic lateral sclerosis assessment questionnaire: development and validation of the ALSAQ-5. J. Neurol. Neurosurg. Psychiatry. 70, 70–73.

Jenkinson, C., Fitzpatrick, R., Swash, M., et al., 2007. Comparison of the 40-item Amyotrophic Lateral Sclerosis Assessment Questionnaire (ALSAQ-40) with a short-form five-item version (ALSAQ-5) in a longitudinal survey. Clin. Rehabil. 21, 266–272.

Julian, T.H., Glascow, N., Barry, A.D.F., et al., 2021. Physical exercise is a risk factor for amyotrophic lateral sclerosis: convergent evidence from Mendelian randomisation, transcriptomics and risk genotypes. EBioMed. 68, 103397.

Keller, S., Bann, C.M., Dodd, S.L., et al., 2004. Validity of the brief pain inventory for use in documenting the outcomes of patients with noncancer pain. Clin. J. Pain. 20, 309–318.

Kloos, A., et al., 2004. Interrater and intrarater reliability of the Tinetti Balance Test. for individuals with amyotrophic lateral sclerosis. J. Neurol. Phys. Ther. 28, 12–19.

Körner, S., et al., 2011. Onset and spreading patterns of upper and lower motor neuron symptoms in amyotrophic lateral sclerosis. Muscle Nerve 43, 636–642.

Kostek, M.C., Gordon, B., 2018. Exercise is an adjuvant to contemporary dystrophy treatments. Exerc. Sport Sci. Rev 46, 34–41.

Kwak, S., 2022. Pain in amyotrophic lateral sclerosis: a narrative review. J. Yeungnam Med. Sci. 39, 181–189.

Lechtzin, N., et al., 2001. Hospitalization in amyotrophic lateral sclerosis: causes, costs, and outcomes. Neurology. 56, 753–757.

Leighton, D.J., Newton, J., Stephenson, L.J., et al.; CARE-MND Consortium, 2019. Changing epidemiology of motor neurone disease in Scotland. J. Neurol. 266, 817–825.

Lin, S.S., Sabharwal, S., Bibbo, C., 2000. Orthotic and bracing principles in neuromuscular foot and ankle problems. Foot Ankle Clin. 5, 235–264.

Longinetti, E., Fang, F., 2019. Epidemiology of amyotrophic lateral sclerosis: an update of recent literature. Curr. Opin. Neurol. 32, 771–776.

Lou, J.S., 2008. Fatigue in amyotrophic lateral sclerosis. Phys. Med. Rehabil. Clin. North Am. 9, 533–543.

Mackay, D.F., Russell, E.R., Stewart, K., et al., 2019. Neurodegenerative disease mortality among former professional soccer players. N. Engl. J. Med. 381, 1801–1808.

McCartney, N., Moroz, D., Garner, S.H., McComas, A.J., 1988. The effects of strength training in patients with selected neuromuscular disorders. Med. Sci. Sports Exerc. 20 (4), 362–368.

Mellies, U., Goebel, C., 2014. Optimum insufflation capacity and peak cough flow in neuromuscular disorders. Ann. Am. Thorac. Soc. 11, 1560–1568.

Miller, R.G., Mitchell, J.D., Moore, D.H., 2012. Riluzole for amyotrophic lateral sclerosis (ALS)/motor neurone disease (MND). Cochrane Database Syst. Rev. 3, CD001447.

Montes, J., et al., 2007. The Timed Up and Go test: predicting falls in ALS. Amyotroph. Lateral Scler. 8, 292–295.

Morrice, J.R., Gregory-Evans, C.Y., Shaw, C.A., 2017. Necroptosis in amyotrophic lateral sclerosis and other neurological disorders. Biochim. Biophys. Acta Mol. Basis Dis. 1863, 347–353.

Motor Neurone Disease Association (MNDA), 2017

Motor Neurone Disease Association (MNDA), 2015. Wheelchairs for people with motor neurone disease. Available at: https://www.mndassociation.org/app/uploads/2021/08/information-sheet-p2-wheelchairs-for-people-with-mnd.pdf.

Motor Neurone Disease Association & Royal College of General Practitioners, 2022. Red flag diagnosis tool for MND. Available at: https://www.mndassociation.org/app/uploads/2022/11/Red-Flag-tool-for-MND.pdf. Accessed 2 November 2022.

Musson, L.S., Collins, A., Opie-Martin, S., et al., 2022. Impact of the Covid-19 pandemic on amyotrophic lateral sclerosis care in the UK. Amyotroph. Lateral Scler. Frontotemporal. Degener. 24, 91–99.

National Institute for Health and Care Excellence (NICE), 2016. Motor neurone disease: assessment and management (NG42). NICE Guideline, London.

National Wheelchair Leadership Alliance, 2022 Wheelchair economic study [online] (Viewed November 2022). Available from: https://wheelchair-alliance.co.uk/app/uploads/2022/09/Wheelchair-economic-study-final-report.pdf

O'Brien, D., Stavroulakis, T., Baxter, S., et al., 2019. The optimisation of noninvasive ventilation in amyotrophic lateral sclerosis: a systematic review. Eur. Respir. J. 54, 1900261.

Okamoto, K., et al., 2009. Lifestyle factors and risk of amyotrophic lateral sclerosis: a case–control study in Japan. Ann. Epidemiol. 19, 359–364.

Oliver, D., 2016. Palliative care for patients with motor neurone disease: current challenges. Degener. Neurol. Neuromuscul. Dis. 6, 65–72.

Oliver, D.J., 2019. Palliative care in motor neurone disease: where are we now? Palliat. Care. 12 1178224218813914

Opie-Martin, S., Ossher, L., Bredin, A., et al., 2021. Motor Neuron Disease Register for England, Wales and Northern Ireland—an analysis of incidence in England. Amyotroph. Lateral Scler. Frontotemporal. Degener. 22, 86–88.

Park, J., Kim, J.E., Song, T.J., 2022. The global burden of motor neuron disease: an analysis of the 2019 Global Burden of Disease Study. Front. Neurol. 13, 864339.

Podsiadlo, D., Richardson, S., 1991. The timed "Up and Go": a test of basic functional mobility for frail elderly persons. J. Am. Geriatr. Soc. 39, 142–148.

Polkey, M.I., Lyall, R.A., Yang, K., et al., 2017. Respiratory muscle strength as a predictive biomarker for survival in amyotrophic lateral sclerosis. Am. J. Respir. Crit. Care Med. 195, 86–95.

Poponick, J.M., et al., 1997. Effect of upper respiratory tract infection in patients with neuromuscular disease. Am. J. Respir. Crit. Care. Med. 156, 659–664.

Prigent, H., Lejaille, M., Falaize, L., et al., 2004. Assessing inspiratory muscle strength by sniff nasal inspiratory pressure. Neurocrit. Care. 1, 475–478.

Pupillo, E., Bianchi, E., Vanacore, N., et al., 2020. Increased risk and early onset of ALS in professional players from Italian soccer teams. Amyotroph. Lateral Scler. Frontotemporal Degener. 21, 403–409.

Rafiq, M.K., 2018. The latest in motor neurone disease. Geriatr. Med. J. 48 (12) Available at: https://www.gmjournal.co.uk/motor-neurone-disease-a-clinical-overview. Accessed 23 May 2022.

Rafiq, M.K., et al., 2015. A preliminary randomised trial of the mechanical insufflators-exsufflator versus breath-stacking technique in patients with amyotrophic lateral sclerosis. Amyotroph. Lateral Scler. Frontotemporal Degener. 16, 448–455.

Rafiq, M.K., et al., 2016a. Mechanical cough augmentation techniques in amyotrophic lateral sclerosis/motor neuron disease (protocol). Cochrane Database Syst. Rev. 12, CD012482.

Rafiq, M.K., Bradburn, M., Mustfa, N., et al., 2016b. Mechanical cough augmentation techniques in amyotrophic lateral sclerosis/motor neuron disease. Cochrane Database Syst. Rev. 12, CD012482.

Richards, D., Morren, J.A., Pioro, E.P., 2020. Time to diagnosis and factors affecting diagnostic delay in amyotrophic lateral sclerosis. J. Neurol. Sci. 417, 117054.

Rooney, J., et al., 2015. A multidisciplinary clinic approach improves survival in ALS: a comparative study of ALS in Ireland and Northern Ireland. J. Neurol. Neurosurg. Psychiatry. 86, 496–503.

Sancho, J., Burés, E., Ferrer, S., et al., 2019. Usefulness of oscillations added to mechanical in-exsufflation in amyotrophic lateral sclerosis. Respir. Care. 65, 596–602.

Sancho, J., et al., 2004. Efficacy of mechanical insufflation-exsufflation in medically stable patients with amyotrophic lateral sclerosis. Chest. 125, 1400–1405.

Sharma, K.R., et al., 1995. Physiology of fatigue in amyotrophic lateral sclerosis. Neurology. 45, 733–740.

Sheers, N., Howard, M.E., Berlowitz, D.J., 2019. Respiratory adjuncts to NIV in neuromuscular disease. Respirology. 24, 512–520.

Shoesmith, C., Abrahao, A., Benstead, T., et al., 2020. Canadian best practice recommendations for the management of amyotrophic lateral sclerosis. CMAJ. 192, E1453–E1468.

Simmons, Z., et al., 2006. The ALSSQOL: balancing physical and non-physical factors in assessing quality of life in ALS. Neurology. 67, 1659–1664.

Su, W.M., Cheng, Y.F., Jiang, Z., Duan, Q.Q., Yang, T.M., Shang, H.F., Chen, Y.P., 2021. Predictors of survival in patients with amyotrophic lateral sclerosis: A large meta-analysis. EBioMedicine. 74, 103732.https://doi.org/10.1016/j.ebiom.2021.103732 Epub 2021 Dec 1. PMID: 34864363; PMCID: PMC8646173.

Stefanetti, R.J., Blain, A., Jimenez-Moreno, C., et al., 2020. Measuring the effects of exercise in neuromuscular disorders: a systematic review and meta-analyses. Wellcome Open Res. 5, 84.

Su, W.-M., Cheng, Y.-F., Jiang, Z., et al., 2021. Predictors of survival in patients with amyotrophic lateral sclerosis: a large meta-analysis. eBioMed. 74, 103732.

Sukockienė, E., Ferfoglia, R.I., Poncet, A., et al., 2021. Longitudinal Timed Up and Go assessment in amyotrophic lateral sclerosis: a pilot study. Eur. Neurol. 84, 375–379.

Sutedja, N.A., et al., 2009. What we truly know about occupation as a risk factor for ALS: a critical and systematic review. Amyotroph. Lateral Scler. 10, 295–301.

Sweeney, P., Park, H., Baumann, M., et al., 2017. Protein misfolding in neurodegenerative diseases: implications and strategies. Transl. Neurodegener. 6, 6.

Takei, K., Watanabe, K., Yuki, S., et al., 2017. Edaravone and its clinical development for amyotrophic lateral sclerosis. Amyotroph. Lateral Scler. Frontotemporal Degener. 18 (Suppl 1), 5–10.

Tinetti, M.E., 1986. Performance-oriented assessment of mobility problems in elderly patients. J. Am. Geriatr. Soc. 34, 119–126.

Tomik, B., Guiloff, R.J., 2010. Dysarthria in amyotrophic lateral sclerosis: a review. Amyotroph. Lateral Scler. 11 (1-2), 4–15.

Toussaint, M., et al., 2009. Limits of effective cough-augmentation techniques in patients with neuromuscular disease. Respir. Care. 54, 359–366.

Toussaint, M., Chatwin, M., Gonzales, J., et al.; ENMC Respiratory Therapy Consortium. 2018. 228th ENMC International Workshop: airway clearance techniques in neuromuscular disorders. Naarden, The Netherlands, 3–5 March, 2017. Neuromuscul. Disord. 28, 289–298.

Toussaint, M., et al., 2015. Cough augmentation in subjects with Duchene Muscular Dystrophy: comparison of air stacking via resuscitator bag versus mechanical ventilation. Respir. Care. 61 (1), 61–77.

Trebbia, G., Lancombe, M., et al., 2005. Cough determinants in patients with neuromuscular disease. Respir. Physiol. Neurobiol. 146, 291–300.

Tzeng, A.C., Bach, J.R., 2000. Prevention of pulmonary morbidity for patients with neuromuscular disease. Chest. 118, 1390–1396.

Vianello, A., Corrado, A., Arcaro, G., et al., 2005. Mechanical insufflation–exsufflation improves outcomes for neuromuscular disease patients with respiratory tract infections. Am. J. Med. Rehabil. 84, 83–88.

Voet, N.B.M., et al., 2013. Strength training and aerobic exercise training for muscle disease. Cochrane Database Syst. Rev. 7, CD003907.

Voet, N.B., van der Kooi, E.L., van Engelen, B.G., Geurts, A.C., 2019. Strength training and aerobic exercise training for muscle disease. Cochrane Database Syst. Rev. 12, CD003907.

Walsh, L.J., Deasy, K.F., Gomez, F., et al., 2021. Use of non-invasive ventilation in motor neuron disease—a retrospective cohort analysis. Chron. Respir. Dis. 18 14799731211063886

Westeneng, H.J., Debray, T.P.A., Visser, A.E., et al., 2018. Prognosis for patients with amyotrophic lateral sclerosis: development and validation of a personalised prediction model. Lancet Neurol. 17, 423–433.

Wijesekera, L.C., Leigh, P.N., 2009. Amyotrophic lateral sclerosis. Orphanet J. Rare. Dis. 4, 3.

Polyneuropathies

Gita Ramdharry, Aisling Carr, and Matilde Laurá

OUTLINE

Introduction, 355
Anatomy and Physiology, 356
Causes of Neuropathy, 356
Specific Types of Neuropathy, 357
Acquired Neuropathies, 357
Guillain–Barré Syndrome, 358
Chronic Demyelinating Polyradiculoneuropathy, 361
Diabetic Neuropathy, 362
Hereditary Neuropathies, 363
Charcot–Marie–Tooth Disease, 363
Assessment of People With Polyneuropathies, 366
**Physical Management and Rehabilitation Approaches
for People with Polyneuropathies, 369**
Acute Rehabilitation of Acquired Polyneuropathies, 370
Long-Term Physical Management and
Rehabilitation, 370
Self-management, 370
*Exercise and Physical Activity Interventions in
Polyneuropathy, 370*
Balance Interventions, 371
Orthotic Management, 372
Management of the Neuropathic Hand, 372
Pain and Fatigue Management, 372
Case Study, 372

Presenting Impairments, 373
Musculoskeletal Integrity and Alignment, 373
Muscle Strength and Sensation, 373
Observation of Activities, 373
Upper Limb Function, 373
Gait, 374
Mr V's Reported Problems and Impact on
Participation, 374
Fatigue, 374
Balance, 374
Pain, 374
Physiotherapy Options for Mr V, 374
Orthotic Prescription, 374
Range of Movement, 375
Muscle Strength and Aerobic Exercise, 375
Balance, 375
Outcome, 375
Management of Upper Limb Function: Exercise, 375
Hand Splints and Equipment, 376
Outcome, 363
Management of Fatigue, 376
Outcome, 376
Self-management, 376
Follow up and Remote Support , 376

INTRODUCTION

Polyneuropathies are generalised disorders of the peripheral nerves and a common neurological problem. The cause, pathology and presentation of this group of diseases are wide ranging and variable (England & Asbury 2004). Some neuropathies have an acute onset and presentation, whereas others have a more chronic, slowly progressing picture. This chapter outlines some common polyneuropathies, with examples given of acquired and hereditary causes. Evidence and best practice for rehabilitation interventions will be illustrated with a case study.

Polyneuropathies affect both motor and sensory neurones and are described as mixed, but some can have a predilection for one modality of neurones with predominantly, or exclusively, motor or sensory deficits. The key pathology is an impairment of transmission of nerve action potentials caused by disruption of either the axon or the myelin sheath (Fig. 14.1). Myelin and axonal damage can occur for

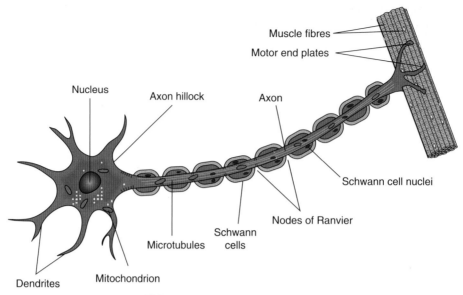

FIG. 14.1 Normal motor neurone.

a variety of reasons, such as infection, drug or environmental toxicity, metabolic and autoimmune disorders, malignancy and genetic factors (Hughes 2008).

ANATOMY AND PHYSIOLOGY

To understand the pathology of nerve disease, a basic understanding of nerve physiology helps to explain the deficits and symptoms experienced by people with neuropathy (see Fig. 14.1) (England & Asbury 2004). The health of the neurone from the proximal to the distal end is maintained by axonal transport. The process of axonal transport aims to move organelles, proteins, lipids, RNA and metabolic by-products up and down the long axons. The cytoskeleton of the axon has three structures along the length: actin microfilaments, neurofilaments and microtubules. Kinesin and dynein are proteins known as 'motor proteins' that anchor to the microtubules and transport organelles and lysosomes along the axon in anterograde and retrograde directions (Prior et al 2017). Transport of mitochondria is important to meet the energy requirements of nerve conduction at the periphery.

Peripheral nervous system myelination occurs in early development through a process of spiral wrapping of Schwann cells' plasma membrane around the axon (Taveggia 2016). In fast conducting myelinated neurones, propagation of the action potential relies on the interaction between the nerve axon and myelin. In motor neurones, an action potential is triggered at the axon hillock when a stimulus is received from the central nervous system. In sensory neurones, depolarisation occurs through stimulation of the sensory end organ. Action potentials are generated by the opening of clustered voltage-gated sodium (Na^+) channels, leading to an influx of Na^+ ions which depolarises the membrane. Closure of the Na^+ channels terminates the action potential by restoring the resting membrane potential (Vucic et al 2009). Clusters of channels also exist at the nodes of Ranvier in myelinated fibres. A process called saltatory conduction allows the current to spread farther and quicker between nodes, thus speeding up the action potential.

CAUSES OF NEUROPATHY

Neuropathies occur when there is damage to the axon or myelin of a neurone. The factors which make peripheral nerves vulnerable to damage are their long length and the high-energy requirements of constant, bidirectional axonal transport. Environmental insults affect function by permeating the incomplete blood–nerve barrier surrounding each neurone (Prior et al 2017).

Axonal neuropathies are the most common type of polyneuropathy. They are characterised by abnormality and degeneration of the nerve axons and can affect nerves of any diameter or modality. Degeneration of the axon results in prevention of propagation of the nerve action potentials manifesting as reductions in amplitude of compound motor action potentials (CMAPs) on electrophysiological testing. The causes vary from metabolic disorders, such as chronic renal failure and malignancy, to genetic mutations or toxicity from chemical agents (England & Asbury 2004).

Demyelination occurs when there is degeneration or destruction of myelin. Myelinated nerves are the larger and faster conducting neurones (e.g., motor neurones and 1a sensory afferents), and a predilection for large-fibre dysfunction is seen in demyelinating neuropathies (England & Asbury 2004). In simple terms, this results in slowing of action potential conduction because of loss of the saltatory spread from node to node. On electrophysiological testing, this results in reduced conduction velocity with relative sparing of the amplitude (or size) of the action potential. It is worth noting, however, that prolonged periods of demyelination can lead to axonal degeneration at which point the action potential amplitude will drop. It has been hypothesised that metabolic regulators and mitochondrial function of Schwann cells are crucial to axonal health, so Schwann cell destruction can lead to axonopathy (Taveggia 2016). Demyelination could cause an alteration of axonal ion channels, increased energy requirements and downregulation of neurotrophic factors from within Schwann cells that lead to disturbances in axonal transport and subsequent axonal degeneration (Nicholson 2006, Pisciotta et al 2021).

SPECIFIC TYPES OF NEUROPATHY

Polyneuropathies can be classified as acquired or inherited, pertaining to the cause of the disease process. Differentiating between the causes is of high importance at diagnosis because some acquired neuropathies are amenable to medical treatment. Four common neuropathies will be presented in detail and are summarised in Table 14.1.

Acquired Neuropathies

There are multiple insults which can cause previously normal nerves to dysfunction, including toxin exposure, mechanical injury, infection, nutritional deficiency, autoimmune attack or metabolic derangement secondary to another medical condition. Defective axonal transport has been implicated as a key pathological process in many, but not all, acquired neuropathies leading to axon degeneration and the subsequent motor and sensory symptoms observed clinically (Prior et al 2017).

Poisons such as heavy metals have a toxic effect on nerve function, with particular impact on motor nerves, but drug toxicity is more common overall. Many cancer chemotherapeutic agents are neurotoxic, but close clinical monitoring and dose adjustment or changing drug can limit nerve damage. Critical care–associated neuropathies have complex pathology and may be partly caused by neuromuscular blocking agents administered during critical illness, but the direct link is unclear and many other factors are also implicated, such as infection and sepsis (Hermans & Van den Berghe 2015). The most common cause of peripheral nerve involvement after Covid-19 infection is critical care–related polyneuropathy and/or myopathy, but compressive, focal damage to sciatic nerve or brachial plexus related to prolonged immobility and complications of prone positioning have been reported (Taga & Lauria 2022). Certain infectious agents have a predilection for nerve-causing injury either by direct infection (leprosy, *Borrelia* spp., brucellosis, tuberculosis, rabies, leptospirosis, cytomegalovirus, and herpes viruses) (Neal & Gasque 2016)) or via postinfection inflammatory insult (*Campylobacter jejuni* and Guillain–Barré syndrome [GBS] or hepatitis C and vasculitic neuropathy). Many of these infectious agents are rare in the developed world but remain common or endemic in geographical hotspots, such as leprosy/*Mycobacterium leprae* in Brazil and Bangladesh. Inflammatory neuropathies may be precipitated by a preceding infection (see Guillain–Barré Syndrome section) or a spontaneous loss of self-regulation leading to autoimmune attack (see Chronic Inflammatory Demyelinating Polyradiculoneuropathy section). Polyneuropathy can also be caused by nutritional deficiencies, affecting the sensory nerves more so than motor pathways. Vitamin B12 deficiency is a common cause of neuropathy and can often be observed in people with chronic alcohol abuse because of problems absorbing the vitamin, as well as reduced intake. Thiamine, pyridoxal and copper should also be considered because malnutrition or malabsorption can result in multiple nutritional deficiencies. Diabetes is a medical condition that can lead to nerve damage as a secondary symptom and is the most common cause of neuropathy in adults in high income countries. Prolonged elevation in blood sugar concentration is the primary pathological process and is neurotoxic via a

TABLE 14.1   **Summary of Four Common Types of Polyneuropathy**

Name of Neuropathy	Cause	Timing of Onset	Rate of Progression	Presentation	Medical Management
Guillain–Barré syndrome	Acquired Inflammatory Autoimmune damage to the myelin	Acute	Rapid, ≤6 weeks to nadir	Ascending sensory impairment motor paralysis	Intravenous immunoglobulin Plasma exchange
Chronic inflammatory demyelinating polyradiculoneuropathy	Acquired Inflammatory Autoimmune damage to the myelin	Chronic	Slow, >8 weeks to nadir	Patchy presentation of sensorimotor impairment	Intravenous immunoglobulin Steroids
Diabetic neuropathy	Acquired axonal neuropathy Metabolic dysfunction secondary to diabetes mellitus	Chronic	Slow, over years	Distal, sensory predominant; mainly affecting small fibres	Control of blood sugar, foot care and pain management
Charcot–Marie–Tooth disease	Hereditary, from mutations in genes affecting peripheral nerve function (myelin or axon)	Chronic	Very slow, over decades	Distal, symmetrical sensorimotor impairment	No disease-modifying medical therapies Focus on symptom management

range of mechanisms (Prior et al 2017). The most common manifestation is a length-dependent anaesthetic neuropathy which results in ulceration of the extremities, leading to amputation.

The commonality of all the acquired neuropathies is their potential for treatment. With correct identification of the underlying cause and appropriate management, the nerve damage can be halted or even reversed in some cases.

Guillain–Barré Syndrome

GBS is an umbrella term for acute-onset, postinfectious inflammatory neuropathies. GBS is a rare, sporadically occurring disease, and incidence rates range from 0.8 to 1.9 (median 1.1) cases per 100,000 people each year (Willison et al 2016). It can affect any age group but is more prevalent in men and in older people, for whom the long-term outcome can be worse (Vucic et al 2009). The most common form in Europe and North America is acute inflammatory demyelinating polyradiculoneuropathy (AIDP) in which patchy inflammatory attack of myelin occurs along the length of the nerves, at both proximal and distal ends. In

Asia, other variants are seen more frequently, such as acute motor axonal neuropathy and acute motor sensory axonal neuropathy which is now believed to represent antibody-mediated destruction of paranodal structures rather than true primary axonal pathology (Fehmi et al 2021).

GBS is an autoimmune disorder where a preceding infection triggers an immune response directed towards neuronal antigens. In about two-thirds of cases, the preceding infectious agent can be identified (Lehmann et al 2012, Vucic et al 2009); *Campylobacter jejuni*, cytomegalovirus, Epstein–Barr and influenza A viruses have been implicated (Willison et al 2016). During the Covid-19 pandemic there were concerns that GBS was a neurological complication of Covid-19 infection, but no link has been found (Keddie et al 2021). A temporal relationship with GBS cases was found, however, after administration of the first dose of Covid-19 vaccines using adenoviral vectors (Keh et al 2023). The risk was 5 cases per 1,000,000 doses, tending to affect older men, and the effect was not observed after repeat doses or with mRNA vaccines.

In AIDP, the immune response to the original infection leads to an inflammatory process mediated by antibodies

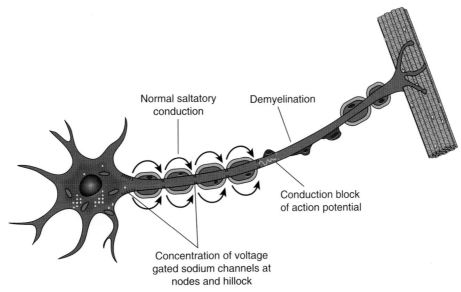

Normal saltatory conduction

Demyelination

Conduction block of action potential

Concentration of voltage gated sodium channels at nodes and hillock

FIG. 14.2 Acute demyelination and conduction block.

which cross-react with specific bacterial epitopes and similar proteins on the surface of neuronal myelin, typically gangliosides on the Schwann cell surface. This molecular mimicry leads to destruction of the myelin sheath and disruption of saltatory conduction leading to a slowing or block of nerve conduction (Fig. 14.2). The impaired function of large-diameter, myelinated motor and sensory neurones results in weakness, numbness and loss of vibration and proprioception as the hallmarks of the clinical syndrome.

Presentation. The AIDP form of GBS presents with lower motor neurone weakness and sensory loss that progresses to nadir (maximum severity) within 6 weeks of onset. Because of the patchy nature of the inflammatory attack, the initial symptoms can begin distal or proximal, upper or lower limbs, cranial nerves and spread from there. The characteristic syndrome is lower back pain, caused by nerve root inflammation, followed by ascending numbness, paraesthesia and weakness. Cranial nerves are affected in 50%, with diplopia and facial and bulbar weakness (Lehmann et al 2012, Vucic et al 2009). Autonomic involvement is commonplace in AIDP, causing fluctuations in blood pressure and cardiac arrhythmias. Symptoms can affect functional abilities such as walking, standing or even sitting in severe cases. Severity is marked by extensive truncal weakness, bulbar dysfunction, dysautonomia and neuromuscular respiratory failure (vital capacity <20 mL/kg). In up to one-third of cases respiratory support is required to maintain lung volumes and manage secondary respiratory infections (England & Asbury 2004, Vucic et al 2009). Secondary complications such as pneumonia and tracheobronchial infections can lead to extended periods of ventilation (Netto et al 2017).

Tracheostomy is common in this scenario and associated with extended critical care admission (Ali et al 2006).

Early recognition of the clinical syndrome is the key to prompt diagnosis because all supportive tests lack sensitivity and specificity. Key examination findings include hypotonia, weakness, areflexia and evidence of large-fibre sensory loss with reduced pinprick, vibration and proprioception in a generally length-dependent pattern. In 25% of patients with GBS, ganglioside antibodies are present in the blood. A combination of elevated cerebrospinal fluid (CSF) protein and fewer than 10 white cells is seen in approximately 80% of cases, although it may not be apparent in the first week (Hughes 2008). In the very early stages, electrophysiology can be unhelpful. Eventually nerve conduction studies show decreased conduction velocity and partial conduction block (see Fig. 14.2).

Medical Management. GBS not affecting mobility is managed conservatively, and recovery is spontaneous albeit gradual. Severe disease is defined as loss of independent ambulation and is the indicator used to initiate treatment. Both intravenous immunoglobulin (IVIg) and plasma exchange (PE) are effective treatments for GBS. They do not alter the endpoint but simply accelerate recovery (Hughes et al 2014). PE hastens recovery compared with supportive treatment alone. There are no adequate comparisons of IVIg with placebo in adults, but there is evidence that in severe disease, IVIg started within 2 weeks from onset hastens recovery as much as PE (Hughes et al 2014). Mainly for practical reasons, IVIg usually is the preferred treatment. Rather surprisingly, given the inflammatory nature of the disease, steroids alone are ineffective. Whether GBS patients with severe disease or poor prognostic markers could benefit from intensified immunomodulation has been debated for many years.

The International GBS Outcome Study is a worldwide prognostic study that aims to get further insight into the pathogenesis of GBS and help develop better prognostic scales (van Doorn 2013). Despite treatment, GBS can be a severe disease, as about 25% of patients require artificial ventilation during a period of days to months, about 20% of patients are still unable to walk after 6 months and 3%–10% of patients die. The Erasmus GBS Respiratory Insufficiency Score uses a combination of factors including age, preceding diarrhoeal illness and muscle weakness at admission to hospital to identify patients at risk of severe disease, prolonged disability and at high risk of intubation (Walgaard et al 2010). A recently published randomised controlled trial compared outcome between a subgroup who received standard of care (IVIg 2 g/kg) versus standard of care plus a second dose of IVIg at 7–10 days (Walgaard et al 2021). No difference was found on any of the clinical outcomes measured at 6 months, but there was a significantly higher rate of complications in those who received a second dose of IVIg. This included thrombosis and haemolytic anaemia, well-recognised IVIg-related adverse events. Therefore in severely affected individuals, high-quality supportive care is paramount, and further immunosuppression or immunomodulation beyond the acute, postinfectious stage is more harmful than beneficial to the patient.

Ventilator and circulatory support is essential for those with significant respiratory failure or dysautonomia and must be managed in a critical care setting. Close clinical monitoring of patients at ward level is vitally important for early identification of those who require increased support. Supported nutrition and protection against aspiration are part of managing those with bulbar involvement. Speech and language therapy and physiotherapy are as important during acute management as during the rehabilitation phase.

In addition, many patients have pain, fatigue or other residual complaints that may persist for months or years. Pain was reported as an initial symptom in 36% of a sample of people with GBS, with 66% reporting pain during the acute phase that persisted during the first year in 38% (Merkies & Kieseier 2016). Medical management of pain includes simple analgesics or opioids, but more often antidepressants such as gabapentin or amitriptyline are required to manage the neuropathic discomfort.

Disease Course and Prognosis. GBS typically runs a monophasic course. Severity is variable, but weakness reaches nadir within 6 weeks (Fig. 14.3). About 5% of patients initially diagnosed with GBS turn out to have acute-onset chronic inflammatory demyelinating polyradiculoneuropathy (CIDP); this manifests as deterioration more than 6 weeks from onset after initial response to treatment. It is sensible to test for paranodal antibodies (contactin, Caspr2, neurofascin) in this scenario because these patients do very well with rituximab. About 10%–20% of cases are left with disabling symptoms (Vucic et al 2009). Recovery will depend on the degree of axonal damage during the earlier stages of the disease. Certain factors have been associated to the degree of secondary axonal loss, such as older age and high levels of impairment at the nadir (Vucic et al 2009).

Although weakness and sensory loss are the major impairments, persistent fatigue is a common feature in the more chronic stage, with 50%–60% reporting severe fatigue after a year (Davidson & Parker 2022, Merkies & Faber 2012). Poor conditioning and fatigue have been associated with worse psychosocial performance after recovery (Khan & Amatya 2012). The severity of fatigue, however, does not correlate with disease severity at the nadir, peripheral nerve function, previous infections or degree of weakness. Instead, relationships with the social and emotional domains of the Short Form 36 (SF-36) were observed (Merkies & Kieseier 2016). Fatigue is more prevalent in females and people older than 50 years (Garssen et al 2006). A relationship was found between fatigue and central activation with repeated muscle contraction that may be caused by changes in motor unit size and myelination pattern on recovery from GBS (Garssen et al 2007). Falls have been found to occur more frequently in the chronic

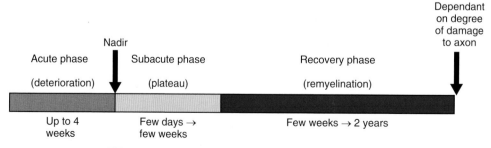

FIG. 14.3 Disease course of Guillain–Barré syndrome.

phase which could be related to body pain and fatigue (Davidson & Parker 2022).

Chronic Demyelinating Polyradiculoneuropathy

CIDP is the most common acquired chronic demyelinating neuropathy affecting approximately 3 per 100,000 people (England & Asbury 2004, Hughes 2008). It occurs more frequently in adults aged 40–60 years with a slightly higher prevalence in men (Westblad et al 2009).

CIDP has similarities to GBS in that it is an immunologically mediated demyelinating neuropathy. It presents with multifocal demyelination affecting spinal nerve roots, proximal nerve trunks and plexuses, predominantly leading to patchy regions of demyelination with some inflammatory infiltrates (Said 2006). The exact cause or trigger for CIDP is not known and is likely to be multifactorial; there is no genetic predisposition, but several studies have suggested an infective episode or vaccination in the weeks before onset of the neuropathy. Approximately half of patients have antibodies against myelin-associated glycoprotein, and protein levels in the CSF are raised with albuminocytologic dissociation similar to GBS (Said 2006).

Presentation. Unlike most inherited and metabolic polyneuropathies, CIDP is not length dependent. A symmetrical, motor-predominant, sensorimotor neuropathy with proximal and distal weakness in the lower limbs is characteristic (Hughes 2008). Although a sensorimotor neuropathy is most common, pure sensory and pure motor forms are reported (Rajabally et al 2009). Most people have absent tendon reflexes and 4%–15% have a facial palsy (Said 2006). The presentation of CIDP is highly variable, but slow progression (to nadir >8 weeks) differentiates it from GBS (Hughes 2008).

Electrophysiology is much more helpful than in diagnosis of GBS, and there are several diagnostic criteria based on electrophysiological abnormalities. The European Federation of Neurological Societies (EFNS) and the Peripheral Nerve Society (PNS) have recently revised diagnostic criteria with widespread clinical application (Van den Bergh et al 2021). Testing reveals slowing and multifocal conduction block as indicative of an acquired demyelinating neuropathy (England & Asbury 2004, Said 2006). Reports of activity-dependent conduction block in CIDP could be functionally important because paresis can increase with repeated use (Pollard 2002). The degree of secondary axonal loss at presentation predicts poor outcome.

People with CIDP report problems with mobility, balance and manual dexterity. In a study describing physical functioning, nearly 50% of subjects (n = 21) reported that balance and walking difficulties were the worst consequences of having CIDP (Westblad et al 2009). The same

study found deficits in balance scores, Timed Up and Go test, manual dexterity and the physical functioning domains of the SF-36 health status questionnaire. Draak and colleagues have developed and validated a Rasch-built, CIDP-specific, patient-rated, disability score: CIDP Rasch-built Overall Disability Scale for inflammatory neuropathy (Draak et al 2014). This score is now in wide clinical use because it correlates well with disease activity and CIDP impact of disease on the individual. Other responsive clinical outcome measures include grip strength and 10-metre timed walk.

Fatigue is reported as severe in people with CIDP and is one of the three most disabling symptoms in most patients (Merkies & Faber 2012). The level of fatigue does not correlate with impairment measures of muscle strength and sensation or disease severity, but does seem to relate to the physical functioning and general health domains of the SF-36 general health measure (Merkies & Kieseier 2016). The consequence of fatigue in this population, however, is the potential for a reduction in daily activity and secondary deconditioning.

CIDP was thought to be a painless condition; however, there have been some reports of mild to moderate pain in some cohorts. The distribution appears to be distal, suggesting a neuropathic origin (Merkies & Kieseier 2016).

Disease Course and Prognosis. The disease course can vary. In a UK population, 52% of cases were relapsing-remitting, 35% had a progressing disease and 13% had a single-incident/monophasic course (Rajabally et al 2009). Response to treatment will also have an important influence in how the disease manifests and changes. In the same UK study, there was a response to immunotherapy in more than 80% of cases, between 15% and 30% may require only one treatment, and of those requiring longer-term treatment initially, natural history studies reveal up to 40% are in remission at 2 years (Rajabally et al 2009).

Medical Management. Patients with mild symptoms without functional impairment do not require treatment. Treatment with corticosteroids or IVIg should be offered to those with moderate or severe disability (Joint Task Force of the EFNS and the PNS 2010, Van den Bergh et al 2021). PE is similarly effective but less readily available and more difficult to deliver. IVIg is usually the first choice because improvement can be fast. The usual first dose of IVIg is 2 g/kg given over 4–5 days at 4–6 weekly intervals until improvement plateaus. Dose and frequency can then be titrated to an optimal individualised regimen according to clinical response measured by disease-specific clinical outcome measurement. Contraindications to corticosteroids will influence the choice towards IVIg and vice versa. For motor CIDP, IVIg is recommended because corticosteroids can result in worsening of the weakness. In the 20% of cases which do not adequately respond to first-line treatments, the addition of a steroid-sparing agent can be considered. Approximately 15% of patients fail to respond to treatment, and lack of response should trigger consideration of CIDP mimics and further investigation (Kuitwaard & van Doorn 2009).

Diabetic Neuropathy

In people older than 40 years, the incidence of peripheral axonal neuropathy is approximately 14%. Of these cases, half have neuropathy caused by diabetes mellitus and almost all the other half are idiopathic. Of the idiopathic group, it is now being suggested that prediabetes or impaired glucose tolerance is a possible cause of neuropathy (Smith & Singleton 2008).

The pathological process is initiated through hyperglycaemia which has a toxic effect on the nerves via oxidative stress, impaired axonal transport and accumulation of end products from glycation (Smith & Singleton 2008). There is also an effect on the microvascular structures supporting the nerves with defects in the capillary endothelia (Smith & Singleton 2008).

Dyslipidaemia has also been implicated, in particular triglyceridaemia, as a possible trigger for diabetic neuropathy (DN) through oxidative stress mechanisms causing neurovascular injury. In mouse models, high-fat feeding results in glucose intolerance and the development of neuropathy (Vincent et al 2009). High levels of serum triglycerides in humans correlate with the progression of DN (Vincent et al 2009).

Presentation. Diagnosis of DN is from neurological examination, indicating the existence of a peripheral neuropathy, and glucose tolerance testing (Hughes 2008). The progression is slow, and prognosis often depends on diabetic management.

DN has several different presentations. Most common is a length-dependent, small-fibre neuropathy. The patient reports burning and numbness in the feet because of the involvement of the smaller-diameter, unmyelinated fibres from the cutaneous pain receptors (England & Asbury 2004). Skin biopsies reveal reduced density of unmyelinated fibres in the epidermis indicating degeneration (England & Asbury 2004).

Next is a length-dependent, sensory-predominant neuropathy characterised by loss of sensation spreading proximally over years; weakness is not typically seen until sensory loss reaches midthigh. The autonomic nervous system is commonly affected but typically subclinical in adult-onset, or type 2, diabetes. Dysautonomia can be extremely bothersome in type 1 with orthostatic hypotension and gastroparesis having significant impact on function. Rare presentations include painful lumbosacral plexopathy or Bruns Garland syndrome, which presents with proximal lower limb pain followed by weakness and marked weight loss. There may be gradual recovery over months in the presence of normalised blood sugar levels, but this is not always the case. Diabetes also puts the individual at risk from focal neuropathies such as compressive mononeuropathies, cranial neuropathies and truncal radiculopathies (Llewelyn 2003).

Where there is a loss of protective sensation, particularly in the foot, plantar ulceration is an unwelcome complication which can lead to partial foot or major lower extremity amputation (Kanade et al 2006, van Deursen 2008). Increases in pressure over the plantar surface can occur because of changes in the gait pattern and increased double support. Elevated plantar pressures can increase the risk of injury to the skin and plantar ulceration. Some concerns have been raised that if walking is encouraged as part of exercise and lifestyle advice, there could be an increase in plantar pressures, so protective footwear is recommended in conjunction with walking and exercise (Kanade et al 2006). A decline in physical fitness and activity levels has been observed with increased foot complications, so prevention is also important for general management of diabetes through an active lifestyle (Kanade et al 2006).

Another consequence of sensory loss is postural instability and falls caused by reduced proprioception and cutaneous sensation. Increased incidence of falls was highlighted in people with diabetes, with and without neuropathy, in a review of evidence (Khan & Andersen 2022). Posturography studies have highlighted an increase in postural sway in people with DN during static standing. One study found a modest correlation between sway and measures of sensation over the plantar surface (Ducic et al 2004). A comparison with people with diabetes but no neuropathy demonstrated a deterioration in balance performance with static standing but no difference with dynamic balance tests (Emam et al 2009). This may be because of the various roles of the different-sized sensory afferents.

Deficits in temporal and spatial gait parameters are also reported because of sensorimotor impairment (Khan & Andersen 2022, Paul et al 2009). A study of muscle activation patterns in people with DN revealed a delay in the first activation peaks of tibialis anterior, the peronei and soleus with treadmill walking, leading to a longer support phase (Sacco & Amadio 2003). The investigators hypothesised that reduced sensation would lead to a delay in the loading response after initial contact. Cognitive and motor load during walking caused deterioration in temporal spatial gait parameters in people with diabetes and a group with DN (Paul et al 2009). This implies that gait impairment and falls risk may increase under dual-task situations.

Medical Management. The mainstay of management is optimal blood sugar control, but fastidious foot care and pain management are important.

Neuropathic pain and dysaesthesia can be difficult to treat but are an important focus of medical management for people with DN. Gabapentin and amitriptyline may reduce pain, but the side effect of weight gain is best avoided in patients with diabetes so pregabalin and duloxetine are recommended as alternative neuropathic pain medications (Llewelyn 2003). Topical lidocaine can be useful when there are discreet areas of dysaesthesia (Hughes 2008). Refractory pain may respond to mexiletine, selective serotonin reuptake inhibitors (citalopram or paroxetine), anticonvulsants (lamotrigine or topiramate), opioids or spinal cord stimulators. Acupuncture and clinical psychologists can also play an important role.

Hereditary Neuropathies

Charcot–Marie–Tooth Disease

The most common hereditary neurological condition is a polyneuropathy called Charcot–Marie–Tooth disease (CMT), which causes degeneration of the peripheral nerves. It has a prevalence of 1 per 2500, although this varies among reported epidemiology studies between 9.7 and 82.3 per 100,000 (Barreto et al 2016, Laurá et al 2019). The name originates from the three neurologists who described it in 1886. The first gene causing the CMT phenotype was mapped in 1989. Since then many more have been identified, and more than 100 genes have been found to cause CMT (Laurá et al 2019, Reilly & Rossor 2020). The most common types of CMT show a slow decline in distal muscle strength and sensation that predominantly affects the longer peripheral nerves. Most genes causing CMT have autosomal dominant inheritance, although there are rarer autosomal recessive types. Family history is an important step in deciding if and how a neuropathy is inherited (Rossor et al 2017).

Type 1 CMT (CMT1) presents with demyelination of the more thickly myelinated, fast-conducting axons, for example, the alpha motor neurones and 1a afferent sensory neurones. As with other demyelinating polyneuropathies, axonal loss occurs with prolonged demyelination. In CMT1 there is an increase in the motor unit size, that is, an increase in the number of muscle fibres supplied by one motor axon. This occurs during the chronic, slow denervation process when unaffected motor axons can produce collateral sprouts that reinnervate previously denervated muscle fibres (Ericson et al 2000).

Type 1 A CMT (CMT1A) refers to a type of CMT1 caused by the most common gene mutation. It accounts for up to 80% of people with CMT1 and is caused by duplication of the *PMP22* gene on the short arm of chromosome 17. Duplication of this gene affects the stability of the myelin sheath, causing progressive demyelination (Pareyson et al 2006).

The genetic test for CMT1A became available in the 1990's, allowing diagnosis of a whole family with a simple blood test from one affected member. On electrophysiological examination, people with CMT1 have symmetrical, distal slowing of peripheral nerve conduction velocities caused by a reduction in saltatory conduction (Fig. 14.4). They may also present with a reduction in the amplitude of CMAP and sensory nerve action potentials (SNAPs), which will reflect the degree of secondary axonal degeneration.

Type 2 CMT (CMT2) presents with degeneration of the nerve axon. The axonal forms of CMT are rarer than type 1. The most common mutation is of the *mitofusin 2* gene, causing type 2 A CMT, which accounts for about 20% of cases (Cartoni & Martinou 2009). Mitofusin 2 is a mitochondrial protein that plays an important role in the process of mitochondrial fusion within a cell. In nerves, the long axon has high-energy requirements far away from the nerve cell body, which is provided by the mitochondria. Deficiency of mitofusin 2 affects the transport of mitochondria down the axon (Cartoni & Martinou 2009, Gutmann & Shy 2015). This can result in degeneration of the distal axon that is initially seen in longer nerves such as those supplying the foot and ankle muscles. The response to denervation seems to differ to CMT1 because people with CMT2 show a compensatory increase in contractile tissue as reflected by muscle fibre hypertrophy. The reasons for the differences are not clear, but it is suggested that in CMT2 there may be a reduced ability to form collateral sprouts (Ericson et al 2000).

As with CMT1, family history is an important step to determine the inheritance, but there are fewer opportunities for diagnostic genetic testing because the genes known for CMT2 can diagnose only around 30% of cases. Electrophysiology aids differentiation between CMT types because people with CMT2 have normal conduction velocities but show a symmetrical reduction in the amplitude of distal CMAPs and SNAPs because of primary axonal degeneration.

There are other types of CMT that vary in inheritance and genetic cause (e.g., X linked and recessive). Other complex genetic subtypes presenting with neuropathy also show upper motor neurone features, such as hereditary spastic paraparesis, ataxias (Laurá et al 2019, Rossor et al 2017), vestibular involvement (Cortese et al 2020, Reilly & Rossor 2020) and multiple other systems (Rossor et al 2017).

Presentation. Muscle wasting is one of the key signs described for people with CMT with the classic 'inverted champagne bottle' appearance of the distal lower limb

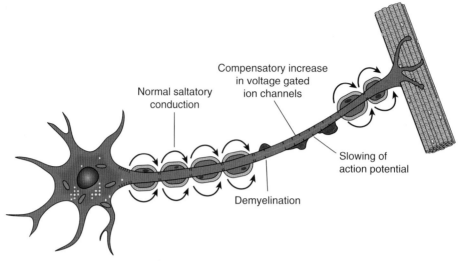

Normal saltatory
conduction

Compensatory increase
in voltage gated
ion channels

Slowing of
action potential

Demyelination

FIG. 14.4 Chronic demyelination.

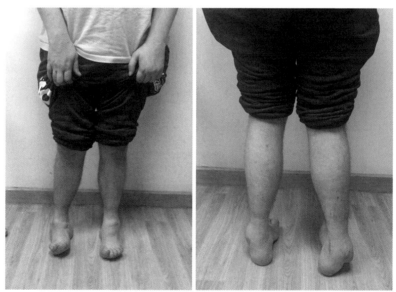

FIG. 14.5 Distal wasting and pes cavus foot deformity in a person with Charcot–Marie–Tooth disease.

(Fig. 14.5) and wasting of the intrinsic hand muscles (Fig. 14.6). Magnetic resonance imaging reveals that atrophy of the distal lower limb muscles can occur even when an individual appears unaffected on clinical examination (Gallardo 2005). The distal lower and upper limb muscles tend to weaken first, showing a slow decline in strength over decades. The degree and extent of weakness have been correlated with axonal loss rather than demyelination in studies of the hand (Videler et al 2008b). The proximal limb muscles are less affected, but some studies have found they are still weak compared with normative data (Morrow et al 2015).

In addition to weakness and wasting, a length-dependent gradual loss of sensation occurs. People with CMT1 show a principal impairment of the thickly myelinated large-diameter sensory nerves that mediate the sensations

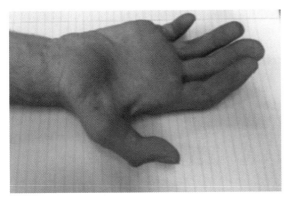

FIG. 14.6 Wasting of the intrinsic hand muscles in a person with Charcot–Marie–Tooth–disease.

of light touch and vibration (Nardone et al 2000). However, sensations conveyed by smaller-diameter fibres (e.g., pain, temperature or pinprick) may also be reduced (Carter et al 1995).

Little has been written about hand deformity in people with CMT, but there has been interest in the presentation and evolution of foot deformity. Pes cavus is a common foot posture observed in people with CMT1 when the condition starts early in life and is described as a foot type with an excessively high longitudinal arch and foot supination (see Fig. 14.5). Pes cavus is often associated with hind foot varus, toe clawing and dorsiflexion of the metatarsophalangeal joints (MTPJs). These deformities are thought to evolve through muscle imbalances over time (Gallardo 2005, Guyton & Mann 2000). In support of this theory, a significant correlation was found between a pes cavus foot structure and ankle dorsiflexion range in children with CMT (Burns et al 2009). People with CMT2 have a very similar phenotype as people with CMT1 with slow progression of distal weakness, wasting and sensory loss. The onset of symptoms, however, may be later in life, so the pes cavus foot type is not always present.

Exploration of upper limb function has revealed that people with CMT can have impaired manual dexterity and upper limb functional tasks (Burns et al 2008, Videler et al 2008a, 2008b) that are related to muscle weakness (Selles et al 2006). In the lower limb, distal weakness has been related to foot drop and failure of the plantarflexors (Vinci & Perelli 2002), which influences the gait pattern as people with CMT walk. Gait analysis has revealed primary distal gait impairments with problems with foot clearance during swing, and reduced contribution of the plantarflexor muscles to progression of the trunk and swing leg (Newman et al 2007).

Fatigue is well documented in people with CMT, and 67% report severe fatigue (Kalkman et al 2005). People with CMT describe normal fatigue caused by activity but also fatigue that is more chronic and is not refreshed by rest (Ramdharry et al 2012c). As a group, people with CMT have been found to be less active than the general population (Kalkman et al 2007, Ramdharry et al 2016) and are deconditioned, as measured by oxygen uptake during exercise (Carter et al 1995, Ramdharry et al 2021c). Aerobic deconditioning and disuse muscle atrophy are a likely consequence of reduced activity levels, which may also affect fatigue and prolonged performance of daily tasks.

People with CMT report more pain than the general population (Padua et al 2008), although it is unclear whether the pain directly results from the neuropathy or secondary musculoskeletal deformities. Axonal CMT (type 2) can affect the smaller pain fibres leading to neuropathic pain, but it has also been reported in a small percentage of people with demyelinating CMT. Laurá and colleagues reported neuropathic pain in 18% of a cohort of people with CMT1A, resulting from the involvement of thinly myelinated Aδ fibres, but they acknowledged that the overall experience of pain was likely to be multifactorial (Laurá et al 2014).

Problems with balance are reported in the clinic by people with CMT. There is an increased prevalence of falls (Eichinger et al 2016, Ramdharry et al 2017), with balance impairment attributed to both motor and sensory impairment (Tozza et al 2016, van der Linden et al 2010). A posturography study of people with different types of CMT found that those with a more axonal presentation had increased postural sway during quiet standing. In dynamic balance situations, people with both types of CMT demonstrated delays in segment coordination (Nardone et al 2006). Dysfunction of myelinated 1A and group II muscle spindle afferents can be associated with balance impairment in CMT (Nardone et al 2000, van der Linden et al 2010), but stability is also challenged with distal motor weakness, particularly of the plantarflexor muscles (Hachisuka et al 1997, Rossor et al 2012).

Medical Management. Currently no medical treatments for CMT are available; however, the current focus is on symptomatic management which includes general advice on foot care, pain management and rehabilitation.

Pain is a frequent complaint in CMT, although it is likely to be multifactorial and mainly related to altered gait or foot deformities. A small proportion of patients have neuropathic pain characteristics that could be amenable to specific drug treatment. Clinical assessment is important in establishing pain characteristics to guide appropriate therapy (Laurá et al 2014).

Orthopaedic interventions are often required in patients with CMT and are indicated for corrections of severe foot deformities, severe scoliosis, hip dysplasia and patellofemoral instability. Scoliosis is observed in 26%–37% and seldom requires surgery unless very severe. Hip dysplasia is rare, and the prevalence in CMT is about 8% (Walker et al 1994). Patellofemoral dislocation has been observed in paediatric (Main et al 2012) and adult cohorts, where morphological changes in the patellofemoral joint, female sex and hypermobility may present risk factors (Leone et al 2020). Anecdotally, people with CMT who have recurrent patellofemoral dislocation can undergo surgical procedures to stabilise the joint (Tan et al 2020). Orthopaedic surgery is frequently performed to correct severe foot deformities, and it is usually indicated when pain and decreased function do not respond to conservative measures, such as physiotherapy and the use of orthosis. Several types of foot operations have been described, and they include soft tissue procedures (tendon lengthening and tendon transfers), osteotomies and fusions such as triple arthrodesis (Laura et al 2017). Foot realignment surgery can have positive outcomes on pain and alignment with interventions from experienced surgeons (Ramdharry et al 2021b), but a possible risk of Charcot neuroarthropathy has been a suggested risk factor (Singh et al 2021).

Disease Course and Prognosis. CMT is a slowly progressive disease which usually does not affect life expectancy. Some types (e.g., CMT1A and CMT2A) start in childhood. It is a very heterogenous condition, and clinical severity may vary even in the same family. People with CMT tend to notice progression slowly over years, rather than months. Most will not fully lose the ability to walk, although they may require orthoses and walking aids to mobilise as they age (Table 14.2).

ASSESSMENT OF PEOPLE WITH POLYNEUROPATHIES

There is no specific guidance or consensus on assessment of people with polyneuropathies, so this section will suggest an approach depending on the setting and disease course, including disease-specific outcome measures that have been validated in these conditions. A summary overview is provided in Table 14.3.

When assessing people with polyneuropathy in the acute setting, for example, for someone with GBS, a respiratory assessment may be necessary. Monitoring vital capacity is important to ascertain the extent, progression and severity of respiratory muscle involvement. If the person with GBS is in a critical care setting, there needs to be an evaluation of ventilatory requirements and possible respiratory complications. A daily assessment of joint range of motion while the person is in critical care will identify any risks of

soft tissue shortening or joint contracture so decisions can be made on splinting.

If the person is awake, a full assessment of muscle strength, sensory impairment and joint range will ascertain a baseline for monitoring improvement as the person starts to recover from the acute episode. It is important to note any reports or indications of pain, particularly if the person is intubated. Liaison with nursing staff is essential to ascertain if there are autonomic symptoms, skin integrity issues and planned pain management because all these factors can alter rehabilitation interventions.

For chronic polyneuropathies, such as CIDP, CMT and DN, ascertaining the degree of lower motor neurone impairment is important. Assessment of muscle strength, using the Medical Research Council (MRC) score, and sensation help to build a picture of how impairments affect functional status. A version of the MRC score has been modified and validated for use in peripheral neuropathies, encompassing four categories instead of five, but it is not in wide clinical use at present (Vanhoutte et al 2012). Joint deformity and pain should be noted. For foot deformity, the Foot Posture Index is a useful tool to record and monitor the foot shape (Redmond et al 2006). Pain can be scored and monitored using a visual analogue score, but it is helpful to ascertain severity, site and triggers. Descriptions of pain are helpful to ascertain if there is a neuropathic or musculoskeletal cause, the latter being more amenable to physiotherapy interventions. Fatigue severity can be measured using a short, validated Fatigue Severity Scale (van Nes et al 2009), but it is also helpful to understand the pattern of fatigue and impact on daily life.

Several functional rating scales have been validated for different neuropathies: the CMT Functional Outcome Measure (Bray et al 2020, Eichinger et al 2018), the Rasch-built Overall Disability Scale for inflammatory neuropathy (van Nes et al 2011) and the Overall Neuropathy Limitation scale, which can be used more generally (Graham & Hughes 2006a). When assessing function and activities, it is important to consider that some of the polyneuropathies are lifelong conditions for which people will have adapted and compensated for impairments over many years. Asking patients what their current challenges are related to their condition is a useful way to direct clinical reasoning and treatment planning. Based on this, a core outcome set has been coproduced with people living with rare neurological conditions, including polyneuropathies, for physical activity interventions that include participation and well-being measures in addition to function (Ramdharry et al 2021a).

Gait assessment should include observation of walking pattern, gait speed (using the 10-metre timed walk) and endurance using the 6-minute timed walk (Padua et al 2016). The Walk-12 scale has also been validated for people

TABLE 14.2 **Summary of Common Physical Presentations of the Main Categories of Peripheral Neuropathy**

Type of Peripheral Neuropathy	Progression Rate	Motor Deficit	Sensory Deficit	Pain	Musculoskeletal	Skin
Guillain–Barré syndrome	Rapid progression to nadir followed by recovery period	Ascending, lower motor neurone muscle weakness	Ascending large-fibre sensory impairment	MSK and neuropathic	Risk of contractions in severe cases with prolonged periods of immobility	Risk of pressure sores in severe cases with prolonged periods of immobility
CIDP	Relapse-remitting course; can "burn out"	Patchy lower motor neurone weakness	Patchy large-fibre sensory impairment	Uncommon but can have MSK pain	Risk of joint instability and injury with muscle weakness	Not common
Diabetic neuropathy	Slowly progressive but can depend on glycaemic control	Mild to moderate, distal lower limb weakness	Glove and stocking small- and large-fibre sensory impairment	Neuropathic pain; can have MSK pain	Charcot joints	High risk of distal ulceration
Charcot–Marie–Tooth disease type 1	Slowly progressive	Mild to moderate distal lower limb weakness	Distal large-fibre sensory impairment	MSK pain	Foot deformity, occasional scoliosis and hip dysplasia; infrequent incidents of Charcot joints	Foot callosities are common; ulceration can occur less frequently
Charcot–Marie–Tooth disease type 2	Slowly progressive	Mild to severe global weakness	Distal small- and large-fibre sensory impairment	Neuropathic pain, may have MSK pain	Risk of joint instability and injury with muscle weakness	Not common

CIDP, Chronic inflammatory demyelinating polyradiculoneuropathy; *MSK*, musculoskeletal.

with neuropathy and ascertains a person's perception of their walking ability (Graham & Hughes 2006b). With balance and falls, ascertain the frequency and common causes of falling (e.g., trips). A modified Clinical Test of Sensory Integration and Balance is a useful way of exploring visual dependence (Shumway-Cook & Horak 1986). Varying the base of support with Romberg's stance, step or tandem standing and single-leg stance will also help to assess the severity of balance impairment, and when self-generated perturbations such as head turning are added, this reveals anticipatory responses. To test reactive responses, pushing on the sternum or fourth thoracic vertebra while watching the distal motor responses will reveal if they are delayed or absent. Established balance measures such as the Berg Balance Scale and the Tinetti test have been found to be reliable for inherited neuropathies (Monti Bragadin et al 2015).

Hand function can be a problem for some people with polyneuropathy. Observe for wasting and any joint limitations. Grip patterns can be altered, and this can be noted

TABLE 14.3 Guidance for Assessment and Outcome Measures for People With Polyneuropathy

Assessment Scenario	Body Functions	Activities	Participation
Acute (e.g., Guillain–Barré syndrome)	Respiratory assessment • Vital capacity • Ventilation Muscle strength • Medical Research Council score Sensory impairment • Site and modality Joint range of motion Pain • Visual analogue scale Skin integrity	Sitting ± assistance Standing ± assistance Walking ± assistance	Premorbid occupation Social situation
Chronic (e.g., chronic inflammatory demyelinating polyradiculoneuropathy, diabetic neuropathy, Charcot–Marie–Tooth disease)	Muscle strength • Medical Research Council score Sensory impairment • Site and modality Joint range of motion Foot deformity • Foot Posture Index Pain • Visual analogue scale Fatigue • Fatigue severity scale	Gait assessment • Observation • 10-metre timed walk • 6-minute walk • Walk-12 scale Balance • Romberg's test • Timed tandem or single leg • Clinical Test of Sensory Integration and Balance • Berg Balance Scale • Tinetti balance assessment Physical activity levels • International Physical Activity Questionnaire • Activity monitors and apps Hand function • Nine-hole peg test • Functional dexterity test Disease-specific composite measures: • Overall Neuropathy Limitation Scale • Rasch-built Overall Disability Scale for inflammatory neuropathy • Charcot–Marie–Tooth disease Examination score	Community mobility Occupation Social situation Leisure

when watching specific tasks such as picking up an object or tying shoelaces. Find out whether people are using splints, supports or adaptive equipment. Assessment tools such as the nine-hole peg test and functional dexterity test have been found to be reliable and sensitive for monitoring hand function in people with neuropathy (Piscosquito et al 2015, Videler et al 2008b).

It is also of major importance to explore how the person's diagnosis of polyneuropathy affects their participation, although there are no formal measures of participation

TABLE 14.4 Summary of Treatment Approaches and Considerations for People With Polyneuropathies

	Treatment Approaches	Considerations
Acute (e.g., Guillain–Barré syndrome)	Respiratory interventions Positioning Splinting and stretching Early mobilisation Strength training	Rehabilitation approach and goals Communication if intubated Pain Fatigue
Chronic (e.g., chronic inflammatory demyelinating polyradiculoneuropathy, diabetic neuropathy, Charcot–Marie–Tooth disease)	Exercise • Aerobic exercise • Strength training • Stretching Balance training • Self-generated movements • Reacting to perturbations • Multisensory proprioceptive training • Divided attention Orthotic management • Foot orthoses and insoles • Off-the-shelf or custom-made ankle–foot orthoses • Vibrating insoles (when commercially available) Pain and fatigue management • Exercise • Education • Pacing • Multidisciplinary team involvement: occupational therapy and psychology Self-management • Education • Goal setting • Modelling and mastery • Reflection on success • Resources such as NM Bridges*	Management approach and goals Delivery within self-management frameworks • Coaching to problem-solve and make choice • Facilitating exploration and taking action

*NM Bridges: https://nmd.bridgesselfmanagement.org.uk/

in nerve diseases. Aim to understand how living with the conditions affects work, study or family life. Physical activity can be limited in some people (Ramdharry et al 2016), so ascertain if they participate in leisure activities or exercise. Self-monitoring of physical activity can provide useful information to both patient and therapist using now readily available activity monitors or questionnaires such as the International Physical Activity Questionnaire (Jimenez-Moreno et al 2017).

PHYSICAL MANAGEMENT AND REHABILITATION APPROACHES FOR PEOPLE WITH POLYNEUROPATHIES

Currently there are no specific guidelines for rehabilitation of people with polyneuropathy. This section presents a summary of available literature on physical management interventions. A summary overview is provided in Table 14.4.

Acute Rehabilitation of Acquired Polyneuropathies

There are no studies of the efficacy of early rehabilitation approaches in GBS. At present intervention is based on experience with other neurological conditions, although the need for therapy input is recognised (Vucic et al 2009). Physical management in the acute stage focuses on respiratory interventions and prevention of secondary complications (Khan 2004). Respiratory treatments include sputum clearance techniques, maintenance of lung volumes and breathing exercises when the person can participate (see Chapter 18). Other interventions advocated are early mobilisation, splinting, positioning, stretches to maintain joint range of motion and exercises to increase strength and endurance (Hughes 2008, Khan & Amatya 2012, Meythaler 1997). A pilot study of electrical stimulation to the quadriceps showed safety of the technique for people in the acute stage, but efficacy needs to be determined in larger trials (Harbo et al 2019). Fear, anxiety and sleep deprivation are common problems experienced by people with GBS in the early stages. Good two-way communication between the multidisciplinary team and patient and carers is vital to ensure they are informed at every stage. This may be challenging if a person is intubated, but it can be supported by speech and language therapy intervention.

Approximately 40% of all people with GBS will need a period of multidisciplinary inpatient rehabilitation with the aim of maximising functional recovery and participation (Khan & Amatya 2012, Meythaler 1997). Good functional improvements were observed in a retrospective study of 45 people admitted for an average of 62 days from first symptoms (Novak et al 2017). Two studies have found that the more severely affected people tend to access rehabilitation or physiotherapy services (Carroll et al 2003, Davidson et al 2009). The impact of therapy input may be important because a survey of people with GBS (>800 participants) found that 90% of people were treated by a physiotherapist, but this decreased to 75% of people after discharge from hospital. The survey found that people who did not receive physiotherapy treatment as an outpatient or in the community had greater levels of disability than those who did (Davidson et al 2009), but overall there is satisfaction with physiotherapy treatment (Dennis & Mullins 2013). Although GBS is a monophasic disease, long-term issues and impact are felt by people living with the condition (Akanuwe et al 2020). They identify rehabilitation and physical activity as important factors affecting recovery (Siriwardena et al 2022).

Long-Term Physical Management and Rehabilitation

Self-management

Self-management approaches for people with long-term neurological conditions have been developed and are gathering good evidence of effect in supporting people make choices to be active in decisions about their health (see Chapter 19). It must be a core approach of physiotherapists to facilitate and support decision making on positive lifestyle behaviours and build confidence in problem-solving the challenges presented by these conditions. Neuromuscular Bridges is a self-management intervention codesigned with people with neuromuscular diseases, including polyneuropathy (Postges et al 2020) (https://nmd.bridgesselfmanagement.org.uk/). The feasibility of the intervention delivered through a specialist service is currently under investigation (Lee et al 2022).

Exercise and Physical Activity Interventions in Polyneuropathy

Ascertaining the evidence for the efficacy of exercise training in people with polyneuropathy is challenging for several reasons. Some neuropathies are relatively rare conditions, so many studies are small, leading to risk of type 2 error (false-negative findings). The Cochrane Library has two reviews that explore exercise in peripheral neuropathy. The first was a review of exercise for people with peripheral neuropathy (White et al 2004), and the second was a review of treatment for people with CMT (Young et al 2008). Both reviews found only a small body of literature on exercise in neuropathies, and they both identified the same randomised control trial as being the only study of sufficient quality for consideration (Lindeman et al 1995). This was the first randomised controlled trial of 24 weeks of resistance training for people with CMT focusing on hip extensors, abductors and knee flexors and extensors at 60%–80% of one repetition max. Significant improvements in isokinetic knee torque and gait speed were observed in the training group.

Other systematic reviews have been conducted focusing on exercise. For GBS, seven studies met the review criteria and included one randomised controlled trial. In total 133 subjects were included in these trials, but the designs and interventions were very heterogeneous, so no pooled analysis could be performed. Five studies included varying aerobic or endurance exercise, one was a balance training protocol and one was a mixed resistance and stretching physiotherapy programme. The authors concluded that the studies to date showed a link between mixed exercise programmes and improved functional outcome but called for higher quality study designs in future trials (Simatos Arsenault et al 2016).

For DN, exercise could have two major positive effects. There is evidence that a 6-month programme of twice-weekly aerobic exercise could regenerate nerve endings in the skin before a person becomes fully diabetic, and walking activities can slow the progression of DN. A review of exercise highlighted these exciting findings and also suggested that reducing sedentary periods could be more effective than short bursts of intensive exercise (Singleton et al 2015). Systematic reviews have also identified positive effects of exercise on gait function in people with DN (Melese et al 2020) and intensity of neuropathic pain (Zhang et al 2021).

For CMT, a systematic review identified nine studies of moderate quality overall that examined 134 people. They reported significant improvements in strength and function, but it was noted that there were few studies of aerobic training (Sman et al 2015). The results of three additional trials have recently been reported since this review. Strength training of the dorsiflexion muscles, in 60 children and adolescents, was compared with sham training in a 12-week intervention (Burns et al 2017). Quantitative strength testing showed a maintenance of dorsiflexor strength over 24 months, whereas children who underwent sham training deteriorated, as expected with disease progression. Of note, all children had baseline strength MRC scores >4 to be able to train, so the implications for weaker adults remain unclear, but this study suggests that strength training could be protective when targeted early enough. A trial of treadmill training in 53 people with CMT1A showed improvements in 6-minute walk distance and balance (Mori et al 2019), and bicycle ergometer training for 28 people led to increases in aerobic fitness (Wallace et al 2019).

These studies highlight the need for further investigation, but positive benefits of exercise for people with polyneuropathy are becoming more apparent. There is mounting evidence that people with polyneuropathy are a sedentary group, and this leads to increased risks of noncommunicable diseases (World Health Organization 2010). One of the traditional barriers to exercise for people with some neuropathies is a concern that exercise will worsen their condition. In the past, people were actively discouraged from exercising. People with CIDP were advised not to exercise during the inflammatory phase of the condition, although evidence for increased deterioration has not been presented. For DN, it was thought that greater physical activity could increase the risk of foot ulcers (Crews et al 2016). For CMT, a specific pathological mechanism has not been suggested (Vinci et al 2003). For other conditions with enlarged motor units (e.g., postpolio syndrome), there are concerns that oxidative stress during exercise can damage already overburdened motor units (Tews 2002). Many of these concerns have been overturned, and the recommendations are that exercise is safe for people with polyneuropathy (Chan et al 2003, Crews et al 2016, van Pomeren et al 2009).

The weight of evidence to date involves trials of structured exercise, and a recent Cochrane Review of physical activity interventions in neuromuscular diseases (including polyneuropathy) highlighted fewer studies supporting engagement in physical activity more generally (Jones et al 2021). With evidence of reduced engagement on the cessation of structured exercise trials (Elsworth et al 2011, Wallace et al 2019), perhaps our focus should now be on behaviour change interventions with the goal of increase physical activity and reducing sedentary time (Busse & Ramdharry 2020, Veenhuizen et al 2019, 2021).

Balance Interventions

Evidence of effective balance interventions is available in people with DN. A systematic review of exercise interventions showed positive effects on static balance, gait and lower limb strength. The 10 trials included tested interventions such as tai chi, proprioceptive balance training, gait training and lower limb resistance training administered two or three times weekly, but there was a larger range of intervention duration (4–52 weeks) (Chapman et al 2017).

Balance training has also been explored in people with CMT. A small randomised controlled trial (n = 16) investigated a 12-day programme using a mechanical balance trainer or dynamic standing frame (Matjačić & Zupan 2006). The exercise group demonstrated significant improvements in the Berg Balance Score, the Timed Up and Go test and the 10-metre timed walk. The control group also significantly improved their Berg Balance Score but to a lesser degree.

A study of multisensory balance training in 30 people with sensory ataxic neuropathy showed improved functional balance. This group had varied pathology but included people with CIDP, idiopathic and hereditary neuropathies. The training was administered three times a week for 5 weeks, and included balance training with vision excluded or disturbed, divided attention with balance task and vibration stimulation to the foot sole (Missaoui & Thoumie 2013). Delivering a combination of multisensory balance training and proximal strength training at home may also be effective. A small feasibility study in CMT1A showed large effect sizes for functional balance (Ramdharry et al 2018), and larger trials of efficacy are required to confirm this.

Vibration input as an intervention has also been explored in a pilot study of 13 people with CMT. Vibration was applied to the quadriceps and triceps surae for 3 days.

There was some indication of improvement in functional and static balance 1 month after, but there was no control group to rule out learning and Hawthorne effect (Pazzaglia et al 2016). The rationale for vibration therapy is to drive central changes in the sensorimotor system through peripheral stimulation via the 1a afferent spindle fibres, but a greater body of work is required to test this theory and ascertain whether there is a significant long-term effect.

Orthotic Management

The main purpose of orthotic intervention for people with neuropathy is to improve gait and balance, through one or more of the following biomechanical aims:

- Redistribution of pressure under the foot;
- Realignment and correction of foot deformities;
- Reduction of foot drop;
- Stabilisation of the ankle joint; and
- Increasing sensory feedback to the foot and/or ankle.

Redistribution of pressure and realignment of the foot and ankle can be a way to reduce pain and the risk of ulceration and skin breakdown. By supporting and stabilising the ankle joint, gait and balance function can be improved.

There is a growing body of evidence for the use of orthoses in neuropathy, but the studies tend to be small, uncontrolled and with little longitudinal follow-up. Part of the challenge is the wide range of custom-made or off-the-shelf devices that can be used to give the biomechanical effects outlined above. Scheffers and colleagues proposed in a study of children with CMT that prescription algorithms should be considered to match devices that give specific biomechanical effects to the presenting impairments of patients (Scheffers et al 2013). This is an innovative approach to manage this issue, but prescription algorithms would need to be developed carefully and tested as an intervention in their own right.

In terms of the biomechanical aims outlined, there is some evidence of effect of in-shoe foot orthoses in reducing pain and redistributing pressure in different polyneuropathies (Burns et al 2006, Ulbrecht et al 2014) but less on the realignment of foot deformities. Several small studies have shown a positive effect on gait and balance when foot drop is supported by ankle–foot orthoses of different types (Dufek et al 2014, Guillebastre et al 2011, Menotti et al 2014, Paton et al 2016, Phillips et al 2012, Ramdharry et al 2012b), but there are fewer trials investigating stabilisation of the ankle (Hachisuka et al 1997). There has been more interest, however, in the sensory effects of orthoses, either through shaped devices or active vibration input (Hijmans et al 2008, Paton et al 2016, Wegener et al 2016). With all these studies there is insufficient size and quality of research in a variety of devices to ascertain overall effect (Paton et al 2016, Sackley et al 2009), but there is observed

potential that needs to be explored in a more pragmatic way that resembles real-life, individualised prescription (Scheffers et al 2013).

In view of the limited evidence for the efficacy of orthotic provision, clinicians should review any devices prescribed with appropriate outcome measures, depending on the aim of the device. People with polyneuropathy may be reluctant to accept orthoses (O'Connor et al 2015, Phillips et al 2011, Ramdharry et al 2012a, Zuccarino et al 2021), so consideration of the person's opinion and inclusion in decision making will help to ensure that a device is prescribed that is acceptable to that individual. Measures of comfort should also be recorded over time because ill-fitting splints can be another reason for nonuse.

Management of the Neuropathic Hand

There has been less attention given to the management of hand weakness. Hand orthoses have been recommended in opinion pieces and guidance (Charcot Marie Tooth Association 2018, Ramdharry et al 2020), but to date there has been only one trial in CMT disease. A trial of a thumb opposition splint showed improvements in dexterity in 13 people with CMT (Videler et al 2012). Similarly, there is a paucity of studies exploring rehabilitation of the hand. A pilot study of a 4-week exercise intervention in nine people with CMT showed improvements in hand grip, tripod grip and function, but this requires comparison with a control group in a larger trial to ascertain efficacy (Prada et al 2018).

Pain and Fatigue Management

Pain is a recognised issue that can adversely affect quality of life. Musculoskeletal pain may be ameliorated with physiotherapy interventions and neuropathic pain with drugs, but many people live with persistent pain. Pain management principles of education, exercise and support are beneficial. Referral to a multidisciplinary pain management programme may be warranted but has not been investigated as a specific approach in the literature (for further information see Chapter 23). Similarly, referrals to fatigue management by occupational therapy colleagues may be helpful. The 16-week 'Energetic' intervention comprises fatigue management sessions and aerobic exercise. It was trialled in a mixed study of people with neuromuscular disorders, including polyneuropathy, resulting in improvements with participation (Veenhuizen et al 2019, 2021).

CASE STUDY

A case history is outlined to explore intervention strategies for a person with CMT. Relevant evidence and clinical reasoning are presented to support the rehabilitation approaches.

Mr V is a 32-year-old man who presented to a neurological outpatient clinic via referral from a neurologist. He was diagnosed with CMT1A from family history, clinical examination, electrophysiological tests and genetic testing. Neurophysiological testing revealed slowed nerve conduction velocity in the bilateral median, ulnar and common peroneal nerves with reductions in the amplitude of the CMAPs and SNAPs. Genetic testing of Mr V and his family revealed that he had a duplication of *PMP22* on chromosome 17.

He is from a mixed South Asian and White background and lives with his husband in a house with internal stairs. No adaptations have been made to the home. He works for a recruitment company and switched to working from home during the Covid-19 pandemic. He has now returned to a hybrid working pattern of working from home and the office.

Presenting Impairments
Musculoskeletal Integrity and Alignment

Mr V had distal upper limb muscle wasting in the thenar eminences and intrinsic hand muscles. The hand adopted a slight 'claw'-like posture with flexion of the proximal and distal interphalangeal joints (PIPs and DIPs) and hyperextension of the metacarpophalangeal joints (MCPJs). In the lower limb, there was wasting of the tibialis anterior, gastrocnemius, peroneal and intrinsic foot muscles, as well as extensor digitorum brevis on the dorsum of the foot. The feet adopted a pes cavus position with calcaneal varus, dorsiflexed MTPJs and clawed toes. Thick callus had formed

on the plantar aspect under the metatarsal heads and under the lateral border of the foot (Fig. 14.7). He had tight Achilles tendons and calf muscles bilaterally with restricted passive dorsiflexion of the right ankle to 2° plantar flexion (knee flexed), 5° plantar flexion (knee extended), and the left ankle to 0° (knee flexed), 2° plantar flexion (knee extended). The lunge test in standing showed 0° dorsiflexion on the right and 3° dorsiflexion on the left.

Muscle Strength and Sensation

MRC muscle testing revealed relatively symmetrical, distal weakness of the hands and feet (Table 14.5). Mr V was unable to stand on his heels but could just raise them from the floor by 1–2 cm. Sensory testing revealed reduced light touch cutaneous sensation in the fingers and feet. Pinprick was reduced up to the mid-palm and just above the ankle. Vibration sense was reduced to the MCPs in the hands and the knees, indicating peripheral dysfunction of the 1 A muscle spindle afferents. He had reduced joint position sense up to the DIPs of the hand and up to the ankle. In standing, Romberg's test revealed a moderate increase in body sway with the eyes closed.

Observation of Activities
Upper Limb Function

Mr V demonstrated difficulties with pinch grip and power grip with the palmar aspect remaining flattened during many dexterity tasks. He demonstrated difficulty managing small fastenings and tied shoelaces by using his thumbs as a hook.

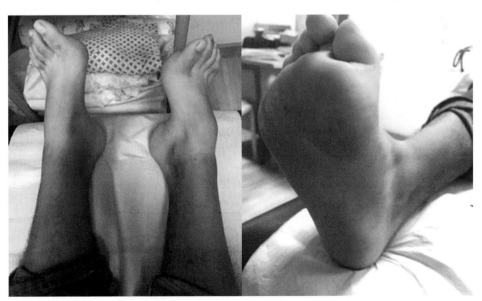

FIG. 14.7 Case study: photograph of Mr V's feet.

TABLE 14.5   Summary of Manual Muscle Strength Testing Using the Medical Research Council Scale

Upper Limb	MRC Grading		Lower Limb	MRC Grading	
	L	R		L	R
Thumb abduction	2	3	Extensor halluces longus	1	0
First dorsal interosseous	3	4	Long toe flexors	4+	4+
Abductor digiti minimi	3	3			
Long finger flexors	5	5	Dorsiflexion	1	2
Long finger extensors	5	5	Plantarflexion	4+	4+
Wrist flexors	5	5	Quadriceps	5	5
Wrist extensors	5	5	Hamstrings	5-	5-
Biceps	5	5	Hip flexors	5	5
Triceps	5	5	Hip extensors	5-	5-

MRC, Medical Research Council.

Gait

Mr V walked with reduced step length, velocity and cadence. His gait pattern was high stepping with bilateral foot drop and delayed heel rise at preswing. Initial contact was with the lateral border of the midfoot. His knees hyperextended during midstance, and there was increased lateral trunk sway. Objective tests demonstrated that Mr V walked at a comfortable speed of 1.19 m/s, over 10 metres, and he covered 356 metres during 6 minutes of walking. During the 6-minute walk, he reported his level of effort as 11 out of 20 on the Borg perceived exertion scale (Borg 1970).

Mr V's Reported Problems and Impact on Participation

Fatigue

Mr V worked full time for the recruitment company. He reported general fatigue where he would wake still tired and not be refreshed by rest. He felt exhausted after a day's work and did little in the evening as a result. His fatigue levels were improved when working from home during the Covid-19 pandemic, but he also acknowledged being less physically active on those days. Mr V reported increased fatigue related to activity (e.g., prolonged walking or standing) and needed to take breaks on shopping trips. He scored 37 out of 63 of the Fatigue Severity Scale, indicating moderate levels of self-reported fatigue (Krupp 2003).

Balance

Mr V. reported difficulty standing for long periods on the spot (e.g., at work-related functions and when queuing for a bus) (Hachisuka et al 1997, Rossor et al 2012). He reported falling approximately four or five times per month. On assessment, Mr V achieved 48 out of 56 on the Berg Balance Scale (Monti Bragadin et al 2015).

Pain

Mr V reported episodic pain anterior to the right lateral malleolus and under the metatarsal heads with prolonged walking that reached 4 of 10 on a visual analogue scale.

Physiotherapy Options for Mr V

To ascertain the best interventions for the problems Mr V presented with, we must turn to the literature exploring rehabilitation for people with polyneuropathy (see earlier).

Orthotic Prescription

Foot orthoses have been seen to be effective for reducing pain for people with pes cavus (Burns et al 2006). Mr V was prescribed full foot orthoses with medial, lateral and transverse arch pads to support the plantar surface and spread weight bearing. The insoles also had a small, 5° lateral wedge under the calcaneus and midfoot to deweight the lateral border of the foot.

Mr V was also prescribed bilateral Push ankle braces (Nea International, Maastricht, Netherlands), which are braces originally designed for ankle instability. Push braces are made of neoprene with calcaneal and lateral support. Preliminary studies have found that Push braces reduce foot drop without compromising the action of the plantarflexor muscles (Ramdharry et al 2012b). Mr V had grade 4+ strength of his plantarflexor muscles that could contribute to gait (Neptune et al 2001), so this benefit was a consideration. It was also believed that the lateral support would be helpful when walking for longer distances in view of the right foot and ankle pain. Mr V preferred the appearance of the Push braces because they looked more 'sporty' than plastic ankle–foot orthoses he had tried previously. He reported they were more comfortable and caused less rubbing because of the softer materials, an important consideration for people with sensory impairment. He was also issued carbon fibre ankle–foot orthoses (Matrix Max, Trulife Limited, Sheffield, UK) that increased his stride length and gait speed. Currently only small studies are available on the effect of carbon fibre ankle–foot orthoses in patients with neuromuscular disorders (Brehm et al 2007, Dufek et al 2014, Eagle et al 2001). He found them beneficial when walking outdoors but cumbersome when driving or negotiating stairs. He uses them when going out for walks or needing to stand for longer periods at functions because they provide more support to the ankle.

Range of Movement

It was theorised that the knee hyperextension and early heel raise Mr V experienced while walking was mainly because of tightness of the Achilles tendon and calf muscles in addition to weakness. It was deemed safe to stretch the calf because he had reasonable strength of the calf muscles. There are some concerns about overstretching muscles in people with severe weakness because the soft tissue tightness may have a role in supporting the ankle during mid to late stance phase (Salsich & Mueller 2000). He was given weight-bearing gastrocnemius and Achilles/soleus stretches with the knee in extension and flexion with 1-minute holds. Mr V was instructed to do the calf stretches while wearing shoes and foot orthoses because the wedging would bring the subtalar joint into a more neutral position and thus avoid overstretching of adjacent structures because of poor alignment. In view of Mr V's busy work schedule, he was advised to stand and do the stretches every time he made himself a cup of tea while he waited for the kettle to boil. This amounted to approximately four times per day.

Muscle Strength and Aerobic Exercise

Strengthening exercises were prescribed for his proximal lower limb muscles because the evidence demonstrates improvements in strength and gait function (Chetlin et al 2004, Lindeman et al 1995, Ramdharry et al 2014). The slight weakness in the hamstrings and hip extensors (see Table 14.1) is likely caused by secondary disuse atrophy because his condition was primarily affecting only strength and sensation below the knees. Mr V joined a gym near work and went two or three times per week. He was prescribed a programme of resistance training for the proximal lower limb muscles starting at 8 repetitions at a 12-repetition maximum, progressing to 12 repetitions, and then gradually increasing the load to a 10-repetition maximum. This prescription was based on recommendations

for improving muscle strength and endurance (American College of Sports Medicine, 2009). He was also cautiously given a heel-raise exercise at five to eight repetitions but was instructed to stop if he experienced excessive muscle soreness, muscle tightness or increased weakness. Because the evidence is not yet clear about strengthening muscles with primary weakness, this was closely monitored. In addition, combining this exercise with his stretching regime would ensure that the repeated heel-raise exercise did not further tighten the plantarflexor muscles. He also participated in exercise bike training to increase his cardiopulmonary fitness and to determine whether this would help to reduce his fatigue (El Mhandi et al 2008, Wallace et al 2019).

Balance

Mr V was given a tandem standing exercise to challenge his balance when standing near a support (Ramdharry et al 2018). He added this to his calf-stretching programme. In addition, he had identified difficulty with prolonged standing in queues, etc. On discussion with Mr V, it was believed a collapsible walking stick would be helpful to carry in his workbag so he could use it for support and to stabilise him in standing as required.

Outcome

Mr V gradually increased the length of time that he wore the orthotic devices over 1 week, culminating in them being worn for most of his active day. He reported a marked reduction in pain to 1 out of 10 on a visual analogue scale with prolonged walking.

After 12 weeks of his exercise programme and new orthoses, improvements in gait quality were observed with better heel strike on initial contact and improved knee alignment on midstance (wearing orthoses). His gait speed improved slightly to 1.22 m/s, but most improvement was seen in the 6-minute test where he walked 402 m. He reported a Borg level 9 out of 20 for exertion during the test using the Borg Rating of Perceived Exertion (Borg 1970).

His Berg Balance Score slightly improved to 50 out of 56 and he reported tripping less when wearing the ankle braces, resulting in significantly fewer falls. The strategy of using the collapsible walking stick proved helpful for periods of prolonged standing, but Mr V admitted he would also find other external supports if available (e.g., walls or rails).

Management of Upper Limb Function: Exercise

A programme of strengthening exercises for the intrinsic hand muscles was recommended using a soft 'stress reliever' ball (lumbricals), elastic bands (finger abduction) and clothes pegs (tripod grip for thumb abduction/opposition). In addition, he was encouraged to strengthen the less-affected long finger flexors, using a gel ball, and extensors, using elastic bands, because they will help with his compensatory strategies. He was advised to do these exercises in short bursts to avoid muscle fatigue, and he kept the equipment on his work desk to enable him to work on the exercises little and often through the day. He was taught stretches on a tabletop to extend the DIPs and PIPs, while maintaining MCPJ flexion, and encouraged to perform this through the day while at work.

Hand Splints and Equipment

Mr V was referred to the occupational therapy service. Mr V trialled a neoprene thumb spica splint, applied to bring the thumb into abduction and flexion (Videler et al 2012). This aided opposition with the other fingers and allowed a pinch grip with medium-sized objects. The occupational therapist obtained a button hook and elastic laces to help with his dressing issues.

Outcome

Mr V found the equipment useful to aid dressing. He decided to stop using the thumb spica because he believed it interfered with how he had learned to do particular tasks. CMT is a slowly progressing condition and people problem-solve tasks, developing compensatory strategies over time. In this case, the change imposed by the splint altered his movement strategies and impaired function.

Management of Fatigue

The referral to occupational therapy also included fatigue management to address issues such as pacing and strategies to manage activities with limited energy resources. Aerobic exercise and engagement in physical activity also formed part of the fatigue management strategy (see earlier).

Outcome

Mr V said he found the fatigue management advice helpful and had trialled some of the strategies. He enjoyed using the exercise bike in the gym and reported feeling more energetic since getting into a regular routine. He started walking from his train stop to work each morning rather than getting the bus, but he felt too tired to do this in the evening. On reassessment, he scored 30 out of 63 using the Fatigue Severity Score.

Self-management

Mr V was introduced to the Neuromuscular Bridges Self-Management programme (https://nmd.bridgesselfmanagement.org.uk/) to explore how other people living with neuromuscular disorders problem-solve some of the issues he has encountered. He was encouraged to reflect on his success and set goals to increase engagement in physical activities he enjoys at levels he will benefit from.

Follow up and Remote Support

Mr V was followed to monitor progress with his programme of intervention. During the Covid-19 pandemic, follow-up sessions were done remotely through videoconferencing. Strategies were discussed on how to continue his management strategies during lockdown restrictions. He purchased an exercise bicycle to use at home and made a point of walking around the block with his carbon fibre ankle braces in the morning, during what would have previously been his morning commute. In addition, he kept exercise bands and dumbbells at his home desk to allow him to engage in small bursts of strengthening exercises through the day, in-between video meetings. Online resources for exercises were also sent for him to try, such as Pilates for people with rare neuromuscular diseases (https://www.youtube.com/playlist?list=PLazCbfp_tqxyve043vSch45aPfMzFfHxX).

He is now on a 'patient-initiated follow-up' system, which is an open access to the service for the next 4 years. This enables him to self-refer in the future. People with progressive conditions often benefit from open access and self-referral systems so they can reenter services quickly as new issues occur. When educated about their condition and therapy interventions that could help them in the future, they have more control over when and what assistance to seek.

■ SELF-ASSESSMENT QUESTIONS

1. Describe the classification of neuropathy according to time of onset, aetiology and anatomy.
2. The disruption of which of the following physiological functions is implicated in the pathology of axonal neuropathy?
   a. Saltatory conduction
   b. Axonal transport
   c. Generation of action potentials
   d. Release of acetyl choline at neuromuscular junction
3. Which of the following is NOT a primary symptom of polyneuropathy?
   a. Lower motor neurone weakness
   b. Loss of proprioception
   c. Muscle wasting
   d. Spasticity
4. True or false: Exercise causes overwork weakness for people with polyneuropathy. Briefly consider the evidence for and against the statement.
5. Describe five potential effects of orthoses for people with polyneuropathy.

REFERENCES

Akanuwe, J.N.A., Laparidou, D., Curtis, F., Jackson, J., Hodgson, T.L., Siriwardena, A.N., 2020. Exploring the experiences of having Guillain-Barré Syndrome: a qualitative interview study. Health Expect. 23, 1338–1349.

Ali, M.I., Fernández-Pérez, E.R., Pendem, S., Brown, D.R., Wijdicks, E.F.M., Gajic, O., 2006. Mechanical ventilation in patients with Guillain-Barré syndrome. Respir. Care. 51, 1403–1407.

American College of Sports Medicine, 2009. ACSM's Guidelines for Exercise Testing and Prescription, 8th Revised edition. ed. Lippincott Williams and Wilkins.

Barreto, L.C.L.S., Oliveira, F.S., Nunes, P.S., et al., 2016. Epidemiologic study of Charcot-Marie-Tooth disease: a systematic review. Neuroepidemiology. 46, 157–165.

Borg, G., 1970. Psychophysical basis of perceived exertion. Med. Sci. Sports Exerc. 14, 377–381.

Bray, P., Cornett, K.M.D., Estilow, T., et al., 2020. Reliability of the Charcot-Marie-Tooth functional outcome measure. J. Peripher. Nerv. Syst. 25, 288–291.

Brehm, M.-A., Beelen, A., Doorenbosch, C.A.M., Harlaar, J., Nollet, F., 2007. Effect of carbon-composite knee-ankle-foot orthoses on walking efficiency and gait in former polio patients. J. Rehabil. Med. 39, 651–657.

Burns, J., Bray, P., Cross, L.A., North, K.N., Ryan, M.M., Ouvrier, R.A., 2008. Hand involvement in children with Charcot-Marie-Tooth disease type 1A. Neuromuscul. Disord. 18, 970–973.

Burns, J., Crosbie, J., Ouvrier, R., Hunt, A., 2006. Effective orthotic therapy for the painful cavus foot: a randomized controlled trial. J. Am. Podiatr. Med. Assoc. 96, 205–211.

Burns, J., Ryan, M.M., Ouvrier, R.A., 2009. Evolution of foot and ankle manifestations in children with CMT1A. Muscle Nerve. 39, 158–166.

Burns, J., Sman, A., Cornett, K., et al., 2017. Safety and efficacy of progressive resistance exercise for Charcot-Marie-Tooth disease in children: a randomised, double-blind, sham-controlled trial. Lancet Child Adolesc. Health. 1, 106–113.

Busse, M., Ramdharry, G., 2020. Targeting sedentary behaviour in neurological disease. Pract. Neurol. 20, 187–188.

Carroll, A., McDonnell, G., Barnes, M., 2003. A review of the management of Guillain-Barré syndrome in a regional neurological rehabilitation unit. Int. J. Rehabil. Res. 26, 297–302.

Carter, G.T., Abresch, R.T., Fowler Jr, W.M., Johnson, E.R., Kilmer, D.D., McDonald, C.M., 1995. Profiles of neuromuscular diseases. Hereditary motor and sensory neuropathy, types I and II. Am. J. Phys. Med. Rehabil. 74, S140–149.

Cartoni, R., Martinou, J.-C., 2009. Role of mitofusin 2 mutations in the physiopathology of Charcot-Marie-Tooth disease type 2A. Exp. Neurol. 218, 268–273.

Chan, K.M., Amirjani, N., Sumrain, M., Clarke, A., Strohschein, F.J., 2003. Randomized controlled trial of strength training in post-polio patients. Muscle Nerve. 27, 332–338.

Chapman, A., Meyer, C., Renehan, E., Hill, K.D., Browning, C.J., 2017. Exercise interventions for the improvement of falls-related outcomes among older adults with diabetes mellitus: a systematic review and meta-analyses. J. Diabetes. Complications. 31, 631–645.

Charcot Marie Tooth Association., 2018. A Guide to Physical and Occupational Therapy for CMT.

Chetlin, R.D., Gutmann, L., Tarnopolsky, M., Ullrich, I.H., Yeater, R.A., 2004. Resistance training effectiveness in patients with Charcot-Marie-Tooth disease: recommendations for exercise prescription. Arch. Phys. Med. Rehabil. 85, 1217–1223.

Cortese, A., Tozza, S., Yau, W.Y., et al., 2020. Cerebellar ataxia, neuropathy, vestibular areflexia syndrome due to RFC1 repeat expansion. Brain J. Neurol. 143, 480–490.

Crews, R.T., Schneider, K.L., Yalla, S.V., Reeves, N.D., Vileikyte, L., 2016. Physiological and psychological challenges of increasing physical activity and exercise in patients at risk of diabetic foot ulcers: a critical review. Diabetes. Metab. Res. Rev. 32, 791–804.

Davidson, I., Parker, Z.J., 2022. Falls in people post-Guillain-Barré syndrome in the United Kingdom: a national cross-sectional survey of community-based adults. Health Soc. Care. Community. 30, e2590–e2603.

Davidson, I., Wilson, C., Walton, T., Brissenden, S., 2009. Physiotherapy and Guillain-Barré syndrome: results of a national survey. Physiotherapy. 95, 157–163.

Dennis, D., Mullins, R., 2013. Guillain-Barré syndrome patient's satisfaction with physiotherapy: a two-part observational study. Physiother. Theory. Pract. 29, 301–308.

Draak, T.H.P., Vanhoutte, E.K., van Nes, S.I., et al., 2014. Changing outcome in inflammatory neuropathies: Rasch-comparative responsiveness PeriNomS Study Group. Neurology. 83, 2124–2132.

Ducic, I., Short, K.W., Dellon, A.L., 2004. Relationship between loss of pedal sensibility, balance, and falls in patients with peripheral neuropathy. Ann. Plast. Surg. 52, 535–540.

Dufek, J.S., Neumann, E.S., Hawkins, M.C., O'Toole, B., 2014. Functional and dynamic response characteristics of a custom composite ankle foot orthosis for Charcot-Marie-Tooth patients. Gait Posture. 39, 308–313.

Eagle, M., Peacock, C., Bushby, K., Major, R., 2001. Facioscapulohumeral muscular dystrophy: gait analysis and effectiveness of ankle foot orthoses (AFOs). Neuromuscul. Disord. 11, 631.

Eichinger, K., Burns, J., Cornett, K., et al., 2018. The Charcot-Marie-Tooth Functional Outcome Measure (CMT-FOM). Neurology. 91, e1381–e1384.

Eichinger, K., Odrzywolski, K., Sowden, J., Herrmann, D.N., 2016. Patient reported falls and balance confidence in individuals with Charcot-Marie-Tooth disease. J. Neuromuscul. Dis. 3, 289–292.

El Mhandi, L., Millet, G.Y., Calmels, P., et al., 2008. Benefits of interval-training on fatigue and functional capacities in Charcot-Marie-Tooth disease. Muscle Nerve. 37, 601–610.

Elsworth, C., Winward, C., Sackley, C., et al., 2011. Supported community exercise in people with long-term neurological conditions: a phase II randomized controlled trial. Clin. Rehabil. 25, 588–598.

Emam, A.A., Gad, A.M., Ahmed, M.M., Assal, H.S., Mousa, S.G., 2009. Quantitative assessment of posture stability using computerised dynamic posturography in type 2 diabetic patients with neuropathy and its relation to glycaemic control. Singapore Med. J. 50, 614–618.

England, J.D., Asbury, A.K., 2004. Peripheral neuropathy. Lancet. 363, 2151–2161.

Ericson, U., Borg, J., Borg, K., 2000. Macro-EMG and muscle biopsy of paretic foot dorsiflexors in Charcot-Marie-Tooth disease. Muscle Nerve. 23, 217–222.

Fehmi, J., Vale, T., Keddie, S., Rinaldi, S., 2021. Nodal and paranodal antibody-associated neuropathies. Pract. Neurol. 21, 273.

Gallardo, E., 2005. Charcot-Marie-Tooth disease type 1A duplication: spectrum of clinical and magnetic resonance imaging features in leg and foot muscles. Brain. 129, 426–437.

Garssen, M.P.J., Schillings, M.L., Van Doorn, P.A., Van Engelen, B.G.M., Zwarts, M.J., 2007. Contribution of central and peripheral factors to residual fatigue in Guillain-Barré syndrome. Muscle Nerve. 36, 93–99.

Garssen, M.P.J., Van Koningsveld, R., Van Doorn, P.A., 2006. Residual fatigue is independent of antecedent events and disease severity in Guillain-Barré syndrome. J. Neurol. 253, 1143–1146.

Graham, R.C., Hughes, R.A.C., 2006a. A modified peripheral neuropathy scale: the Overall Neuropathy Limitations Scale. J. Neurol. Neurosurg. Psychiatry. 77, 973–976.

Graham, R.C., Hughes, R.A.C., 2006b. Clinimetric properties of a walking scale in peripheral neuropathy. J. Neurol. Neurosurg. Psychiatry. 77, 977–979.

Guillebastre, B., Calmels, P., Rougier, P.R., 2011. Assessment of appropriate ankle-foot orthoses models for patients with Charcot-Marie-Tooth disease. Am. J. Phys. Med. Rehabil. 90, 619–627.

Gutmann, L., Shy, M., 2015. Update on Charcot-Marie-Tooth disease. Curr. Opin. Neurol. 28, 462–467.

Guyton, G.P., Mann, R.A., 2000. The pathogenesis and surgical management of foot deformity in Charcot-Marie-Tooth disease. Foot Ankle Clin. 5, 317–326.

Hachisuka, K., Ohnishi, A., Yamaga, M., Dozono, K., Ueta, M., Ogata, H., 1997. The role of weakness of triceps surae muscles in astasia without abasia. J. Neurol. Neurosurg. Psychiatry. 62, 496–500.

Harbo, T., Markvardsen, L.K., Hellfritzsch, M.B., Severinsen, K., Nielsen, J.F., Andersen, H., 2019. Neuromuscular electrical stimulation in early rehabilitation of Guillain-Barré syndrome: a pilot study. Muscle Nerve. 59, 481–484.

Hermans, G., den Berghe, G., Van, 2015. Clinical review: intensive care unit acquired weakness. Crit. Care. 19, 274.

Hijmans, J.M., Geertzen, J.H.B., Zijlstra, W., Hof, A.L., Postema, K., 2008. Effects of vibrating insoles on standing balance in diabetic neuropathy. J. Rehabil. Res. Dev. 45, 1441–1449.

Hughes, R., 2008. Peripheral nerve diseases: the bare essentials. Pract. Neurol. 8, 396–405.

Hughes, R.A.C., Swan, A.V., van Doorn, P.A., 2014. Intravenous immunoglobulin for Guillain-Barré syndrome. Cochrane Database Syst. Rev. 9, CD002063

Jimenez-Moreno, A.C., Newman, J., Charman, S.J., et al., 2017. Measuring habitual physical activity in neuromuscular disorders: a systematic review. J. Neuromuscul. Dis. 4, 25–52.

Joint Task Force of the EFNS and the PNS, 2010. European Federation of Neurological Societies/Peripheral Nerve Society guideline on management of multifocal motor neuropathy. Report of a joint task force of the European Federation of Neurological Societies and the Peripheral Nerve Society–first revision. J. Peripher. Nerv. Syst. 15, 295–301.

Jones, K., Hawke, F., Newman, J., et al., 2021. Interventions for promoting physical activity in people with neuromuscular disease. Cochrane Database Syst. Rev. 5, CD013544

Kalkman, J.S., Schillings, M.L., van der Werf, S.P., et al., 2005. Experienced fatigue in facioscapulohumeral dystrophy, myotonic dystrophy, and HMSN-I. J. Neurol. Neurosurg. Psychiatry. 76, 1406–1409.

Kalkman, J.S., Schillings, M.L., Zwarts, M.J., van Engelen, B.G.M., Bleijenberg, G., 2007. The development of a model of fatigue in neuromuscular disorders: a longitudinal study. J. Psychosom. Res. 62, 571–579.

Kanade, R.V., van Deursen, R.W.M., Harding, K., Price, P., 2006. Walking performance in people with diabetic neuropathy: benefits and threats. Diabetologia. 49, 1747–1754.

Keddie, S., Pakpoor, J., Mousele, C., et al., 2021. Epidemiological and cohort study finds no association between COVID-19 and Guillain-Barré syndrome. Brain. J. Neurol. 144, 682–693.

Keh, R.Y.S., Scanlon, S., Datta-Nemdharry, P., et al., 2023. COVID-19 vaccination and Guillain-Barré syndrome: analyses using the National Immunoglobulin Database BPNS/ABN COVID-19 Vaccine GBS Study Group. Brain J. Neurol. 146, 739–748.

Khan, F., 2004. Rehabilitation in Guillian Barre syndrome. Aust. Fam. Physician. 33, 1013–1017.

Khan, F., Amatya, B., 2012. Rehabilitation interventions in patients with acute demyelinating inflammatory polyneuropathy: a systematic review. Eur. J. Phys. Rehabil. Med. 48, 507–522.

Khan, K.S., Andersen, H., 2022. The impact of diabetic neuropathy on activities of daily living, postural balance and risk of falls–a systematic review. J. Diabetes Sci. Technol. 16, 289–294.

Krupp, 2003. Measurement of fatigue Fatigue. Butterworth Heineman, Philadelphia.

Kuitwaard, K., van Doorn, P.A., 2009. Newer therapeutic options for chronic inflammatory demyelinating polyradiculoneuropathy. Drugs. 69, 987–1001.

Laurá, M., Hutton, E.J., Blake, J., et al., 2014. Pain and small fiber function in Charcot-Marie-Tooth disease type 1A. Muscle Nerve. 50, 366–371.

Laurá, M., Pipis, M., Rossor, A.M., Reilly, M.M., 2019. Charcot-Marie-Tooth disease and related disorders: an evolving landscape. Curr. Opin. Neurol. 32, 641–650.

Laura, M., Singh, D., Ramdharry, G., et al., 2017. Prevalence and orthopedic management of foot and ankle deformities in Charcot Marie Tooth disease. Muscle Nerve. 57, 255–259.

Lee, L.E., Kulnik, S.T., Curran, G., Boaz, A., Ramdharry, G., 2022. Protocol for a hybrid II study exploring the feasibility of delivering, evaluating, and implementing a self-management programme for people with neuromuscular diseases at a specialist neuromuscular centre (ADAPT-NMD) [preprint]. https://doi.org/10.21203/rs.3.rs-1292582/v1

Lehmann, H.C., Hughes, R.A.C., Kieseier, B.C., Hartung, H.-P., 2012. Recent developments and future directions in Guillain-Barré syndrome. J. Peripher. Nerv. Syst. 17 (Suppl. 3), 57–70. https://doi.org/10.1111/j.1529-8027.2012.00433.x.

Leone, E., Davenport, S., Robertson, C., Laura, M., Ramdharry, G.M., 2020. Incidence and risk factors for patellofemoral dislocation in adults with Charcot-Marie-Tooth disease: an observational study. J. Peripher. Nerv. Syst. 25, 491.

Lindeman, E., Leffers, P., Spaans, F., et al., 1995. Strength training in patients with myotonic dystrophy and hereditary motor and sensory neuropathy: a randomized clinical trial. Arch. Phys. Med. Rehabil. 76, 612–620.

Llewelyn, J.G., 2003. The diabetic neuropathies: types, diagnosis and management. J. Neurol. Neurosurg. Psychiatry. 74 (Suppl. 2), ii15–ii19.

Main, M., Hiscock, A., Muntoni, F., 2012. Dislocating patellae in children with CMT1a. Neuromuscul. Disord. 22, 869.

Matjacić, Z., Zupan, A., 2006. Effects of dynamic balance training during standing and stepping in patients with hereditary sensory motor neuropathy. Disabil. Rehabil. 28, 1455–1459.

Melese, H., Alamer, A., Hailu Temesgen, M., Kahsay, G., 2020. Effectiveness of exercise therapy on gait function in diabetic peripheral neuropathy patients: a systematic review of randomized controlled trials. Diabetes Metab. Syndr. Obes. Targets Ther. 13, 2753–2764.

Menotti, F., Laudani, L., Damiani, A., Mignogna, T., Macaluso, A., 2014. An anterior ankle-foot orthosis improves walking economy in Charcot-Marie-Tooth type 1A patients. Prosthet. Orthot. Int. 38, 387–392.

Merkies, I.S.J., Faber, C.G., 2012. Fatigue in immune-mediated neuropathies. Neuromuscul. Disord. 22 (Suppl. 3), S203–207.

Merkies, I.S.J., Kieseier, B.C., 2016. Fatigue, pain, anxiety and depression in Guillain-Barré syndrome and chronic inflammatory demyelinating polyradiculoneuropathy. Eur. Neurol. 75, 199–206.

Meythaler, J.M., 1997. Rehabilitation of Guillain-Barré syndrome. Arch. Phys. Med. Rehabil. 78, 872–879.

Missaoui, B., Thoumie, P., 2013. Balance training in ataxic neuropathies. Effects on balance and gait parameters. Gait Posture. 38, 471–476.

Monti Bragadin, M., Francini, L., Bellone, E., et al., 2015. Tinetti and Berg balance scales correlate with disability in hereditary peripheral neuropathies: a preliminary study. Eur. J. Phys. Rehabil. Med. 51, 423–427.

Mori, L., Signori, A., Prada, V., et al., 2019. Treadmill training in patients affected by Charcot-Marie-Tooth neuropathy: results of a multicenter, prospective, randomized, single-blind, controlled study TreSPE study group. Eur. J. Neurol. 27, 280–287.

Morrow, J.M., Sinclair, C.D.J., Fischmann, A., et al., 2015. MRI biomarker assessment of neuromuscular disease progression: a prospective observational cohort study. Lancet Neurol. 15, 65–77.

Nardone, A., Grasso, M., Schieppati, M., 2006. Balance control in peripheral neuropathy: are patients equally unstable under static and dynamic conditions? Gait Posture. 23, 364–373.

Nardone, A., Tarantola, J., Miscio, G., Pisano, F., Schenone, A., Schieppati, M., 2000. Loss of large-diameter spindle afferent fibres is not detrimental to the control of body sway during upright stance: evidence from neuropathy. Exp. Brain Res. 135, 155–162.

Neal, J.W., Gasque, P., 2016. The role of primary infection of Schwann cells in the aetiology of infective inflammatory neuropathies. J. Infect. 73, 402–418.

Neptune, R.R., Kautz, S.A., Zajac, F.E., 2001. Contributions of the individual ankle plantar flexors to support, forward progression and swing initiation during walking. J. Biomech. 34, 1387–1398.

Netto, A.B., Taly, A.B., Kulkarni, G.B., Uma Maheshwara Rao, G.S., Rao, S., 2017. Complications in mechanically ventilated patients of Guillain-Barre syndrome and their prognostic value. J. Neurosci. Rural Pract. 8, 68–73.

Newman, C.J., Walsh, M., O'Sullivan, R., et al., 2007. The characteristics of gait in Charcot-Marie-Tooth disease types I and II. Gait Posture. 26, 120–127.

Nicholson, G.A., 2006. The dominantly inherited motor and sensory neuropathies: clinical and molecular advances. Muscle Nerve. 33, 589–597.

Novak, P., Šmid, S., Vidmar, G., 2017. Rehabilitation of Guillain-Barré syndrome patients: an observational study. Int. J. Rehabil. Res. 40, 158–163.

O'Connor, J., McCaughan, D., McDaid, C., et al., 2015. Orthotic management of instability of the knee related to neuromuscular and central nervous system disorders: a mixed methods study. Draft report to Health Technology Agency (under review). University of York.

Padua, L., Cavallaro, T., Pareyson, D., Quattrone, A., Vita, G., Schenone, A., 2008. Charcot-Marie-Tooth and pain: correlations with neurophysiological, clinical, and disability findings. Neurol. Sci. 29, 193–194.

Padua, L., Pazzaglia, C., Pareyson, D., et al., 2016. Novel outcome measures for Charcot-Marie-Tooth disease: validation and reliability of the 6-min walk test and StepWatch(TM) Activity Monitor and identification of the walking features related to higher quality of life CMT-TRIAAL Group. Eur. J. Neurol. 23, 1343–1350.

Pareyson, D., Scaioli, V., Laurá, M., 2006. Clinical and electrophysiological aspects of Charcot-Marie-Tooth disease. Neuromolecular Med. 8, 3–22.

Paton, J., Hatton, A.L., Rome, K., Kent, B., 2016. Effects of foot and ankle devices on balance, gait and falls in adults with sensory perception loss: a systematic review. JBI Database Syst. Rev. Implement. Rep. 14, 127–162.

Paul, L., Ellis, B.M., Leese, G.P., McFadyen, A.K., McMurray, B., 2009. The effect of a cognitive or motor task on gait parameters of diabetic patients, with and without neuropathy. Diabet. Med. J. 26, 234–239.

Pazzaglia, C., Camerota, F., Germanotta, M., Di Sipio, E., Celletti, C., Padua, L., 2016. Efficacy of focal mechanic vibration treatment on balance in Charcot-Marie-Tooth 1A disease: a pilot study. J. Neurol. 263, 1434–1441.

Phillips, M., Radford, K., Wills, A., 2011. Ankle foot orthoses for people with Charcot Marie Tooth disease – views of users and orthotists on important aspects of use. Disabil. Rehabil. Assist. Technol. 6, 491–499.

Phillips, M.F., Robertson, Z., Killen, B., White, B., 2012. A pilot study of a crossover trial with randomized use of ankle-foot orthoses for people with Charcot–Marie–Tooth disease. Clin. Rehabil. 26, 534–544.

Pisciotta, C., Saveri, P., Pareyson, D., 2021. Challenges in treating Charcot-Marie-Tooth disease and related neuropathies: current management and future perspectives. Brain Sci. 11, 1447.

Piscosquito, G., Reilly, M.M., Schenone, A., et al., 2015. Responsiveness of clinical outcome measures in Charcot-Marie-Tooth disease CMT-TRIAAL Group, CMT-TRAUK Group. Eur. J. Neurol. 22, 1556–1563.

Pollard, J.D., 2002. Chronic inflammatory demyelinating polyradiculoneuropathy. Curr. Opin. Neurol. 15, 279–283.

Postges, H., Jones, F., Lee, L., et al., 2020. Neuromuscular bridges: outcome of the development phase of a self-management programme for people with neuromuscular diseases. J. Peripher. Nerv. Syst. 554.

Prada, V., Schizzi, S., Poggi, I., et al., 2018. Hand rehabilitation treatment for Charcot-Marie-Tooth disease: an open label pilot study. J. Neurol. Neurophysiol. 9.

Prior, R., Van Helleputte, L., Benoy, V., Den Bosch, L.V., 2017. Defective axonal transport: a common pathological mechanism in inherited and acquired peripheral neuropathies. Neurobiol. Dis. 105, 300–320.

Rajabally, Y.A., Simpson, B.S., Beri, S., Bankart, J., Gosalakkal, J.A., 2009. Epidemiologic variability of chronic inflammatory demyelinating polyneuropathy with different diagnostic criteria: study of a UK population. Muscle Nerve. 39, 432–438.

Ramdharry, G., Bull, K., Jeffcott, R., Frame, A., 2020. An expert opinion: rehabilitation options for people with polyneuropathy. Adv. Clin. Neurosci. Rehabil. 19, 17–19.

Ramdharry, G., Buscemi, V., Boaz, A., et al., 2021a. Proposing a core outcome set for physical activity and exercise interventions in people with rare neurological conditions. Front. Rehabil. Sci. 2, 62.

Ramdharry, G., Dudziec, M., Lee, L., Massey, C., Reilly, M.M., 2018. Balance training in people with Charcot-Marie-Tooth 1A (BALTiC trial) improves balance and gait. Presented at the Peripheral Nerve Society. J. Peripher. Nerv. Syst., 268.

Ramdharry, G.M., Pollard, A.J., Marsden, J.F., Reilly, M.M., 2012a. Comparing gait performance of people with Charcot-Marie-Tooth disease who do and do not wear ankle foot orthoses. Physiother. Res. Int. 17, 191–199.

Ramdharry, G., Singh, D., Gray, J., et al., 2021b. A prospective study on surgical management of foot deformities in Charcot Marie tooth disease. J. Peripher. Nerv. Syst. 26, 187–192.

Ramdharry, G.M., Day, B.L., Reilly, M.M., Marsden, J.F., 2012b. Foot drop splints improve proximal as well as distal leg control during gait in Charcot-Marie-Tooth Disease. Muscle Nerve. 46, 512–519.

Ramdharry, G.M., Pollard, A., Anderson, C., et al., 2014. A pilot study of proximal strength training in Charcot-Marie-Tooth disease. J. Peripher. Nerv. Syst. 19, 328–332.

Ramdharry, G.M., Pollard, A.J., Grant, R., et al., 2016. A study of physical activity comparing people with Charcot-Marie-Tooth disease to normal control subjects. Disabil. Rehabil. 39, 1753–1758.

Ramdharry, G.M., Reilly-O'Donnell, L., Grant, R., Reilly, M.M., 2017. Frequency and circumstances of falls for people with Charcot-Marie-Tooth disease: a cross sectional survey. Physiother. Res. Int. 23, e1702.

Ramdharry, G.M., Thornhill, A., Mein, G., Reilly, M.M., Marsden, J.F., 2012c. Exploring the experience of fatigue in people with Charcot-Marie-Tooth disease. Neuromuscul. Disord 22 (Suppl. 3), S208–213.

Ramdharry, G.M., Wallace, A., Hennis, P., et al., 2021c. Cardiopulmonary exercise performance and factors associated with aerobic capacity in neuromuscular diseases. Muscle Nerve. 64, 683–690.

Redmond, A.C., Crosbie, J., Ouvrier, R.A., 2006. Development and validation of a novel rating system for scoring standing foot posture: the Foot Posture Index. Clin. Biomech. 21, 89–98.

Reilly, M.M., Rossor, A.M., 2020. Humans: the ultimate animal models. J. Neurol. Neurosurg. Psychiatry. 91, 1132–1136.

Rossor, A.M., Carr, A.S., Devine, H., et al., 2017. Peripheral neuropathy in complex inherited diseases: an approach to diagnosis. J. Neurol. Neurosurg. Psychiatry. 88, 846–863.

Rossor, A.M., Murphy, S., Reilly, M.M., 2012. Knee bobbing in Charcot–Marie–Tooth disease. Pract. Neurol. 12, 182–183.

Sacco, I.C.N., Amadio, A.C., 2003. Influence of the diabetic neuropathy on the behavior of electromyographic and sensorial responses in treadmill gait. Clin. Biomech. 18, 426–434.

Sackley, C., Disler, P.B., Turner-Stokes, L., Wade, D.T., Brittle, N., Hoppitt, T., 2009. Rehabilitation interventions for foot drop in neuromuscular disease. Cochrane Database Syst. Rev. 3 CD003908.

Said, G., 2006. Chronic inflammatory demyelinating polyneuropathy. Neuromuscul. Disord. 16, 293–303.

Salsich, G.B., Mueller, M.J., 2000. Effect of plantar flexor muscle stiffness on selected gait characteristics. Gait Posture. 11, 207–216.

Scheffers, G., Hiller, C., Refshauge, K., Burns, J., 2013. Prescription of foot and ankle orthoses for children with Charcot–Marie–Tooth disease: a review of the evidence. Phys. Ther. Rev. 17, 79–90.

Selles, R.W., van Ginneken, B.T.J., Schreuders, T.A.R., Janssen, W.G.M., Stam, H.J., 2006. Dynamometry of intrinsic hand muscles in patients with Charcot-Marie-Tooth disease. Neurology. 67, 2022–2027.

Shumway-Cook, A., Horak, F.B., 1986. Assessing the influence of sensory interaction of balance. Suggestion from the field. Phys. Ther. 66, 1548–1550.

Simatos Arsenault, N., Vincent, P.-O., Yu, B.H.S., Bastien, R., Sweeney, A., 2016. Influence of exercise on patients with Guillain-Barré syndrome: a systematic review. Physiother. Can. 68, 367–376.

Singh, D., Gray, J., Laura, M., Reilly, M.M., 2021. Charcot neuroarthropathy in patients with Charcot Marie Tooth disease. Foot Ankle Surg. 27, 865–868.

Singleton, J.R., Smith, A.G., Marcus, R.L., 2015. Exercise as therapy for diabetic and prediabetic neuropathy. Curr. Diab. Rep. 15, 120.

Siriwardena, A.N., Akanuwe, J.N.A., Botan, V., et al., 2022. Patient-reported symptoms and experience following Guillain-Barré syndrome and related conditions: questionnaire development and validation. Health Expect. Int. J. 25, 223–231.

Sman, A.D., Hackett, D., Fiatarone Singh, M., Fornusek, C., Menezes, M.P., Burns, J., 2015. Systematic review of exercise for Charcot-Marie-Tooth disease. J. Peripher. Nerv. Syst. 20, 347–362.

Smith, A.G., Singleton, J.R., 2008. Impaired glucose tolerance and neuropathy. Neurologist. 14, 23–29.

Taga, A., Lauria, G., 2022. COVID-19 and the peripheral nervous system. A 2-year review from the pandemic to the vaccine era. J. Peripher. Nerv. Syst. 27, 4–30.

Tan, S.H.S., Chua, C.X.K., Doshi, C., Wong, K.L., Lim, A.K.S., Hui, J.H., 2020. The outcomes of isolated lateral release in patellofemoral instability: a systematic review and meta-analysis. J. Knee Surg. 33, 958–965.

Taveggia, C., 2016. Schwann cells–axon interaction in myelination. Curr. Opin. Neurobiol. 39, 24–29.

Tews, D.S., 2002. Apoptosis and muscle fibre loss in neuromuscular disorders. Neuromuscul. Disord. 12, 613–622.

Tozza, S., Aceto, M.G., Pisciotta, C., et al., 2016. Postural instability in Charcot-Marie-Tooth 1A disease. Gait Posture. 49, 353–357.

Ulbrecht, J.S., Hurley, T., Mauger, D.T., Cavanagh, P.R., 2014. Prevention of recurrent foot ulcers with plantar pressure-based in-shoe orthoses: the CareFUL prevention multicenter randomized controlled trial. Diabetes Care. 37, 1982–1989.

Van den Bergh, P.Y.K., van Doorn, P.A., Hadden, R.D.M., et al., 2021. European Academy of Neurology/Peripheral Nerve Society guideline on diagnosis and treatment of chronic inflammatory demyelinating polyradiculoneuropathy: report of a joint task force–second revision. J. Peripher. Nerv. Syst. 26, 242–268.

van der Linden, M.H., van der Linden, S.C., Hendricks, H.T., van Engelen, B.G.M., Geurts, A.C.H., 2010. Postural instability in Charcot-Marie-Tooth type 1A patients is strongly associated with reduced somatosensation. Gait Posture. 31, 483–488.

van Deursen, R., 2008. Footwear for the neuropathic patient: offloading and stability. Diabetes Metab. Res. Rev. 24 (Suppl. 1), S96–S100.

van Doorn, P.A., 2013. Diagnosis, treatment and prognosis of Guillain-Barré syndrome (GBS). Presse Med. 42, e193–201.

van Nes, S.I., Vanhoutte, E.K., Faber, C.G., Garssen, M., van Doorn, P.A., Merkies, I.S.J., 2009. Improving fatigue assessment in immune-mediated neuropathies: the modified Rasch-built fatigue severity scale. J. Peripher. Nerv. Syst. 14, 268–278.

van Nes, S.I., Vanhoutte, E.K., van Doorn, P.A., et al., 2011. Rasch-built Overall Disability Scale (R-ODS) for immune-mediated peripheral neuropathies. Neurology. 76, 337–345.

van Pomeren, M., Selles, R.W., van Ginneken, B.T.J., Schreuders, T.A.R., Janssen, W.G.M., Stam, H.J., 2009. The hypothesis of overwork weakness in Charcot-Marie-Tooth: a critical evaluation. J. Rehabil. Med. 41, 32–34.

Vanhoutte, E.K., Faber, C.G., van Nes, S.I., et al., 2012. Modifying the Medical Research Council grading system through Rasch analyses. Brain J. Neurol. 135, 1639–1649.

Veenhuizen, Y., Cup, E.H.C., Jonker, M.A., et al., 2019. Self-management program improves participation in patients with neuromuscular disease: a randomized controlled trial. Neurology. 93, e1720–e1731.

Veenhuizen, Y., Satink, T., Graff, M.J., et al., 2021. Mixed methods evaluation of a self-management group programme for patients with neuromuscular disease and chronic fatigue. BMJ Open. 11, e048890.

Videler, A., Eijffinger, E., Nollet, F., Beelen, A., 2012. A thumb opposition splint to improve manual dexterity and upper-limb functioning in Charcot-Marie-Tooth disease. J. Rehabil. Med. 44, 249–253.

Videler, A.J., Beelen, A., Nollet, F., 2008a. Manual dexterity and related functional limitations in hereditary motor and sensory neuropathy. An explorative study. Disabil. Rehabil. 30, 634–638.

Videler, A.J., Beelen, A., van Schaik, I.N., de Visser, M., Nollet, F., 2008b. Manual dexterity in hereditary motor and sensory neuropathy type 1a: severity of limitations and feasibility and reliability of two assessment instruments. J. Rehabil. Med. 40, 132–136.

Vincent, A.M., Hinder, L.M., Pop-Busui, R., Feldman, E.L., 2009. Hyperlipidemia: a new therapeutic target for diabetic neuropathy. J. Peripher. Nerv. Syst. 14, 257–267.

Vinci, P., Esposito, C., Perelli, S.L., Antenor, J.A.V., Thomas, F.P., 2003. Overwork weakness in Charcot-Marie-Tooth disease. Arch. Phys. Med. Rehabil. 84, 825–827.

Vinci, P., Perelli, S.L., 2002. Footdrop, foot rotation, and plantarflexor failure in Charcot-Marie-Tooth disease. Arch. Phys. Med. Rehabil. 83, 513–516.

Vucic, S., Kiernan, M.C., Cornblath, D.R., 2009. Guillain-Barré syndrome: an update. J. Clin. Neurosci. 16, 733–741.

Walgaard, C., Jacobs, B.C., Lingsma, H.F., et al., 2021. Second intravenous immunoglobulin dose in patients with Guillain-Barré syndrome with poor prognosis (SID-GBS): a double-blind, randomised, placebo-controlled trial Dutch GBS Study Group. Lancet Neurol. 20, 275–283.

Walgaard, C., Lingsma, H.F., Ruts, L., et al., 2010. Prediction of respiratory insufficiency in Guillain-Barré syndrome. Ann. Neurol. 67, 781–787.

Walker, J.L., Nelson, K.R., Heavilon, J.A., et al., 1994. Hip abnormalities in children with Charcot-Marie-Tooth disease. J. Pediatr. Orthop. 14, 54–59.

Wallace, A., Pietrusz, A., Dewar, E., et al., 2019. Community exercise is feasible for neuromuscular diseases and can improve aerobic capacity. Neurology. 92, e1773–e1785.

Wegener, C., Wegener, K., Smith, R., Schott, K.-H., Burns, J., 2016. Biomechanical effects of sensorimotor orthoses in adults with Charcot-Marie-Tooth disease. Prosthet. Orthot. Int. 40, 436–446.

Westblad, M.E., Forsberg, A., Press, R., 2009. Disability and health status in patients with chronic inflammatory demyelinating polyneuropathy. Disabil. Rehabil. 31, 720–725.

White, C.M., Pritchard, J., Turner-Stokes, L., 2004. Exercise for people with peripheral neuropathy. Cochrane Database Syst. Rev. 4, CD003904

Willison, H.J., Jacobs, B.C., van Doorn, P.A., 2016. Guillain-Barré syndrome. Lancet. 388, 717–727.

World Health Organization, 2010. WHO Global status report on noncommunicable diseases. World Health Organization, Geneva.

Young, P., De Jonghe, P., Stögbauer, F., Butterfass-Bahloul, T., 2008. Treatment for Charcot-Marie-Tooth disease Cochrane Database of Systematic Reviews. John Wiley & Sons, Ltd, Hoboken.

Zhang, Y.-H., Hu, H.-Y., Xiong, Y.-C., et al., 2021. Exercise for neuropathic pain: a systematic review and expert consensus. Front. Med. 8, 756940.

Zuccarino, R., Anderson, K.M., Shy, M.E., Wilken, J.M., 2021. Satisfaction with ankle foot orthoses in individuals with Charcot-Marie-Tooth disease. Muscle Nerve. 63, 40–45.

Neuromuscular Disorders

Anna Mayhew, Gita Ramdharry, Aleksandra Pietrusz,
Meredith James, Jane Newman, and Charlotte Massey

OUTLINE

Introduction, 383
Anatomy and Physiology of Neuromuscular
  Disorders, 383
Overview of Causes of Neuromuscular Disorders, 385
  Acquired Neuromuscular Disorders, 386
  Genetic Neuromuscular Disorders, 386
Principles of Assessment and Management, 387
  Assessment, 387
  Physical Management and Rehabilitation, 387
Specific Types of Neuromuscular Disorders, 387
  Idiopathic Inflammatory Myopathies, 387
    Disease Course and Prognosis, 387
    Presentation, 387
    Assessment and Outcome Measures, 388
    Medical Management, 388
    Physical Management, 388
  Muscular Dystrophies, 388
    Duchenne Muscular Dystrophy, 388
    Facioscapulohumeral Muscular Dystrophy, 393

  Limb Girdle Muscular Dystrophy, 394
Myotonic Dystrophy Type 1, 395
  Disease Course and Prognosis, 395
  Assessment and Outcome Measures, 397
  Medical Management, 398
  Physical Management, 398
Spinal Muscular Atrophy, 399
  Presentation, 399
  Disease Course and Prognosis, 400
  Medical Management, 401
  Physical Management, 401
Mitochondrial Diseases, 401
  Presentation, 401
  Disease Course and Prognosis, 402
  Assessment and Outcome Measures, 402
Case Studies, 405
  Spinal Muscular Atrophy, 405
  Limb Girdle Muscular Dystrophy, 406

INTRODUCTION

Neuromuscular disorders (NMDs) are a heterogenous group of diseases that are characterised by muscle weakness and atrophy (Swash & Schwartz 2013). The neuromuscular umbrella includes conditions that involve the peripheral neuromuscular system, from the anterior horn cell body in the spinal cord to the muscle membrane. This includes the diseases of the peripheral nerves, or polyneuropathies, which are addressed in more detail in Chapter 14. Anterior horn cell diseases include motor neurone disease (e.g., amyotrophic lateral sclerosis) and are addressed in more detail in Chapter 13. Significant variation exists in onset, severity and progression rate between the different conditions, with some causing death in infancy and other types experienced as lifelong conditions into older age.

ANATOMY AND PHYSIOLOGY OF NEUROMUSCULAR DISORDERS

To understand the pathology of NMDs, a basic understanding of the structures and physiology involved helps to explain the deficits and symptoms experienced by people living with NMD. The peripheral neuromuscular motor system starts at the anterior horn cell in the spinal cord that exits as a motor neurone. This terminates at the neuromuscular junction where release of the neurotransmitter acetyl choline (ACh) occurs once the presynaptic membrane is hyperpolarised by an action potential. ACh receptors are sited on the postsynaptic membrane and bind with ACh that is released into the synaptic cleft. Binding to the receptors results in an influx of sodium ions and expulsion of potassium ions which alters the membrane potential. This activates voltage-gated sodium ion channels that then propagate the action potential through the t-tubules of the muscle fibre. This stimulates voltage-gated calcium ion channels that cause calcium ions to flood into the sarcoplasmic reticulum of the muscle fibre causing excitation contraction coupling (ECC) (Mukund & Subramaniam 2020).

The sarcomere (Fig. 15.1) is composed of two alternating sets of protein filaments: thin filaments (α-actin and associated proteins) and thick filaments (myosin and associated proteins). Calcium ions released during ECC bind to the protein troponin within the sarcomere causing the shape of the troponin-tropomyosin to change, exposing the head of the myosin molecules and allowing binding of actin. The muscle contraction occurs to a repeated cycle of actin and myosin engagement, gradually shifting the filaments over each other (Mukund & Subramaniam 2020).

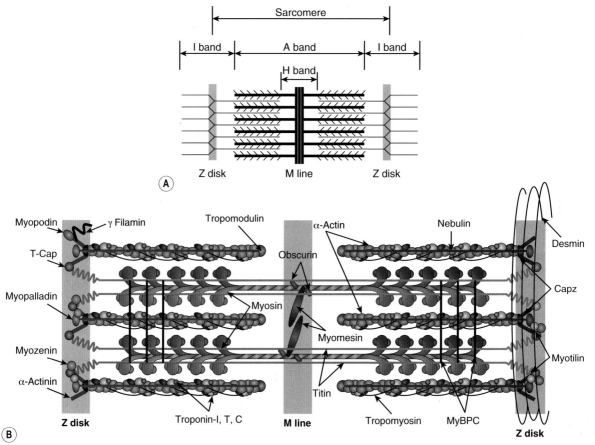

FIG. 15.1 (A) Schematic representation of the striated skeletal muscle sarcomere showing the arrangement of thick and thin filaments in the sarcomere and identifying bands of overlap between them. (B) Schematic diagram of the sarcomere summarising organisation and location of major sarcomeric proteins. Cytosolic Ca2+ brings about a conformational change in the structure of troponin C, revealing myosin binding sites. Myosin heads successively bind and crawl along the length of actin, bringing about sarcomeric contraction. (Reprinted with permission from Mukund & Subramaniam 2020.)

Several additional processes relating to stimulation, metabolism, structure and regeneration are crucial to the integrity of the sarcomere (Fig. 15.2) (Mukund & Subramaniam 2020). Disruption to any of these processes can lead to loss of muscle function and degeneration and atrophy of muscle tissue, a key feature of NMDs. This can be primary atrophy, where the degeneration is within the muscle tissue itself, or secondary atrophy, with denervation for example. Atrophy of skeletal muscle tissue has been observed using magnetic resonance imaging (MRI) in both primary muscle disease and denervation. It presents as fatty infiltration of the muscle fibres, and the percentage intramuscular fat has been correlated with strength, but the distribution of fatty infiltration and atrophy can vary between muscles for different conditions (Alic et al 2021, Morrow et al 2015, Mul et al 2017). In some NMDs, degeneration is also observed in smooth muscle (Mary et al 2018).

OVERVIEW OF CAUSES OF NEUROMUSCULAR DISORDERS

NMDs can be classified as **acquired or inherited**, pertaining to the cause of the disease process affecting muscle structure and function (Fig. 15.3).

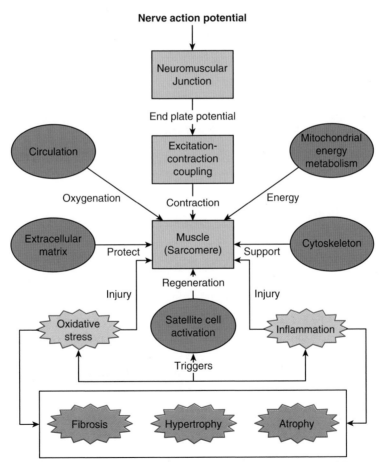

FIG. 15.2 Schematic representation of dystrophin-glycoprotein complex (DGC) and of other sarcoplasmic associated proteins involved in muscular dystrophies. (Reprinted with permission from Mukund & Subramaniam 2020).

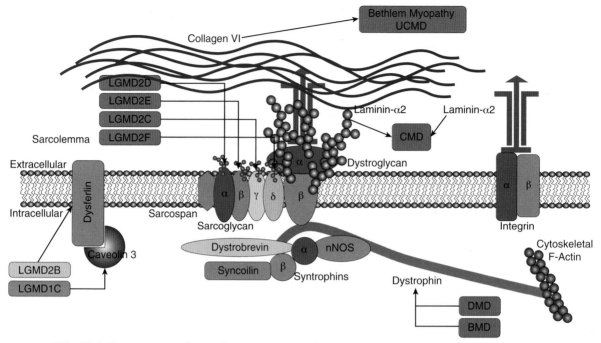

FIG. 15.3 Components of muscle structure and function—a schematic representation of the various functional components necessary for or arising as a consequence of muscle function, in health and disease. *BMD*, Becker's muscular dystrophy; *CMD*, congenital muscular dystrophy; *DMD*, Duchenne muscular dystrophy; *LGMD*, limb girdle muscular dystrophy; *UCMD*, Ullrich congenital muscular dystrophy. (Reprinted with permission from Nigro & Piluso 2015.)

Acquired Neuromuscular Disorders

Acquired NMDs can be caused by external factors (e.g., infection or toxicity) or are idiopathic in nature. Poliomyelitis is caused by a viral infection affecting the anterior horn cell of the spinal cord. Critical illness myopathies and neuropathies may be in part caused by toxicity of sedation and paralysing agents on the neuromuscular system in intensive care, but the risk factor also increases with prolonged stay where there is sepsis and multiorgan dysfunction. The Covid-19 pandemic saw high numbers of admission to critical care units and increased numbers of people with associated NMDs (Bagnato et al 2021, Cabañes-Martínez et al 2020). The largest group of idiopathic diseases affecting muscle tissue is the inflammatory neuropathy group which can overlap with rheumatological conditions, such as Sjogren's disease (see Idiopathic Inflammatory Myopathies section).

Genetic Neuromuscular Disorders

The muscle membrane is a complex structure of proteins with specific roles in the function and integrity of the structure. Genetic mutations of any of these proteins can cause instability in the structure and function of the sarcolemma membrane, leading to cell death, degeneration and muscle atrophy (Nigro & Piluso 2015). They are collectively known as the **muscular dystrophies** and are inherited and progressive (see Muscular Dystrophies section). Figure 15.3 summarises the primary structural issue for involvement of different muscular dystrophies. Some types of muscular dystrophy also involve cardiac and respiratory muscles (Nigro & Piluso 2015).

KEY POINTS

- Understanding the pathology of NMDs helps to explain the deficits and symptoms experienced by people living with NMD.
- NMDs can be classified as **acquired or inherited**. Acquired NMDs can be caused by external factors or are idiopathic in nature. Inherited NMDs are a heterogeneous group of rare genetic diseases that involve muscles, motor neurones, peripheral nerves or the neuromuscular junction.

PRINCIPLES OF ASSESSMENT AND MANAGEMENT

Assessment

At the heart of assessment is the patient and their concerns, and this will assist in building a picture of priorities in the clinic. Here we are dealing with a set of distinct diseases; however, assessments can be grouped according to the World Health Organization *International Classification of Functioning, Disability & Health Framework* (WHO 2001) of **body functions and structure:** measures of muscle strength and weakness, posture, range of motion, respiratory function, pain and fatigue; **activities:** measures of motor performance, gait and activities of daily living; **participation:** impact on home, work and social participation. In the disease-specific sections that follow more detail will be given about the precise assessments suitable for the different disorders. Assessment should be focused, when possible, on information useful for management and monitoring any intervention of changes.

Physical Management and Rehabilitation

NMDs are rare which can mean they take a significant time to reach the right clinic for care and diagnosis. For many of these conditions there are no or limited therapeutic drugs and there is no cure, so management focuses on maintaining and promoting function for as long as possible and managing decline with dignity. This can feel uncomfortable for therapists used to patients responding to treatment and requires an adjustment of expectations. However, the field is changing rapidly, and genetic advances are leading to revolutionary therapeutic treatments for some of these diseases, such as spinal muscular atrophy. The role of physiotherapy and helping individuals stay active regardless of ambulatory status cannot be over-emphasised. Limited resources for adults can make accessing therapy challenging.

The following sections provide more detail of management principles for specific conditions, but there are some cross-cutting approaches that apply to all people living with NMDs. People with NMDs as a group tend to be more sedentary than the general population (Jones et al 2021) so support and online resources to increase engagement in physical activity can be introduced, for example, exercise videos (Scottish Muscle Network videos: https://www.smn.scot.nhs.uk/videos-and-podcasts/; Neuromuscular Centre UK videos: https://www.nmcentre.com/therapies-exercise-at-home). Bespoke programmes to assist engagement in activity are emerging (Veenhuizen et al 2019). People living with these long-term conditions also benefit from self-management support. Resources and approaches specific to NMDs have been developed to empower people to make positive life choices, set goals and increase confidence (Postges et al 2020).

SPECIFIC TYPES OF NEUROMUSCULAR DISORDERS

The following sections will focus on specific NMDs or groups of diseases that may be encountered in neurology or rehabilitation clinics.

Idiopathic Inflammatory Myopathies

Idiopathic inflammatory myopathies (IIMs) are a heterogenous group of **acquired** diseases, falling into subsets with varying clinical and pathophysiological features: dermatomyositis (DM), inclusion body myositis (IBM), immune-mediated necrotising myopathy (IMNM) and polymyositis (PM) (Dalakas 2020, Lazarou & Guerne 2013).

Disease Course and Prognosis

Acute or subacute onset is observed in IMNM, PM or DM with muscle weakness and wasting feature clinically or sometimes subclinically in DM. This is usually in adulthood, but there is a juvenile form of DM (Dalakas 2020). People usually present with IBM in the fifth or sixth decade and report an insidious onset with progressive muscle weakness and wasting.

Presentation

Systemic and local inflammation in the acute phase impairs muscle contraction, causing fatigability and reduced function, although the correlation between weakness and disease activity is not clearly related (Munters et al 2014). MRI analysis reveals increasing percentage fat fraction in PM, DM (Qi et al 2008, Yao et al 2016) and IBM (Morrow et al 2015a). This represents primary atrophy of the muscle fibres that correlates with muscle function and disability, explaining more prolonged presentations of weakness. Primary weakness tends to present in the proximal lower limbs in PM, and there is a specific pattern of weakness in IBM affecting the forearm flexors, quadriceps, tibialis anterior and bulbar muscles.

Physical inactivity and sedentary lifestyles can lead to disuse muscle atrophy that could cause additional detriment in conditions where primary muscle weakness and wasting are features (Busse & Ramdharry 2020, Ramdharry 2010). People living with IIM show lower levels of physical activity compared with control subjects (Pinto et al 2016, Ramdharry et al 2021), and there are correlations between physical activity levels and disease severity (Landon-Cardinal et al 2020, Pinto et al 2016, Ramdharry et al 2021). There is evidence of deconditioning in some IIM cohorts. MRI demonstrated volume loss in muscles less affected by fatty atrophy owing to primary disease in IBM, indicating secondary disuse atrophy (Morrow et al 2015b).

Assessment and Outcome Measures

A core outcome set for exercise trials in IIM was developed by the International Myositis Assessment and Clinical Studies (IMACS) group (Isenberg et al 2004) that can be applied to in-clinic assessment. This includes manual muscle testing (MMT), a patient and physical global disease activity rating using a 100-point visual analogue scale (VAS) and Health Assessment Questionnaire (HAQ). There are also disease-specific scales such as the Inclusion Body Myositis Functional Rating Scale (IBMFRS) (Jackson et al 2008, Ramdharry et al 2019) and the Myositis Activities Profile (MAP) (Alexanderson et al 2012).

Medical Management

High-dose steroids and other immunotherapies are offered to people with DM, PM and IMNM. People with IBM do not usually respond to immunosuppression, with physical therapy recommended as the main management strategy (Dalakas 2020). Trials of myostatin inhibitors so far have failed to increase muscle mass and function in IBM patients but research continues (Ahmed et al 2016).

Physical Management

A primary strategy in the management of IIM is exercise. Strength and aerobic training is safe and can target deconditioning and disuse atrophy (Alemo Munters et al 2014, Ramdharry & Anderson 2022, Voet et al 2019). There is an emerging body of work exploring the effect of resistance exercise on inflammation using tests of inflammatory markers and muscle biopsy (Talotta et al 2022). If exercise is shown to have an effect on the disease process, this may have potential to affect progression and disease course.

Clinical management also includes orthotics if foot drop presents in persons with IBM, and knee braces may help when there is significant quadriceps weakness. A small trial of knee–ankle–foot orthoses (KAFOs) showed improved gait parameters for a cohort of people with IBM, but the practicality of wearing these bulky braces was questioned (Bernhardt et al 2011).

KEY POINTS

- Idiopathic inflammatory neuropathies cause progressive primary muscle weakness but can also be affected by secondary disuse weakness and deconditioning.
- Exercise is safe in these conditions and may slow progression of the myopathy.
- Orthotics may also assist function in the presence of significant weakness and mobility impairment.

Muscular Dystrophies

Inherited or spontaneous mutations of genes coding for proteins in the muscle membrane cause different types of muscular dystrophies (see Fig. 15.3). Three of the most common types are described in more detail in the following sections.

Duchenne Muscular Dystrophy

Duchenne muscular dystrophy (DMD) is caused by a mutation in the dystrophin gene resulting in deficit or complete absence of dystrophin protein in skeletal muscle tissue. DMD is characterised by rapid, progressive muscle degeneration leading to loss of ambulation in early teens, respiratory and cardiac complications, and premature death. Skeletal, respiratory and cardiac muscles are involved as are the extramuscular systems (brain).

DMD is the most common form of childhood-onset muscular dystrophy with incidence of 1 per 3,500–6,000 live male births (Bushby et al 2010, Mah et al 2014, Ryder et al 2017). It is estimated to affect about 2,500 boys and men living in the United Kingdom with prevalence being reported as 19.5 cases per 100,000 (Mendell et al 2012, Moat et al 2013, Ryder et al 2017).

Presentation. Progressive muscle weakness starts in early childhood and leads to a significantly shortened life expectancy resulting from fatal respiratory complications or cardiac failure (Ryder et al 2017). Table 15.1 outlines motor function progression of the disease through life.

The disease severity at the time of transition to adult services varies greatly. Corticosteroid (CS)-naïve patients will have been wheelchair bound for several years and have profound muscle weakness, whereas those treated with CS will generally have preserved upper limb function, with a few transitioning still ambulant (Matthews et al 2016, McDonald et al 2018, Ricotti et al 2013).

Respiratory muscles are affected and involved in all disease stages. However, the weakness is never significant in ambulant individuals, whose forced vital capacity (FVC) remains above 70% of predicted value for age (normal values >80%).

Lung function progression can be divided into three stages. In the early years of life there is an improvement, which starts plateauing during early nonambulatory stage and begins to decline during late nonambulatory phase (LoMauro et al 2018, Trucco et al 2020). Table 15.2 outlines stages of pulmonary decline from the onset of respiratory decline to FVC below 1 litre.

The onset and rate of decline can vary depending on CS therapy with evidence showing higher peak pulmonary function, delayed onset of the respiratory decline and NIV requirements in long-term CS users (Butterfield et al 2022, Connolly et al 2016, Henricson et al 2013, LoMauro et al 2018,

TABLE 15.1 Characteristics of Different Stages of Progression in Duchenne Muscular Dystrophy Through Life (Emery et al 2015)

Disease Stage	Clinical Presentation
Onset in early childhood	• Commonly presenting with delay in walking at about 18 months of age • Increased falls • Tiptoe gait • Pseudohypertrophy of calf muscles • Inability to hop on one leg, run or jump properly • Waddling gait • Difficulty lifting head off the bed, rising from the floor and climbing stairs
Early stages	• Bilateral and symmetrical muscle weakness more prominent proximally than distally and in lower more than upper limbs manifesting as the classical Gower's manoeuvre – child using thighs to climb up to extend the hips and push up the trunk
As the disease advances	• Waddling gait becomes more prominent leading to the development of Achilles tendon contractures and eventually equinovarus deformity – more apparent when individuals become wheelchair bound • Activity limitation already occurs in the early ambulatory stage of DMD (Ricotti et al 2019)
Loss of ambulation (LOA)	• LOA on average by 12 years of age in CS-naïve boys (never had CS treatment) with DMD (Emery et al 2015, Ricotti et al 2013) • Introduction of CS therapy delays LOA to between 12.5 and 14 years (Ricotti et al 2013)
Later stages of the disease	• Development of upper limb (UL) and lower limb (LL) contractures • Development of talipes equinovarus deformity of the feet, which can cause pain and difficulties with wearing footwear • If wheelchair support is insufficient – an individual at risk of developing severe kyphoscoliosis posing serious problem by restricting pulmonary airflow to the compressed side • UL strength declines continuously, independent of the ambulatory status (significant loss can occur before LOA) • Pain and contractures limit function despite preserved strength

Mayer et al 2015, McDonald et al 2018). CS therapy is also associated with significant reduction in occurrence and severity of scoliosis (Alman et al 2004, Lebel et al 2013, Sussman et al 2020).

Cognitive. One-third of patients have cognitive impairments, including learning disability, autistic spectrum disorder, attention deficit/hyperactivity and emotional and behavioural problems (Emery et al 2015, Hoskin 2018).

Disease Course and Prognosis. The life expectancy of persons with DMD has increased significantly thanks to improvements in standards of care (SOC) (Birnkrant et al 2018). Subsequently, DMD has evolved from a paediatric disease to a chronic, severe, multisystem, adult condition.

Cardiac and respiratory failure are considered the main causes of mortality (Landfeldt et al 2020, Van Ruiten et al 2016) with cardiac disease being regarded currently as the major cause of death (Birnkrant & Carter 2021).

Assessment and Outcome Measures. Considering the progressive nature of DMD, the international SOC recommend 6-monthly, standardised, routine assessments to monitor disease progression and capture any changes over time to guide management (Birnkrant et al 2018a, 2018b).

Measurements of muscle strength and motor and pulmonary function are the main aspects of physiotherapy assessment of those with DMD. With improving survival and increasing number of clinical trials, there have been several disease-specific outcome measures (OMs) developed in the past 10 years (Table 15.3).

Adult DMD North Star Network (ANSN) is a network of specialists who look after adults with DMD within the

TABLE 15.2 Stages of Pulmonary Decline in People With Duchenne Muscular Dystrophy From the Onset of Respiratory Decline to Forced Vital Capacity < 1 Litre

Stages of Respiratory Function Decline	Clinical Presentation
Onset of pulmonary decline	• Associated with early stages of loss of ambulation (LOA) (LoMauro et al 2018, McDonald et al 2018) • Dyspnoea may not be evident as by the time of significant decline in lung function; individuals tend to be wheelchair bound with lesser physiological need
As DMD progresses	• Respiratory muscle weakness leads to ineffective cough and development of sleep-disordered breathing (SDB) (LoMauro et al 2018) • Lower diaphragmatic contribution to tidal volume gradually progressing into restrictive lung disease • Forced vital capacity (FVC)% predicted (FVC%p) ≤60% predicted for age is associated with impaired cough strength, impaired secretion clearance, atelectasis, recurrent respiratory infections and nocturnal and diurnal hypoventilation (LoMauro et al 2018)
Onset of respiratory failure	• Varies between FVC%p <50% and 35% • The first sign is the night-time hypoventilation (FVC < 50% increases risk of SDB) (LoMauro et al 2018) • The early respiratory failure phase can last several months and longer, until the symptoms of abnormal gas tensions start manifesting during the day • The survival prognosis becomes poor with average survival <9.7 months unless noninvasive ventilation (NIV) is initiated (Emery et al 2015, Rall & Grimm 2012)
FVC < 1 L	• Associated with higher risk mortality in DMD (Eagle et al 2002, LoMauro et al 2018, Mayer et al 2015, Sheehan et al 2018) • Median survival of 3.1 years (without intervention) and 5-year survival of only 8% • Individuals who reached FVC < 1 L are 4.1 times more likely to die (McDonald et al 2018)

United Kingdom. It was founded in 2017 to advance care of this patient population and to develop a prospective clinical database which includes a set of standardised OMs to be used with all patients across the United Kingdom.

Timed function tests like 10-metre walk, 6-minute walk and the timed raise from the floor from supine lying are more commonly performed with children. Muscle strength assessment is important to monitor pattern and progression of muscle weakness to guide therapy management. Joint range of motion (ROM) should be measured regularly to assess for contracture development (Table 15.4). Assessing spinal posture and positioning in wheelchair is important to ensure comfort and facilitate activities and participation.

Adults with DMD should be assessed at least annually for support and advice on ventilation and airway clearance to prevent and treat chest infections (Narayan et al 2022). FVC is considered the most important negative predictor of survival and is monitored annually in persons with DMD from the day of diagnosis (Table 15.5) (Eagle et al 2002, Maye et al 2015, LoMauro et al 2018, McDonald et al 2018, Sheehan et al 2018).

Medical Management. Currently there is no cure for DMD. ANSN recently published the *ANSN: Consensus Guideline for the Standard of Care of Adults With DMD* document outlining recommendations for medical care of this population (Quinlivan et al 2021).

CS therapy is started in most children to improve muscle strength and function and delay the loss of ambulation (LOA) (Matthews et al 2016, McDonald et al 2018). The CS benefits are internationally recognised (Matthews et al 2016), and the international

TABLE 15.3 Outcome Measures Currently Used to Monitor Disease and Measure Changes Over Time in People With Duchenne Muscular Dystrophy

Outcome Measure	Description
Functional performance and motor ability tests	
Brooke (Brooke et al 1981)	• Developed for DMD • Measure of upper limb function • Fast and easy to complete • Modified version is the entry item to the Performance of Upper Limb (PUL)
Vignos (Vignos et al 1963)	• Developed for DMD • Measure of lower limb function • Fast and easy to complete
North Star Ambulatory Assessment (NSAA) (Mayhew et al 2013a, 2020, Mazzone et al 2009, Ricotti et al 2013, Ridout et al 2016, Scott et al 2012)	• Developed for ambulant children with DMD • Includes 17 items • Validated and sensitive to change
Transition Assessment North Star Worksheet (TANS)	• Developed for DMD to use during transition from ambulant to nonambulant disease stage • Novel outcome measure, currently being validated • Includes items to capture transfer ability and trunk function
Performance of Upper Limb 2.0 (PUL 2.0) (Mayhew et al 2013b, 2020, Mazzone et al 2012, Pane et al 2018, Ricotti et al 2019)	• Developed for assessing upper limb function in ambulant and nonambulant people with DMD • 23 items (including entry item), structured for assessment of proximal to distal upper limb function
Patient-reported outcome measures (PROMs)	
DMD Functional Ability Self-Assessment Tool (DMDSAT) (Landfeldt et al 2015)	• Designed to measure functional ability in ambulant and nonambulant people with DMD • Also linked to cost of illness and health-related quality of life data, mapped well onto health economic outcomes • Includes 8 items in 4 domains: arm function, mobility, transfers and ventilation status
PROM for Upper Limb Function in Duchenne Muscular Dystrophy (DMD Upper Limb PROM) (Klingels et al 2017)	• Designed specifically for DMD to assess upper limb function • Applicable across a wide age range and in the different stages of the disease • Related to activities of daily living (ADLs) that cannot be observed in a clinical setting
Egen Klassifikation Scale Version 2 (EK2) (Steffensen et al 2001)	• Designed to measure functional ability in nonambulant DMD and spinal muscular atrophy (SMA) • Examines activities and abilities such as transfers, trunk mobility, wheelchair use, bed mobility, cough, well-being, feeding, bulbar issues and distal hand function • 17 items (15 self-reported, 2 observed items)
Quality of Life Measure for People With Slowly Progressive and Genetic Neuromuscular Disease (QoL-gNMD 1.0) (Dany et al 2015, 2017)	• Validated questionnaire to assess health-related quality of life (HRQL) in patients with slowly progressive NMD • Composed of 2 general items and 24 items classified in 3 domains: (1) impact of physical symptoms, (2) self-perception and (3) activities and social participation

TABLE 15.4   Specific Joints Commonly Measured in Adults With Duchenne Muscular Dystrophy

Body Part	Specific Area Commonly Measured in Adults With DMD
Lower limb	Ankle dorsiflexion
	Knee extension ambulant (supine with full knee extension)
	Knee extension nonambulant (sitting at 90° hip flexion)
	Hip extension (Thomas test)
	Iliotibial band (ITB)
Upper limb	Long finger flexors
	Wrist extension with fingers flexed
	Supination (with elbow flexed in 90°)
	Elbow extension
	Shoulder in flexion and abduction/scapular plane
Neck	Neck flexion
	Neck extension
	Neck rotation
	Neck side flexion

TABLE 15.5   Respiratory Assessment Items Included in the Adult North Star Respiratory Assessment Form for Duchenne Muscular Dystrophy

Respiratory assessment	• Number of respiratory infections • Symptoms of nocturnal hypoventilation or other sleep-disordered breathing (fatigue, dyspnoea, morning headache, excessive daytime sleepiness, frequent nocturnal awakenings or difficult arousal, difficulty concentrating, awakening with dyspnoea and tachycardia, frequent nightmares) • Presence of awake dyspnoea. • Experience coughing with/after food or drink • Pulmonary function testing (FVC, FVC% pred, PCF, PEF, SNIP) • Ventilation (night-time/daytime use [hours/day], compliance) • Secretion clearance techniques (breathing exercises [including breath stacking], LVR bags, MI:E [cough-assist machine], HFCWO [recruitment with Percussionaire/vest], suction, manual assisted cough, mucolytic, other)

FVC, Forced vital capacity; *FVC% pred*, percent predicted forced vital capacity; *HFCWO*, high-frequency chest wall oscillation; *LVR*, lung volume recruitment bag; *MI:E*, mechanical insufflation-exsufflation; *PCF*, peak cough flow; *PEF*, peak expiratory flow; *SNIP*, sniff nasal inspiratory pressure.

SOC recommend continuation of CS treatment in persons with DMD throughout life (Birnkrant et al 2018a, 2018b). However, use of CS in adults still varies because of complexity of the disease and relatively limited experience and expertise in the management of this group in later stages of the disease.

Additionally, in the United Kingdom, ataluren, which targets a specific type of mutation, is available to a small number of individuals with DMD.

Physical Management. Therapy for DMD starts immediately after the diagnosis is made and is critical for symptom management with the aim to improve function, participation and effectively quality of life (QoL).

Considering most people with DMD transition to adult services after ambulation is lost, upper limb function becomes essential to independence and QoL in a population that spends most of their lives wheelchair bound. Functional activities such as self-feeding or ability to perform transfers are clinically meaningful. Maintaining them or slowing the progression leading to their loss is crucial for ADLs and overall QoL of individuals with DMD.

Appropriate physical activities and management of joint ROM with stretching, orthotics, positioning, correct wheelchair setup and sleeping system for each individual are essential to promote function and participation, manage pain and maintain best possible QoL (Narayan et al 2022).

The role of physiotherapists in respiratory management of adults with DMD is to anticipate pulmonary decline by maximising ventilation and airway clearance to prevent chest infection, acute exacerbations and hospital admissions. Individuals should be reviewed at least annually, and carers should be trained in airway clearance techniques (e.g., assisted inspiration like breath stacking, operating manual assisted cough) (Chatwin & Simonds 2009, Hull et al 2012, Kravitz 2009).

The North Star Network therapists have recently published a detailed *ANSN Consensus Document for Therapists Working With Adults With DMD – Therapy Guidelines*, which aims to help guide therapists to best support adults living with DMD (Narayan et al 2022). This publication and a detailed manual were developed with a multidisciplinary team and holistic approach, written by UK neuromuscular specialist therapists working in UK Centres of Excellence for NMDs and rehabilitation therapists with a special interest in neuromuscular conditions. Specific sections on respiratory management, rehabilitation physiotherapy (including contracture management and wheelchair considerations), exercise therapy, occupational therapy and speech and language therapy (including assessment and management of oropharyngeal dysphagia) can be found in the manual. The document was published in conjunction with the *ANSN: Consensus Guideline for the Standard of Care of Adults With DMD* (Quinlivan et al 2021).

KEY POINTS

- Six-monthly, standardised, routine assessments to monitor disease progression and capture any changes over time to guide management are recommended for patients with Duchenne muscular dystrophy.
- Individualised physical activities and management of joint range of motion (with stretching, orthotics, positioning, correct wheelchair setup and sleeping system) are essential to improve function and increase participation, manage pain and maintain and improve best possible quality of life.
- Regular monitoring of respiratory function and cough strength are vital to anticipate deterioration and to prevent hospital admissions.

Facioscapulohumeral Muscular Dystrophy

Facioscapulohumeral muscular dystrophy (FSHD) is a muscle disease typically causing weakness of the muscles of the face, shoulder and legs. FSHD is caused by complex genetic changes that lead to abnormal production of the DUX4 protein with toxic effect on muscle cells. It is the third most common muscular dystrophy with a prevalence of nearly 1 per 15,000 (Flanigan et al 2001), but there is high clinical variability, with some people presenting very mildly, so this may be an underestimation (Deenen et al 2014).

FSHD is an autosomal dominant disease. Ninety-five percent of patients have mutation of the *D4Z4* gene causing abnormal production of the DUX4 protein with a toxic effect on muscle cells. This subtype is FSHD-1 with the remaining 5% of cases (FSHD-2) caused by a mutation in *SMCHD1* that leads to abnormal DUX4 production (Statland & Tawil 2016).

Presentation. Clinically, FSHD presents a broad variability even within the same family. The range of severity starts from asymptomatic individuals to severe infantile forms. In general, symptoms begin by the end of second decade, and typically affected individuals have asymmetric involvement of facial, shoulder and arm muscles followed by lower leg and hip girdle ('descending pattern') (Statland & Tawil 2014).

Disease Course and Prognosis. Usually people with the condition initially seek medical help when they notice difficulty in lifting their arms overhead because of weakness of scapular fixators. The disease is progressive, and approximately 20% of individuals become wheelchair dependent. Life expectancy is not reduced in most cases; however, disability caused by physical limitation is significant with negative effect on QoL (Statland & Tawil 2014). In addition to upper limb impairment, balance and gait are affected by involvement of the trunk and limb muscles (Horlings et al 2009), with foot drop commonly presenting. Facial weakness can affect expression, affecting communication, social participation and eating (Sezer et al 2021).

Assessment and Outcome Measures. The focus of functional assessment is upper limb range, scapular stability and gait performance. Upper limb function can be measured using scales such as the Performance of Upper Limb (PUL) (Gandolla et al 2020). There are also disease-specific OMs measuring wider presentation and function, such as the FSHD Clinical Score (Lamperti et al 2010) and the FSHD functional composite score (FSHD-COM) (Eichinger et al 2018).

Medical Management. There are currently no curative medical interventions, although therapeutics to target DUX4 protein expression are currently under trial, with promising early phase trials of losmapimod (Mellion et al 2021) that are moving to phase 3, investigating effectiveness.

Until efficacious therapies are adopted, interventions focus on symptom relief, for example, pain management. Scapular fixation is a surgical technique that can be used for some people with FSHD. The procedure fixes the scapula to the chest wall and is one option to improve upper limb function and manage shoulder pain for people with FSHD. Several case series have suggested that scapular fixation is safe and can be effective in increasing shoulder ROM (Demirhan et al 2009); however, anecdotally the results of this type of surgery are often mixed.

Physical Management. Exercise interventions are important for the management of people with FSHD. Strength and aerobic training are safe (Voet et al 2019), can reverse deconditioning and may affect longer-term outcomes. A small but interesting study explored the rate of change of fatty infiltration of the muscles over time using MRI. This is an indicator of primary muscle destruction and atrophy. They found a reduction in rate of fatty infiltration over 6 months in a group that exercised and a group that increased general physical activity compared with a no-exercise control group (Janssen et al 2016).

Orthotic management is an important consideration. For the lower limbs, ankle–foot orthoses (AFOs) can improve walking function (Aprile et al 2013, Eagle et al 2001). There have been small, uncontrolled studies of Lycra vests used to stabilise the scapulae and reduce pain (Drivsholm et al 2018).

KEY POINTS

- Facioscapulohumeral muscular dystrophy (FSHD) is an inherited disease resulting from a mutation causing production of the DUX4 protein. People with FSHD usually present first with weakness and wasting of the scapular muscles. The disease can then progress to the upper arms, axial muscles, proximal and distal lower limb muscles.
- Exercise is safe for people with FSHD, and there is some early evidence that it may slow progression.
- Scapular fixation surgery can aid upper limb function and shoulder supports may also assist function, but evidence is limited.
- Orthotic devices and walking aids are useful adjuncts to support independent mobility.

Limb Girdle Muscular Dystrophy

Limb girdle muscular dystrophy (LGMD) is a heterogeneous group of rare, inherited muscle diseases which present with progressive weakness affecting proximal muscles to a greater extent than distal muscles. The pelvic and shoulder girdle muscles are most affected, although one of the presenting features of LGMD is that individuals achieve independent walking ability (Walton & Nattrass 1954). The inheritance patterns are most commonly autosomal recessive, but dominant inheritance is also seen. There are numerous genetic mutations. Table 15.6 lists the most common genotypes, the protein involved and the original classification where LGMD1s are autosomal dominant and LGMD2s are autosomal recessive (Bushby 1995b). Therefore, for calpain the original classification was LGMD2A. However, a more recent classification has been created to accommodate a greater number of subtypes which defines dominant LGMD as 'D' and recessive as 'R' followed by a number which defines the order in which diseases were identified (Straub et al 2018). Therefore, for calpain the new classification is LGMDR1.

Table 15.6 also describes the common patterns of muscle weakness seen in the subtypes, the likelihood of cardiac and respiratory muscles also being involved, and notes other common presenting features. This table can assist clinicians with diagnosis. Age of onset for LGMD2 (R) is typically teenage years to early adulthood, although the sarcoglycanopathies are often present in childhood, and for LGMD1 (D) typically adulthood. For adults presenting phenotypically as LGMD a genetic diagnosis may not always be possible.

Disease Course and Prognosis. The disease course is variable but usually slowly progressive, although some individuals can have a severe and rapid deterioration of function. Ability to walk may or may not be lost over many years, and individuals often report periods of stability followed by points of progression which may be associated with significant events such as trauma or birth of a child. Figure 15.4 illustrates disease progression in relationship to mobility. More recently large natural history studies have described subtype progression in more detail (Jacobs et al 2021).

Assessment and Outcome Measures. Assessment should include surveillance of potentially affected systems, including musculoskeletal and respiratory function. Respiratory function can be monitored with a simple FVC, adding in a peak cough flow as a measure in individuals reporting difficulties with cough or secretion clearance. Cough can be monitored via patient-reported outcome measures (PROMs) such as the Egan Klassifikation Scale (EK2) (Steffensen et al 2001, 2002), which although not originally designed for use in LGMD has proved to be a useful and meaningful measure in nonambulant individuals with dysferlinopathy (Mayhew et al 2022). It also captures ability to use arms, eat, transfer and stand and is a valuable tool to identify areas in which a therapist can help an individual maintain function and independence.

The North Star Assessment for Limb Girdle Type Muscular Dystrophies (NSAD) is suitable for ambulant and nonambulant individuals with LGMD and covers many items which directly relate to ADLs (Jacobs et al 2021). Alongside these, PROMs such as the ACTIVLIM and Quality of Life measure for slowly progressive muscle disease (QOLgNMD) can capture ADLs in the home (Batcho et al 2016, Dany et al 2015, 2017). Assessment should include checking joint ranges with measurement of specific joints in which you may want to monitor intervention. Simple timed tests such as a 10-metre walk/run test or a Timed Up and Go test can also be a way to monitor progression and evaluate gait patterns (Dunaway et al 2014, Murphy et al 2019). Other symptoms may require more careful assessment such as pain, which can be common in LGMDR9 in particular (Richardson et al 2021).

Medical Management. Currently no drug treatments exist for LGMD although gene therapy is currently being investigated for this population (Bittel et al 2022, Potter et al 2018, 'Safety, β-sarcoglycan Expression, and Functional Outcomes from Systemic Gene Transfer of rAAVrh74.

MHCK7.SGCB in Limb Girdle Muscular Dystrophy Type 2E', MDA Clinical & Scientific Conference 2022, n.d.). Management is focused on multidisciplinary and symptomatic care. If cardiac issues are part of subtype presentation, cardiac monitoring is required and intervention may be appropriate. The use of CS is not usually indicated (Walter et al 2013).

Physical Management. Management aims to promote function and prolong independence as well as anticipate decline. It also aims to minimise secondary complications such as contractures and pain. As disease progresses it is key to ensure individuals stay active and can participate in family and social life as well as have good access to work and study environments. The role of a specially trained physiotherapist is vital to ensure the correct treatment for individuals with neuromuscular conditions, such as develop individually designed exercise and stretching programmes, identify and prescribe aids and equipment (e.g., orthoses, calipers, wheelchairs and standing frames), advise on moving and handling issues, monitor respiratory function and advise on techniques to assist with breathing exercises and methods of clearing secretions. Equipment and aids for the home are essential as the disease progresses and should be anticipated. It is not uncommon for a house move to be required to achieve accessibility as stairs become harder and more bathroom adaptations are required. Falls management is another key consideration and ensuring individuals have an emergency plan and the necessary equipment to get back up off the floor. Although currently no SOC exist for LGMD they are under development for some subtypes, and standards for other diseases such as DMD can be a useful starting point.

> **KEY POINTS**
>
> - Specific subtypes may need particular monitoring for respiratory and cardiac involvement or hand involvement (see Table 15.6).
> - Assessment should include measures of upper and lower limb functional ability because upper limb involvement does not necessarily present only after lower limbs are involved.
> - Anticipating issues based on stage of decline can help promote independence and maintain function.

Myotonic Dystrophy Type 1

Myotonic dystrophy type 1 (DM1) is the most common form of adult muscular dystrophy with a European prevalence of 3–15 per 100,000 (Turner & Hilton-Jones 2014); however, a recent study in the USA has suggested prevalence could be as much as 4.8 per 10,000 (Johnson et al 2021). It is an autosomal dominant inherited condition with multisystem involvement, namely, brain, heart, endocrine system, eyes and both small and skeletal muscle. There is currently no disease-modifying therapy available, and management is symptomatic.

DM1 is caused by an expansion of an unstable CTG trinucleotide repeat in the myotonic dystrophy protein kinase (DMPK) gene, located on chromosome 19. This gene codes for myosin kinase expressed in skeletal muscle. Unaffected individuals will have between 5 and 37 CTG repeats; anyone with 38–49 repeats is considered to have a 'premutation' allele but will not be symptomatic, and more than 50 repeats is nearly always associated with symptomatic disease. This is important because DM1 involves genetic anticipation, a phenomenon in which signs and symptoms become more severe and/or appear at an earlier age. This is because the DMPK alleles greater than 37 repeats are unstable and may expand in length during meiosis and mitosis, meaning children may inherit considerably longer repeats, increasing disease severity (Ashizawa et al 2000). The severity of anticipation is dependent on the size of the repeat and sex of the parent. Men and women are equally likely to pass on the gene to their children; however, an affected woman is more likely to have a severely affected child than a man (Whelan et al 2002).

Disease Course and Prognosis

DM1 is usually characterised by phenotype into adult onset, childhood onset and congenital(Table 15.7). In general, longer CTG repeats correlate with an earlier age of onset and more severe disease; this is more significant with repeats below 400 (Hamshere et al 1999). With more than 400 repeats the CGT length is mitotically unstable, leading to somatic mosaicism for the size of the expansion, meaning repeat length may be different in different tissues. In clinical practice CTG expansion is measured in the blood.

Muscle weakness occurs most frequently in facial muscles, sternocleidomastoid and distal muscles of the forearms, and ankle dorsiflexors. It can also be present in the quadriceps, respiratory muscles, pharyngeal muscles, tongue and extraocular muscles (Bouchard et al 2015). Movements showing the greatest rate of change in strength over a year are ankle dorsiflexion and pinch grip (Whittaker et al 2006). Myotonia, a slowed relaxation following a normal muscle contraction, is common. It is most prominent in the early stages of the disease and is seen most consistently in facial, jaw and intrinsic hand muscles (Logigian et al 2010). There is an increased risk of cardiomyopathy, conduction disorder and arrythmias in DM1. The risk of a cardiac condition disorder is 60 times greater than in the general population (Johnson et al 2015). Respiratory muscle weakness and decreased cough capacity are the main causes of morbidity

TABLE 15.6 Common Presenting Features for Common Limb Girdle Muscular Dystrophy Subtypes

Subtype	Thigh Muscle Involvement	Leg	Shoulder Girdle	Distal Upper Limb
LGMD2A/R1 calpain	Adductors/semi-membranosus Preserved sartorius and gracilis Posterior > anterior thigh involved	Tib ant, Gastrocs, soleus	Yes, winging	No
LGMD2B/R2 dysferlin	Adductors/hamstring Abductors well preserved Vastus involved	Gastrocs and soleus	Yes	Long finger flexors
LGMD2I/R9 FKRP	Hamstrings/adductors/ rec femoris/ quads	Calf hypertrophy but gastrocs preserved	Yes	No
LGMD2C/R5 2D/R3 2E/R4 2F/R6 Sarcoglycans	Thigh adductors, glutei and posterior thigh muscles	Relatively spared	Yes	No
LGMD2L/R12 ANO5	Hamstrings/adductors worse than anterior thigh	Posterior calf, possible hypertrophy	Mild involvement	No
LGMD1D/D1 DNAJB6	Variable Hamstrings > quads Rec fem and sartorius often preserved	Variable, medial gastrocs and soleus	Variable	No

Please note these are general subtype features and characteristics. Individual patients may present differently.
1/D, dominant; *2/R*, recessive; *LGMD*, limb girdle muscular dystrophy.
(Source: Bushby, 1995; Gorman Grainne et al ,2015; Kierkegaard et al, 2011a; Kierkegaard et al 2011b; Kierkegaard et al 2018; Kierkegaard and Tollbäck 2007; Mayhew et al 2013a; Mayhew et al 2013b; McFarland et al 2002; Ng et al 2021a; Ng et al 2021b; Ricotti et al 2016.)

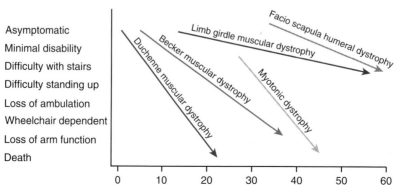

FIG. 15.4 Disease progression in relationship to mobility for muscular dystrophies. (Image courtesy of Anna Mayhew.)

Respiratory	Cardiac	Presents With Contractures	Pain As a Presenting Feature	Age of Onset	Other Features
Yes	No	Yes, calf and possibly elbow	No	Childhood/ teens	Lordosis, possible hypertrophy
No	No	No	Possible in calves	Late teens/ early 20s	Often sporty teenagers cannot stand on tip toes
Yes	Yes	No	Variable	Late teens, can be younger	High variability, jack-knife method for sit to stand
Yes	Yes	No	No	Childhood	Scoliosis and contractures possible Variability in presentation Childhood onset has rapid progression and similar to DMD
No	Yes	No	Exercise induced	Late onset in 30s but distal weakness can start earlier	Slowly progressive Can be asymmetrical
Variable	Variable	No	No	Often >40 years	

and mortality in those with DM1 (Hartog et al 2021). This is likely because of a combination of central dysfunction to respiratory drive, respiratory muscle weakness, notably the diaphragm, and upper airway and pharyngeal muscle dysfunction leading to increased risk of aspiration (Benditt & Boitano 2013, Hartog et al 2021). Executive, visuospatial, arithmetic, attention and speed dependent ability have all been shown to be reduced in patients with DM1 when compared with healthy control subjects (Winblad et al 2016). As the disease progresses issues with fluid intelligence (abilities to acquire new concepts and to adapt to unfamiliar situations) may manifest, alongside apathy and anosognosia (Winblad et al 2016). Gastrointestinal problems are

common with reduced peristalsis in the hypopharynx and proximal oesophagus leading to dysphagic symptoms. Reports of irritable bowel-type symptoms are also common, with 28% of patients reporting slow gastric emptying, 50% reporting diarrhoea and 30% reporting occasional faecal incontinence (Turner & Hilton-Jones 2014).

Assessment and Outcome Measures

Assessment should include a full social history to establish any functional areas of difficulty, including activity levels and exercise activities, and a strength assessment focusing on distal muscles of the forearm, ankles, neck flexors and orofacial muscles. A comprehensive assessment of balance

TABLE 15.7 **Phenotypical Characteristics of Myotonic Dystrophy (adapted from Turner & Hilton-Jones 2014)**

Phenotype	Clinical Signs	CTG Repeat Size	Age of Onset	Average Age of Death
Premutation	None	38–49	NA	NA
Mild, late onset, asymptomatic	Mild myotonia Cataracts	50–100	20–70	60–normal lifespan
Classic	Weakness Myotonia Cataracts Insulin insensitivity Conduction deficits Frontal balding Respiratory failure	50–1,000	10–30	48–60
Childhood onset	Facial weakness Myotonia Psychosocial problems Low IQ Conduction deficits	50–1,000	1–10	As above
Congenital	Infantile hypotonia Respiratory failure Learning disability Cardiorespiratory complications	>1,000	Birth	45

NA, Not applicable.

and gait should be undertaken focusing on dynamic balance but including static balance, and a detailed assessment of falls incidence and mechanism of falls (Hammeran et al 2015). Respiratory assessment is important for all patients because many have respiratory impairment despite being mobile. This should include FVC, sniff nasal inspiratory pressure (SNIP), peak cough flow (PCF) and a subjective assessment for signs of hypoventilation. It is important to consider the impact of dysphagia on risk of chest infections (Allen & O'Leary 2018). Because of apathy and cognitive impairments discussed earlier, these patients are often poor symptom reporters so this must be considered during assessment. Table 15.8 may support assessment.

Medical Management

Medical management consists of monitoring respiratory and cardiac function. There are currently no disease-modifying drugs and symptomatic management can be given pharmacologically. Respiratory failure can be managed with NIV and cough can be augmented with numerous devices including lung volume recruitment and manual insufflation-exsufflation (Chatwin et al 2018, Hartog et al 2021, Toussaint et al 2009).

Physical Management

Physiotherapy input should promote function and independence. Treatment and management should focus on the impairments seen on assessment. Cognitive changes described earlier mean there is a clear need for education on how impairments do and will affect them and how to manage risk. Treatments can include:

- Provision of orthotics for foot drop
- Provision of gait aids
- Education and advice about maintaining activity levels. Moderate- or low-intensity aerobic and resistance exercise is recommended and advice regarding reducing the amount of time sedentary (Gionola et al 2013, Duong and Eichinger 2020). It is important to note cardiac involvement in this condition which must be considered when prescribing exercise interventions
- Balance training programme focusing on balance impairments found in assessment (Hammeran et al 2015)
- Distal upper limb weakness and myotonia can affect function; therefore referral to occupational therapy and linking to adaptive equipment for upper limb function is important

TABLE 15.8 Recommended Assessment Procedures for Myotonic Dystrophy (Hammeran et al 2015, Jimenez-Moreno et al 2019, Wood et al 2018)

Muscle Function
Prioritise assessment of:
- Neck flexors
- Ankle dorsiflexors and plantar flexors
- Wrist flexors and extensors
- Hand grip (finger flexors)
- Knee extensors
- Proximal muscles less likely to be affected initially but likely to be more affected as the disease progresses
- Handheld dynamometry is preferred to manual muscle testing

Functional Assessments
- 10-metre walk test
- 9-hole peg test
- Sit to stand (30 s)
- Getting in/out of bed, especially lie to sit

Balance
- Dynamic tests better than static
- Step test
- 10-metre max/run
- Timed Up and Go

Respiratory
- Forced vital capacity
- Sniff inspiratory pressure
- Peak cough flow

KEY POINTS
- Symptoms can be variable. Distal muscle weakness tends to occur first affecting day-to-day functioning.
- Cognitive impairment is common and can affect management plans and should be considered.
- Physiotherapy input should be guided by problems identified on assessment and include respiratory monitoring.
- Activity, exercise, orthotics and adaptations can improve physical functioning and independence.

- Cough augmentation and chest management plan as indicated

Consensus-based care guidelines were published in 2018 which can support and guide assessment and management (Ashizawa et al 2018). They include monitoring guides for respiratory care presented in flowchart form and guide to physical management including exercise and adaptations (https://www.myotonic.org/sites/default/files/pages/files/MDF_Consensus-basedCareRecsAdultsDM1_1_21.pdf).

Spinal Muscular Atrophy

SMA is the most common disease of the spinal motor neurone occurring in 1 in approximately 10,000 births with a carrier frequency of 1 in 35–70 (Farrar et al 2013, Kolb & Kissel 2011, Sugarman et al 2012). SMA is an autosomal recessive condition caused in most cases by the homozygous deletion of the *SMN1* gene (Kolb & Kissel 2011). This causes a loss of motor neurones in the anterior horn of the spinal cord and results primarily in muscle weakness.

There are four types of *SMN1*-related SMA, with types 1, 2 and 3 manifesting during infancy/childhood, while type 4 onset is in adulthood (Mercuri et al 2012). Classification of SMA type depends on the age of onset and highest level of motor function achieved (Wang et al 2012), and severity, in some part, is influenced by the presence of a second similar protein, SMN2, and how many copies of this are also present (more copy numbers lead to a milder phenotype).

Presentation

SMA presents very differently depending on the severity of muscle weakness, which is its main symptom. Traditionally the disease was classified based on this severity:
- Type 1 – Those who never achieve sitting, presents at birth or soon after.
- Type 2 – Those who achieve sitting but never walk, usually presents by 18 months of age.
- Type 3 – Achieve walking, presents in childhood.
- Type 4 – Walkers with an adult presentation.

However, with treatments this classification may cease to be helpful, and a category based on current best function (e.g., nonsitter, sitter, walker) may be more appropriate. Weakness also occurs in the respiratory muscles with relative preservation of the diaphragm. This weakness affects motor function and can lead to a mixture of hypermobility and joint contractures, scoliosis, reduced lung volume and poor cough. There is also some autonomic involvement, especially evident in types 1 and 2, which can lead to hypersensitivity and excessive sweatiness. Table 15.9 outlines the key presenting features of the different types. Bear in mind that this classification is for a clinician's benefit and represents a continuum. Cognitive ability is not impaired in SMA.

TABLE 15.9	**Presenting Features of Spinal Muscular Atrophy**			
	SMA Type 1	**SMA Type 2**	**SMA Type 3**	**SMA Type 4**
Age of onset	Birth to 6 months	<18 months	>18 months	Adulthood
Highest function	Never sits unsupported	Never walks	Walks	Walks
SMN2 copy number	2	3–4	3–4	4 or more
Presenting features	Poor head control Profound weakness, froglike posture	Able to sit but will have lost this ability without treatment by adulthood Reduced trunk and arm function Complications of weakness and its impact on the skeleton leads to scoliosis and joint contractures	Able to walk in childhood but this may well have been lost by adulthood because of growth and progression May avoid significant scoliosis if they remain on their feet during puberty	May present as difficulty climbing stairs and with running in adulthood Gait abnormalities Proximal weakness greater than distal involvement
Respiratory features	Weak intercostal muscles, relative strong diaphragm, bell-shaped chest, paradoxical breathing Usually leads to early death by 2 years of age without treatment	Intercostal weakness and scoliosis cause restrictive lung disease	May have respiratory compromise in adulthood	Not usually
Additional features	Swallowing and feeding issues because of bulbar involvement Autonomic symptoms of sweatiness of hands and feet Tongue fasciculations	Swallowing may become an issue in adulthood; also autonomic related sweatiness and hypersensitivity particularly in the feet SMA tremor usually present (polyminimyoclonus) Jaw tightness possible (trismus)	May develop bulbar issues in adulthood Tremor may be present	Not usually

Disease Course and Prognosis

For those presenting in childhood, best function is often followed by deterioration, not necessarily because weakness progresses but because the muscle strength that is present needs to work over longer levers as a child grows. The impact of respiratory weakness also progresses and in the most severe type (type 1) used to be the main cause of death.

The good news is that this traditional presentation is now being altered by the advent of significant therapies that can alter the course of the disease (Ojala et al 2021), so much so that early treatment (especially in asymptomatic infants) can mean those who would never have sat, sit unaided and even walk. For this reason, it makes sense to define severity by current function with an expectation that new skills may be achieved or at least maintained for longer. For those receiving treatment as adults, therapies may slow the rate of decline or halt progression which is itself a significant gain for many of these individuals. The mechanism of action of these therapies may also affect strength and fatigue.

Assessment and Outcome Measures. Based on Table 15.9 one can identify the key needs of any assessment. Which assessments will depend on the age of the individual, and in adults this will include respiratory function (FVC and PCF), a measure of motor performance, assessing joint range given the significant presence of contractures and assessment of the spine given the high incidence of scoliosis.

Many measures of motor performance exist for SMA. Remember the key is to use the right one – one that is sensitive to change (and the patient does not reach a ceiling if they get stronger or reach a floor if they get weaker) and which captures function important to the individual. For adults who can sit, walk and have a high level of function, the Revised Hammersmith Scale (RHS) is recommended (Ramsey et al 2017). For those where arm function is key the revised upper limb module (RULM) can be implemented (Mazzone et al 2016) alongside the EK2 (Steffensen 2008, Werlauff & Fynbo Steffensen 2014). The 6-minute walk test can be considered for walkers and can also capture endurance based on comparisons of distance travelled in each minute (Dunaway Young et al 2016).

Medical Management

For many individuals, treatment is now becoming a reality with drug therapies targeting presentation of the SMN2 protein to promote muscle strength (Ojala et al 2021). Management consists of monitoring respiratory, cardiac and bulbar function and orthopaedic complications. Most orthopaedic surgeries will have taken place during childhood. NIV and cough assist devices can help manage reduced lung and cough function.

Physical Management

The aim is to promote function, mobility and independence. Exercise and activity are key to delivering this and SOC offer guidance to clinicians and individuals (Mercuri et al 2017, Wang et al 2007). Other key areas of management centre around managing joint contractures, and this can include stretches, orthotics and braces, although in adults orthotics are less commonly used because contractures often remain very stable. Seating and mobility devices including mobile arm supports can promote function in the nonambulant group. Specific stretching devices such as a jaw jack can assist those with jaw tightness (trismus). Exercise and activity play an important role in this group and should be promoted (Anziska & Inan 2014, Lewelt et al 2015, Voet et al 2019). It is important that activity is seen as exercise, especially in the nonambulant population, and should focus on aerobic and strengthening exercise at

> ### KEY POINTS
> - Measurement of function should be linked to an individual's current issues and concerns.
> - Respiratory function, motor performance, bulbar function and fatigue should all be evaluated, and the choice of measures will depend on the functional level of the individual.
> - Exercise can help to slow decline in muscle function, improve physical and mental well-being, and enhance quality of life.

a submaximal level as well as being tailored for individual muscle group strength.

Mitochondrial Diseases

Mitochondria are organelles within the cell whose primary role is the production of energy in the form of adenosine triphosphate (ATP) via the process of oxidative phosphorylation. Mitochondrial diseases (MD) are a group of neurometabolic disorders that affect the ability of mitochondria to produce energy with a prevalence estimated at 1 in 4,300 (Gorman et al 2015).

Subtypes of mitochondrial disease are classified based on the genetic defect or a recognised clinical syndrome. Mitochondrial disease can be a result of a mutation within the mitochondrial genome such as a point mutation (m.3243 A<G), a single large-scale deletion or nuclear gene defects such as *RRM2B* and *POLG*. Mitochondrial diseases can also be described as recognised syndromes such as Leigh syndrome and MELAS (mitochondrial encephalomyoathy, lactic acidosis and strokelike episodes), although most patients do not have a syndromic presentation (Gorman et al 2016, Ng et al 2021a).

The genetics and inheritance of these diseases are complex and can occur due to any pattern of inheritance owing to the involvement of two genomes, nuclear and mitochondrial DNA (mtDNA) (Fig. 15.5).

Presentation

Mitochondrial diseases can present at any age with a wide spectrum of symptoms that are variable in severity. Symptoms occur in multiple systems but are predominantly seen in tissues with a high-energy demand such as brain, heart and muscles (Fig. 15.6) (McFarland & Turnbull 2009).

Mitochondrial DNA disease presentation is not only dependent on the genotype but also on a threshold effect. All nucleated cells contain numerous mitochondria with multiple copies of mtDNA. Disease occurs when all copies of mtDNA are affected (homoplasmy) or when the

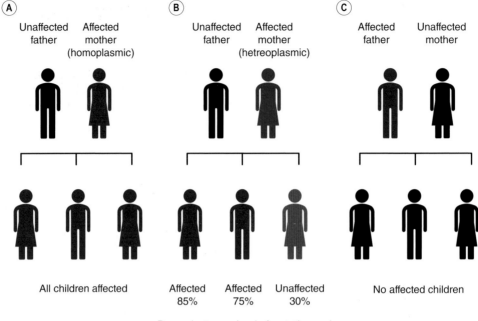

FIG. 15.5 Diagrammatic representation of the strict maternal inheritance of mitochondrial DNA disease. (Image courtesy of Jane Newman, created with Biorender.com.)

number of mutated versus wild-type mtDNA (heteroplasmy) exceeds a threshold, often between 60% and 80% (de Laat et al 2012, Shoffner et al 1990, White et al 1999) (Fig. 15.7).

Disease Course and Prognosis

The disease course and prognosis are difficult to predict and in part are dependent on the underlying genotype, disease onset and the extent of multisystem involvement. Children can present very early in life with severe neurodegenerative symptoms that fluctuate with high morbidity and mortality (Lake et al 2016, Lim et al 2022, Sofou et al 2014), whereas adult patients can present with slowly progressive symptoms such as eyelid ptosis, chronic progressive external ophthalmoplegia, sensorineural deafness, ataxia, neuropathy and myopathy. However, acute neurological presentation such as seizures and strokelike episodes (SLEs) can occur in any age group and are common in subgroups of adult mitochondrial disease and can progress to neurodegeneration with cognitive impairment (Lax et al 2017, Ng et al 2021b, McFarland 2002).

Assessment and Outcome Measures

A thorough musculoskeletal and neurological assessment is essential to identify all symptoms affecting function. Currently there are no validated outcomes specifically for mitochondrial disease. However, many routine timed tests have been used within research and have the potential to assess physiotherapy intervention such as timed tests (Koene et al 2018, Mancuso et al 2017, Newman et al 2015). Developments in the use of gait measurements (Galna et al 2013) and real world data via accelerometery (Apabhai et al 2011, Hickey et al 2016) may prove useful in the future.

Recommended outcomes were outlined in an international workshop report (Mancuso et al 2017) and are listed via Appendix 1 of physiotherapy guidelines at https://www.newcastle-mitochondria.com/wp-content/uploads/2019/09/Final-version-Mito-Physio-guidance-for-3-centre-website.pdf.

Medical Management. Currently there is no cure for mitochondrial disease with medical management being surveillance and supportive in nature (Pfeffer et al 2012). Numerous treatments are being researched to improve

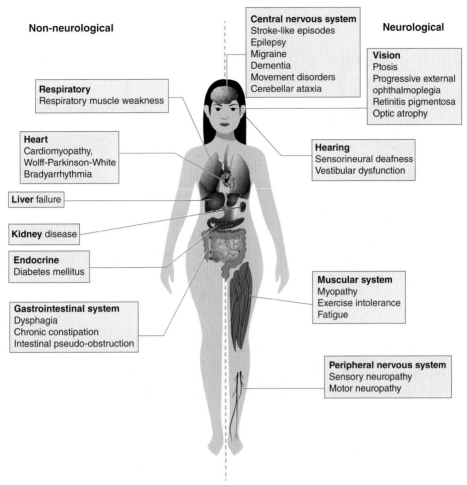

Non-neurological

Central nervous system
Stroke-like episodes
Epilepsy
Migraine
Dementia
Movement disorders
Cerebellar ataxia

Neurological

Vision
Ptosis
Progressive external
ophthalmoplegia
Retinitis pigmentosa
Optic atrophy

Respiratory
Respiratory muscle weakness

Heart
Cardiomyopathy,
Wolff-Parkinson-White
Bradyarrhythmia

Hearing
Sensorineural deafness
Vestibular dysfunction

Liver failure

Kidney disease

Endocrine
Diabetes mellitus

Muscular system
Myopathy
Exercise intolerance
Fatigue

Gastrointestinal system
Dysphagia
Chronic constipation
Intestinal pseudo-obstruction

Peripheral nervous system
Sensory neuropathy
Motor neuropathy

FIG. 15.6 Clinical presentations of mitochondrial disease. (Image courtesy of Jane Newman, created with Biorender.com.)

symptoms and provide reproductive options to reduce disease transmission (Craven et al 2017, Ng et al 2022).

Acute hospital admissions for adult patients occur for a variety of reasons such as seizures, confusion (encephalopathy), SLEs, aspiration pneumonia or intestinal pseudo-obstruction. For further information regarding medical management, see https://www.newcastle-mitochondria.com/clinical-professional-home-page/clinical-publications/clinical-guidelines.

An SLE is unlike a vascular stroke because it is not caused by a thrombosis of vascular territory and is driven by seizure activity (Ng et al 2019). Physiotherapy may need to be delayed because of medical intervention to reduce seizures.

Physical Management. Physiotherapy intervention can occur in a variety of medical locations from intensive care to outpatient and community settings. For further information, the authors refer the reader to https://mitochondrialdisease.nhs.uk/media//documents/final_version_mito_physio_guidance_for_3_centre_website.pdf.

Physiotherapy during an acute admission will likely be supportive in nature. During a metabolic crisis, excessive physical activity should be avoided and close liaison with medical staff is crucial to avoid further depletion of energy supplies.

Reasons for referral to physiotherapy are varied and include those described later in text.

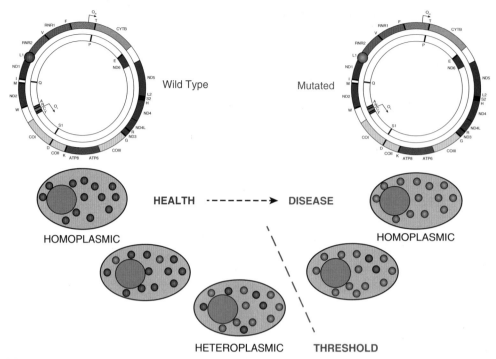

FIG. 15.7 Schematic diagram of the mtDNA within a cell. (Image courtesy of Professor R McFarland, Wellcome Centre for Mitochondrial Research, Newcastle University.)

TABLE 15.10   Key Points to Consider Before Prescribing Exercise to Patients With Mitochondrial Disease

- Cardiac function should be known before undertaking structured exercise.
- Severe muscle symptoms with increased heart rate at rest and symptoms of lactic acidaemia after low-intensity activities are rare.

In these cases, energy conservation may be required, and exercise undertaken with caution.

- Diabetes mellitus is a common feature in mtDNA disease (e.g., m.3243A>G) and should be monitored before and after exercise.
- A formal cardiopulmonary exercise test can help physiotherapists to understand the exercise limitations and be beneficial in guiding exercise prescription.

Exercise intolerance and muscle symptoms can result from primary disease and/or deconditioning because of reduced levels of activity (Apabhai et al 2011, Gorman et al 2015, Grady et al 2014). Exercise (aerobic and resistance) is safe and beneficial in enabling optimisation of aerobic capacity and muscle strength (Table 15.10) (Stefanetti et al 2020, Tarnopolsky 2014).

Fatigue is a common and complex symptom (Gorman et al 2015, Mancuso et al 2012). Physiotherapy input can include energy conservation, pacing, aids provision,

individualised exercise interventions and liaison with occupational therapists.

Respiratory muscles can be affected and NIV support may be required in severe cases (Lim et al 1993, Sahni & Wolfe 2018).

Numerous neurological symptoms can affect balance and can result in difficulties with mobility and result in falls (Fig. 15.6). A detailed assessment will determine the most relevant factors and therefore direct treatment. Intervention is dependent on

KEY POINTS

- Mitochondrial diseases are often multisystemic and can present at any age.
- Symptoms predominantly present in tissues with a high energy demand (such as brain, cardiac, muscle) and are variable in severity.
- Exercise is safe and beneficial for most people with mitochondrial disease although caution is advised for a small group of patients (e.g., high lactate levels at rest, cardiac involvement).
- Physiotherapy input should be guided by problems identified on assessment, not diagnosis.

the symptom, not the disease, and can include exercise, aid provision and splinting (Holmes et al 2019, Martikainen et al 2016, Ng et al 2021).

CASE STUDIES

Spinal Muscular Atrophy

Introduction: Barbara is a young 28-year-old woman who lives with her parents. She is employed in IT and works from home. She was diagnosed as a toddler with type 2 SMA with two copies of *SMN2* gene.

Because of her muscle weakness Barbara is fully dependent on a wheelchair and its support; however, she can sit independently for a few seconds on the edge of the bed at home and she practices this. Barbara remains in her wheelchair for most of the day, but she leads an active and motivated lifestyle. Her goal is to stand again in a standing frame, but at this moment she does not have the right equipment or enough support from her local therapy team. She does struggle with fatigue but manages it by pacing her activity. She enjoys eating, but it takes her a long time, and she needs some assistance. She uses a fork or a spoon with her elbow held up on a high table. She uses a cup with a long straw for drinking. Chewing is hard for Barbara, and she avoids certain foods because they are a choking hazard. She has reduced lung function and uses a cough assist device because of more frequent chest infections and is due to start using NIV soon. Barbara has over time developed joint contractures in her upper and lower limbs which she manages with regular stretching by family and carers. Her muscle weakness, growth and postural asymmetry led to scoliosis at an early age which was managed conservatively for many years before spinal surgery at age 12 years. She has recently started risdiplam therapy which aims to increase the expression of *SMN2* genes and thereby improve muscle function.

Assessment: When she attends clinic (every 6 months) the **EK2** helps assess both her arm function and how she

specifically feeds herself. It also captures her ability to manage different foods and whether she has difficulty swallowing and chewing. Joint ranges are reviewed before conducting functional scales. This allows us to ensure she has sufficient range for function as well as ensuring personal hygiene can be maintained. Some joints are measured to monitor change more accurately, but this is not necessary for all joint ranges. She has some jaw tightness (measures in millimetres with a Willis bite gauge). The **Adaptive Test for Neuromuscular Disorders (ATEND)** captures her motor performance because it is more appropriate for very weak adult individuals. Arm function is captured in more detail using the **RULM**. These tools help monitor the impact of drug therapy but importantly help identify areas in which we can help Barbara maintain and potentially improve function. The plan for her next clinic visit is to add an assessment of her sitting ability (using early items on RHS). This will require hoisting but could well be a step to assessing functional improvements on a therapy. Respiratory function is evaluated using **forced vital capacity, peak cough flow** and **overnight pulse oximetry** under supervision of the respiratory specialist team. Her wheelchair and equipment are also reviewed when she attends clinic, and she has a separate appointment for respiratory support and cough assist and ventilatory equipment. She is also asked to fill in some PROMs relating to bulbar function, fatigue and will be asked specifically about any other changes she has noticed since she was last seen in clinic.

Therapy: She manages her contractures with stretches from her family and carers and she uses a jaw jack to manage her jaw tightness which really helps. She also does muscle strengthening exercises using a light resistance band and practices sitting on the edge of her bed at home. She does some seated Pilates exercises which she was given some instruction on whilst in clinic alongside access to some online video material. She does not use any specific orthotics. We are working with local providers to see if a standing frame could be supplied to help her stretch, practice her motor skills as well as aid digestion and bone health.

Equipment: She has an electric wheelchair with tilt and recline, riser and tray and a profiling bed and specialist mattress for pressure. She has a ceiling tracking hoist and multiple home adaptations.

Key Messages:

- Functional outcome measures should be chosen based on the issues that the patient is having, and they should be appropriate to capture changes over time.
- Patients may have limited local support and should therefore be thoroughly instructed and supported at each clinic appointment; followups through phone or video calls should be considered.
- Adults with SMA may have different expectations of therapy and these should be carefully discussed.

Limb Girdle Muscular Dystrophy

Introduction: Sarah is 54 years old and she lives with her husband and two children. She is employed in management, working in a primarily desk-based role. She was diagnosed with LGMD2B/R2 when she was 25. Sarah lives in a typical two-storey terrace house with a single flight of stairs, and bedroom and bathroom located upstairs. Sarah attends clinic on a yearly basis. At her most recent clinic the main concern was a significant deterioration in mobility.

- Now walking only short distances with two elbow crutches
- Losing independence in ADLs: work, driving, mobility
- Struggling with prolonged writing
- Struggles to get out of a chair
- Increased falls
- Swims once a week, with family member to assist

Assessment: The North Star Assessment for limb girdle type muscular dystrophies (NSAD), PUL, ACTIVLIM patient report outcome measure, lower limb range of motion, visual gait analysis.

Respiratory function evaluated using FVC in sitting and supine and PCF.

Equipment needs: Sarah will require an electric wheelchair with seat riser to assist transfers and recline.

Seating and bed in the home need to be raised to assist transfers. Additional banister or possibly a stair lift. Onward referral to occupational therapist, wheelchair services and driving assessment centre.

As transfers become more difficult, a sit-to-stand transfer hoist could be used and has the option to be used as a standing frame for therapy.

Longer term, given the inability to adapt the current house, a move to a more suitable house with ground floor bedroom and bathroom, wheelchair-accessible entrance, bathroom with wash/dry toilet and either a roll-in shower/shower chair or hoist accessible bath.

Therapy option:

- Review provision of lower limb orthoses and mobility aides. If issues with foot clearance, see if providing orthotic at ankle may assist. Wheeled walker may be more suitable than crutches.
- Together with her family's assistance, routine use of the sit-to-stand hoist as a standing frame with the aim of providing weight-bearing exercise, reduce risk of contractures secondary to prolonged wheelchair use, and aid digestion.
- Ensure pool access is appropriate because walking into the pool may not be possible in the future.
- Create falls management plan because Sarah is unable to rise from floor independently. This could include removing trip hazards, introducing lifting cushion, having voice-activated options for calling for assistance.

Key Messages:

- The assessment of a patient with LGMD is guided by their current concerns and functional status: ambulant, transitioning or nonambulant. Appropriate outcome measures should be sensitive to change over time in this slowly deteriorating disease, and we are measuring to guide our clinical management.
- Clinic visits are the opportunity to monitor and address loss of function and prepare patients for their future with timely intervention. LOA and transition to wheelchair use are common in persons with these conditions and require significant time to prepare and adapt home, work and social environments.

SELF-ASSESSMENT QUESTIONS

1. How would you assess and manage jaw tightness in an adult with spinal muscular dystrophy?
2. What body systems may be involved in limb girdle muscular dystrophy?
3. What do you need to consider when advising exercise in myotonic dystrophy?
4. What pieces of information would you as a physiotherapist like to know before assessing a patient with mitochondrial disease?
5. What is the difference between primary muscle atrophy and secondary muscle atrophy in people with NMDs

REFERENCES

Ahmed, M., Machado, P.M., Miller, A., et al., 2016. Targeting protein homeostasis in sporadic inclusion body myositis. Sci. Transl. Med. 8, 331ra41.

Alemo Munters, L., Alexanderson, H., Crofford, L.J., Lundberg, I.E., 2014. New insights into the benefits of exercise for muscle health in patients with idiopathic inflammatory myositis. Curr. Rheumatol. Rep. 16, 429.

Alexanderson, H., Reed, A.M., Ytterberg, S.R., 2012. The Myositis Activities Profile -- initial validation for assessment of polymyositis/dermatomyositis in the USA. J. Rheumatol. 39, 2134–2141.

Alic, L., Griffin, J.F., Eresen, A., Kornegay, J.N., Ji, J.X., 2021. Using MRI to quantify skeletal muscle pathology in Duchenne muscular dystrophy: a systematic mapping review. Muscle Nerve. 64, 8–22.

Allen, J.E., O'Leary, E.L., 2018. Considerations for chest clearance and cough augmentation in severe bulbar dysfunction: a case study. Can. J. Respir. Ther. 54, 66.

Alman, B., Raza, S., Biggar, W., 2004. Steroid treatment and the development of scoliosis in males with Duchenne muscular dystrophy. J. Bone Joint Surg. 86, 519–524.

Anziska, Y., Inan, S., 2014. Exercise in neuromuscular disease. Semin. Neurol. 34, 542–556.

Apabhai, S., Gorman, G.S., Sutton, L., et al., 2011. Habitual physical activity in mitochondrial disease. PLoS One. 6, e22294.

Aprile, I., Bordieri, C., Gilardi, A., et al., 2013. Balance and walking involvement in facioscapulohumeral dystrophy: a pilot study on the effects of custom lower limb orthoses. Eur. J. Phys. Rehabil. Med. 49, 169–178.

Ashizawa, T., Gagnon, C., Groh, W.J., et al., 2018. Consensus-based care recommendations for adults with myotonic dystrophy type 1. Neurol. Clin. Pract. 8, 507–520.

Ashizawa, T., Gonzales, I., Ohsawa, N., et al., 2000. New nomenclature and DNA testing guidelines for myotonic dystrophy type 1 (DM1). Neurology., 54.

Bagnato, S., Ferraro, M., Boccagni, C., et al., 2021. COVID-19 neuromuscular involvement in post-acute rehabilitation. Brain Sci. 11, 1611.

Batcho, C.S., van den Bergh, P.Y., van Damme, P., et al., 2016. How robust is ACTIVLIM for the follow-up of activity limitations in patients with neuromuscular diseases? Neuromuscul. Disord. 26, 211–220.

Benditt, J.O., Boitano, L.J., 2013. Pulmonary issues in patients with chronic neuromuscular disease. Am J Resp Crit Care Med. 187, 1046–1055.

Bernhardt, K., Oh, T., Kaufman, K., 2011. Stance control orthosis trial in patients with inclusion body myositis. Prosthet. Orthot. Int. 35, 39–44.

Birnkrant, D.J., Bushby, K., Bann, C.M., et al., 2018a. Diagnosis and management of Duchenne muscular dystrophy, part 2: respiratory, cardiac, bone health, and orthopaedic management. Lancet Neurol. 17, 347–361.

Birnkrant, D.J., Bushby, K., Bann, C.M., et al., 2018b. Diagnosis and management of Duchenne muscular dystrophy, part 1: diagnosis, and neuromuscular, rehabilitation, endocrine, and gastrointestinal and nutritional management. Lancet Neurol. 17, 251–267.

Birnkrant, D.J., Carter, J.C., 2021. Cardiopulmonary phenotypic variability and discordance in Duchenne muscular dystrophy: implications for new therapies. Pediatr. Pulmonol. 56, 738–746.

Bittel, D.C., Sreetama, S.C., Chandra, G., et al., 2022. Secreted acid sphingomyelinase as a potential gene therapy for limb girdle muscular dystrophy 2B. J. Clin. Invest. 132, 1.

Bouchard, J.P., Cossette, L., Bassez, G., Puymirat, J., 2015. Natural history of skeletal muscle involvement in myotonic dystrophy type 1: a retrospective study in 204 cases. J. Neurol. 262, 285–293.

Brooke, M.H., Griggs, R.C., Mendell, J.R., et al., 1981. Clinical trial in Duchenne dystrophy. I. The design of the protocol. Muscle Nerve. 4, 186–197.

Bushby, K., Finkel, R., Birnkrant, D.J., et al., 2010. Diagnosis and management of Duchenne muscular dystrophy, part 1: diagnosis, and pharmacological and psychosocial management. Lancet Neurol. 9, 77–93.

Bushby, K.M.D., 1995. Diagnostic criteria for the limb-girdle muscular dystrophies: report of the ENMC Consortium on Limb-Girdle Dystrophies. Neuromuscul. Disord. 5, 71–74.

Busse, M., Ramdharry, G., 2020. Targeting sedentary behaviour in neurological disease. Pract. Neurol. 20, 187–188.

Butterfield, R.J., Kirkov, S., Conway, K.M., et al., 2022. Evaluation of effects of continued corticosteroid treatment on cardiac and pulmonary function in non-ambulatory males with Duchenne muscular dystrophy from MD STARnet. Muscle Nerve. 66, 15–23.

Cabañes-Martínez, L., Villadóniga, M., González-Rodríguez, L., et al., 2020. Neuromuscular involvement in COVID-19 critically ill patients. Clin. Neurophysiol. 131, 2809–2816.

Chatwin, M., Simonds, A.K., 2009. The addition of mechanical insufflation/exsufflation shortens airway-clearance sessions in neuromuscular patients with chest infection. Respir. Care. 54, 1473–1479.

Chatwin, M., Toussaint, M., Gonçalves, M.R., et al., 2018. Airway clearance techniques in neuromuscular disorders: a state of the art review. Respir. Med. 136, 98–110.

Connolly, A.M., Florence, J.M., Zaidman, C.M., et al., 2016. Clinical trial readiness in non-ambulatory boys and men with duchenne muscular dystrophy: MDA-DMD network follow-up. Muscle Nerve. 54, 681–689.

Craven, L., Tang, M.-X., Gorman, G.S., et al., 2017. Novel reproductive technologies to prevent mitochondrial disease. Hum. Reprod. Update. 23, 501–519.

Dalakas, M.C., 2020. Inflammatory myopathies: update on diagnosis, pathogenesis and therapies, and COVID-19-related implications. Acta Myol. 39, 289–301.

Dany, A., Barbe, C., Rapin, A., et al., 2015. Construction of a Quality of Life Questionnaire for slowly progressive neuromuscular disease. Qual. Life Res. 24, 2615–2623.

Dany, A., Rapin, A., Lavrard, B., et al., 2017. The quality of life in genetic neuromuscular disease questionnaire: Rasch validation of the French version. Muscle Nerve. 56, 1085–1091.

Dany, A., Rapin, A., Réveillère, C., et al., 2017. Exploring quality of life in people with slowly-progressive neuromuscular disease. Disabil. Rehabil. 39, 1262–1270.

Deenen, J.C.W., Arnts, H., Van Der Maarel, S.M., et al., 2014. Population-based incidence and prevalence of facioscapulohumeral dystrophy. Neurology. 83, 1056–1059.

de Laat, P., Koene, S., van den Heuvel, L.P.W.J., et al., 2012. Clinical features and heteroplasmy in blood, urine and saliva in 34 Dutch families carrying the m.3243A > G mutation. J. Inherited Metab. Dis. 35, 1059–1069.

Demirhan, M., Uysal, O., Atalar, A.C., et al., 2009. Scapulothoracic arthrodesis in facioscapulohumeral dystrophy with multifilament cable. Clin. Orthop. Relat. Res. 467, 2090–2097.

Drivsholm, P., Busk, L., Nybro, T., Werlauff, U., 2018. Evaluation of dynamic movement orthoses (DMO) as a means to relieve pain and fatigue in patients with facio-scapulo-humeral muscular dystrophy. Neuromuscul. Disord. 28, S138.

Dunaway, S., Montes, J., Garber, C.E., et al., 2014. Performance of the timed "up & go" test in spinal muscular atrophy. Muscle Nerve. 50, 273–277.

Dunaway Young, S., Montes, J., Kramer, S.S., et al., 2016. Six-minute walk test is reliable and valid in spinal muscular atrophy. Muscle Nerve. 54, 836–842.

Duong, T., Eichinger, K., 2020. Role of physical therapy in the assessment and management of individuals with myotonic dystrophy. Myotonic Dystrophy Foundation. Available on MDF_RoleofPhysicalTherapy_1_21.pdf (myotonic.org). Accessed on 25 July 2023.

Eagle, M., Baudouin, S., Chandler, C., et al., 2002. Survival in Duchenne muscular dystrophy: improvements in life expectancy since 1967 and the impact of home nocturnal ventilation. Neuromusc. Dis. 12, 926–929.

Eagle, M., Peacock, C., Bushby, K., Major, R., 2001. Facioscapulohumeral muscular dystrophy: gait analysis and effectiveness of ankle foot orthoses (AFOs). Neuromuscul. Disord. 11, 631.

Eichinger, K., Heatwole, C., Iyadurai, S., et al., 2018. Facioscapulohumeral muscular dystrophy functional composite outcome measure. Muscle Nerve. 58, 72–78.

Emery, A.E.H., Muntoni, F., Quinlivan, R.C.M., 2015. Duchenne muscular dystrophy. 4th ed. Oxford University Press.

Farrar, M.A., Vucic, S., Johnston, H.M., et al., 2013. Pathophysiological insights derived by natural history and motor function of spinal muscular atrophy. J. Pediatr. 162, 155–159.

Flanigan, K.M., Coffeen, C.M., Sexton, L., et al., 2001. Genetic characterization of a large, historically significant Utah kindred with facioscapulohumeral dystrophy. Neuromusc. Disord. 11, 525–529.

Galna, B., Newman, J., Jakovljevic, D., et al., 2013. Discrete gait characteristics are associated with m.3243A>G and m.8344A>G variants of mitochondrial disease and its pathological consequences. J. Neurol. 1–10.

Gandolla, M., Antonietti, A., Longatelli, V., et al., 2020. Test-retest reliability of the Performance of Upper Limb (PUL) module for muscular dystrophy patients. PloS One. 15, e0239064.

Gianola, S., Pecoraro, V., Lambiase, S., et al., 2013. Efficacy of muscle exercise in patients with muscular dystrophy: a systematic review showing a missed opportunity to improve outcomes. PLoS One. 8, e65414.

Gorman Grainne, S., Blakely, E.L., Hornig-Do, H.-T., et al., 2015. Novel MTND1 mutations cause isolated exercise intolerance, complex I deficiency and increased assembly factor expression. Clin. Sci. 128, 895–904.

Gorman, G.S., Chinnery, P.F., DiMauro, S., et al., 2016. Mitochondrial diseases. Nat. Rev. Dis. Prim. 2, 16080.

Gorman, G.S., Elson, J.L., Newman, J., et al., 2015. Perceived fatigue is highly prevalent and debilitating in patients with mitochondrial disease. Neuromusc. Disord. 25, 563–566.

Gorman, G.S., Schaefer, A.M., Ng, Y., et al., 2015. Prevalence of nuclear and mitochondrial DNA mutations related to adult mitochondrial disease. Ann. Neurol. 77, 753–759.

Grady, J.P., Campbell, G., Ratnaike, T., et al., 2014. Disease progression in patients with single, large-scale mitochondrial DNA deletions. Brain. 137, 323–334.

Hammarén, E., Kjellby-Wendt, G., Lindberg, C., 2015. Muscle force, balance and falls in muscular impaired individuals with myotonic dystrophy type 1: a five-year prospective cohort study. Neuromusc. Disord. 25, 141–148.

Hamshere, M.G., Harley, H., Harper, P., et al., 1999. Myotonic dystrophy: the correlation of (CTG) repeat length in leucocytes with age at onset is significant only for patients with small expansions. J. Med. Genet. 36, 59–61.

Hartog, L., Zhao, J., Reynolds, J., et al., 2021. Factors influencing the severity and progression of respiratory muscle dysfunction in myotonic dystrophy type 1. Front. Neurol. 12, 658532.

Henricson, E.K., Abresch, R.T., Cnaan, A., et al., 2013. The cooperative international neuromuscular research group Duchenne natural history study: glucocorticoid treatment preserves clinically meaningful functional milestones and reduces rate of disease progression as measured by manual muscle testing and other commonly used clinical trial outcome measures. Muscle Nerve. 48, 55–67.

Hickey, A., Gunn, E., Alcock, L., et al., 2016. Validity of a wearable accelerometer to quantify gait in spinocerebellar ataxia type 6. Physiol. Meas. 37, N105–N117.

Holmes, S., Male, A.J., Ramdharry, G., et al., 2019. Vestibular dysfunction: a frequent problem for adults with mitochondrial disease. J. Neurol. Neurosurg. Psychiatry. 90, 838–841.

Horlings, C.G.C., Munneke, M., Bickerstaffe, A., et al., 2009. Epidemiology and pathophysiology of falls in facioscapulohumeral disease. J. Neurol. Neurosurg. Psychiatry. 80, 1357–1363.

Hoskin, J., 2018. A Guide to Duchenne Muscular Dystrophy: Information and Advice for Teachers and Parents. Jessica Kingsley Publishers, London and Philadelphia.

Hull, J., Aniapravan, R., Chan, E., et al., 2012. British Thoracic Society guideline for respiratory management of children with neuromuscular weakness. Thorax. 67 (Suppl. 1), i1–40.

Isenberg, D.A., Allen, E., Farewell, V., et al., 2004. International consensus outcome measures for patients with idiopathic inflammatory myopathies. Development and initial validation of myositis activity and damage indices in patients with adult onset disease International Myositis and Clinical Studies Group (IMACS). Rheumatology. 43, 49–54.

Jackson, C.E., Barohn, R.J., Gronseth, G., et al., 2008. Inclusion body myositis functional rating scale: a reliable and valid measure of disease severity Muscle Study Group. Muscle Nerve. 37, 473–476.

Jacobs, M.B., James, M.K., Lowes, L.P., et al., 2021. Assessing dysferlinopathy patients over three years with a new motor scale. Ann. Neurol. 89, 967–978.

Janssen, B., Voet, N., Geurts, A., et al., 2016. Quantitative MRI reveals decelerated fatty infiltration in muscles of active FSHD patients. Neurology. 86, 1700–1707.

Jimenez-Moreno, A.C., Nikolenko, N., Kierkegaard, M., et al., 2019. Analysis of the functional capacity outcome measures for myotonic dystrophy. Ann. Clin. Transl. Neurol. 6, 1487–1497.

Johnson, N.E., Butterfield, R.J., Mayne, K., et al., 2021. Population-based prevalence of myotonic dystrophy type 1 using genetic analysis of statewide blood screening program. Neurology. 96, e1045–e1053.

Jones, K., Hawke, F., Newman, J., et al., 2021. Interventions for promoting physical activity in people with neuromuscular disease. Cochrane Database Syst. Rev. 5, CD013544

Kierkegaard, M., Harms-Ringdahl, K., Edström, L., et al., 2011a. Feasibility and effects of a physical exercise programme in adults with myotonic dystrophy type 1: a randomized controlled pilot study. J. Rehabil. Med. 43 , 695–702.

Kierkegaard, M., Harms-Ringdahl, K., Holmqvist, L.W., Tollbck, A., 2011b. Functioning and disability in adults with myotonic dystrophy type 1. Disabil. Rehabil. 33, 1826–1836.

Kierkegaard, M., Petitclerc, É., Hébert, L.J., et al., 2018. Responsiveness of performance-based outcome measures for mobility, balance, muscle strength and manual dexterity in adults with myotonic dystrophy type 1. J. Rehabil. Med. 50, 269–277.

Kierkegaard, M., Tollbäck, A., 2007. Reliability and feasibility of the six-minute walk test in subjects with myotonic dystrophy. Neuromusc. Disord. 17, 943–949.

Klingels, K., Mayhew, A.G., Mazzone, E.S., et al., 2017. Development of a patient-reported outcome measure for upper limb function in Duchenne muscular dystrophy: DMD Upper Limb PROM. Dev. Med. Child Neurol. 59, 224–231.

Koene, S., van Bon, L., Bertini, E., et al., 2018. Outcome measures for children with mitochondrial disease: consensus recommendations for future studies from a Delphi-based international workshop. J. Inherit. Metab. Dis. 41, 1267–1273.

Kolb, S.J., Kissel, J.T., 2011. Spinal muscular atrophy: a timely review. Arch. Neurol. 68, 979–984.

Kravitz, R.M., 2009. Airway clearance in Duchenne muscular dystrophy. Pediatrics. 123, S231–S235.

Lake, N.J., Compton, A.G., Rahman, S., Thorburn, D.R., 2016. Leigh syndrome: one disorder, more than 75 monogenic causes. Ann. Neurol. 79, 190–203.

Lamperti, C., Fabbri, G., Vercelli, L., et al., 2010. A standardized clinical evaluation of patients affected by facioscapulohumeral muscular dystrophy: the FSHD clinical score. Muscle Nerve. 42, 213–217.

Landfeldt, E., Mayhew, A., Eagle, M., et al., 2015. Development and psychometric analysis of the Duchenne muscular dystrophy Functional Ability Self-Assessment Tool (DMDSAT). Neuromuscul. Disord. 25, 937–944.

Landfeldt, E., Thompson, R., Sejersen, T., et al., 2020. Life expectancy at birth in Duchenne muscular dystrophy: a systematic review and meta-analysis. Eur. J. Epidemiol. 35, 643–653.

Landon-Cardinal, O., Bachasson, D., Guillaume-Jugnot, P., et al., 2020. Relationship between change in physical activity and in clinical status in patients with idiopathic inflammatory myopathy: a prospective cohort study. Semin. Arthritis Rheum. 50, 1140–1149.

Lax, N.Z., Gorman, G.S., Turnbull, D.M., 2017. Review: central nervous system involvement in mitochondrial disease. Neuropathol. Appl. Neurobiol. 43, 102–118.

Lazarou, I.N., Guerne, P.-A., 2013. Classification, diagnosis, and management of idiopathic inflammatory myopathies. J. Rheumatol. 40, 550–564.

Lebel, D.E., Corston, J.A., McAdam, L.C., et al., 2013. Glucocorticoid treatment for the prevention of scoliosis in children with Duchenne muscular dystrophy: long-term follow-up. J. Bone Joint Surg. Am. 95, 1057–1061.

Lewelt, A., Krosschell, K.J., Stoddard, G.J., et al., 2015. Resistance strength training exercise in children with spinal muscular atrophy. Muscle Nerve 52, 559–567.

Lim, A.Z., McFarland, R., Taylor, R.W., et al., 1993. RRM2B mitochondrial DNA maintenance defects. In: Adam, M.P., Ardinger, H.H., Pagon, R.A. (Eds.), GeneReviews(*). University of Washington, SeattleCopyright ©, Seattle (WA), pp. 1993–2022. University of Washington, Seattle. GeneReviews is a registered trademark of the University of Washington, Seattle. All rights reserved

Lim, A.Z., Ng, Y.S., Blain, A., et al., 2022. Natural history of Leigh syndrome: a study of disease burden and progression. Ann. Neurol. 91, 117–130.

Logigian, E.L., Martens, W.B., Moxley, R.T., et al., 2010. Mexiletine is an effective antimyotonia treatment in myotonic dystrophy type 1. Neurology. 74, 1441–1448.

LoMauro, A., Romei, M., Gandossini, S., et al., 2018. Evolution of respiratory function in Duchenne muscular dystrophy from childhood to adulthood. Eur. Respir. J. 51.

Mah, J.K., Korngut, L., Dykeman, J., et al., 2014. A systematic review and meta-analysis on the epidemiology of Duchenne and Becker muscular dystrophy. Neuromuscul. Disord. 24, 482–491.

Mancuso, M., Angelini, C., Bertini, E., et al., 2012. Fatigue and exercise intolerance in mitochondrial diseases. Literature revision and experience of the Italian Network of mitochondrial diseases. Neuromusc. Disord. 22 (Suppl. 3), S226–S229.

Mancuso, M., McFarland, R., Klopstock, T., Hirano, M., 2017. International workshop: outcome measures and clinical trial readiness in primary mitochondrial myopathies in children and adults. Consensus recommendations. 16–18 November 2016, Rome, Italy. Neuromusc. Disord. 27, 1126–1137.

Martikainen, M.H., Ng, Y., Gorman, G.S., et al., 2016. Clinical, genetic, and radiological features of extrapyramidal movement disorders in mitochondrial disease. JAMA Neurol. 73, 668–674.

Mary, P., Servais, L., Vialle, R., 2018. Neuromuscular diseases: diagnosis and management. Orthop. Traumatol. Surg. Res. 104, S89–S95.

Matthews, E., Brassington, R., Kuntzer, T., et al., 2016. Corticosteroids for the treatment of Duchenne muscular dystrophy. Cochrane Database Syst. Rev. 5, CD003725

Mayer, O.H., Finkel, R.S., Rummey, C., et al., 2015. Characterization of pulmonary function in Duchenne muscular dystrophy. Pediatr. Pulmonol. 50, 487–494.

Mayhew, A.G., Cano, S.J., Scott, E., et al., 2013a. Detecting meaningful change using the North Star Ambulatory Assessment in Duchenne muscular dystrophy. Dev. Med. Child Neurol. 55, 1046–1052.

Mayhew, A.G., Coratti, G., Mazzone, E.S., et al., 2020. Performance of upper limb module for Duchenne muscular dystrophy. Dev. Med. Child Neurol. 62, 633–639.

Mayhew, A.G., James, M.K., Moore, U., et al., 2022. Assessing the relationship of patient reported outcome measures with functional status in dysferlinopathy: a Rasch analysis approach. Front. Neurol. 13, 828525.

Mayhew, A., Mazzone, E.S., Eagle, M., et al., 2013b. Development of the Performance of the Upper Limb module for Duchenne muscular dystrophy. Dev. Med. Child Neurol. 55, 1038–1045.

Mazzone, E.S., Mayhew, A., Montes, 2016. Revised upper limb module for spinal muscular atrophy: development of a new module. Muscle Nerve. 55, 869–874.

Mazzone, E.S., Messina, S., Vasco, G., et al., 2009. Reliability of the North Star Ambulatory Assessment in a multicentric setting. Neuromuscul. Disord. 19, 458–461.

Mazzone, E.S., Vasco, G., Palermo, C., et al., 2012. A critical review of functional assessment tools for upper limbs in Duchenne muscular dystrophy. Dev. Med. Child Neurol. 54, 879–885.

McDonald, C.M., Gordish-Dressman, H., Henricson, E.K., et al., 2018. Longitudinal pulmonary function testing outcome measures in Duchenne muscular dystrophy: long-term natural history with and without glucocorticoids. Neuromuscul. Disord. 28, 897–909.

McDonald, C.M., Henricson, E.K., Abresch, R.T., et al., 2018. Long-term effects of glucocorticoids on function, quality of life, and survival in patients with Duchenne muscular dystrophy: a prospective cohort study. Lancet. 391, 451–461.

McFarland, R., Taylor, R.W., Turnbull, D.M., 2002. A neurological perspective on mitochondrial disease. Lancet Neurol. 9, 829–840.

McFarland, R., Turnbull, D.M., 2009. Batteries not included: diagnosis and management of mitochondrial disease. J. Intern. Med. 265, 210–228.

Mellion, M.L., Ronco, L., Berends, C.L., et al., 2021. Phase 1 clinical trial of losmapimod in facioscapulohumeral dystrophy: safety, tolerability, pharmacokinetics, and target engagement. Br. J. Clin. Pharmacol. 87, 4658–4669.

Mendell, J.R., Shilling, C., Leslie, N.D., et al., 2012. Evidence-based path to newborn screening for Duchenne muscular dystrophy. Ann. Neurol. 71, 304–313.

Mercuri, E., Bertini, E., Iannaccone, S.T., 2012. Childhood spinal muscular atrophy: controversies and challenges. Lancet Neurol. 11, 443–452.

Mercuri, E., Finkel, R.S., Muntoni, F., et al., 2017. Diagnosis and management of spinal muscular atrophy: part 1: recommendations for diagnosis, rehabilitation, orthopedic and nutritional care. Neuromusc. Disord. 28, 103–115.

Moat, S.J., Bradley, D.M., Salmon, R., et al., 2013. Newborn bloodspot screening for Duchenne muscular dystrophy: 21 years experience in Wales (UK). Eur. J. Hum. Genet. 21, 1049–1053.

Morrow, J.M., Sinclair, C.D.J., Fischmann, A., et al., 2015. MRI biomarker assessment of neuromuscular disease progression: a prospective observational cohort study. Lancet Neurol. 15, 65–77.

Mukund, K., Subramaniam, S., 2020. Skeletal muscle: a review of molecular structure and function, in health and disease. Wiley Interdisciplinary Reviews. Syst. Biol. Med. 12, e1462.

Mul, K., Vincenten, S.C.C., Voermans, N.C., et al., 2017. Adding quantitative muscle MRI to the FSHD clinical trial toolbox. Neurology. 89, 2057.

Murphy, A.P., Morrow, J., Dahlqvist, J.R., et al., 2019. Natural history of limb girdle muscular dystrophy R9 over 6 years: searching for trial endpoints. Ann. Clin. Transl. Neurol. 6, 1033–1045.

Narayan, S., Pietrusz, A., Allen, J., et al., 2022. Adult North Star Network (ANSN): Consensus Document for Therapists Working with Adults with Duchenne Muscular Dystrophy (DMD) – Therapy Guidelines. J Neuromuscul Dis. 9, 365–381.

Newman, J., Galna, B., Jakovljevic, D.G., et al., 2015. Preliminary evaluation of clinician rated outcome measures in mitochondrial disease. J. Neuromusc. Dis. 2, 157–165.

Ng, Y.S., Bindoff, L.A., Gorman, G.S., et al., 2019. Consensus-based statements for the management of mitochondrial stroke-like episodes. Wellcome Open Res. 4.

Ng, Y.S., Bindoff, L.A., Gorman, G.S., et al., 2021a. Mitochondrial disease in adults: recent advances and future promise. Lancet Neurol. 20, 573–584.

Ng, Y.S., Lax, N.Z., Blain, A.P., et al., 2022. Forecasting stroke-like episodes and outcomes in mitochondrial disease. Brain. 145, 542–554.

Ng, Y.S., Lim, A.Z., Panagiotou, G., et al., 2021b. Endocrine manifestations and new developments in mitochondrial disease. Endocrine Rev. 43, 583–609.

Nigro, V., Piluso, G., 2015. Spectrum of muscular dystrophies associated with sarcolemmal-protein genetic defects. Biochim. Biophys. Acta. 1852, 585.

Ojala, K.S., Reedich, E.J., Didonato, C.J., Meriney, S.D., 2021. In search of a cure: the development of therapeutics to alter the progression of spinal muscular atrophy. Brain Sci. 11, 1–39.

Pane, M., Coratti, G., Brogna, C., et al., 2018. Upper limb function in Duchenne muscular dystrophy: 24 month longitudinal data. PLoS One. 13, e0199223.

Pfeffer, G., Majamaa, K., Turnbull, D.M., et al., 2012. Treatment for mitochondrial disorders. Cochrane Database Syst. Rev., 4.

Pinto, A.J., Yazigi Solis, M., de Sá Pinto, 2016. Physical (in)activity and its influence on disease-related features, physical capacity, and health-related quality of life in a cohort of chronic juvenile dermatomyositis patients. Semin. Arth. Rheum. 46, 64–70.

Postges, H., Jones, F., Lee, L., et al., 2020. Neuro-muscular bridges: outcome of the development phase of a self-management programme for people with neuromuscular diseases. J. Peripheral Nerv. Syst. 554.

Potter, R.A., Griffin, D.A., Sondergaard, P.C., et al., 2018. Systemic delivery of dysferlin overlap vectors provides long-term gene expression and functional improvement for dysferlinopathy. Hum. Gene Ther. 29, 749.

Qi, J., Olsen, N.J., Price, R.R., et al., 2008. Diffusion-weighted imaging of inflammatory myopathies: polymyositis and dermatomyositis. J. Magn. Reson. Imag. 27, 212–217.

Quinlivan, R., Messer, B., Murphy, P., et al., 2021. Adult North Star Network (ANSN): Consensus Guideline for the Standard of Care of Adults With Duchenne Muscular Dystrophy. J. Neuromuscul. Dis. 8, 899–926.

Rall, S., Grimm, T., 2012. Survival in Duchenne muscular dystrophy. Acta Myol. 31, 117–120.

Ramdharry, G., Morrow, J., Hudgens, S., et al., 2019. Investigation of the psychometric properties of the inclusion body myositis functional rating scale with Rasch analysis. Muscle Nerve. 60, 161–168.

Ramdharry, G.M., 2010. Rehabilitation in practice: management of lower motor neuron weakness. Clin. Rehabil. 24, 387–397.

Ramdharry, G.M., Wallace, A., Hennis, P., et al., 2021. Cardiopulmonary exercise performance and factors associated with aerobic capacity in neuromuscular diseases. Muscle Nerve. 64, 683–690.

Ramsey, D., Scoto, M., Mayhew, A., et al., 2017. Revised Hammersmith Scale for spinal muscular atrophy: a SMA specific clinical outcome assessment tool. PLOS One. 12, e0172346.

Richardson, M., Mayhew, A., Muni-Lofra, R., et al., 2021. Prevalence of pain within limb girdle muscular dystrophy R9 and implications for other degenerative diseases. J. Clin. Med. 10, 5517.

Ricotti, V., Ridout, D.A., Pane, M., et al., 2016. The NorthStar Ambulatory Assessment in Duchenne muscular dystrophy: considerations for the design of clinical trials. J. Neurol. Neurosurg. Psychiatry. 87, 149–155.

Ricotti, V., Ridout, D.A., Scott, E., et al., 2013. Long-term benefits and adverse effects of intermittent versus daily glucocorticoids in boys with Duchenne muscular dystrophy. J. Neurol. Neurosurg. Psychiatry. 84, 698–705.

Ricotti, V., Selby, V., Ridout, D., et al., 2019. Respiratory and upper limb function as outcome measures in ambulant and non-ambulant subjects with Duchenne muscular dystrophy: a prospective multicentre study. Neuromusc. Disord. 29, 261–268.

Ryder, S., Leadley, R.M., Armstrong, N., et al., 2017. The burden, epidemiology, costs and treatment for Duchenne muscular dystrophy: an evidence review. Orphanet J. Rare Dis. 12, 79.

Safety, β-sarcoglycan Expression, and Functional Outcomes from Systemic Gene Transfer of rAAVrh74.MHCK7.SGCB in Limb Girdle Muscular Dystrophy Type 2E | MDA Clinical & Scientific Conference 2022, n.d. Available at: https://mdaconference.org/node/1170. Accessed 16 May 2022.

Sahni, A.S., Wolfe, L., 2018. Respiratory care in neuromuscular diseases. Respir. Care. 63, 601–608.

Scott, E., Eagle, M., Mayhew, A., et al., 2012. Development of a functional assessment scale for ambulatory boys with Duchenne muscular dystrophy. Physiother. Res. Int. 17, 101–109.

Sezer, S., Cup, E.H.C., Roets-Merken, 2021. Experiences of patients with facioscapulohumeral dystrophy with facial weakness: a qualitative study. Disabil. Rehabil. 1–8.

Sheehan, D., Birnkrant, D., Benditt, J., et al., 2018. Respiratory management of the patient with Duchenne muscular dystrophy. Pediatrics. 142, S62–S71.

Shoffner, J.M., Lott, M.T., Lezza, A.M.S., et al., 1990. Myoclonic epilepsy and ragged-red fiber disease (MERRF) is associated with a mitochondrial DNA tRNALys mutation. Cell. 61, 931–937.

Sofou, K., De Coo, I.F.M., Isohanni, P., et al., 2014. A multicenter study on Leigh syndrome: disease course and predictors of survival. Orphanet J. Rare Dis. 9, 52.

Statland, J., Tawil, R., 2014. Facioscapulohumeral muscular dystrophy. Neurol. Clin. 32, 721–728. ix

Statland, J.M., Tawil, R., 2016. Facioscapulohumeral muscular dystrophy. Contin. Minneap. Minn 22, 1916–1931.

Stefanetti, R., Blain, A., Jimenez-Moreno, C., et al., 2020. Measuring the effects of exercise in neuromuscular disorders: a systematic review and meta-analyses [version 1; peer review: 2 approved]. Wellcome Open Res. 5.

Steffensen, B.F., Mayhew, A., 2008. Egen Klassifikation (EK) revisited in spinal musculara trophy. Neuromusc. Disord. 18, 740–741.

Steffensen, B., Hyde, S., Lyager, S., Mattsson, E., 2001. Validity of the EK scale: a functional assessment of non-ambulatory individuals with Duchenne muscular dystrophy or spinal muscular atrophy. Physiother. Res. Int. 6, 119–134.

Steffensen, B.F., Hyde, S.A., Attermann, J., Mattsson, E., 2002. Reliability of the EK scale, a functional test for non-ambulatory persons with Duchenne dystrophy. Adv. Physiother. 4, 37–47.

Straub, V., Murphy, A., Udd, B., 2018. 229th ENMC international workshop: limb girdle muscular dystrophies – Nomenclature and reformed classification Naarden, the Netherlands, 17–19 March 2017. Neuromuscul Disord 28, 702–710.

Sugarman, E.A., Nagan, N., Zhu, H., et al., 2012. Pan-ethnic carrier screening and prenatal diagnosis for spinal muscular atrophy: clinical laboratory analysis of >72,400 specimens. Eur. J. Hum. Genet. 20, 27–32.

Sussman, M.D., Sienko, S.E., Buckon, C.E., et al., 2020. Efficacy of corticosteroid in decreasing scoliosis and extending time to loss of ambulation in a single clinic: an effectiveness trial. J. Child Orthop. 14, 421–432.

Swash, M., Schwartz, M.S., 2013. Neuromuscular Diseases: A Practical Approach to Diagnosis and Management. Springer Science & Business Media.

Talotta, R., Porrello, I., Restuccia, R., Magaudda, L., 2022. Physical activity in idiopathic inflammatory myopathies: two intervention proposals based on literature review. Clin. Rheumatol. 41, 593–615.

Tarnopolsky, M.A., 2014. Exercise as a therapeutic strategy for primary mitochondrial cytopathies. J. Child Neurol. 29, 1225–1234.

Toussaint, M., Boitano, L.J., Gathot, V., et al., 2009. Limits of effective cough-augmentation techniques in patients with neuromuscular disease. Respir. Care. 54, 359–366.

Trucco, F., Domingos, J.P., Tay, C.G., et al., 2020. Cardiorespiratory progression over 5 years and role of corticosteroids in Duchenne muscular dystrophy: a single-site retrospective longitudinal study. Chest. 158, 1606–1616.

Turner, C., Hilton-Jones, D., 2014. Myotonic dystrophy: diagnosis, management and new therapies. Curr. Opin. Neurol. 27, 599–606.

Van Ruiten, H.J., Marini Bettolo, C., Cheetham, T., et al., 2016. Why are some patients with Duchenne muscular dystrophy dying young: an analysis of causes of death in North East England. Eur. J. Paediatr. Neurol. 20, 904–909.

Veenhuizen, Y., Cup, E.H.C., Jonker, M.A., et al., 2019. Self-management program improves participation in patients with neuromuscular disease: a randomized controlled trial. Neurology. 93, E1720–E1731.

Vignos, P., Spencer, G., Archibald, K., 1963. Management of progressive muscular dystrophy in childhood. JAMA. 13, 89–96.

Voet, N.B., Kooi, E.L., van der Engelen, B.G., van Geurts, A.C., 2019. Strength training and aerobic exercise training for muscle disease. Cochrane Database Syst. Rev. 12.

Walter, M.C., Reilich, P., Thiele, S., et al., 2013. Treatment of dysferlinopathy with deflazacort: a double-blind, placebo-controlled clinical trial. Orphanet J. Rare Dis. 8, 1–15.

Walton, J.N., Nattrass, F.J., 1954. On the classification, natural history and treatment of the myopathies. Brain. 77, 169–231.

Wang, C.H., Dowling, J.J., North, K., et al., 2012. Consensus statement on standard of care for congenital myopathies. J. Child Neurol. 27, 363–382.

Wang, C.H., Finkel, R.S., Bertini, E.S., et al., 2007. Consensus statement for standard of care in spinal muscular atrophy. J. Child Neurol. 22, 1027–1049.

Werlauff, U., Steffensen, B., Fynbo, 2014. The applicability of four clinical methods to evaluate arm and hand function in all stages of spinal muscular atrophy type II. Disabil. Rehabil. 36, 2120–2126.

Whelan, D.T., Carson, N., Zeesman, S., 2002. Paternal transmission of the congenital form of myotonic dystrophy type 1: a new case and review of the literature. Am. J. Med. Genet. 107, 222–226.

White, S.L., Collins, V.R., Wolfe, R., et al., 1999. Genetic counseling and prenatal diagnosis for the mitochondrial DNA mutations at nucleotide 8993. Am. J. Hum. Genet. 65, 474–482.

Whittaker, R.G., Ferenczi, E., Hilton-Jones, D., 2006. Myotonic dystrophy: practical issues relating to assessment of strength. J. Neurol. Neurosurg. Psychiatry. 77, 1282–1283.

WHO, 2001. The International Classification of Functioning, Disability and Health. Available at: https://doi.org/10.1097/01.pep.0000245823.21888.71. Accessed on 21 July 2021.

Winblad, S., Samuelsson, L., Lindberg, C., Meola, G., 2016. Cognition in myotonic dystrophy type 1: a 5-year follow-up study. Eur. J. Neurol. 23, 1471–1476.

Wood, L., Bassez, G., van Engelen, B., et al., 2018. 222nd ENMC International Workshop: Myotonic dystrophy, developing a European consortium for care and therapy, Naarden, The Netherlands, 1–2 July 2016. Neuromusc. Disord. 28, 463–469.

Yao, L., Yip, A.L., Shrader, J.A., et al., 2016. Magnetic resonance measurement of muscle T2, fat-corrected T2 and fat fraction in the assessment of idiopathic inflammatory myopathies. Rheumatology. 55, 441–449.

Functional Motor Disorders

Glenn Nielsen and Kate Holt

OUTLINE

Key Points, 413
Introduction, 414
Historical Perspective, 414
Epidemiology, 415
Pathophysiology, 415
    A Biopsychosocial Formulation, 417
Diagnosis, 418
Prognosis, 418
Clinical Presentations, 418
    Functional Weakness, 418
    Functional Gait Disorder, 419
    Functional Tremor, 419
    Functional Jerks, 419
    Functional Dystonia, 420
    Fixed Functional Dystonia, 420
    Persistent Postural-Perceptual Dizziness, 420
    Other Categories, 420
    Other Common Symptoms and Comorbidities in
        Patients With Functional Motor Disorder, 421
Role of the Multidisciplinary Team, 421
    Neurology, 421
    Psychiatry, 421
    Psychological Therapy, 421
    Occupational Therapy, 421
    Speech and Language Therapy, 421
    Other Treatments, 422

Evidence for Rehabilitation of Functional Motor
    Disorder, 422
Before Commencing Rehabilitation, 422
Assessment, 423
    Subjective Assessment, 423
    Physical Assessment, 423
    Outcome Measures, 423
Physiotherapy Interventions, 423
    Education, 425
    Movement Retraining, 425
    Addressing Persistent Pain and Fatigue, 426
    Self-Management, 426
Considerations for Treatment, 426
    Recognising Comorbidities, 426
    Medications, 429
    Nonepileptic Seizures and Physiotherapy, 429
    Adaptive Aids, Equipment and Environmental
        Modifications, 429
    Functional Motor Disorder and Falls, 429
    Treatment Intensity, Duration and Setting, 429
    Concluding Treatment, 429
Conclusion, 430
Case Study, 430

KEY POINTS

- Functional motor disorder (FMD) is the motor dominant variant of functional neurological disorder (FND).
- Patients experience motor symptoms such as weakness, tremor, dystonia and/or altered gait patterns. These typically occur alongside nonmotor symptoms including but not limited to somatosensory disturbance.
- FND is best understood within a biopsychosocial framework. Symptoms occur in the absence of structural disease, and can be explained using predictive models of brain function.

- Once considered a diagnosis of exclusion, FMD is now diagnosed based on the clinical examination, using 'rule-in' signs such as Hoover's sign for leg weakness.
- There is a growing evidence base for the effectiveness of physiotherapy and multidisciplinary rehabilitation for FMD.
- Physiotherapy treatment aims to restore normal automatic movement patterns, using a motor relearning approach, while redirecting the patient's focus of motor attention.

INTRODUCTION

Functional neurological symptoms have been broadly defined as genuine neurological symptoms that are associated with alternation in functioning of brain networks rather than a structural disease process (Hallett et al 2022). It is a diagnosis that exists on the boundary between the disciplines of neurology and psychiatry. Symptoms are diverse and can include disorders of movement, sensation and awareness. Although overlap is common, this chapter is concerned with functional symptoms affecting movement, which will be referred to as functional motor disorder (FMD). Patients with FMD typically present with one or a combination of weakness, tremor, jerks, spasms, dystonic postures or an altered gait pattern.

Over the years, many different terms have been used to describe patients with FMD, including hysteria, conversion disorder, dissociative motor disorder, psychogenic, nonorganic, pseudoneurological and medically unexplained (Edwards et al 2014). There is ongoing disagreement over the most appropriate terminology, which reflects the complexity, heterogeneity and limited understanding of the condition. The term 'functional' has been gaining traction as the preferred term amongst medical professionals, although some have rejected this term, arguing that it is ambiguous (Fahn & Olanow 2014). The term functional is used to imply a change in the function of the nervous system rather than structure (Trimble 1982). Surveys of the lay public indicate that 'functional' is less likely to imply *not real* or *put on*, compared with other commonly used terms and therefore is less likely to be offensive to patients (Stone et al 2002). Official classification systems are beginning to reflect the increasing use of the term functional. The most recent version of the *Diagnostic Statistical Manual of Mental Disorders* (DSM-5-TR) updated its terminology to 'Functional Neurological Symptoms Disorder (Conversion Disorder)', where previously the latter term was placed first (American Psychiatric Association 2022).

HISTORICAL PERSPECTIVE

It is likely that FMD has always been an ailment of the human condition. Early descriptions appear in ancient Greek and Roman texts describing symptoms of choking, mutism and paralysis, and were believed to be caused by spontaneous movement of the uterus within the body. The association of functional symptoms with the uterus continued until well into the 19th century (Pearce 2014). This belief obviously confined the diagnosis to women and gave rise to the label 'hysteria', derived from the Greek and Latin words for *uterus*. During the Middle Ages (5th–15th centuries), beliefs about the uterus were often replaced by beliefs of demonic possession and witchcraft. 'Hysterical' women were subjected to exorcisms, torture and sometimes put to death (Tasca et al 2012).

The 19th century has been described as the heyday of hysteria, when great interest and time was devoted to the subject by the pioneers of neurology and psychiatry (Micale 1993). French neurologist Jean-Martin Charcot (1825–1893) was an extremely influential figure in the history of FMD. Under his influence, FMD (then hysteria) became a specific and defined neurological diagnosis (Goetz 2016). Neurologist Sigmund Freud (1856–1939) may be the most famous early clinician in the field of hysteria. Despite being a neurologist, Freud's work and his role in the development of psychoanalysis was influential in moving hysteria towards the field of psychiatry in the 20th century, and consequently it effectively became excluded from the field of neurology (Kanaan 2016). Freud's ideas regarding hysteria centred on repression of a traumatic event, and its subsequent conversion into physical symptoms. He highlighted the role of the unconscious to differentiate hysteria from feigning and considered sexual abuse to be an important trigger.

The onset of World War I saw an epidemic of FMD with what became known as shell shock. In reaction to trench warfare, soldiers presented with a variety of physical and psychological symptoms, including gait disorders, tremors, nightmares and panic attacks (Stone 2016a). In modern times, the incidence of FMD remains higher in the armed forces compared with the general population (Garrett et al 2020).

Following World War I, there was a common perception that hysteria had disappeared from medicine, being replaced by more elusive symptoms such as pain and fatigue. Stone et al (2008) have argued that FMD has remained largely unchanged in incidence and presentation over time, but patients became effectively invisible because of a reluctance of neurologists to make the diagnosis (Stone et al 2008). This appeared to lead to the disappearance of FMD from neurological curricula and textbooks (Stone

2016a), which may help to explain the current lack of awareness of the diagnosis. The 'disappearance' of FMD appeared to last until the mid 1990's, when a resurgence of interest in the topic can be seen in the scientific literature, in part fuelled by advances in modern imaging techniques. The past decade in particular has seen important milestones, such as the first large powered randomised controlled trials of treatment (Goldstein et al 2020; Nielsen et al 2019) and the inauguration of an international society devoted to the study of FND (Functional Neurological Disorder Society 2020).

EPIDEMIOLOGY

Reported rates of incidence of FMD range from 4 to 12 per 100,000 population per year (Carson et al 2012). To put this into context, the incidence of multiple sclerosis is estimated to be 4–6 per 100,000 in northern parts of North America and Europe (Goodin 2014), and estimates of the incidence of Parkinson's range from 8 to 18 per 100,000 (de Lau & Breteler 2006). Studying the incidence of FMD is complicated by problems with inconsistent application of diagnostic criteria and inaccurate coding of the diagnosis in medical records (Carson & Lehn 2016). For these reasons, it is assumed that reported rates of incidence are likely to be underestimates.

Functional symptoms are very common in clinical neurology settings. The Scottish Neurological Symptoms Study recruited 36 of 38 neurologists working in the Scottish National Health Service and asked them to record the diagnosis made in all new referrals over a 15-month period. In addition, the neurologists were asked to rate the degree to which they considered the patient's symptoms could be explained by disease. They found that FND (both motor and nonmotor symptoms) was the second most common diagnosis made, comprising 16% of patients, second only to headache (19%). In addition, 30% of patients had neurological symptoms that were considered to be either 'not at all' or only 'somewhat' explained by neurological disease (Stone et al 2010).

Across studies there is a unified agreement that FMD is more common in women than men, with figures ranging from 60% to 75% female (Carson & Lehn 2016). However, some motor phenotypes (Parkinson-like symptoms and jerks) are more common in men (Lidstone et al 2022). The most common age of FMD onset occurs in midlife, 35–45 years, with a second peak in late adolescence, but onset can occur across all ages, from young children to the elderly (Lidstone et al 2022).

Corresponding to the high incidence and disability caused by FMD is a substantial economic burden. Costs are associated with extensive health and social care utilisation,

as well as high rates of unemployment and receipt of disability benefits (Carson et al 2011).

PATHOPHYSIOLOGY

The pathophysiology of FMD is complex and multifactorial. Pathophysiological models used to explain FMD have, up until recently, primarily focused on psychological stress factors and have been heavily influenced by the Freudian theory. However, converging lines of evidence from contemporary clinical, laboratory and epidemiological research support the need for a broad multifactorial biopsychosocial model to understand the complexity and heterogeneity of FMD.

A range of psychological and sociological theories have been suggested to explain FMD, but no unified psychological theory exists (Carson et al 2016b). Psychological explanations for functional symptoms include the concepts of primary and secondary gain, where the conversion of psychological distress into physical symptoms is considered the primary gain, and secondary gain is the benefits or material advantage (either conscious or unconscious) of being ill (Carson et al 2016b). Sociological theories of FMD include the sick role, where the patient is unconsciously motivated to seek legitimisation from a doctor to access the sick role, which affords them an exemption from societal responsibilities and other secondary gain, such as disability benefits (Carson et al 2016b). A criticism of these explanations is that these forces are not unique to FMD and arguably apply to all health conditions to varying extents.

The concepts of classical and operant conditioning have been used to explain how symptoms are developed and maintained. Learning theories help to explain fear avoidance behaviours and underpin the use of cognitive behavioural therapy (CBT) (Carson et al 2016b). The psychological experience of dissociation is a commonly cited theoretical aetiological mechanism of FMD. The term *dissociation* refers to two phenomena: detachment, which describes a sense of separation from the self or the world, and compartmentalisation, a reversible loss of voluntary control of an intact function (Brown 2016).

It has been well established that psychological problems such as anxiety, depression and stressful life events are more common in people with FMD compared with the general population and patients with neurological disease (Kranick et al 2011). A systematic review and meta-analysis of studies of adverse life events in people with FND (motor and nonmotor symptoms) found that the odds of being diagnosed with FND was 5.6 times higher in people who experienced emotional neglect in childhood, 3.9 times higher following physical abuse and 3.3 times higher following sexual abuse (Ludwig et al 2018). In a multicentre case-control study of 696 patients with FMD, higher rates of lifetime sexual abuse were reported in women (35.3%) and men (11.5%) with FMD compared with other neurological disease controls (10.6% of women and 5.6% of men) (Kletenik et al 2022). Lifetime rates of physical abuse were also higher in FMD compared with controls (36.5% of women and 27.8% of men with FMD compared with 17.0% of women and 19.4% of men in the control group). Although more common, these data show that the majority of patients are unaffected by these adverse life events. The relationship between anxiety, depression and FMD is also unclear. For instance, average self-reported anxiety scores are higher in groups of patients with FMD compared with other diagnoses, but many patients with FMD score within the normal (subclinical) range (Kranick et al 2011). Taken together, these data suggest that psychological comorbidity and trauma are relevant to many patients but not necessarily all, and that psychological factors may be best considered as risk factors for developing FMD rather than the cause.

Factors other than psychological have become increasingly recognised as an important part of the aetiology. For example, there are several studies that demonstrate a relationship between FMD and physical precipitating events, including injury, adverse drug reactions, surgery and neurological disease (Pareés et al 2014b; Stone et al 2009a).

Research into the neurobiological basis for FMD has become a topic of increasing interest. This research is based on the logic that if we assume that FMD is a genuine problem and that patients are not feigning their symptoms, then symptoms must have neurological correlates that can be objectively measured. Neuroimaging studies, although limited by small subject numbers and differing paradigms, have shown several interesting findings. Patients with FMD appear distinct from those asked to feign neurological symptoms (Voon et al 2010); patients with FMD have shown abnormal recruitment of limbic areas and an abnormal functional connectivity between the amygdala and motor areas (Aybek & Vuilleumier 2017); finally, activity in areas associated with a normal sense of self-agency appear to be different in patients versus controls, which may be related to the patients' reported experience that symptoms feel involuntary (Aybek & Vuilleumier 2017). Neurophysiological studies have also found differences in sensorimotor processing in patients with FMD when compared with health controls (Macerollo et al 2015, Pareés et al 2014a, Teodoro et al 2018).

Edwards et al (2012) described a hypothetical neurobiological model for FMD that has gained increasing traction and evidence-based support in the scientific literature. The model highlights key mechanisms that may account for how functional motor symptoms are generated; these include an abnormal attentional focus and erroneous illness beliefs/expectations (Edwards et al 2012). The role of attention in FMD can be easily demonstrated because functional motor symptoms require attention to manifest. When the patient's attention is distracted away from their symptoms, there is a reduction or disappearance of the movement disorder (Edwards et al 2013). Expectation as a symptom mechanism relates to the patient's expectation or belief that their movement will be abnormal. Edwards et al (2012) described the mechanism by which belief and expectation may result in functional symptoms in regards to the theory of active inference of brain function and the *free energy principle* (Friston 2010). In brief, active inference refers to

---

KEY POINTS

- Psychological comorbidity is common in patients with FMD but does not appear to be universal (Kranick et al 2011).
- Several studies demonstrate a relationship between FMD and physical precipitating events, including injury, adverse drug reactions, surgery and neurological disease (Pareés et al 2014b, Stone et al 2009).
- Functional motor symptoms require attention to manifest. When the patient's attention is distracted away from their symptoms, there is a reduction or disappearance of the movement disorder (Edwards et al 2013).
- Conversely, directing the patient's attention towards their body and their symptoms exacerbates abnormal movement (Edwards et al 2013).
- Illness beliefs, specifically the expectation that movement will be abnormal, is thought to be an important mechanism that drives functional neurological symptoms (Edwards et al 2013).

how the brain operates using predictive models rather than attempting to process *in real time* the potentially infinite amount of afferent and efferent information available when performing functions such as controlling movement. The predictive models are based on our previous experiences of interacting with the world. In the context of FMD, an expectation of abnormal movement related to a particular illness belief (e.g., I have paralysis) is thought to act as a movement prior that influences motor output at a preconscious level. The concept of active inference can explain the experience of picking up an object that you expect to be heavy but turns out to be light, with a resulting overshoot of the movement. Another example is the experience of stepping onto a stationary escalator resulting in unsteady movement. In both examples, the expectations associated with the task resulted in motor output that was unplanned.

A Biopsychosocial Formulation

From a clinical perspective, it is recommended that the patient and their problem should be considered within a biopsychosocial framework, with the understanding that there is considerable heterogeneity amongst patients and that there is no one common aetiology. Within a biopsychosocial framework, the aetiology of FMD is often considered in regards to predisposing factors – things that make a person vulnerable to developing FMD; precipitating factors – things that may have triggered the movement problem; and perpetuating factors – things that work to maintain the status quo (Table 16.1). This framework can be helpful to understand the broader context of a patient's problem, to formulate an understanding of relevant issues and plan an intervention.

From a physiotherapy perspective, we recommend conceptualising symptoms of FMD as learnt patterns of movement, driven by illness belief/expectation and an abnormal amount of attention directed towards the body. Multiple additional factors may also affect a patient's movement, such as a fear of falling, antalgic movement patterns, fear avoidance and loss of physical fitness.

The physiotherapist should recognise that multiple comorbidities are common in patients with FMD, and this

---

TABLE 16.1 A Range of Potential Mechanisms and Aetiological Factors in Patients With Functional Movement Disorder

Factors	Biological	Psychological	Social
Factors acting at all stages	'Organic' disease (including underlying neurological disease and hypermobility syndromes) History of previous functional symptoms Chronic pain and fatigue	Emotional disorder Personality disorder	Socioeconomic/deprivation Life events and difficulties
Predisposing factors	Genetic factors affecting personality Biological vulnerabilities in the nervous system	Adverse childhood experiences Personality traits Poor attachment/coping style	Childhood neglect/abuse Poor family functioning Symptom modelling of others
Precipitating factors	Abnormal physiological event or state (e.g., drug side effect, hyperventilation, sleep deprivation, sleep paralysis) Physical injury/pain	Adverse life events Acute dissociative episode/panic attack	
Perpetuating factors	Plasticity in central nervous system motor and sensory (including pain) pathways leading to habitual abnormal movement Deconditioning Neuroendocrine and immunological abnormalities similar to those seen in depression and anxiety	Illness beliefs (patient and family) Perception of symptoms as being irreversible Not feeling believed Perception that movement causes damage Avoidance of symptom provocation Fear of falling	Social benefits of being ill Availability of legal compensation Ongoing medical investigations and uncertainty Employment and financial issues Disability support

Adapted from Stone et al (2012) and Nielsen et al (2015b).

can include psychological problems such as anxiety and depression. Life events, emotional disorder and personality traits are relevant in understanding and treating some patients with FMD, in which case treatment may be best placed within a multidisciplinary team. However, in some cases, physiotherapy as a standalone intervention may be appropriate and effective.

DIAGNOSIS

In the past, FMD has been described as a diagnosis of exclusion, but in recent times there has been a move towards making a positive (rule-in) diagnosis. A positive diagnosis can be made based on specific clinical signs of FMD, incongruity with recognised neurological disease and internal inconsistency during the physical examination (Edwards & Bhatia 2012). Many clinical signs have been described to positively identify FMD (Aybek & Perez 2022). Perhaps the most clinically useful is Hoover's sign for functional lower limb weakness, which has been shown to have high specificity (99%) and sensitivity (94%) (Daum et al 2014). A selection of clinical signs for FMD are described in Table 16.2. An example of incongruity with recognised clinical disease is midline splitting of sensory disturbance, where there is an exact demarcation of reduced sensation at the midline of the trunk. This is said to be a functional sign because cutaneous branches of the intercostal nerves cross the midline, although midline splitting is a possible consequence of a thalamic stroke (Stone 2009). Other examples of symptoms that are incongruous with recognised disease include a global pattern of limb weakness, a nonpyramidal pattern of weakness (which does occur in some types of neuromuscular disease) and a tubular visual field (Stone & Carson 2015). An example of internal inconsistency during physical examination is when the patient is unable to actively plantarflex their ankle against resistance but can stand on their toes.

In addition to clinical signs, key features of the history may support the diagnosis. This can include a history of other functional symptoms, rapid onset and progression of symptoms to peak disability (e.g., occurring over a period of hours) and physical precipitating factors. Psychological problems such as anxiety, depression, trauma and recent stress are generally more common in FMD than other neurological diagnoses, but they are not universal and therefore are an unreliable basis for the diagnosis (Stone et al 2013). It is also generally recommended that specific and targeted investigations should be conducted to rule out other potential causes for symptoms; this may include MRI and nerve conduction testing (Edwards & Bhatia 2012).

It is often suggested that the diagnosis of FMD should be made by a neurologist (Espay & Lang 2015). This is because of the potential complexity of ruling out rare neurological conditions that may mimic FMD, such as alien hand phenomenon in corticobasal degeneration (Stone et al 2013). In addition, on rare occasions, FMD may exist as a prodromal state for neurological disease. For example, a functional gait disturbance and psychiatric symptoms may occur before the onset of firm signs of motor neurone disease, multiple system atrophy or Parkinson's (Stone et al 2013). Despite these complexities, in modern neurological practice the diagnosis of FMD is stable, with studies showing a misdiagnosis rate of between 1% and 4%, which is in line with other neurological diagnoses (Stone et al 2009b).

PROGNOSIS

The prognosis of FMD is generally considered poor. A systematic review of long-term follow-up studies found that approximately 40% of patients with FMD were the same or worse at a mean follow up of 7 years (Gelauff et al 2014). However, this review excluded studies of outcome after specific interventions for FMD; therefore treatment may lead to better outcomes. In addition, these data are based on a broad cross-section of patients with FMD, including those who had chronic symptoms at baseline assessment. There are limited data on the prognosis of first episode acute-onset FMD, a group that may have a higher rate of symptom resolution.

Several prognostic indicators have been identified. Longer duration of symptoms before diagnosis and the presence of personality disorder are among the most powerful predictors of poor outcome. High satisfaction with care has been shown to predict positive outcome (Gelauff et al 2014).

The poor prognosis of FMD may reflect the lack of availability of specific treatments and also the disjointed way that treatment services have been structured, where patients can fall through that gap between physical and mental health services. On a more optimistic note, recent studies of physical-based rehabilitation have reported promising outcomes, with treatment effects lasting at follow-up periods of 1 and 2 years (Czarnecki et al 2012, Jordbru et al 2014).

CLINICAL PRESENTATIONS

Functional neurological symptoms rarely occur in isolation. Functional motor, sensory and cognitive symptoms commonly coexist together, often alongside fatigue and persistent pain (Butler et al 2021). Several specific presentations of FMD have been described; the most common are discussed in the following sections.

Functional Weakness

Functional weakness most commonly presents as weakness or paralysis of the limbs. It may occur in any combination

TABLE 16.2   Clinical Signs of Functional Motor Disorder

Clinical Sign	Description
Hoover's sign	Hip extension weakness that returns to normal when the contralateral hip is flexed against resistance
Give-way weakness/collapsing weakness	Muscle power is initially generated on testing, which quickly gives way or collapses
Hip abductor sign	Hip abduction power is tested bilaterally in a patient with unilateral weakness. The patient is supine. Power in both limbs is generated in a positive test
Clear signs of inconsistency	For example, weak ankle plantarflexion on testing but the patient can walk on their toes
Hemifacial muscle overactivity presenting with unilateral limb symptoms	Overactivity of orbicularis oculus, orbicularis oris and/or platysma giving the appearance of a facial droop
Sternomastoid test	Weakness of head turning to affected arm and leg in functional hemiparesis
Drift without pronation test	During a 'pronator drift' test, the forearm may not pronate in a functional hemiparesis
Global pattern of weakness	Flexors and extensors equally affected, e.g., wrist flexion and wrist extension
Tremor entrainment or distractibility	When tapping an unaffected limb at a set frequency, the affected limb entrains to the set frequency of tapping or the tremor stops
Dragging monoplegic gait	The leg is dragged at the hip behind the body
Walking on ice gait	Exaggerated postural responses (e.g., pivoting at the waist with a narrow base of support) whilst still managing to maintain a standing position

From Daum et al (2014), Edwards & Bhatia (2012) and Nielsen et al (2017b).

including monoparesis, hemiparesis, paraparesis and tetraparesis (Stone & Aybek 2017). The weakness is characterised by internal inconsistency, such as an inability to actively move the lower limbs on command, while retaining some ability to weight bear. Clinical signs used to identify functional weakness are described in Table 16.2.

Patients presenting with sudden onset of functional weakness are often mistakenly directed through emergency stroke treatment pathways. In this context patients are often referred to as stroke mimics (other conditions that can also mimic stroke include migraine and brain tumours). Within specialist stroke services, functional stroke mimic represents a reported range of 1.4%–8.4% of all admissions and 0.5%–5% of all patients who receive intravenous thrombolysis for presumed stroke (Nielsen et al 2017a).

Functional Gait Disorder

A functional gait disorder can present as part of a mixed functional movement disorder picture (because of functional weakness, dystonia, tremor, altered sensation, pain, etc.) or as an isolated problem (Fung 2016). Common patterns of functional gait disorder have been described, including dragging leg gait, walking on ice gait (reduction in step height as if ice skating), astasia-abasia (inability to stand or walk despite normal power when tested on the bed, often with exaggerated postural adjustments), excessive slowness, uneconomic postures, knee buckling and scissoring-leg gait (Daum et al 2014, Fung, 2016).

Functional Tremor

Functional tremor most commonly affects upper limbs but can also affect lower limbs, head and neck, and even the soft palate (Edwards & Bhatia 2012). Functional tremor is characterised by distractibility and entrainability (see Table 16.2). Functional tremor may occur at rest and/or with movement (action tremor). The tremor may be generated by alternating contraction of agonist-antagonist muscles or by cocontraction (Edwards & Bhatia 2012).

Functional Jerks

Functional jerks are intermittent jerking movements that can affect any part of the body, although jerks affecting the trunk are probably the most common (axial jerks) (Dreissen et al 2016). Because functional jerks are intermittent with variable frequency, it is difficult to assess the effect of distraction, which makes diagnosis complex. A clinical diagnostic test has been devised for functional myoclonus, which involves electroencephalogram-electromyography (EEG-EMG) back averaging to assess for cortical activity before movement. In patients with functional myoclonus and in normal voluntary movement, there is a premovement potential (also known as a *Bereitschaftspotential*) arising approximately 1.5 seconds before activity (Edwards & Bhatia 2012). The test is not suitable for all cases; it requires at least 30 recorded measurements and may not be possible when jerks occur at a frequency greater than 3–5 per second (Edwards & Bhatia 2012). Many patients with functional jerks were previously diagnosed with myoclonus that was presumed to originate from the spinal cord, often called *propriospinal myoclonus*. The development of EEG-EMG back averaging to assess for premovement potentials has resulted in many patients being rediagnosed with an FMD, and the existence of structurally caused propriospinal myoclonus has been questioned (Erro et al 2014).

Functional Dystonia

Functional dystonia presents as dystonic postures and movement that can affect virtually any body part, including the limbs, facial muscles, head, neck and the tongue. Functional dystonia may present with other functional symptoms such as tremor, weakness and altered sensation.

Fixed Functional Dystonia

Fixed functional dystonia (FFD) is characterised by fixed posturing of usually a distal limb, often developing after a relatively minor initial injury. See Figure 16.1 for an example of bilateral ankle FFD. The clinical picture and symptoms that ensue become disproportionate to the initial injury where a pattern of cocontraction of muscles around a joint creates a fixed position (Schrag et al 2004). Pain is often a dominant symptom. Altered skin temperature, colour, and hair and nail growth are common and are related to reduced movement and blood circulation. Other motor signs are sometimes present such as cocontraction tremor and muscle wasting in more severe long-term cases (Ganos et al 2014). This clinical picture often fits the diagnostic criteria of complex regional pain syndrome type 1 (CRPS-1), and in these cases the problem is sometimes referred to as *CRPS-dystonia* (Schrag et al 2004). Despite the different diagnostic labels, contemporary opinion is that CRPS-1 and FFD are conditions that probably occupy points on a spectrum of the same disorder (Popkirov et al 2018). Depending on severity and duration of symptoms, patients can develop debilitating joint contractures because of joint immobility and muscle overactivity. An evaluation under anaesthetic can help to differentiate a fixed

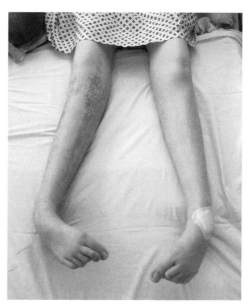

FIG. 16.1 Example of bilateral ankle fixed functional dystonia (FFD19).

contracture from active posturing. At the more severe end of the spectrum, it is not uncommon for patients to seek amputation of the limb, the result of which is often unfavourable (Edwards et al 2011).

Persistent Postural-Perceptual Dizziness

Persistent postural-perceptual dizziness (PPPD) is a functional vestibular disorder characterised by persistent dizziness, nonspinning vertigo and often unsteadiness in standing and walking (Staab et al 2017). In hospital-based settings, PPPD accounts for 20% of patients with vestibular symptoms and 40% in dedicated vestibular services (Hallett et al 2022).

Traditional vestibular rehabilitation therapy (VRT) has been recommended for PPPD, but more targeted psychologically informed VRT is an interesting development (Herdman et al 2022).

Other Categories

Other categories of FMD have been described in the literature and used in clinical descriptions for research cohorts. Mixed movement disorder is often used to describe a mixture of motor symptoms including dystonia, weakness and tremor. FMD can mimic Parkinson's and is sometimes reported as the specific category functional parkinsonism. These patients can exhibit a functional tremor (usually at rest and during action), slow and effortful movement, abnormal response to postural stability testing and resistance to passive movement (Jankovic 2011).

Other Common Symptoms and Comorbidities in Patients With Functional Motor Disorder

Dissociative seizures (DSs) (also called nonepileptic/psychogenic/functional seizures) are a specific presentation of FND characterised by episodes of decreased awareness and often associated with movement resembling tonic-clonic epileptic seizures (Brown & Reuber 2016). DSs are not considered part of the spectrum of functional *movement* disorders because of the predominant characteristic of reduced awareness. However, symptom crossover is common, and many patients with a primary complaint of DS will also experience functional motor symptoms and vice versa. In general, patients with a predominant problem of DS differ from those with FMD in several ways. They are more likely to be younger, more likely to report childhood abuse and more likely to report adverse life events before the onset of their symptoms (Brown & Reuber 2016). Specialist CBT and psychodynamic psychotherapy are recognised as the main types of treatment for DS (Goldstein et al 2020).

It is common for patients with FMD to experience functional symptoms in other body systems. Among the most commonly reported are gastrointestinal complaints (many are diagnosed with irritable bowel syndrome), bladder problems (including urinary retention and frequency) and pain syndromes (such as pelvic pain or fibromyalgia). Some patients will have other medical conditions and complaints that may need separate diagnosis and treatment, for example, migraine, hypermobile Ehlers Danlos syndrome and psychiatric diagnoses such as obsessive-compulsive disorder.

ROLE OF THE MULTIDISCIPLINARY TEAM

There is limited but growing evidence for treatment of FMD, and there are no formal treatment guidelines. Most of the literature suggests that management should involve a multidisciplinary team, which may involve neurology, psychiatry, physiotherapy, occupational therapy, speech therapy, psychology, specialist nurses and the patient's general practitioner.

Neurology

As described above, neurologists are usually the clinicians responsible for making the diagnosis of FMD. In addition, neurologists have a key role in treatment of FMDs, starting with effective communication and explanation of the diagnosis (Edwards & Bhatia 2012, Stone & Carson 2015). Other roles of the neurologist may include treating comorbidity such as migraine and chronic pain, rationalising medications and referral to other medical specialities for assessment. In some cases, a neurologist may oversee rehabilitation.

Psychiatry

The role of psychiatry will differ between patients and may be dependent on how services are commissioned within the relevant healthcare system. The key role of a psychiatrist is to assess and treat psychiatric morbidity. Psychiatrists may also oversee rehabilitation in a multidisciplinary team (Demartini et al 2014, McCormack et al 2013).

Psychological Therapy

Psychological therapies are an important part of the treatment of FMD for many patients. There are two main approaches to treatment: psychodynamic therapy and CBT, the latter having the largest evidence base (Gutkin et al 2021). There are a number of promising pilot and cohort studies of psychological therapy for FMD, but to date there are no adequately powered randomised controlled trials (RCTs). An RCT of a CBT-based, guided self-help intervention for patients with a wide range of functional neurological symptoms, including motor symptoms, showed benefits in subjective health at 3 months and the physical function domains of the Short Form 36 (SF-36) questionnaire at 3 and 6 months (Sharpe et al 2011). A single-blind pilot study of 29 patients found benefit for CBT and CBT plus physical activity compared with standard medical care (Dallocchio et al 2016). There is also some evidence for psychodynamic interpersonal therapy combined with neurological consultation (Hubschmid et al 2015, Kompoliti et al 2014).

Occupational Therapy

Occupational therapy is recognised as an integral part of multidisciplinary rehabilitation for people with FMD. Nicholson et al (2020) published consensus recommendations for treatment, highlighting the dual training of occupational therapists in physical and mental health (Nicholson et al 2020). The recommendations are structured around a biopsychosocial aetiological framework, including advice around education and rehabilitation within functional activity. There is also a focus on self-management strategies relating to problems such as fatigue and pain.

Speech and Language Therapy

Speech and language therapy (also known as speech pathology) can help to address a range of functional symptoms such as dysphonia, dysfluency and language articulation disorders, swallowing disorders such as dysphagia and globus, cough and upper airway symptoms. Treatment has been described in a recent publication, *Management of Functional Communication, Swallowing, Cough and Related Disorders: Consensus Recommendations for Speech and Language Therapy* (Baker et al 2021). The theoretical underpinnings of treatment mirror that described in this chapter.

Other Treatments

A range of other treatments have been described for FMD. This includes transcranial magnetic stimulation (Pollak et al 2014), therapeutic sedation (Stone et al 2014) and hypnosis (Phillips et al 2022). Although controlled evidence for efficacy of these treatments is currently lacking, they may prove to be useful treatment adjuncts in some patients.

Alternative therapies such as reflexology are popular amongst some patients, and often patients turn to alternative therapies when they have been unable to find support from the conventional healthcare system. Alternative therapies can be a contentious issue, particularly in a cohort of patients who are vulnerable to iatrogenic harm.

EVIDENCE FOR REHABILITATION OF FUNCTIONAL MOTOR DISORDER

There is growing evidence that physical-based rehabilitation can be effective for selected patients with FMD (Nielsen et al 2013). To date, there is evidence from a randomised feasibility study (Nielsen et al 2017a), a delayed-start controlled trial (Jordbru et al 2014) and several large cohort studies (Czarnecki et al 2012, Dallocchio et al 2010). A multicentre single-blind RCT of physiotherapy for FMD is currently underway and due for completion in 2023 (Nielsen et al 2019).

A recent randomised, controlled study assessed the feasibility of conducting a large trial of specialist physiotherapy for FMD (Nielsen et al 2017a). Sixty patients were randomised to receive either a specialist physiotherapy intervention or a standard community neurophysiotherapy control. The intervention was a specific treatment protocol composed of education, movement retraining and development of a self-management plan, which was delivered over 5 consecutive days. Patients with severe pain, fatigue and psychiatric comorbidity were excluded. At 6 months follow up, 72% of the intervention group rated their symptoms as improved compared with 18% in the control group. There was a moderate to large treatment effect across a range of physical outcome measures and a quality-adjusted life-year gain that was suggestive of a cost-effective intervention. The promising outcomes from this study should be interpreted with caution because the study was designed to assess feasibility and was not powered to detect a treatment effect. The powered version of this trial is due to be completed in 2023.

Jordbru et al (2014) completed a delayed-start controlled trial of physical rehabilitation in patients with functional gait disorder. Patients were randomised to receive a 3-week inpatient rehabilitation programme immediately or after a 4-week delay (waiting list control). The multidisciplinary team included a physician, physiotherapist, occupational therapist, nurse and an educator in adapted physical activity. The intervention was described as adapted physical activity with an education and cognitive-behavioural frame of reference. Important elements of the intervention included the symptom explanation (disconnect between the nervous system and muscles); positively reinforcing normal function (such as an improvement in gait or posture) while avoiding reinforcement of dysfunction; and activities such as bicycle riding, outdoor canoeing and indoor climbing, which aimed to shift focus from disability to mastering the activity. At the end of treatment, the intervention group had a significant improvement in the Functional Independence Measure, Functional Mobility Scale and Short Form-12 (SF-12). Improvement was carried over 12 months, except for the mental health domain of the SF-12.

Physical rehabilitation is also supported by evidence from large cohort studies. Czarnecki et al (2012) reported outcomes from an intensive 5-day outpatient treatment programme. In this programme, patients were assessed by a psychiatrist, but the intervention was carried out by physiotherapists and occupational therapists. Treatment was described as relearning normal movement, with use of distraction strategies, repetition and positive reinforcement. At the end of treatment, 70% of 60 patients rated themselves as markedly improved or almost completely normal; this decreased to 60% at 2-year follow up. Dallocchio et al (2010) report the outcomes of a progressive group-walking programme for patients with mild to moderate FMD. This straightforward intervention resulted in an improvement in symptom severity in 60% of patients (Dallocchio et al 2010). Several other cohort studies support the use of physiotherapy for FMD, including a study of patients admitted to an acute neurology ward (Matthews et al 2016, Nielsen et al 2013, 2015a). There is also uncontrolled evidence for physical rehabilitation from multidisciplinary rehabilitation programmes involving psychological and physical treatments (Demartini et al 2014, McCormack et al 2013, Moene et al 2002).

The evidence base for physical rehabilitation is growing, but there are significant gaps. The generalisability of this literature is limited by the eligibility criteria of the studies; for example, it is common to exclude patients with more severe comorbidity (including psychopathology) and those who do not accept the diagnosis. Comparing the different study outcomes is challenging because of the heterogeneity of the patient population and the study interventions, as well as the inconsistent use of objective outcome measures. Finally, there are limited data on long-term outcomes.

BEFORE COMMENCING REHABILITATION

Before commencing treatment, it is usually recommended that the patient's medical investigations have been completed and that a diagnosis has been made and explained to the patient by their physician (Nielsen et al 2015b). The physician's initial diagnostic explanation is often regarded as an essential platform for further treatment, and there is some evidence that a successful consultation is associated with an improved patient outcome (Carson et al 2016a, Thomas et al 2006).

It has been recommended that the terms of treatment should be negotiated before commencing intervention (Nielsen et al 2015b). A treatment agreement that defines parameters such as the number of sessions and expectations of the patient can provide an impetus for change and may preempt difficulties in discharging the patient at the conclusion of rehabilitation.

ASSESSMENT

Subjective Assessment

In addition to gathering information, the subjective assessment of the patient with FMD has been described as an opportunity to develop trust and rapport, and the assessment itself may have therapeutic value (Stone 2016b). A comprehensive subjective assessment will guide the treatment plan and identify issues that need to be considered when supporting the patient to self-manage. The subjective assessment should consider the following elements:

- The circumstances under which the symptoms developed: Does the patient recognise a precipitating event?
- A comprehensive list of symptoms: For each symptom, ascertain variability, severity, frequency, impact on daily life and exacerbating and easing factors.
- Typical 24-hour routine, including support required for activities of daily living: This may reveal perpetuating factors such as boom-bust activity patterns, poor sleep hygiene and excessive support from carers.
- Use of adaptive aids and equipment
- Activity limitations and participation restrictions
- Social history, including employment/education status: If the patient is currently working/in school, are they experiencing any difficulties and are there opportunities to help them maintain their employment?
- Explore the patient's understanding of their diagnosis: Ask the patient what they have been told about their diagnosis. Explore their understanding of the results of medical investigations. For example, what do they understand by an MRI report finding of 'degenerative disc disease'. Do they believe their diagnosis of FMD, or do they have concerns that they have an underlying disease that has not been properly investigated?
- Goals for rehabilitation

Physical Assessment

Completing a neuroassessment is important, but findings of assessment at the level of impairment (e.g., muscle power and sensation) will not necessarily correlate with disability in patients with FMD. For example, a patient may be unable to initiate lower limb movement when assessed in supine but may be able to stand and step unsupported. This type of inconsistency is a diagnostic feature of FMD and should not be interpreted as deception or lack of effort on behalf of the patient. Assessment at the level of activity (e.g., habitual resting postures, upper limb tasks, transfers, mobility, gait pattern, getting on and off the floor) is arguably more informative to understand disability and plan treatment.

The symptoms of FMD are often amplified during examination because the patient's attention is drawn towards their body. The physiotherapist should note and explore the variability of the patient's symptoms with distraction and redirection of attention. Novel movement, such as walking backwards, is often asymptomatic and therefore useful in movement retraining. The assessment can also include clinical signs listed in Table 16.2, such as Hoover's sign and tremor entrainment.

Outcome Measures

Measuring treatment outcome in FMD can be complex. Measurement at the level of impairment (e.g., weakness) and activity limitation (e.g., gait speed) have questionable test–retest reliability because of the inherent variability of FMD symptoms over short periods. Generic quality of life measures may lack of sensitivity in this population because of the multiple health domains affected by FMD (e.g., physical disability, fatigue, cognitive symptoms and psychological distress) (Nielsen et al 2017a). Specific assessments for FMD have been described; however, these have important limitations, including the time taken to complete, and therefore have limited clinical utility (Hinson et al 2005, Nielsen et al 2017a). Pick et al (2020) systematically reviewed the use of outcome measures in treatments for FMD (Pick et al 2020). The authors found an absence of validated and widely endorsed clinically useful assessment tools. It was highlighted that patient-reported outcomes are important. An interim recommendation was made to select a range of outcome measures covering the domains of the core symptom (e.g., gait), other physical symptoms (e.g., pain or fatigue), psychological symptoms (e.g., anxiety and depression), life impact (quality of life scale) and health economics. See Table 16.3 for a selection of potentially useful outcome measures.

PHYSIOTHERAPY INTERVENTIONS

There are currently no evidence-based guidelines for the treatment of FMD. Most interventional studies describe

TABLE 16.3   Potentially Useful Outcome Measures for Functional Motor Disorder

Outcome Measure	Measurement Domain	Description
Administered Physical Assessments		
10-metre timed walk (Peters et al 2013)	Walking speed	A quick and reliable test of gait speed and step length over 10 m (Peters et al 2013)
Berg Balance Scale (Berg et al 1992)	Balance	A widely used measure of balance shown to have good reliability and validity (La Porta et al 2012) Alternative balance and gait assessments may be of equal or greater value
Patient-Reported Questionnaires		
Clinical Global Impression Scale (CGI) (Busner & Targum 2007)	Patient perception of change	Patient-rated perception of improvement on a 5- or 7-point Likert scale. CGI scales are commonly used clinically and in research for FMD (Czarnecki et al 2012, Nielsen et al 2017a, Sharpe et al 2011)
Functional Mobility Scale (Graham et al 2004)	Mobility-related disability	Very brief scale that quantifies functional mobility by determining assistance required when walking 5, 50 and 500 m. The scale has been shown to have good validity and reliability in children with cerebral palsy (Graham et al 2004) and has been used in studies of adults with FMD (Jordbru et al 2014, Nielsen et al 2017a)
Disabilities of the Arm Shoulder and Hand (DASH) (Hudak et al 1996)	Upper limb disability	A measure of upper limb function that is not disease specific
Short Form 36 (Jenkinson et al 1994)	Health-related quality of life	A quality of life scale that yields eight health domain scores covering aspects of physical and mental health
Hospital Anxiety and Depression Scale (HADS) (Zigmond & Snaith 1983)	Anxiety and depression	A psychological screening tool that has shown to be a valid and reliable measure of anxiety and depression in and out of the hospital environment (Zigmond & Snaith 1983).
Brief Illness Perception Questionnaire (B-IPQ) (Broadbent et al 2006)	Illness beliefs	A quantitative measure of illness beliefs, shown to be valid and reliable. It produces eight dimensions that can be analysed separately or as a total score (Broadbent et al 2006).
Functional Motor Disorder Specific Outcome Measure		
Psychogenic Movement Disorders Rating Scale (Hinson et al 2005) or Simplified Functional Movement Disorders Rating Scale (S-FMDRS) (Nielsen et al 2017c)	Observed severity of movement impairment	A standardised rating scale to assess and score the severity of FMD via video. The original scale was simplified by Nielsen et al (2017c) and found to have good inter-rater reliability, validity and sensitivity. This assessment tool was designed for research and may have little clinical utility
Health Economic Analysis and Quality of Life		
EQ-5D-5L (Herdman et al 2011)	Health-related quality of life	A simple quality of life measure that is commonly used to generate quality-adjusted life years

important overarching treatment principles (Nielsen et al 2015b). These include:

- Create an expectation of improvement.
- Promote open and consistent communication between the multidisciplinary team and patient.
- Involve family and carers in treatment.
- Avoid passive treatments. When handling the patient, the aim should be to redirect attention and facilitate movement rather than support.
- Encourage early weight bearing.
- Foster independence and self-management.
- Use goal-directed rehabilitation focusing on function and automatic movement (e.g., walking) rather than the impairment (e.g., weakness) and controlled movement (e.g., strengthening exercises).
- Minimise reinforcement of maladaptive movement patterns and postures.
- Avoid use of adaptive equipment and mobility aids, although these are not always contraindicated, particularly in patients who have completed rehabilitation without improvement.
- Avoid use of splints and devices that immobilise joints.
- Recognise and challenge unhelpful thoughts and behaviours.

In the absence of sufficient evidence to produce treatment guidelines, a multidisciplinary group of clinicians with expertise in FMD produced consensus recommendations for physiotherapy intervention for FMD (Nielsen et al 2015b). The recommendations are based on a physically biased aetiological model for FMD, which conceives of the motor symptoms as involuntary but learnt patterns of movement that are driven by abnormal self-directed attention and erroneous illness beliefs. Psychosocial factors are recognised but are not the specific focus of the intervention. The authors state that the important components of physiotherapy are education, movement retraining, addressing secondary problems associated with FMD (e.g., pain and fatigue) and supporting the patient to self-manage. These components are described in the following sections.

Education

Patients with FMD commonly report confusion and a lack of understanding of their diagnosis (Nettleton et al 2005). This is problematic when it is considered that erroneous illness beliefs may be an important factor in developing and driving symptoms. Helping the patient to understand their problem in a biopsychosocial context and teaching them strategies to manage their symptoms should therefore be considered an essential part of treatment (Nielsen et al 2015b).

Jon Stone (neurologist) and Alan Carson (neuropsychiatrist) from Edinburgh have produced a large body of work describing methods of communicating the diagnosis

of FMD to patients (Carson et al 2016a, Stone 2009, Stone & Edwards 2012). Their work has been influential and widely adopted in clinical practice. Physiotherapy provides an opportunity for patients to develop further insight into their symptoms. Patient education should consider the following ingredients:

1. Use of the term *functional*, with an explanation that this refers to there being a problem with the function of the nervous system, rather than structure.
2. Acknowledge that the symptoms are real and are not imagined or 'put on'.
3. Acknowledge that FMD is a common cause of disability.
4. Explain that symptoms can improve because they are not caused by irreversible damage. However, acknowledge that improvement can take effort and time.
5. Explain how FMD is diagnosed; this may include demonstrating to the patient that their movement can be normal with distractions or explain clinical signs (such as Hoover's sign or tremor entrainment, see Table 16.2).
6. Explain that a wide variety of factors may be involved in triggering symptoms, including injury, illness and/or psychological factors.
7. Introduce the role of physical rehabilitation in 'retraining' the nervous system to help regain control over movement.
8. It may be important to discuss other terms sometimes used for FMD and the fact that some health professionals have ambivalent or negative attitudes to FMD (Ahern et al 2009, Espay et al 2009).
9. This information should be backed up with written or online information (e.g., http://www.neurosymptoms.org).

Movement Retraining

Movement retraining aims to restore normal movement patterns. The mechanisms by which movement retraining may work include:

- Altering unhelpful beliefs and expectations about movement;
- Reducing abnormal self-focus during movement and restoring 'automatically' generated movement; and
- Changing maladaptive compensatory habitual postures, movement patterns and behaviours.

Movement retraining can address unhelpful beliefs by demonstrating to the patient that their movement can be normal. This is also a powerful way to help the patient understand the diagnosis and convince them that it is correct. Stone and Edwards (2012) suggest explaining to patients with a positive Hoover's sign that this demonstrates that the 'wiring is intact' despite the patient being unable to move normally on command (Stone & Edwards 2012). During physiotherapy, normal movement can be produced in the context of meaningful activity. The key to normalise movement is to redirect the patient's focus of motor attention. For example, a functional gait disturbance often normalises when the patient is asked to walk backwards, walk up a set of stairs or during supported heel-toe stepping. Tasks that normalise movement usually involve novel or unfamiliar movements where redirection of attention away from the body/symptom is required to achieve the task. Normal movement can be demonstrated to the patient with the aid of mirrors and video.

Movement retraining usually follows a sequential approach, where elementary symptom-free components of movement are established, and built upon in successive stages to gradually reshape normal movement patterns (Czarnecki et al 2012, Trieschmann et al 1970). Asking patients to watch themselves in the mirror as they move may help to redirect attention away from their body (towards their reflection). The mirror provides feedback to help the patient shape movement, as well as providing them with evidence of normal movement (which may influence beliefs and expectations).

Movement retraining in the context of meaningful tasks, such as standing up from a chair and transferring from a chair to a bed (as opposed to, for example, hip and knee flexion-extension exercises) can helpfully direct the patient's focus towards the goal of the movement, rather than the components of movement. In this way, task practice is less likely to promote unhelpful self-focussed attention and symptom exacerbation. General principles of motor learning and skill acquisition apply to rehabilitation of patients with FMD (Nielsen 2016). These include task-orientated practice, repetition, task shaping and feedback.

Strategies that normalise movement by redirecting the patient's focus of motor attention and elicit more automatic movement can be explored during physiotherapy sessions. Often the patient has developed their own strategies. The patient is then encouraged to use strategies that normalise their movement throughout their day. Consolidation and generalisation of movement retraining is achieved by gradually increasing the difficulty of tasks, changing the environment (e.g., outdoors, busy environments), varying speeds and multitasking. Table 16.4 lists treatment ideas and movement strategies for different functional motor symptoms.

Addressing Persistent Pain and Fatigue

Comorbid chronic pain and chronic fatigue are common in patients with FMD, affecting up to 90% (Butler et al 2021). Pain and fatigue may act as predisposing, precipitating or perpetuating factors in FMD and therefore should be addressed as part of physical rehabilitation. Evidence-based treatments for both pain and fatigue include a combination of education, exercise and self-management (Butler & Moseley 2003, Hansen et al 2010, Lamb et al 2010, Moss-Morris et al 2013). Treatment is well described in the literature, and further discussion is beyond the scope of this chapter.

Self-Management

A self-management approach to treatment recognises that FMDs are often chronic conditions with multiple contributing factors that can require ongoing treatment and that setbacks and symptom relapses are common. Self-management ensures the patient is empowered to put knowledge and skills into practice to improve their health and well-being. For the patient to understand and accept the value of a self-management approach to treatment, they may require a shift in their concept of illness from a traditional biomedical model, where the patient is a passive recipient of treatment, to a biopsychosocial model, where the patient is considered an active partner in the management of their health (Boger et al 2015). Also see Chapter 19 on self-management in this textbook.

The key to fostering self-management is to help the patient to understand their problem and to learn strategies that can improve their symptoms. Self-management should be seen as an enhancement to active treatment, as opposed to handing back responsibility to patients who may already feel abandoned by the healthcare profession. One specialist centre describes the use of a rehabilitation workbook to support self-management within physiotherapy (Nielsen et al 2015a, 2017a). The workbook is completed with support from the clinician during the course of treatment and contains information regarding FMD, goal setting, markers of progress (e.g., charting progression on an outcome measure score), personalised treatment strategies, the patient's personal reflections on treatment sessions and plans for managing difficult days and setbacks.

CONSIDERATIONS FOR TREATMENT

Recognising Comorbidities

Coexisting symptoms make a significant contribution to the illness burden of most patients with FMD. Common comorbidities include migraine, chronic pain, fatigue, anxiety, depression, urinary retention and gastrointestinal symptoms. An improvement in FMD with physical rehabilitation may have a positive impact on other health problems. Conversely, there may be some situations where the comorbidity needs to be addressed, either before or in parallel to FMD for progress to be made.

In this chapter we have suggested that psychopathology should be considered a risk factor for developing

TABLE 16.4	**Symptom-Specific Treatment Ideas**
Functional gait disorder and lower limb weakness	Following a sequential motor learning approach is a well-described treatment strategy for functional gait disorder and lower limb weakness. This involves helping the patient to master simple elements of movement and gradually building the complexity as treatment progresses.
	If the patient can take some weight through their lower limbs, retraining sit to stand is a good starting place. Sit to stand often improves within a single session, which can be motivating for the patient. The fear of falling can be reduced by practicing in a safe environment, such as between two raised plinths. A mirror positioned in front of the patient can help to redirect their attention, discourage them from looking down and provide visual feedback.
	Early standing with rhythmical weight shift in a safe environment can help to trigger automatic muscle recruitment. Encourage rhythmical lateral and/or anterior-posterior weight shift, aiming to redirect the patient's focus of attention away from their legs and towards the action of weight shifting. This can be progressed to stepping and walking.
	Novel walking movements such as stepping backwards, sideways, or turning in circles can trigger more appropriate movement patterns in problems of gait coordination. Asking a patient to walk by sliding their feet along the floor (as if wearing skis) can sometimes trigger ankle dorsiflexor muscle activity in patients with a functional-foot drop presentation.
	Treadmill walking with feedback from a mirror can help to generate more automatic stepping. The use of a body weight support harness may be helpful initially to build confidence where fear of falling is part of the problem.
Upper limb weakness	Dense upper limb weakness is rare, but when present a good starting point is weight bearing to generate automatic muscle activity.
	A more common presentation is mild weakness with a common complaint being a tendency to drop things. Start by helping the patient to minimise habitual nonuse by identifying unhelpful habits (such as hiding the affected hand in a pocket) and instead maximising opportunities to use the affected limb.
	Practice bilateral hand tasks that are familiar or important to the patient that may not be associated with their symptoms (e.g., use of mobile telephone or computer tablet). Use speed, rhythm and weight bearing to encourage activity.
	Electrical muscle stimulation can be a useful adjunct in treatment sessions for upper limb or lower limb weakness.
Tremor	Minimise unhelpful coping strategies, such as sitting on the hand or tensing the muscles in an attempt to suppress the tremor.
	There is often a pattern of excessive proximal muscle activity in the limb which might be driving the tremor. In this case learning to relax the proximal muscles can be a good starting point.
	Moving in front of a mirror can help to shift attentional focus away from the internal sensory experience of the tremor. Experiment with competing movements that require a redirection of motor attention, or imposing an active movement on top of the tremor (e.g., shoulder rolling, clapping to a rhythm or moving the arms in large fluid movements as if conducting an orchestra).
	Breathing exercises for relaxation is useful for some patients, particularly when a resting tremor interferes with the ability to get to sleep.

(Continued)

TABLE 16.4 Symptom-Specific Treatment Ideas—cont'd

Fixed functional dystonia	If pain and allodynia are present, then this will need to be considered throughout treatment. Pain physiology education along with a graded desensitisation and movement/activity plan may be required.
	Addressing unhelpful habitual resting postures is an important starting point and often a continuing focus for therapy. Patients typically rest with the affected limb in the dystonic position, reinforcing the abnormal posture and movement. Ask the patient to think about all of their resting positions over a 24-hour period and help them to find ways to maximise time spent in positions of more optimal joint alignment. When trying to achieve resting postures with relaxed muscles, surface contact is desirable as opposed to the limb hanging. It can be helpful to explain why neutral positions might feel unpleasant or unnatural with reference to changes in perceptual brain-body maps (i.e., cortical representation of the body (Stone et al 2012).
	Experiment with different ways to normalise muscle activity around a joint. Weight bearing with rhythmical movement can help to trigger reciprocal muscle activation and relaxation around the joint, thereby helping to turn down overactive muscles. For example, anterior-posterior weight shift in standing may reduce plantarflexor muscle activity, or the action of sit to stand can help to relax ankle equinovarus posturing through reciprocal muscle inhibition. Electrical muscle stimulation of the antagonist muscles can sometimes be helpful in achieving improved limb posture during therapy and may be useful to retrain movement if the patient is able to tolerate the sensation.
	Passive stretching, splinting and any form of immobilisation can exacerbate the posturing activity and therefore have detrimental effects in some cases. Instead, if possible, the patient should be supported to move the joint through available range within activity and through therapeutic resting postures.
	Although there is limited evidence, botulinum toxin injections are often used in patients with fixed functional dystonia and muscle pain. Although the evidence suggests that the mode of action is likely to be mostly placebo (Dreissen et al 2019), it may be a reasonable treatment adjunct to consider if other approaches to treatment have failed.
Jerks/myoclonus/ functional tics	In the case of paroxysmal symptoms, it can be helpful to explore with the patient any premonitory sensations, feelings or urges they might experience just before the unwanted movement. Patients can sometimes learn to effectively use a therapeutic strategy such as a competing movement, distraction or mindful activity before the unwanted movement occurs. Self-focus and hypervigilance are typically part of functional jerks, but patients often do not initially recognise that they are overattending to their body.
	Other treatment strategies include addressing habitual postures and behaviours that might be feeding into overactive muscle groups. Breath holding and abdominal bracing are common.
	Experiment with opposing movements that interfere with the abnormal movement pattern (e.g., deep breathing exercises or trunk rotations for abdominal jerks, scapula retraction exercises for upper limb or head/neck functional tics). Desensitise and lengthen overactive tight muscles through therapeutic resting postures and movement rather than aggressive stretching.
Persistent postural perceptual dizziness (PPPD)	Patients with PPPD often present with balance and gait problems. The already described approach to functional gait can be helpful. Set up the environment to make the patient feel safe to explore movement while gradually breaking maladaptive habits such as a fixed head position and fixed gaze to avoid provoking dizziness.
	There is emerging evidence for a CBT informed physiotherapy approach for PPPD (Herdman et al 2022). In addition to movement retraining, this approach integrates the CBT model to address avoidance behaviours with behavioural experiments and graded exposure. Patients may not tolerate eye-tracking exercises, in which case they may not achieve desensitisation using traditional vestibular rehabilitation approaches.

Adapted from Nielsen et al (2015b).

FMD rather than a primary cause. This may include complex problems such as personality disorder and self-harm (Binzer et al 1997). When such problems are present, in the interest of safety, rehabilitation may be best placed under the supervision of a psychiatrist or within a multidisciplinary team.

Medications

Often patients with FMD take high doses of sedating medications, including benzodiazepines, opioids and muscle relaxants such as baclofen. This may be a barrier to successful rehabilitation when concentration, attention and muscle power are affected. Commencing physical rehabilitation may be an opportunity to reduce and come off unnecessary medications.

Nonepileptic Seizures and Physiotherapy

As described earlier in the chapter, some patients with FMD also experience DSs. If a patient referred for physical rehabilitation has a history of DS, it is recommended that a plan of what to do in the event of a seizure is arranged in advance with the patient. In most cases this includes ensuring the patient is safe, removing objects from the surrounding environment that may cause harm, not restraining the patient, placing a pillow under their head if appropriate and remaining calm. Often it can be helpful to talk the patient calmly through the event (for more information, see http://www.neurosymptoms.org). It is usually not appropriate to call an ambulance for a DS, unless the patient sustains an injury, the attack is unusually prolonged or there are other signs of danger.

Adaptive Aids, Equipment and Environmental Modifications

It is generally recommended that aids and adaptations should be avoided in the rehabilitation of patients with FMD. Adaptations can prevent the return of normal movement patterns and result in secondary problems such as pain and deconditioning. Splints, orthoses and casts can draw attention to the body and therefore often exacerbate functional motor symptoms. Joint immobilisation in casts and splints has been associated with the onset and exacerbation of FFD and therefore may be directly harmful (Schrag et al 2004).

In some cases it may be appropriate or necessary to provide adaptive equipment. For example, if a patient has not made progress after completing suitable treatment, it may be appropriate to issue a wheelchair or other mobility aids to enable discharge from hospital, increase independence and improve quality of life. In this case, the patient should be involved in the decision, having been made aware of the benefits and potential for harm. A plan can be put in place

to limit the potential negative impact, such as identifying opportunities for a wheelchair-using patient to engage in daily weight-bearing activity. Decisions and advice should be well documented, and the patient should be followed up to monitor use of the equipment.

Functional Motor Disorder and Falls

It is generally considered that patients with FMD are at low risk for falls and injury, despite movement patterns (such as walking on ice gait) that may suggest otherwise. It may therefore be appropriate to take greater apparent risks in this population while progressing independent ambulation. Often low confidence and a fear of falling is a limiting factor, which may need to be addressed. However, injuries including fractures are reported in some patients with FMD (Nielsen et al 2017a), and the situation may be more complicated if there is a history of self-harming behaviour. In this situation, rehabilitation decisions should be supported by a multidisciplinary team.

Treatment Intensity, Duration and Setting

There is insufficient evidence to determine the most effective treatment parameters and they are likely to differ between patients. Some treatment programmes report benefit from short-duration, high-intensity treatment over consecutive days in patients without irritable pain and fatigue (Czarnecki et al 2012, Nielsen et al 2015a, Nielsen 2016). Inpatient interventions have the advantage of removing the patient from social and environmental factors that may be perpetuating their problem to focus on treatment, although domiciliary interventions have the advantage of being able to address relevant environmental issues and may be able to provide less intensive treatment over a longer duration. Specialist inpatient multidisciplinary treatments for FMD are described in the literature, with admission times reported from 4 weeks to several months (Demartini et al 2014, McCormack et al 2013, Moene et al 2002).

Concluding Treatment

Symptom relapse and setbacks are common after improvement with rehabilitation for FMD (Nielsen et al 2013). It is therefore important to prepare the patient for this event before concluding treatment. For example, the therapist can explain that setbacks are common and reassure the patient that they are usually transitory. A relapse management plan can include identifying potential factors that may precipitate a setback, such as ill health, exacerbation of chronic pain/fatigue, overdoing things, stress and anxiety. The plan to address a setback may include encouraging relative rest, identifying and addressing issues that may have triggered the setback, graded return to normal activity and revisiting the movement strategies that were part of the initial treatment plan.

It is important to recognise that some patients may not improve with rehabilitation. In this case, the focus of treatment may need to be directed towards disability management and adaptations to improve quality of life. Offering some patients intermittent follow up may help to limit deterioration over time. In reality, complete symptom resolution in patients with chronic FMD symptoms is rare, and there are other markers of a good treatment outcome that should be acknowledged, for example, reduced health service use, avoidance of iatrogenic harm by prevention of unnecessary medical procedures, improved quality of life and reduced distress from symptoms.

CONCLUSION

FMD is a common cause of disability and distress amongst patients seen in neurological practice. Prognosis is considered poor, although there is growing evidence that rehabilitation based on movement retraining is effective for many patients. Current evidence and expert opinion suggest that physical rehabilitation should be informed by a biopsychosocial understanding of the patient's problem and include education, movement retraining and self-management skills, ideally within a multidisciplinary team. An understanding that functional motor symptoms are driven by self-focused attention should underpin physiotherapy interventions. More research is required to define the mechanisms responsible for symptoms, develop specific treatment strategies and allow for the production of evidence-based treatment guidelines.

CASE STUDY

Jenny was referred to physiotherapy with a diagnosis of functional weakness. She is 42 years old, a mother of two school-aged children and has a partner who works full time.

Jenny's problem started 6 months previously during a particularly busy day at work. She had been suffering from a migraine but felt she could not take any more time off. Her colleagues noticed that her speech was slurred, and Jenny had a feeling of numbness down her left side. Concerned that she was having a stroke, her colleagues called an ambulance and she was rushed to hospital. She was admitted to the acute stroke ward and had an MRI, which was reported as normal. Following this, she had several other investigations including a lumber puncture, which she remembers being a particularly unpleasant experience. Immediately after the lumbar puncture, she noticed her left arm and leg felt weak, and Jenny remembers feeling very frightened.

After 2 days in hospital, Jenny was told by a doctor that all her tests were normal, that there was nothing wrong with her and she could go home. She was told that her symptoms were probably brought on by stress, which confused Jenny, as she did not feel as though she was any more stressed than usual when her symptoms started. She was discharged from hospital, walking with a quad-stick. Over the following weeks her speech returned to normal, but there was no significant change to the left-sided weakness.

The physiotherapist completed a thorough subjective assessment, documenting the onset of symptoms. It was clear that this had been a very frightening experience for Jenny and that she did not have a good understanding of what was wrong. Jenny reported left-sided weakness, right hip pain and fatigue. She required assistance with washing and dressing and meal preparation, and she had started to rely on an attendant-propelled wheelchair for outdoor mobility. She had not fallen but had experienced several near falls, which left her frightened of falling.

On physical assessment, Jenny had a positive Hoover's sign (see Table 16.5). She walked with a quad-stick in her right hand and her left leg dragged behind her. She was dependent on right upper limb support to stand and transfer. When the physiotherapist assisted Jenny to step backwards, her movement appeared less symptomatic.

Jenny completed a block of treatment, which included physiotherapy and occupational therapy. Treatment started with education about the diagnosis of FMD. Jenny reported feeling relieved to finally have some understanding of what was wrong and that FMD was a real problem and not just 'all in her head'. The therapist showed Jenny how certain manoeuvres seemed to trigger automatic normal movement, such as walking backwards and side-to-side weight shift. This made Jenny feel that further improvement was possible and helped to rebuild her confidence. Movement retraining started with sit to stand, practicing in a safe environment between two raised plinths and in front of a mirror. Within a single session, Jenny's sit to stand improved significantly. Having the raised plinths on either side of the chair for upper limb support gave Jenny the confidence to take more weight through her left leg and use momentum and forward weight transference. Gait retraining also started in the safe environment between two raised plinths. Initially Jenny practiced standing with rhythmical side-to-side weight shift, with only fingertip support on the plinths. This was progressed to taking very small steps while maintaining the side-to-side weight shift rhythm, stepping with facilitatory support from the physiotherapist. Treadmill training was also used. At times Jenny's gait pattern would break down or she would experience difficulty initiating steps. On these occasions, initiating movement through

TABLE 16.5 **Case Study Problem List, Goals and Plan**

Problem List	Goals	Plans
Lack of knowledge and understanding of the diagnosis	For Jenny and her husband to have a better understanding of the diagnosis of FMD	Education about FMD: This includes helping Jenny to make sense of the events leading up to the onset of her symptoms and the role of self-directed attention in exacerbating functional symptoms. This information will be documented in her physiotherapy workbook.
Asymmetrical sit to stand movement pattern	To be able to stand up and sit down with an efficient, symmetrical movement pattern from a variety of different chair heights	Retrain sit to stand movement in front of a mirror. Focus on starting posture, forward weight transfer, symmetry and momentum.
Altered walking pattern	To be able to walk unaided with a symmetrical pattern	Retrain simple elements of gait between two raised plinths. Experiment with strategies to trigger automatic muscle activity in the left leg (e.g., using weight shift, different speeds, sliding feet). Build the complexity of the movement elements and gradually shape into an appropriate walking pattern. Progress to treadmill training and then walking in more challenging environments.
Fatigue and pain	To create a self-management plan for fatigue and pain	Education about pain and fatigue, including the role of boom-bust patterns of activity and the importance of graded exercise, activity and relative rest. Help Jenny to create an activity plan by setting a baseline level of activity. Jenny should be encouraged to plan to complete a similar level of activity each day of the week and schedule regular rest periods. She should plan to increase the activity level very slowly in an incremental fashion over the coming months.

slow, gentle weight shift was a useful strategy to trigger automatic movement. In occupational therapy, Jenny practiced movement strategies during activities of daily living, which included washing and dressing, meal preparation and shopping.

During rehabilitation, Jenny completed a workbook. This included information about FMD and specific examples of how she could integrate physiotherapy and occupational therapy strategies into everyday life. Jenny wrote out a graded activity plan to help increase her activity slowly while avoiding boom-bust activity cycles. She also wrote out a plan for what she would do on difficult days, when her movement was worse. By the end of Jenny's block of treatment, her movement appeared to return to normal, although she reported feeling some residual left-sided numbness and weakness after overdoing things. Her right hip pain had improved now that she was weight bearing more equally. She scored full marks on the Berg Balance Scale and made a significant improvement in her 10-metre walk time. Jenny had ongoing support from occupational therapy for negotiating a graded return to work plan with her employers.

SELF-ASSESSMENT QUESTIONS

1. Describe the aetiology of FMD in terms of a biopsychosocial framework.
2. Describe the rationale for physical rehabilitation of FMD.
3. Identify important overarching principles for the treatment of FMD.
4. Identify the roles of the multidisciplinary team in the treatment of FMD.
5. Discuss the risks associated with mobility aids, adaptations, splints and casts in FMD.

REFERENCES

Ahern, L., Stone, J., Sharpe, M.C., 2009. Attitudes of neuro-science nurses toward patients with conversion symptoms. Psychosomatics. 50, 336–339.

American Psychiatric Association, 2022. Diagnostic and Statistical Manual of Mental Disorders: DSM-5-TR. American Psychiatric Publishing, Arlington.

Aybek, S., Perez, D.L., 2022. Diagnosis and Management of Functional Neurological Disorder. BMJ. 376, o64.

Aybek, S., Vuilleumier, P., 2017. Imaging studies of functional neurologic disorders. In: Hallett, M., Stone, J., Carson, A. (Eds.), Functional Neurologic Disorders, Vol 139 of the Handbook of Clinical Neurology Series. Elsevier, Amsterdam, pp. 73–84.

Baker, J., Barnett, C., Cavalli, L., et al., 2021. Management of functional communication, swallowing, cough and related disorders: consensus recommendations for speech and language therapy. J. Neurol. Neurosurg. Psychiatry. 92, 1112–1125.

Berg, K.O., Wood-Dauphinee, S.L., Williams, J.I., Maki, B., 1992. Measuring balance in the elderly: validation of an instrument. Can. J. Public. Health. 83 (Suppl. 2), S7–S11.

Binzer, M., Andersen, P.M., Kullgren, G., 1997. Clinical characteristics of patients with motor disability due to conversion disorder: a prospective control group study. J. Neurol. Neurosurg. Psychiatry. 63, 83–88.

Boger, E., Ellis, J., Latter, S., et al., 2015. Self-management and self-management support outcomes: a systematic review and mixed research synthesis of stakeholder views. PLoS One. 10, e0130990.

Broadbent, E., Petrie, K.J., Main, J., Weinman, J., 2006. The brief illness perception questionnaire. J. Psychosom. Res. 60, 631–637.

Brown, R., Reuber, M., 2016. Psychological and psychiatric aspects of psychogenic non-epileptic seizures (PNES): a systematic review. Clin. Psychol. Rev. 45, 157–182.

Brown, R.J., 2016. Dissociation and functional neurologic disorders. In: Hallett, M., Stone, J., Carson, A. (Eds.), Functional Neurologic Disorders, Vol 139 of the Handbook of Clinical Neurology Series. Elsevier, Amsterdam, pp. 85–94.

Busner, J., Targum, S.D., 2007. The clinical global impressions scale: applying a research tool in clinical practice. Psychiatry (Edgmont). 4, 28–37.

Butler, M., Shipston-Sharman, O., Seynaeve, 2021. International online survey of 1048 individuals with functional neurological disorder. Eur. J. Neurol. 28, 3591–3602.

Butler, D.S., Moseley, G.L., 2003. Explain Pain. Noigroup. Publications, Adelaide.

Carson, A., Brown, R., David, A.S., et al., 2012. Functional (conversion) neurological symptoms: research since the millennium. J. Neurol. Neurosurg. Psychiatry. 83, 842–850.

Carson, A., Lehn, A., 2016. Epidemiology. In: Hallett, M., Stone, J., Carson, A. (Eds.), Functional Neurologic Disorders, Vol 139 of the Handbook of Clinical Neurology Series. Elsevier, Amsterdam, pp. 47–60.

Carson, A., Lehn, A., Ludwig, L., Stone, J., 2016a. Explaining functional disorders in the neurology clinic: a photo story. Pract. Neurol. 16, 56–61.

Carson, A., Ludwig, L., Welch, K., 2016b. Psychologic theories in functional neurologic disorders. In: Hallett, M., Stone, J., Carson, A. (Eds.), Functional Neurologic Disorders, Vol 139 of the Handbook of Clinical Neurology Series. Elsevier, Amsterdam, pp. 105–120.

Carson, A., Stone, J., Hibberd, C., et al., 2011. Disability, distress and unemployment in neurology outpatients with symptoms "unexplained by organic disease.". J. Neurol. Neurosurg. Psychiatry. 82, 810–813.

Czarnecki, K., Thompson, J.M., Seime, R., Geda, Y.E., Duffy, J.R., Ahlskog, J.E., 2012. Functional movement disorders: successful treatment with a physical therapy rehabilitation protocol. Parkinsonism. Relat. Disord. 18, 247–251.

Dallocchio, C., Arbasino, C., Klersy, C., Marchioni, E., 2010. The effects of physical activity on psychogenic movement disorders. Mov. Disord. 25, 421–425.

Dallocchio, C., Tinazzi, M., Bombieri, F., Arnó, N., Erro, R., 2016. Cognitive behavioural therapy and adjunctive physical activity for functional movement disorders (Conversion Disorder): a pilot, single-blinded, randomized study. Psychother. Psychosom. 85, 381–383.

Daum, C., Hubschmid, M., Aybek, S., 2014. The value of "positive" clinical signs for weakness, sensory and gait disorders in conversion disorder: a systematic and narrative review. J. Neurol. Neurosurg. Psychiatry. 85, 180–190.

de Lau, L.M., Breteler, M.M., 2006. Epidemiology of Parkinson's disease. Lancet. Neurol. 5, 525–535.

Demartini, B., Batla, A., Petrochilos, P., Fisher, L., Edwards, M.J., Joyce, E., 2014. Multidisciplinary treatment for functional neurological symptoms: a prospective study. J. Neurol. 261, 2370–2377.

Dreissen, Y.E.M., Cath, D.C., Tijssen, M.A.J., 2016. Functional jerks, tics, and paroxysmal movement disorders. In: Hallett, M., Stone, J., Carson, A. (Eds.), Functional Neurologic Disorders, Vol 139 of the Handbook of Clinical Neurology Series. Amsterdam, pp. 247–258.

Dreissen, Y.E.M., Dijk, J.M., Gelauff, J.M., et al., 2019. Botulinum neurotoxin treatment in jerky and tremulous functional movement disorders: a double-blind, randomised placebo-controlled trial with an open-label extension. J. Neurol. Neurosurg. Psychiatry. 90, 1244–1250.

Edwards, M.J., Adams, R.A., Brown, H., Parees, I., Friston, K.J., 2012. A Bayesian account of "hysteria. Brain. 135, 3495–3512.

Edwards, M.J., Alonso-Canovas, A., Schrag, A., Bloem, B.R., Thompson, P.D., Bhatia, K., 2011. Limb amputations in fixed dystonia: a form of body integrity identity disorder? Mov. Disord. 26, 1410–1414.

Edwards, M.J., Bhatia, K.P., 2012. Functional (psychogenic) movement disorders: merging mind and brain. Lancet. Neurol. 11, 250–260.

Edwards, M.J., Fotopoulou, A., Parees, I., 2013. Neurobiology of functional (psychogenic) movement disorders. Curr. Opin. Neurol. 26, 442–447.

Edwards, M.J., Stone, J., and Lang, A.E., 2014. From psychogenic movement disorder to functional movement disorder: It's time to change the name. Mov Disord. 29, 849–852.

Erro, R., Edwards, M.J., Bhatia, K.P., Esposito, M., Farmer, S.F., Cordivari, C., 2014. Psychogenic axial myoclonus: clinical features and long-term outcome. Parkinsonism. Relat. Disord. 20, 596–599.

Espay, A.J., Goldenhar, L.M., Voon, V., Schrag, A., Burton, N., Lang, A.E., 2009. Opinions and clinical practices related to diagnosing and managing patients with psychogenic movement disorders: an international survey of movement disorder society members. Mov. Disord. 24, 1366–1374.

Espay, A.J., Lang, A.E., 2015. Phenotype-specific diagnosis of functional (psychogenic) movement disorders. Curr. Neurol. Neurosci. Rep. 15, 32.

Fahn, S., Olanow, C.W., 2014. "Psychogenic movement disorders": they are what they are. Mov. Disord. 29, 853–856.

Friston, K., 2010. The free-energy principle: a unified brain theory? Nat. Rev. Neurosci. 11, 127–138.

Functional Neurological Disorder Society, 2020. Functional Neurological Disorder Society (FNDS). Available at: https://www.fndsociety.org/. Accessed April 20, 2022.

Fung, V.S.C., 2016. Functional gait disorder. In: Hallett, M., Stone, J., Carson, A. (Eds.), Functional Neurologic Disorders, Vol 139 of the Handbook of Clinical Neurology Series. Elsevier, Amsterdam, pp. 263–270.

Ganos, C., Edwards, M.J., Bhatia, K.P., 2014. The phenomenology of functional (psychogenic) dystonia. Mov. Disord. Clin. Pract. 1, 36–44.

Garrett, A.R., Hodges, S.D., Stahlman, S., 2020. Epidemiology of functional neurological disorder, active component, U.S. Armed Forces, 2000-2018. MSMR. 27, 16–22.

Gelauff, J., Stone, J., Edwards, M.J., Carson, A., 2014. The prognosis of functional (psychogenic) motor symptoms: a systematic review. J. Neurol. Neurosurg. Psychiatry. 85, 220–226.

Goetz, C.G., 2016. Charcot, hysteria, and simulated disorders. In: Hallett, M., Stone, J., Carson, A. (Eds.), Functional Neurologic Disorders, Vol 139 of the Handbook of Clinical Neurology Series. Elsevier, Amsterdam, pp. 11–23.

Goldstein, L.H., Robinson, E.J., Mellers, J.D.C., et al., 2020. Cognitive behavioural therapy for adults with dissociative seizures (CODES): a pragmatic, multicentre, randomised controlled trial. Lancet. Psychiatry. 7, 491–505.

Goodin, D., 2014. The epidemiology of multiple sclerosis: insights to disease pathogenesis. In: Goodin, D. (Ed.), Multiple Sclerosis and Related Disorders, Vol 122 of the Handbook of Clinical Neurology. Elsevier, Amsterdam, pp. 231–266.

Graham, H.K., Harvey, A., Rodda, J., Nattrass, G.R., Pirpiris, M., 2004. The functional mobility scale (FMS). J. Pediatr. Orthop. 24, 514–520.

Gutkin, M., McLean, L., Brown, R., Kanaan, R.A., 2021. Systematic review of psychotherapy for adults with functional neurological disorder. J. Neurol. Neurosurg. Psychiatry. 92, 36–44.

Hallett, M., Aybek, S., Dworetzky, B.A., McWhirter, L., Staab, J.P., Stone, J., 2022. Functional neurological disorder: new subtypes and shared mechanisms. Lancet. Neurol. 21, 537–550.

Hansen, Z., Daykin, A., Lamb, S.E., 2010. A cognitive-behavioural programme for the management of low back pain in primary care: a description and justification of the intervention used in the Back Skills Training Trial (BeST; ISRCTN 54717854). Physiotherapy. 96, 87–94.

Herdman, D., Norton, S., Murdin, L., Frost, K., Pavlou, M., Moss-Morris, R., 2022. The INVEST trial: a randomised feasibility trial of psychologically informed vestibular rehabilitation versus current gold standard physiotherapy for people with Persistent Postural Perceptual Dizziness. J. Neurol. 269, 4753–4763.

Herdman, M., Gudex, C., Lloyd, A., et al., 2011. Development and preliminary testing of the new five-level version of EQ-5D (EQ-5D-5L). Qual. Life. Res. 20, 1727–1736.

Hinson, V.K., Cubo, E., Comella, C.L., Goetz, C.G., Leurgans, S., 2005. Rating scale for psychogenic movement disorders: scale development and clinimetric testing. Mov. Disord. 20, 1592–1597.

Hubschmid, M., Aybek, S., Maccaferri, G.E., et al., 2015. Efficacy of brief interdisciplinary psychotherapeutic intervention for motor conversion disorder and nonepileptic attacks. Gen. Hosp. Psychiatry. 37, 448–455.

Hudak, P.L., Amadio, P.C., Bombardier, C., 1996. Development of an upper extremity outcome measure: the DASH (disabilities of the arm, shoulder and hand) [corrected]. The Upper Extremity Collaborative Group (UECG). Am. J. Ind. Med. 29, 602–608.

Jankovic, J., 2011. Diagnosis and treatment of psychogenic parkinsonism. J. Neurol. Neurosurg. Psychiatry. 82, 1300–1303.

Jenkinson, C., Wright, L., Coulter, A., 1994. Criterion validity and reliability of the SF-36 in a population sample. Qual. Life Res. 3, 7–12.

Jordbru, A.A., Smedstad, L.M., Klungsøyr, O., Martinsen, E.W., 2014. Psychogenic gait disorder: a randomized controlled trial of physical rehabilitation with one-year follow-up. J. Rehabil. Med. 46, 181–187.

Kanaan, R.A.A., 2016. Freud's hysteria and its legacy. In: Hallett, M., Stone, J., Carson, A. (Eds.), Functional Neurologic Disorders, Vol 139 of the Handbook of Clinical Neurology Series. Elsevier, Amsterdam, pp. 37–44.

Kletenik, I., Holden, S.K., Sillau, S.H., et al., 2022. Gender disparity and abuse in functional movement disorders: a multicenter case-control study. J. Neurol. 269, 3258–3263.

Kompoliti, K., Wilson, B., Stebbins, G., Bernard, B., Hinson, V., 2014. Immediate vs. delayed treatment of psychogenic movement disorders with short term psychodynamic psychotherapy: randomized clinical trial. Parkinsonism. Relat. Disord. 20, 60–63.

Kranick, S., Ekanayake, V., Martinez, V., Ameli, R., Hallett, M., Voon, V., 2011. Psychopathology and psychogenic movement disorders. Mov. Disord. 26, 1844–1850.

La Porta, F., Caselli, S., Susassi, S., Cavallini, P., Tennant, A., Franceschini, M., 2012. Is the Berg Balance Scale an internally valid and reliable measure of balance across different etiologies in neurorehabilitation? A revisited Rasch analysis study. Arch. Phys. Med. Rehabil. 93, 1209–1216.

Lamb, S.E., Lall, R., Hansen, Z., et al., 2010. A multicentred randomised controlled trial of a primary care-based cognitive behavioural programme for low back pain. The Back Skills

Training (BeST) trial. Health. Technol. Assess. (Rockv). 14, 1–128.

Lidstone, S.C., Costa-Parke, M., Robinson, E.J., Ercoli, T., Stone, J., 2022. Functional movement disorder gender, age and phenotype study: a systematic review and individual patient meta-analysis of 4905 cases. J. Neurol. Neurosurg. Psychiatry. 93, 609–616.

Ludwig, L., Pasman, J.A., Nicholson, T., et al., 2018. Stressful life events and maltreatment in conversion (functional neurological) disorder: systematic review and meta-analysis of case-control studies. Lancet. Psychiatry. 5, 307–320.

Macerollo, A., Chen, J.-C., Pareés, I., Kassavetis, P., Kilner, J.M., Edwards, M.J., 2015. Sensory attenuation assessed by sensory evoked potentials in functional movement disorders. PLoS One. 10, 1–6.

Matthews, A., Brown, M., Stone, J., 2016. Inpatient physiotherapy for functional (psychogenic) gait disorder: a case series of 35 patients. Mov. Disord. Clin. Pract. 28, 93–96.

McCormack, R., Moriarty, J., Mellers, J.D., et al., 2013. Specialist inpatient treatment for severe motor conversion disorder: a retrospective comparative study. J. Neurol. Neurosurg. Psychiatry. 85, 895–900.

Micale, M.S., 1993. On the "disappearance" of hysteria. A study in the clinical deconstruction of a diagnosis. Isis. 84, 496–526.

Moene, F.C., Spinhoven, P., Hoogduin, K.A.L., van Dyck, R., 2002. A randomised controlled clinical trial on the additional effect of hypnosis in a comprehensive treatment programme for in-patients with conversion disorder of the motor type. Psychother. Psychosom. 71, 66–76.

Moss-Morris, R., Deary, V., Castell, B., 2013. Chronic fatigue syndrome. Handbook. Clin. Neurol. 110, 303–314.

Nettleton, S., Watt, I., O'Malley, L., Duffey, P., 2005. Understanding the narratives of people who live with medically unexplained illness. Patient. Educ. Couns. 56, 205–210.

Nicholson, C., Edwards, M.J., Carson, A.J., et al., 2020. Occupational therapy consensus recommendations for functional neurological disorder. J. Neurol. Neurosurg. Psychiatry. 91, 1037–1045.

Nielsen, G., 2016. Physical treatment of functional neurologic disorders. In: Hallett, M., Stone, J., Carson, A. (Eds.), Functional Neurologic Disorders, Vol 139 of the Handbook of Clinical Neurology Series. Elsevier, Amsterdam, pp. 555–569.

Nielsen, G., Buszewicz, M., Stevenson, F., et al., 2017a. Randomised feasibility study of physiotherapy for patients with functional motor symptoms. J. Neurol. Neurosurg. Psychiatry. 88, 484–490.

Nielsen, G., Edwards, M.J., Stone, J., 2017b. Functional disorders presenting to the stroke service. In: Caplan, L., Biller, J., Leary, M., Thomas, A., Lo, E., Yenari, M., John, Z. (Eds.), Primer on Cerebrovascular Diseases. Elsevier, Amsterdam, pp. 623–630.

Nielsen, G., Ricciardi, L., Demartini, B., Hunter, R., Joyce, E., Edwards, M.J., 2015a. Outcomes of a 5-day physiotherapy programme for functional (psychogenic) motor disorders. J. Neurol. 262, 674–681.

Nielsen, G., Ricciardi, L., Meppelink, A., Holt, K., Teodoro, T., Edwards, M.J., 2017c. A simplified version of the Psychogenic Movement Disorders Rating Scale: The Simplified Functional

Movement Disorders Rating Scale (S-FMDRS). Mov. Disord. Clin. Pract. 4, 710–716.

Nielsen, G., Stone, J., Buszewicz, M., et al., 2019. Physio4FMD: protocol for a multicentre randomised controlled trial of specialist physiotherapy for functional motor disorder. BMC Neurol. 19, 242.

Nielsen, G., Stone, J., Edwards, M.J., 2013. Physiotherapy for functional (psychogenic) motor symptoms: a systematic review. J. Psychosom. Res 75, 93–102.

Nielsen, G., Stone, J., Matthews, A., et al., 2015b. Physiotherapy for functional motor disorders: a consensus recommendation. J. Neurol. Neurosurg. Psychiatry. 86, 1113–1119.

Pareés, I., Brown, H., Nuruki, A., et al., 2014a. Loss of sensory attenuation in patients with functional (psychogenic) movement disorders. Brain. 137, 2916–2921.

Pareés, I., Kojovic, M., Pires, C., et al., 2014b. Physical precipitating factors in functional movement disorders. J. Neurol. Sci. 338, 174–177.

Pearce, J.M.S., 2014. Before Charcot. Front. Neurol. Neurosci. 35, 1–10.

Peters, D.M., Fritz, S.L., Krotish, D.E., 2013. Assessing the reliability and validity of a shorter walk test compared with the 10-meter walk test for measurements of gait speed in healthy, older adults. J. Geriatr. Phys. Ther. 36, 24–30.

Phillips, W., Price, J., Molyneux, P.D., Deeley, Q., 2022. Hypnosis. Pract. Neurol. 22, 42–47.

Pick, S., Anderson, D.G., Asadi-Pooya, A.A., et al., 2020. Outcome measurement in functional neurological disorder: a systematic review and recommendations. J. Neurol. Neurosurg. Psychiatry. 91, 638–649.

Pollak, T.A., Nicholson, T.R., Edwards, M.J., David, A.S., 2014. A systematic review of transcranial magnetic stimulation in the treatment of functional (conversion) neurological symptoms. J. Neurol. Neurosurg. Psychiatry. 85, 191–197.

Popkirov, S., Hoeritzauer, I., Colvin, L., Carson, A.J., Stone, J., 2018. Complex regional pain syndrome and functional neurological disorders: time for reconciliation. J. Neurol. Neurosurg. Psychiatry. 90, 608–614.

Schrag, A., Trimble, M., Quinn, N., Bhatia, K., 2004. The syndrome of fixed dystonia: an evaluation of 103 patients. Brain 127, 2360–2372.

Sharpe, M., Walker, J., Williams, C., et al., 2011. Guided self-help for functional (psychogenic) symptoms: a randomized controlled efficacy trial. Neurology. 77, 564–572.

Staab, J.P., Eckhardt-Henn, A., Horii, A., Jacob, R., Strupp, M., Brandt, T., Bronstein, A., 2017. Diagnostic criteria for persistent postural-perceptual dizziness (PPPD): consensus document of the committee for the classification of vestibular disorders of the barany society. J. Vestib. Res. Equilib. Orientat. 27, 191–208.

Stone, J., 2016a. Neurologic approaches to hysteria, psychogenic and functional disorders from the late 19th century onwards. In: Hallett, M., Stone, J., Carson, A. (Eds.), Functional Neurologic Disorders, Vol 139 of the Handbook of Clinical Neurology Series. Elsevier, Amsterdam, pp. 25–36.

Stone, J., 2016b. Functional neurological disorders: the neurological assessment as treatment. Pract. Neurol. 16, 7–17.

Stone, J., 2009. The bare essentials: functional symptoms in neurology. Pract. Neurol. 9, 179–189.

Stone, J., Aybek, S., 2017. Functional limb weakness and paralysis. In: Hallett, M., Stone, J., Carson, A. (Eds.), Functional Neurologic Disorders, Vol 139 of the Handbook of Clinical Neurology Series. Elsevier, Amsterdam, pp. 213–228.

Stone, J., Carson, A., 2015. Functional neurologic disorders. Continuum. (Minneap Minn). 21, 818–837.

Stone, J., Carson, A., Aditya, H., Prescott, R., Zaubi, M., Warlow, C., Sharpe, M., 2009a. The role of physical injury in motor and sensory conversion symptoms: a systematic and narrative review. J. Psychosom. Res. 66, 383–390.

Stone, J., Carson, A., Duncan, R., et al., 2009b. Symptoms "unexplained by organic disease" in 1144 new neurology outpatients: how often does the diagnosis change at follow-up? Brain. 132, 2878–2888.

Stone, J., Carson, A., Duncan, R., et al., 2010. Who is referred to neurology clinics? The diagnoses made in 3781 new patients. Clin. Neurol. Neurosurg. 112, 747–751.

Stone, J., Edwards, M.J., 2012. Trick or treat? Showing patients with functional (psychogenic) motor symptoms their physical signs. Neurology. 79, 282–284.

Stone, J., Gelauff, J., Carson, A., 2012. A "twist in the tale": altered perception of ankle position in psychogenic dystonia. Mov. Disord. 27, 585–586.

Stone, J., Hewett, R., Carson, A., Warlow, C., 2008. The "disappearance"of hysteria: historical mystery or illusion? J. R. Soc. Med. 101, 12–18.

Stone, J., Hoeritzauer, I., Brown, K., Carson, A., 2014. Therapeutic sedation for functional (psychogenic) neurological symptoms. J. Psychosom. Res. 76, 165–168.

Stone, J., Reuber, M., Carson, A., 2013. Functional symptoms in neurology: mimics and chameleons. Pract. Neurol. 13, 104–113.

Stone, J., Wojcik, W., Durrance, D., et al., 2002. What should we say to patients with symptoms unexplained by disease? The "number needed to offend." BMJ. 325, 1449–1450.

Tasca, C., Rapetti, M., Carta, M.G., Fadda, B., 2012. Women and hysteria in the history of mental health. Clin. Pract. Epidemiol. Ment. Heal. 8, 110–119.

Teodoro, T., Anne, M.M., Little, S., et al., 2018. Abnormal beta power is a hallmark of explicit movement control in functional movement disorders. Neurology. 90, e247–e253.

Thomas, M., Vuong, K.D., Jankovic, J., 2006. Long-term prognosis of patients with psychogenic movement disorders. Parkinsonism. Relat. Disord. 12, 382–387.

Trieschmann, R.B., Stolov, W.C., Montgomery, E.D., 1970. An approach to the treatment of abnormal ambulation resulting from conversion reaction. Arch. Phys. Med. Rehabil. 51, 198–206.

Trimble, M.R., 1982. Functional diseases. Br. Med. J. (Clin. Res. Ed). 285, 1768.

Voon, V., Gallea, C., Hattori, N., Bruno, M., Ekanayake, V., Hallett, M., 2010. The involuntary nature of conversion disorder. Neurology. 74, 223–228.

Zigmond, A.S., Snaith, R.P., 1983. The hospital anxiety and depression scale. Acta. Psychiatr. Scand. 67, 361–370.

Vestibular Rehabilitation

*Dara Meldrum, Lisa Burrows, David Herdman,
and Rory McConn-Walsh*

The overwhelming vertigo, the awful sickness and the turbulent eye movements – all enhanced by the slightest movement of the head, combine to form a picture of helpless misery that has few parallels in the whole field of injury and disease.

—*Terence Cawthorne 1945*

OUTLINE

Introduction, 438
Epidemiology, 438
Anatomy and Physiology of the Vestibular System, 438
Vestibular Ocular Reflex and Vestibulospinal Reflex, 440
Pathophysiology, 441
Peripheral Disorders, 441
Central Disorders, 443
Other Causes of Dizziness, 445
Diagnosis, 446
Medical and Surgical Management, 446
   Ménière's Disease, 447
   Persistent Benign Paroxysmal Positional Vertigo, 447
   Vestibular Schwannoma, 447
Assessment, 447
   Physical Impairments, 448
   Functional Ability, 448
   Outcome Measures, 448
Prognosis, 450
Interventions, 453
   Gaze Stability Exercises, 454

Habituation Exercises, 454
Visual Desensitisation Exercises, 454
Balance and Gait Reeducation, 454
Management of Benign Paroxysmal Positional Vertigo, 456
Horizontal Canal Benign Paroxysmal Positional Vertigo, 456
Secondary Problems, 457
Other Considerations, 459
   Covid-19 and the Vestibular System, 459
   Remote and Digital Vestibular Rehabilitation, 459
   Multidisciplinary Team, 459
   Specialist Centres and Support Groups, 459
   Support Groups, 460
   Useful Resources, 460
Conclusion, 460
Case Studies, 460
   Case 1: Peripheral Vestibular Neuritis, 460
   Case 2: Benign Paroxysmal Positional Vertigo, 461

INTRODUCTION

Normal postural stability, or 'balance' as it is commonly known, is fundamental to activities of daily living. Visual, vestibular and somatosensory systems have important and integrated roles in the maintenance of balance, and the neurological patient can present with problems in any or all of these components. This chapter will focus on the assessment and treatment of patients who have a primary problem in the vestibular system. Vestibular dysfunction is characterised by several signs and symptoms including vertigo, dizziness, oscillopsia (a false sensation that the visual surround is oscillating), gait and balance impairment, nausea and nystagmus (Table 17.1). Patients with such dysfunction present the physiotherapist with specific problems and require specialised assessment and treatment techniques, collectively referred to as *vestibular rehabilitation*. Vestibular rehabilitation has its roots in the empirical work of Cawthorne and Cooksey, who in the 1940's first documented the important role of exercise in recovery after a vestibular injury (Cooksey 1946). The evidence base is now well established for the effective role of physiotherapy in the management of patients with vestibular disorders (Hansson 2007, Hillier & McDonnell 2011, Porciuncula et al 2012, Ricci et al 2010), and vestibular rehabilitation is recognised as a specialist area within physiotherapy (http://www.csp.org.uk/professional-networks/acpivr). Independent prescriber physiotherapy posts within vestibular rehabilitation have also recently emerged (Burrows et al 2017). Historically, vestibular rehabilitation has been associated with the ear, nose and throat (ENT) medical specialty, but it is now practiced across many others (e.g., neurology, care of the elderly, paediatrics, musculoskeletal,

sports medicine), with only 25% of clinicians practicing in a dedicated vestibular rehabilitation service (Meldrum et al 2020). Considering that vestibular dysfunction is so highly prevalent, it is important for all physiotherapists to acquire clinical skills to evaluate the vestibular system.

KEY POINTS

Vertigo is the sensation of self-motion (of head/body) when no self-motion is occurring or the sensation of distorted self-motion during an otherwise normal head movement (Bisdorff et al 2015). Dizziness is the sensation of disturbed or impaired spatial orientation without a false or distorted sense of motion (Bisdorff et al 2015).

Dizziness and vertigo are further classified into being spontaneous or triggered (Bisdorff et al 2009).

EPIDEMIOLOGY

Vertigo and dizziness are common but distinct symptoms that can be caused by many disease processes. The 1-year prevalence of moderate or severe vertigo or dizziness in adults is 25% (Grill et al 2018), and 50% of those with dizziness report postural unsteadiness (Yardley et al 1998a). In a large cross-sectional study including a random sample of more than 6500 community-dwelling Americans older than 40 years, 27% reported dizziness and 35.4% were unable to stand on foam with eyes closed for 30 seconds, indicating problems with using vestibular information for balance (Agrawal et al 2009). Prevalence of dizziness increases to one in three in those older than 65 years (Colledge et al 1994), and dizziness is the most common complaint of patients presenting to primary care in those older than 75 years (Sloane 1989). There is a very low prevalence of dizziness in people younger than 25 years. Vestibular vertigo (arising from disease or disorder affecting the inner ear) affects more than 5% of adults each year with a lifetime prevalence of 7.8% (Neuhauser et al 2005) and is more common in females (Agus et al 2013). It is estimated that vestibular hypofunction affects between 53 and 95 million adults in Europe and the USA (Grill et al 2018). More than 60% of those with vestibular vertigo report decreased work productivity in the form of lost working days (Benecke et al 2013), and healthcare use costs are high, with 80% seeking a medical consultation (Neuhauser et al 2005) and most requiring medication (Kovacs et al 2019).

ANATOMY AND PHYSIOLOGY OF THE VESTIBULAR SYSTEM

The anatomy and physiology of the vestibular system are complex, but an understanding is crucial for successful

TABLE 17.1 Signs and Symptoms of Vestibular Disorders That Should Be Evaluated During History Taking	
Primary Symptoms and Signs	**Associated Problems**
Vertigo	Neck and back pain
Dizziness/light-headedness	Physical
Nausea and vomiting	deconditioning
Oscillopsia	Agoraphobia
Nystagmus	Hyperventilation
Disequilibrium/impaired	Falls
balance	Hearing loss/tinnitus
Panic/anxiety	Aural fullness
Gait abnormality	Headache
Fatigue	

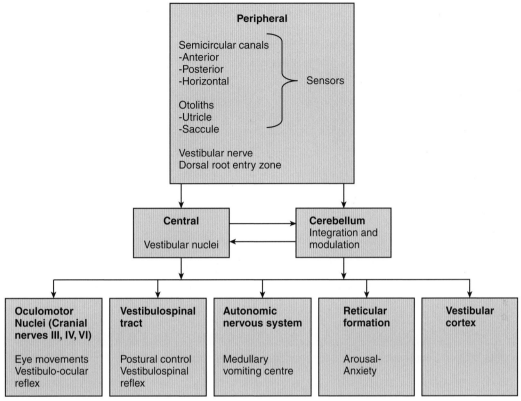

FIG. 17.1 Functional organization of the vestibular system and vestibular labyrinth.

treatment of vestibular disorders. A brief organisational overview is shown in Fig. 17.1. The vestibular system has both *sensory* and *motor* functions and is generally divided into peripheral and central components. The peripheral system consists of the vestibular end organ (housed in the petrous temporal bone of the skull) and the vestibular nerve up to and including the dorsal root entry zone. The central system includes the vestibular nuclei in the brainstem and their central connections.

The vestibular end organ includes the semicircular canals (SCCs) and the otoliths (utricle and saccule). The SCCs consist of three canals on each side (horizontal, anterior and posterior) which are orientated at 90° angles to each other (Figs. 17.1 and 17.2). Each canal is coupled functionally with a canal in the opposite end organ with both horizontal canals, the left anterior and right posterior and the right posterior and left anterior canals, coupled together (see Fig. 17.2). Specialised sensors known as hair cells are located in the SCCs in a region known as the cupula and respond to *angular velocity* of head movement in different planes. Each canal responds best to movement in its own

plane. For example, when the head rotates to the right, the hair cells in the right horizontal SCC increase their firing rate and those in the left horizontal SCC decrease their firing rate (Fig. 17.3). Thus the central nervous system (CNS) gains information relating to the velocity and direction of head movement from both sides. This means that if one side is damaged and no longer providing input, the contralateral side can provide information about head movement (but only at lower velocity head movements). The otoliths have different hair cells in a region known as the macula. Hair cells in the maculae are covered by a layer of calcium carbonate crystals called *otoconia*. They respond to the force of gravity and thus can provide the CNS with information on *head tilt* and *linear acceleration* (i.e., going up and down in a lift or going forwards or backwards in a car).

The peripheral system is a tonically active system, that is, it always has a certain firing level (approximately 40–90 spikes per second which can increase or decrease with head movement) (Goldberg & Fernandez 1971, Lacour et al 2009). Symmetrical firing is interpreted by the brain as no movement, and the CNS interprets any asymmetry in the

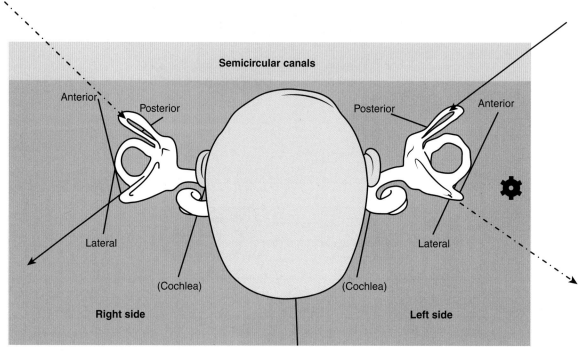

FIG. 17.2 Arrangement of the semicircular canals and their pairings. (Adapted from aVOR app.)

firing rate as movement. This fact is of utmost importance when considering a patient who has loss of vestibular function on one side (i.e., decrease or absence of firing) because there will be a *relative* increase of firing on the intact side even when the head is not moving (see Fig. 17.3). This asymmetry and the resultant disturbance in cortical spatial orientation are thought to form the basis of vertigo and produce the nystagmus seen in unilateral peripheral vestibular disease (Brandt 2000).

The vestibular nerve sends fibres to two main areas: the vestibular nuclei and the cerebellum (see Fig. 17.1). The vestibular nuclei are responsible for integrating information received from the end organ with that received from other sensory systems and the cerebellum. Vestibular nuclei send fibres to the oculomotor nuclei, vestibulospinal tracts, contralateral vestibular nuclei, reticular formation, cerebellum, autonomic nervous system and the cortex. The symptoms of nausea, vomiting and anxiety associated with vestibular disorders are as a result of abnormal activation of the autonomic and reticular pathways, respectively (see Fig. 17.1). For a more detailed description of vestibular anatomy and physiology, the reader is referred to Hain and Helminski (2007) and Kingma and van de Berg (2016).

VESTIBULAR OCULAR REFLEX AND VESTIBULOSPINAL REFLEX

The motor functions of the vestibular system include the vestibular ocular reflex (VOR) and the vestibulospinal reflex (VSR). The function of the VOR is to maintain stable vision when the head is moving. A good example of this is being able to focus on an object when walking. If the eyes moved with the head as it goes up and down when a person is walking, it would be impossible to see clearly. The VOR enables the eyes (through activation of the appropriate ocular muscles) to move in the opposite direction and at an equal velocity to the head. The image of the object thus remains stable on the retina. For the VOR to function normally, velocity of eye movement must be equal to and in the opposite direction to the head movement. This is known as the 'gain' of the VOR. Patients who have problems with the vestibular system have impairment of the gain of the VOR and therefore demonstrate problems with gaze stability. They often describe that during self-motion objects seem as if they are moving. The function of the VSR is primarily to maintain and regain postural control, and it does this through monosynaptic and polysynaptic vestibulospinal pathways. Clinical and laboratory testing of the function

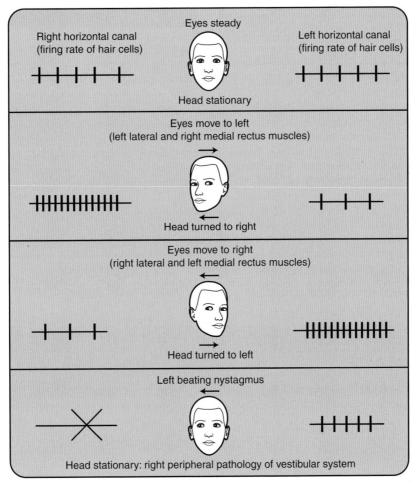

FIG. 17.3 Function of the horizontal canals in generating a vestibular ocular reflex (VOR).

of the VOR is described later in the section on diagnosis and Table 17.4.

PATHOPHYSIOLOGY

Vestibular disorders can broadly be classified anatomically into peripheral or central, depending on which area pathology affects. They are further classified by duration: acute, episodic or chronic (Bisdorff et al 2009, 2015). Common peripheral and central vestibular disorders are shown in Table 17.2. 'Functional' neurovestibular disorders are also common, which represent perceptual dysregulation of the balance system that is unconnected to any damage or alteration in structure (Staab 2012). It is important to note that vertigo and dizziness are not always caused by pathology affecting the vestibular system; there may be many other causes, including orthostatic hypotension, cardiac disorders, psychiatric disorders and hyperventilation, and these should be evaluated before referral to physiotherapy. The exact cause of dizziness frequently remains uncertain, and a trial of vestibular rehabilitation may be suggested in the absence of a specific diagnosis. The pathology of disorders that can affect the central vestibular system (e.g., cerebrovascular accidents, traumatic brain injury and multiple sclerosis) is considered in other chapters.

PERIPHERAL DISORDERS

Vestibular neuritis (also called *neuronitis*) is a common peripheral vestibular problem thought to be caused by a

TABLE 17.2   Peripheral and Central Vestibular Disorders

Peripheral	Central
Viral: Vestibular neuritis/ labyrinthitis	Ischaemia, e.g., lateral medullary syndrome (Wallenberg's syndrome)
Benign paroxysmal positional vertigo	Vertebrobasilar insufficiency
Perilymph fistula	Infection
Ménière's disease	Head injury
Vascular occlusion	Degenerative disease, e.g., multiple sclerosis, Friedreich's ataxia
Iatrogenic (ototoxic drugs, surgery)	
Head injury (labyrinthine concussion)	Base of skull abnormalities, e.g., Arnold–Chiari malformation
Vestibular schwannoma (may have a central component)	Tumours of the cerebellopontine angle
	Drugs
	Epilepsy
	Migraine

KEY POINTS

Nystagmus is a rhythmical oscillation of the eyes. There is a slow movement or 'phase' in one direction and a fast corrective movement in the opposite direction. By convention, nystagmus is named by the direction of the fast phase. For example, left beating horizontal nystagmus is one in which the slow phase of the nystagmus is horizontal movement of the eyes towards the right and the fast phase of the nystagmus is horizontal eye movement towards the left. There are many causes of nystagmus. In the patient with an acute peripheral vestibular disorder, a spontaneous nystagmus can be seen with its fast phase beating away from the side of the lesion. After a few days the nystagmus is not visible in room light but may be evident indefinitely with infrared goggles (visual fixation is removed: see Fig. 17.5).

virus (Strupp & Brandt 2010). It results in varying degrees of hair cell loss and unilateral vestibular paresis (or hypofunction). Patients present with an acute onset of vertigo, nausea and vomiting that are severely incapacitating and worsened by head and eye movements. On examination, a spontaneous horizontal nystagmus can be seen, the fast phase of which beats away from the involved side. This is caused by the asymmetrical tonic firing of the vestibular nerves (see Fig. 17.3). Balance and gait abnormalities are also evident (Allum & Adkin 2003, Fetter et al 1990). Hearing is not generally affected, but if it is the condition is called *labyrinthitis*. Symptoms generally resolve over 2–6 weeks but not always completely (Cousins et al 2017, Strupp & Brandt 2013).

Benign paroxysmal positional vertigo (BPPV) is the most common cause of episodic vertigo in peripheral vestibular disorders (Bhattacharyya et al 2017). It has a lifetime prevalence of 2.4% and a 1-year incidence of 0.6% (von Brevern et al 2007). Prevalence increases with age and is almost seven times higher in those older than 60 years compared with those aged 18–39 years (von Brevern et al 2007). In elderly people BPPV is often undiagnosed (Oghalai et al 2000). The name encompasses the associated features:
- *Benign*: the prognosis for recovery is favourable
- *Paroxysmal*: the associated vertigo is short-lived, generally less than 1 minute

- *Positional*: the vertigo is provoked by certain head positions
- *Vertigo*: a spinning sensation is experienced

In addition, nausea and anxiety can be reported, and occasionally vomiting occurs. Imbalance is reported in 50% of patients, and most patients report vertigo when turning over in bed (von Brevern et al 2007).

BPPV is thought to be caused by detached utricular otoconia entering one of the SCCs and either floating free in the canal (canalithiasis) or adhering to the cupula (cupulolithiasis) (Epley 1980). This has the effect of making the SCCs responsive to gravity when they normally are not. The SCCs usually respond to head movement in their respective planes and increase their firing rate during head movement, returning to normal tonic firing level when the head has stopped moving. However, if the head moves into a dependent position and then stops, the displaced otoconia are heavier and will continue to move in the canal, stimulating the hair cells in the canal to continue firing. The central vestibular system interprets this as further movement and generates a VOR for that canal, and the patient develops nystagmus and vertigo. This nystagmus has a latency of 1–50 seconds, is generally transient in nature (it stops when the otoconia come to a resting position) and, in the case of posterior semicircular canal (PSCC), BPPV is torsional towards the affected ear. If the patient repeatedly moves into the provoking position, the vertigo and nystagmus will decrease because of habituation of the response (Baloh et al 1987). The diagnosis of BPPV is generally made using the Hallpike–Dix manoeuvre (Fig. 17.4) in which the head is moved into a provocative position (Bhandari et al 2021). BPPV most commonly affects the PSCC (approximately 85%–95% of cases) but

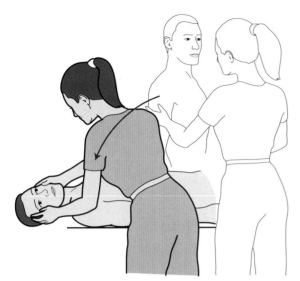

FIG. 17.4 The Hallpike–Dix test.

can also affect the horizontal (5%–15% of cases) (Parnes et al 2003, White et al 2005) and very rarely the anterior canal (Baloh et al 1993, De La Meilleure 1996). Multiple canal involvement can also occur.

Patients with BPPV report vertigo associated with certain head movements, that is, rolling over in bed, looking up or bending down, and will usually avoid these movements. Treatment consists of physical manoeuvres, sometimes repeated a few times during one session (Gordon & Gadoth 2004), that aim to reposition the displaced otoconia back into the utricle (Gold et al 2014, Hilton & Pinder 2004b). These manoeuvres are highly effective in most cases and lead to full resolution of symptoms (Bhattacharyya et al 2017, Hilton & Pinder 2004a). BPPV has a high recurrence rate of 25% (von Brevern et al 2007), necessitating further treatment.

Ménière's disease is thought to be caused by an increase in the volume of and/or a problem with absorption of the endolymph (the fluid in the inner ear). This results in dilation of the endolymphatic spaces (endolymphatic hydrops) (Lopez-Escamez et al 2017). This happens episodically and unpredictably, and an attack is characterised by a complaint of a fullness in the ear, reduction of hearing, and tinnitus (a ringing sound in the ear). This is followed by vertigo, vomiting and postural imbalance, and nystagmus is observed. The episodes may last from 30 minutes to 72 hours and then the patient gradually improves (Committee on Hearing and Equilibrium 1995). Episodes are generally managed with medication, diet and rest, but in severe cases surgery may be indicated (see later). Vestibular rehabilitation can

be helpful for patients with Ménière's disease if symptoms of disequilibrium and dizziness continue between attacks (Clendaniel & Tucci 1997, Garcia et al 2013, Gottshall et al 2005).

Bilateral vestibular hypofunction is relatively uncommon. It can be caused by infections (e.g., meningitis), tumours (e.g., bilateral vestibular schwannoma [VS] in neurofibromatosis), Ménière's disease, autoimmune diseases and ototoxic drugs (e.g., aminoglycoside antibiotics) (Lucieer et al 2016, Rinne et al 1998). In some cases, the cause is unknown. Patients with bilateral vestibular hypofunction do not usually report vertigo when vestibular loss is symmetrical. Their main problems include balance and gait impairments. They also have decreased gaze stability caused by loss of VOR function, report that they cannot see clearly during head movements and describe their surroundings as bouncing or jumping. This is termed *oscillopsia*. Vestibular rehabilitation is indicated for patients with bilateral vestibular loss, but outcomes are not as favourable (Brown et al 2001, Herdman et al 2015, Krebs et al 2003, Porciuncula et al 2012).

Presbyvestibulopathy is defined as an age-related, chronic vestibular disorder presenting with unsteadiness, gait abnormalities and/or recurrent falls in the presence of mild bilateral vestibular hypofunction (Agrawal et al 2019). Diagnostic criteria incorporate symptom history, bedside examination and vestibular testing to aid diagnosis, and it requires bilaterally reduced function of the VOR. VOR function can be assessed using the video head impulse test (vHIT; high frequency range), rotatory chair (middle frequency range) or caloric testing (low frequency range) (Agrawal et al 2019). Age-related changes to vision, proprioception and central functions may be comorbid and contribute to age-related balance system dysfunction known as *presbystasis* (Rogers 2010). There is growing evidence of an association between cognitive performance and vestibular function which can affect way finding, speed of cognition and decision making (Bouny et al 2022, Pineault et al 2020).

CENTRAL DISORDERS

Vestibular migraine (VM) is a primary headache disorder considered when recurrent, intermittent dizziness is the predominant, most disabling symptom experienced. However, VM is not always accompanied by a headache. The diagnostic criteria from the Barany Society (Lempert et al 2012, 2022) and the International Classification of Headache Disorders (IHS 2018) require a current or past history of migraine with or without aura and vestibular symptoms of moderate to severe intensity lasting 5 minutes to 72 hours. At least five episodes should have occurred,

50% of episodes should have at least one of three migrainous symptoms (headache, phonophobia and photophobia or visual aura) and episodes should not be better accounted for by another vestibular disorder. VM is underdiagnosed particularly at the primary care level (Formeister et al 2018, Sohn 2016). Trauma and genetics are understood to cause VM (Oh et al 2001), and it is hypothesised to be a CNS disorder mediated by the trigeminal complex and cortical spreading depression, but exact mechanisms remain unclear (Nowaczewska 2020, Sohn 2016). Cho et al (2016) found a 10.3% prevalence of VM in migraineurs, and Neuhauser et al (2006) estimated a lifetime prevalence of 1% and a 1-year prevalence of 0.9%, affecting up to 2.7% of the general population (Formeister et al 2018). Those most affected are more likely to be female (>80%), 40–49 years of age and have a history of motion sickness, imbalance and food-trigger headaches (Beh et al 2019, Li et al 2022). Significantly more anxiety and depression have been found in those with VM compared with healthy controls or those with nonvestibular migraine (Kutay et al 2017). Common triggers include stress (39%), bright lights (26%), weather changes (26%), sleep deprivation (26%) and hormonal fluctuations (Beh et al 2019). Overuse of pain relief or acute attack medication (e.g., paracetamol, ibuprofen, codeine, triptans) can cause medication overuse headaches (MOH) with dizziness (IHS 2018). Current evidence (in the form of retrospective and observational studies) supporting vestibular rehabilitation for improving the physical symptoms associated with VM is weak (Alghadir et al 2018, Sugaya et al 2017, Whitney et al 2000, Wrisley et al 2002). Motion sensitivity is experienced by 56% of VM patients but only 16% are referred to vestibular rehabilitation (Power et al 2018), although emerging evidence for vestibular rehabilitation in VM patients shows improved self-reported dizziness and functional gait on the Dizziness Handicap Inventory and Functional Gait Assessment outcome measures, respectively (Stancel-Lewis et al 2022).

Dizziness and balance disorders are common after a *traumatic brain injury* (TBI) with head injury and concussion (Akin et al 2017, Marcus et al 2019). As many as half of patients with a TBI will be affected by vestibular symptoms, which may last for 6 months or longer (Maskell et al 2006). Because the vestibular system lies in the temporal bone, any temporal skull fracture increases the risk of damage. However, dizziness can be triggered regardless of any structural damage because there is often a lack of correlation between objective and subjective features of vestibular dysfunction (Sargeant et al 2018).

With acute TBI, patients may develop 'vestibular agnosia' (Calzolari et al 2021). Patients cannot perceive any dizziness despite having signs of vestibular disorders such as BPPV. For this reason, it is a good idea to check for signs of imbalance and BPPV testing in patients after head injury because they may not readily report feeling dizzy (Smith et al 2020).

Vestibular schwannoma is a benign growth on the vestibulocochlear nerve (eighth cranial nerve). It presents with unilateral hearing loss (94%), unilateral constant tinnitus (83%), vestibular hypofunction symptoms and imbalance (17%–75%) and rarely trigeminal or facial neuropathies and cerebellar ataxia (Goldbrunner et al 2020). There is a genetic predisposition and link to neurofibromatosis 2. Observation and monitoring with MRI of the internal acoustic meatus (IAM) in specialist multidisciplinary team (MDT) skull-based clinics is recommended because surgery and radiotherapy are considered for larger tumours or tumours with cystic degeneration. Vestibular rehabilitation including VOR retraining, strength, sensory and functional balance training and falls risk management may improve symptoms, reduce anxiety and falls risk while improving balance and vertigo (Vereeck et al 2008). Although there is little published evidence to support this, vestibular rehabilitation approaches in the management of unilateral vestibular hypofunction are transferable.

Vascular vertigo (VV) refers to dizziness and vertigo with a vascular cause (Kim et al 2022). Assessment and management of modifiable cardiovascular risk factors should be addressed (e.g., arrhythmias, cholesterol, blood pressure, exercise, diabetes, smoking, alcohol). VV can be episodic or prolonged, and differential diagnosis between an acute vestibulopathy (vestibular neuritis or labyrinthitis) and stroke is time critical.

Stroke can cause dizziness, nausea, vomiting, motion intolerance and postural instability. Commonly the anterior inferior cerebellar artery (AICA) is involved, resulting in lesions (ischaemic or haemorrhagic) in the medial longitudinal fasciculus, vestibular nuclei, posterior fossa, cerebellum, brainstem, parietotemporal cerebral areas and labyrinthine structures (all supplied by the AICA) and may result in impairments of VOR gain, coordination, smooth pursuit, saccades and cochlear or vestibular function (Sayed et al 2021). Diagnostic criteria propose acute dizziness, vertigo or unsteadiness for 24 hours or more. An examination protocol called the HINTS+, which incorporates the *Head Impulse Test* (HIT), gaze-evoked *Nystagmus, Test of Skew,* and hearing loss or neurological deficit, can help to differentiate acute stroke and a peripheral vestibulopathy. Vestibular rehabilitation including VOR training, sensory balance exercises and gait training improves gait speed, dynamic balance and stride length (Balci et al 2013, Mitsutake et al 2020, Tramontano et al 2018); however, more randomised controlled trials are needed.

Vertebral (and/or subclavian) artery compression syndrome (occlusion or stenosis), previously known as bow hunter's syndrome (Lida et al 2018) or rotational vertebral artery syndrome (occlusion/compression), presents with symptoms of dizziness or vertigo with or without tinnitus produced by sustained neck positions into either rotation, extension and/or side flexion and can be sensitised with shoulder abduction. After ruling out conditions which better account for symptoms (e.g., BPPV, posterior fossa and cerebellar pontine angle tumours/cysts, multiple sclerosis, vestibular paroxysmia and Chiari malformation), evidence of either vertebral artery compression on dynamic angiography or reduced blood flow on transcranial Doppler is required for diagnosis. Nystagmus is rarely present during provocation (Kim et al 2021, Schubert et al 2021), and referral to a neurovascular specialist is recommended.

Vestibular paroxysmia (VP) is a neurovascular cross-compression of the eighth cranial nerve, and diagnosis is mainly based on a history of frequent spontaneous attacks of vertigo, typically lasting less than 1 minute, and radiological evidence. Patients usually respond to carbamazepine or oxcarbazepine (Strupp et al 2016). *Persistent postural perceptual dizziness* (PPPD) is a recently agreed term for a functional vestibular disorder that is an amalgamation of previously described conditions such as space and motion discomfort, phobic postural vertigo, visual vertigo or chronic subjective dizziness (Staab et al 2017). The core features that suggest a diagnosis include prolonged symptoms of dizziness, unsteadiness or nonspinning vertigo that are present on most days for more than 3 months (Staab et al 2017). Patients usually feel worse when they are upright, either sitting unsupported or standing and walking. They also feel worse when in motion, either moving themselves or passively such as when riding a lift or in a vehicle. Patients also feel worse when exposed to visually complex or moving stimuli.

The disorder can be precipitated by any event that triggers dizziness and disrupts balance function, such as another vestibular disorder, other neurological or medical illness or psychological distress (Habs et al 2020). Therefore people with PPPD may have more than one diagnosis, but PPPD persists for longer than the triggering illness. PPPD can also occur spontaneously, although caution should be exercised in the case of a slow progressive onset because of the possibility of an emerging neurodegenerative disorder. The prevalence of PPPD in people presenting with dizziness is around 20% (Adamec et al 2020, Staibano et al 2019) but may be even higher in specialist clinics.

PPPD is often perpetuated by anxiety-related features, such as focusing on symptoms, negative illness- and symptom-related beliefs and avoidance behaviour (Whalley et al 2017). Patients will often overestimate the degree of harm caused by dizziness and may consciously process

walking movements to avoid falling. This disrupts normal 'automatic' postural control processes, and their muscles stiffen up resulting in a gait pattern akin to 'walking on ice' (Holmberg et al 2009, Schniepp et al 2013). There is also a functional shift in multisensory processing of spatial orientation whereby patients with PPPD rely more on visual input. This produces vulnerability to disorienting effects of complex or moving visual stimuli, such as walking through a supermarket aisle, scrolling on a phone or e-tablet or watching fast-moving scenes on television.

Vestibular rehabilitation (habituation exercises and balance retraining), along with cognitive behavioural therapy and medication (selective serotonin reuptake inhibitors or serotonin-norepinephrine reuptake inhibitors), has shown some promise for this patient group (Bittar & Lins 2015, Herdman et al 2022, Popkirov et al 2018, Schaaf & Hesse 2015, Thompson et al 2015).

OTHER CAUSES OF DIZZINESS

Cervical dizziness (CD), formally known as cervicogenic dizziness, is a controversial term used to describe dizziness associated with cervical spine dysfunction. It is a complex and difficult condition to classify and understand because these symptoms overlap with many other pathologies (Devaraja 2018, Reiley et al 2017), and at present there is no single diagnostic test. It is characterised by symptoms of imbalance and dizziness with nonspinning vertigo or dizziness that is associated with cervical spine movement. There must also be cervical spine pain and limited range of movement and sometimes associated headache. It can be considered a diagnosis only when all other causes are excluded. The cause is proposed to be abnormal neck proprioceptive information arising as a result of injury or pain that creates a sensory mismatch during cervical spine movement (Devaraja 2018, Reiley et al 2017).

Orthostatic blood pressure impairment is a common non-vestibular cause of dizziness, light-headedness, unsteadiness or vertigo occurring on standing up. It can be related to orthostatic hypotension, postural orthostatic tachycardia syndrome (POTS) and dysautonomia. Orthostatic blood pressure is defined by a significant reduction in systolic (>20 mm Hg) and/or diastolic (>10 mm Hg) blood pressure within 3 minutes upon standing from lying/sitting or during a head-up tilt table test. POTS is defined by development of orthostatic symptoms with a heart rate increment of 30 or more beats/min on being upright (or 40 beats/min in people younger than 20 years). Management strategies include a medication review with the general practitioner, independent prescriber or pharmacist; falls prevention; hydration; regular mealtimes; movement before standing (e.g., repeated alternate crossing and uncrossing legs); slow movement into standing; and isometric buttock squeezes while standing (Sheikh et al 2022).

DIAGNOSIS

Patients presenting with vertigo, imbalance and dizziness may be referred for specialised audiovestibular testing to evaluate whether a central or peripheral vestibular disorder is the cause of their symptoms. The following list provides an overview of diagnostic testing for vestibular disorders.

1. *Audiology screening:* This includes pure tone audiogram/speech discrimination, tympanogram (tympanic membrane pressure test), tinnitus screening questions and otoscopy. Certain conditions causing dizziness may result in hearing loss across different frequencies. These include Ménière's disease, ototoxic medications, head trauma, VS and previous middle ear surgery. Audiology screening will provide important information about the audiovestibular pathway and middle ear function and can inform further investigations and management.

2. *Caloric/oculomotor testing:* This is the most used test of peripheral vestibular function and provides a quantitative measure of lateral SCC function in each inner ear (Jacobson & Shepard 2021). It is performed by measuring the response of the VOR (nystagmus) to the instillation of cold and warm water down the external ear canal. As well as assessing peripheral vestibular function, oculomotor testing can also detect oculomotor disturbance (abnormal saccades, smooth pursuit) suggestive of a central disorder.

3. *vHIT:* This is a computerised head-impulse test which measures the gain of the VOR (i.e., the ratio of the velocity of head movement to the velocity of eye movement) during a task where the patient is instructed to fixate on a target while the examiner moves the patient's head with small amplitudes and high accelerations of movement in different planes. The vHIT can assess the individual function of all six SCCs. It can be useful when caloric testing is contraindicated (e.g., narrow external ear canal or tympanic membrane perforation) and is considered complementary to the current 'gold standard' caloric testing (Vallim et al 2021). However, emerging evidence suggests vHIT may be more accurate at discriminating stroke from vestibular neuritis in patients with acute dizziness and therefore may be a valuable first-line investigation (Morrison et al 2022).

4. *Vestibular evoked myogenic potentials (VEMPs):* VEMPs testing can be performed at different frequencies to detect abnormalities of inner ear function. Cervical and ocular VEMPs (cVEMPs and oVEMPs) test the function of the saccule and utricle, respectively (Rosengren

et al 2019). VEMPs can also be used in the diagnosis of SCC dehiscence (an opening in the temporal bone covering the SCC) in conjunction with computed tomography imaging (Noji & Rauch 2020).

5. *Magnetic resonance imaging (MRI):* Any patient who presents with unexplained dizziness that is persistent or progressive should have an MRI scan (preferably with gadolinium enhancement) of the brain and cerebellopontine angle to exclude lesions such as a brain tumour, multiple sclerosis or embolic/haemorrhagic events. If unilateral hearing loss or constant unilateral tinnitus is reported, the IAM should also be scanned using MRI to exclude compression of the vestibular nerve from a VS or vascular structure.

6. *Skull vibration-induced nystagmus testing (SVINT):* SVINT uses a 100-Hz bone-conducted vibration tool applied to either mastoid. In healthy asymptomatic people it has little or no effect, but in people with a unilateral vestibular hypofunction it will induce a (predominantly horizontal) nystagmus with a quick phase beating away from the affected side. It is a simple noninvasive and reliable indicator of vestibular function asymmetry and side of vestibular loss which can be used in a variety of clinical settings (Dumas et al 2017, 2021).

7. *Posturography:* Mainly used as a research tool, posturography provides a quantitative measure of certain functional aspects of dynamic equilibrium (Di Fabio 1995, Fetter et al 1990, Visser et al 2008). It potentially has a role in the assessment of dizziness and can also be used to monitor the effects of rehabilitation. Adding low-frequency head movements on an unstable surface improves sensitivity and specificity in persons with chronic unilateral vestibular lesions (Janc et al 2021).

MEDICAL AND SURGICAL MANAGEMENT

The acute rotatory vertigo suffered during acute peripheral vestibular dysfunction is caused by sudden asymmetry in vestibular input to the CNS. Vestibular sedatives are a group of drugs that have a well-established record of controlling such attacks. These drugs have variable anticholinergic, antiemetic and sedative properties. They include phenothiazines (e.g., prochlorperazine,), antihistamines (e.g., cinnarizine, dimenhydrinate, promethazine, meclizine) and benzodiazepines (e.g., diazepam, lorazepam) (Joint Formulary Committee 2022). These drugs are valuable for the management of acute vertigo, and they can be administered by intramuscular or intravenous injection, suppository, buccal absorption or orally, depending on the individual drug. However, they should ideally be restricted to short-term use (3 days) and avoided for the management of chronic peripheral labyrinthine disorders because they may suppress central vestibular activity, thereby delaying compensation and symptomatic recovery.

Ménière's Disease

Recommended first-line management of Ménière's disease includes lifestyle management, hydration, reduced caffeine intake, exercise, vestibular rehabilitation, cognitive behavioural therapy and acute attack management with prochlorperazine, cinnarizine or betahistine (Clyde et al 2017, Espinosa-Sanchez & Lopez-Escamez 2020, Jiang et al 2021, Nevoux et al 2018, NICE CKS 2017, Zhang et al 2022). Evidence for prolonged daily use of medication is weak (Devantier et al 2020); however, in severe cases using daily betahistine at increased doses may be considered before surgical intervention because this is thought to increase microcirculation of the inner ear.

For those patients with unilateral Ménière's disease who are symptomatic for 6 months to 1 year despite conservative management, surgery can be considered as a last resort (Dorion 1998, Nevoux et al 2018). This entails a mastoidectomy and drilling out the three SCCs under general anaesthesia. This approach is effective at treating the vertiginous episodes by destroying all peripheral vestibular function, although all residual hearing is destroyed.

If the hearing is useful, surgery should attempt to preserve the remaining hearing. This can be done by means of topical gentamicin injection (ITG), intratympanic steroid injection (ITS), endolymphatic sac decompression or vestibular neurectomy. Intratympanic injections involve the intratympanic instillation of gentamicin or steroid solution into the middle ear (Jiang et al 2021, Nedzelski et al 1992). Medication diffuses into the inner ear across the round window membrane where ITG selectively destroys vestibular and not cochlear hair cells and ITS reduces inflammation. Success rates of greater than 80% have been reported for ITG with higher success in reducing vertigo attack frequency compared with ITS (Jiang et al 2020). The main disadvantage is a risk of sensorineural hearing loss, although this is similar for ITS and ITG (Jiang et al 2021, Zhang et al 2022). Endolymphatic sac decompression entails a mastoidectomy with removal of all bone over the endolymphatic sac/duct and possibly inserting a drain into it (Moffat 1994). The sac is the proposed site of obstruction of endolymphatic reabsorption in Ménière's disease, and this procedure enables the sac to expand during the active disease process. Vestibular neurectomy entails transecting the vestibular nerves in the posterior cranial fossa. The main disadvantages are damage to the facial and cochlear nerves together with intracranial complications. Vestibular rehabilitation is important after these procedures.

Persistent Benign Paroxysmal Positional Vertigo

Surgery is rare because of the high success rates of canal repositioning manoeuvres (Bhattacharyya et al 2017). Cases of intractable (> 1 year) and incapacitating BPPV can be treated by occlusion of the PSCC (Parnes & McClure 1990). This approach involves a mastoidectomy with isolation and then occlusion of the PSCC. This is a safe and effective operation with success rates greater than 90%–95% (Walsh et al 1999). Before this operation, singular neurectomy was advocated, but this is a technically more demanding operation with a risk of sensorineural hearing loss.

Vestibular Schwannoma

There are currently three methods of managing VS. These include conservative management, surgery (combined ENT and neurosurgery) and stereotactic radiosurgery. Conservative management is reserved for small tumours that are not growing or for patients who are unfit or express a desire not to have surgery (Walsh et al 2000). For those tumours that are growing, causing symptoms and are larger than 1–2 cm in diameter, then surgery should be considered. The aim of surgery is to remove the tumour without traumatising the facial nerve and, when indicated, to preserve hearing. Three surgical approaches are possible, and the type used depends on the level of remaining hearing. If the hearing is not serviceable or useful, a translabyrinthine approach is performed (House & Hitselberger 1985, Schwartz et al 2018). The main advantage of this technique is there is minimal brain retraction with easy surgical access, although all remaining hearing is sacrificed. If the hearing is useful, the tumour is approached either via a retrosigmoid or a middle cranial fossa approach in an attempt to preserve the hearing (Sekhar et al 1996). The main disadvantage of the former is there is cerebellar retraction, whereas the latter is technically demanding. Stereotactic radiosurgery entails the accurate application of radiotherapy from an external source to the site of the VS with minimal surrounding tissue damage. Treatment success with stereotactic radiosurgery has been reported as 97.7% with an acceptable toxicity profile (Patel et al 2017).

ASSESSMENT

A thorough assessment of the vestibular patient is a crucial prerequisite to any treatment. Although many aspects of the examination are similar to that of any physiotherapy assessment, there are specific tests that should be performed. The patient should be made aware that aspects of the examination often provoke symptoms and leave the patient feeling unwell. It is advisable to request the patient have someone with them on the first assessment who can accompany them home if required. A history is taken of the present complaint, the onset, nature, severity, duration and irritability of symptoms, and the aggravating and alleviating factors. True vertigo (asking 'Do you spin?' or 'Does the room spin?') should be differentiated from nonspinning vertigo (asking 'Does the world seem like it is moving when it is not' or 'Do you feel like you are moving when you are not?'). These should also be differentiated from dizziness, light-headedness, giddiness and disequilibrium (Bisdorff et al 2009). A history should be taken of other associated symptoms (see Table 17.1). It should be ascertained how long the patient has had the symptoms and what was their initial presentation. The history relating to the very first episode, if there has been more than one, and although it may have been a long time previously, is critically important. These previous episodes and their outcomes should be explored. Pertinent past medical history includes problems with vision, other peripheral or CNS disorders (e.g., migraine, epilepsy, previous head injury), cardiorespiratory disease (low or high blood pressure), endocrinological diseases (e.g., diabetes) or musculoskeletal problems (particularly cervical spine problems) and any previous vestibular surgery. The effects of the problem on the patient's occupational and leisure activities should also be noted. Medications – type, dosage, effect and plans for cessation – should also be discussed. Results of any investigations should be noted. Special questions are shown in Table 17.3.

Physical Impairments

The examination of the vestibular patient commences with a screening of the cervical spine (range of movement and any symptoms with movement). After this, the oculomotor examination is performed (Table 17.4). The patient is firstly examined for the presence of spontaneous nystagmus and

TABLE 17.3   Special Questions During History Taking

Have you noticed any loss of hearing?

Have you any ringing in your ears or a feeling of fullness?

Have you ever fallen?

Have you ever lost consciousness?

Have you any double vision, trouble swallowing or speaking during an attack?

Any other neurological symptoms such as weakness, numbness or pins and needles?

Do you have a history of migraine or other headaches?

Have you any neck pain or stiffness?

the direction (of the fast phase) noted. Nystagmus can be upbeating, downbeating, horizontal, torsional or a mixture (e.g., upbeating torsional). It is not always visible in room light when the patient can fixate on something and suppress it. Specialised infrared goggles (Fig. 17.5) can be used to view the eyes with fixation removed. Nystagmus of peripheral origin is generally direction fixed and increases when the patient gazes in the direction of the fast phase. Spontaneous upbeating, downbeating or a pure torsional nystagmus indicates a CNS lesion (Kerber & Baloh 2011). Ocular range of movement (gaze up, down, left and right), smooth pursuit and saccadic eye movements, and the ability to cancel the VOR are then assessed (Table 17.4). These eye movements are centrally programmed, and deficits observed are indicative of CNS disorders (Tusa 2010). Specific tests of peripheral vestibular loss include the head impulse test (Kerber & Baloh 2011).

The assessment of posture, tone, strength, sensation, proprioception, coordination, and reflexes provides useful information (particularly when a central lesion is suspected or known). A musculoskeletal examination is carried out on the trunk and extremities if indicated. Particular attention should be directed to the cervical spine and the feet because these have important roles in balance.

Functional Ability

Dynamic visual acuity is a functional measure of the VOR and objectively quantifies how visual acuity degrades during head movement (Badke et al 2004, Herdman et al 1998). The patient sits in front of a visual acuity chart (e.g., an Early Treatment of Diabetic Retinopathy Study chart) (Fig. 17.6). They are asked to verbalise the letters on the chart, starting at the top of the chart and working their way down. The lowest line at which they can accurately identify three of (usually) five letters is noted as their static visual acuity. The examiner stands behind the patient and holds the patient's head while rotating it leftwards and rightwards in the horizontal plane at a rate of 2 Hz and at an amplitude of about 30°. The patient repeats the task of reading the letters aloud. If the VOR is functioning normally, visual acuity will not degrade more than two lines on the chart. Gait and balance are then assessed (Table 17.5).

Outcome Measures

A systematic review of outcome measures used in vestibular rehabilitation research found a total of 50 (Fong et al 2015). Of these, the top four most commonly reported were the Dizziness Handicap Inventory (DHI) (Jacobson & Newman 1990), the Activities-specific Balance Confidence (ABC) (Legters et al 2005, Marchetti et al 2011, Powell & Myers 1995), the Vertigo Symptom Scale (VSS) (Yardley et al 1992) and the Visual Analogue Scale (VAS) of dizziness,

TABLE 17.4 Key Assessment Findings

Oculomotor Examination	Details

Spontaneous nystagmus
  Room light (visual fixation)
  Frenzel lenses (no visual fixation)
Gaze-evoked nystagmus[a]
Smooth Pursuit[a]
Saccades[a]
VOR cancellation[a]
VOR
  Gaze stabilisation with head movement
  Slow head movement
  Fast head movement
Positional tests
	Patient looks straight ahead. The eyes are observed for a nystagmus, and the direction is noted. Frenzel lenses both remove visual fixation and magnify the eyes (see Fig. 17.6). Nystagmus arising from a peripheral vestibular disorder can be suppressed by visual fixation.
	Ability to hold eyes steady on a stationary object. If abnormal, the eyes will make jerky movements to remain on the object.
	Ability to track a moving object with the eyes when the head is stationary. When normal, the eyes make smooth movements; abnormalities include jerky movements of the eyes.
	Ability to move the eyes from one stationary target to another when the head is stationary. When abnormal, the eyes may over- or under-shoot the target.
	Ability to suppress the VOR and move the eyes in phase with the head. Patient is asked to follow a moving target as the examiner moves the head in the same direction.
	A normal VOR is when the eyes can make a compensatory movement to stay on a stationary target when the head moves. Patient is asked to keep eyes steady on a target whilst the examiner moves patient's head in a small range of movement from side to side and then up and down slowly. This is repeated with faster movements of the head. Abnormalities would involve a saccadic movement of the eyes to stay on the target.

Hallpike–Dix test (see Fig. 17.4) Horizontal roll test	The patient is long sitting on plinth with eyes open. The head is turned 45° to the side that is being tested. The patient is brought quickly into a lying position with the head in 30° extension by the examiner. This position is maintained for 50 seconds, and the presence, duration and direction of nystagmus is noted. Symptoms are also noted. This test is diagnostic for BPPV. The nystagmus observed will usually be upbeating and torsional towards the affected side, i.e., towards the left in the left Hallpike–Dix position. This indicates a posterior semicircular canal BPPV. In extremely rare cases, the anterior canal can be affected and the nystagmus will be downbeating and torsional towards the affected side. The patient lies supine, the examiner rolls the head to the left, and the patient's eyes are examined for nystagmus, direction and intensity. The head is then rolled to the right, and the patient's eyes are examined for nystagmus, direction and intensity. If the nystagmus is horizontal and the fast phase is towards the ground (geotropic nystagmus) when the head is turned to either side, this is likely to be canalithiasis of the horizontal canal. Usually the nystagmus is more intense on one side, and this is the affected side. If the nystagmus is horizontal and the fast phase is away from the ground (apogeotropic) when the head is turned to either side, this is likely to be cupulolithiasis of the horizontal canal. Usually the nystagmus is more intense on the unaffected side.

BPPV, Benign paroxysmal positional vertigo; *VOR*, vestibular ocular reflex.
[a]If this test is abnormal, it is indicative of central nervous system pathology.

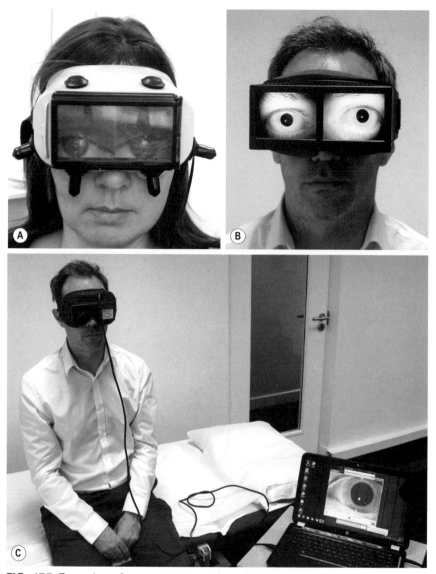

FIG. 17.5 Examples of eye movement observing and recording systems. These are used to remove visual fixation and magnify the eyes for ease of observation.

imbalance and oscillopsia (Herdman et al 2012). A recent survey of vestibular rehabilitation practice in Europe confirmed that the DHI, VAS and ABC were most used for patient-reported outcome measures, and the modified Clinical Test of Sensory Interaction of Balance (Fig. 17.7), Functional Gait Assessment, Dynamic Gait Index, Romberg and tandem Romberg tests were the most used outcome measures of balance and gait (Meldrum et al 2020) (see Table 17.5). Reliability has been established for

most of the commonly used outcome measures (Hall & Herdman 2006, Herdman 2010).

PROGNOSIS

In most cases, the symptoms of patients with a unilateral peripheral vestibular loss spontaneously ameliorate in about six weeks. The process by which the patient recovers is called *vestibular compensation*. The spontaneous

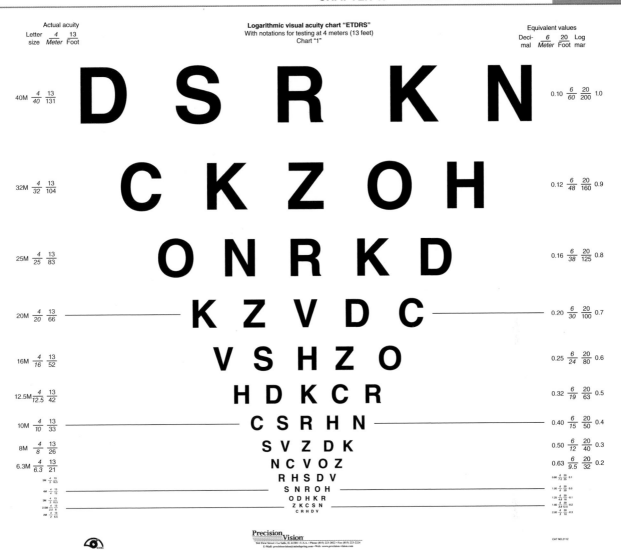

FIG. 17.6 An Early Treatment for Diabetic Retinopathy Study (ETDRS) chart.

nystagmus disappears by 2–3 days (static compensation) and the symptoms associated with movement (vertigo, visual blurring and postural unsteadiness) by 6 weeks (dynamic compensation). Hair cells have not been shown to regenerate in humans; therefore the patient must recover by other means. Research has shown that plastic changes occur in the CNS in response to peripheral vestibular pathology which are responsible for vestibular compensation (Curthoys & Halmagyi 2007, Lacour & Bernard-Demanze 2014, Macdougall & Curthoys 2012). Three processes are thought to contribute. Initially the cerebellum inhibits firing of the vestibular nuclei of the unaffected side, probably to reduce the asymmetry produced by the

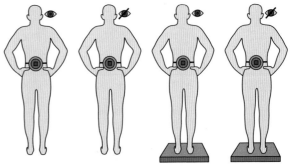

FIG. 17.7 The Modified Clinical Test of the Sensory Interaction of Balance (mCTSIB).

TABLE 17.5 Balance and Gait Assessment and Outcome Measures

Balance and Gait Outcome Measures	Details
Romberg (Black et al 1982)	Patient stands with feet close together and eyes closed. This test can also be performed with eyes open in very severely impaired patients.
Tandem Romberg	Patient stands heel to toe with preferred foot in front.
Eyes open	Patient is asked to stand on one leg with eyes open and then closed.
Eyes closed	Patient is asked to walk heel to toe on a line for a distance of 3 feet, and the number of steps off the line is counted.
One-leg stance (Bohannon et al 1984)	This is the farthest distance that the patient can reach without moving their feet.
Eyes open	A 14-item functional balance assessment.
Eyes closed	A 13-item functional balance assessment and a 9-item gait assessment.
Tandem walking	A six-item test of balance involving manipulation of visual, vestibular and somatosensory systems.
Functional reach test (Duncan 1990, Mann et al 1996)	The visual conflict dome is a modified Japanese lantern placed over the patient's head which gives erroneous information about the vertical and thus reduces the ability of the patient to use visual cues for balance. This test has been modified to contain items 1, 2, 4 and 5 (mCTSIB) (see Fig. 17.7).
Berg Balance Scale (Berg et al 1989)	
Tinetti's Balance Performance Assessment (Tinetti 1986)	
Clinical Test of Sensory Interaction and Balance (CTSIB) (Cohen et al 1993, Shumway-Cook & Horak 1986)	
1. Stand with feet together eyes open.	Computerised system using a specialised force plate and visual surround which measures postural sway in conditions similar to the CTSIB.
2. Stand with feet together eyes closed.	Gait speed over 10 m; gait speed is a sensitive marker of overall gait function.
3. Stand with feet together and visual conflict dome.	An eight-item rating of gait function including a timed walk, changing speed, walking with head turns, walking over and around obstacles and up a staircase. Maximum score of 21.
4. Stand on foam eyes open.	
5. Stand on foam eyes closed.	
6. Stand on foam with visual conflict dome.	
Posturography	Time taken to rise from a chair and sit down again five times. Normative data are available.
Gait Measures	
10-m walk test	This tests the ability of the person to step over objects in forwards, sideways and backwards directions.
Dynamic Gait Index Long and short form (Hall & Herdman 2006, Hall et al 2004, Marchetti & Whitney 2006, Whitney et al 2003)	Similar to the DGI, this test incorporates items from the DGI and scores them in a similar way. It includes additional tests such as walking with eyes closed and walking backwards. There is a total of 10 items and a maximum score of 30.
Five times sit to stand (Meretta et al 2006)	This is an amalgamation of balance and gait tests, incorporating Timed Up and Go, some items from the DGI and also measures of anticipatory and reactive balance. There is a total of 14 items and a maximum score of 28.
Four Square Step Test (Whitney et al 2007)	
Functional Gait Assessment (Wrisley et al 2004)	
Mini-Balance Evaluation Systems Test (Franchignoni et al 2010, Godi et al 2013)	Concussion-specific measure: Patient scores symptoms during tests of smooth pursuit, horizontal and vertical saccades, convergence, VOR horizontal, VOR vertical, and visual motion sensitivity.
Vestibular ocular motor screening (Mucha et al 2014)	

Balance tests are timed for a period of up to 30 seconds, and the best of three attempts is recorded for assessment of change over time.

CTSIB, Clinical Test of Sensory Interaction in Balance; *DGI*, Dynamic Gait Index; *VOR*, vestibular ocular reflex.

lesion. The vestibular nucleus of the affected side begins to spontaneously tonically fire again probably because of neurochemical changes produced by the loss of input (denervation supersensitivity) (Curthoys 2000).

The second process is known as sensory substitution. In this process the CNS reorganises to substitute or use inputs more efficiently from intact systems including vision and somatosensory and cervical proprioceptive systems. The intact vestibular end organ can compensate for loss on the other side because both sides respond to head movement in any direction. It is important to note also that if there is some remaining vestibular function on the pathological side, the CNS will use it.

Lastly the process of habituation is thought to play a role in vestibular compensation. Habituation is generally defined as a reduction in response over time with repeated exposure to a specific stimulus. This is the process thought to underpin improvement with vestibular exercises in which the patient repeatedly performs head and/or eye movements that provoke symptoms of vertigo.

The reasons why some patients fail to compensate are not always clear but may be a result of abnormality in the CNS, visual, somatosensory or musculoskeletal systems. Also the lesion may be too large or is fluctuating. Animal studies have shown that compensation is delayed by immobilisation or reduced or absent visual inputs and is promoted by exercise (Courjon et al 1977, Fetter et al 1988, Igarashi et al 1988, Lacour et al 1981). It is thought that the CNS needs to experience the *error* signals for vestibular compensation to occur. It is possible that psychological factors that result in excessive vigilance and avoidance of head and body movements can impede vestibular compensation. Certain medications, including those used in the treatment of vestibular problems, can also delay compensation (Zee 1985). An intact CNS is vitally important for the process of vestibular compensation, and human and animal studies have shown that central vestibular problems will have a slower and more incomplete recovery (Aleisa et al 2007, Shepard et al 1993). Recently it has been shown that vestibular rehabilitation which is provided early after a vestibular neuritis (within the first 2 weeks) results in superior recovery of dynamic visual acuity (Lacour et al 2020). In bilateral vestibular loss, there may be no remaining VOR function with which to compensate, so the process of sensory substitution plays a major role in the recovery of these patients. Recovery will always be incomplete.

KEY POINTS

Most patients with unilateral peripheral vestibular pathology spontaneously recover in a few weeks through a process known as *vestibular compensation*. Patients who do not spontaneously recover present for treatment and benefit from vestibular rehabilitation.

INTERVENTIONS

Vestibular rehabilitation aims to educate the patient; maximise vestibular compensation, thus reducing vertigo,

TABLE 17.6 Patient Groups That Benefit From Vestibular Rehabilitation (Shepard & Telian 1995)

Patients with noncompensated peripheral vestibular disorders

Benign paroxysmal positional vertigo

Stable central vestibular lesions or mixed central and peripheral lesions (e.g., head injury)

Multifactorial balance abnormalities (e.g., elderly)

Postablative surgery (e.g., vestibular schwannoma resection, labyrinthectomy)

TABLE 17.7 Treatment Plan and Goals

Education

Habituation exercises

Adaptation exercises

Balance and gait reeducation

Particle repositioning manoeuvres (e.g., Modified Epley's; see Fig. 17.9)

Physical conditioning

Relaxation

Breathing exercises

Treatment of neck and back pain

Correction of postural abnormalities

Goals of Treatment

Encourage and educate regarding importance of head movement and physical exercise for vestibular compensation

Reduce subjective symptoms of dizziness, vertigo, anxiety, oscillopsia, imbalance and nausea

Improve gaze stability

Improve static and dynamic balance with particular attention to improving the use of vestibular cues (i.e., exercises with eyes closed and on an unstable surface)

Reduce fall risk

Improve balance control during gait

Maintain or improve fitness levels

dizziness and nausea; improve balance and gait; and reduce or alleviate secondary problems such as physical deconditioning and neck or back pain. Patient groups that benefit most from vestibular rehabilitation are shown in Table 17.6, and there are now many texts on this subject alone (Herdman & Clendaniel 2015, Jacobson & Shephard 2021).

A vestibular rehabilitation programme will likely target several impairments, and these are summarised in Table 17.7. Patients commonly report that they believe their symptoms are too severe to have a benign cause and fear a more sinister pathology (most commonly a brain tumour) despite the latter being excluded by the medical team. Practically without exception, the first encounter with the patient thus requires education and reassurance about the problem. It is important that the patient receives an explanation about the principles of vestibular compensation and the importance of movement for this process because patients have usually been avoiding symptom-provoking movements and postures. Written information is very useful (see recommended literature at the end of the chapter).

Gaze Stability Exercises

The patient with unilateral vestibular hypofunction who has not been able to compensate usually has three main problems: decreased gain of the VOR leading to decreased gaze stability during head movement (oscillopsia), vertigo or associated symptoms at rest or during head/self-movement (often termed *motion sensitivity*) and impaired balance and gait. Clinical guidelines are now available for the treatment of unilateral vestibular hypofunction (Hall et al 2021). Each of these requires separate treatment approaches. Gaze stability is promoted with eye–head coordination exercises (Enticott et al 2008, Herdman et al 1995, Meldrum & Jahn 2019, Szturm et al 1994, Venosa & Bittar 2007). For example, the patient is asked to look at a stationary object (this could be a letter pinned to a wall) and rotate their head in the horizontal plane and then up and down keeping the letter in focus (known as VORx1 exercises) (Fig. 17.8). The patient is instructed to do the exercise for up to a minute but only as tolerated. The speed and duration of the exercise are increased progressively. A metronome can be used (aiming for 120 beats/min), and the exercise can be made more difficult by having the object move out of phase with the head. The patient moves an object they are holding to the left and their head to the right, keeping their eyes on the object at all times, and then performs the opposite movement (known as VORx2 exercises). A progressive 6-week programme of gaze stabilisation exercises has been described by Meldrum et al (2015).

Habituation Exercises

Motion sensitivity is decreased by exercises that aim to habituate the patient to movement (Clendaniel 2010, Norre & Beckers 1989, Shepard & Telian 1995). It is first determined what head, eye or body movements cause vertigo or dizziness. Patients are then instructed to carry out these movements for short periods three to four times a day. Each movement or exercise is repeated just to the point where symptoms begin to come on. Gradually over time the patient habituates to the movement, and the duration, frequency or complexity can be increased (e.g., decreasing the base of support when doing the exercises). It is important

that the patient is warned that they should not feel excessively symptomatic after performing the exercises because this may decrease compliance. Exercises should be graded gently and performed only as tolerated. In the early stages, patients may be able to perform only one exercise at a time. Alternatively, the Motion Sensitivity Quotient (Smith-Wheelock et al 1991) or the modified Motion Sensitivity Quotient (Heusel-Gillig et al 2022), both validated measures, can be used as a basis for habituation exercises. The patient performs tests of head and body movements (e.g., getting into the HPD position, rolling over in bed and rotating 180° in standing) and rates the intensity and duration of their symptoms. Those movements that cause mild to moderate symptoms are used as the basis for the exercise programme and progressed as tolerated.

Visual Desensitisation Exercises

People with chronic vestibular disorders often experience dizziness triggered by movement of the visual environment (so-called visually induced dizziness, or ViD for short) (Bisdorff et al 2009). ViD is believed to be caused by a reliance on visual cues for spatial orientation, although the mechanisms are still poorly understood. Questionnaires such as the Situational Characteristics Questionnaire (Dannenbaum & Chilingaryan 2011) and Visual Vertigo Analogue Scale can be helpful to identify ViD (Guerraz et al 2001, Jacob et al 1989, Pavlou et al 2006).

Vestibular rehabilitation for ViD usually includes graded exposure to visual motion, often using optokinetic stimulus. This can be in a simulator or using virtual reality (Alahmari et al 2014, Gottshall & Sessoms 2015, Pavlou 2004, Pavlou et al 2012). It can also be achieved with low-cost methods such as using a disco ball or watching visual motion videos on YouTube (see the excellent YouTube channel by Gabrielle Pierce https://www.youtube.com/channel/UCwDX4UUxFH7BZhs2gFYw6oA) (Pavlou et al 2013).

Optokinetic stimulation can be provocative; consequently it is usually introduced later into a person's vestibular rehabilitation programme. Visual stimuli that trigger mild or moderate, rather than severe, symptoms are usually selected. Factors to consider include the screen size, duration, varying distances from the screen, progressing from fixating in the middle of the screen to practicing saccades and scanning, and progressing from sitting to standing/walking. Caution should be exercised for people with a history of migraine to avoid triggering headache. For these patients, a more conservative approach is needed, usually beginning with a short duration (i.e., 15 seconds) and fewer repetitions.

Balance and Gait Reeducation

Balance exercises are customised to the patient depending on the findings of the balance assessment and are

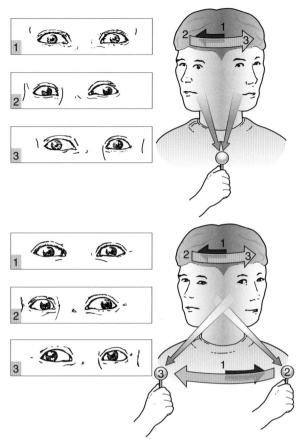

Instructions for vestibular adaptation exercises

Tape a business card on the wall in front of you so that you can read it

Move your head back and forth sideways, keep the words in focus

Move your head faster but keep the words in focus. Continue to do this for 1 or 2 minutes without stopping

Repeat the exercise moving your head up and down

Repeat the exercises using a large pattern such as a checkerboard (full-field stimulus)

Initially, this exercise can be performed in a sitting position. To increase the difficulty of the exercise and to work on static postural stability, this exercise can be performed while standing. Initially start with your feet apart, and gradually work toward standing with one foot in front of the other

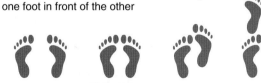

FIG. 17.8 Adaptation exercises.

included in the home exercise programme. For example, if a patient has a particular dependence on vision and it is known that there is some remaining vestibular function, the therapist might choose to include exercises that minimise visual inputs for the patient to use and 'strengthen' remaining vestibular function. Exercises with eyes closed and/or on an unstable surface (such as a foam cushion or wobble board or moveable platform) would be included in such a programme. Balance exercises can be graded by progressively decreasing the area of the base of support, increasing the height of the centre of gravity from the supporting surface, or manipulation of the environment by the removal or alteration of visual (e.g., eyes closed or head moving) or somatosensory (e.g., on foam or on a uneven surface) cues.

The complexity of balance tasks is progressively increased over time as the patient improves. For example, when a patient is able to walk on a flat surface with good postural control, they can be asked to walk at a faster pace, walk on an incline or walk while talking or moving their head up and down or from side to side. Care should be taken particularly in the initial stages to avoid falls. This is best achieved by having another person supervise or by having a supportive surface such as a wall or chair nearby.

Balance has been shown to improve with vestibular rehabilitation in several randomised controlled studies using various approaches such as force plates, gaming technologies, virtual reality, tai chi or more conventional approaches (Cakrt et al 2010, McGibbon et al 2005, Meldrum et al 2015, Sparrer et al 2013, Strupp et al 1998, Teggi et al 2009, Xie et al 2021).

Gait and postural reeducation are also important because patients may adopt abnormal postures whilst moving and decrease the amplitude of head movement (Mijovic et al 2014, Wang et al 2021). They may turn en bloc rather than dissociating their head from their trunk. Retraining can include use of verbal and visual feedback. Gait aids may be necessary in the acute stages.

The patient with a central vestibular loss requires a similar therapeutic approach, but recovery will be slower and more incomplete (Balci et al 2013, Shepard & Telian 1995). Recent randomised controlled trials investigating vestibular rehabilitation in patients with multiple sclerosis have demonstrated a positive benefit in improving balance, dizziness and fatigue (Garcia Munoz et al 2020, Hebert et al 2011, Ozgen et al 2016). Also vestibular rehabilitation can have positive benefits for those with dizziness and balance disorders after concussion (Alsalaheen et al 2010, Kleffelgaard et al 2019, Kontos et al 2021, Murray et al 2017, Schneider et al 2014).

The mainstay of treatment for the patient with bilateral vestibular loss is to encourage substitution of visual

and proprioceptive systems for vestibular function (Herdman et al 2003, 2007, Krebs et al 1993). It is thought that these patients may be able to substitute pursuit and saccadic eye movements (generated by the CNS) and the cervico-ocular reflex to maintain gaze stability. Thus balance exercises and functional activities incorporating saccadic and pursuit eye movements are included in programmes for these patients. Results from a systematic review concluded that there is moderate strength evidence that gaze stability and balance can be improved in adults with bilateral vestibular hypofunction (Porciuncula et al 2012). However, well-designed large clinical trials are needed.

Management of Benign Paroxysmal Positional Vertigo

The management of the patient with BPPV is based on manoeuvres (called canal repositioning manoeuvres or liberatory manoeuvres) or exercises which move the otoconia responsible for the vertiginous episodes from the involved canal back into the utricle (Bhattacharyya et al 2017, Hilton & Pinder 2004). In most cases the otoconia are in the PSCC. For canalithiasis (the crystals are free floating), Epley's manoeuvre (Epley 1992) or a modified version is commonly used (Fig. 17.9). The head is moved through different positions so that the otoconia move out of the involved SCC. After Epley's manoeuvre has been performed, the HPD test is repeated and, if still positive, the manoeuvre can be repeated within a treatment session up to four times, as long as the patient can tolerate it (Korn et al 2007). Patients can be taught to self-perform the manoeuvre. If severe nausea or vomiting occurs because of BPPV, medication can be taken before or after treatment (e.g., cinnarizine); however, medication use is not generally advised in the management of BPPV, and vestibular suppressants can reduce nystagmus during testing, making diagnosis less certain (Gurumukhani et al 2021).

Horizontal Canal Benign Paroxysmal Positional Vertigo

Although there are several liberatory manoeuvres for horizontal canal BPPV, the most used and effective manoeuvres are the roll manoeuvre (360° degrees) and Gufoni manoeuvre (Fig. 17.10 A and B) (Fu et al 2020, Mandala et al 2013, 2019, 2020, Zuma et al 2020). In systematic reviews and a meta-analysis, the BBQ roll and Gufoni manoeuvre have a 95%–100% success rate (van den Broek et al 2014). The Gufoni manoeuvre is shown to have a more immediate resolution compared with a roll manoeuvre, but both have similar efficacy at 30-day follow-up evaluation. The Gufoni manoeuvre may be preferable when treating elderly or

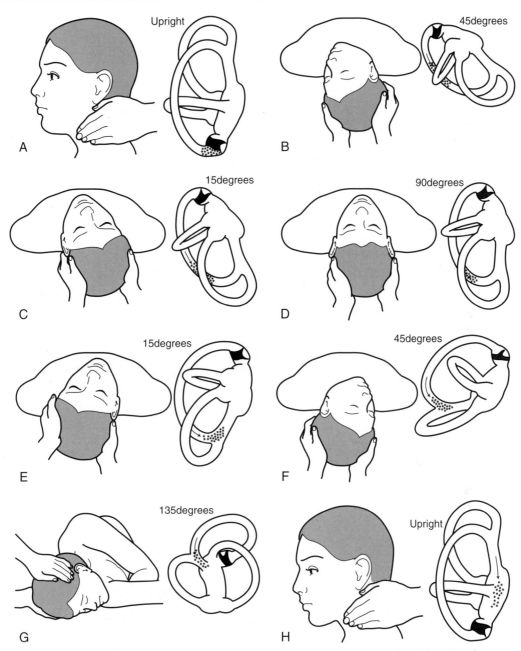

FIG. 17.9 Modified Epley's manoeuvre for left-sided benign paroxysmal positional vertigo.

obese patients or those with mobility issues. If an individual is unable to tolerate a manoeuvre or prefers not to have one performed, an alternative is forced prolonged positioning and involves lying on the opposite side to the problem for 12 hours (Kinne et al 2021).

Secondary Problems

Patients will often complain of neck pain and less commonly back pain associated with vertigo. Stiffness of the cervical spine caused by avoidance of head movements is frequently observed, and these patients often benefit

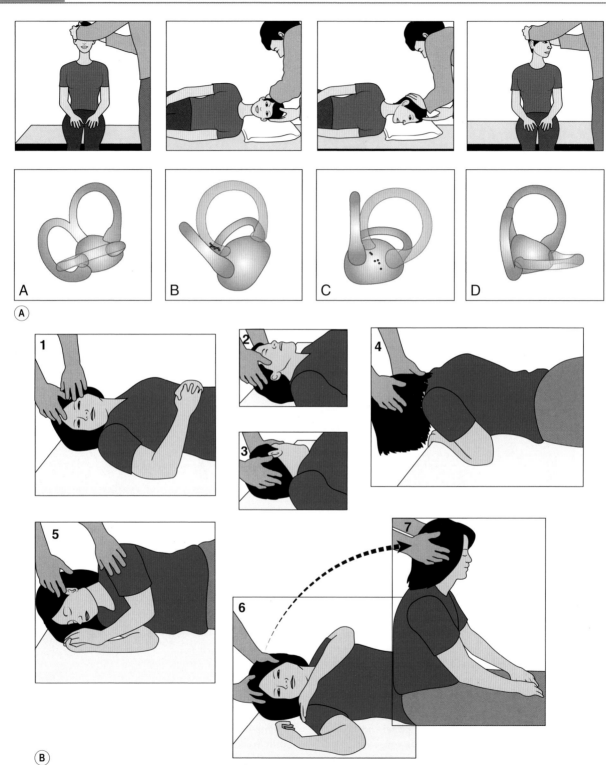

FIG. 17.10 Gufoni (A) and BBQ roll (B) for horizontal canal benign paroxysmal positional vertigo.

from joint mobilisations, electrotherapy and heat therapy. Physical deconditioning can also occur because patients understandably limit any activity that causes an increase in their symptoms. Promoting exercise through a graduated walking programme is usually the easiest and most acceptable way for patients to increase their exercise tolerance again (Meldrum et al 2015). Walking is also a functional and relevant context for the patient (e.g., as opposed to a static exercise bike), and head movements and visual stimulation during walking probably assist the process of vestibular compensation (Asai et al 2022). As the patient improves, they should be encouraged to resume their normal sporting or leisure activities as tolerated.

The physiotherapist can also intervene in the symptoms of anxiety and hyperventilation. Simple education on breathing, control of breathing (breathing exercises), the adverse effects of hyperventilation on cerebral blood flow and recognition of hyperventilation can help the patient recognise and control the problem. Relaxation classes or tapes can be used to teach the patient control of anxiety and associated muscular tension. Where significant anxiety exists or the patient describes agoraphobia, psychological evaluation and treatment are indicated, and there is evidence that cognitive behavioural therapy is an effective treatment when included as part of a vestibular rehabilitation programme (Herdman et al 2022, Schaaf & Hesse 2015, Yardley et al 2012).

OTHER CONSIDERATIONS

Covid-19 and the Vestibular System

The severe acute respiratory syndrome coronavirus 2 (SARS-CoV-2, Covid-19) was first reported in the latter part of 2019 and was officially declared a pandemic by the World Health Organization in March 2020. Studies of the effects of Covid-19 on the audiovestibular system are emerging. Dizziness is reported by up to 16.6% of patients in the first 21 days of infection, but for most dizziness resolves quickly (Alde et al 2022). A recent systematic review reported a pooled estimate of 7.2% of rotatory vertigo (Lough et al 2022). Studies that have measured vestibular function after Covid-19 infection have found varying results. One study reported low incidences of abnormalities in the Video Head Impulse test (Gallus et al 2021), but another found significant impairments in VOR gains after Covid-19 infection (Yilmaz et al 2022). The latter study also found that 20% of patients complained of balance problems after Covid-19 infection with significantly worse balance performance on computerised dynamic posturography when compared with controls. Clinicians evaluating dizziness, vertigo and imbalance should include questions about Covid-19 infection and any temporal associations with audiovestibular problems.

Remote and Digital Vestibular Rehabilitation

Digital health is a rapidly growing area, facilitating remote management and oversight of vestibular rehabilitation. The Covid-19 pandemic has accelerated adoption of a digital and remote approach to vestibular rehabilitation with more than 80% of physical therapists agreeing that telehealth was an effective platform for vestibular rehabilitation (Harrell et al 2021). Evidence is now emerging that digital approaches are effective for vestibular rehabilitation (Geraghty et al 2017, van Vugt et al 2020). Van Vugt et al (2020) in a three-arm randomised controlled trial found that internet-based vestibular rehabilitation was more effective than standard medical care. Moreover, there were no significant differences in outcomes between those who received solely an internet-based vestibular rehabilitation intervention and those who had two home visits during the internet-based programme. Meldrum et al (2022) recently reported significant improvements in subjective outcomes of dizziness, vertigo, imbalance, oscillopsia and anxiety in patients with vestibular dysfunction who used an app-based programme to perform and track their exercises and symptoms remotely. It is envisaged that digital vestibular rehabilitation will become more widespread in the future.

Multidisciplinary Team

Patients with vestibular problems can be seen by a variety of members of the MDT, and communication between them facilitates optimum management. Diagnosis can be made at the level of primary care, and it must be emphasised that most patients are managed at this level because vestibular problems are generally associated with a favourable prognosis and spontaneous resolution. Patients who continue to experience problems can be referred for assessment and diagnosis to ENT physicians, audiovestibular physicians (neuro-otologists), physiotherapists who may or may not prescribe medications (Burrows et al 2017, Kasbekar et al 2014), audiologists (Tavora-Vieira et al 2022), neurologists and neurosurgeons. Audiologists and audiological scientists carry out vestibular function testing, and audiologists and physiotherapists undertake vestibular rehabilitation and falls management. Psychiatrists and psychologists are involved in the management of psychological problems associated with vestibular problems.

Specialist Centres and Support Groups

Vestibular rehabilitation is a specialist area within physiotherapy, although vestibular and balance rehabilitation is relevant across a lifespan within all specialties. There are now many centres worldwide that specialise in vestibular rehabilitation, and there is a physiotherapy special interest group – the Association of Physiotherapists Interested in Vestibular Rehabilitation (ACPIVR) – in the United Kingdom that provides support, education materials, resources, patient information leaflets and training opportunities (http://www.acpivr.com). There are competency documents from the Bárány Society (van de Berg et al 2022) (www.thebaranysociety.org) and the ACPIVR framework for physiotherapists working within vestibular and balance system healthcare. Both can be used to identify individual learning needs and develop competency. The Royal Institute for Deaf People (http://www.rnid.org.uk), the British Brain and Spine Foundation (www.brainandspine.org.uk), the American Physical Therapy Association (http://www.APTA.org) and the Vestibular Disorders Association (http://www.vestibular.org) are useful websites that have patient information leaflets on different aspects of vestibular and hearing problems. The American Physical Therapy Association website and Vestibular First (http://www.vestibularfirst.com) also host journal clubs and podcasts on different aspects of vestibular rehabilitation.

Support Groups

Royal National Institute for Deaf People
   19-23 Featherstone Street
   London EC1 Y8SL
   www.rnid.org.uk
Ménière's Society
   The Atrium
   Curtis Road, Dorking
   Surrey RH4 1XA
   https://www.menieres.org.uk/

Useful Resources

The free aVOR app can be downloaded from the Apple app store and is useful for teaching and demonstrating aspects of vestibular rehabilitation to patients. It consists of a three-dimensional 'virtual' head and labyrinths. It generates ocular movements in response to head movement and can be programmed to have a central or peripheral vestibular disorder such as BPPV, unilateral hypofunction or cerebellar involvement. The resultant nystagmus is generated.

An educational website with a step-by-step guide to examination of eye movements and the vestibular system and interpretation of results with video examples can be found at https://novel.utah.edu/Gold.

CONCLUSION

The strength of scientific evidence supporting physical management of vestibular disease is growing and validates the inclusion of vestibular rehabilitation in most rehabilitation settings. An MDT approach with specialised therapists is likely to provide optimal outcomes. Although gaps remain in the knowledge relating to specific types and intensity of exercises, particularly in the area of visually induced dizziness and functional vestibular disorders, it is likely that future research will enhance knowledge and further improve outcomes.

CASE STUDIES

Case 1: Peripheral Vestibular Neuritis

Mr V, a 68-year-old man, presented with a 6-month history of vertigo that was aggravated by walking, bending down, looking up and turning around. He described that his head constantly felt 'all mixed up and muzzy'. His symptoms began with a sudden onset of severe vertigo, vomiting and unsteadiness. He was then unable to walk unaided and was confined to bed for 4 days. Over the following few weeks his symptoms gradually decreased in severity but remained problematic. An MRI scan was normal. Hearing was normal. Electronystagmography showed no positional nystagmus, and all tests of smooth pursuit and saccades were normal. Caloric testing demonstrated a 100% right canal paresis with an 88% directional preponderance to the left. A diagnosis of a right peripheral vestibular neuritis was made. His medications were betahistine (Serc) and prochlorperazine (Stemetil) twice a day. Medical history included prostate surgery 2 years ago. He had no previous history of vertigo. Mr V was a retired accountant and was unable to pursue his usual hobbies of gardening and walking since the onset of his symptoms. Findings were normal on examination of tone, power, sensation, proprioception, reflexes and coordination. There were no cervical spine symptoms, and the range of movement of the cervical spine was pain free and within normal limits. On oculomotor examination there was no spontaneous nystagmus (in room light or with fixation removed by infrared goggles) (see Fig. 17.6). Smooth pursuit and saccadic eye movements were normal. The VOR cancellation test was normal. VOR testing revealed a catch-up saccadic movement of the eyes to the left during a right clinical head impulse test. Positional tests (HPD test) were negative bilaterally. A normal gait pattern was observed. The Romberg test was normal. Mr V was unable to maintain tandem Romberg with his eyes closed. One-leg stance (OLS) test times were normal with eyes open but were decreased with eyes closed (left OLS, 3 seconds; right OLS, 2 seconds). He could tandem walk a 1-metre line but took four steps off the line. Mr V had difficulty with item 5 (he was able to maintain the position for only 5 seconds) of the Clinical Test for Sensory

Interaction in Balance (CTSIB). When Mr V performed repeated tracking movements with his eyes, he reported moderate vertigo. He also reported severe vertigo with repeated head movements in all planes with eyes open and closed, bending down to touch the floor and turning on the spot. Mr V was firstly given an explanation of why he was experiencing his symptoms and the process of vestibular compensation. He agreed that his main problems were motion sensitivity (i.e., vertigo provoked by movement) and balance impairment. His treatment programme aimed to increase the gain of the VOR through adaptation exercises and to decrease motion sensitivity. Mr V carried out an exercise programme four times daily. Initially exercises consisted of focusing on a business card in his hand whilst moving his head from side to side and then up and down at a speed that kept the letters in focus. He also carried out habituation exercises. These included visually tracking his own thumb as he moved it from side to side and then up and down while keeping his head steady. Other exercises included head and cervical spine movements (rotation and flexion and extension), which were performed with his eyes open and closed. Each exercise was performed only until vertigo began to develop. Over 4 months, the speed, complexity and duration of exercises were gradually increased as symptoms lessened. Mr V was also provided with a balance exercise programme that he performed daily. He was encouraged to discuss cessation of betahistine and prochlorperazine with his doctor and decrease use over time. He had discontinued all use of vestibular medications 2 months later.

Mr V steadily improved and had five sessions of treatment over 6 months. Two months into treatment, he developed a common cold and reported that his symptoms temporarily worsened. At his final visit, he reported he felt '85% of normal'. His VSS and Vertigo Handicap Questionnaire scores demonstrated a significant improvement. His balance had improved, demonstrated by an increase in time on balance tests. He had resumed his hobbies.

Case 2: Benign Paroxysmal Positional Vertigo

Mrs F was a 76-year-old woman who presented with a lightheaded, spinning sensation and described being off balance during walking but has no symptoms when still. Her symptoms worsen when she turned quickly, looked up to get things out of the cupboard, got in and out of bed and when she rolled over in bed to the right. The spinning sensation lasted less than 1 minute and could trigger nausea. Her symptoms started 6 weeks ago when she was getting up out of bed and suddenly she became very dizzy, lost her balance and had to lie down. There were no symptoms when lying still, and although symptoms had reduced in intensity with time, they remained. The general practitioner prescribed prochlorperazine and referred her for vestibular rehabilitation; medication was stopped because it did not help.

There were no other associated symptoms of hearing loss, tinnitus, aural fullness, ear discharge, headaches, visual disturbance or falls and no focal neurological deficit. Good general health was described with no other health problems; Mrs F was in a safe relationship, lived an active healthy lifestyle, exercised regularly, did not smoke and only occasionally drank alcohol. She had not driven since the onset of dizziness.

On examination, she had full cervical spine range of movement with no pain or symptom provocation. All ocular motor screening, including saccades, smooth pursuit, convergence/divergence, VOR cancellation and head impulse testing, was normal. Video-oculography examining gaze evoked nystagmus, and head shaking nystagmus was normal. Dynamic visual acuity testing resulted in a two-line discrepancy within normal ranges. Gait was normal, and balance testing using the modified CTSIB and five times sit to stand were normal, highlighting a low falls risk. The HPD test with infrared video goggles was normal on the left but on the right produced a latent (5 seconds) sensation of dizziness associated with an upbeating, right torsional nystagmus lasting 20 seconds. Supine rolls tests were negative bilaterally, and there was no adverse reaction to testing procedures.

A positive right HPD is indicative of a right posterior canalithiasis BPPV which is best treated with Epley's or Semont's manoeuvre. A right Epley's manoeuvre was performed with informed verbal consent and without adverse reaction. A second Epley's manoeuvre was performed to improve efficacy, an information leaflet was provided, and falls and fracture risk, safety, recurrence rates and not to drive if dizzy were discussed. Normal activity including walking with head movements and visual targeting was encouraged, no movement restriction was advised, and the consultation was accurately documented. During a review 1 week later, Mrs F reported symptoms had resolved and all provoking activities previously described were normal. Further treatment in the event of recurrence was advised to reduce falls and fracture risk, and she was discharged.

Clinical note: This is a straightforward case of BPPV with no complicating features. BPPV affects the posterior canal in 80% of cases, and appropriate canal repositioning manoeuvres are the most effective management, with more than 90% of cases resolving after one treatment session. Medication in most cases is not recommended unless there is extreme nausea, vomiting or severe anxiety. Further investigation with MRI is recommended only if symptoms do not resolve within three treatment sessions because a central abnormality (e.g., stroke or aneurysm) can (rarely) mimic BPPV. Careful counselling and demonstration of the testing and treatment manoeuvres can help reduce anxiety and improve patient participation. Dizziness and imbalance usually resolve within 48 hours of a successful treatment as the balance system recalibrates. A clear indication of success is no symptoms in provoking positions and clear HPD and supine roll tests.

SELF-ASSESSMENT QUESTIONS

1. What is vestibular neuritis? Explain how vestibular neuritis leads to the loss of body functions, and list the body functions that can be affected by vestibular neuritis.
2. What is vestibular compensation? Give the main reasons why a patient may fail to compensate after a peripheral vestibular lesion.
3. Vestibular disorders are classified as central or peripheral. Apart from vestibular neuritis, list three peripheral and three central disorders.
4. Nystagmus is observed in unilateral peripheral vestibular loss. Define nystagmus. In a patient with right unilateral vestibular loss, describe both the direction of nystagmus and the reason for this.
5. What does BPPV stand for? List the main signs and symptoms of BPPV. What SCC is affected most commonly, and name a treatment for BPPV of this canal?

REFERENCES

Adamec, I., Juren Meaški, S., Krbot Skorić, M., et al., 2020. Persistent postural-perceptual dizziness: clinical and neurophysiological study. J. Clin. Neurosci. 72, 26–30.

Agrawal, Y., Carey, J.P., Della Santina, C.C., et al., 2009. Disorders of balance and vestibular function in us adults: data from the national health and nutrition examination survey, 2001–2004. Arch. Int. Med. 169, 938–944.

Agrawal, Y., Van de Berg, R., Wuyts, F., et al., 2019. Presbyvestibulopathy: diagnostic criteria consensus document of the classification committee of the Bárány Society. J. Vestib. Res. 29, 161–170.

Agus, S., Benecke, H., Thum, C., Strupp, M., 2013. Clinical and demographic features of vertigo: findings from the REVERT registry. Front. Neurol. 4, 48.

Akin, F.W., Murnane, O.D., Hall, C.D., Riska, K.M., 2017. Vestibular consequences of mild traumatic brain injury and blast exposure: a review. Brain Inj. 31, 1188–1194.

Alahmari, K.A., Sparto, P.J., Marchetti, G.F., et al., 2014. Comparison of virtual reality based therapy with customized vestibular physical therapy for the treatment of vestibular disorders. IEEE Trans. Neural. Syst. Rehabil. Eng. 22, 389–399.

Aldè, M., Barozzi, S., Di Berardino, F., et al., 2022. Prevalence of symptoms in 1512 COVID-19 patients: have dizziness and vertigo been underestimated thus far? Int. Emerg. Med. 17, 1343–1353.

Aleisa, M., Zeitouni, A.G., Cullen, K.E., 2007. Vestibular compensation after unilateral labyrinthectomy: normal versus cerebellar dysfunctional mice. J. Otolaryngol. 36, 315–321.

Alghadir, A.H., Anwer, S., 2018. Effects of vestibular rehabilitation in the management of a vestibular migraine: a review. Front. Neurol. 9, 440.

Allum, J.H., Adkin, A.L., 2003. Improvements in trunk sway observed for stance and gait tasks during recovery from an acute unilateral peripheral vestibular deficit. Audiol. Neurotol. 8, 286–302.

Alsalaheen, B.A., Mucha, A., Morris, L.O., et al., 2010. Vestibular rehabilitation for dizziness and balance disorder after concussion. J. Neurol. Phys. Ther. 34, 87–93.

Asai, H., Murakami, S., Morimoto, H., et al., 2022. Effects of a walking program in patients with chronic unilateral vestibular hypofunction. J. Phys. Ther. Sci. 34, 85–91.

Badke, M.B., Shea, T.A., Miedaner, J.A., Grove, C.R., 2004. Outcomes after rehabilitation for adults with balance dysfunction. Arch. Phys. Med. Rehabil. 85, 227–233.

Balci, B.D., Akdal, G., Yaka, E., Angin, S., 2013. Vestibular rehabilitation in acute central vestibulopathy: a randomized controlled trial. J. Vestib. Res. 23, 259–267.

Baloh, R.W., Honrubia, V., Jacobson, K., 1987. Benign positional vertigo: clinical and oculographic features in 240 cases. Neurology. 37, 371–378.

Baloh, R.W., Jacobson, K., Honrubia, V., 1993. Horizontal semicircular canal variant of benign positional vertigo. Neurology. 43 2542–2542

Beh, S.C., Masrour, S., Smith, S.V., Friedman, D.I., 2019. The spectrum of vestibular migraine: clinical features, triggers, and examination findings. Headache J. Head Face Pain. 59, 727–740.

Benecke, H., Agus, S., Kuessner, D., et al., 2013. The burden and impact of vertigo: findings from the REVERT patient registry. Front. Neurol. 4, 136.

Berg, K., Wood-Dauphine, S., Williams, J.I., Gayton, D., 1989. Measuring balance in the elderly: preliminary development of an instrument. Physiother. Canada. 41, 304–311.

Bhandari, A., Kingma, H., Bhandari, R., 2021. BPPV simulation: a powerful tool to understand and optimize the diagnostics and treatment of all possible variants of BPPV. Front. Neurol. 12, 632286.

Bhattacharyya, N., Gubbels, S.P., Schwartz, S.R., et al., 2017. clinical practice guideline: benign paroxysmal positional vertigo (update). Otolaryngol. Head Neck Surg. 156, S1–S47.

Bisdorff, A., Von Brevern, M., Lempert, T., Newman-Toker, D.E., 2009. Classification of vestibular symptoms: towards an international classification of vestibular disorders. J. Vestib. Res. 19, 1–13.

Bisdorff, A.R., Staab, J.P., Newman-Toker, D.E., 2015. Overview of the international classification of vestibular disorders. Neurol. Clin. 33, 541–550.

Bittar, R.S., Lins, E.M., 2015. Clinical characteristics of patients with persistent postural-perceptual dizziness. Braz. J. Otorhinolaryngol. 81, 276–282.

Black, F.O., Wall III, C., Rockette Jr, H.E., Kitch, R., 1982. Normal subject postural sway during the Romberg test. Am. J. Otolaryngol. 3, 309–318.

Bohannon, R.W., Larkin, P.A., Cook, A.C., et al., 1984. Decrease in timed balance test scores with aging. Phys. Ther. 64, 1067–1070.

Bouny, P., Trousselard, M., Jacob, S., et al., 2022. Environment and body-brain interplay affect inhibition and decision-making. Sci. Rep. 12, 1–14.

Brandt, T., 2000. Management of vestibular disorders. J. Neurol. 247, 491–499.

Brown, K.E., Whitney, S.L., Wrisley, D.M., Furman, J.M., 2001. Physical therapy outcomes for persons with bilateral vestibular loss. Laryngoscope. 111, 1812–1817.

Burgess, A., Kundu, S., 2006. Diuretics for Ménière's disease or syndrome. Cochrane Database Syst. Rev. 3, CD003599.

Burrows, L., Lesser, T., Kasbekar, A., et al., 2017. Independent prescriber physiotherapist led balance clinic: the Southport and Ormskirk pathway. J. Laryngol. Otol. 131, 417–424.

Cakrt, O., Chovanec, M., Funda, T., et al., 2010. Exercise with visual feedback improves postural stability after vestibular schwannoma surgery. Eur. Arch. Otorhinolaryngol. 267, 1355–1360.

Calzolari, E., Chepisheva, M., Smith, R.M., et al., 2021. Vestibular agnosia in traumatic brain injury and its link to imbalance. Brain. 144, 128–143.

Cawthorne, T., 1946. Vestibular Injuries. SAGE Publications.

Cho, S.J., Kim, B.K., Kim, B.S., et al., 2016. Vestibular migraine in multicenter neurology clinics according to the appendix criteria in the third beta edition of the International Classification of Headache Disorders. Cephalalgia. 36, 454–462.

Chu, E.C., Al Zoubi, F., Yang, J., 2021. Cervicogenic dizziness associated with craniocervical instability: a case report. J. Med. Cases. 12, 451.

Clendaniel, R.A., 2010. The effects of habituation and gaze stability exercises in the treatment of unilateral vestibular hypofunction: a preliminary results. J. Neurol. Phys. Ther. 34 111–6

Clendaniel, R.A., Tucci, D.L., 1997. Vestibular rehabilitation strategies in Meniere's disease. Otolaryngol. Clin. North Am. 30, 1145–1158.

Clyde, J.W., Oberman, B.S., Isildak, H., 2017. Current management practices in Meniere's disease. Otol. Neurotol. 38, e159–e167.

Colledge, N.R., Wilson, J.A., Macintyre, C.C., Maclennan, W.J., 1994. The prevalence and characteristics of dizziness in an elderly community. Age Ageing. 23, 117–120.

Committee on Hearing and Equilibrium, 1995. Committee on Hearing and Equilibrium guidelines for the diagnosis and evaluation of therapy in Meniere's disease. Otolaryngol. Head Neck Surg. 113, 181–185.

Cooksey, F.S., 1946. Rehabilitation in vestibular injuries. Proc. R. Soc. Lond. B. Biol. Sci. 39, 273–278.

Courjon, J.H., Jeannerod, M., Ossuzio, I., Schmid, R., 1977. The role of vision in compensation of vestibulo ocular reflex after hemilabyrinthectomy in the cat. Exp. Brain Res. 28, 235–248.

Cousins, S., Kaski, D., Cutfield, N., et al., 2017. Predictors of clinical recovery from vestibular neuritis: a prospective study. Ann. Clin. Transl. Neurol. 4, 340–346.

Curthoys, I.S., 2000. Vestibular compensation and substitution. Curr. Opin. Neurol. 13, 27–30.

Curthoys, I.S., Halmagyi, G.M., 2007. Vestibular compensation: clinical changes in vestibular function with time after unilateral vestibular loss. In: Herdman, S.J. (Ed.), Vestibular Rehabilitation, 3rd ed. F.A. Davis, Philidephia.

Dannenbaum, E., Chilingaryan, G., Fung, J., 2011. Visual vertigo analogue scale: an assessment questionnaire for visual vertigo. J. Vestib. Res. 21, 153–159.

De La Meilleure, G., Dehaene, I., Depondt, M., et al., 1996. Benign paroxysmal positional vertigo of the horizontal canal. J. Neurol. Neurosurg. Psychiatry. 60, 68–71.

Devantier, L., Hougaard, D., Händel, M.N., et al., 2020. Using betahistine in the treatment of patients with Ménière's disease: a meta-analysis with the current randomized-controlled evidence. Acta Otolaryngol. 140, 845–853.

Devaraja, K., 2018. Approach to cervicogenic dizziness: a comprehensive review of its aetiopathology and management. Eur. Arch. Otorhinolaryngol. 275, 2421–2433.

Dieterich, M., Staab, J.P., 2017. Functional dizziness: from phobic postural vertigo and chronic subjective dizziness to persistent postural-perceptual dizziness. Curr. Opin. Neurol. 30, 107–113.

Di, Fabio, R.P., 1995. Sensitivity and specificity of platform posturography for identifying patients with vestibular dysfunction. Phys. Ther. 75, 290–305.

Dorion, D., 1998. Scott-Brown's otolaryngology. J. Otolaryngol. Head Neck Surg. 27, 309.

Dumas, G., Curthoys, I.S., Lion, A., et al., 2017. The skull vibration-induced nystagmus test of vestibular function—a review. Front. Neurol. 8, 41.

Dumas, G., Fabre, C., Charpiot, A., et al., 2021. Skull vibration-induced nystagmus test in a human model of horizontal canal plugging. Audiol. Res. 11, 301–312.

Duncan, P.W., Weiner, D.K., Chandler, J., Studenski, S., 1990. Functional reach: a new clinical measure of balance. J. Gerontol. 45, M192–M197.

Enticott, J.C., Vitkovic, J.J., Reid, B., et al., 2008. Vestibular rehabilitation in individuals with inner-ear dysfunction: a pilot study. Audiol. Neurootol. 13, 19–28.

Epley, J.M., 1980. New dimensions of benign paroxysmal positional vertigo. Otolaryngol. Head Neck Surg 88, 599–605.

Epley, J.M., 1992. The canalith repositioning procedure: for treatment of benign paroxysmal positional vertigo. Otolaryngol. Head Neck Surg. 107, 399–404.

Espinosa-Sanchez, J.M., Lopez-Escamez, J.A., 2020. The pharmacological management of vertigo in Meniere disease. Expert Opin. Pharmacother. 21, 1753–1763.

Fetter, M., Diener, H.C., Dichgans, J., 1990. Recovery of postural control after an acute unilateral vestibular lesion in humans. J. Vestib. Res. 1, 373–383.

Fetter, M., Zee, D.S., Proctor, L.R., 1988. Effect of lack of vision and of occipital lobectomy upon recovery from unilateral labyrinthectomy in rhesus monkey. J. Neurophysiol. 59, 394–407.

Fleming, J.B., Vora, T.K., Harrigan, M.R., 2013. Rare case of bilateral vertebral artery stenosis caused by C4–5 spondylotic changes manifesting with bilateral bow hunter's syndrome. World Neurosurg. 79, 799.E1–799.E5.

Fong, E., Li, C., Aslakson, R., Agrawal, Y., 2015. Systematic review of patient-reported outcome measures in clinical vestibular research. Arch. Phys. Med. Rehabil. 96, 357–365.

Formeister, E.J., Rizk, H.G., Kohn, M.A., et al., 2018. The epidemiology of vestibular migraine: a population-based survey study. Otol. Neurotol. 39, 1037–1044.

Franchignoni, F., Horak, F., Godi, M., et al., 2010. Using psychometric techniques to improve the Balance Evaluation Systems Test: the mini-BESTest. J. Rehabil. Med. 42, 323–331.

Fu, W., Han, J., Chang, N., et al., 2020. Immediate efficacy of Gufoni maneuver for horizontal canal benign paroxysmal positional vertigo (HC-BPPV): a meta-analysis. Auris Nasus Larynx. 47, 48–54.

Gallus, R., Melis, A., Rizzo, D., et al., 2021. Audiovestibular symptoms and sequelae in COVID-19 patients. J. Vestib. Res. 31, 381–387.

Garcia, A.P., Gananca, M.M., Cusin, F.S., et al., 2013. Vestibular rehabilitation with virtual reality in Meniere's disease. Braz. J. Otorhinolaryngol. 79, 366–374.

García-Muñoz, C., Cortés-Vega, M.D., Heredia-Rizo, A.M., et al., 2020. Effectiveness of vestibular training for balance and dizziness rehabilitation in people with multiple sclerosis: a systematic review and meta-analysis. J. Clin. Med. 9, 590.

Geraghty, A.W.A., Essery, R., Kirby, S., et al., 2017. Internet-based vestibular rehabilitation for older adults with chronic dizziness: a randomized controlled trial in primary care. Ann. Fam. Med. 15, 209–216.

Gerlier, C., Hoarau, M., Fels, A., et al., 2021. Differentiating central from peripheral causes of acute vertigo in an emergency setting with the HINTS, STANDING, and ABCD2 tests: a diagnostic cohort study. Acad. Emerg. Med. 28, 1368–1378.

Godi, M., Franchignoni, F., Caligari, M., et al., 2013. Comparison of reliability, validity, and responsiveness of the mini-BESTest and Berg Balance Scale in patients with balance disorders. Phys. Ther. 93, 158–167.

Gold, D.R., Morris, L., Kheradmand, A., Schubert, M.C., 2014. Repositioning maneuvers for benign paroxysmal positional vertigo. Curr. Treat. Options Neurol. 16, 307.

Goldberg, J.M., Fernandez, C., 1971. Physiology of peripheral neurons innervating semicircular canals of the squirrel monkey. I. Resting discharge and response to constant angular accelerations. J. Neurophysiol. 34, 635–660.

Goldbrunner, R., Weller, M., Regis, J., et al., 2020. EANO guideline on the diagnosis and treatment of vestibular schwannoma. Neuro-oncology. 22, 31–45.

Gordon, C.R., Gadoth, N., 2004. Repeated vs single physical maneuver in benign paroxysmal positional vertigo. Acta Neurol. Scand. 110, 166–169.

Gottshall, K.R., Hoffer, M.E., Moore, R.J., Balough, B.J., 2005. The role of vestibular rehabilitation in the treatment of Meniere's disease. Otolaryngol. Head Neck Surg. 133, 326–328.

Gottshall, K.R., Sessoms, P.H., 2015. Improvements in dizziness and imbalance results from using a multidisciplinary and multisensory approach to vestibular physical therapy – a case study. Front. Syst. Neurosci. 9, 106.

Grill, E., Heuberger, M., Strobl, R., et al., 2018. Prevalence, determinants, and consequences of vestibular hypofunction. Results from the KORA-FF4 survey. Front. Neurol. 9, 1076.

Guerraz, M., Yardley, L., Bertholon, P., et al., 2001. Visual vertigo: symptom assessment, spatial orientation and postural control. Brain. 124, 1646–1656.

Gurumukhani, J.K., Patel, D.M., Shah, S.V., et al., 2021. Negative impact of vestibular suppressant drugs on provocative positional tests of BPPV: a study from the western part of India. Ann. Indian Acad. Neurol. 24, 367.

Habs, M., Strobl, R., Grill, E., et al., 2020. Primary or secondary chronic functional dizziness: does it make a difference? A DizzyReg study in 356 patients. J. Neurol. 267, 212–222.

Hain, T.C., Helminski, J.O., 2007. Anatomy and physiology of the vestibular system. In: Herdman, S.J. (Ed.), Vestibular Rehabilitation, 3rd ed. F.A. Davis, Philadelphia.

Hall, C.D., Herdman, S.J., 2006. Reliability of clinical measures used to assess patients with peripheral vestibular disorders. J. Neurol. Phys. Ther. 30, 74–81.

Hall, C.D., Herdman, S.J., Whitney, S.L., et al., 2021. Vestibular rehabilitation for peripheral vestibular hypofunction: an updated clinical practice guideline from the American Physical Therapy Association. J. Neurol. Phys. Ther. 40, 124–155.

Hall, C.D., Schubert, M.C., Herdman, S.J., 2004. Prediction of fall risk reduction as measured by dynamic gait index in individuals with unilateral vestibular hypofunction. Otol. Neurotol. 25, 746–751.

Hammerle, M., Swan, A.A., Nelson, J.T., Treleaven, J.M., 2019. Retrospective review: effectiveness of cervical proprioception retraining for dizziness after mild traumatic brain injury in a military population with abnormal cervical proprioception. J. Manipul. Physiol. Ther. 42, 399–406.

Hansson, E.E., 2007. Vestibular rehabilitation – For whom and how? A systematic review. Adv. Physiother. 9, 106–116.

Harrell, R.G., Schubert, M.C., Oxborough, S., Whitney, S.L., 2021. Vestibular rehabilitation telehealth during the SARS-CoV-2 (COVID-19) pandemic. Front. Neurol. 12, 781482.

Hebert, J.R., Corboy, J.R., Manago, M.M., Schenkman, M., 2011. Effects of vestibular rehabilitation on multiple sclerosis-related fatigue and upright postural control: a randomized controlled trial. Phys. Ther. 91, 1166–1183.

Herdman, D., Norton, S., Murdin, L., et al., 2022. The INVEST trial: a randomised feasibility trial of psychologically informed vestibular rehabilitation versus current gold standard physiotherapy for people with persistent postural perceptual dizziness. J. Neurol. 10, 1–11.

Herdman, S.J., 2010. Computerized dynamic visual acuity test in the assessment of vestibular deficits. In: Scott, D.Z.E., David, S.Z. (Eds.), Handbook of Clinical Neurophysiology. Elsevier, London.

Herdman, S.J., Clendaniel, R., 2015. Vestibular Rehabilitation. F.A. Davis, Philadelphia.

Herdman, S.J., Clendaniel, R.A., Mattox, D.E., et al., 1995. Vestibular adaptation exercises and recovery: acute stage after acoustic neuroma resection. Otolaryngol. Head Neck Surg. 113, 77–87.

Herdman, S.J., Hall, C.D., Delaune, W., 2012. Variables associated with outcome in patients with unilateral vestibular hypofunction. Neurorehabil. Neural Repair. 26, 151–162.

Herdman, S.J., Hall, C.D., Maloney, B., et al., 2015. Variables associated with outcome in patients with bilateral vestibular hypofunction: preliminary study. J. Vestib. Res. Equil. Orient. 25, 185–194.

Herdman, S.J., Hall, C.D., Schubert, M.C., et al., 2007. Recovery of dynamic visual acuity in bilateral vestibular hypofunction. Arch. Otolaryngol. Head Neck Surg. 133, 383–389.

Herdman, S.J., Schubert, M.C., Das, V.E., Tusa, R.J., 2003. Recovery of dynamic visual acuity in unilateral vestibular hypofunction. Arch. Otolaryngol. Head Neck Surg. 129, 819–824.

Herdman, S.J., Tusa, R.J., Blatt, P., et al., 1998. Computerized dynamic visual acuity test in the assessment of vestibular deficits. Am. J. Otol. 19, 790–796.

Heusel-Gillig, L., Santucci, V., Hall, C.D., 2022. Development and validation of the modified motion sensitivity test. Otol. Neurotol. 43, 944–949.

Hillier, S.L., McDonnell, M., 2011. Vestibular rehabilitation for unilateral peripheral vestibular dysfunction. Cochrane Database Syst. Rev. 2, CD005397.

Hilton, M., Pinder, D., 2004. The Epley (canalith repositioning) manoeuvre for benign paroxysmal positional vertigo. Cochrane Database Syst. Rev. 12, CD003162.

Holmberg, J., Tjernström, F., Karlberg, M., et al., 2009. Reduced postural differences between phobic postural vertigo patients and healthy subjects during a postural threat. J. Neurol. 256, 258–262.

House, W.F., Hitselberger, W.F., 1985. The neurotologist view of the surgical management of acoustic neuromas. Clin. Neurosurg. 32, 214–222.

Igarashi, M., Ishikawa, K., Ishii, M., Yamane, H., 1988. Physical exercise and balance compensation after total ablation of vestibular organs. Prog. Brain Res. 76, 395–401.

IHS Headache Classification Committee of the International Headache Society (IHS)., 2018. The International Classification of Headache Disorders, 3rd ed. Cephalalgia. 38, 1–211.

Iida, Y., Murata, H., Johkura, K., et al., 2018. Bow hunter's syndrome by nondominant vertebral artery compression: a case report, literature review, and significance of downbeat nystagmus as the diagnostic clue. World Neurosurg. 111, 367–372.

Jacob, R.G., Lilienfeld, S.O., Furman, J.M.R., Turner, S.M., 1989. Space and motion phobia in panic disorder with vestibular dysfunction. J. Anxiety Disord. 3, 117–130.

Jacobson, G.P., Newman, C.W., 1990. The development of the Dizziness Handicap Inventory. Arch. Otolaryngol. Head Neck Surg. 116, 424–427.

Jacobson, G.P., Shephard, N.T., 2021. Balance Function Assessment and Management. Plural Publishing, San Diego.

Janc, M., Sliwinska-Kowalska, M., Politanski, P., et al., 2021. Posturography with head movements in the assessment of balance in chronic unilateral vestibular lesions. Sci. Rep. 11, 1–8.

Jiang, M., Zhang, Z., Zhao, C., 2021. What is the efficacy of gentamicin on the incidence of vertigo attacks and hearing in patients with Meniere's disease compared with steroids? A meta-analysis. J. Neurol. 268, 3717–3727.

Joint Formulary Committee., 2022. British National Formulary, 83rd ed. BMJ Group and Pharmaceutical Press, London.

Kasbekar, A.V., Mullin, N., Morrow, C., et al., 2014. Development of a physiotherapy-led balance clinic: the Aintree model. J. Laryngol. Otol. 128, 966–971.

Kerber, K.A., Baloh, R.W., 2011. The evaluation of a patient with dizziness. Neurol. Clin. Pract. 1, 24–33.

Kim, J.S., Newman-Toker, D.E., Kerber, K.A., et al., 2022. Vascular vertigo and dizziness: diagnostic criteria. J. Vestib. Res. 32, 205–222.

Kingma, H., Van De Berg, R., 2016. Anatomy, physiology, and physics of the peripheral vestibular system. Handbook Clin. Neurol. 137, 1–16.

Kinne, B.L., Harless, M.G., Lauzon, K.A., Wamhoff, J.R., 2021. Roll maneuvers versus side-lying maneuvers for geotropic horizontal canal BPPV: a systematic review. Phys. Ther. Rev. 26, 439–446.

Kleffelgaard, I., Soberg, H.L., Tamber, A.L., et al., 2019. The effects of vestibular rehabilitation on dizziness and balance problems in patients after traumatic brain injury: a randomized controlled trial. Clin. Rehabil. 33, 74–84.

Knapstad, M.K., Nordahl, S.H.G., Goplen, F.K., 2019. Clinical characteristics in patients with cervicogenic dizziness: a systematic review. Health Sci. Rep. 2, e134.

Kontos, A.P., Eagle, S.R., Mucha, A., et al., 2021. A randomized controlled trial of precision vestibular rehabilitation in adolescents following concussion: preliminary findings. J. Pediatr. 239, 193–199.

Korn, G.P., Dorigueto, R.S., Gananca, M.M., Caovilla, H.H., 2007. Epley's maneuver in the same session in benign positional paroxysmal vertigo. Braz. J. Otorhinolaryngol. 73, 533–539.

Kovacs, E., Wang, X., Grill, E., 2019. Economic burden of vertigo: a systematic review. Health Econ. Rev. 9, 1–14.

Krebs, D.E., Gill-Body, K.M., Parker, S.W., et al., 2003. Vestibular rehabilitation: useful but not universally so. Otolaryngol. Head Neck Surg. 128, 240–250.

Krebs, D.E., Gill-Body, K.M., Riley, P.O., Parker, S.W., 1993. Double-blind, placebo-controlled trial of rehabilitation for bilateral vestibular hypofunction: preliminary report. Otolaryngol. Head Neck Surg. 109, 735–741.

Kutay, Ö., Akdal, G., Keskinoğlu, P., et al., 2017. Vestibular migraine patients are more anxious than migraine patients without vestibular symptoms. J. Neurol. 264 (Suppl. 1), 37–41.

Lacour, M., Bernard-Demanze, L., 2014. Interaction between vestibular compensation mechanisms and vestibular rehabilitation therapy: 10 recommendations for optimal functional recovery. Front. Neurol. 5, 285.

Lacour, M., Dutheil, S., Tighilet, B., et al., 2009. Tell me your vestibular deficit, and I'll tell you how you'll compensate. Ann. N.Y. Acad. Sci. 1164, 268–278.

Lacour, M., Laurent, T., Alain, T., 2020. Rehabilitation of dynamic visual acuity in patients with unilateral vestibular hypofunction: earlier is better. Eur. Arch. Otorhinolaryngol. 277, 103–113.

Lacour, M., Vidal, P.P., Xerri, C., 1981. Visual influences on vestibulospinal reflexes during vertical linear motion in normal and hemilabyrinthectomized monkeys. Exp. Brain Res. 43, 383–394.

Legters, K., Whitney, S.L., Porter, R., Buczek, F., 2005. The relationship between the Activities-specific Balance Confidence Scale and the Dynamic Gait Index in peripheral vestibular dysfunction. Physiother. Res. Int. 10, 10–22.

Lempert, T., Olesen, J., Furman, J., et al., 2012. Vestibular migraine: diagnostic criteria. J. Vestib. Res. 22, 167–172.

Lempert, T., Olesen, J., Furman, J., et al., 2022. Vestibular migraine: diagnostic criteria1. J. Vestib. Res. 32, 1–6.

Li, Z.Y., Shen, B., Si, L.H., et al., 2022. Clinical characteristics of definite vestibular migraine diagnosed according to criteria jointly formulated by the Bárány Society and the International Headache Society. Braz. J. Otorhinolaryngol. 88 (Suppl. 3), S147–S154.

Lida, Y., Murata, H., Johkura, K., et al., 2018. Bow hunter's syndrome by nondominant vertebral artery compression: a case report, literature review, and significance of downbeat nystagmus as the diagnostic clue. World Neurosurg. 111, 367–372.

Lough, M., Almufarrij, I., Whiston, H., Munro, K.J., 2022. Revised meta-analysis and pooled estimate of audio-vestibular symptoms associated with COVID-19. Int. J. Audiol. 61, 705–709.

Lopez-Escamez, J., Carey, J., Chung, W., et al., 2017. Diagnostic criteria for Meniere's disease according to the Classification Committee of the Barany Society. HNO. 65, 887–893.

Lucieer, F., Vonk, P., Guinand, N., et al., 2016. Bilateral vestibular hypofunction: insights in etiologies, clinical subtypes, and diagnostics. Front. Neurol. 7, 26.

Macdougall, H.G., Curthoys, I.S., 2012. Plasticity during vestibular compensation: the role of saccades. Front. Neurol. 3, 21.

Mandalà, M., Califano, L., Casani, A.P., et al., 2020. Double-blind randomized trial on the efficacy of the forced prolonged position for treatment of lateral canal benign paroxysmal positional vertigo. Laryngoscope. 131, E1296–E1300.

Mandalà, M., Pepponi, E., Santoro, G.P., et al., 2013. Double-blind randomized trial on the efficacy of the Gufoni maneuver for treatment of lateral canal BPPV. Laryngoscope. 123, 1782–1786.

Mandalà, M., Salerni, L., Nuti, D., 2019. Benign positional paroxysmal vertigo treatment: a practical update. Curr. Treat. Options Neurol. 21, 66.

Mann, G.C., Whitney, S.L., Redfern, M.S., et al., 1996. Functional reach and single leg stance in patients with peripheral vestibular disorders. J. Vestib. Res. 6, 343–353.

Marchetti, G.F., Whitney, S.L., 2006. Construction and validation of the 4-item dynamic gait index. Phys. Ther. 86, 1651–1660.

Marchetti, G.F., Whitney, S.L., Redfern, M.S., Furman, J.M., 2011. Factors associated with balance confidence in older adults with health conditions affecting the balance and vestibular system. Arch. Phys. Med. Rehabil. 92, 1884–1891.

Marcus, H.J., Paine, H., Sargeant, M., et al., 2019. Vestibular dysfunction in acute traumatic brain injury. J. Neurol. 266, 2430–2433.

Maskell, F., Chiarelli, P., Isles, R., 2006. Dizziness after traumatic brain injury: overview and measurement in the clinical setting. Brain Inj. 20, 293–305.

Mcgibbon, C.A., Krebs, D.E., Parker, S.W., et al., 2005. Tai chi and vestibular rehabilitation improve vestibulopathic gait via different neuromuscular mechanisms: preliminary report. BMC Neurol. 5, 3.

Meldrum, D., Burrows, L., Cakrt, O., et al., 2020. Vestibular rehabilitation in Europe: a survey of clinical and research practice. J. Neurol. 267 (Suppl. 1), 24–35.

Meldrum, D., Herdman, S., Vance, R., et al., 2015. Effectiveness of conventional versus virtual reality-based balance exercises in vestibular rehabilitation for unilateral peripheral vestibular loss: results of a randomized controlled trial. Arch. Phys. Med. Rehabil. 96, 1319–1328.

Meldrum, D., Jahn, K., 2019. Gaze stabilisation exercises in vestibular rehabilitation: review of the evidence and recent clinical advances. J. Neurol. 266, 11–18.

Meldrum, D., Murray, D., Vance, R., et al., 2022. Toward a digital health intervention for vestibular rehabilitation: usability and subjective outcomes of a novel platform. Front. Neurol. 13, 836796.

Meretta, B.M., Whitney, S.L., Marchetti, G.F., et al., 2006. The five times sit to stand test: responsiveness to change and concurrent validity in adults undergoing vestibular rehabilitation. J. Vestib. Res. 16, 233–243.

Mijovic, T., Carriot, J., Zeitouni, A., Cullen, K.E., 2014. Head movements in patients with vestibular lesion: a novel approach to functional assessment in daily life setting. Otol. Neurotol. 35, e348–e357.

Mitsutake, T., Imura, T., Tanaka, R., 2020. The effects of vestibular rehabilitation on gait performance in patients with stroke: a systematic review of randomized controlled trials. J. Stroke Cerebrovasc. Dis. 29, 105214.

Moffat, D.A., 1994. Endolymphatic sac surgery: analysis of 100 operations. Clin. Otolaryngol. Allied Sci. 19, 261–266.

Morrison, M., Korda, A., Zamaro, E., et al., 2022. Paradigm shift in acute dizziness: is caloric testing obsolete? J. Neurol. 269, 853–860.

Mucha, A., Collins, M.W., Elbin, R.J., et al., 2014. A Brief Vestibular/Ocular Motor Screening (VOMS) assessment to evaluate concussions: preliminary findings. Am. J. Sports Med. 42, 2479–2486.

Murdin, L., Schilder, A.G., 2015. Epidemiology of balance symptoms and disorders in the community: a systematic review. Otol. Neurotol. 36, 387–392.

Murray, D.A., Meldrum, D., Lennon, O., 2017. Can vestibular rehabilitation exercises help patients with concussion? A systematic review of efficacy, prescription and progression patterns. Br. J. Sports Med. 51, 442–451.

Nacci, A., Ferrazzi, M., Berrettini, S., et al., 2011. Vestibular and stabilometric findings in whiplash injury and minor head trauma. Acta Otorhinolaryngol. Ital. 31, 378–389.

Nedzelski, J.M., Schessel, D.A., Bryce, G.E., Pfleiderer, A.G., 1992. Chemical labyrinthectomy: local application of gentamicin for the treatment of unilateral Meniere's disease. Am. J. Otol. 13, 18–22.

Neuhauser, H.K., Radtke, A., Von Brevern, M., et al., 2006. Migrainous vertigo: prevalence and impact on quality of life. Neurology. 67, 1028–1033.

Neuhauser, H.K., Von Brevern, M., Radtke, A., et al., 2005. Epidemiology of vestibular vertigo: a neurotologic survey of the general population. Neurology. 65, 898–904.

Nevoux, J., Barbara, M., Dornhoffer, J., et al., 2018. International consensus (ICON) on treatment of Ménière's disease. Eur. Ann Otorhinolaryngol. Head Neck Dis. 135, S29–32.

NICE CKS., 2017. Meniere's disease. Available at: https://cks.nice.org.uk/topics/menieresdisease/. Accessed 14 June 2022.

Noij, K.S., Rauch, S.D., 2020. Vestibular evoked myogenic potential (VEMP) testing for diagnosis of superior semicircular canal dehiscence. Front. Neurol. 11, 695.

Norre, M.E., Beckers, A., 1989. Vestibular habituation training: exercise treatment for vertigo based upon the habituation effect. Otolaryngol. Head Neck Surg. 101, 14–19.

Nowaczewska, M., 2020. Vestibular migraine – an underdiagnosed cause of vertigo. Diagnosis and treatment. Neurol. Neurochir. Polska. 54, 106–115.

Oghalai, J.S., Manolidis, S., Barth, J.L., et al., 2000. Unrecognized benign paroxysmal positional vertigo in elderly patients. Otolaryngol. Head Neck Surg. 122, 630–634.

Oh, A.K., Lee, H., Jen, J.C., et al., 2001. Familial benign recurrent vertigo. Am. J. Med. Genet. 100, 287–291.

Ozgen, G., Karapolat, H., Akkoc, Y., Yuceyar, N., 2016. Is customized vestibular rehabilitation effective in patients with multiple sclerosis? A randomized controlled trial. Eur. J. Phys. Rehabil. Med. 52, 466–478.

Parnes, L.S., Agrawal, S.K., Atlas, J., 2003. Diagnosis and management of benign paroxysmal positional vertigo (BPPV). CMAJ. 169, 681–693.

Parnes, L.S., Mcclure, J.A., 1990. Posterior semicircular canal occlusion for intractable benign paroxysmal positional vertigo. Ann. Otol. Rhinol. Laryngol. 99, 330–334.

Patel, M.A., Marciscano, A.E., Hu, C., et al., 2017. Long-term treatment response and patient outcomes for vestibular schwannoma patients treated with hypofractionated stereotactic radiotherapy. Front. Oncol. 7, 200.

Pavlou, M., Bronstein, A.M., Davies, R.A., 2013. Randomized trial of supervised versus unsupervised optokinetic exercise in persons with peripheral vestibular disorders. Neurorehabil. Neural Repair. 27, 208–218.

Pavlou, M., Davies, R.A., Bronstein, A.M., 2006. The assessment of increased sensitivity to visual stimuli in patients with chronic dizziness. J. Vestib. Res. 16, 223–231.

Pavlou, M., Kanegaonkar, R.G., Swapp, D., et al., 2012. The effect of virtual reality on visual vertigo symptoms in patients with peripheral vestibular dysfunction: a pilot study. J. Vestib. Res. 22, 273–281.

Pavlou, M., Lingeswaran, A., Davies, R.A., et al., 2004. Simulator based rehabilitation in refractory dizziness. J. Neurol. 251, 983–995.

Pineault, K., Pearson, D., Wei, E., et al., 2020. Association between saccule and semicircular canal impairments and cognitive performance among vestibular patients. Ear Hear. 41, 686.

Popkirov, S., Stone, J., Holle-Lee, D., 2018. Treatment of persistent postural-perceptual dizziness (PPPD) and related disorders. Curr. Treat. Options Neurol. 20, 50.

Porciuncula, F., Johnson, C.C., Glickman, L.B., 2012. The effect of vestibular rehabilitation on adults with bilateral vestibular hypofunction: a systematic review. J. Vestib. Res. 22, 283–298.

Powell, L.E., Myers, A.M., 1995. The Activities-specific Balance Confidence (ABC) scale. J. Gerontol. Sci. 50A, M28–M34.

Power, L., Shute, W., McOwan, B., et al., 2018. Clinical characteristics and treatment choice in vestibular migraine. J. Clin. Neurosci. 52, 50–53.

Reiley, A.S., Vickory, F.M., Funderburg, S.E., et al., 2017. How to diagnose cervicogenic dizziness. Arch. Physiother. 7, 12.

Ricci, N.A., Aratani, M.C., Doná, F., et al., 2010. A systematic review about the effects of the vestibular rehabilitation in middle-age and older adults. Braz. J. Phys. Ther. 14, 361–371.

Rinne, T., Bronstein, A.M., Rudge, P., et al., 1998. Bilateral loss of vestibular function: clinical findings in 53 patients. J. Neurol. 245, 314–321.

Rogers, C., 2010. Presbyastasis: a multifactorial cause of balance problems in the elderly. South African. Fam. Pract. 52, 431–434.

Rosengren, S.M., Colebatch, J.G., Young, A.S., et al., 2019. Vestibular evoked myogenic potentials in practice: methods, pitfalls and clinical applications. Clin. Neurophysiol. Pract. 4, 47–68.

Sargeant, M., Sykes, E., Saviour, M., et al., 2018. The utility of the Sports Concussion Assessment Tool in hospitalized traumatic brain injury patients. J. Concussion, 2.

Sayed, S.Z., Wahat, N.A., Raymond, A.A., et al., 2021. Quantitative vestibular function tests in posterior circulation stroke patients: a review. Med. J. Malaysia. 76, 898–905.

Schaaf, H., Hesse, G., 2015. Patients with long-lasting dizziness: a follow-up after neurotological and psychotherapeutic inpatient treatment after a period of at least 1 year. Eur. Arch. Otorhinolaryngol. 272, 1529–1535.

Schneider, K.J., Meeuwisse, W.H., Nettel-Aguirre, A., et al., 2014. Cervicovestibular rehabilitation in sport-related concussion: a randomised controlled trial. Br. J. Sports Med. 48, 1294–1298.

Schniepp, R., Wuehr, M., Pradhan, C., et al., 2013. Nonlinear variability of body sway in patients with phobic postural vertigo. Front. Neurol. 4, 115.

Schubert, M.C., Carter, N., Lo, S., 2021. Case report: bow hunter syndrome—one reason to add non-gravity dependent positional nystagmus testing to your clinical neuro-otologic exam. Front. Neurol. 12, 814998.

Schwartz, M.S., Lekovic, G.P., Miller, M.E., 2018. Translabyrinthine microsurgical resection of small vestibular schwannomas. J. Neurosurg. 129, 128–138.

Sekhar, L.N., Gormley, W.B., Wright, D.C., 1996. The best treatment for vestibular schwannoma (acoustic neuroma): microsurgery or radiosurgery? Otol. Neurotol. 17, 676–682.

Sheikh, N.A., Ranada, S., Lloyd, M., et al., 2022. Lower body muscle preactivation and tensing mitigate symptoms of initial orthostatic hypotension in young females. Heart Rhythm. 19, 604–610.

Shepard, N.T., Telian, S.A., 1995. Programmatic vestibular rehabilitation. Otolaryngol. Head Neck Surg. 112, 173–182.

Shepard, N.T., Telian, S.A., Smith-Wheelock, M., Raj, A., 1993. Vestibular and balance rehabilitation therapy. Ann. Otol. Rhinol. Laryngol. 102, 198–205.

Shumway-Cook, A., Horak, F.B., 1986. Assessing the influence of sensory interaction on balance: suggestion from the field. Phys. Ther. 66, 1548–1550.

Sloane, P.D., 1989. Dizziness in primary care. Results from the National Ambulatory Medical Care Survey. J. Fam. Pract. 29, 33–38.

Smith, R.M., Marroney, N., Beattie, J., et al., 2020. A mixed methods randomised feasibility trial investigating the management of benign paroxysmal positional vertigo in acute traumatic brain injury. Pilot Feasibility Stud. 6, 130.

Smith-Wheelock, M., Shepard, N.T., Telian, S.A., 1991. Long-term effects for treatment of balance dysfunction: utilizing a home exercise approach. Semin. Hearing. 12, 297–301.

Sohn, J.H., 2016. Recent advances in the understanding of vestibular migraine. Behav. Neurol. 2016, 1801845.

Sohsten, E., Bittar, R.S., Staab, J.P., 2016. Posturographic profile of patients with persistent postural-perceptual dizziness on the sensory organization test. J. Vestib. Res. 26, 319–326.

Sparrer, I., Duong Dinh, T.A., Ilgner, J., Westhofen, M., 2013. Vestibular rehabilitation using the Nintendo® Wii Balance Board – a user-friendly alternative for central nervous compensation. Acta Otolaryngol. 133, 239–245.

Staab, J.P., 2012. Chronic subjective dizziness. Continuum (Minneap Minn). 18, 1118–1141.

Staab, J.P., Eckhardt-Henn, A., Horii, A., et al., 2017. Diagnostic criteria for persistent postural-perceptual dizziness (PPPD): Consensus document of the committee for the Classification of Vestibular Disorders of the Bárány Society. J. Vestib. Res. 27, 191–208.

Staibano, P., Lelli, D., Tse, D., 2019. A retrospective analysis of two tertiary care dizziness clinics: a multidisciplinary chronic dizziness clinic and an acute dizziness clinic. J. Otolaryngol. Head Neck Surg. 48, 11.

Stancel-Lewis, J., Lau, J.W.L., Male, A., et al., 2022. Vestibular rehabilitation therapy for the treatment of vestibular migraine, and the impact of traumatic brain injury on outcome: a retrospective study. Otol. Neurotol. 43, 359–367.

Strupp, M., Arbusow, V., Maag, K.P., et al., 1998. Vestibular exercises improve central vestibulospinal compensation after vestibular neuritis. Neurology. 51, 838–844.

Strupp, M., Brandt, T., 2010. Vestibular neuritis. In: Scott, D.Z.E., David, S.Z. (Eds.), Handbook of Clinical Neurophysiology. Elsevier.

Strupp, M., Brandt, T., 2013. Peripheral vestibular disorders. Curr. Opin. Neurol. 26, 81–89.

Strupp, M., Lopez-Escamez, A., Kim, J.-S., et al., 2016. Vestibular paroxysmia: diagnostic criteria. Consensus document of the committee for the classification of vestibular disorders of the Barany Society. J. Vestib. Res. 26, 409–415.

Sugaya, N., Arai, M., Goto, F., 2017. Is the headache in patients with vestibular migraine attenuated by vestibular rehabilitation? Front. Neurol. 8, 124.

Szturm, T., Ireland, D.J., Lessing-Turner, M., 1994. Comparison of different exercise programs in the rehabilitation of patients with chronic peripheral vestibular dysfunction. J. Vestib. Res. 4, 461–479.

Távora-Vieira, D., Voola, M., Majteles, L., et al., 2022. Extended scope of practice audiology in the ENT outpatient clinic – a pilot study. Int. J. Audiol. 61, 29–33.

Teggi, R., Caldirola, D., Fabiano, B., et al., 2009. Rehabilitation after acute vestibular disorders. J. Laryngol. Otol. 123, 397–402.

Thompson, K.J., Goetting, J.C., Staab, J.P., Shepard, N.T., 2015. Retrospective review and telephone follow-up to evaluate a physical therapy protocol for treating persistent postural-perceptual dizziness: a pilot study. J. Vestib. Res. 25, 97–103. quiz 103–104

Tinetti, M.E., 1986. Performance-oriented assessment of mobility problems in elderly patients. J. Am. Geriatr. Soc. 34, 119–126.

Tramontano, M., Bergamini, E., Iosa, M., et al., 2018. Vestibular rehabilitation training in patients with subacute stroke: a preliminary randomized controlled trial. NeuroRehabilitation. 43, 247–254.

Tusa, R.J., 2010. Bedside assessment of the dizzy patient. In: Scott, D.Z.E., David, S.Z. (Eds.), Handbook of Clinical Neurophysiology. Elsevier.

Vallim, M.G.B., Gabriel, G.P., Mezzalira, R., et al., 2021. Does the video head impulse test replace caloric testing in the assessment of patients with chronic dizziness? A systematic review and meta-analysis. Braz. J. Otorhinolaryngol. 87, 733–741.

Van de Berg, R., Murdin, L., Whitney, S.L., et al., 2022. Curriculum for vestibular medicine (vestmed) proposed by the Barany society. J. Vestib. Res. 32, 89–98.

van den Broek, E.M.J.M., van der Zaag-Loonen, H.J., Bruintjes, T.D., 2014. Systematic review: efficacy of gufoni maneuver for treatment of lateral canal benign paroxysmal positional vertigo with geotropic nystagmus. Otolaryngol. Head Neck Surg. 150, 933–938.

Van Vugt, V.A., Bosmans, J.E., Finch, A.P., et al., 2020. Cost-effectiveness of internet-based vestibular rehabilitation with and without physiotherapy support for adults aged 50 and older with a chronic vestibular syndrome in general practice. BMJ Open. 10, e035583.

Venosa, A.R., Bittar, R.S., 2007. Vestibular rehabilitation exercises in acute vertigo. Laryngoscope. 117, 1482–1487.

Vereeck, L., Wuyts, F.L., Truijen, S., et al., 2008. The effect of early customized vestibular rehabilitation on balance after acoustic neuroma resection. Clin. Rehabil. 22, 698–713.

Visser, J.E., Carpenter, M.G., Van Der Kooij, H., Bloem, B.R., 2008. The clinical utility of posturography. Clin. Neurophysiol. 119, 2424–2436.

Von Brevern, M., Radtke, A., Lezius, F., et al., 2007. Epidemiology of benign paroxysmal positional vertigo: a population based study. J. Neurol. Neurosurg. Psychiatry. 78, 710–715.

Walsh, R.M., Bath, A.P., Bance, M.L., et al., 2000. The role of conservative management of vestibular schwannomas. Clin. Otolaryngol. Allied Sci. 25, 28–39.

Walsh, R.M., Bath, A.P., Cullen, J.R., Rutka, J.A., 1999. Long-term results of posterior semicircular canal occlusion for intractable benign paroxysmal positional vertigo. Clin. Otolaryngol. Allied Sci. 24, 316–323.

Wang, L., Zobeiri, O.A., Millar, J.L., et al., 2021. Head movement kinematics are altered during gaze stability exercises in vestibular schwannoma patients. Sci. Rep. 11, 7139.

Whalley, M.G., Cane, D.A., 2017. A cognitive-behavioral model of persistent postural-perceptual dizziness. Cogn. Behav. Pract. 24, 72–89.

White, J.A., Coale, K.D., Catalano, P.J., Oas, J.G., 2005. Diagnosis and management of lateral semicircular canal benign paroxysmal positional vertigo. Otolaryngol. Head Neck Surg. 133, 278–284.

Whitney, S., Wrisley, D., Furman, J., 2003. Concurrent validity of the Berg Balance Scale and the Dynamic Gait Index in people with vestibular dysfunction. Physiother. Res. Int. 8, 178–186.

Whitney, S.L., Marchetti, G.F., Morris, L.O., Sparto, P.J., 2007. The reliability and validity of the Four Square Step Test for people with balance deficits secondary to a vestibular disorder. Arch. Phys. Med. Rehabil. 88, 99–104.

Whitney, S.L., Wrisley, D.M., Brown, K.E., Furman, J.M., 2000. Physical therapy for migraine-related vestibulopathy and vestibular dysfunction with history of migraine. Laryngoscope. 110, 1528–1534.

Wrisley, D.M., Marchetti, G.F., Kuharsky, D.K., Whitney, S.L., 2004. Reliability, internal consistency, and validity of data obtained with the functional gait assessment. Phys. Ther. 84, 906–918.

Wrisley, D.M., Whitney, S.L., Furman, J.M., 2002. Vestibular rehabilitation outcomes in patients with a history of migraine. Otol. Neurotol. 23, 483–487.

Xie, M., Zhou, K., Patro, N., et al., 2021. Virtual reality for vestibular rehabilitation: a systematic review. Otol. Neurotol. 42, 967–977.

Yardley, L., Barker, F., Muller, I., et al., 2012. Clinical and cost effectiveness of booklet based vestibular rehabilitation for chronic dizziness in primary care: single blind, parallel group, pragmatic, randomised controlled trial. BMJ. 344, e2237.

Yardley, L., Burgneay, J., Andersson, G., et al., 1998a. Feasibility and effectiveness of providing vestibular rehabilitation for dizzy patients in the community. Clin. Otolaryngol. Allied. Sci. 23, 442–448.

Yardley, L., Masson, E., Verschuur, C., et al., 1992. Symptoms, anxiety and handicap in dizzy patients: development of the vertigo symptom scale. J. Psychosom. Res. 36, 731–741.

Yardley, L., Owen, N., Nazareth, I., Luxon, L., 1998b. Prevalence and presentation of dizziness in a general practice community sample of working age people. J. Royal Coll. Gen. Pract. 48, 1131–1135.

Yilmaz, O., Mutlu, B.Ö., Yaman, H., et al., 2022. Assessment of balance after recovery from Covid-19 disease. Auris Nasus Larynx. 49, 291–298.

Zee, D.S., 1985. Perspectives on the pharmacotherapy of vertigo. Arch. Otolaryngol. 111, 609–612.

Zhang, S., Guo, Z., Tian, E., et al., 2022. Meniere disease subtyping: the direction of diagnosis and treatment in the future. Expert. Rev. Neurother. 22, 115–127.

Zuma e Maia, F., Ramos, B.F., Cal, R., et al., 2020. Management of lateral semicircular canal benign paroxysmal positional vertigo. Front. Neurol. 11, 1040.

Specific Management

Respiratory Management

Louise Platt and Ailsa Carmichael

OUTLINE

Introduction, 473
Central Nervous Control of Breathing, 474
Respiratory Assessment of the Neurological
    Patient, 474
    Lung Function, 474
        *Maximal Inspiratory Pressure and Maximal
            Expiratory Pressure, 476*
    Peak Cough Flow, 477
    Arterial Blood Gases, 478
    Chest Radiographs, 478
    Respiratory Pattern, 478
    Respiratory Reserve, 478
Early Mobilisation, 479
Respiratory Treatment and Management, 479
    Maintenance of a Patent Airway, 479
    Maximal Insufflation Capacity, 481
    Manual Cough, 482

Mechanical Insufflation and Exsufflation, 482
Other Considerations, 482
Respiratory Muscle Training, 483
Management of Acute Respiratory Failure, 483
Tracheostomy and Weaning, 483
Respiratory Function in Neurological
    Conditions, 484
    Central Conditions, 484
    Subarachnoid Haemorrhage, 484
    Spinal Cord Injury and Disease, 484
    Anterior Horn Cell Conditions, 486
    Neuropathy, 487
    Neuromuscular Junction, 487
    Muscle Conditions, 487
Management of Traumatic Brain Injury, 488
Conclusion, 492

INTRODUCTION

An acute neurological insult or neurological disease may affect breathing through injury to the respiratory control centres (RCC) or to one or more of the respiratory system sensors leading to altered rate, depth and pattern of breathing. Associated muscle weakness and fatigue will further contribute to respiratory compromise and dysfunction. Initially, this will result in dysfunction of gas exchange, which can, if left uncorrected, lead to respiratory failure. If swallowing, cough and airway clearance are affected, then airway protection will be compromised, resulting in possible aspiration and leading to further dysfunction of gas exchange. Changes in blood gas chemistry can lead to changes within the cerebral vasculature, which can lead to brain hypoxia and secondary brain injury. Neurological patients can also acquire respiratory infections through immobility. It is therefore vital that a full respiratory assessment is completed and close liaison with the medical team and other members of the multiprofessional team (e.g., medical team, nursing team, physiotherapist and speech and language therapist [SLT] colleagues) is sought.

This chapter will review the central nervous system control of breathing. It will then focus on respiratory assessment of the neurological patient, ending with respiratory management and considerations in specific neurological conditions.

COMMON PROBLEMS IN NEUROLOGICAL CONDITIONS THAT AFFECT RESPIRATION (RACCA ET AL 2020)

- Injury to respiratory control centres (brainstem)
- Respiratory muscle weakness
- Fatigue
- Impaired swallowing (aspiration)
- Impaired ability to cough (sputum retention/infection)
- Hypoxia
- Hypercapnia
- Autonomic nervous system dysfunction

CENTRAL NERVOUS CONTROL OF BREATHING

Breathing is coordinated through a number of cortical areas primarily located within the medulla oblongata (inspiratory and expiratory centres) and the pons (pneumotaxic and apneustic centres). Collectively they are known as the RCCs and control breathing through activation and modulation of the muscles that drive respiration (Ikeda et al 2017). Neurones within the medulla trigger inspiration, providing signals to the phrenic and intercostal nerves. The pneumotaxic centre determines the frequency of respiration, whereas the apneustic centre controls the intensity of breathing (Fig. 18.1).

The RCC can be influenced by higher cortical areas to temporarily increase, decrease or cease respiratory frequency to hyperventilate, hypoventilate or breath hold. Hypoventilation and apnoea (absence of breathing) are commonly seen in traumatic brain injury (TBI), raised intracranial pressure (ICP; >20 mmHg; Stocchetti et al 2017) and cerebrovascular accident. Ventilation may also vary depending on the level of arousal; hypoxia is a major contributory factor to secondary brain damage in TBI, especially in individuals with a decreased level of consciousness (LOC).

The RCC is responsible for the basic rhythm and control of breathing; however, this is modulated by sensory feedback mechanisms to ensure that breathing meets the dynamic oxygen requirements placed on the body. Central and peripheral chemoreceptors, mechanoreceptors, irritant receptors, juxtacapillary receptors, proprioceptors, spinal cord reflexes and nasopulmonary reflexes all modulate patterns of breathing, and all can be affected by acute neurological insult, as well as in neurological long-term conditions. The relationship between brain function and lung function is critical because the brain requires adequate oxygenation to function, and the respiratory system relies on drive from the brain to control ventilation. In neurological conditions, cerebral blood flow can be altered by oedema,

a change in blood pressure (BP) or direct injury. Likewise, lung function may be affected by damage to the RCC.

Many neurological conditions have a direct influence on the respiratory system, leading to an acute deterioration of respiratory function. Because neurological deterioration can occur quickly, careful monitoring is essential during the acute phase. Patients with neurological conditions may be intubated and ventilated, sedated, possibly paralysed and admitted to intensive care during the acute phase. The management aim in the acute phase is to ensure adequate oxygenation is maintained to the brain and vital organs to avoid secondary ischaemic changes; therefore, treatment aims should be directed at:

- Preventing sputum retention;
- Optimising lung volume;
- Maintaining a patent airway;
- Ensuring adequate ventilation; and
- Preserving the integrity of the musculoskeletal system.

Once the patient is stable, early mobilisation can commence, which will further enhance lung function, cardiovascular function and neuromusculoskeletal integrity.

RESPIRATORY ASSESSMENT OF THE NEUROLOGICAL PATIENT

In conjunction with a full respiratory assessment (see Elements of Respiratory Assessment Box; Bruton 2011), particular attention should be given to lung function, peak cough flow (PCF), arterial blood gases (ABGs), chest radiographs, respiratory patterns and respiratory reserve considerations for early mobilisation. If any red flags are noticed, the assessment may need to be adapted or shortened (see Respiratory Red Flags Box; Bruton 2011).

Lung Function

Inspiratory muscle weakness leads to a reduction in VC. VC is the volume change at the mouth between full inspiration and complete expiration (Fig. 18.2). VC is measured using a spirometer and may be considered an aerosol-generating procedure (AGP). Local policies and guidance should be adhered to regarding protection of patients and devices secondary to the Covid-19 pandemic. Patients are required to completely fill and empty their lungs whilst wearing a nose clip and using a mouthpiece; this can be difficult for patients with neurological weakness. A normal VC in supine position indicates that respiratory muscle weakness is unlikely. However, in many neurological conditions weakness can fluctuate; therefore, the VC and SpO_2 should be checked at regular intervals (Mangera et al 2012).

Significant diaphragm weakness is associated with a decline in VC by more than 25% when going from an upright to a supine position (Mezidi & Guérin 2018). This

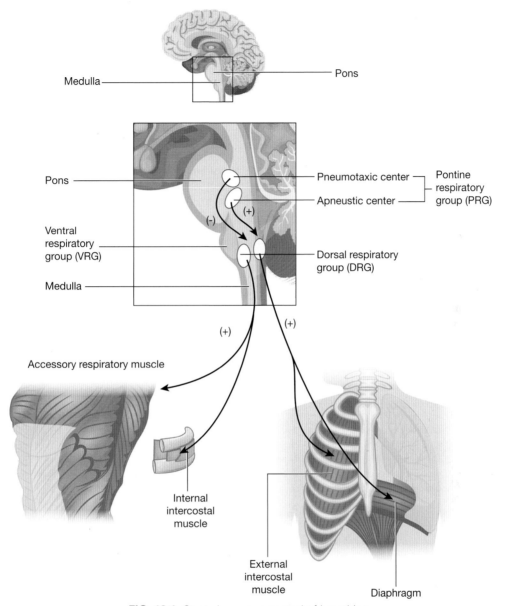

FIG. 18.1 Central nervous control of breathing.

is because of the abdominal contents pushing up on the weakened diaphragm. It should be noted that in the presence of mild muscle weakness, lung function may appear to be normal.

Monitoring of VC is essential in progressive conditions, such as Guillain–Barré syndrome, to indicate when ventilatory support is required. Mechanical ventilation is often required when VC declines to less than 15 mL/kg body weight (Rabinstein 2005, Singh and Widjicks 2021) or when VC is less than 1 L (Singh & Widjicks 2021). Functional residual capacity will be reduced if there is weakness in the respiratory muscles that keep the chest wall expanded at the end of expiration.

There are other tests of respiratory muscle strength such as the sniff test. A sniff nasal inspiratory pressure (SNIP) manoeuvre is a short, voluntary inspiratory manoeuvre

ELEMENTS OF A RESPIRATORY ASSESSMENT (BRUTON 2011, WITH PERMISSION)

General End-of-Bed Observations
Breathing pattern, cyanosis, distress, accessory muscle use, swallowing, speech pattern, posture

History (From Patient/Relatives/Friends)
Past medical history of present complaint, recent symptoms (cough/sputum/chest tightness/breathlessness), smoking history, environmental exposures (pollution/occupational), family health history, travel history, social history, drug history

Clinical Examination
Inspection – hands (finger clubbing, tremor, temperature); chest shape; breathing rate, depth, frequency, symmetry (left:right) and regularity; sputum (quantity, colour, smell); cough competence

Palpation checking for – tracheal centrality; chest pulsations/tenderness/depressions/bulges/movements/scars; tactile/vocal fremitus
Percussion – to detect chest resonance/dullness
Auscultation – to listen for presence/absence normal or added lung sounds

Current General Status
Body temperature, BP, pulse rate, fluid balance, blood chemistry, ICP

Respiratory Bedside/Laboratory Testing
Chest X-rays/other imaging, sputum culture, ABGs, pulse oximetry, lung function tests (e.g., vital capacity), PCF, inspiratory/expiratory pressures (mouth/sniff/transdiaphragmatic)

ABGs, Arterial blood gases; *BP*, blood pressure; *ICP*, intracranial pressure; *PCF*, peak cough flow.

RESPIRATORY RED FLAGS (BRUTON 2011, WITH PERMISSION)

- General (e.g., chest pain/haemoptysis) – always need further investigation because of potential to indicate serious pathology
- Breathlessness or inability to talk in complete sentences at rest – breathlessness may be of sudden onset or gradual; if related to muscle weakness, it may initially be more apparent at night when lying down/sleeping
- Accessory muscle use while at rest – normal breathing requires minimal effort, so use of additional muscles (e.g., sternocleidomastoid) indicates respiratory distress
- Weak cough or inability to clear secretions – suggests weakness of expiratory muscles
- Cyanosis (dusky or bluish tinge to skin) – seen round lips/tongue = central cyanosis. Usually occurs only

once arterial oxygen tension decreases to less than 8 kPa (60 mmHg) and oxygen saturation (SpO_2) less than 90%. Can be difficult to reliably detect in artificial lighting
- Altered mental status – agitation/drowsiness. Acute confusion with breathlessness may indicate severe hypoxaemia (or sepsis/metabolic disturbance)
- Exhaustion and shallow breathing – may follow a period of 'distressed' breathing, when work of breathing overwhelms the patient and fatigue leads to ventilatory failure
- Altered arterial blood gases – hypoxaemia with hypercapnia indicates ventilatory failure
- Vital capacity declining to less than 15 mL/kg body weight indicates respiratory muscle weakness requiring ventilator support (Lawn et al 2001)

that is measured in one occluded nostril using a portable commercial system; however, it is not suitable in patients with nasal congestion. The sniff test has the advantage that it is easy to administer; however, it is a global measure of respiratory muscle strength and does not differentiate between weakness in different respiratory muscles (ATC/ERS 2002, Laveneziana et al 2019).

Maximal Inspiratory Pressure and Maximal Expiratory Pressure

Mouth pressures represent global inspiratory and expiratory muscle strength. Maximal inspiratory pressure (MIP) reflects the strength of the diaphragm, external intercostal muscles and accessory muscles, whereas maximal expiratory pressure (MEP) represents expiratory muscle and cough strength. Mouth pressures can be measured via a device through the mouth or via an endotracheal tube (ETT)/tracheostomy to establish a baseline respiratory function in those with neuromuscular disorders affecting respiratory muscle strength (Mangera et al 2012). It can also be used to support the weaning process of those liberating from ventilators in the intensive care unit (ICU) (Bissett et al 2019). They are particularly useful as objective indicators of the inability to breathe in patients who are

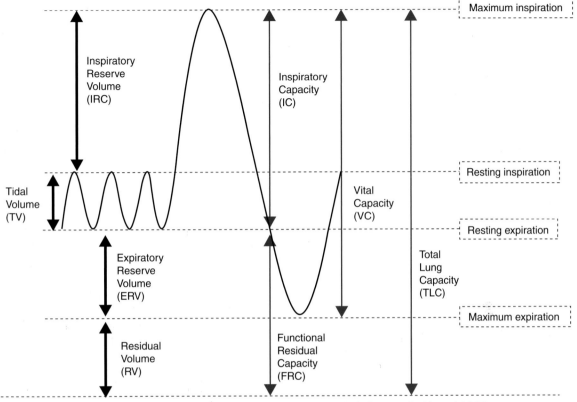

FIG. 18.2 Lung volumes and capacities in neurological disease (Lufti et al 2017).

CRITICAL VALUES OF VITAL CAPACITY

- Normal values are calculated from the patient age, height and gender.
- A decline in VC by more than 25% in supine indicates significant diaphragm weakness.
- When VC declines to less than 1.5 L, careful monitoring is required.
- When VC declines to less than 1 L, ventilation may be required (Rabinstein 2005, Bird & Levine 2022).

CRITICAL VALUES OF PEAK COUGH FLOW (BTS/ACPRC 2009, MOSES ET AL 2018)

- 360–840 L/min is normal
- <270 L/min at risk for serious infection; therefore teach airway clearance strategies
- <160 L/min may require ventilation
- Peak expiratory flow of 60 L/min as demonstrated on the ventilator flow waveform (for intubated/tracheostomised patients)

without obvious respiratory distress (Bird & Levine 2022). Several expert-based threshold values for these parameters have been proposed (Morgan et al 2005, NICE NG42 2016, Janssens et al 2019).

Peak Cough Flow

PCF is a measure of maximal airflow during a cough. It can be measured through a mouthpiece or a face mask attached to a peak flow meter, and patient cooperation is essential. PCF is a useful indicator of cough strength and effectiveness.

When it is equal to or less than 270 L/min, strategies should be implemented to assist airway clearance (see Critical Values of Peak Cough Flow box). If it declines to 160 L/min and the use of physiotherapy adjuncts and treatment is ineffective, then medical advice regarding consideration of ventilation should be sought (BTS/ACPRC 2009). Individuals with weak or impaired inspiratory and/or expiratory muscles, with or without glottis closure issues (bulbar insufficiency, tracheostomy), will have a decreased PCF (Chatwin et al 2018).

Arterial Blood Gases

Arterial blood gas measurement is essential; both partial pressure of oxygen (PaO_2) and partial pressure of carbon dioxide ($PaCO_2$) can be affected by respiratory muscle weakness. Pulse oximetry is useful, providing a noninvasive measure of SpO_2. It can help identify problems such as atelectasis and pneumonia (see Critical Blood Gas Values box).

CRITICAL BLOOD GAS VALUES (BTS 2017)

- Normal value for PaO_2: 75–100 mmHg (10–13.3 kPa),
- <60 mmHg <8 kPa indicates hypoxaemia
- Normal value for $PaCO_2$: 34–46 mmHg (4.6–6.1 kPa),
- <35 mmHg indicates hypercapnia
- Normal value for SpO_2: 95%–98%, to <95% requires careful monitoring, <90% indicates hypoxia

---

Hypercapnia (increased levels of carbon dioxide) and associated acidosis (increased acidity) will often develop in the presence of significant respiratory muscle weakness with associated hypoventilation (Main & Denehy 2016). For those with chronic hypoventilation, a raised arterial bicarbonate level is often found. This is a compensating mechanism and may be more pronounced in the morning or after periods of sleep (Hillman et al 2014).

Chronic nocturnal hypoventilation may occur in patients with neuromuscular and chest wall disease. Symptoms suggestive of nocturnal hypoventilation include poor sleep quality, hypersomnia, morning headaches, nightmares, waking with breathlessness and enuresis (urinary incontinence). A patient with a VC of less than 50% of predicted value may be at risk for nocturnal hypoventilation and may benefit from further investigation and instigation of noninvasive ventilation (NIV). If effective, resolution of clinical symptoms is expected. Overnight respiratory sleep study will assist in diagnosis by showing derangement of ABGs and reduced SpO_2 (Annane et al 2014).

Chest Radiographs

Chest radiographs will show volume loss associated with generalised weakness. A raised hemidiaphragm may indicate unilateral diaphragm weakness, and a bilateral raised hemidiaphragm should be further investigated to establish diaphragmatic weakness/paralysis (Mangera et al 2012, Nason et al 2012).

Respiratory Pattern

Respiratory pattern is subjective; however, it may give an indication of the degree of respiratory muscle weakness. Respiratory pattern can be affected by damage to the RCC in the pons and upper midbrain, respiratory muscle weakness and fatigue, or abnormal alterations in ABG tensions. If respiratory pattern changes during mobilisation, it may indicate deterioration in respiratory function (Gosselink 2008, Stiller & Phillips 2003). The degree in fluctuation from the baseline needs to be assessed and also how quickly the patient returns to baseline.

Respiratory Reserve

The PaO_2 in arterial blood declines steadily with age, reaching approximately 10.3 kPa by the age of 60 years (West 2001). The fraction of inspired oxygen (FiO_2) can assist in the assessment of suitability for rehabilitation. This should be considered in conjunction with PaO_2 and reflects the respiratory reserve (Fig. 18.3).

$$\frac{\text{Partial pressure of arterial oxygen kPa (PaO}_2\text{)}}{\text{Fraction of inspired oxygen (FiO}_2\text{)}} \times 7.5 = \text{Respiratory Reserve}$$

Examples

Normal breathing room air

$$\frac{13.3 \text{ kPa}}{0.21} \times 7.5 = 475 \text{ High respiratory reserve}$$

Head injury with tracheostomy

$$\frac{10.2 \text{ kPa}}{0.30} \times 7.5 = 255 \text{ Marginal respiratory reserve}$$

FIG. 18.3 Calculation for respiratory reserve (Stiller & Phillips 2003). Examples are shown for a healthy person breathing room air and a patient with head injury.

CRITICAL VALUES OF THE PAO2/FIO2 RATIO

- >300 indicates that a patient is likely to have sufficient respiratory reserve to tolerate rehabilitation
- 200–300 indicates marginal respiratory reserve
- <200 indicates low respiratory reserve

The PaO_2/FiO_2 ratio can be calculated easily and used to give an indication of a patient's ability to tolerate rehabilitation (Stiller & Phillips 2003).

If the benefit of mobilising a patient who has marginal respiratory reserve outweighs the potential risks, then increasing respiratory support or additional supplemental oxygen should be considered. The use of respiratory reserve should be used in conjunction with all available parameters to assess suitability for early rehabilitation.

Oxygen uptake needs to be considered because there will be increased oxygen consumption because of increased muscle activities such as turning and mobilising. At rest, minimal levels of oxygen consumption are required for vital functions (aerobic metabolism). Metabolic demands change with the surface area of the body, lean muscle mass, gender and age. Oxygen consumption and metabolic demands will be affected by sepsis, temperature and BP. Liaison with the dietician is important to ensure appropriate nutrition is provided to meet any changes in metabolic demands to ensure effective oxygen uptake (Preiser et al 2015).

EARLY MOBILISATION

Early mobilisation in critical care has been shown to be both safe and feasible (Adler & Malone 2012, Nydahl et al 2017, Stiller 2013). The clinician must assess whether there is sufficient respiratory and cardiovascular reserve and neurological stability before mobilising a patient (Hodgson et al 2014). It is beyond the scope of this chapter to comprehensively review early mobilisation, but the key cardiorespiratory parameters that should be considered are variations in BP being less than 20% of baseline and resting heart rate (HR) less than 50% age-predicted maximal heart rate (Stiller & Phillips 2003). There are limited published clinical data concerning resting HR and BP. Fig. 18.4 outlines an example of a clinical algorithm for early rehabilitation used for neurosurgical patients in intensive care.

It is important to ensure that oxygenation is maximised to avoid or limit ischaemia. The balance between rehabilitation activity and the demands on the cardiorespiratory system from any residual neurological deficit must be maintained. If there has been a period of immobility caused by the neurological insult, then systemic changes will have

occurred. This includes cardiorespiratory deconditioning, muscle weakness from immobility, alignment changes of joints and muscle plus potential secondary conditions not associated with the primary illness, such as critical illness polyneuropathy. It is therefore important to monitor patients for signs of fatigue or deterioration during early mobilisation. This may indicate that the intervention is not being tolerated and needs to be adapted. It is also important to establish whether the response to mobilisation is an anticipated or normal physiological response to exercise.

Progressive neurological disorders may exhibit a gradual deterioration in function, including the respiratory system; therefore, physiotherapy interventions should be aimed at maximising available function within the limits of the cardiorespiratory system (Hodgson et al 2014).

RESPIRATORY TREATMENT AND MANAGEMENT

Maintenance of a Patent Airway

Patients with neurological weakness often present with an ineffective cough. An effective cough is essential to clear airway secretions from the proximal airways and minimise the risk of atelectasis, reduced alveolar ventilation, mucus plugging and respiratory tract infections (RTIs) (Stehling et al 2015). For an effective cough one needs firstly to take a deeply sufficient breath in; the glottis needs to close briefly to allow an increase in intrathoracic pressure, followed by an explosive glottis opening together with abdominal contraction (Chatwin et al 2018). In the presence of an ETT because of an open glottis and therefore limited pressure and flow generation, results may need to be adjusted for comparison (Moses et al 2018).

Insufficient cough strength has a significant impact on effective sputum clearance for patients with neuromuscular weakness. Patients may have difficulty with sputum clearance as a result of inspiratory or expiratory muscle weakness or impaired bulbar function. It is important to ascertain the specific component of the cough with which a patient is having difficulty. If both inspiratory and expiratory weakness have been ruled out, then referral to an SLT should be considered for the joint assessment of bulbar function (Simonds 2017). It should be remembered that an ineffective cough may be a result of a combination of issues.

There is an emerging evidence base that bulbar impairment has a more severe impact on the respiratory function than previously acknowledged, which may directly affect physiotherapy intervention (Allen & O'Leary, 2018, Anderson 2021).

Airway clearance techniques and strategies should be considered to assist with secretion clearance when SpO_2

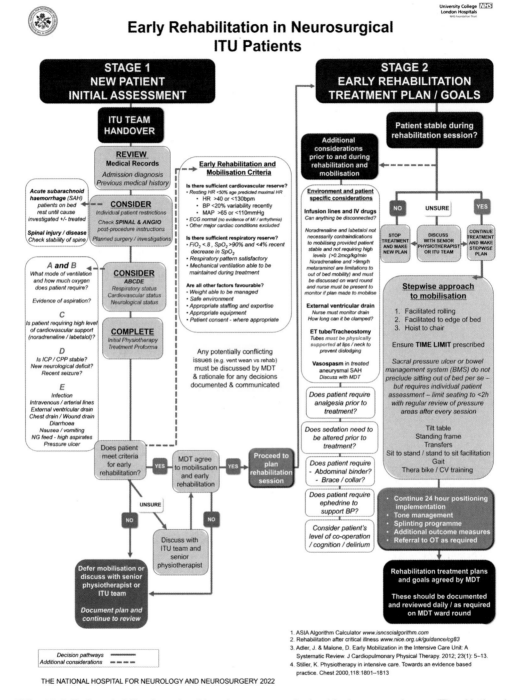

FIG. 18.4 Early rehabilitation algorithm in neurosurgical critical care patients. (The National Hospital for Neurology & Neurosurgery (NHNN) Local Guidelines reproduced with kind permission from Critical Care Unit, NHNN, London, UK.) *BP*, Blood pressure; *CV*, cardiovascular; *ECG*, electrocardiogram; *ET*, endotracheal; *HR*, heart rate; *ICP*, intracranial pressure; *ITU*, intensive care unit; *IV*, intravenous; *MAP*, mean arterial pressure; *MDT*, multidisciplinary team; *NG*, nasogastric; *OT*, occupational therapy.

declines to less than 95%, PCF is equal to or less than 270 L/min and VC declines to less than 1500 mL or 50% predicted value. After careful assessment, treatment can be focused on either specific or all of the phases of the cough cycle (Fig. 18.5).

Maximal Insufflation Capacity

The maximal insufflation capacity (MIC) is the maximal volume of air that can be held in the lungs after breath stacking. Breath stacking is an exercise used to facilitate an increase in inspiratory volume, which is useful when muscles are weak and taking a deep breath is difficult (BTS/ACPRC 2009). The aim of MIC is to increase the inspiratory reserve volume further than the active ability of the inspiratory muscles. It may be possible to teach active breath stacking as part of the active cycle of breathing with an end-inspiratory 'sniff' for those patients without bulbar dysfunction.

Glossopharyngeal breathing (e.g., frog breathing) is a form of positive pressure technique that can be used to assist failing respiratory muscles which may be useful for some patients (Maltais 2011). The technique involves the use of the glottis to add to an inspiratory effort by gulping boluses of air into the lungs. It should be considered for patients with reduced VC and those with decreased voice strength. Lung volume recruitment bags can be used as an adjunct to improve MIC (Chatwin et al 2018, McKim et al 2012). Some of the indications for use are inspiratory weakness, reduced chest wall compliance and retained secretions. There are a number of precautions and contraindications, for example, cognitive impairment, reduced consciousness, pneumothorax and use after meals. Recommendations for interventions are shown in the Key Interventions for Maximal Insufflation Capacity box. Regular breath stacking increases MIC (increased thoracic range of movement) in 70% of patients, resulting in increased cough effectiveness (Sheers et al 2019, Toussaint et al 2018).

KEY INTERVENTIONS FOR MAXIMAL INSUFFLATION CAPACITY

- Start by using lung volume recruitment, then consider using the mechanical insufflation and exsufflation (MI:E) device.
- Consider regular breath stacking (10–15 maximal lung inflations three times a day).

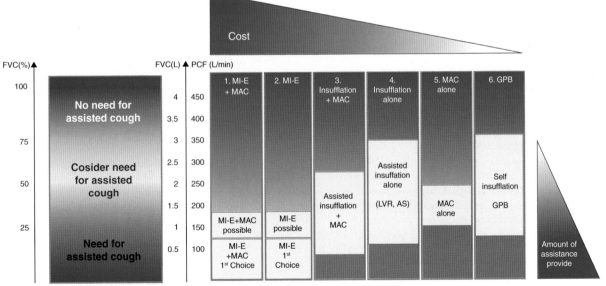

FIG. 18.5 A guide to the use of cough augmentation strategies in the neuromuscular population (Toussaint et al 2018). This figure seeks to integrate the published literature regarding critical values percent predicted FVC (FVC%), vital capacity (FVC) and peak cough flow (PCF), alongside the relative cost and amount of assistance required for the initiation of proximal airway clearance techniques. The clinician can decide on which technique (mechanical in-exsufflation [MI:E], manually assisted cough [MAC], air stacking [AS], lung volume recruitment [LVR] or glossopharyngeal breathing [GPB]) to use depending on the objective markers of FVC%, FVC and PCF.

Manual Cough

A manually assisted cough (MAC) manoeuvre involves the application of an abdominal thrust or costal lateral compression using hand placements after an adequate spontaneous inspiration or maximal insufflation. This technique should be used to increase PCF in patients with neuromuscular disease or those with abdominal weakness secondary to spinal cord injury or under the effects of sedation in the neuro-ICU. The technique can be used in isolation or alongside a MIC strategy (Gosselink et al 2011). The technique may be applied in different positions and with different hand thrusts; the technique should be modified for the patient to ensure an effective result.

Mechanical Insufflation and Exsufflation

Devices such as the NIPPY clearway and the Phillips E70 are noninvasive devices that provide MI:E by applying positive pressure to the airways, then rapidly switching to a negative pressure to stimulate the expiratory flow needed to cough, and thus aid the clearance of secretions (Stehling et al 2015, Swingwood et al 2020). Devices should be considered with patients who are unable to increase their PCF using other strategies (Fig. 18.4). MI:E is indicated when there is inspiratory, expiratory and bulbar dysfunction. Bulbar function needs to be assessed and severe dysfunction may be a contraindication; therefore, close liaison with SLT is advised (Simonds 2017).

MI:E has been shown to assist with recruiting lung volumes, optimising thoracic range of motion and increasing lung compliance (Moses et al 2018). The use of MI:E after extubation may reduce reintubation rates (Gonçalves et al 2012). The device can be applied to the patient by using a face mask, mouthpiece, ETT or via a tracheostomy. MI:E pressures should be titrated to suit the individual patient in the generation of a cough, and consideration should be made for application through artificial airways (Chatwin & Simonds 2020, Moses et al 2018).

Intermittent positive-pressure breathing (IPPB) can be delivered by MI:E machines to deliver inspiratory breaths. The device will provide a patient-triggered passive inspiration, which is larger than that which the patient would be able to generate by themselves.

NIV, the provision of ventilator support via a patient's upper airway, is often used overnight (BTS/ICS 2016). In some centres, physiotherapy will be involved in the setting up of NIV; however, there will be local guidance and governance frameworks regarding this.

When using any adjunct using positive pressure in the neurological population, consideration must be given to the following contraindications:

- Bulbar involvement;
- Neurosurgical procedure (e.g., transsphenoidal approach);
- Inability to protect airway (poor swallow); and
- Vomiting.

Other Considerations

The patient's position needs to be considered to optimise the treatment effect. For example, patients with spinal cord injury may need to be treated in supine to maximise their VC. The patient's VC should be taken in supine and upright, and the treatment should occur in the position with the largest VC, which often is supine (Respiratory Information for Spinal Cord Injury 2023).

Manual techniques such as vibrations can be used in conjunction with the treatment adjuncts to increase peak expiratory flow. By manipulating the chest wall to create a peak expiratory flow bias 10% greater than that of peak inspiratory flow, the proximal movement of mucus occurs through the two-phase gas–liquid flow mechanism (McIlwaine et al 2017, Shannon et al 2010). Chatwin et al (2018) completed a state-of-the-art review of the literature and have classified airway clearance practices into proximal and peripheral airway clearance techniques (Fig. 18.6). This provides a useful tool for the physiotherapist when considering techniques and adjuncts to aid sputum clearance. When using any of the techniques, suctioning equipment should be on hand to assist with airway clearance if required.

Hydration needs to be optimised because systemic hydration improves the viscoelasticity of the sputum, so airway hydration is essential and humidification should be considered (Fisher & Paykel Healthcare 2015, O'Driscoll et al 2017). The type of humidification required is patient dependent, and the physiotherapist should clinically reason what is the optimal delivery method depending on the presentation. Careful consideration must be given in the presence of an artificial airway.

Patients may present with breathlessness, and a full assessment to ascertain cause must be carried out. Where indicated, physiotherapy techniques for the management of this can be used in patients with neurological dysfunction; however, some techniques will need careful consideration and monitoring because they may be contraindicated (e.g., head-down position in acute TBI).

KEY POINTS TO OPTIMISE TREATMENT EFFECTS

- Consider patient position.
- Use treatment adjuncts with manual techniques.
- Have suction equipment readily on hand.
- Consider optimal delivery method for humidification.

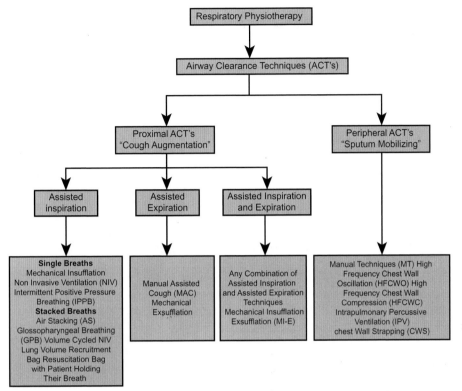

FIG. 18.6 Classification of airway clearance techniques for use in patients with neuromuscular disease (Chatwin et al 2018).

Respiratory Muscle Training

Respiratory muscle weakness is common in patients with neuromuscular dysfunction resulting in inadequate ventilation, nocturnal hypoventilation and ineffective cough. When inspiratory muscles are affected, there will be a reduction in VC and expansion of the chest wall. If the expiratory muscles are affected, then there will be a reduction in cough strength leading to sputum retention, infection and atelectasis. Inspiratory muscle training is recommended in patients with suspected or confirmed respiratory muscle weakness (BTS/ACPRC 2009) and has been shown to improve the outcomes of patients weaning from ventilators in the ICU, either because of underlying neuromuscular disease or simply because of diaphragmatic atrophy after mechanical ventilation (Bissett et al 2019). There is emerging evidence to support the efficacy of inspiratory and expiratory muscle training, with improved outcomes in the neuromuscular disease and spinal cord injury population, both in and out of the ICU (Aslan et al 2014, McDonald & Stiller 2019).

Management of Acute Respiratory Failure

Neurological patients in acute respiratory failure are likely to require some form of mechanical ventilation which will be led by the medical/neurointensive team. This provides many challenges and should be tailored to the unique needs of the patient (Racca et al 2020). The aim of physiotherapy intervention is to optimise respiratory function while maintaining the neuromusculoskeletal system. Common interventions are:

- Suction;
- Cough augmentation and airway clearance strategies;
- Manual techniques;
- Positioning;
- Manual hyperinflation (MHI)/ventilator hyperinflation; and
- Mobilisation.

Tracheostomy and Weaning

A tracheostomy is an artificial airway inserted directly into the trachea to facilitate ventilation and secretion clearance.

Considerations for the insertion of a tracheostomy in patients with neurological impairment include inability to protect and maintain the airway, upper airway obstruction, excessive bronchial secretions, avoidance of laryngeal complications of prolonged ventilation and assistance with ventilator weaning.

It is becoming more common to plan for earlier insertion of a tracheostomy to improve patient comfort and outcome (Keeping 2016), but the timing of the insertion will be directed by patient need and local guidance. With increasing use of tracheostomies, there have been a number of initiatives to improve patient care, for example, the National Tracheostomy Safety Project and National Confidential Enquiry into Patient Outcome and Death Report (2014).

Tracheostomy weaning in the neuroscience population should be through a patient-centred, goal-directed, and multidisciplinary approach. The pathway should be individualised to the patient's need and performed in collaboration with the multidisciplinary team (MDT) (Hirzallah et al 2019, Hunt & McGowan 2015, McClenaghan et al 2021).

An example of a local decision-making tool to help guide the initial cuff deflation of a tracheostomised patient is presented in Fig. 18.7 (McGowan et al 2021).

RESPIRATORY FUNCTION IN NEUROLOGICAL CONDITIONS

Examples are given for each type of neurological condition: central conditions, subarachnoid haemorrhage, spinal cord injury and disease, anterior horn cell conditions, neuropathy, neuromuscular junction and muscle conditions, and ending with the management of TBI.

Central Conditions

Some common central nervous system conditions are presented in Table 18.1.

Neural control of respiration depends on three pathways:
1. Automatic (metabolic) respiration: to maintain acid–base balance (Howard & Davidson 2003);
2. Voluntary (behavioural) respiration: allows modulation of ventilation in response to voluntary acts such as speaking, singing, breath hold and straining (Howard & Davidson 2003); and
3. Limbic (emotional) control: allows respiratory modulation to emotion such as laughing, coughing and anxiety (Howard & Davidson 2003).

Subarachnoid Haemorrhage

Specific BP parameters should be set by the neurosurgeon/intensive care specialist stating the desired systolic and diastolic pressure to maintain adequate cerebral perfusion. In the presence of an unprotected aneurysm, this will be to reduce the risk for rupture. Any intervention that may increase BP should be used with caution. These include coughing, straining (Valsalva manoeuvre) and manual techniques, particularly if they cause a pain response. It is essential to ensure the patient has adequate pain relief before intervention. If the patient is already sedated, then bolus sedation may be indicated. In sedated and ventilated patients, it is important not to prophylactically hyperventilate because of added risk of ischaemia from vasoconstriction (Asehnoune et al 2018).

If vasospasm is present, then BP will need to be maintained to minimise ischaemia of brain tissue. In this case interventions that decrease BP should be used with caution. These may include ventilator hyperventilation, MHI, NIV, cough assist, IPPB and changes in posture from supine to upright. When suctioning, precaution should be taken to avoid hypoxia and hypercapnia and prolonged changes to ICP. Patients must be monitored for any changes in their neurological status, for example, limb weakness, focal deficit, changes in conscious levels or a decline in their Glasgow Coma Score. Patients with vasospasm will usually be on a level of a vasopressor to increase BP, which could prohibit mobilisation. However, asymptomatic vasospasm is not a contraindication to sitting people out of bed. Consideration must be given to the patient's clinical stability and vasopressor requirements and should be discussed daily on the MDT ward rounds. Local policies will apply.

Spinal Cord Injury and Disease

Four common spinal cord conditions are:
- Traumatic spinal cord injury;
- Transverse myelitis;
- Metastatic cord compression; and
- Spinal tumour.

Respiratory function and treatment will depend on the neurological level and whether the lesion is complete or incomplete (Table 18.2).

In the management of patients with spinal cord injury, liaison with the clinical team is essential regarding spinal precautions that will affect physiotherapeutic treatment. Incomplete injuries have a mixed picture of functional level because of areas of respiratory muscle preservation.

The pathophysiology of spinal cord injury is complex, and patients may rapidly deteriorate and require urgent intubation and ventilation (Racca et al 2020). Spinal injuries above the level of T6 are at risk for haemodynamic instability because of the loss of sympathetic outflow. This results in hypotension and bradycardia on suctioning. Intravenous atropine should be available.

In patients with diaphragm and respiratory muscle involvement, continuous positive airway pressure will not improve ventilation and increases carbon dioxide retention. NIV should be considered in conjunction with the MDT.

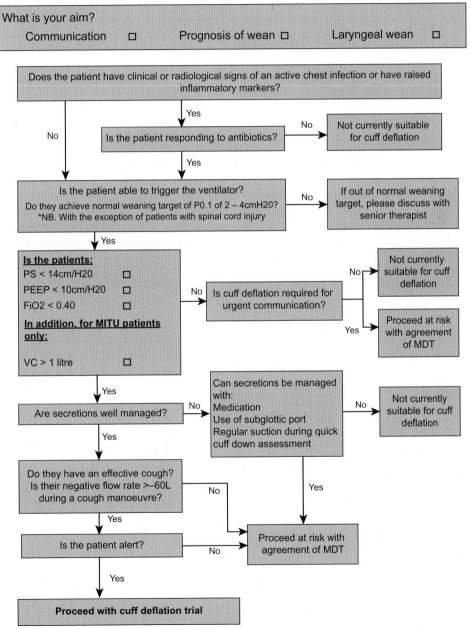

FIG. 18.7 Decision-making tool for initial tracheostomy cuff deflation on patients who are ventilated on the surgical/medical intensive care unit (McGowan et al 2021).

TABLE 18.1   Central Nervous System Conditions (McCool et al 2021, Racca et al 2020)

CNS Conditions	Respiratory Considerations	Treatment Considerations
Unilateral or bilateral tegmental infarcts in the pons	Apneustic breathing (deep, gasping inspiration with a pause at full inspiration, followed by brief insufficient release) Impairment of carbon dioxide responsiveness	Reduced response to demands on cardiorespiratory systems during exercise Any surgical nasal approach should be treated with caution when considering any invasive nasal modality (e.g., nasal suction, intermittent positive-pressure ventilation)
Lateral medullary syndrome	Acute failure of automatic respiration	Requires mechanical ventilation
Basal pons infarcts pyramids and adjacent ventral portion of the medulla	Irregular breathing pattern Inability to initiate volitional breathing	Inability to effectively cough to command Inability to deep breathe to command Inability to breath hold
Lesion in anterior pathways	Loss of automatic control Apnoea (cessation of breathing)	Requires mechanical ventilation

TABLE 18.2   Spinal Cord Level and Respiratory Function (Clapham 2009, Howard & Davidson 2003, Racca et al 2020, Terson de Paleville et al 2011)

Level of Lesion	Affected Respiratory Muscles	Respiratory Considerations	Treatment Options
C2	Diaphragm Intercostals Abdominals, accessory muscles	No respiratory effort Ventilator dependent No cough Fatigue	Suction, manual or ventilator hyperinflation Manual techniques Mechanical cough device Manual assisted cough
C4	Partial diaphragm Partial accessory muscles Intercostals, abdominals	Ventilator independent but may require nocturnal ventilation Paradoxical breathing Ineffective cough Fatigue	Glossopharyngeal breathing Assisted cough machine Manual assisted cough Intermittent positive-pressure breathing Mechanical cough
C6	Partial accessory muscles, intercostals Abdominals	Ventilator independent Ineffective cough Fatigue	As for C4
T1	Intercostals and abdominals	Ineffective cough Fatigue	As for C6
T12	None	Effective cough	All respiratory physiotherapy techniques

Mechanical cough assist machines have been found to be a useful adjunct in the presence of altered or absent cough and may be useful prophylactically.

Anterior Horn Cell Conditions

Three common anterior horn cell conditions are:
- Poliomyelitis;
- Motor neurone disease; and
- Proximal spinal atrophy.

Respiratory insufficiency occurs because of respiratory muscle weakness or associated bulbar weakness leading to aspiration and bronchopneumonia (Howard & Davidson 2003, McCool et al 2021, NICE NG42 2016, Racca et al 2020) (Table 18.3).

TABLE 18.3 Anterior Horn Cell (Aboussouan & Mireles-Cabodevila 2013, McCool et al 2021, Racca 2020)

Common Conditions	Respiratory Considerations	Treatment Considerations
Poliomyelitis	Respiratory muscle weakness Fatigue	All respiratory physiotherapy interventions are appropriate
Motor neurone disease (MND) Spinal muscular atrophy (SMA)	Respiratory muscle weakness Bulbar impairment Fatigue Weak intercostal muscles/relative strong diaphragm, bell-shaped chest, paradoxical breathing Restrictive lung disease Bulbar impairment	May require noninvasive ventilatory support with deterioration May require tracheostomy All respiratory physiotherapy interventions may be appropriate once full assessment is completed, e.g., impact of bulbar dysfunction on use of adjuncts Full assessment in specialist clinic should be undertaken All respiratory physiotherapy interventions may be appropriate

TABLE 18.4 Neuropathy (Khanna et al 2017, Prasad et al 2021, Rabinstein 2005)

Common Condition	Respiratory Considerations	Treatment Considerations
Guillain–Barré syndrome (GBS)	Primarily inspiratory muscle weakness Weakness of abdominal muscles Weakness of accessory muscles Impaired cough Bulbar weakness Retained secretions Aspiration pneumonia Atelectasis (collapsed lung) Fatigue	One-third will require mechanical ventilation A decline in tidal volume of <15 mL/kg indicates the need for ventilatory support May require prolonged weaning All physiotherapy techniques appropriate

Neuropathy

Guillain–Barré syndrome is a neuropathy which often is associated with respiratory insufficiency (Table 18.4).

Respiratory insufficiency occurs because of respiratory muscle weakness or associated bulbar weakness leading to possible respiratory failure, aspiration or bronchopneumonia (Howard & Davidson 2003, Racca et al 2020). VC monitoring is useful in determining both deterioration and resolution of respiratory function. Patients who present with bulbar dysfunction and bilateral facial weakness have an increased likelihood to deteriorate and require mechanical ventilation (Lawn et al 2001, Rabinstein 2005).

Neuromuscular Junction

Three common neuromuscular conditions are:
- Myasthenia gravis (Table 18.5);
- Lambert–Eaton myasthenic syndrome; and
- *Clostridium botulinum*.

Muscle fatigue may occur in patients with pathologies that affect the neuromuscular junction. A graded regimen of rehabilitation should be used with additional ventilatory support when rehabilitating in the early stages, including the use of noninvasive ventilation (Rabinstein 2005).

Muscle Conditions

Muscular dystrophies and metabolic myopathies are common; some examples are presented in Table 18.6:
- Muscular dystrophies; and
- Metabolic myopathies.

Respiratory insufficiency caused by respiratory muscle weakness or associated bulbar weakness can lead to possible respiratory failure, aspiration or bronchopneumonia (McCool et al 2021, Racca et al 2020). Associated skeletal changes may further affect respiratory function and compliance of the chest wall.

TABLE 18.5   Neuromuscular Junction (Prasad et al 2021, Racca 2020)

Common Condition	Respiratory Considerations	Treatment Considerations
Myasthenia gravis	Diaphragm weakness may occur with mild peripheral weakness Fatigue	Long-term ventilation All physiotherapy techniques appropriate

TABLE 18.6   Muscle (LoMauro et al 2018, Narayan et al 2022, Racca 2020, Ryder et al 2017, Trucco et al 2020)

Common Conditions	Respiratory Considerations	Treatment Considerations
Duchenne muscular dystrophy	Respiratory failure develops late Intercostal and expiratory muscle weakness Scoliosis Kyphosis Bulbar weakness Fatigue	Aspiration (the entry of secretions or foreign material into the trachea or lungs) Reduced lung compliance All physiotherapy techniques are appropriate Breath stacking techniques including lung volume recruitment bags
Becker's muscular dystrophy	Scoliosis Respiratory muscle weakness Fatigue	All physiotherapy techniques are appropriate
Fascioscapulohumeral dystrophy	May have selective diaphragm weakness Fatigue	All physiotherapy techniques are appropriate
Acid maltase deficiency	Early selective diaphragm weakness Fatigue	All physiotherapy techniques are appropriate

TABLE 18.7   Classification of Brain Injury

Primary Brain Injury	Secondary Brain Injury
Focal: Disruption of brain vessels Haematoma formation Contusions Traumatic subarachnoid haemorrhage Diffuse: Diffuse axonal injury	Extracranial causes: Systemic hypotension Hypoxaemia (reduced oxygen levels) Hypercapnia (excess carbon dioxide) Disturbances of blood coagulation Intracranial causes: Haematoma brain swelling Disturbances in the microvascular circulation Infection

MANAGEMENT OF TRAUMATIC BRAIN INJURY

The classification of the pathophysiology of brain injury is shown in Table 18.7. In reality, both primary focal and diffuse brain injury coexist. Primary brain injury occurs at the time of injury and is irreversible.

The management of TBI is aimed at prevention of secondary brain injury (Coles 2004, Marik 2002). Secondary damage occurs to neurones because of physiological responses after the initial injury leading to cerebral ischaemia (Marik 2002). Terminology associated with cerebral pressures and blood flow with normal ranges are listed in Table 18.8.

TABLE 18.8 Definitions and Normal Values Relating to Cerebral Haemodynamics (Clapham 2009, Coles 2004)

Term	Definition	Normal Range
Intracranial pressure	Pressure within the cranial cavity	0–10 mmHg
Cerebral perfusion pressure	Net pressure of blood flow to the brain	60–100 mmHg
Cerebral blood flow	Amount of blood that passes through the brain per minute	50 mL/100 g/min of brain tissue

TABLE 18.9 Signs and Symptoms of Raised Intracranial Pressure

Early Signs and Symptoms	Late Signs and Symptoms
Headache	Severe headache
Confusion	Projectile vomiting
Convulsions	Reduced level of consciousness
Irritability	Irregular breathing
Lethargy	Abnormal limb posturing
Restlessness	Flexion/extension
Focal neurology	Cushing's response
Pupil dysfunction	Impaired brainstem function

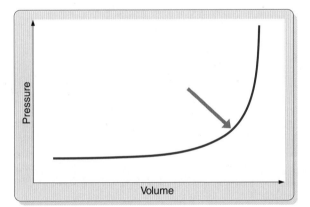

FIG. 18.8 Monroe Kellie Doctrine. Graph showing the normal volume–pressure relationship within the cranial vault. Arrow indicates point where brain compliance is lost because of all compensatory mechanisms within the cranial vault being exhausted. After this point on the graph, a small rise in intracranial volume will cause an exponential rise in intracranial pressure. (From Lindsay & Bone 2004, with permission.)

Because of the limited space within the cranial vault, if there is a rise in volume (e.g., from a haematoma, space-occupying lesion or increase in cerebral blood volume), then there will be a subsequent rise in ICP. In Fig. 18.8 the point marked on the curve indicates the point when the brain's compliance stops, leading to a large increase in pressure with a small increase in volume (Lindsay & Bone 2004). The signs and symptoms of raised ICP are shown in Table 18.9.

It is important for the therapist to consider any potential effects an intervention may have on cerebral perfusion pressure (CPP) (Roth et al 2012) because an increasing ICP or a declining mean arterial pressure (MAP) can have detrimental effects which, if sustained, will lead to cerebral ischaemia (CPP = MAP – ICP). The cerebral vasculature is highly responsive to changes in the $PaCO_2$, metabolic by-products, level of blood acidity or alkalinity and PaO_2. This can result in increased cerebral blood volume leading to an increase in ICP or cerebral ischaemia (Fig. 18.9).

Patients who have undergone a TBI commonly present with a reduced LOC; respiratory problems associated with this are outlined in Table 18.10.

Cardiorespiratory interventions may themselves have a detrimental effect on cerebral oxygenation which could potentially contribute to the secondary cerebral ischaemia. Therefore a risk assessment before every respiratory intervention should be carried out involving ICP and CPP (Table 18.11).

Liaising with the clinical team can give important information regarding patient response to handling or interventions. Local policies should be checked regarding monitors, equipment, patient parameters and postsurgical procedures.

If therapy is indicated and the risk of treatment is deemed acceptable, the potential detrimental effects associated with individual treatment modalities need to be carefully considered (Table 18.12).

Extraventricular drains should be managed according to departmental policies during treatment sessions (Young et al 2019). Awareness of surgical procedures such as craniectomy (removal of bone flap) and ICP must be considered in all treatment planning.

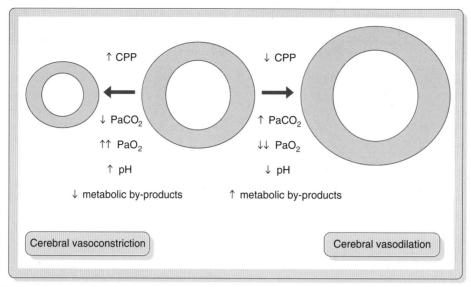

FIG. 18.9 Factors affecting cerebral vasculature. Diagram showing the effect of the reactivity of the cerebral vasculature to the partial pressure of carbon dioxide ($PaCO_2$), partial pressure of oxygen (PaO_2), blood acidity/alkalinity (pH) and metabolic by-products. *CPP*, Cerebral perfusion pressure. (From Lindsay & Bone 2004, with permission.)

TABLE 18.10   Common Problems With a Reduced Consciousness Level (Clapham 2009, Pryor & Prasad 2008)

Common Problems	Treatment Considerations
Reduced airway protection Sputum retention	• Use of airway protection techniques • Insertion of nasopharyngeal airway (if nonintubated or had a tracheostomy [opening through the trachea to create an airway]) • Insertion of oral airway (if nonintubated or had a tracheostomy) • Suction • Gravity-assisted positioning • Manual hyperinflation • Manual techniques, e.g., chest vibrations/shaking, percussion • Cough augmentation strategies, e.g., MI:E, IPPB, manual assisted cough
Hypoventilation	• Manual hyperinflation • IPPB • NIV
Atelectasis (collapsed lung)	• Manual hyperventilation • IPPB
Type II respiratory failure (low oxygen with high carbon dioxide)	• Liaise with critical care specialist • May require intubation or NIV

IPPB, Intermittent positive-pressure breathing; *NIV*, noninvasive ventilation.

TABLE 18.11 Risk Assessment (Clapham 2009)

Intracranial Pressure	Cerebral Perfusion Pressure	Risk
<15 mmHg	70 mmHg (stable)	Low
15–20 mmHg	70 mmHg (settles quickly after treatment within 5 minutes)	Moderate
>20 mmHg	Low	High

TABLE 18.12 Effects of Respiratory Intervention (Capp & Platt 2018, Clapham 2009, Newman et al 2018, Pryor & Prasad 2008)

Physiotherapy Technique	Potential Treatment Effects
MHI	↑ Intrathoracic pressure leading to: ↓ venous return to the heart leading to ↑ cerebral blood volume and ↑ ICP ↓ filling pressure to the right atrium from the inferior vena cava leading to ↓ in stroke volume and drop in blood pressure The depth and rate of manual hyperventilation will affect the cerebral vasculature as a result of carbon dioxide retention or removal. This can either reduce or increase ICP If ICP is high, then rapid small-volume breaths will reduce ICP by removal of CO_2 to allow intermittent manual hyperinflation breaths Intersperse this with large-volume MHI breath for therapeutic effect
Positioning	Treatment position may be limited to 15–30° head-up position to reduce ICP Head must be kept aligned in midline (chin in line with sternum) to reduce pooling of venous blood within the brain from neck vein obstruction in patients with a raised ICP Patients may not tolerate turning. Bolus sedation may be required When changing patients' position, do so slowly in patients with raised ICP. Risk for aspiration if bulbar weakness
Manual techniques (shaking, vibrations, percussion)	Noxious stimulation, therefore: Ensure adequate analgesia May require bolus sedation Note: Bolus sedation may drop blood pressure. Bronchospasm Slow, single-handed percussion may reduce ICP
Intermittent positive-pressure breathing/the BIRD/noninvasive ventilation	↑ Intrathoracic pressure therefore may have similar effects to MHI May reduce mean arterial pressure
Suction	Hypoxia Hypercapnia leading to ↑ ICP ↑ intrathoracic pressure caused by coughing leading to increased ICP Valsalva manoeuvre (forced exhalation against closed vocal cords) Vasovagal response (cardioinhibitory and vasodepressor responses) leading to bradycardia (heart rate <60 beats/min)

ICP, Intracranial pressure; *MHI*, manual hyperinflation.

Remember, to minimise the detrimental effects of physiotherapy intervention:

- Keep treatment time short (Clapham 2009);
- Increase the patient's level of sedation; and
- Ideally do one intervention at a time to observe how the patient responds and to assess the efficacy of the intervention.

CONCLUSION

Patients with neurological conditions often have associated cardiorespiratory impairment either as a direct result of their condition or as secondary complications (Mangera et al 2012).

Common clinical problems in this patient group are:

- Injury to the brainstem RCC resulting in impaired LOC;
- Respiratory muscle weakness;
- Fatigue;
- Breathlessness;
- Impaired swallowing (aspiration);
- Impaired ability to cough (sputum retention/infection);
- Hypoxia;
- Raised ICP; and
- Hypercapnia.

Respiratory physiotherapy is indicated within this patient group; however, careful clinical reasoning is essential to ensure effectiveness of treatment and that patient safety is maintained at all times. A holistic assessment of function is essential with liaison with MDT colleagues to ensure that patient's outcome is optimised.

SELF-ASSESSMENT QUESTIONS

1. At which point would you consider stopping a physiotherapy intervention in a patient with acute TBI who is intubated and has ICP monitoring in situ? What parameters would you consider acceptable?
2. What objective measure would you consider in assessing cough strength? When would you commence physiotherapy intervention, and what would this be?
3. What are the RCCs, and what are their functions?

REFERENCES

Aboussouan, L., Mireles-Cabodevila, E., 2013. Respiratory support in patients with amyotrophic lateral sclerosis. Respir. Care. 58, 1555–1558.

Adler, J., Malone, D., 2012. Early mobilization in the intensive care unit: a systematic review. Cardiopulmon. Phys. Ther. J. 23, 5–13.

Allen, J.E., O'Leary, E.L., 2018. Considerations for chest clearance and cough augmentation in severe bulbar dysfunction: a case study. Can. J. Resp. Ther. 54, 66–70. https://doi.org/10.29390/cjrt-2018-014

American Thoracic Society/European Respiratory Society, 2002. 'ATS/ERS Statement on Respiratory Muscle Testing'. Am. J. Respir. Crit. Care Med. 166, 518–624.

Andersen, T.M., Hov, B., Halvorsen, T., Røksund, O.D., Vollsæter, M., 2021. Upper airway assessment and responses during mechanically assisted cough. Respir. Care. 66, 1196–1213.

Annane, D., Orlikowski, D., Chevret, S., 2014. Nocturnal mechanical ventilation for chronic hypoventilation in patients with neuromuscular and chest wall disorders. Cochrane. Database. Syst. Rev. 12, CD001941.

Asehnoune, K., Roquilly, A., Cinotti, R., 2018. Respiratory management in patients with severe brain injury. In: Vincent, J.L. (Ed.), Annual Update in Intensive Care and Emergency Medicine. Springer, Cham.

Aslan, G., Gurses, H.N., Issever, H., Kiyan, E., 2014. Effects of respiratory muscle training on pulmonary functions in patients with slowly progressive neuromuscular disease: a randomised controlled trial. Clin. Rehabil. 28, 573–581.

Bird, S.J., Levine, J.M., 2022. Overview of the treatment of myasthenic gravis. In: Shefner, J.M., Goddeau, R.P. (Eds.) Up to Date. Available at: https://www.uptodate.com/contents/overview-of-the-treatment-of-myasthenia-gravis#H696671084. Accessed April 2022.

Bissett, B., Leditschke, I.A., Green, M., Marzano, V., Collins, S., Van Haren, F., 2019. Inspiratory muscle training for intensive care patients: a multidisciplinary practical guide for clinicians. Aust. Crit. Care. 32, 249–255.

Bruton, A., 2011. Respiratory management in neurological rehabilitation. In: Stokes, M., Stack, E. (Eds.), Physical Management for Neurological Conditions. Elsevier Science, London.

BTS, 2017. Guideline for oxygen therapy use in adults in healthcare and emergency settings. Thorax. 72 (Suppl. 1), i1–i90.

BTS/ACPRC, 2009. Guidelines: physiotherapy management of the adult, medical, spontaneously breathing patient. Thorax. 64 (Suppl. 1), i1–i51.

BTS/ICS, 2016. Guidelines for the ventilatory management of acute hypercapnic respiratory failure in adults. Thorax. 71 (Suppl. 2), ii1–ii35.

Capp A., Platt, L., 2018. Respiratory management. In: Lennon, S., Ramdharry, G., Verheyden, G. (Eds.) The Neurological Physiotherapy Pocketbook, 2nd Ed., p. 121.

Chatwin, M., Simonds, A.K., 2020. Long-term mechanical insufflation-exsufflation cough assistance in neuromuscular disease: patterns of use and lessons for application. Respir. Care. 65, 135–143.

Chatwin, M., Toussaint, M., Goncalves, M.R., et al., 2018. Airway clearance techniques in neuromuscular disorders: a state of the art review. Resp. Med. 136, 98–110.

Clapham, L., 2009. Calls to the neurology/neurosurgical unit. In: Harden, B., Cross, J., Broad, M., Quint, M., Ritson, P., Thomas, S. (Eds.), Emergency Physiotherapy, 2nd Ed. Churchill Livingstone, Edinburgh.

Coles, J.P., 2004. Regional ischemia after head injury. Curr. Opin. Crit. Care. 10, 120–125.

Fisher & Paykel Healthcare (Fphcare), 2015. Essential humidity for a successful non-invasive ventilation strategy. Available at: www.fphcare.com. Accessed on 1 Feb 2022.

Gonçalves, M.R., Honrado, T., Winck, J.C., Paiva, J.A., 2012. Effects of mechanical insufflation-exsufflation in preventing respiratory failure after extubation: a randomized controlled trial. Crit. Care. 16, 1–8.

Gosselink, R., Bott, J., Johnson, M., et al., 2008. Physiotherapy for adult patients with critical illness: recommendations of the European Respiratory Society and European Society of Intensive Care Medicine Task Force on physiotherapy for critically ill patients. Intens. Care. Med. 34, 1188–1199.

Gosselink, R., Clerckx, B., Robbeets, C., Vanhullebusch, T., Vanpee, G., Segers, J., 2011. Physiotherapy in the intensive care unit. Neth. J. Crit. Care. 15, 66–75.

Hillman, D., Singh, B., McArdle, N., Eastwood, P., 2014. Relationships between ventilatory impairment, sleep hypoventilation and type 2 respiratory failure. Respirology. 19, 1106–1116.

Hirzallah, F.M., Alkaissi, A., do Céu Barbieri-Figueiredo, M., 2019. A systematic review of nurse-led weaning protocol for mechanically ventilated adult patients. Nurs. Crit. Care. 24, 89–96.

Hodgson, C.L., Stiller, K., Needham, D.M., et al., 2014. Expert consensus and recommendations on safety criteria for active mobilization of mechanically ventilated critically ill adults. Crit. Care. 18, 658–667.

Howard, R.S., Davidson, C., 2003. Long term ventilation in neurogenic respiratory failure. J. Neurol. Neurosurg. Psychiatry. 74 (Suppl. 3), iii24–iii30.

Hunt, K., McGowan, S., 2015. Tracheostomy management. BJA Educ. 15, 149–153.

Ikeda, K., Kawakami, K., Onimaru, H., et al., 2017. The respiratory control mechanisms in the brainstem and spinal cord: integrative views of the neuroanatomy and neurophysiology. J. Physiol. Sci. 67, 45–62.

Janssens, J.P., Adler, D., Ferfoglia, R.I., et al., 2019. Assessing inspiratory muscle strength for early detection of respiratory failure in motor neuron disease: should we use MIP, SNIP, or both? Respiration. 98, 114–124.

Keeping, A., 2016. Early versus late tracheostomy for critically ill patients: a clinical evidence synopsis of a recent Cochrane Review. Can. J. Resp. Ther. 52, 27–28.

Khanna, M., Rawat, N., Gupta, A., et al., 2017. Pulmonary involvement in patients with Guillain-Barré syndrome in subacute phase. J. Neurosci. Rural. Pract. 8, 412–416.

Laveneziana, P., Albuquerque, A., Aliverti, A., et al., 2019. ERS statement on respiratory muscle testing at rest and during exercise. Eur. Respir. J. 5, 1801214.

Lawn, N.D., Fletcher, D.D., Henderson, R.D., Wolter, T.D., Wijdicks, E.F., 2001. Anticipating mechanical ventilation in Guillain-Barré syndrome. Arch. Neurol. 58, 893–898.

Lindsay, K., Bone, I., 2004. Neurology and Neurosurgery Illustrated, 3rd Ed. Churchill Livingstone, New York.

LoMauro, A., Romei, M., Gandossini, S., Pascuzzo, R., Vantini, S., D'Angelo, M.G., Aliverti, A., 2018. Evolution of respiratory function in Duchenne muscular dystrophy from childhood to adulthood. Eur. Respir. J. 51, 1701418.

Main, E., Denehy, L., 2016. Cardiorespiratory Physiotherapy. Elsevier, London.

Maltais, F., 2011. Glossopharyngeal breathing. Am. J. Resp. Crit. Care. Med. 184, 381.

Mangera, Z., Panesar, G., Makker, H., 2012. Practical approach to management of respiratory complications in neurological disorders. Int. J. Gen. Med. 5, 255–263.

Marik, P.E., Varon, J., Trask, T., 2002. Management of head trauma. Chest. 122, 699–711.

McClenaghan, F., McGowan, S., Platt, L., Hunt, K., Fishman, J., 2021. Multidisciplinary team management of tracheostomy procedures in neurocritical care patients: our experience over 17 years in a quaternary centre. J. Laryngol. Otol. 1–21.

McCool, D., Hilbert, J., Wolfe, L.F., Benditt, J.O., 2021. The respiratory system and neuromuscular diseases. In: Broaddus, C., Ernst, J., King, T., Lazarus, S., Sarmiento, K., Schnapp, L., Stapleton, R. (Eds.), Murray & Nadel's Textbook of Respiratory Medicine, 7th Ed. Elsevier Health Science, pp. 1812–1828.

McDonald, T., Stiller, K., 2019. Inspiratory muscle training is feasible and safe for patients with acute spinal cord injury. J. Spinal. Cord. Med. 42220–227.

McGowan, S., Potter, L., Carmichael, A., Ritchie, J., Khan, J., 2021. A decision making tool and protocol for early cuff deflation and one way valve inline for patients who are ventilated with a tracheostomy – a case series report. ICS State of the Art Virtual Conference, December 2021. J. Intensive. Care. Soc. 23 (Suppl 1), 1–210.

McKim, D.A., Katz, S.L., Barrowman, N., Ni, A., LeBlanc, C., 2012. Lung volume recruitment slows pulmonary function decline in Duchenne muscular dystrophy. Arch. Phys. Med. Rehabil. 93, 1117–1122.

McIlwaine, M., Bradley, J., Elborn, J.S., Moran, F., 2017. Personalising airway clearance in chronic lung disease. Eur. Respir. Rev. 26, 160086.

Mezidi, M., Guérin, C., 2018. Effects of patient positioning on respiratory mechanics in mechanically ventilated ICU patients. Ann. Transl. Med. 6, 384.

Morgan, R.K., McNally, S., Alexander, M., Conroy, R., Hardiman, O., Costello, R.W., 2005. Use of Sniff nasal-inspiratory force to predict survival in amyotrophic lateral sclerosis. Am. J. Resp. Crit. Care. Med. 171, 269–274.

Moses, R., Morris, K., Ronson, L., 2018. The use of mechanical insufflation exsufflation for adults invasively ventilated a guide to aid practical application. Available at: https://twitter.com/nhsleader/status/995745313423069185?lang=en-GB. Accessed on 24 Feb 2022.

Narayan, S., Pietrusz, A., Allen, J., et al., 2022. Adult North Star Network (ANSN): consensus document for therapists working with adults with Duchenne muscular dystrophy (DMD) – therapy guidelines. J. Neuromusc. Dis. 9, 365–381.

Nason, L.K., Walker, C.M., McNeeley, M.F., Burivong, W., Fligner, C.L., Godwin, J.D., 2012. Imaging of the diaphragm: anatomy and function. Radiographics. 32, E51–E70.

National Confidential Enquiry into Patient Outcome and Death, 2014. On The Right Trach? Available at: http://www.ncepod.org.uk/2014report1/downloads/OnTheRightTrach_FullReport.pdf. Accessed on 7 Dec 2021.

National Institute for Health and Care Excellence, 2016. Motor neurone disease: assessment and management. NICE guideline [NG42]. Available at: https://www.nice.org.uk/guidance/ng42. Accessed on 1 Feb 2022.

Newman, A., Gravesande, J., Rotella, S., et al., 2018. Physiotherapy in the neurotrauma intensive care unit: a scoping review. J. Crit. Care. 48, 390–406.

Nydahl, P., Sricharoenchai, T., Chandra, S., Kundt, F.S., Huang, M., Fischill, M., Needham, D., 2017. Safety of patient mobilization and rehabilitation in the intensive care unit. Ann. Am. Thorac. Soc. 14, 766–777.

O'Driscoll, B.R., Howard, L.S., Earis, J., Mak, V., 2017. BTS Guideline for oxygen therapy use in adults in healthcare and emergency settings British Thoracic Society Emergency Oxygen Guideline Group, BTS Emergency Oxygen Guideline Development Group. Thorax. 72 (Suppl. 1), i1–i90.

Prasad S., Pal K., Chen R., 2021. Breathing and the nervous system. In: Aminoff, M., Josephson, A. (Eds). Aminoff's Neurology and General Medicine, 6th Ed., pp. 3–19.

Preiser, J.C., van Zanten, A.R., Berger, M.M., et al., 2015. Metabolic and nutritional support of critically ill patients: consensus and controversies. Crit. Care. 191–11.

Pryor, J.A., Prasad, A.S., 2008. Physiotherapy for Respiratory and Cardiac Problems: Adults and Paediatrics, 4th Ed. (Physiotherapy Essentials) Elsevier Health Sciences.

Rabinstein, A.A., 2005. Update on respiratory management of critically ill neurologic patients. Curr. Neurol. Neurosci. Rep. 5, 476–482.

Racca, F., Vianello, A., Mongini, T., Ruggeri, P., Versaci, A., Vita, G.L., Vita, G., 2020. Practical approach to respiratory emergencies in neurological diseases. Neurol. Sci. 41, 497–508.

Respiratory Information for Spinal Cord Injury (RISCI), 2023. Weaning guidelines for adult spinal cord injured patients in critical care units. Available at: http://risci.org.uk/resources/. Accessed on 19 June 2023.

Roth, C., Stitz, H., Kalhout, A., Kleffmann, J., Deinsberger, W., Ferbert, A., 2012. Effect of early physiotherapy on intracranial pressure and cerebral perfusion pressure. Neurocrit. Care. 18, 33–38.

Ryder, S., Leadley, R.M., Armstrong, N., Westwood, M., de Kock, S., Butt, T., Jain, M., Kleijnen, J., 2017. The burden, epidemiology, costs and treatment for Duchenne muscular dystrophy: an evidence review. Orphanet. J. Rare. Dis. 12, 79.

Shannon, H., Stiger, R., Gregson, R.K., Stocks, J., Main, E., 2010. Effect of chest wall vibration timing on peak expiratory flow and inspiratory pressure in a mechanically ventilated lung model. Physiotherapy. 96, 344–349.

Sheers, N., Howard, M.E., Berlowitz, D.J., 2019. Respiratory adjuncts to NIV in neuromuscular disease. Respirology. 24, 512–520.

Simonds, A.K., 2017. Progress in respiratory management of bulbar complications of motor neuron disease/amyotrophic lateral sclerosis. Thorax. 72, 199–201.

Singh, T.D., Wijdicks, E.F., 2021. Neuromuscular respiratory failure. Neurol. Clin. 39, 333–353.

Stehling, F., Bouikidis, A., Schara, U., Mellies, U., 2015. Mechanical insufflation/exsufflation improves vital capacity in neuromuscular disorders. Chron. Resp. Dis. 12, 31–35.

Stiller, K., 2013. Physiotherapy in intensive care: an updated systematic review. Chest. 144, 825–847.

Stiller, K., Phillips, A., 2003. Safety aspects of mobilising acutely ill inpatients. Physiother. Theory. Pract. 19, 239–257.

Stocchetti, N., Carbonara, M., Citerio, G., et al., 2017. Severe traumatic brain injury: targeted management in the intensive care unit. Lancet. Neurol. 16, 452–464.

Swingwood, E., Stilma, W., Tume, L., et al., 2020. The use of mechanical insufflation-exsufflation in invasively ventilated critically ill adults: a scoping review protocol. Syst. Rev. 9, 1–5.

Terson de Paleville, D.G., McKay, W.B., Folz, R.J., Ovechkin, A.V., 2011. Respiratory motor control disrupted by spinal cord injury: mechanisms, evaluation, and restoration. Transl. Stroke. Res. 2, 463–473.

Toussaint, M., Chatwin, M., Gonzales, J. et al, 2018. 228th ENMC International Workshop: airway clearance techniques in neuromuscular disorders Naarden, The Netherlands, 3–5 March, 2017. Neuromusc. Dis. 28, 289–298.

Trucco, F., Domingos, J.P., Tay, C.G., et al., 2020. Cardiorespiratory progression over 5 years and role of corticosteroids in Duchenne muscular dystrophy: a single-site retrospective longitudinal study. Chest. 158, 1606–1616.

West, J., 2001. Pulmonary Physiology and Pathophysiology. An Integrated, Case-Based Approach. Lippincott Williams & Wilkins, Philadelphia.

Young, B., Moyer, M., Pino, W., Kung, D., Zager, E., Kumar, M.A., 2019. Safety and feasibility of early mobilization in patients with subarachnoid hemorrhage and external ventricular drain. Neurocrit. Care. 31, 88–96.

Self-Management

Fiona Jones and Fiona Leggat

OUTLINE

Introduction, 495
Self-Management: What is it and Why Now? 496
  Defining Self-Management, 497
  Self-Management Is Not New, 499
Self-Management Programmes: Theory and
Research, 499
  Understanding Responses to Neurological
    Disability, 499
    Social Cognitive Theory and Self-Efficacy – A Critical
      Factor in Self-Management, 500
    Stress Coping Model, 501
    Transtheoretical Model of Behaviour Change and
      Motivational Interviewing, 502
  Components of Self-Management Programmes, 502

Self-Management Programmes: the Evidence Base
  for Neurological Conditions, 503
  Adapting the Self-Management Approach to
    Neurological Conditions, 503
  Issues in Self-Management Research, 505
  Self-Management and Stroke, 505
  Measurement of Self-Management, 506
Supporting Self-Management: Providing Information
  Alone Is Not Enough, 507
  Lessons Learnt From Long Covid: How Can Self-
    Management Be Supported?, 508
Conclusion, 510

INTRODUCTION

Self-management as a term can be contentious. For some people it conveys a sense of being left to get on with it. For most individuals living with a neurological condition, good self-management is getting on with everyday life and doing the things that are meaningful and important. Self-management is also not purely about complying with advice or following instructions. Rather, it is having the freedom, confidence and knowledge to manage in a way that works for each individual. To focus purely on disease self-management, such as managing medication, is now recognised to be a narrow approach (Morgan et al 2017). Although a neurological condition is only one part of an individual's life, gaining confidence to cope with a symptom such as spasticity can have a profound impact on many social, functional and emotional issues. In addition, everyone can and will react differently to a sudden event such as stroke or an exacerbation of multiple sclerosis (MS), and patterns of adjustment and coping are often uncertain. Self-management as a term is therefore complex, and individuals require a continuum of support rather than a 'one size fits all' approach.

One way to understand self-management is to recognise that many individuals are already very resourceful in the face of different challenges associated with their neurological condition. Consider, for example, the person with stroke who works out a way to open a yoghurt pot with one hand or plans a trip across town in a wheelchair. Nevertheless, there will be times, often in the early weeks and months, that an individual and their family will require guidance and support from a health professional. Yet the way in which the support is given could have a profound effect on how successful a person is at being able to self-manage. We know from research that the way a therapist starts off a session or introduces the aim of the treatment can affect how an individual perceives their role and responsibility (Jones et al 2017). As rehabilitation professionals, we have a unique opportunity to enable individuals to control their symptoms and develop a range of skills and strategies to live in an optimum way with their condition. But paradoxically, we also have the potential to disempower and inhibit individuals from developing self-management skills, and to become more reliant on our help and expertise. To facilitate a departure from reliance on the 'expert therapy clinician' towards a more collaborative approach which will sustain successful self-management is now becoming central to many areas of health policy and national guidelines (Intercollegiate Stroke Working Party 2016, NHS England 2019).

The evidence relating to successful self-management support consistently demonstrates the value of an individualised, tailored and interactive approach (de Silva 2011, National Voices 2014). The health professional and individual share their ideas and decide on actions together. What constitutes a good outcome is also defined and agreed collaboratively (Légaré & Thompson-Luduc 2014). Actions by therapists, such as providing information in one format with no opportunity to ask questions or providing a home exercise programme just before discharge, show no evidence of effectiveness. Consequently, tailoring self-management support requires an appreciation of factors that act as barriers to or enablers of behaviour change and action. We can learn what works best and for whom from a growing body of research evidence (Kidd et al 2017). But we can also learn from the experiences of those individuals and their families whom we see every day in practice. This experiential learning can be especially vital when learning more about what works for people experiencing new and emerging neurological conditions. For instance, for people living with post-Covid-19 syndrome, often known as long Covid, lived experience may provide rich insight into how people are self-managing while the academic and clinical field plays catch up (Ladds et al 2020).

This chapter will explore self-management and provide an overview of the key areas of research and discourses relevant to neurorehabilitation. The chapter is organised in four sections. First, we describe definitions and conceptualisations of self-management and its place in healthcare policy and research today. Second, we consider how self-management can be understood based on individual responses to neurological disability and related psychological theory. Third, we provide an overview of the evidence base for self-management programmes for people with neurological conditions. Lastly, we discuss some of the skills healthcare professionals require to provide effective self-management support for people with neurological conditions. A focus on the new and emerging neurological condition, long Covid, is given here.

SELF-MANAGEMENT: WHAT IS IT AND WHY NOW?

To understand self-management and how the term has evolved, it may be helpful to consider its reference in healthcare policy and research. Self-management discourses are often situated in the context of changing demographics, increasing pressures on resources and implications associated with an ageing population (Ellis et al 2017, Fletcher et al 2019). As life expectancy increases globally, more people are likely to be living with the consequences and challenges of a long-term condition; as such, demand on healthcare and other public systems is likely to grow (Bloom et al 2015). Estimates attribute 23% of the global burden of disease (disability-adjusted life-years) to disorders in people aged 60 years and older, 49% of the burden in high-income regions and 20% in low- and middle-income regions (Prince et al 2015). The leading contributing disease clusters are cardiovascular conditions (including stroke), cancer, chronic respiratory disease, musculoskeletal conditions and, ranked fifth, mental and neurological conditions (Prince et al 2015). The increasing impact of noncommunicable disease and degenerative long-term conditions such as Parkinson's or dementia on our ageing societies requires some significant changes in health policy and economics (Bloom et al 2015).

Sceptics have suggested that the economic pressures associated with large numbers of people living longer and requiring healthcare have driven the advancement and popularity of self-management programmes (Fletcher et al 2019, Kendall & Rogers 2007). As mentioned earlier, at face value the term 'self-management' lends itself to the interpretation that it is about getting patients to 'manage by themselves'. It is evident how these understandings can play to a political rhetoric of reducing public health service spending through an emphasis on individuals' personal responsibility for their health. This neoliberal appropriation and moralisation of the self-management approach has been criticised not only in the academic arena (Ellis et al 2017, Kendall et al 2011, Kendall & Rogers 2007, Morgan et al 2017, Rogers et al 2009) but also by people who live with long-term conditions and who are sensitive to and experience the implications of these political developments in their daily lives (Kulnik et al 2017).

The complexity and tensions related to the term self-management have been highlighted by several groups, how it can convey to individuals they have a moral responsibility to actively manage their condition and lifestyle (Ellis et al 2017, Fletcher et al 2019). However, a self-management support model works alongside individuals to support their skills, such as problem solving and resource utilisation, and fosters collective and social action (Kendall et al 2011, Kendall & Rogers 2007, Lorig & Holman 2003, Vassilev et al 2019). Since the emergence of self-management as a concept, we now recognise that it is broader and more nuanced, underpinned by values of collective responsibility, empowerment, person-centeredness, mutuality and citizenship, and realised through collaboration between users of health services and health service providers (Jones et al 2016a).

Research exploring self-management support for individuals with neurological conditions is now catching up with a large body of work in other chronic diseases such as arthritis and diabetes. But what self-management means to someone living with a life-limiting condition, such as motor neurone disease, could be different to someone managing life after a spinal cord injury. Context is crucial, not only in relation to the type of condition but also with respect to other social determinants such as family networks, economic status, health literacy, religion, culture and ethnicity (Bate et al 2014, Moore et al 2015). We could learn from social scientists who describe context as a fluid and changeable process, depending on both inner influences (health condition, personal agency) and outer influences (services, therapeutic care and family support). This should help us understand why someone appears not to engage in self-management, or when it seems as if their family are doing too much. In this chapter we want to emphasise that as healthcare professionals we must reflect on our own practice and find ways to support self-management, rather than the responsibility of the individual living with a neurological condition.

Defining Self-Management

Many current and older definitions of self-management reflect both the medical and social aspects of living with and managing a chronic condition. A seminal definition given by Barlow et al. (2002, p. 178) referred to self-management as:

...an individual's ability to manage the symptoms, treatment, physical and psychosocial consequences and lifestyle changes inherent in living with a chronic condition. Efficacious self-management encompasses ability to monitor one's condition and to affect the cognitive, behavioural and emotional responses necessary to maintain a satisfactory quality of life, thus, a dynamic and continuous process of self-regulation is established.

Self-management can also be used interchangeably with the term 'self-management education', as defined in a recent report by NHS England (2016, p. 15):

...any form of formal education or training for people with long-term conditions that focuses on helping people to develop the knowledge, skills and confidence to manage their own health and care effectively.

What these definitions suggest is that self-management means greater responsibility on the part of the individual, and that skills and knowledge can to a degree be taught. Thus self-management is seen as a move towards encouraging and supporting patients to play a more active role in their own health, and this aligns with other healthcare policy in the United Kingdom and globally, which emphasises people-centred care and engagement:

Given the right guidance and support, empowered people can address damaging health behaviours and/ or challenges in their environment that prevent healthy lifestyles. Supporting self-management will be critical for many countries where ageing populations and the growing burden of noncommunicable disease means that there is ever greater demand for health services. (World Health Organization 2015, p. 22)

But to achieve engagement in self-management practices, it could be argued that there needs to be greater concordance with the way healthcare professionals are working with individuals. As we have already mentioned, the transition towards successful self-management will happen at different time points for each person. This means an important role for therapists is being able to gauge an individual's readiness to take on more responsibility. This may be difficult when the amount of treatment and timing is predetermined. More involvement, self-responsibility and shared decision making may be key components of self-management, but in some cases organisations and services are unable to adapt and tailor their support to what is needed.

If we take the example of how stroke rehabilitation services often end abruptly after an intensive first few weeks or months, a continued body of evidence reveals how individuals can experience isolation and lack of psychological, emotional and social support, leading to a sense of abandonment and limited social participation (Pearce et al 2015, Woodman et al 2014). This could also suggest that rehabilitation services fail to adequately prepare individuals and their families for the transition from poststroke rehabilitation to community living. Early introduction of self-management support within an integrated, pathway-wide focus on self-management could bridge this gap by fostering individuals' self-management skills and creating supportive communities of practice (Jones et al 2013, Mäkelä et al 2014).

Experts on self-management may not fully agree on all its components, but most agree on what it is not. What can be misleading about using the term 'self-management education' is the focus on providing information, which when used alone has very little impact on behaviour change. Also, an individual's involvement in self-management is likely to fluctuate over time and will depend on several factors, for example, the stage of life when a person receives their diagnosis and acknowledgement that the neurological condition is only one part of the person's life. This will doubtless influence how much time, priority and importance a person gives to self-management – indeed what they can or want to do. People's responses to self-management are therefore unique (Corben & Rosen 2005).

Self-management has also been defined according to a specified outcome, for example, practicing specific health behaviours such as diet control. In some long-term conditions, specific technical skills may play an important part of self-management, such as inhaler management for people with respiratory disease or blood glucose monitoring in people with diabetes (Newman et al 2004). These aspects may be appropriate for more didactic self-management education interventions, which are relatively straightforward to design. But the specific health behaviours needed to self-manage a neurological condition are more difficult to specify and generalise. Over the past decade, there has been an encouraging growth in research that seeks to adapt the concept of self-management to neurological patient groups, which is testament to the promise this approach holds in the future.

Kate Lorig, pioneer and founder of the generic group-based Chronic Disease Self-management Programme (CDSP), described self-management as distinct from medical care and involving 'learning and practicing skills necessary to carry an active and emotionally satisfying life in the face of a chronic condition' (Lorig 1993). What this definition adds is the aspect of learning, with the unique difference between self-management programmes and educational programmes being the need to facilitate behaviour change through different means.

Clearly, much of health policy on self-management shows an emphasis on partnership and empowerment, and this approach has been cited as one of the key components of an integrated and person-centred health service (World Health Organization 2015). But it has been argued that if self-management programmes are provided in clinical settings by health professionals, then the balance of power still lies with the professional and not the individual (Wilson et al 2007). It has also been suggested that implicit in many self-management programmes is an assumption that the best regimes are those suggested by a clinician, and that the best outcome is achieved through optimum compliance (Kendall & Rogers 2007).

Do therapists and patients see a good outcome in the same way, and does it always involve the individual adhering to advice and following treatment plans? Early research by Maclean and colleagues (2002) found that stroke patients perceived by health professionals to be highly motivated were more compliant with the aims and expectations of rehabilitation and more likely to understand and follow the advice of professionals. However, some patients perceived to have low motivation described the mixed messages given by therapists in discouraging their individual efforts. This highlighted concerns about which patient is doing 'better' and is more likely to learn the skills of self-management, the patient not complying with treatment and trying activities independently, or the patient following advice and complying with rehabilitation (Maclean et al 2002). In a later systematic review, Boger and colleagues (2015) explored what outcomes of self-management programmes were considered important by different stakeholders. They found that views of patients, families, professionals and other stakeholders about what constitutes a good outcome have not been elicited, and programmes often measure success according to clinical measures and rarely consider the impact on psychosocial outcomes.

If an individual feels obliged to take part in and comply with a specified treatment strategy, is this compliance a successful outcome? This could create a contradiction with the new group of self-managers, described as reflexive autonomous individuals and not passively accepting medical advice (Wilson et al 2007). Against the rather negative predictions of growing numbers of people living with chronic disease and likely to need medical care, the self-care and self-help traditions described by sociologists demonstrate that many adults are comfortable taking responsibility for their long-term conditions (Kendall et al 2011). It is worth remembering that many individuals self-manage without the support of a clinician or self-management training, as in the example of Lee:

Lee, a 77-year-old stroke survivor, lived at home with his wife and no longer received regular physiotherapy. He described his paretic leg as being unpredictable and no longer under his control, but he dealt with this by 'learning not to panic and rely so much on my powerful stronger leg'. He achieved this by setting small tasks where the likelihood of success was high 'giving my leg a chance to succeed' (Jones 2004). Self-management strategies in Lee's case involved decision making, setting targets and reflecting on progress. He explained, 'Doing more walking at home is my goal, you must have a goal, and have measures which you can check against which are fairly objective, and I do roughly do that, how many yards I have walked each day, I use notebooks and diaries to record how I am doing'.

The key to incorporating shared decision making into rehabilitation involves creating space and opportunity to participate in decision making and problem solving, and not asking the individual to comply with an exercise or treatment. Caroline Ellis-Hill has highlighted the importance of the shared discourse between the therapist and patient, to facilitate self-discovery and problem solving on behalf of the patient. In this way, the therapist is acting more as a guide or coach, rather than an expert. From this insight, Ellis-Hill developed the Life Thread Model, based on narrative theory and focusing on interpersonal relationships (Ellis-Hill et al 2008). In using this model, the balance of power between professionals and patients is recognised. It includes endorsing a positive view of self, 'being' with somebody, as well as 'doing' things for them, and seeing acquired disability as a time of transition rather than simply of loss. As with much of the literature concerning self-management, this emphasises the need for healthcare professionals to avoid giving answers too readily, and the need to really pay attention to individuals' stories, preferences and ideas.

Self-Management Is Not New

If we consider self-management as being about the individual, their story and their ideas, we can easily see that much of self-management is not necessarily new. Individuals with chronic conditions have always found ways of coping, showing resourcefulness both at an individual and community level. In some way the concept of self-management represents the realisation that people, not healthcare services, are at the centre of managing their long-term condition. As Lorig and Holman (2003) put it: 'One cannot not manage'. Sociologists such as Mike Bury and others have highlighted that models of coping with a chronic condition, based on resilience and self-responsibility, have existed for many decades. They also argue that healthcare professionals would make a case that they have long promoted self-management (Bury et al 2005). There are a great many examples of how people with a neurological condition self-manage, not only at a personal level but also at a more collective, societal level. Peer support is one way. Support from peers can facilitate exchanges of ideas, experiences and advice (Sadler et al 2017), and impacts of peer support can include learning, enhanced motivation and emotional comfort (Clark et al 2020). Peer support can consist of groups held in local communities such as a stroke club, and there is a growth of online support groups, particularly when the neurological condition is less common and individuals are not easily able to meet. Facilitated through the continuous development and spread of online and interactive technology, there are now many good examples of this, such as the UK-based online platform HealthUnlocked (available at https://healthunlocked.com). Peer support can be particularly relevant when considering the Covid-19

pandemic and the rise in social isolation which has led to new, differing challenges for people, including a rise in poststroke anxiety and stroke prevalence (Ahmed et al 2020, Gronewold & Hermann 2021).

As a therapy profession providing a service for patients with many different neurological conditions, maybe we should question whether our starting point always needs to be health. After stroke, self-management behaviours are often promoted to prevent a second event and reduce risk factors through strategies such as increasing activity. But exercise and access to community groups can be challenging for stroke survivors even if they wish to adopt a healthier lifestyle (Rimmer et al 2008). In this way, social isolation from an inaccessible environment may be more of a barrier to successful self-management. The role of community in both formal and informal self-help activities, such as stroke clubs, is a vital aspect of a more collective approach to self-management (Ch'ng et al 2008, Vassilev et al 2014).

Facilitating peer support amongst individuals sharing similar neurological conditions can be a relatively easy way to encourage an exchange of ideas, knowledge and plans, all components of active self-management. Clark and colleagues found that to develop such peer support groups, we also need to involve those they seek to help in the planning and content (Clark et al 2018). Exploring the concept of peer support amongst stroke survivors, participants said the space to share was important; they wanted to fit in with the group, involve family and friends if possible and the logistics of travel and facilitation needed to be considered. Importantly they wanted the opportunity to personalise and tailor the content to their own needs. Critical to this is the idea of having a shared experience in a group setting whilst not losing sight of the fact that everyone is an individual. Notwithstanding the potential benefit of groups, we also know they are not right for everyone and the term 'self-management group' may be off-putting for some (Satink et al 2015). We also need to consider how inclusive groups are to people who have cognitive and communication problems and consider individual responses to self-management to know how to tailor support (Wray et al 2018).

SELF-MANAGEMENT PROGRAMMES: THEORY AND RESEARCH

Understanding Responses to Neurological Disability

Traditionally therapists have always supported individuals to learn and to gain confidence in dealing with their neurological condition. However, the expectation that individuals will follow the advice offered does not fully consider motivation, fears, beliefs and other difficulties, which might influence how this advice will be incorporated into individuals' daily lives.

Why is it important to gain more understanding of motivation, fears and beliefs? Before examining some of the psychological theories underpinning self-management programmes, it is worth reviewing some qualitative research related to these concepts. Taking the experience of stroke as the main example, for which there is now an extensive body of qualitative evidence (Pearce et al 2015), it becomes clear how confidence and beliefs about self-management will be based on a diverse range of events occurring in the poststroke period. These may be personal experiences as a result of a change in independence and life circumstances, but equally could be shaped by external factors such as the environment and structure of rehabilitation, and the nature of interactions with professionals and family.

Fear and uncertainty perceived by individuals are also well documented in studies exploring the early poststroke period (Pearce et al 2015). Anxiety about bringing on a second stroke or feeling out of control may act as a barrier to setting goals and taking action. The sudden loss of independence and changes in identity associated with acute stroke also heighten individual concerns about potential losses and the restriction of future roles. This early period of instability and uncertainty poststroke may have a profound influence on forming judgements and beliefs about the future. In addition, the high levels of depression and anxiety experienced by stroke survivors may be compounded by these feelings of dependency and loss of control. Some of the practices in early stroke care could reinforce feelings of helplessness and dependency, which are not conducive to developing self-management skills (Pearce et al 2015, Woodman et al 2014).

Stroke is usually a sudden-onset event, but with neurological conditions such as MS, the onset is more gradual but potentially less predictable. For many, diagnosis is a protracted experience with the challenge of making sense of the long-term implications of living with a changeable chronic condition. The need to get a named diagnosis, lack of psychosocial support and concerns about the consequences on lifestyle often dominate early stages, along with stress and fear about the unpredictability and coping with major challenges. Nevertheless, with time, individuals can develop more proactive attitudes and strategies, gaining more knowledge about their own disease progression and accessing formal and informal support networks (Kirkpatrick Pinson et al 2009, Malcomson et al 2008).

What these qualitative studies tell us is that individuals living with a neurological condition will experience numerous beliefs, emotional responses and barriers that could influence successful rehabilitation and self-management.

FACTORS INFLUENCING REHABILITATION AND SELF-MANAGEMENT AFTER STROKE (JONES ET AL 2008A, PEARCE ET AL 2015, WOODMAN ET AL 2014)

- Fear and uncertainty about a second event or dependency on others
- Worry about unpredictability of disease
- Recovery is personal and perceived within a personal narrative
- Concerns for the future challenges
- Feelings of discontinuity with previous life
- Personal benchmarks which may not match therapy goals
- Importance of hope and the possibility of further improvement

Social Cognitive Theory and Self-Efficacy – A Critical Factor in Self-Management

What then is the best way of helping an individual to learn more about their own beliefs and responses to rehabilitation? Psychological theories can provide a framework for understanding human behaviour, and many self-management interventions are developed based on different theories. The most commonly cited in the development of self-management programmes is social-cognitive theory (SCT), in which an individual's belief in their own capability to produce a change in a specific behaviour (self-efficacy) is said to be critical to the success (Bandura 1989, 1997). Self-efficacy is a construct introduced by Albert Bandura and defined as 'people's beliefs about their capabilities to produce designated levels of performance that exercise influence over events that affect their lives' (Bandura 1994). Self-efficacy beliefs can determine how people feel, think, motivate themselves and behave with regards to their health. For example, self-efficacy influences motivation and health behaviours, by determining the goals people set, how much effort they invest in achieving those goals and their resilience when faced with difficulties or failure (Dixon et al 2007). Individuals with strong self-efficacy tend to select challenging goals and approach difficult tasks as challenges to overcome, rather than as threats to avoid. In the face of failure, such individuals may heighten and sustain their efforts, quickly recover their sense of efficacy and even attribute failure to insufficient effort or deficient knowledge and skills that can be acquired (Bandura 1994).

The difference between SCT and other theories is that Bandura provides a clear direction regarding how to influence self-efficacy, which can inform therapeutic interaction and self-management programmes. The construct of self-efficacy also appears to provide resonance with many aspects of sustaining progress and coping with setbacks whilst living with a neurological condition. The information and feedback that an individual obtains from the performance of a task are the sources of self-efficacy.

There are four main sources of self-efficacy (Bandura 1997):
1. Mastery experiences
2. Vicarious experiences
3. Verbal persuasion
4. Physiological feedback

Mastery experiences include positive experiences in a task or skill. As people's experiences of success may improve their self-efficacy, breaking the task into smaller achievable components may be useful to build up and accumulate confidence (van de Laar & van der Bijl 2001). For people with stroke, this could be gained after accomplishment of a small personal goal through independent effort (Jones et al 2008a). Mastery experiences are said to be the most reliable source of efficacy information (Schwarzer 1992) and have been targeted in neurological rehabilitation through a variety of methods (Johnston et al 2007, Kendall et al 2007, Watkins et al 2007).

Vicarious experience is gained through the comparison and modelling of others, as it can be beneficial to observe someone perceived to be similar successfully performing the task, for example, learning from another individual's experience of the recovery period poststroke. Seeing others' achievements, especially for individuals who are uncertain of their capabilities to perform certain tasks, may help the observers believe that they also possess capabilities to perform the same tasks (Bandura 1997).

Verbal persuasion serves to increase an individual's belief about their personal level of skill using persuasion and verification from a significant other, such as a health professional, family member or friend. However, verbal persuasion needs to be directed in such a way that it enables the individual to interpret the experience of performing the skills as a success (Bandura 1997).

Feedback is where the efficacy beliefs are formed from feedback produced by an individual's own psychological or physiological state. Self-efficacy may be increased by asking the individual doing a new task or trying something for the first time how it felt, and then encouraging reflection on how nervous they felt when first doing the task. In this way even the most subtle changes and progress are confirmed together and used as an opportunity for learning and reflection (Bandura 1997, Ewart 1992).

Neurological rehabilitation provides an ideal opportunity to address a combination of these four sources of self-efficacy and continually enhance an individual's self-management. Accordingly, some self-management

interventions developed specifically for people with neurological conditions are informed by SCT (Fryer et al 2016, Jones & Riazi 2011). If there are multiple components of a personal goal such as walking, individuals are likely to have several distinct, interrelated self-efficacy beliefs. Practice to ensure transference of beliefs regarding capability to different situations and settings therefore requires a dynamic cognitive process. Although some authors take the view that dedicated self-management support should focus on the period after discharge from inpatient rehabilitation to the community (Satink et al 2016), it may be important to provide patients with the widest possible window of opportunity to practice tasks and simultaneously receive sustained support to build self-efficacy. Earliest possible development of effective self-management skills leads to greater service efficiency and enhanced patient preparation for transition to community living, and there are examples of how self-management support can successfully be provided in acute hospital and inpatient settings (Jones et al 2016a, Mäkelä et al 2014). A recent trial of a 12-week stroke self-management programme confirmed the key role played by self-efficacy as a mediator that affected patient-perceived performance and satisfaction. The authors recommended that through stroke rehabilitation which focuses on shared goal setting and problem solving gains can be made in both patient competence and confidence (Nott et al 2021).

Stress Coping Model

Another theory used to inform self-management programmes is the stress coping model (Lazarus 1990), which can be used to explain the strategies people use to overcome the challenges and stresses of living with a chronic disease. Programmes based on this model usually incorporate the use of cognitive behavioural techniques to encourage individuals to develop more positive and active coping strategies. Passive and avoidant behaviours (such as evading activity or not taking medication) will usually have detrimental effects on health outcomes, so it will be important for therapists to recognise and explore unhelpful

---

STAGES OF CHANGE (PROCHASKA & VELICER 1997)

Precontemplation: no intention to take any action
Contemplation: intends to take action within the next few month
Preparation: intends to take action within the next few days
Action: change in behaviour which has been sustained for less than 6 months
Maintenance: change in behaviour which has been sustained for more than 6 months

beliefs and anxieties that might be impeding progress. An example can be taken from cardiac rehabilitation, where self-management programmes involve individuals learning to perceive feelings of breathlessness and raised heart rate as a positive and necessary step towards fitness, as opposed to a negative experience indicative of a possible medical complication (Ewart 1992).

Transtheoretical Model of Behaviour Change and Motivational Interviewing

The Transtheoretical Model of Behaviour Change (Prochaska & Velicer 1997) has been used in a large number of self-management programmes and makes an assumption that behaviour changes involve movement through a specified number of stages (Serlachius & Sutton 2009). The likelihood of change is also influenced by factors related to motivation and readiness to change.

Interventions should match the participant's stage of change. However, the model has been criticised in recent years because of problems defining the stages and following suggestions that the stages are not real time periods and are difficult to operationalise. Nonetheless, a technique known as motivational interviewing (MI) based on the Transtheoretical Model of Change has been used successfully in the acute stroke care setting (Watkins et al 2007). MI uses a counselling technique based on four principles.

The principles of MI are to:
1. Express empathy;
2. Develop a discrepancy between unhealthy behaviour and patients' goals;
3. Work with resistance by inviting new perspectives; and
4. Support self-efficacy.

MI requires therapeutic skills of reflective listening, asking open questions, affirming and summarising (Levensky et al 2007). By adopting these principles and skills, practitioners focus on encouraging patients to explore their reasons for behaviour change and help them to develop their own strategies to enable this change. The patient is empowered to make their own decisions, thereby maintaining self-efficacy and increasing their confidence in their abilities to make a change (Levensky et al 2007).

The move away from didactic expert-led treatments for people with neurological conditions to a more collaborative problem-solving approach is a positive step towards supporting self-management. But the theoretical basis of each approach requires careful consideration. SCT theory is the most used theory, but in practice it is likely that there is overlap between the different theories and self-management programmes.

Components of Self-Management Programmes

Theoretical influences guide the delivery and content of many self-management programmes. An understanding of theory also enables the variables and outcomes to be defined and tested using the relevant measures, as well as the specific content of programmes. Some key components of self-management are presented in Fig. 19.1.

Problem solving involves the individual deciding on the problem, breaking it down into smaller parts, thinking of various solutions, selecting a course of action, trying out the action or strategy and evaluating success, or choosing an alternative action if necessary.

Target or goal setting involves translating thoughts into actions, or the difference between what people say and what they do, and requires a selection of strategies, which if successful can provide mastery experiences.

Resource utilisation involves making use of what other resources may be available to sustain participation or enable further progress. It could include accessing local self-help groups, seeking expert advice if a problem emerges or using friends or family to support access to services or activities.

Collaboration involves working together with a healthcare professional to decide together on a course of action or preferred direction to rehabilitation. The therapist and the individual share their expertise. This can be a shift from traditional thinking whereby the therapist is perceived as the expert.

Knowledge is critical because living with a neurological condition involves a continuous process of learning from new experiences, particularly when the condition can fluctuate and change over time. Increased knowledge

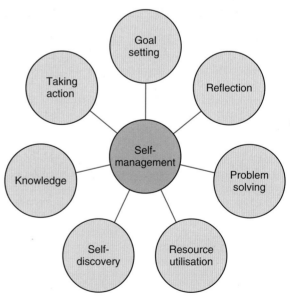

FIG. 19.1 Key strategies associated with successful self-management (based on Jones et al 2016a, 2016b).

about the condition, symptoms and treatment is an important aspect of self-management but should represent a more active process than just gaining knowledge. A key skill is being able to gather, process and evaluate the information.

It is worth restating that successful self-management involves 'doing' and 'taking action'. Whether it is mobilising support or finding a new way of doing something, the action is on the part of the individual. Put more simply, if we are to promote self-management as part of rehabilitation, we need to consider ways of individuals discovering their own strengths and difficulties, experimenting and trying out different strategies and activities. Inevitably this requires an element of risk taking.

The above provides some idea of the complexity and range of skills promoted and facilitated through self-management programmes. But if we remember that a self-management intervention does not mean simply imparting and providing information but is an active collaborative process, then we can start to understand how a behaviour change may be possible. However, there can be many different interpretations of each process and skill. Table 19.1 highlights two alternative approaches to goal setting, and it is clear that process B may take more time and skill. But if the key outcome is to enable confidence to self-manage, then the interaction is not straightforward and requires active listening skills and patience on the part of the therapist.

SELF-MANAGEMENT PROGRAMMES: THE EVIDENCE BASE FOR NEUROLOGICAL CONDITIONS

Avenues of delivery and design features of self-management programmes can vary, but there is now a growing body of evidence for and against different types of interventions in relation to conditions of sudden onset, such as stroke and traumatic brain injury. The development of programmes for the more progressive and unpredictable conditions such as MS has been slower to advance, but they are also now emerging (Busse et al 2021). In principle, self-management programmes can be (Table 19.2):

- Designed for a generic group or disease specific;
- Delivered by healthcare professionals or by trained lay leaders; and
- Group based or individualised.

Adapting the Self-Management Approach to Neurological Conditions

Self-management programmes are clearly distinct from simple patient education or skills training, in that they are designed to encourage and support people with chronic diseases in taking an active part in the management of their own condition. Kate Lorig and researchers at Stanford University are the main pioneers of self-management research and developed what is perhaps the most well-known programme, the CDSP. The programme is a 6-week,

TABLE 19.1 Alternative Approaches to Goal Setting	
Process A	**Process B**
1. Goals are discussed between therapist and patient based on what they enjoy doing and what is important to them.	1. The patient's story (narrative) is discussed. What do they enjoy doing, and what is important to them?
2. A suitable goal is decided upon and written in the therapy notes.	2. A list of long-term goals and hopes is written down (by the patient, if possible).
3. Patient works with therapist to achieve goal within a predetermined therapy time (no time is spent independently practicing activities outside of therapy).	3. Patient is encouraged to think of what they would like to work on first, what could be something a little smaller but still meaningful that they would like to do in the next few days.
4. Patient achieves goal with the help of the therapist.	4. A smaller target or goal is written down with a timeframe.
5. 'Goal achieved' recorded in the therapy notes.	5. Patient is asked how confident they feel about achieving the goal within the next few days, and if possible confidence is scored using a self-efficacy scale.
	6. The action needed by the therapist and the patient is agreed upon together after each therapy session; the patient is asked how they feel they are progressing towards their own goal and asked to rate their confidence.
	7. Patient records when they have achieved the target, and a record of successes is kept with the patient at all times.
	8. Families are invited to read the targets and progress made.

TABLE 19.2	Strengths and Limitations of Selected Self-Management Interventions	
Intervention	Strengths	Limitations
Group-based interventions	• More cost-effective • Value of group learning, social and peer support	• Better attendance from women and individuals with higher health literacy; poorer attendance from underprivileged groups • No scope for individuals learning and changing behaviour at different rates • Practical difficulties accessing group venues, in particular for individuals with mobility restrictions
One-to-one interventions	• Tailoring to individual needs • Some barriers to self-management cannot be shared in a group setting • Can be delivered in nonclinical setting and incorporated into rehabilitation	• More time needed, reduced opportunity for modelling and vicarious learning • Less cost-effective
Layperson leaders	• Can act as role models • Less costly • May not have to relearn an approach to chronic disease self-management • Could be in a good position to encourage others to join groups	• Information about training and skills required by lay leader not reported • Some difficulties recruiting suitable leaders and providing the infrastructure for support
Professional leaders	• More able to address factual issues relating to condition and treatment • Easier to integrate into rehabilitation	• Healthcare professionals traditionally deliver more didactic approaches, e.g., medical advice • Training needs often not recognised
Disease specific	• Allows more focus on specific skills required for different conditions	• Emphasis on disease-specific skills first rather than general skills, could reduce learning and management of subsequent health challenges
Generic	• More cost-effective and encourages practice of more generic problem-solving skills • Effective for individuals with multiple comorbidities	• Difficulties of facilitating a group with wide-ranging conditions, symptoms and disease trajectories • No disease-specific advice

layperson-led self-management skills training course for people with generic long-term physical conditions. Early evaluations suggested improved outcomes and some cost reductions for chronic care following the programme. Main outcomes included increase in exercise, improved coping strategies and symptom management, reduced fatigue, fewer hospital visits and fewer medical consultations at 6-month follow-up, as well as at 1- and 2-year follow-up (Lorig et al 2001). Lorig and others have argued that the most empowering aspect of CDSP-based courses is that they are not facilitated by a health professional but by a lay volunteer who has a long-term condition themselves (Kennedy et al 2005); however, the evidence for this is limited. In the UK, the CDSP was initially adopted as the Expert Patient Programme, but attempts to integrate it into the National Health Service had limited success (Bury & Pink 2005), possibly because of the lack of engagement by healthcare professionals, particularly general practitioners (Kennedy et al 2005). Furthermore, trials have not provided convincing evidence of the generalisability of the program, given that men and ethnic groups are greatly underrepresented in most studies (Jordan & Osborne 2007). One reason for this could be that active self-management is such a complex set of skills that generic approaches are unlikely to reach the depth required to develop these skills, particularly in individuals with more complex conditions such as stroke (Davidson 2005).

Arguably, many key components of programmes such as the CDSP could be adapted for people with neurological conditions, and there has been some success with disease-specific self-management initiatives. A self-management programme developed to encourage exercise behaviours for people with mild to moderate MS showed significant improvements in walking speed and quality of life in the study group (Hartley 2009). Despite the lack of a control group, the authors suggest this model provides evidence of the potential benefits of introducing an earlier self-management intervention for encouraging exercise for people with MS. Qualitative evidence from people with stroke, MS and spinal cord injury who took part in the CDSP demonstrated the positive impact of the programme, but also highlighted how self-management training needs may differ between the three groups, with respect to timing, content and delivery of sessions (Hirsche et al 2011). Owing to the Covid-19 pandemic, self-management support interventions are now being adapted for virtual delivery (Lowe et al 2021). Such delivery may help to reach people with neurological conditions who face physical barriers to participation in self-management programmes.

Issues in Self-Management Research

The main methodological issues associated with self-management research are:

- Underlying theory poorly developed or not made explicit;
- Complex intervention not comprehensively described, and therefore difficult to replicate;
- Importance of context not acknowledged or given insufficient consideration;
- Intervention is not self-management training but has a more educational focus;
- High levels of attrition, particularly from group-based programmes;
- Some seminal research is questionable; it lacked a control group and samples were self-selecting;
- Some groups such as those with lower educational level and men tend not to access self-management programmes; and
- Many of the results report short-term benefits, but few studies report long-term outcomes.

Despite these issues, there are several positive outcomes from well-designed programmes, particularly those with a clear theoretical framework and well-described components.

Self-Management and Stroke

Although stroke is underrepresented in self-management research compared with chronic diseases such as asthma and diabetes, it nevertheless leads the way in bringing the self-management approach to the neurological field. This may also be related to a shift in our understanding of stroke more as a long-term condition than an acute event. Traditionally, the medical and research communities have viewed acquired brain injuries such as stroke and traumatic brain injury as acute events, and much of the focus has been on acute medical management and early rehabilitation. But individuals affected by stroke often experience long-term consequences and express concerns about the lack of social and community support once the early period of rehabilitation is completed (Pearce et al 2015, Woodman et al 2014). Compared with cardiac events, there is also a noticeable difference in the management after stroke, with a much more coordinated programme of self-management education and staged rehabilitation available for cardiac patients. This is puzzling considering that the causes of stroke mirror those of chronic heart disease and that the controllable risk factors such as diet, activity and smoking are identical. Increasingly, there is greater understanding of the ongoing impact of stroke and also acknowledgement of the lasting potential for functional improvement in the longer term. A view of stroke more as a chronic condition allows an appreciation of how self-management interventions can lead to long-term benefits for individuals poststroke.

The growing evidence base in stroke self-management research is reflected in the number of systematic reviews that have been published in recent years (Fryer et al 2016, Jones et al 2015, Jones & Riazi 2011, Lennon et al 2013, Parke et al 2015, Warner et al 2015) and in high-profile opinion pieces and clinical guidelines that endorse the introduction of a self-management approach to neurological rehabilitation (Dobkin 2016, Intercollegiate Stoke Working Party 2016). The most recent systematic review and meta-analysis by Fryer and colleagues (2016), for example, used robust Cochrane methodology and included 14 randomised controlled trials with 1863 participants in total. Combined data from six studies provided moderate-quality evidence that stroke self-management programmes compared with usual care improved quality of life, and provided low-quality evidence of improvements in self-efficacy. Individual studies reported benefits for health-related behaviours such as reduced use of health services, smoking and alcohol intake, as well as improved diet and attitude (Fryer et al 2016). Although these findings are positive and encouraging, it must also be considered that evidence syntheses through systematic review and meta-analysis provide a level of abstraction at which individual study details often remain hidden. Study heterogeneity, and specifically variation in the types and delivery of self-management programmes, is an acknowledged limitation of pooling evidence. Furthermore, most self-management interventions can be considered complex interventions (Craig et al 2008), developed within a specific context and tailored for a particular group. The review by Fryer et al (2016), for example, included self-management interventions as diverse as:

- Delivery of individual self-management support integrated within the usual practice of stroke rehabilitation therapist, supported through use of a stroke-specific workbook (Jones et al 2016b);

- Provision of written resources and telephone support from trained professionals for people with stroke and their family members (Bishop et al 2014);
- An internet-based information programme, delivered by a health professional at the homes of people with stroke and their family members (Kim et al 2013);
- Individual self-management support tailored to the Maori community of New Zealand and delivered by a representative from that community (Harwood et al 2012); and
- A stroke-specific modification of the Stanford CDSP delivered to groups of 10–15 participants (Kendall et al 2007)

The evidence landscape is complicated further by studies of interventions, which were not explicitly conceptualised and labelled as 'self-management' interventions, but which some review authors nevertheless consider adequate for inclusion in evidence syntheses of self-management (Parke et al 2015). This reflects the general complex nature of self-management interventions bringing together several components, or 'active ingredients', some of which may also form part of more narrow patient education interventions or even generic good rehabilitation practice, such as person-centred goal setting and collaborative decision making. Therefore, although systematic reviews and meta-analyses of controlled trials provide a helpful strand of high-level evidence, leading researchers in the field will also emphasise that it is important to appreciate the specific content of different self-management programmes, characteristics and whole system dynamics of implementation settings, and the internal validity of individual controlled trials.

Measurement of Self-Management

Measuring self-management is not straightforward because the behaviours that contribute are multifaceted and depend largely on each individual and the challenges of the particular condition. The most important consideration is to define the outcome of interest, for example, activity or levels of fatigue, and then find a valid and reliable measure of the target outcome (DeVellis & Blalock 2009). Work is also being conducted to identify self-management outcomes that are relevant to and considered important by the respective stakeholders in the topic, that is, patients, their families, health professionals and commissioners of health services (Boger et al 2015). There are potentially many outcome measurements that can be used to evaluate self-management, and it may not always be possible to gain direct observed evidence of change in target behaviour. Some measures are self-reported because direct observation is

difficult, and these can include scales that test more factual information, for example, knowledge about the condition, or measurement of a more subjective state, such as perceived competency or mood. Many measures require a degree of cognitive competency, for example, recalling past events or rating one's own ability in a certain task such as 'walk across the room without falling'.

There are several scales to specifically measure self-management behaviours, and these can be both generic and disease specific. The Self-Management Behaviours scale is a generic measure developed by Lorig and colleagues to evaluate the effectiveness of their CDSP (Lorig et al 1996). The scale has also been adopted for disease-specific programmes such as the Arthritis Self-Management Programme (Barlow & Barefoot 1996). It captures responses relating to different self-management behaviours such as managing medication and self-exercise (Lorig et al 1996). The more recently developed Patient Activation Measure is a generic self-reported questionnaire that assesses an individual's understanding of their role in the care process and their knowledge, skills and confidence to manage their health and healthcare, a construct described as 'patient activation' (Hibbard et al 2004). It is proposed that individuals can be categorised into four 'levels of activation', to facilitate tailored interactions between patients and health professionals, although some authors suggest caution in neurological patient groups. Compared with those chronic conditions that are generally very responsive to lifestyle modification such as asthma and diabetes, unpredictable and progressive neurological conditions such as MS and Parkinson's will likely require a more nuanced and differentiated understanding of a person's capacity and ability to self-manage (Packer et al 2015).

The effectiveness of programmes underpinned by SCT is often measured by change in self-efficacy. A generic self-reported self-efficacy scale has been developed and validated by Schwarzer and colleagues (Luszczynska et al 2005). However, Bandura supports a model of measurement in which it is suggested that efficacy beliefs should be measured in terms of specific judgements within the chosen area of activity (Bandura 1997). Therefore it is important to use a self-efficacy scale that is relevant to the target behaviours and specific to the context of living with the particular chronic condition. Examples of such scales within neurological rehabilitation are the Stroke Self-Efficacy Questionnaire (Jones et al 2008b) and the MS Self-Efficacy Scale (Airlie et al 2001).

Overall, self-management for people with neurological conditions is spearheaded by work in stroke, which has provided a remarkable success story. The field has developed from the first mention of 'self-management' in the UK national clinical guideline for stroke (Intercollegiate Stroke

> **SELECTED SELF-MANAGEMENT OUTCOME TOOLS**
>
> - Self-Management Behaviours Scale (Lorig et al 1996)
> - Patient Activation Measure (Hibbard et al 2004)
> - Stroke Self-Efficacy Questionnaire (Jones et al 2008b)
> - Multiple Sclerosis Self-Efficacy Scale (Airlie et al 2001)

Working Party 2008) to the first Cochrane systematic review of self-management programmes for people with stroke (Fryer et al 2016). Stroke self-management holds a firm place in clinical guidelines, and researchers are now focusing on the finer details of programme components, processes of implementation and whole system dynamics within stroke care pathways (Jones et al 2016a). There is great opportunity to build on this evidence and expertise in stroke self-management, to replicate and further the field with respect to other neurological conditions as well.

SUPPORTING SELF-MANAGEMENT: PROVIDING INFORMATION ALONE IS NOT ENOUGH

Listening is without doubt the most important skill for therapists to use when supporting self-management. Not just listening with one eye on the time, but actively hearing and capitalising on ideas, information or concerns an individual might tell us. This is not always easy when faced with a long assessment schedule or when time is limited. In fact, we know that when time is limited healthcare professionals will use more didactic methods, telling and teaching rather than sharing and collaborating (Mudge et al 2015). As previously mentioned, it is important to consider that the nature of our therapeutic relationships can be established from the first contact. The way in which we communicate can determine how much or how little an individual will feel 'led' or 'involved' in their care, as this quote from a stroke survivor illustrates:

> 'Well, every time she came in she would say 'can you do this' and 'can you do that' and if there was an improvement – because she would count the seconds that I did it in, on one foot, so many seconds – and then she would tick it off on her list.' (Jones et al 2017)

A key term already mentioned in this chapter is the concept of shared decision making. Often used interchangeably with self-management support, individuals are actively encouraged to make decisions and choices about their care and reflect on what is important to them (Ahmad et al 2014). As expected, evidence shows that when individuals are more involved, they are also more satisfied with their care, and this way of working can also create real efficiencies in already time-limited services (Lewis-Barned 2016). Therapists should have a vested interest in learning the skills to support shared decision making and self-management, which can maximise the potential of every interaction, as well as creating efficiencies within our services.

Achieving shared decision making requires skill and effort by both the professional and individual patient. It is easy to see how the provision of self-management information could be a quicker, more convenient method. Partnership is at the heart of working in this way, and success requires the ability for professionals to relinquish some control and not be concerned if the route to a goal might not be their chosen one. Norris and Kilbride (2014) interviewed physiotherapists and occupational therapists who received training to integrate a self-management approach in a stroke pathway. Participants described the shift in their thinking, from comfortably controlling what happened towards a more uncertain way of working full of potential risks and unknowns. This article and others describe the many barriers and obstacles to fully sharing decision making. If someone tries to walk unaided and learns from the experience that they need more support, that in itself might be a good outcome, but it comes with a possible risk. These concerns often come into sharp focus whilst working with individuals who have cognitive and/or communication problems. One of the most common questions asked by participants in self-management training is 'what if the person lacks cognitive insight?' Clearly, to fully support self-management with as many individuals as we can, we should explore the specific skills and strategies that can be used to overcome these challenges.

Consider the example of a young woman recovering from acute traumatic brain injury. She cannot engage in therapy, she cannot sleep; in fact she cannot even fully remember or understand that she has had a brain injury. She is hospitalised in an acute neurosurgery ward that has a large throughput of patients. Nurses and therapists have very limited time, and she has no immediate friends or family members who can support.

This example has many obstacles to supporting self-management and sharing decision making. There are some key principles associated with self-management, such as problem solving, reflection, knowledge and goal setting. But these all require some cognitive ability. Below are some ideas about where we could start.

- Encourage her to write down what is on her mind to get down her thoughts and ideas.

- Encourage her to talk to other patients – Is there someone she could sit with who has been through a similar experience?
- Spend time finding out what is most important to her, and get to know what motivates her.
- Encourage her to write her own record of small successes and help her to see how she has made an important contribution to her progress.
- Do not use the word 'goals' because she does not understand what this means – Say, 'What is important to you now and in the future?'
- Integrate these strategies into your everyday interactions with this individual and encourage other staff to do the same.

These are relatively small steps that can start to prioritise self-management as part of therapy and care, but they may not be commonly used, especially when time is limited. Yet if we describe a good self-manager as someone who is able to find solutions to problems and set goals, it begs the question as to how best we can support individuals to get to this point. By looking outside of self-management literature to that of palliative care or dementia care, we can also learn what skills are relevant in these more complex situations. Atul Gawande in his seminal text 'Being Mortal' (2014) asks a woman in the end stage of her cancer, 'What would make a good day for you?' Tom Kitwood (1997) in his work in dementia highlights the importance of personhood, which he described as 'a standing or status that is bestowed upon one human being, by others, it implies recognition, respect and trust'. Through this recognition, respect and trust, the personhood of an individual will be enhanced, as well as their well-being. Both of these authors highlight the need to get to know the person and what is important to them, and for that we need mutual trust and respect. These are solid principles for good self-management support in any setting or context.

Lessons Learnt From Long Covid: How Can Self-Management Be Supported?

Beyond getting to know a person with a neurological condition and giving them space to share experiences and allocating time to listen, our recent work with people living with long Covid has given us fresh insight into how self-management can be supported.

The context surrounding a person and their neurological condition is crucial. Covid-19, the predisposing illness to long Covid, was considered an unexpected and unknown phenomenon to most. Although many people across the UK felt the impact of the Covid-19 pandemic, some people with long Covid feel that political action or inaction contributed to their long-term condition. This has led to feelings of injustice, anger and frustration. Others have felt

a sense of guilt and blame from others in their personal community around developing the condition (Macpherson et al 2022, Taylor et al 2021). For instance, people have been interpreted as those who broke lockdown rules and thus are somewhat deserving of their illness, despite that often not being the case. With a prolonged period before a formal recognition of the condition by the World Health Organization, the long Covid community has felt isolated, silenced and unsupported by healthcare professionals and by some friends, family and employers (Callan et al 2022, Humphreys et al 2021, Kingstone et al 2021, Ladds et al 2020).

Some people with other neurological conditions, as well as people with long Covid, have taken a dislike to the term 'self-management'. People with the condition have described how self-management feels like DIY – being left to just 'do it yourself'. With experiences of being passed around healthcare services, or an inability to access services (Macpherson et al 2022), 'self-management' can feel like they are being passed the responsibility to manage their own condition. In that sense, self-management can appear to be unsupportive, contributing to aloneness and helplessness. We have observed how the term 'self-management', and the appearance of having to 'go it alone', can immediately influence motivation to participate in self-management activities, as well as motivation to enhance self-management skills (e.g., problem solving). As a result, an explanation of what is meant by self-management, not merely use of the term, should be adopted by healthcare professionals. Working with people with long Covid, we have found a phrase to explain 'self-management', overcoming this possible barrier to engagement. Similar to the NHS England (2016) definition, we now explain self-management as 'enhancing a person's knowledge, skills and confidence in their condition through personalised support from a healthcare professional'. Use of this language or providing some clarification of self-management to people with a neurological condition may help to mitigate any unrealistic expectations of what they are about to receive.

Emerging research indicates that long Covid comprises many neurological symptoms (e.g., short-term memory loss, confusion, sensory sensitivity and cognitive processing difficulty). Although some people have described their neurological symptoms as 'brain fog' (Graham et al 2021), others have explained how this terminology does not do the plethora of varying symptoms justice (Callan et al 2022). For example, although easy to refer to, 'brain fog' clusters together specific domains of cognitive function, including executive function, attention, memory and language. Therefore, for some people, this term does not always convey the specific nature of their symptom (Callan et al 2022). People with long Covid have further explained how their neurological symptoms interact with numerous physiological challenges, which contributes to the extreme unpredictability of their condition (Callan et al 2022). Without a knowledge base or medical answers, such unpredictability has led to fear and an inability to envisage a return to peoples' former selves (Burton et al 2022). Although common symptoms are now coming to the forefront (Ladds et al 2020), the symptoms experienced appear unique to each person; severity and prevalence of symptoms fluctuate differently for different people. This means that for healthcare professionals, people with long Covid who sit before them will not be the same, so they cannot and should not be treated the same.

In neurological conditions comprising a plethora of symptoms, each likely presenting differently, healthcare professionals should allocate time and space to listen to each person's unique experience of the condition. A person's ability to feel understood can be a powerful experience, and therefore assumptions gained from other individuals or personal experience should be left aside. A person experiencing an unpredictable illness may not understand their experience themselves. For example, people with neurological conditions such as long Covid can struggle to communicate their symptoms because of the word-finding and memory issues they are experiencing (Callan et al 2022). Therefore, giving a person time and space to find their words, vocalise their experience and have such experience listened to can be an extremely positive encounter. It can allow the person to make sense of their condition, foster a blossoming relationship between the person and healthcare professional and lead to a more positive care experience (Atherton et al 2021, Callan et al 2022, Ladds et al 2021).

Our work with long Covid sufferers has further challenged our view of what constitutes progress in physical and neurological rehabilitation. Traditionally progress is conceptualised as taking a forward or onward movement towards something that is desired, such as 'full recovery'. In rehabilitation, this has been no different. Yet, with long Covid, what constitutes recovery and the progressive steps needed to move towards recovery are still relatively unclear. Some people with long Covid question whether complete medical recovery will ever be possible. With the unpredictable nature of long Covid symptoms, trying to make forward progress and cure each symptom could lead to consistent failure and low mood if not achieved. Similarly, with the term 'better', the fluctuation of symptoms means that people are not able to engage in their typical everyday activities. Thus they feel unable to describe themselves as better. This inability to feel 'better' or make traditional forward 'progress' can reduce motivation and confidence to engage in self-management.

Instead of conceptualising progress as recovery and a forward motion, in long Covid a plateau or maintaining symptom stability has been described as progress. In that sense, being 'better' is not conceptualised as having less prevalent or severe symptoms, but as having a greater ability to control symptoms that are present. By reframing 'progress' to include plateaus and emphasising the importance of knowledge and control, it can allow people with a neurological condition a wider, more achievable margin in which to experience 'progress'. Likewise, with 'better', by altering a person's focus of better from being more of a long-term entity (e.g., a day) to a temporary feeling that they might feel for an hour, it may restore feelings of confidence and well-being. These views may contradict the traditional view of progress in self-management and rehabilitation but may offer more attractive propositions for healthcare professionals working with people with unpredictable physical and neurological conditions.

Through an iterative process of codesign, and by working with and not 'on' people with lived experience, we have slowly developed an understanding of people's need and priorities. In the self-management literature base, it is highlighted that self-management interventions can take many forms (Fryer et al 2016). However, the high attrition and low reach of programmes can pose challenges. This suggests that although self-management interventions can be moulded and adapted, this may not be being done to an adequate standard to meet the needs of the target population. Instead, codesign or coproduction can offer a process to develop self-management programmes that are rooted in the desires and practicalities of those living with a particular condition. Such collaborative practices have been advocated in long Covid. For example, the term 'long Covid' was born from those suffering with the illness (Callard & Perego 2021), and people with lived experience have provided a wealth of understanding into the condition. As Macpherson and colleagues (2022) stated "people with long Covid are well placed to cocreate this understanding and communication" (p. 8).

In our own long Covid research, we have undertaken an iterative codesign process with people living with the condition. During the process, the lived experience group has made key decisions about what the personalised self-management resources should look like, discussing and selecting the format and content. Among a plethora of content, sections to note included building joy, a long Covid first aid kit and the context of the Covid-19 pandemic. Before the codesign activities, such self-management strategies had received only limited attention in the literature and thus may not have featured in the resources without the input of people with lived experience. For example, although Burton et al (2022) identified that adapting hobbies and activities was important for well-being in the self-management of long Covid, the concept of a long Covid self-management first aid kit presented a novel, practical desire by people living with the condition. Therefore attention should be paid to the needs of people with different neurological conditions so that resources and self-management programmes can offer valuable, insightful support and to ensure care is tailored appropriately to maximise outcome improvement.

In summary, our work with long Covid patients has taught us the following neurological self-management lessons:

- Appreciate the context of a condition and the person;
- Do not just say 'self-management' – Clarify and explain what self-management means;
- Put aside your assumptions of a person's condition and validate their personal experience;
- 'Brain fog' and 'cognitive difficulty' may not always be adequate descriptors of a person's neurological symptoms;
- Be aware of using the terms 'better', 'progress' and recovery'; and
- Work with people with lived experience to understand their self-management needs.

CONCLUSION

In this chapter we have attempted to provide a balanced overview of self-management and the issues of importance when working with individuals with neurological conditions. We have not included reference to digital forms of self-management support and fully recognise that there are a great many resources accessed online which can support key areas such as knowledge, problem solving and goal setting. Equally, it is important to acknowledge that many resources will be found by individuals through their own efforts rather than those suggested by therapists. Self-management is also about an individual selecting the right resource for them, and there are many excellent websites which have sought to pool resources, such as the my-therappy.co.uk website which houses links to more than 75 apps suitable for rehabilitation and self-management after stroke and brain injury (https://www.my-therappy.co.uk).

Self-management is now firmly embedded in our policy and practice, not only for individuals living with long-term conditions in the community but also the principles can equally and successfully be applied in acute settings. We can learn lessons from self-management programmes that have worked and not worked using outcome data, as well as synthesising experiences from people living with long-term conditions and healthcare professionals supporting self-management. A useful guide in this respect can be found in one of many relevant publications from the

UK-based charity The Health Foundation (de Longh et al 2015). This practical guide highlights key lessons for integrating self-management into any service, which are summarised in Fig. 19.2.

In summary, supporting individuals to self-manage may require a change in how therapists currently work in neurorehabilitation. In addition to the key skills required to deliver self-management programmes, it is also necessary to reflect on the values that underpin our practice. National Voices (2014, p. 2) in their review on self-management define person-centred care as:

KEY POINTS

- As healthcare professionals, it is incumbent on us to reflect on our own practice and find ways to support self-management, rather than viewing it solely as the responsibility of the individual living with a neurological condition.
- We need to be able to gauge an individual's readiness to take on more responsibility, as people's responses to self-management are unique.
- The unique difference between an educational and a self-management programme is that the latter facilitates behaviour change through different means.
- Many individuals self-manage without the support of a clinician or self-management training. To support a person's self-management, health professionals need to avoid giving answers too readily, and need to tune into individuals' stories, preferences and ideas.
- Useful practical strategies for building up confidence to self-manage include supporting an individual to break down tasks into smaller achievable components.
- It can be beneficial to observe someone who is perceived to be similar successfully performing tasks, for example, learning from another individual's experience of recovery after stroke.
- Self-efficacy beliefs should be measured in terms of specific judgements within the chosen area of activity.
- There are a number of positive outcomes from well-designed self-management programmes, particularly those with a clear theoretical framework and well-described 'active ingredients'.
- Listening is the most important skill for health professionals when supporting self-management – not just listening with one eye on the time, but actively hearing and capitalising on ideas, information or concerns an individual might tell us.

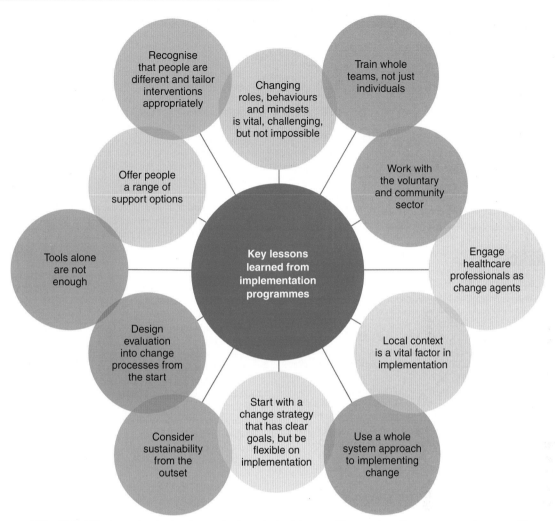

FIG. 19.2 What works to implement shared decision making and self-management support? Lessons learned from implementation programmes. (Reproduced with permission from Ahmand et al 2014, p. 6).

'placing people at the forefront of their health and care. This ensures people retain control, helps them make informed decisions and supports a partnership between people, families and health and social services.'

Overall, policy and research strongly support the need for healthcare professionals working with individuals with long-term conditions to adopt a more collaborative approach. Therapists working in neurorehabilitation should be no different and need to be ready to learn new skills, work in different ways and challenge practice that is not consistent with these principles. As Terry, a stroke survivor, explained: 'I mean sometimes physiotherapy can be a very passive thing, but I enjoyed it the most when I was putting equal into it as well, and I felt we, things were being achieved'.

SELF-ASSESSMENT QUESTIONS

1. What are some of the ways you could define self-management?
2. What is the difference between patient education or information provision and a self-management programme?
3. What is self-efficacy, and which psychological processes can strengthen a person's self-efficacy?
4. What skills do therapists require to support patient self-management?
5. What are some of the most common methods of delivering self-management programmes, and what ingredients are thought to be most effective?

REFERENCES

Ahmad, N., Ellins, J., Krelle, H., Lawrie, M., 2014. Person-centred care: from ideas to action. Bringing together the evidence on shared decision making and self-management support. The Health Foundation, London.

Ahmed, Z.M., Khalil, M.F., Kohail, A.M., et al., 2020. The prevalence and predictors of post-stroke depression and anxiety during COVID-19 pandemic. J. Stroke. Cerebrovasc. Dis. 29, 105315.

Airlie, J., et al., 2001. Measuring the impact of multiple sclerosis on psychosocial functioning: the development of a new self-efficacy scale. Clin. Rehabil. 15, 259–265.

Atherton, H., Briggs, T., Chew-Graham, C., 2021. Long COVID and the importance of the doctor–patient relationship. Br. J. Gen. Pract. 71, 54–55.

Bandura, A., 1989. Human agency in social cognition theory. Am. Psychol. 44, 1175–1184.

Bandura, A., 1994. Self-efficacy. In: Ramachaudran, V. (Ed.), Encyclopedia of Human Behavior. Academic Press, New York, pp. 71–81.

Bandura, A., 1997. The nature and structure of self-efficacy. In: Bandura, A. (Ed.), Self-Efficacy: The Exercise of Control. W.H Freeman and Company, New York.

Barlow, J., Sturt, J., Hearnshaw, H., 2002. Self-management interventions for people with chronic conditions in primary care: examples from arthritis, asthma and diabetes. Health. Educ. J. 61, 365–378.

Barlow, J.H., Barefoot, J., 1996. Group education for people with arthritis. Patient. Educ. Counsel. 27, 257–267.

Bate, P., Robert, G., Fulop, N., Øvretveit, J., Dixon-Woods, M., 2014. Perspectives on context. A selection of essays considering the role of context in successful quality improvement. The Health Foundation, London.

Bishop, D., Miller, I., Weiner, D., et al., 2014. Family Intervention: Telephone Tracking (FITT): a pilot stroke outcome study. Top. Stroke. Rehabil. 21, S63–74.

Bloom, D.E., et al., 2015. Macroeconomic implications of population ageing and selected policy responses. Lancet. 385, 649–657.

Boger, E., et al., 2015. Self-management and self-management support outcomes: a systematic review and mixed research synthesis of stakeholder views. PLoS ONE. 10, e0130990

Burton, A., Aughterson, H., Fancourt, D., Philip, K.E.J., 2022. Factors shaping the mental health and well-being of people experiencing persistent COVID-19 symptoms or 'long COVID': qualitative study. BJPsych. Open. 8, 1–8.

Bury, M., Newbould, J., Taylor, D., 2005. A Rapid Review of the Current State of Knowledge Regarding Lay-Led Self-Management of Chronic Illness. National Institute for Clinical Excellence, London.

Bury, M., Pink, D., 2005. The HSJ debate: self-management of chronic disease doesn't work. Health. Serv. J. 115, 18–19.

Busse, M., Latchem-Hastings, J., Button, K., et al., 2021. Web-based physical activity intervention for people with progressive multiple sclerosis: application of consensus-based intervention development guidance. BMJ Open. 11, e045378

Callan, C., Ladds, E., Husain, L., et al., 2022. 'I can't cope with multiple inputs': a qualitative study of the lived experience of 'brain fog' after COVID-19. BMJ Open. 12, e056366

Callard, F., Perego, E., 2021. How and why patients made long Covid. Soc. Sci. Med. 268, 113426.

Ch'ng, A., French, D., Maclean, N., 2008. Coping with the challenges of recovery from stroke. J. Health. Psychol. 13, 1136–1146.

Clark, E., Bennett, K., Ward, N., Jones, F., 2018. One size does not fit all – stroke survivor's views on group self-management interventions. Disabil. Rehabil. 40, 569–576.

Clark, E., MacCrosain, A., Ward, N.S., Jones, F., 2020. The key features and role of peer support within group self-management interventions for stroke? A systematic review. Disabil. Rehabil. 42, 307–316.

Corben, S., Rosen, R., 2005. Self-management for long-term conditions: patients' perspectives on the way ahead. King's Fund, London.

Craig, P., Dieppe, P., Macintyre, S., Michie, S., Nazareth, I., Petticrew, M., 2008. Developing and evaluating complex interventions: the new Medical Research Council guidance. BMJ. 29, a1655

Davidson, L., 2005. Recovery, self management and the expert patient – changing the culture of mental health from a UK perspective. J. Ment. Health. 14, 25–35.

de Longh, A., Fagan, P., Fenner, J., Kidd, L., 2015. A practical guide to self-management support. Key components for successful implementation. The Health Foundation, London.

de Silva, D., 2011. Helping people help themselves. A review of the evidence considering whether it is worthwhile to support self-management. The Health Foundation, London.

DeVellis, R., Blalock, S., 2009. Outcomes of self-management interventions. In: Newman, S., Steed, L., Mulligan, K. (Eds.), Chronic Physical Illness: Self-Management and Behavioural Interventions. Open University Press, Berkshire, pp. 148–169.

Dixon, G., Thornton, E., Yound, C., 2007. Perceptions of self-efficacy and rehabilitation among neurologically disabled adults. Clin. Rehabil. 21, 230–240.

Dobkin, B.H., 2016. Behavioural self-management strategies for practice and exercise should be included in neurologic rehabilitation trials and care. Curr. Opin. Neurol. 29, 693–699.

Ellis, J., Boger, E., Latter, S., et al., 2017. Conceptualisation of the 'good' self-manager: a qualitative investigation of stakeholder views on the self-management of long-term health conditions. Soc. Sci. Med. 176, 25–33.

Ellis-Hill, C., Payne, S., Ward, C., 2008. Using stroke to explore the Life Thread Model: an alternative approach to understanding rehabilitation following an acquired disability. Disabil. Rehabil. 30, 150–159.

Ewart, C., 1992. The role of physical self efficacy in the recovery from a heart attack. In: Schwarzer, R. (Ed.), Self-Efficacy: Thought Control of Action. Taylor and Francis, Philadelphia, pp. 287–305.

Fletcher, S., Kulnik, S.T., Demain, S., Jones, F., 2019. The problem with self-management: Problematising self-management and power using a Foucauldian lens in the context of stroke care and rehabilitation. PLOS ONE. 14, e0218517.

Fryer, C.E., et al., 2016. Self management programmes for quality of life in people with stroke. Cochrane. Database. Syst. Rev. 8, CD010442.

Gawande, A., 2014. Being mortal: illness, medicine and what matters in the end. Profile Books, London.

Graham, E.L., Clark, J.R., Orban, Z.S., et al., 2021. Persistent neurologic symptoms and cognitive dysfunction in non-hospitalized Covid-19 "long haulers". Annu. Clin. Transl. Neurol. 8, 1073–1085.

Gronewold, J., Hermann, D.M., 2021. Social isolation and risk of fatal cardiovascular events. Lancet. Public. Health. 6, e197–198.

Hartley, S., 2009. Developing a self-management and exercise model for people with multiple sclerosis. Int. J. Ther. Rehabil. 16, 34–42.

Harwood, M., Weatherall, M., Talmaitoga, A., et al., 2012. Taking charge after stroke: promoting self-directed rehabilitation to improve quality of life – a randomised controlled trial. Clin. Rehabil. 26, 493–501.

Hibbard, J.H., et al., 2004. Development of the Patient Activation Measure (PAM): conceptualizing and measuring activation in patients and consumers. Health. Serv. Res. 39 (4 Pt 1), 1005–1026.

Hirsche, R.C., et al., 2011. Chronic disease self-management for individuals with stroke, multiple sclerosis and spinal cord injury. Disabil. Rehabil. 33, 1136–1146.

Humphreys, H., Kilby, L., Kudiersky, N., et al., 2021. Long COVID and the role of physical activity: a qualitative study. BMJ Open. 11, e047632.

Intercollegiate Stroke Working Party, 2008. National Clinical Guideline for Stroke, 3rd ed. Royal College of Physicians, London.

Intercollegiate Stroke Working Party, 2016. National Clinical Guideline for Stroke, 5th ed. Royal College of Physicians, London. Available at: https://www.strokeaudit.org/SupportFiles/Documents/Guidelines/2016-National-Clinical-Guideline-for-Stroke-5t-(1).aspx. Accessed June 15, 2022.

Johnston, M., et al., 2007. Recovery from disability after stroke as a target for a behavioural intervention: results of a randomized controlled trial. Disabil. Rehabil. 29, 1117–1127.

Jones, F., 2004. A memorable patient: an individual approach to stroke recovery. Physiother. Res. Int. 9, 147–148.

Jones, F., Gage, H., Drummond, A., et al., 2016b. Feasibility study of an integrated stroke self-management programme: a cluster-randomised controlled trial. BMJ Open. 6, e008900.

Jones, F., Mandy, A., Partridge, C., 2008a. Reasons for recovery after stroke: a perspective based on personal experiences. Disabil. Rehabil. 30, 507–516.

Jones, F., McKevitt, C., Riazi, A., Liston, M., 2017. How is rehabilitation with and without an integrated self-management approach perceived by UK community-dwelling stroke survivors? A qualitative process evaluation to explore implementation and contextual variations. BMJ Open. 7, e014109.

Jones, F., Pöstges, H., Brimicombe, L., 2016a. Building Bridges between healthcare professionals, patients and families: a coproduced and integrated approach to self-management support in stroke. NeuroRehabilitation. 39, 471–480.

Jones, F., Reid, F., Partridge, C., 2008b. The Stroke Self-Efficacy Questionnaire (SSEQ): measuring individual confidence in functional performance after stroke. J. Nurs. Healthcare. Chron. Ill 17, 244–252.

Jones, F., Riazi, A., 2011. Self-efficacy and self-management after stroke: a systematic review. Disabil. Rehabil. 33, 797–810.

Jones, F., Riazi, A., Norris, M., 2013. Self-management after stroke: time for some more questions? Disabil. Rehabil. 35, 257–264.

Jones, T., et al., 2015. A systematic review of the efficacy of self-management programs for increasing physical activity in community-dwelling adults with acquired brain injury (ABI). Syst. Rev. 4, 51.

Jordan, J., Osborne, R., 2007. Chronic disease self-management education programs: challenges ahead. Med. J. Aust. 186, 84–87.

Kendall, E., Rogers, A., 2007. Extinguishing the social? State sponsored self-care policy and the Chronic Disease Self-Management Programme. Disabil. Soc. 22, 129–143.

Kendall, E., et al., 2007. Recovery following stroke: the role of self-management education. Soc. Sci. Med. 64, 735–746.

Kendall, E., et al., 2011. Self-managing versus self-management: reinvigorating the socio-political dimensions of self-management. Chron. Illn. 7, 87–98.

Kennedy, A., Rogers, A., Gately, C., 2005. From patients to providers: prospects for self-care skills trainers in the National Health Service. Health. Soc. Care. Commun. 13, 431–440.

Kidd, T., Carey, N., Mold, F., et al., 2017. A systematic review of the effectiveness of self-management interventions in people with multiple sclerosis at improving depression, anxiety and quality of life. PLoS One. 11, e0185931.

Kim, J., Lee, S., Kim, J., 2013. Effect of a web-based stroke education program on recurrence prevention behaviours among stroke patients: a pilot study. Health. Educ. Res. 28, 488–501.

Kingstone, T., Campbell, P., Andras, A., et al., 2021. Exploring the impact of the first wave of COVID-19 on social work practice: a qualitative study in England. UK. Br. J. Soc. Work. 52, 2043-2062.

Kirkpatrick Pinson, D.M., Ottens, A.J., Fisher, T.A., 2009. Women coping successfully with multiple sclerosis and the precursors of change. Qual. Health. Res. 19, 181–193.

Kitwood, T., 1997. Dementia reconsidered; the person comes first. Open University Press, London.

Kulnik, S.T., Pöstges, H., Brimicombe, L., Hammond, J., Jones, F., 2017. Implementing an interprofessional model of self-management support across a community workforce: a mixed-methods evaluation study. J. Interprof. Care. 31, 75–84.

Ladds, E., Rushforth, A., Wieringa, S., et al., 2020. Persistent symptoms after Covid-19: qualitative study of 114 "long Covid" patients and draft quality principles for services. BMC Health. Serv. Res. 20, 1144.

Ladds, E., Rushforth, A., Wieringa, S., et al., 2021. Developing services for long COVID: lessons from a study of wounded healers [published correction appears in Clin Med (Lond). Mar;21(2):160]. Clin. Med. (Lond) 21, 59–65.

Lazurus, R., 1990. Stress, coping and illness. In: Friendman, H. (Ed.), Personality and Disease. John Wiley and Sons, Oxford, pp. 97–120.

Légaré, F., Thompson-Leduc, P., 2014. Twelve myths about shared decision making. Patient. Educ. Couns. 96, 281–286.

Lennon, S., McKenna, S., Jones, F., 2013. Self-management programmes for people post stroke: a systematic review. Clin. Rehabil. 27, 867–878.

Levensky, E., et al., 2007. Motivational interviewing: an evidence based approach to counselling helps patients follow treatment recommendations. Am. J. Nurs. 107, 50–58.

Lewis-Barned, N., 2016. Shared decision making and support for self-management: a rationale for change. Fut. Hosp. J 3, 117–120.

Lorig, K., 1993. Self-management of chronic illness: a model for the future. Generations. 17, 11–14.

Lorig, K., et al., 1996. Outcome measures for Health Education and Other Health Care Interventions. V. Baker. SAGE Publications.

Lorig, K., et al., 2001. Effect of a self-management program on patients with chronic disease. Eff. Clin. Pract. 4, 256–262.

Lorig, K., Holman, H.R., 2003. Self-management education: history, definition, outcomes and mechanisms. Ann. Behav. Med. 26, 1–7.

Lowe, R., Barlow, C., Lloyd, B., et al., 2021. Lifestyle, Exercise and Activity Package for People living with Progressive Multiple Sclerosis (LEAP-MS): adaptions during the COVID-19 pandemic and remote delivery for improved efficiency. Trials. 22, 286.

Luszczynska, A., Scholz, U., Schwarzer, R., 2005. The general self-efficacy scale: multicultural validation studies. J. Psychol. 139, 439–457.

Maclean, N., et al., 2002. The concept of patient motivation. A qualitative analysis of stroke professionals' attitudes. Stroke. 33, 444–448.

Macpherson, K., Cooper, K., Harbour, J., Mahal, D., Miller, C., Nairn, M., 2022. Experiences of living with long COVID and of accessing healthcare services: a qualitative systematic review. BMJ Open. 11, e050979.

Mäkelä, P., Gawned, S., Jones, F., 2014. Starting early: integration of self-management support into an acute stroke service. BMJ Qual. Improv. Rep. 3, u202037.w1759.

Malcomson, K., Lowe-Strong, A., Dunwoody, L., 2008. What can we learn from the personal insights of individuals living and coping with multiple sclerosis? Disabil. Rehabil. 30, 662–674.

Moore, L., Frost, J., Britten, N., 2015. Context and complexity: the meaning of self-management for older adults with heart disease. Soc. Health. Ill. 37, 1254–1269.

Morgan, H.M., et al., 2017. We need to talk about purpose: a critical interpretive synthesis of health and social care professionals' approaches to self-management support for people with long-term conditions. Health Expect. 20, 243–259.

Mudge, S., Kayes, N., McPherson, K., 2015. Who is in control? Clinicians' view on their role in self-management approaches: a qualitative metasynthesis. BMJ Open. 5, e007413.

National Voices., 2014. Supporting Self-Management. A Summary of the Evidence. National Voices, London. Available at: www.nationalvoices.org.uk/publications/our-publications/supporting-self-management. Accessed April 27, 2017.

Newman, S., Steed, L., Mulligan, K., 2004. Self-management interventions for chronic illness. Lancet. 364, 1523–1537.

NHS England, 2016. Realising the value. Ten key actions to put people and communities at the heart of health and wellbeing. NHS England, London.

NHS England., 2019. The NHS Long Term Plan. NHS England, London. Available at: https://www.longtermplan.nhs.uk/wp-content/uploads/2019/08/nhs-long-term-plan-version-1.2.pdf. June 15, 2022.

Norris, M., Kilbride, C., 2014. From dictatorship to a reluctant democracy: stroke therapists talking about self-management. Disabil. Rehabil. 36, 32–38.

Nott, M., Wiseman, L., Seymour, T., Pike, S., Cuming, T., Wall, G., 2021. Stroke self-management and the role of self-efficacy. Disabil. Rehabil. 43, 1410–1419.

Packer, T.L., et al., 2015. The Patient Activation Measure: a validation study in a neurological population. Qual. Life Res. 24, 1587–1596.

Parke, H.L., et al., 2015. Self-management support interventions for stroke survivors: a systematic meta-review. PLoS ONE. 10, e0131448.

Pearce, G., et al., 2015. Experiences of self-management support following a stroke: a meta-review of qualitative systematic reviews. PLoS ONE. 10, e0141803.

Prince, M.J., et al., 2015. The burden of disease in older people and implications for health policy and practice. Lancet. 385, 549–562.

Prochaska, J., Velicer, W., 1997. The transtheoretical model of health behaviour change. Am. J. Health. Promot. 12, 38–48.

Rimmer, J., Wang, E., Smith, D., 2008. Barriers associated with exercise and community access for individuals after stroke. J. Rehabil. Res. Develop. 45, 315–322.

Rogers, A., et al., 2009. Are some more equal than others? Social comparison in self-management skills training for long-term conditions. Chron. Illn. 5, 305–317.

Sadler, E., et al., 2017. Developing a novel peer support intervention to promote resilience after stroke. Health. Soc. Care. Commun. 25, 1590–1600.

Satink, T., Cup, E.H., de Swart, B.J., Nijhuis-van der Sanden, M.W., 2015. How is self-management perceived by community living people after a stroke? A focus group study. Disabil. Rehabil. 37, 223–230.

Satink, T., et al., 2016. Self-management develops through doing of everyday activities – a longitudinal qualitative study of stroke survivors during two years post-stroke. BMC Neurol. 16, 221.

Serlachius, A., Sutton, S., 2009. Self-management and behavioural change: theoretical models. In: Newman, S., Steed, L., Mulligan, K. (Eds.), Chronic Physical Illness: Self-Management and Behavioural Interventions. Open University Press, Berkshire, pp. 47–63.

Schwarzer, R., 1992. Self-efficacy in the adoption and maintenance of health behaviours: theoretical approaches and a new model. In: Schwarzer, R. (Ed.), Self-Efficacy: Thought Control of Action. Taylor and Francis, Philadelphia, pp. 217–245.

Taylor, A.K., Kingstone, T., Briggs, T.A., et al., 2021. 'Reluctant pioneer': A qualitative study of doctors' experiences as patients with long COVID. Health. Expect. 24, 833–842.

van de Laar, K.E., van der Bijl, J.J., 2001. Strategies enhancing self-efficacy in diabetes education: a review. Sch. Inq. Nurs. Pract. 15, 235–248.

Vassilev, I., Band, R., Kennedy, A., James, E., Rogers, A., 2019. The role of collective efficacy in long-term condition management: a metasynthesis. Health. Soc. Care. Commun. 27, e588–e603.

Vassilev, I., Rogers, A., Kennedy, A., Koetsenruijter, J., 2014. The influence of social networks on self-management support: a metasynthesis. BMC Public. Health. 14, 719.

Watkins, C., et al., 2007. Motivational interviewing early after acute stroke: a randomized, controlled trial. Stroke. 38, 1004–1009.

Warner, G., et al., 2015. A systematic review of the effectiveness of stroke self-management programs for improving function and participation outcomes: self-management programs for stroke survivors. Disabil. Rehabil. 37, 2141–2163.

Wilson, P., Kendall, S., Brooks, F., 2007. The Expert Patients Programme: a paradox of patient empowerment and medical dominance. Health. Soc. Care. Commun. 15, 426–438.

Woodman, P., et al., 2014. Social participation post stroke: a meta-ethnographic review of the experiences and views of community-dwelling stroke survivors. Disabil. Rehabil. 36, 2031–2043.

World Health Organization, 2015. WHO global strategy on people-centred and integrated health service: interim report. World Health Organization, Geneva.

Wray, F., Clarke, D., Forster, A., 2018. Post-stroke self-management interventions: a systematic review of effectiveness and investigation of the inclusion of stroke survivors with aphasia. Disabil. Rehabil. 40, 1237–1251.

Neurorehabilitation Technologies

Belinda Lange, José Eduardo Pompeu, and Paolo Bonato

OUTLINE

Introduction, 515
Role of Technologies in Neurological Rehabilitation, 516
Types of Technologies Used in the Rehabilitation
    Setting, 517
    Technologies for Home-Based Rehabilitation, 519
      Sensor-Based Systems, 519
      Video Analysis, 521
      Virtual Reality Headsets,, 523
    Robot-Assisted Motor Training, 525

Wearable Technology for Field Assessments and
    Interventions, 528
Current Evidence, 533
Practical Tips for Choosing Technologies, 534
    Choosing Technology, 534
    Choosing an Activity/Task/Game, 534
    Client Considerations, 535
Conclusion, 535
Case History, 535

INTRODUCTION

Virtual rehabilitation, the use of interactive technologies with clinical populations, has gained momentum in recent years. Interactive technologies are applications that involve real-time two-way flow of information based on user input (e.g., gestures, touch screen, sensors) and a response output from the system (in the form of visual, audio, haptic and/or assistive feedback). A range of interactive technologies can be leveraged to support, guide and enhance rehabilitation. These technologies can be used in clinic, community and/or home settings. Gamification or game-based rehabilitation has emerged as a key strategy to enhance motor and cognitive interventions applied to assessment, rehabilitation and training across a wide range of age groups and conditions. Extended reality (XR) encompasses virtual reality (VR) and augmented reality (AR) applications (Andrews et al 2019) and involves the use of interactive technologies that encourage activity through realistic interactions with virtual environments. There has been a rapid increase in research since the late 2000's on the use of interactive technologies such as low-cost video gaming technologies (from companies such as Nintendo and Microsoft), sensor- and

gesture-based applications, wearable technologies (Frisoli et al 2016, Rodgers et al 2019) and robotics in the rehabilitation setting (Keshner et al 2019, Nizamis et al 2021). This chapter aims to provide an overview and examples of existing and new interactive technologies that can be used within neurorehabilitation.

Development of new interactive technologies is moving at such a fast pace that the availability, cost, accessibility and acceptance of technologies has improved rapidly. Technologies that cost tens of thousands of pounds even 5 years ago are now readily available and easily accessible to consumers at a much lower cost. These rapid innovations and developments have been driven by the entertainment industry and a wider acceptance of the use of technologies in the rehabilitation setting. The impact of lockdowns and limited in-person interactions during the Covid-19 pandemic has highlighted the benefits of interactive technologies to support rehabilitation. In this rapidly changing field, a range of different interactive technologies can be used to support care through assessment, monitoring, engaging, motivating and supporting individuals. Interactive technologies have demonstrated potential to improve and augment current rehabilitation practices; however, many of

517

these technologies have been superseded with newer innovations, and more research is required to explore and build supporting evidence (Alashram et al 2021, Calafiore et al 2022, Laver et al 2017, Voinescu et al 2021). This chapter will provide examples of interactive technologies and will also provide guidance for evaluating and choosing technologies that may not yet be available.

ROLE OF TECHNOLOGIES IN NEUROLOGICAL REHABILITATION

The use of interactive technologies in neurorehabilitation is motivated by the observation that these technologies have potential to deliver high-intensity, high-dosage, task-specific interventions. These are key 'ingredients' to achieve neuroplasticity and hence maximise the recovery of motor function in clients with neurological injury or impairment such as stroke and traumatic brain injury. The principles of neuroplasticity and their applicability to neurorehabilitation were first demonstrated in animal experiments, most prominently those carried out by Nudo and colleagues in the early 1990's (Nudo et al 1996). The results of these studies inspired profound changes in the way rehabilitation interventions are designed and deployed (Kleim 2008, Langhorne et al 2011, Maier et al 2019).

Evidence suggests that functional task-specific training within a meaningful context supports neuroplastic changes and skill acquisition (Levac et al 2019, You et al 2005). Innovative technologies can be used to enhance the guiding principles of physiotherapy practice outlined in Chapter 1. Interactive technologies demand focus and attention, and can motivate the user to move by providing them with a sense of achievement, even if they cannot correctly perform a given task in the 'real world' (Lange et al 2009, Rose et al 2005).

Motor learning is defined as a process of acquisition or modification of a motor skill or behaviour (Shishov et al 2017). It can also be defined as relatively permanent internal changes that occur as a function of practice (Lage et al 2015). Practice refers to the repetition of movements and involves a conscious effort of organisation, execution or evaluation, and modification of the motor actions in each attempt (Lage et al 2015). The initial stage of motor learning is defined as the cognitive stage, in which the learner's attention is strongly focused on task performance. In this phase, attention is fundamental to the performance of the task, and there are many errors and variability of the movement. In the early stages of motor learning, the greater variability in motor behaviour is common until a more effective motor strategy is experienced by the learner. Interactive technologies provide an ideal environment in which to explore different motor behaviours, make and correct errors and provide opportunities for repetition of a task in a controlled environment. To the extent that the most effective motor behaviour for task performance is selected, this can lead to a reduction in motor behaviour variability, a decrease in the number of errors, the elimination of unnecessary motor gestures, a reduction in attentional demand for performance of the task and, finally, the reduction of energy expenditure (Shishov et al 2017). The second stage of motor learning is described as the associative stage, in which the need for attention and the variability of movement decreases. During the acquisition phase of the new skill, a decrease in the number of errors, an increase in execution speed and a decrease in the energy expenditure for the performance of the task are observed. The improvement of the motor performance and the variability of the movement decreases as performance of the task becomes more consistent. Interactive technologies have potential to provide a controlled environment in which one can practice a task. The last stage of motor learning is automatic, in which the apprentice can perform the task learned with fewer attentional requirements. At this stage, the learner can perform two or more tasks concomitant with the skill learned (Shishov et al 2017). In this stage, the motor skill can be transferred to similar contexts, which is known as *adaptability*. In this case, when a certain parameter of the task is modified, the performance is still maintained (Lage et al 2015, Levac et al 2016, Makino et al 2016, Shishov et al 2017). For example, when the weight or size of a soccer ball is changed, the individual who has already learned the motor skill of kicking a soccer ball is able to maintain a performance similar to the learned condition. Interactive technologies and game-based tasks provide unique opportunities to modify the environment or context in which a task is performed and add distractions, remove feedback or modify the attentional requirements and cognitive load of the task.

Rehabilitation is based on practical modifications to the learning of motor skills across these three stages of motor learning. The process of motor learning essentially depends on practice. Motor learning is characterised by the slow acquisition of the skill, dependent on the number of repetitions of the motor task and the association between learned ability and the task that is specifically trained. Studies have investigated the factors that may influence the relearning of motor tasks, suggesting it is not only the repetition that contributes to motor learning but also motivation and feedback. Among the tools investigated, interactive technologies can provide systematic feedback and motivate users to engage in highly repetitive tasks that promote motor learning (Darekar et al 2015, Demers et al 2021, Holden, 2005).

The game-based elements of motor skills practiced with interactive technologies can provide meaningful practice of salient tasks. For example, dos Santos Mendes et al (2012) analysed the motor learning of people with Parkinson's using Nintendo Wii Fit games. Participants practiced 10 different games with specific motor and cognitive tasks. Motor learning was assessed by observing the performance of participants during the practice sessions. To assess whether the changes of motor performance of participants were persistent, the authors assessed performance 30 days after the end of the acquisition phase. Results showed that participants improved and maintained skilled performance after 30 days, in 7 of the 10 trained games. Participants were also able to transfer the motor skills to a similar postural task performed in a real environment (dos Santos Mendes et al 2012).

Motor learning is strongly influenced by feedback, characterised as information about the movement performed. Feedback can be extrinsic or intrinsic (Shumway-Cook & Woollacott 2017). The intrinsic feedback comes from an individual's sensory system. Thus somatosensory information such as proprioception, nociception and other sensory modalities are fundamental for movement planning and control (Shumway-Cook & Woollacott 2017). The extrinsic feedback comes from additional environmental sources about the motor act and can be classified as either 'knowledge of performance' or 'knowledge of results' (Shumway-Cook & Woollacott 2017). For example, verbal information about the pattern of the learner's movement is a type of feedback related to performance. Information about the consequences of the motor task refers to knowledge of the results. Motor learning is a process that fundamentally depends on practice, and the type and frequency of feedback can influence the effectiveness of the process (Shumway-Cook & Woollacott 2017). Interactive technologies and game-based tasks can provide many different types of feedback. Players can receive visual, auditory and even tactile feedback regarding their task goals and committed errors. Task progress can be visualised through increasing or decreasing points or game scores. At the end of the trial, the player usually receives information about the results of their performance through the total score. Some applications have the capability to provide a visual replay of the gameplay. Together, both kinds of feedback, knowledge of performance and knowledge of results, have potential to improve the motor learning process. dos Santos Mendes et al (2012) analysed the learning of virtual tasks in individuals with Parkinson's. In this study, participants practiced four games of Microsoft Kinect 'Kinect Adventures' game that contained motivational elements such as visual and auditory stimuli that indicated task progress such as gold coins, real-time scoring, motivational sounds and unlocking advanced game levels. The authors postulate that these elements helped participants to maintain motivation for continued training, minimising the impact of monotonous movements and gameplay. Moreover, in all games, feedback of movement through visual and auditory stimuli was continuously present. Avatars (virtual characters) were used to visualise the movements performed by the player, providing additional real-time performance feedback. Some researchers argue that observing the action of an avatar may increase the effects of training by activating mirror neurones (Borrego et al 2019, Buccino et al 2012, Pelosin et al 2010, 2013). An external focus of attention (attention on the effect of the movement) has been demonstrated to be more effective in motor learning than an internal focus of attention (i.e., focus on own body movements) (Wulf et al 2010).

KEY POINTS

- Interactive technologies involve real-time two-way flow of information based on user input (e.g., gestures, touch screen, sensors) and a response output from the system (in the form of visual, audio, haptic and/or assistive feedback).
- Interactive technologies can encourage and motivate people to move and provide an opportunity to practice meaningful task-specific training activities.
- Interactive technologies can provide multimodal feedback on performance and results.
- There is evidence to support the 'active ingredients' of interactive technologies in rehabilitation to enhance motor learning.
- More investigation to identify and quantify the effect of individual interactive technology intervention features on motor learning and the transfer of learning to real-world activities is needed.

TYPES OF TECHNOLOGIES USED IN THE REHABILITATION SETTING

The makeup of interactive technologies varies, but interactive systems generally consist of hardware and software that provide input into the system and output from the system. Hardware includes both input and output devices. Input devices send information to the system for processing. This can include tracking hardware such as sensors that track the device or the user's head, hand, eyes and/or body as they move and interact with the activity. Tracking can be achieved through various integrated or peripheral devices such as hand controllers, gloves, image processing or eye tracking. Use of buttons or keys on a keyboard, controller or handheld device that send commands to the system can also be used for input. Output hardware is the information displayed or sent by a system. Displays can include physical devices such as monitors, touch-screen tablets, projectors, goggles/glasses or headsets on which the visual content is displayed. Audio output includes sound played through the display hardware or through an additional speaker hardware or device. Haptic output includes sensory feedback provided to the user through controllers, gloves or wearable devices. Active assistance can be provided through robotic devices that can provide body weight support and/or guide movement. Software is the computer programme that contains the two-dimensional (2D), three-dimensional (3D) or video-based environment and the instructions of how it can be interacted with. Software can generally run on a variety of operating systems including Windows, Mac, Android and iOS as well as via a variety of modern web browsers, game systems and/or specialised systems. Content relates to the specific aim or goal of the experience intended for the user. It is the application / game / interaction / experience. Content is the meaning and purpose of the software programme and drives the design of the software and hardware. Content can range from visualisations of movement to game-based activities to complex functional tasks.

Game-based rehabilitation involves the use of commercially available video games (designed for entertainment) or games or activities specifically designed for rehabilitation (Lange et al 2010). Recent generations of commercially available video games are based on virtual scenarios in which the player is encouraged to solve physically and cognitively demanding tasks using physical interaction and/or gestures. Commercially available game consoles have a great variety of movement-based games, each with specific rules and goals that require and encourage coordinated movements of the body in sitting and/or standing positions. One of the main differences between the various video game consoles involves the hardware used to interact with the video game tasks. Some examples are provided in the next section. It is important to understand that these systems have been designed for entertainment and have not been designed specifically for use in the rehabilitation setting. This means that clinicians have limited control over the content and how it is used by clients. Additional challenges exist in the pace at which commercial gaming technologies are updated, making older hardware and software obsolete. Applications that have been designed specifically for rehabilitation can leverage commercially available hardware but present content that is more tailored for rehabilitation goals. Clinicians generally have more control over the content. Although initially many of the tailored systems were developed in the research setting, the growth of the field in recent years has seen more commercially available rehabilitation technologies enter the market. Some of these

systems have been evaluated; however, others have not undergone evaluation or testing.

Extended reality is an overarching term that has been used to describe the use of interactive technologies to enhance, extend or change a person's reality (Andrews et al 2019, Palmas & Klinker 2020). XR encompasses interactive technologies such as VR and AR. VR has been defined as 'an artificial environment which is experienced through sensory stimuli (such as sights and sounds) provided by a computer and in which one's actions partially determine what happens in the environment' (Merriam-Webster, n.d.b). This means that VR places the user in a virtual environment that they can interact with, and VR systems range on a scale of nonimmersive to immersive. VR systems can be made up of a range of different combinations of hardware, software and interaction methods, and examples range from mobile games on tablets and phones, commercially available video game systems, systems viewed through a head-mounted display, fully enclosed platform or room-size tracking systems, and the use of robotic devices to actively assist movement and/or support the user. Nonimmersive VR such as traditional video games can be presented on a monitor or projector and typically use a keyboard or controller to interact with the environment. Immersive VR blocks out the user's view of the real world and transports them to a virtual environment that can be presented through a headset or large enclosed or semi-enclosed set of display monitors such as a Cave Automatic Virtual Environment (CAVE) system. AR has been defined as '…an enhanced version of reality created by the use of technology to overlay digital information on an image of something being viewed through a device (such as a smartphone camera)' (Merriam-Webster, n.d.a). AR senses the real environment using cameras and sensors and projects virtual information visually onto the person's view of the existing environment. One of the benefits of AR is that virtual images are overlayed onto the real environment. XR tools have been used in a range of areas including entertainment and gaming, training for a range of fields including healthcare professionals, and rehabilitation. As the field evolves, some inconsistency exists in the terminology used for virtual rehabilitation, which can make it challenging when reviewing and interpreting the literature. For the purpose of this chapter, we have chosen to use the more general term interactive technologies to describe the range of different technologies, including VR and AR, that can be used in the rehabilitation setting.

Interactive technologies can be used across different settings to support a range of goals throughout the rehabilitation journey. Home-based rehabilitation technologies range from simple digital exercise programmes to more complex and targeted sensor-based technologies. Robotic devices require more complex and often expensive systems that benefit from clinician assistance, support and monitoring. Robotic-assisted training is more commonly used in the inpatient or outpatient settings. Finally, wearable technologies have been used across settings for assessment and monitoring of progress and recovery.

Technologies for Home-Based Rehabilitation

Home-based exercise programmes are an integral part of rehabilitation interventions. Because access to one-on-one outpatient therapy sessions is limited, adherence to home-based exercise programmes is key to achieve mass motor practice and hence clinically significant motor gains. Adherence to home-based exercise programmes is poor, often preventing clients from achieving the amount of practice that is sufficient to maximise motor gains. To encourage adherence, clinicians often provide clients with handwritten notes and/or printouts of the list of prescribed therapeutic exercises. Clinicians have recently started to use electronic platforms that encourage client adherence by relying on electronic calendars, reminders delivered using mobile devices and web-based applications that demonstrate the correct modality of performance of the prescribed exercises via videoclips and educational material. Many of these web-based applications are also used for televisits, which are becoming more common with the impact of Covid-19 on in-person clinic visits.

The simplest of these systems to 'electronically prescribe' a home-based exercise intervention typically allows clinicians to send an email message to their clients with a link to a webpage or mobile application (app) that provides them with the list of exercises that the clinician has chosen for them. Typically, therapeutic exercises are selected from a library of exercises that are part of the web-based platform/app. The exercises are presented via videoclips that demonstrate how to perform the exercises with correct form. Some products also provide videoclips explaining mistakes to avoid and encouraging clients to maintain adherence. Adherence data are available to the clinicians for remote monitoring of their clients. Examples of commercially available systems for home-based rehabilitation interventions include Exercise Pro Live (Exercise Pro Live), MedBridge (MedBridge), Physiotech (Physiotech), Physitrack (Physitrack), Real Time Rehab (Real Time Rehab), Sword Health (Sword Health) and Wellpepper (Wellpepper). The use of these systems has gained momentum as a result of Covid-19 lockdowns and ongoing impacts on in-person clinic and home-based healthcare visits. However, evidence supporting the use of these apps is limited and more research is needed (Bonura et al 2022, Burns et al 2021).

Sensor-Based Systems

A significant shortcoming of simple electronic prescribing systems is that they do not provide appropriate feedback about the exercise form. They might provide instructions about how to avoid common mistakes, but they are not able to 'observe' the client and generate client-specific feedback for each repetition of the exercise routine. In other words, neither the clients nor their clinicians know whether the home-based exercises have been performed in an appropriate manner unless clinicians connect with clients via videocall, which is most often impractical. To address this problem, a second generation of systems for home-based rehabilitation has been developed that uses sensing technology to monitor clients as they perform the exercises. The most traditional among these systems are standalone systems, namely, systems that are not designed for remote connection between the client and clinician. These systems are typically based on interactive games such as gaming systems or VR. They are designed to gather data from peripheral sensors or body-worn sensors as input to control the games. These systems have potential to encourage correct performance of the exercises by relying on elements of the interactive game that discourage, for instance, the performance of compensatory movements to achieve the game goals more easily (Lange et al 2009).

Early examples of standalone game-based systems include video gaming consoles that were designed and marketed for entertainment. Much of the research in interactive technologies for neurorehabilitation has focused on the use of video gaming systems. The Nintendo Wii, Nintendo's fifth console, was released in 2006. Among its features, the Wii introduced an innovative wireless controller, Wii Remote, capable of detecting movements through an accelerometer and infrared sensor. The Wii Remote allows the user to interact with the video game software through upper limb movements and control. One of the most used Nintendo Wii games in research on the use of game-based interactive technologies in upper limb rehabilitation is Wii Sports. Wii Sports includes five distinct sport experiences using the Wii Remote – Tennis, Baseball, Golf, Bowling and Boxing – that can be played in the comfort of one's living room. The player can use the Wii Remote to mimic the actions of the sports and interact with the virtual tasks using upper limb movements. These characteristics of the Nintendo Wii provide opportunities for clinicians to use these games for rehabilitation of the upper limb or to challenge balance in standing or sitting of people with neurological conditions.

The Nintendo Wii Fit was released in 2007. The Wii Fit Balance Board is a sensor-based input device that allows players to perform balance tasks using a balance board that

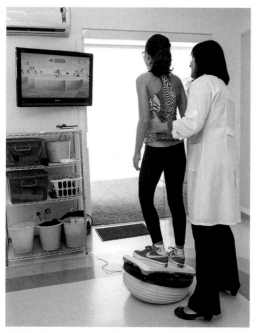

FIG. 20.1 Client playing Nintendo Wii Fit Penguin game. The Wii Fit balance board is being used on an unstable surface to challenge balance.

contains sensors that capture the displacement of the user's centre of pressure and uses this information to control the movements of a virtual avatar or virtual objects in the game environment (Fig. 20.1). Compared with a standard force platform, the Wii Fit Balance Board has been demonstrated to provide a valid and reliable measure of centre of pressure (Clark et al 2010, Holmes et al 2013, Hubbard et al 2012). Depending on the game, fast and controlled body displacements are required to interact with the virtual tasks. Multidirectional displacement of the body's centre of pressure can challenge stability, as well as stimulate and potentially improve postural control responses of the players. Although a large body of research exists supporting the use of the systems in rehabilitation, the Nintendo Wii and WiiFit are no longer supported by Nintendo. Nintendo's latest console, Nintendo Switch, was released in 2017 and does not support motion tracking that can be leveraged in rehabilitation.

More recent examples of standalone systems are shown in Fig. 20.2. Fig. 20.2A shows the ArmeoSenso (Hocoma). The system is designed to facilitate the performance of therapeutic exercises by clients with hemiparesis (e.g., stroke and traumatic brain injury patients). Sensors are used to track the movements of the upper limbs and trunk in 3D. The detected movements are used as input to interactive games. The games are chosen based on the objectives of the prescribed rehabilitation intervention. The ArmeoSenso system (Hocoma 2021) is suitable for use both in the clinic and in the home setting. Although we are not aware of any clinical trial that has explored the use of the ArmeoSenso system for group therapy, a study by Wittmann et al (2016) showed that the ArmeoSenso can be used for self-directed arm therapy, leading to high-dosage interventions. Widmer et al (2022) used the ArmeoSenso for an intervention study in which clinicians provided minimum supervision. The results of these clinical investigations suggest that the ArmeoSenso is suitable for self-directed, home-based therapy and support indirectly the statement that the system is suitable for group therapy.

Fig. 20.2B shows the MusicGlove system (FlintRehab). The system consists of an instrumented glove and a computer system that are used to encourage clients to practice individual finger movements and grasp/release movements as clients play video games. In clinical studies using the system, Friedman and colleagues (2011, 2014) showed improvements in hand function in response to therapy relying on the MusicGlove. Specifically, they showed better results on the Box and Block test (but no difference in Fugl-Meyer Assessment Upper Extremity [FMA-UE] and Wolf Motor Function Test [WMFT] scores) in a group of stroke patients training with the MusicGlove compared with control subjects. The system is designed to be low cost, which is a desirable characteristic when one considers a deployment in the home setting.

Another low-cost system is shown in Fig. 20.2C. It is called FitMi, and it is also a product by FlintRehab (2022). The system is a sensor-based object that clients are encouraged to manipulate as part of a simple game requiring the performance of hand grasp/release movements and forearm pronation/supination movements, as these are movements that stroke patients have significant difficulties performing.

Numerous other sensor-based systems have been developed and tested by researchers for upper limb and gait rehabilitation. Arteaga et al (2008) developed a low-cost prototype system equipped with 10 inertial measurement units (IMUs) to track clients' posture and generate feedback using sound, vibration and light-emitting diode (LED) lights. Dorsch et al (2015) and Byl et al (2015) developed sensor-based systems for gait training and used them in both the inpatient and the outpatient settings. Although these studies were not performed in the home and community settings, the form factor of these systems is suitable for home therapy.

In contrast to standalone systems, systems that have been developed as an evolution of the simple systems (i.e., by adding wearable sensors to systems designed to prescribe

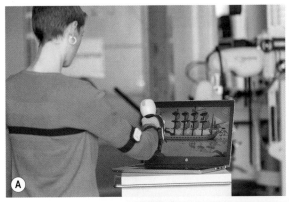
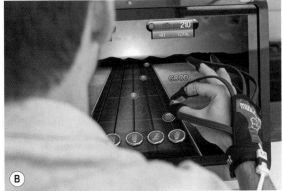
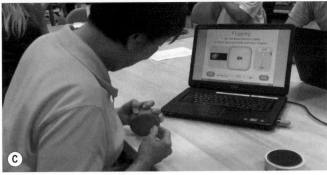

FIG. 20.2 Examples of sensor-based systems for home-based rehabilitation. (A) The ArmeoSenso (Source: Hocoma AG), (B) The MusicGlove (Source: FlintRehab), and (C) FitMi (Source: FlintRehab).

home-based exercises) would typically track exercise form, provide feedback to clients if the exercises are not performed properly and provide regular reporting to clinicians to track progress. However, the activity is not currently integrated into an interactive game (at least not in the products that we have examined as of today). Examples of the systems that provide sensor-based input for feedback on exercises but are more focused on basic exercises rather than game-based interactions are the first-generation Hinge Health system for low back pain (Hinge Health) and the Sword Health system for musculoskeletal pain (Sword Health).

Video Analysis

A third generation of home-based exercise systems is now emerging. This new family of systems leverages recent advances in machine learning that resulted in the development of video analysis techniques with unprecedented performance. Video hardware ranges from low-cost video cameras to more complex infrared depth-sensing cameras (i.e., cameras that provide data fully suitable to derive 3D reconstructions). These techniques can track 'key points' (i.e., anatomical landmarks) and derive skeleton representations of the movements displayed by clients. Several software libraries are currently available for video analysis, including AlphaPose (Fang et al 2017), ArtTrack (Insafutdinov et al 2017), DeeperCut (Insafutdinov et al 2016), DeepLabCut (Mathis et al 2018), DeepPose (Toshev 2014), MediaPipe and OpenPose (Cao et al 2017, 2021). These software libraries rely on deep learning algorithms designed to track key points – such as the ankle, knee and hip joint positions – and derive a simplified (skeleton) representation of the body. This process is referred to as 'pose estimation'. Importantly, the algorithms can rely on data collected using low-cost video cameras.

These motion tracking techniques do not provide estimates of clients' movements as accurately as camera-based motion capture systems typically found in research laboratories. However, they provide estimates marked by accuracy that is sufficient to generate feedback during the performance of home-based exercises. The potential applications of these machine learning algorithms to the field of rehabilitation are countless. Recent reviews have discussed their potential impact on clinical practice (Arac 2020, Cronin 2021, Seethapathi et al 2019).

The release of the Microsoft Xbox 360 with the Microsoft Kinect in 2010 had a significant impact on the use and development of video analysis-based interactive technologies that spanned far beyond the world of video games and has reached into areas of the daily lives of people who are not traditionally identified as 'gamers'. The next versions of the Microsoft Xbox and Kinect sensor were released in 2013: Microsoft Xbox One with Kinect for Xbox One and Kinect for Windows v2. The Microsoft Kinect uses an infrared sensor and video camera to track the user in 3D space within an area of 6 m². Similar technologies have been released by other companies, including Asus XION, Intel RealSense and Leap Motion. The Leap Motion uses infrared cameras and infrared LEDs to track the user's hands and fingers within a smaller volume rather than tracking gross full-body movements. Despite differences in tracking technology for each camera system, hand and full-body tracking can be engaging and intuitive means to interact with games and interactive applications, serving a dual role as input device and data collection tool.

Microsoft Kinect games require postural responses like those of the Nintendo Wii Fit; however, the Nintendo Wii Fit requires more static control because the player must stand or step on/off of the Wii Fit Balance Board to interact with the game task. The Microsoft Kinect games demand fast responses combining movements of multidirectional steps with upper extremity reaching movements (Fig. 20.3). In some Kinect game tasks, players are required to jump and crouch while changing direction of movements. The player is not restricted to one area but can be tracked within an area of 6 m². The accuracy of the Microsoft Kinect's body tracking in 3D space is dependent on the position of the user in front of the sensor, self-occlusion and the presence of other objects within the field of view (Da Gama et al 2015). A range of content using the Microsoft Kinect sensor with game-based applications specifically developed for rehabilitation has been evaluated (Chang et al 2012, Da Gama et al 2015, Lange et al 2010, 2012, Mousavi Hondori & Khademi 2014, Webster & Celik 2014). The Microsoft Kinect sensor is no longer supported by Microsoft Xbox; however, the Microsoft Azure Kinect was released in 2020 as a separate hardware device with a focus on robotics, healthcare and retail sectors instead of gaming and entertainment. The Microsoft Azure Kinect has been used in a range of pilot studies exploring game-based rehabilitation for a range of conditions (Amprimo et al 2022, Belotti et al 2022, Królikowska et al 2023).

Several studies have started to explore the possibility of using these video analysis techniques to derive estimates of clinical assessment measures (Cornman et al 2021, Stenum

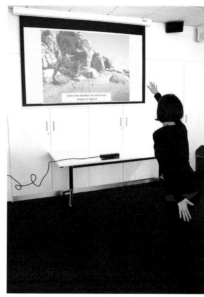

FIG. 20.3 The Microsoft Kinect tracks the user without markers or handheld devices. The user can reach for virtual objects while sitting or standing.

et al 2021). A few studies have explored their use for tracking upper limb and hand movements (Ahmed et al 2021, Zhu et al 2021). Ahmed and colleagues (2021) explored tracking movement during the performance of home-based rehabilitation exercises and outlined work accomplished towards the development of a platform for upper limb home-based exercises named the Semi-Automated Rehabilitation at the Home (SARAH) system. The system relies on OpenPose (Cao et al 2017, 2021) and on the output of an object tracking and recognition algorithm (Ren et al 2015). A substantial body of literature has been focused on the technical validation of these algorithms, especially in the analysis of gait patterns (Mehdizadeh et al 2021, Stenum et al 2021, Takeda et al 2021, Viswakumar et al 2021).

These technical developments – enabled by work recently accomplished in the field of deep learning – have led to several products that not only allow clinicians to electronically prescribe a home-based exercise routine but also track clients using video analysis techniques and generate feedback accordingly. The following are commercially available systems that enable the prescription of exercises for home-based therapy that already provide video tracking capability: BlueJay Mobile Health (2022), Evolv Rehabilitation Technologies (2022), the new Hinge Health product (based on video analysis) (2022), Kaia Health (2022), UINCARE (2022) and WizeCare (2022). Fig. 20.4

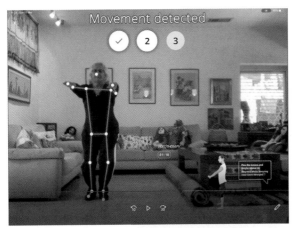

FIG. 20.4 An example (WizeCare) of the video tracking capability embedded in systems for home-based rehabilitation. The system provides therapists with the opportunity to prescribe a battery of home-based exercises. The tracking system provides a skeleton representation from which one can derive adherence and exercise form data. An avatar (bottom right) demonstrates the exercises and encourages patients during the session (Source: https://dev.wizecare.com/).

shows a screen capture of the WizeCare system. The screen capture shows a client (left side of the screen) performing an exercise routine at home, a stick diagram representation of the client based on the key points tracked by the system and an avatar (bottom right of the screen) that guides the client throughout the session.

The deep learning algorithms used by these platforms are often suitable for both standard (i.e., monocular) low-cost cameras and depth cameras (i.e., cameras that provide data fully suitable to derive 3D reconstructions). The availability of sensing technologies, advanced video analysis algorithms and web-based platforms for electronic prescription of home-based exercises is changing dramatically the way rehabilitation interventions are deployed in the home setting.

Virtual Reality Headsets

In recent years, VR headsets have become more affordable and accepted. VR headsets are a goggle-like display device that is worn over the head with small LCD or organic LED (OLED) displays in front of each eye. Different types of headsets are available for use with VR systems, ranging in price from tens of thousands of pounds to around 300 pounds. The VR headsets that are available differ in the display technology (LCD versus OLED display), display resolution (the higher the resolution, the clearer the

image), refresh rate (motion appears smoother with higher refresh rates, typically >60–90 frames per second), latency (time between input and output – the longer the latency, the more lag between input and output), field of view, head tracking (3 degrees of freedom – only tracking head rotation; 6 degrees of freedom – also tracking head translation through additional cameras), eye tracking within headsets (e.g., FOVE, Tobii eye tracker) and input devices (e.g., hand-tracked controllers).

Affordable consumer VR headsets are available. The Oculus Rift, developed by Oculus VR, was released in 2016. It has a 110° field of view and uses a Constellation tracking camera to track the user within an area of 5 feet by 11 feet. The HTC Vive, developed by HTC and Valve, was released in 2016. It has a 110° field of view and sensors located on the headset with a laser-based tracking system to provide room-scale tracking, enabling the user to walk around in an area of approximately 20 m². Two fully tracked, hand-held wireless controllers can be used to interact with virtual objects (Fig. 20.5A). One limitation of the HTC Vive is that the sensors required for tracking the headset need to be mounted on a wall or placed on tripods to form a 4.5 m by 4.5 m tracking space, reducing the portability of the setup. A simpler and more accessible VR headset, Google Cardboard, released in 2015, is a cardboard headset shell in which a smartphone can be mounted. It is made up on a cardboard sheet, two lenses, two magnets, two Velcro strips and one rubber band. An updated version of the headset was released as Google Daydream, offering a more comfortable headset design with padding. When used with stereoscopic display software and specifically developed mobile apps installed on the smartphone, these VR headsets are affordable, accessible VR systems. Like the concept of Google Cardboard and Daydream, the Samsung Gear VR was developed by Samsung and released in 2015 for use with Samsung Galaxy and Note smartphones. The Samsung Gear VR provides a headset shell in which Samsung Galaxy and Note smartphones can be mounted and special software used to provide a passive or interactive VR experience (see Fig. 20.5B). The VR headset technologies are evolving so rapidly that many of these early VR headset systems are no longer supported in 2022. More recent headsets such as the Meta Quest 2 (released in 2020; see Fig. 20.5C), the HP Reverb G2 (released in 2020) and the Meta Quest Pro (released in 2022) are smaller, lighter and contain more features. For example, the Meta Quest Pro includes eye tracking and contains options for presentation of both AR and VR content.

Early research exploring the use of VR headsets in neurorehabilitation describes the development and initial evaluation of customised software to support rehabilitation (Høeg et al 2021a, Shah et al 2022, Shen et al 2020), but

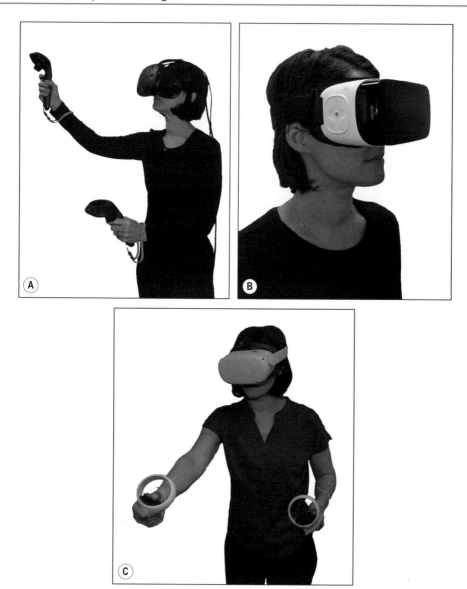

FIG. 20.5 Virtual reality headset. (A) User wearing HTC Vive headset with handheld controllers (Source: HTC Vive). (B) Samsung Gear VR headset uses a smartphone as the screen. The smartphone is inserted inside the headset (Source: Samsung Gear). (C) Meta Quest 2 VR headset with handheld controllers (Source: Meta Quest).

there is limited evidence for the effectiveness of VR headset interventions in neurorehabilitation. In addition to the research-focused systems (e.g., Marin-Pardo et al 2020, Vaezipour et al 2022), several companies have released rehabilitation-specific VR headset systems and software: REALSystem VR (Penumbra 2022, Wu et al 2019), XRHealth (Kalron et al 2022, XRHealth 2022), InMotionVR (2022) and Corpus VR (2022). Many of the claims related to the use of VR headset systems in rehabilitation quote the early literature in virtual rehabilitation that evaluated the use of video game systems (e.g., Nintendo Wii, Microsoft Kinect) and research systems that did not use VR headset hardware (Høeg et al 2021b). Further research is needed to evaluate the effectiveness and safety of the use of VR

KEY POINTS

- Simple home-based exercise interventions provide examples of exercises but do not provide specific feedback on performance.
- Sensor-based systems use sensors worn or held by the user to track movement and provide feedback on performance within an interactive gaming activity.
- Video analysis uses machine learning approaches for motion tracking analysis of data captured from video or infrared depth sensing cameras.
- VR headsets have potential to be used to provide interactive rehabilitation, but more research is needed.

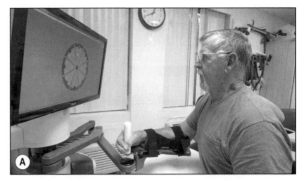

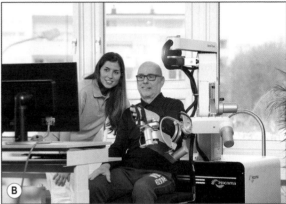

FIG. 20.6 Robotic systems for upper limb rehabilitation. (A) MIT Manus, an end-effector system developed at MIT (Source: www.bioniklabs.com). (B) Armeo Power, an exoskeleton system originally developed at ETH Zurich (as the ARMin robotic system) and later modified to lead to the current product (Source: Hocoma AG).

headset systems in rehabilitation. It is anticipated that the research and development in this area will grow substantially in coming years.

Robot-Assisted Motor Training

Robotic devices provide active assistance to the client to support, assist or drive movement. Robotic devices vary in complexity, setup and amount of assistance provided to the user. These devices can target rehabilitation goals for upper limb, lower limb or gait training. Some robots integrate VR or AR activities to support engagement. Other robots target only the robot-assisted training activity without visual or auditory feedback.

Fig. 20.6 shows two examples of robots for upper limb motor training. Fig. 20.6A shows the MIT Manus, an end-effector system. The robot was originally developed at Massachusetts Institute of Technology (MIT) based on a new approach proposed by Hogan (1987), who pioneered the development of systems for robot-assisted neurorehabilitation. End-effector systems are robots with a single point of contact with the client, typically the distal component of a robotic arm that provides unloading and movement assistance. In contrast, exoskeleton systems are robots with components that are strapped to different body segments. Fig. 20.6B shows an example of such system, namely, the ARMin, a commercially available system based on work carried out in Robert Riener's laboratory at Eidgenössische Technische Hochschule (ETH) Zurich (Nef et al 2007) that eventually led to launching the robot as a Hocoma product and to clinical investigation showing motor gains associated with its use (Klamroth-Marganska et al 2014).

These robotic systems are generally controlled using a control modality called impedance control. Impedance control is a control modality that is based on setting a target trajectory of movement and generating a mechanical effect around the target trajectory that is equivalent to attaching

a spring and a damper to the trajectory of motion. This control modality allowed researchers to explore the use of robotics in motor training of the upper limbs and later to assess its clinical potential in pilot studies (Aisen et al 1997, Krebs et al 1998) that showed great promise. Experiments carried out with rehabilitation robots pointed out the relevance of factors such as unloading and movement assistance, where considerations about unloading were largely inspired by work carried out by Dewald and colleagues (Beer et al 2007, Dewald & Beer 2001, Dewald et al 1995, Miller & Dewald 2012).

End-effector systems are typically easier to use because the setup time is quick. The client holds onto the distal component of the robotic arm, the working volume is calibrated, the clinician chooses the level of unloading and movement assistance and the client is ready to start the training session. Exoskeleton systems are typically more cumbersome to use because they require adjustments in the length of the exoskeleton segments to accommodate for different arm sizes and carefully align the centre of rotation of the anatomical joints with the centre of rotation of the exoskeleton joints. This is critical to avoid excessive loads on the anatomical joints. Then clinicians proceed with the calibration of the working volume, and they choose the level of unloading and movement assistance before the client is ready to start the session. The advantage of exoskeleton systems is that once the robot's joints are carefully aligned with the anatomical joints, the loads on the anatomical joints can be precisely controlled, hence avoiding excessive loads on the anatomical joints. In fact, robotic joints can be selectively locked, leading to 'protecting' individual joints. This is not possible with end-effector systems, which are therefore less desirable when clients present with joint instabilities.

Robotic systems have also been designed for gait training. Fig. 20.7 shows an end-effector system (Fig. 20.7A) called GEO (Reha Technology AG) and an exoskeleton system (Fig. 20.7B) called Lokomat (Hocoma AG) for gait training. End-effector systems for gait training were first proposed by Hesse and colleagues, who pioneered the use of footplates that moved the feet to mimic the trajectory of movement during level-ground walking (Hesse & Uhlenbrock 2000, Schmidt et al 2007) and evaluated them in clinical studies with positive results (Pohl et al 2007). The first commercially available system developed by Hesse's research team was called the Gait Trainer and was somewhat like the GEO shown in Fig. 20.7A. Exoskeleton systems for gait training were pioneered by Colombo and

his colleagues (Colombo et al 2000, Jezernik et al 2003) and later shown to be effective in several client populations (Alashram et al 2021, Belas dos Santos et al 2018, Nam et al 2017). End-effector and exoskeleton systems for gait training have similar advantages and disadvantages as robotic systems for upper limb training. End-effector systems are marked by setup time that is virtually null but would not typically provide effective means to control proximal segments (i.e., movements of the pelvis and trunk). Vice versa, exoskeleton systems require significant setup time but provide accurate control on joint loads.

In addition to facilitating training, robots can be used to track the client's response to the rehabilitation intervention by analysing changes in motor patterns recorded during the training sessions. This has been shown by many authors for upper limb motor training (Merlo et al 2013, Straudi et al 2015, Volpe et al 2009), and results have been summarised in several review papers (de-la-Torre et al 2020, Zariffa et al 2011). Robots typically do not control (i.e., provide actuation) or 'allow' all the degrees of freedom. In other words, gait training robots might restrict movement to the sagittal plane or might provide actuation at the hip and knee but use springs to limit plantarflexion while otherwise not providing other ankle control. Clinicians should carefully consider on a client-by-client basis whether the technology available to them 'controls' all the degrees of freedom relevant to achieving their clinical objectives (Pietrusinski et al 2013).

Robots alone do not have the ability to selectively target all aspects of the biomechanics and neural control of

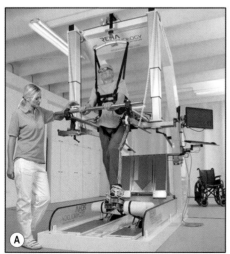
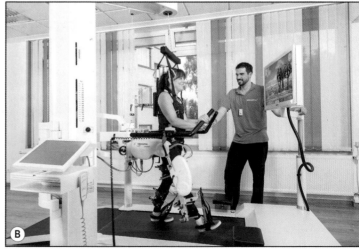

FIG. 20.7 Robotic systems for gait training. (A) GEO, an end-effector system based on footplates whose trajectory simulates ambulatory function (Source: https://www.mossrehab.com/g-eo). (B) Lokomat, an exoskeleton-based system developed by Hocoma AG (Source: Hocoma AG).

movement that are relevant in the context of gait training of neurological clients. In fact, experiments have suggested that it is sometimes difficult to predict what changes in motor patterns will be observed in response to a force field generated by the robot. Certain changes cannot be achieved by solely relying on the haptic feedback generated by the robotic system. It has been suggested that attention should be paid to studying the individual interaction with the robot (Cajigas et al 2017). Not everything can be achieved via haptic feedback, and other input modalities should always be considered. VR and AR as well as interactive games are key to achieving changes in motor patterns that are not 'achievable' using haptic feedback alone (Clark et al 2019, Ferreira dos Santos et al 2016, Kim et al 2020, Makhataeva & Varol, 2020, Mubin et al 2019).

In considering VR and AR as well as interactive games, rehabilitation specialists often put emphasis on achieving a good level of client engagement. Clinicians would go out of their way to achieve client's active participation during the robot-assisted rehabilitation session. That is important because sessions during which clients are not actively engaged will most likely lead to no improvements in motor ability. However, attention should also be paid to the integration between visual input and motor tasks. This is referred to as *visuomotor integration*, which is known to be impaired in many neurological clients (e.g., stroke and traumatic brain injury patients). An example of application of these principles can be found in the study by Mirelman et al (2009) in which the authors trained all the participants using a robotic system, but only a subset of the study participants was challenged with a visuomotor integration task. The authors observed better clinical outcomes in the group who received training that combined robotics and interactive gaming. They argued that this was the case likely because the training addressed visuomotor integration impairments in the study participants even if, unfortunately, data collected during the study did not include the assessment of visuomotor integration impairments.

Robotic systems are an appealing tool when treating clients with severe motor impairments. They provide unloading and movement assistance. Hence clinicians can use them with clients even if they have limited residual motor output. In these clients, one would anticipate that active systems would be required. However, when residual motor abilities make it possible, passive 'robotic' systems should be considered. Properly speaking, robotic systems are devices with actuation, that is, motors that control the mechanical characteristics of the device. However, in the clinical environment, at times people would refer to passive systems as 'robotic systems' because they have similar characteristics to fully actuated systems. Although this is incorrect, it is worth emphasising that passive systems are often designed to be suitable to perform motor training in clients with neurological conditions, but with the ability to generate some residual motor output. In upper limb rehabilitation, systems that provide unloading via a spring-based exoskeleton (Colomer et al 2013, Gijbels et al 2011, Taveggia et al 2016) are sometimes referred to as 'robotic systems'. Again this is incorrect. However, these systems are often suitable to treat clients with moderate to severe motor impairments.

Recent advances in soft robotics have provided additional opportunities to achieve high-intensity, high-dosage, task-specific interventions. Interestingly, because soft robots are often designed to be 'worn', if they are configured for motor training, these systems could be used to deliver therapy all day long. In other words, wearable robots could provide the opportunity to extend rehabilitation beyond the clinical sessions. Fig. 20.8 shows two of the soft robotic systems developed by Walsh and his research team. Fig. 20.8A shows a lower limb exosuit designed to facilitate walking, and Fig. 20.8B shows a pneumatic glove designed to facilitate restoring hand function. This is part of the significant body of work done in this area by Walsh and his team at the Wyss Institute (Asbeck et al 2015, Awad et al 2017, 2020, Ding et al 2018, Kim et al 2019, Mosadegh et al 2014, Polygerinos et al 2015a, 2015b, Shin et al 2022).

Robotic systems should not be a replacement for traditional therapy. They are meant to facilitate motor practice rather than replace traditional one-on-one therapy. Ideally robots should be used to enable group therapy. Robotics is generally thought as most suitable for clients with severe impairments because these clients require assistance to perform motor tasks, whereas clients with mild to moderate impairments can undergo interventions without assistance (e.g., using constraint-induced movement therapy or similar techniques). Because robotics would be primarily used with clients with severe impairments, we would anticipate that robotics would be extensively used during the subacute phase after a neurological injury. However, this does not exclude the use of robotics in the chronic phases if clients experience severe residual impairments. In both the subacute and chronic phases, combining robotics and other intervention strategies should always be given proper consideration. Several techniques could be used in combination with physical therapy, most prominently pharmacotherapies and neuromodulation techniques, although obtaining good clinical outcomes requires identifying clients who could benefit from these techniques (Leon et al 2017, Pennati et al 2015, Tran et al 2016).

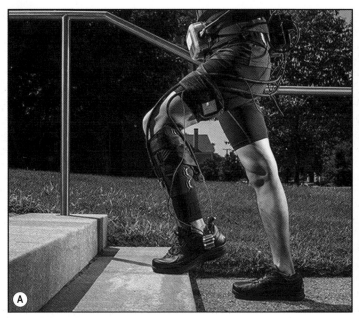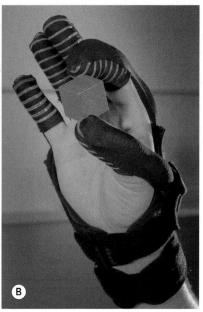

FIG. 20.8 Soft robotic systems to augment gait (A) and to facilitate retraining hand function (B). These systems are examples of wearable robots that could be utilised both to augment function and to extend rehabilitation outside of the clinic (Sources: A, from https://www.rolex.org/rolex-awards/applied-technology/conor-walsh and B, © Wyss Institute at Harvard University).

KEY POINTS

- Two types of robotic devices are used in rehabilitation: end-effector and exoskeleton systems. End-effector systems are marked by a shorter setup time, but exoskeleton systems can more accurately control the loads exerted by the robot on individual joints.
- Therapists should carefully observe changes in motor patterns displayed by neurological clients in response to robot-assisted rehabilitation because such changes are predictive of and correlate with motor gains achieved in response to robot-assisted training.
- VR, AR, and interactive games are an important component of robotic systems for rehabilitation. They are important not only because they encourage clients to be actively engaged during the training session (which is key to achieve motor gains) but also because they challenge the client's ability to perform visuomotor integration tasks.
- Recent advances in soft robotics have paved the way towards the development of robots that clients can wear all day long. If designed for this purpose, these systems could be an effective tool to extend rehabilitation beyond the walls of the clinics.

Wearable Technology for Field Assessments and Interventions

Recent advances in wearable technology have enabled the development of new approaches to monitor clinical outcomes and deploy interventions in the clinic and in the home and community setting (Dobkin & Dorsch 2011, Maceira-Elvira et al 2019, Patel et al 2012). We provide some examples of assessment and intervention techniques that rely on wearable technology and target motor functions; however, the technology provides researchers and clinicians with the ability to monitor the effects of and deploy rehabilitation interventions targeting additional domains (i.e., beyond motor function). Tracking rehabilitation outcomes is important in the context of designing and deploying interventions that maximise motor gains by accounting for the unique characteristics of each client. As they monitor the response to the prescribed rehabilitation intervention, clinicians can periodically assess whether changes in the treatment regime are needed.

A large body of work has been focused on developing techniques to estimate clinical scores via the analysis of wearable sensor data. Data are typically collected using IMUs during the performance of a battery of motor tasks. Various techniques have been developed to generate estimates of the FMA-UE subscale, the Functional Ability Scale (FAS), the Box and Block Test (BBT) and the Action Research Arm Test (ARAT) scores. Among others, Yu et al (2016) collected accelerometer and flex-sensor data from stroke patients as they performed seven movements derived from the items of the FMA-UE subscale. The sensor data were then analysed by developing a novel machine learning-based algorithm that provided accurate estimates of the FMA scores. Del Din et al (2011) gathered data using six accelerometers positioned on the trunk and the hemiparetic arm and hand of stroke and traumatic brain injury patients as they performed eight tasks taken from the item of the WMFT. They developed an algorithm based on an ensemble of decision trees (called random forest) that generated accurate estimates of the FMA scores. Patel et al (2010) took a similar approach to estimate FAS scores. Adans-Dester et al (2020) used the same experimental approach and generated improved estimates of FMA and FAS scores also using accelerometer-based data features that were fed to a random forest-based algorithm. Friedman et al (2011) showed that estimates of the BBT scores can be obtained via the analysis of data collected using a sensorised glove that they used to deploy an interactive gaming-based intervention. Repnik et al (2018) collected IMU and electromyographic data during the performance of the ARAT. The ARAT is a clinical test designed to assess motor capacity. The authors found a high level of correlation between the ARAT scores and the movement time and smoothness as derived using the sensor data.

This summarised body of work shows that sensor data collected during the performance of batteries of motor tasks taken from the items of standardised clinical assessments can be used as input to machine learning-based algorithms and thus generate accurate estimates of clinical scores. These batteries of motor tasks can be performed in the clinic or outside the clinic (via self-administration of the assessment or during a televisit). The estimated clinical scores capture the severity of motor impairments and the capacity for activity. In other words, they capture what clients can do but do not capture what clients actually do outside of the clinic. A significant amount of work has been devoted to addressing the latter issue, namely, to gather measures of the performance of activity. Fig. 20.9 provides a summary of the approach taken by Lang's research group (Bailey & Lang, 2014, Bailey et al 2014, 2015a, 2015b, Doman et al 2016, Lang et al 2013) to address this issue, that is, to derive measures of the performance of activity in the home and community settings. Fig. 20.9A shows the wrist units used to collect accelerometer data. Fig. 20.9B shows an example of raw accelerometer data (collected over 90 minutes). Fig. 20.9C shows six plots representing the upper limb activity of six stroke patients with low (top

plots), moderate (plots in the middle) and high (bottom plots) motor capability as captured by ARAT scores ranging from 10 (top plots) to 48 (bottom plots). The three plots on the left side show the data of individuals whose hemiparetic arm is the dominant arm. The three plots on the right show the data of individuals whose hemiparetic arm is the nondominant arm. Each plot consists of a collection of dots whose position on the horizontal axis represents the ratio of activity detected on the nonparetic side (points on the left) versus the activity detected on the paretic side (points on the right); the vertical axis represents how vigorous was the detected activity; finally, the colour of each dot represents the duration of the activity. These plots (and the parameters derived from these plots) capture the laterality of the activity performed by stroke patients, which is a function of the clients' ARAT scores. Interestingly, because the wrist units capture gross arm movements (as opposed to the fine motor control tasks involving the manipulation of objects), the plots are not affected by hand dominance.

Wearable technology has also been used to derive estimates of clinical scores that capture mobility limitations such the 10-metre walk test (10MWT) and the Timed Up and Go (TUG) test. The work done in this context has been geared towards 'instrumenting' standardised clinical tests for the purpose of collecting more in-depth information than clinical tests would typically do. For instance, Bergamini et al (2017) used a set of five IMUs to collect acceleration and angular velocity data from the pelvis, sternum and head during the performance of the 10MWT. The authors then derived parameters that capture, for instance, symmetry of movement, hence expanding upon the information that is typically collected during the clinical test. Similarly, Garcia et al (2021) collected IMU data during the performance of the 10MWT to derive a metric of gait smoothness (as a proxy measure of lower limb spasticity). Salarian et al (2010) and Wüest et al (2016) developed an instrumented version of the TUG test using IMU that provided the authors with the opportunity to estimate parameters capturing quality of movement during the performance of different phases of the test (e.g., sit to walk, turn to sit).

Wearable technology has been used not only to monitor activities but also to encourage clients to increase upper limb motor practice and increase their mobility. Preliminary studies suggest that promoting an increase in upper limb motor practice might be more challenging than promoting a mobility increase. Goal setting and coaching appear to be more critical when attempting to increase upper limb motor practice. Two different approaches have been tested so far in pilot studies. The first approach consists of providing clients with feedback about upper limb movement counts. Whitford et al (2018) carried out a study in eight chronic stroke patients. They monitored upper limb movements in study participants by using wrist-worn sensor units. Clinicians visited participants' homes three times per week and provided them with feedback about amount and symmetry of the activity detected by the sensor units. The intervention led to an increase in the perception of study participants of their use of the paretic arm. However, analysis of the accelerometer data suggested that no significant change in the amount of use of the paretic arm had occurred. Schwerz de Lucena et al (2021) used a device capable of monitoring the movements of the index finger (by relying on a ring made of ferromagnetic material and a magnetometer embedded in a wrist unit). The

authors recruited 20 chronic stroke patients and randomised them to one of two groups. Participants in the first group received feedback on movement counts and a daily goal chosen according to the severity of their impairment. Participants in the second group were monitored using the same technology but did not receive any feedback. Both groups were asked to perform home-based exercises. The authors observed motor gains in both groups but did not observe any statistically significant difference between the two groups.

An alternative approach to encourage clients to increase upper limb motor practice is to provide them with reminders, typically in the form of vibrations. Fig. 20.10 shows

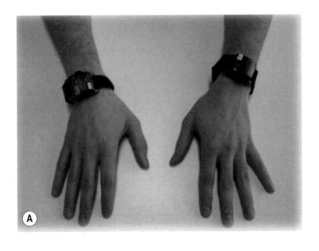

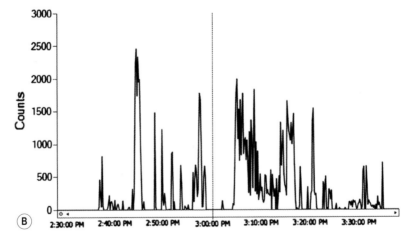

FIG. 20.9 Monitoring activity outside of the clinic. (A) Wrist units equipped with accelerometers used to monitor upper limb movements. (B) Example of raw accelerometer data.

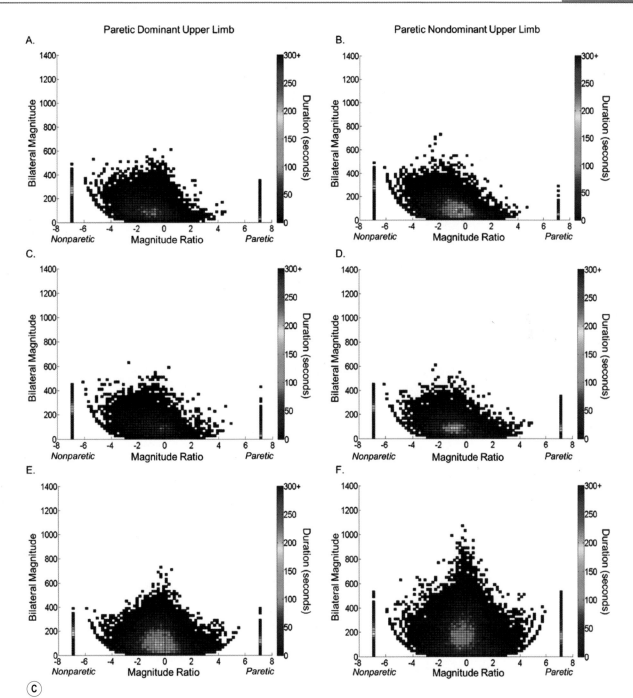

FIG. 20.9—cont'd (C) Examples of graphical representations of the data collected using the sensor units. Plots are shown for patients with different ARAT scores (low scores on top, high scores on the bottom) [Sources: A and B, from Lang et al (2013); C, Bailey et al (2015b).]

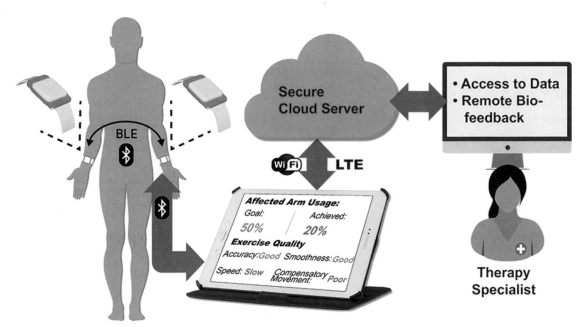

FIG. 20.10 Schematic representation of a system designed to encourage patients with hemiparesis to increase the amount of use of the paretic upper limb. Patients wear wrist units equipped with accelerometers. Data are analysed to derive a use ratio, meaning the amount of use of the affected arm relative to the amount of use detected from the contralateral one. Feedback is provided to encourage an increase in paretic limb use based on a target value set by the treating therapist (Source: Courtesy of BioSensics).

a schematic representation of the system developed by Lee et al (2018). Two wrist-worn units are used to detect goal-directed movements of the paretic and contralateral arm. The clinician and the client set together a target value of the activity of the paretic limb relative to the activity of the contralateral limb. If such target value is not reached, then the unit on the contralateral limb vibrates at intervals agreed upon by the client and clinician. The vibrations serve the purpose of reminding clients that they must increase the level of upper limb motor practice. Signal et al (2020) used a similar system to assess whether clients respond to the reminders by increasing the use of the paretic arm. Data were collected via visual observation of clients' response to the reminders. The results showed an increase in upper limb use in response to the reminders. Da-Silva et al (2018) carried out a similar study to determine how often the vibration-based reminders should be delivered and whether clients would respond by displaying an increase in level of activity in the hour after the reminder. Positive results from the study prompted the authors to launch a follow-up study in which they tested an actual intervention and gathered preliminary positive results. Wei et al (2018) tested the therapeutic efficacy of this reminder-based approach in 84 stroke patients who had the first stroke in the previous 6 months. Participants were randomly allocated to the intervention group (device worn with vibrations delivered), the sham group (device worn with no vibrations) or control group (usual therapy). A small but statistically significant greater improvement in the intervention group in one of the ARAT scores was observed. A significant difference in the amount of arm activity between groups (measured by an accelerometer) was also observed.

A significant number of studies have explored the use of wearable technology to encourage clients to improve their mobility. A 2018 Cochrane review (Lynch et al 2018) found no clear effect of the use of activity monitors on step count in a community setting or an inpatient rehabilitation setting. However, recent studies (Grau-Pellicer et al 2020, Hassett et al 2020) have put more emphasis on coaching and the use of a multimodal approach (e.g., smartphone application with GPS and accelerometer-based sensing to monitor walking distance and speed a pedometer and a WhatsApp group; an exercise programme with aerobic, task-oriented, balance, and stretching components; and a progressive daily ambulation programme monitored by a smartphone application and a pedometer). These studies

- Wearable sensors, called *inertial measurement units*, designed to track the movements of body segments have been used to collect biomechanical data whose characteristics correlate with scores derived using clinical scales that quantify motor impairments and functional limitations.
- The same sensing technology can be used to capture the performance of motor activities in the home and community setting, hence enabling the assessment of what clients actually do as opposed to what they are capable of doing (as typically assessed in the clinic).
- The data collected using wearable sensors can also be used to encourage motor practice outside of the clinic. For instance, wrist-worn units can be used to monitor upper limb use and encourage the use of the hemiparetic limb when appropriate.

showed improvements in community ambulation (Grau-Pellicer et al 2020) and mobility scores (Hassett et al 2020), respectively, for the intervention group. Overall these studies suggest that wearable technology can provide an effective tool to encourage clients to increase their mobility in the home and community settings.

CURRENT EVIDENCE

There has been a rapid increase in research over the past decade on the use of interactive technologies in the rehabilitation setting (Keshner et al 2019, Nizamis et al 2021). With this increase in scientific publications, the number of systematic reviews with meta-analyses exploring the efficacy of interactive technologies for use in different populations has grown considerably in the past 5 years (Keshner et al 2019, Voinescu et al 2021).

Interactive technologies, when used as an adjunct to standard care, have been reported to improve upper limb function in stroke rehabilitation compared with standard care (Laver et al 2017). There is promising but inconclusive evidence to support the use of interactive technologies on balance, mobility and functional activities (Laver et al 2017, Mubin et al 2019, Voinescu et al 2021). Forty-one meta-analyses were included in a recent umbrella review exploring the effectiveness and quality of evidence of interactive technology interventions in stroke (n = 32), traumatic brain injury (n = 3) and cerebral palsy (n = 6) rehabilitation (Voinescu et al 2021). The majority of the 41 studies were evaluated as being of low- or very low-quality evidence with 14 and 3 rated as moderate- or high-quality

evidence, respectively. The interactive technologies ranged from commercial video gaming systems to immersive tailored systems (both commercial and research prototypes). Overall the review supported the potential benefits of interactive technologies to improve "ambulation function of children with cerebral palsy, mobility, balance, upper limb function, and body structure/function and activity of people with stroke, and upper limb function of people with acquired brain injury" (Voinescu et al 2021). The review also highlighted that improvement in outcomes was related to the capacity to customise the intervention for individual needs. The use of interactive technologies has demonstrated potential to improve motor (gait, balance, upper limb) and cognitive outcomes compared with standard care or no intervention for people with multiple sclerosis (Calafiore et al 2021, Maggio et al 2019, Nascimento et al 2021, Webster et al 2021, Yeh et al 2020). A smaller number of studies have reported promising but inconclusive evidence for the use of robotics or VR for people with Parkinson's (Navarro-Lozano et al 2022, Sevcenko & Lindgren 2022). A limited number of studies on the use of interactive technologies for spinal cord injury have demonstrated positive findings; however, small sample sizes and lower quality methodologies suggest more higher quality trials are needed (Alashram et al 2021, De Miguel-Rubio et al 2022, Yeo et al 2019, Zhang et al 2022).

Scientific evidence on the effectiveness of virtual rehabilitation has been strengthened in recent years; however, most studies are pilot studies with small samples (Laver et al 2017, Maggio et al 2019, Voinescu et al 2021, Webster et al 2021, Yeh et al 2020, Zanatta et al 2022). The types of interactive technologies and, more importantly, the content and specificity of the tasks and activities within these applications vary widely. Much of the research has been undertaken on hardware that is no longer supported (such as the Nintendo Wii) and/or has been developed and evaluated in the research setting with no translation into the clinical setting (Garcia-Munoz & Casuso-Holgado 2019, Goble et al 2014, Laver et al 2017, Wardani et al 2021). The methodologies and outcome measures vary across trials, making it difficult to compare and analyse pooled results. Further research in this area should evaluate the safety and effectiveness of interactive technologies for rehabilitation in high-quality trials with a focus on consistent methodologies, common outcome measures and detailed description of the intervention (content, system, prescription). More information is also needed to evaluate the mechanisms through which these technologies support rehabilitation. In the next 5–10 years it is anticipated that the field will continue to evolve from development, user testing and pilot studies to focus on more targeted evaluation of effectiveness.

PRACTICAL TIPS FOR CHOOSING TECHNOLOGIES

Technologies are evolving at a rapid pace, with updated or new hardware and software released regularly. It can be difficult for clinicians and researchers to keep up with this pace, and daunting to novices and experts in the field alike. This rapid release cycle of new hardware creates a discrepancy between modern systems and outdated research results and therapy systems. Research projects, publication timelines and clinical trials often take several years to complete. On the contrary, hardware updates occur much more frequently, with new VR headsets, controllers, sensors and games being released constantly. Relatively recent technologies such as the Nintendo Wii and Microsoft Kinect are already outdated and not commercially available anymore. This can make it difficult for clinicians to keep abreast of the latest evidence and use this information to make choices to implement technology interventions in the clinical setting. It is important for clinicians who are interested in adding interactive technologies into their repertoire of treatment interventions to have a good understanding of the benefits and limitations of the technology they will be using. One of the most important elements of interactive interventions to analyse is the technology's demands on the user's motor and cognitive systems. In this way, when a new technology and/or software is created, clinicians will have the capacity to assess the feasibility of the technology to be applied in the rehabilitation of specific client populations. Of course, the evaluation of the clinician does not replace the need for research to analyse the efficaciousness of each new technology, but it does allow for exploration of the use of technologies in the clinical setting. We strongly recommend that, before using any new system, it is necessary to understand its feasibility, safety and efficaciousness. We further encourage interactive technology developers and researchers to place a stronger focus on the design of hardware-agnostic systems that can easily accommodate new hardware as it becomes available. Such systems are built around carefully designed tasks and therapeutic elements that will function consistently, regardless of the specific hardware that is being used.

Choosing Technology

When making a choice about using a technology within the clinical setting, it is important to determine what the technology adds to clinical practice. Many of the commercially available and customisable interactive technologies can be used as an adjunct to traditional therapy interventions. This means that the technology should be used to complement and enhance the existing clinical interventions or clinical goals. The technology should not detract or distract from the intended clinical goals. When considering using an interactive technology within the clinical setting, the amount and type of equipment needed to support the technology intervention should be well understood. Practical decisions such as where the equipment will be set up, where it will be kept, who has access to the equipment and who will provide the technical support will have an impact on when and how much the system may be used. Anecdotally, the implementation of interactive technologies within a clinical setting has worked well when there is a 'champion' within the department who leads the effort. This is likely because there is a dedicated person who is familiar with the technology and can assist with training and troubleshooting.

Choosing an Activity/Task/Game

It is important to have a good understanding of the physical and cognitive requirements of any technology and gaming intervention that is chosen. Before using an app, game or interactive tool with a client, the clinician must be familiar with the interaction requirements, the progression of the tasks, the available options/task settings, the 'scoring' and the feedback provided. Some games may be suitable only for clients with a particular goal or a certain level of ability. Some games can have complex instructions or interaction requirements that may be too difficult or may not align with clinical goals (Lange et al 2009). It is important to consider the complete experience and take into account the client's cognitive level when choosing an interactive task.

Depending on the aim of the therapy, clinicians can select specific games or activities. For example, if the aim of the therapy is to improve static balance, the clinician could select games that require maintenance of static balance over a force plate performing static tasks (e.g., Nintendo Wii Fit) or games that require reaching out of base of support (e.g., Microsoft Kinect). As the client's performance improves, the clinician can change the level of difficulty of the game or change the task. An example progression could start by using a static posture in bipedal stance and later progressing to a static unipedal posture.

In general, the key aspects to consider when deciding on the interactive task/games to use with clients include the goal of the rehabilitation session (assessment, support, intervention), the core challenge (balance, memory, dual tasking, physical interaction, cognitive interaction), the setting the technology is to be used in (inpatient, outpatient or home) and the intended time anticipated to be spent on the intervention (one session, multiple sessions). The flexibility and continuity across sessions should also be considered: (1) Can the content be used within the time available for a rehabilitation session? (2) Can the content be picked up in a following session where it was left in the previous session? (3) Does the content allow for new tasks to be performed in each session? (4) How will data be recorded, stored and tracked? and (5) Will the system be usable by multiple people?

Cost of the system can include a one-off payment for hardware and software. However, ongoing costs of software/app/game and/or access to an internet connection can add up quickly.

The level of challenge of the game or activity should be carefully considered: How quickly does the level of challenge change? Does the level of challenge change once a certain criterion is met, or does the level of challenge change after a certain period? Is this level of challenge appropriate for my client and our rehabilitation goals? Is the game too frustrating? Can the tasks be customised for my client? If not, can I do something with the environment and setup to customise? Examples of such customisation include standing with tablet mounted on a wall and using Wii Fit board with hands. Can I modify the feedback or scoring?

Client Considerations

To select optimal VR or gaming systems and games or activities, clinicians must analyse their motor and cognitive demands to select the appropriate strategy according to the client's abilities. As clients improve, new levels of difficulties could be selected to impose more challenge on the treatment, and new games with higher motor and cognitive demands can be used.

When the Nintendo Wii was first released, many clinicians adopted interactive gaming technology in their clinical practice. Anecdotal evidence, followed by evidence from qualitative studies (Galvin & Levac 2011, Lange et al 2009, Levac & Miller 2013), suggested that the Nintendo Wii was not appropriate for some clients with moderate to severe cognitive and/or physical impairments.

If the client has any physical impairments, the use of a mouse, touchscreen or physical tracking may be difficult. The clinician could explore options for different starting positions (sitting versus standing) or input methods if possible. If the client has cognitive impairments, interventions with multiple simultaneous commands and complex controls could be too challenging. Screen size and contrast of the game should be carefully considered if the client has visual impairments. The importance and impact of instructions and task feedback for people with hearing, speech and language impairments should also be considered. The goals of the application or game should match the therapeutic goals of the client. Other questions that should be considered: Does the game have a tutorial? Are the (audio/visual) instructions clear? Is the (audio/visual) feedback appropriate? Is the scoring appropriate? Does the game track progress? Are the data meaningful? What is the game

KEY POINTS

- The rapid pace of development of new interactive technologies has improved the availability and cost of technologies.
- The rapid pace of development of new interactive technologies and slower pace of research activities can make it difficult for clinicians to keep up with the latest available technologies and make evidence-based choices about technology options.
- When choosing a technology to use, clinicians should consider the technology, task content and their client's needs and goals.

really requiring my client to do? Are the game's interactions helpful or harmful to the client's rehabilitation? Can the game be played independently, or is supervision required? Who is going to use the system: clinician, client or caregiver? What are the required levels of cognitive ability and technical knowledge? Can the game be played within the duration of a treatment session? How much time will it take in the home setting?

CONCLUSION

There has been a rapid increase in research and development of interactive technologies used for rehabilitation during the past decade. Interactive technologies can encourage and motivate people to move and provide an opportunity to practice meaningful task-specific training activities in a safe and structured environment. It is important to keep in mind that interactive technologies are a tool in the clinician's toolkit of assessment and intervention options in the rehabilitation setting. As with all tools, clinical reasoning is an important part of the decision-making process. Technologies are evolving at a rapid pace, with new hardware and software being released regularly. It can be difficult for clinicians and researchers to keep up with this pace and can be daunting to novices and experts in the field alike. This rapid release cycle of new hardware creates a discrepancy between modern technologies and outdated research results, resources and therapy systems. This means that clinicians need to rely on their clinical judgement when choosing a technology to use in the rehabilitation setting.

CASE HISTORY

A case history is outlined to provide an example of the use of VR as an intervention poststroke. Yamato et al (2016) describe this case history and associated discussion in more detail. Mr S is a 72-year-old man who survived an ischaemic stroke in the middle cerebral artery. Before his stroke, he lived with his wife and was independent with activities of daily living. Two weeks after his stroke, he was admitted to an inpatient stroke rehabilitation unit with normal cognitive function (25 of 30 on the Mini-Mental State Examination). He presented with right-sided weakness (41 of 66 points on the FMA) and moderate limitation in hand function (assessed through the BBT, he moved 23 blocks in 60 seconds). Mr S could walk short distances indoors with the supervision of one person and was unable to walk outdoors. He scored 2 of 12 in the Short Physical Performance Battery. He stood unassisted with feet parallel and shoulder width apart for 8 seconds. Semi-tandem and tandem stances were not attempted. He walked 4 metres in 21 seconds (0.19 m/s) and scored 1 of 4 on the walking subscale. He scored 1 of 4 on the sit-to-stand subscale (stood up without using his hands five times in 17.5 seconds). In the first assessment, Mr S showed interest in new technologies, and his physical clinician decided to include the Nintendo Wii gaming console as an adjunct to his treatment to improve his upper limb function and mobility. The goals of his treatment were to improve upper limb function and increase independence with mobility. The choice to use the Nintendo Wii and Nintendo Wii Fit involved familiarity of the patient with the technology, accessibility of the technology within the clinic, clinician's knowledge of the games available, suitability of the games to target upper limb and hand function and overall mobility, and suitability of the available games to provide an appropriate level of challenge for Mr S and meet the goals of his rehabilitation. The intervention was provided in a private room of the hospital, without any distractions. Mr S completed a programme of 1 hour of supervised VR sessions, five times per week for 3 weeks (15 hours total). The games selected were from the Wii Sports, Wii Fit and Cooking Mama games. The selected games were chosen to focus on improving upper limb function (Wii Sports and Cooking Mama require upper limb activities) and mobility (Penguin game from Wii Fit encourages weight shift to improve loading the right leg for standing and walking). The level of difficulty was adjusted to meet the appropriate level of ability for Mr S (The Tightrope game from Wii Fit changed from a heel toe walking activity to a step-touch exercise using a block). The therapist selected between four and six different games to complete each session, with Mr S playing each game between three and six times, depending on the length and difficulty of the game. In the first session of training, the physical therapist assisted Mr S to interact with the games using his body movements. The physical therapist also assisted Mr S to hold the controls (Wii Remote and Nunchuk) and facilitated the correct movements of his arm and hand when necessary. In addition to the VR intervention, Mr S completed 1–2 hours of conventional physical therapy five times per week and other therapies provided by the multidisciplinary team. After the 3-week combined intervention (VR plus conventional therapy) period, Mr S demonstrated improvement in upper limb function (FMA-UE score improved from 41 to 46 points), hand function (BBT score increased from 23 to 26 blocks) and mobility (Short Physical Performance Battery score increased from two to eight points). He improved from 1 of 4 to 4 of 4 in the balance subscale. His walking subscale score remained at 1 of 4; however, his walking improved from 4 metres in 21 seconds (0.19 m/s) to 4 metres in 11 seconds (0.36 m/s). Mr S improved from 1 of 4 to 3 of 4 in the sit-to-stand subscale (improved from five sit to stands in 17.5 seconds to 11.3 seconds).

SELF-ASSESSMENT QUESTIONS

1. In this case study, the Nintendo Wii was chosen as the interactive technology. What other interactive technologies described in this chapter may be appropriate for use with this patient and why?
2. Commercially available video game technologies have been designed for entertainment. Describe three potential challenges of the use of commercially available video games in rehabilitation.
3. When choosing a technology to use, clinicians should consider the technology, game content and patient needs. List some of the key questions clinicians could ask themselves in each of these areas.
4. List the limitations of the research evaluating the use of interactive technologies in rehabilitation.

REFERENCES

Adans-Dester, C., Hankov, N., O'Brien, A., et al., 2020. Enabling precision rehabilitation interventions using wearable sensors and machine learning to track motor recovery. NPJ Digit. Med. 3, 1–10.

Ahmed, T., Thopalli, K., Rikakis, T., et al., 2021. Automated movement assessment in stroke rehabilitation. Front. Neurol. 12, 1396.

Aisen, M.L., Krebs, H.I., Hogan, N., et al., 1997. The effect of robot-assisted therapy and rehabilitative training on motor recovery following stroke. Arch. Neurol. 54, 443–446.

Alashram, A.R., Annino, G., Padua, E., 2021. Robot-assisted gait training in individuals with spinal cord injury: a systematic review for the clinical effectiveness of Lokomat. J. Clin. Neurosci. 91, 260–269.

Amprimo, G., Masi, G., Priano, L., et al., 2022. Assessment tasks and virtual exergames for remote monitoring of Parkinson's disease: an integrated approach based on Azure Kinect. Sensors. 22, 8173.

Andrews, C., Southworth, M.K., Silva, J.N., Silva, J.R., 2019. Extended reality in medical practice. Curr. Treatment Options Cardiovasc. Med. 21, 1–12.

Arac, A., 2020. Machine learning for 3D kinematic analysis of movements in neurorehabilitation. Curr. Neurol. Neurosci. Rep. 20, 29.

Arteaga, S., Chevalier, J., Coile, A., et al., 2008. Low-cost accelerometry-based posture monitoring system for stroke survivors. Proceedings of the 10th International ACM SIGACCESS Conference on Computers and Accessibility.

Asbeck, A.T., De Rossi, S.M., Holt, K.G., Walsh, C.J., 2015. A biologically inspired soft exosuit for walking assistance. Int. J. Robotics Res. 34 (6), 744–762.

Awad, L.N., Bae, J., O'Donnell, K., et al., 2017. A soft robotic exosuit improves walking in patients after stroke. Sci. Transl. Med. 9, eaai9084

Awad, L.N., Kudzia, P., Revi, D.A., et al., 2020. Walking faster and farther with a soft robotic exosuit: implications for post-stroke gait assistance and rehabilitation. IEEE Open J. Eng. Med. Biol. 1, 108–115.

Bailey, R.R., Birkenmeier, R.L., Lang, C.E., 2015a. Real-world affected upper limb activity in chronic stroke: an examination of potential modifying factors. Top. Stroke Rehabil. 22, 26–33.

Bailey, R.R., Klaesner, J.W., Lang, C.E., 2014. An accelerometry-based methodology for assessment of real-world bilateral upper extremity activity. PloS One. 9, e103135.

Bailey, R.R., Klaesner, J.W., Lang, C.E., 2015b. Quantifying real-world upper-limb activity in nondisabled adults and adults with chronic stroke. Neurorehabil. Neural Repair. 29, 969–978.

Bailey, R.R., Lang, C.E., 2014. Upper extremity activity in adults: referent values using accelerometry. J. Rehabil. Res. Devel. 50, 1213.

Beer, R.F., Ellis, M.D., Holubar, B.G., Dewald, J.P., 2007. Impact of gravity loading on post-stroke reaching and its relationship to weakness. Muscle Nerve. 36, 242–250.

Belas dos Santos, M., Barros de Oliveira, C., 2018. Dos Santos, A., et al., 2018. A comparative study of conventional physiotherapy versus robot-assisted gait training associated to physiotherapy in individuals with ataxia after stroke. Behav. Neurol. 2892065.

Belotti, N., Bonfanti, S., Locatelli, A., et al., 2022. A tele-rehabilitation platform for shoulder motor function recovery using serious games and an Azure Kinect device. Stud. Health Technol. Inform. 293, 145–152.

Bergamini, E., Iosa, M., Belluscio, V., et al., 2017. Multi-sensor assessment of dynamic balance during gait in patients with subacute stroke. J. Biomech. 61, 208–215.

BlueJay Mobile Health., 2022. BlueJay Mobile Health. Available at: https://www.bluejayhealth.com/. Accessed on 5 Dec 2022.

Bonura, A., Motolese, F., Capone, F., et al., 2022. Smartphone app in stroke management: a narrative updated review. J. Stroke. 24, 323–334.

Borrego, A., Latorre, J., Alcañiz, M., Llorens, R., 2019. Embodiment and presence in virtual reality after stroke. A comparative study with healthy subjects. Front. Neurol. 10, 1061.

Buccino, G., Arisi, D., Gough, P., et al., 2012. Improving upper limb motor functions through action observation treatment: a pilot study in children with cerebral palsy. Devel. Med. Child Neurol. 54, 822–828.

Burns, S.P., Terblanche, M., Perea, J., et al., 2021. mHealth intervention applications for adults living with the effects of stroke: a scoping review. Arch. Rehabil. Res. Clin. Trans. 3, 100095.

Byl, N., Zhang, W., Coo, S., Tomizuka, M., 2015. Clinical impact of gait training enhanced with visual kinematic biofeedback: patients with Parkinson's disease and patients stable post stroke. Neuropsychologia. 79, 332–343.

Cajigas, I., Koenig, A., Severini, G., et al., 2017. Robot-induced perturbations of human walking reveal a selective generation of motor adaptation. Sci. Robot. 2, eaam7749

Calafiore, D., Invernizzi, M., Ammendolia, A., et al., 2021. Efficacy of virtual reality and exergaming in improving balance in patients with multiple sclerosis: a systematic review and meta-analysis. Front. Neurol. 12, 773459.

Calafiore, D., Negrini, F., Tottoli, N., et al., 2022. Efficacy of robotic exoskeleton for gait rehabilitation in patients with subacute stroke: a systematic review. Eur. J. Phys. Rehabil. Med. 58,1.

Cao, Z., Martinez, G.H., Simon, T., et al., 2021. OpenPose: real-time multi-person 2D pose estimation using part affinity fields. IEEE Trans. Pattern Anal. Mach. Intell. 43, 172–186.

Cao, Z., Simon, T., Wei, S.-E., Sheikh, Y., 2017. Realtime multi-person 2D pose estimation using part affinity fields. arXiv:1611.08050.

Chang, C.-Y., Lange, B., Zhang, M., et al., 2012. Towards pervasive physical rehabilitation using Microsoft Kinect. 2012 6th international conference on pervasive computing technologies for healthcare (PervasiveHealth) and workshops. San Diego, CA, 2012, 159–162.

Clark, R.A., Bryant, A.L., Pua, Y., et al., 2010. Validity and reliability of the Nintendo Wii Balance Board for assessment of standing balance. Gait Posture. 31, 307–310.

Clark, W.E., Sivan, M., O'Connor, R.J., 2019. Evaluating the use of robotic and virtual reality rehabilitation technologies to improve function in stroke survivors: a narrative review. J. Rehabil. Assist. Technol. Eng. 6, 2055668319863557

Colombo, G., Joerg, M., Schreier, R., Dietz, V., 2000. Treadmill training of paraplegic patients using a robotic orthosis. J. Rehabil. Res. Devel. 37, 693–700.

Colomer, C., Baldoví, A., Torromé, S., et al., 2013. Efficacy of Armeo® Spring during the chronic phase of stroke. Study in mild to moderate cases of hemiparesis. Neurologia. 28, 261–267.

Cornman, H.L., Stenum, J., Roemmich, R.T., 2021. Video-based quantification of human movement frequency using pose estimation: a pilot study. PLoS One. 16, e0261450.

Corpus V.R., 2022. Corpus VR. Available at: https://corpusvr.com/. Accessed on 5 Dec 2022.

Cronin, N.J., 2021. Using deep neural networks for kinematic analysis: challenges and opportunities. J. Biomech. 123, 110460.

Da Gama, A., Fallavollita, P., Teichrieb, V., Navab, N., 2015. Motor rehabilitation using Kinect: a systematic review. Games Health J. 4, 123–135.

Darekar, A., McFadyen, B.J., Lamontagne, A., Fung, J., 2015. Efficacy of virtual reality-based intervention on balance and mobility disorders post-stroke: a scoping review. J. Neuroeng. Rehabil. 12, 46.

Da-Silva, R.H., van Wijck, F., Shaw, L., et al., 2018. Prompting arm activity after stroke: a clinical proof of concept study of wrist-worn accelerometers with a vibrating alert function. J. Rehabil. Assist. Technol. Eng. 5 2055668318761524

de-la-Torre, R., Oña, E.D., Balaguer, C., Jardón, A., 2020. Robot-aided systems for improving the assessment of upper limb spasticity: a systematic review. Sensors. 20, 5251.

De Miguel-Rubio, A., Muñoz-Pérez, L., Alba-Rueda, A., et al., 2022. A therapeutic approach using the combined application of virtual reality with robotics for the treatment of patients with spinal cord injury: a systematic review. Int. J. Environ. Res. Public Health. 19, 8772.

Del Din, S., Patel, S., Cobelli, C., Bonato, P., 2011. Estimating Fugl-Meyer clinical scores in stroke survivors using wearable sensors. Annu. Int. Conf. IEEE Eng. Med. Biol. Soc. 2011, 5839–5842.

Demers, M., Fung, K., Subramanian, S.K., et al., 2021. Integration of motor learning principles into virtual reality interventions for individuals with cerebral palsy: systematic review. JMIR Serious Games. 9, e23822.

Dewald, J.P., Beer, R.F., 2001. Abnormal joint torque patterns in the paretic upper limb of subjects with hemiparesis. Muscle Nerve. 24, 273–283.

Dewald, J.P., Pope, P.S., Given, J.D., et al., 1995. Abnormal muscle coactivation patterns during isometric torque generation at the elbow and shoulder in hemiparetic subjects. Brain. 118, 495–510.

Ding, Y., Kim, M., Kuindersma, S., Walsh, C.J., 2018. Human-in-the-loop optimization of hip assistance with a soft exosuit during walking. Sci. Robot. 3, eaar5438

Dobkin, B.H., Dorsch, A., 2011. The promise of mHealth: daily activity monitoring and outcome assessments by wearable sensors. Neurorehabil. Neural Repair. 25, 788–798.

Doman, C.A., Waddell, K.J., Bailey, R.R., et al., 2016. Changes in upper-extremity functional capacity and daily performance during outpatient occupational therapy for people with stroke. Am. J. Occup. Ther 70 7003290040p7003290041-7003290040p7003290011

Dorsch, A.K., Thomas, S., Xu, X., et al., 2015. SIRRACT: an international randomized clinical trial of activity feedback during inpatient stroke rehabilitation enabled by wireless sensing. Neurorehabil. Neural Repair. 29, 407–415.

dos Santos Mendes, F.A., Pompeu, J.E., Lobo, A.M., et al., 2012. Motor learning, retention and transfer after virtual-reality-based training in Parkinson's disease – effect of motor and cognitive demands of games: a longitudinal, controlled clinical study. Physiotherapy. 98, 217–223.

Evolv Rehabilitation Technologies., 2022. Evolv Rehabilitation Technologies. Available at: https://evolvrehab.com/. Accessed on 5 Dec 2022.

Exercise Pro Live., 2022. Exercise Pro Live. Available at: https://www.exerciseprolive.com/. Accessed on 5 Dec 2022.

Fang, H.-S., Xie, S., Tai, Y.-W., Lu, C., 2017. RMPE: Regional multi-person pose estimation. Proceedings of the IEEE International Conference on Computer Vision. 2017, 2353–2362.

Ferreira dos Santos, L., Christ, O., Mate, K., et al., 2016. Movement visualisation in virtual reality rehabilitation of the lower limb: a systematic review. Biomed. Eng. 15, 75–88.

FlintRehab., 2022. FlintRehab. Available at: https://www.flintrehab.com/. Accessed on 5 Dec 2022.

Friedman, N., Chan, V., Reinkensmeyer, A.N., et al., 2014. Retraining and assessing hand movement after stroke using the MusicGlove: comparison with conventional hand therapy and isometric grip training. . J. Neuroeng. Rehabil. 11, 1–14.

Friedman, N., Chan, V., Zondervan, D., et al., 2011. MusicGlove: motivating and quantifying hand movement rehabilitation by using functional grips to play music. Annu. Int. Conf. IEEE Eng. Med. Biol. Soc. 2011, 2359–2363.

Frisoli, A., Solazzi, M., Loconsole, C., Barsotti, M., 2016. New generation emerging technologies for neurorehabilitation and motor assistance. Acta Myol. 35, 141.

Galvin, J., Levac, D., 2011. Facilitating clinical decision-making about the use of virtual reality within paediatric motor rehabilitation: describing and classifying virtual reality systems. Dev. Neurorehabil. 14, 112–122.

Garcia-Munoz, C., Casuso-Holgado, M., 2019. Effectiveness of Wii Fit Balance board in comparison with other interventions for post-stroke balance rehabilitation. Systematic review and meta-analysis. Rev. Neurol. 69, 271–279.

Garcia, Fd.V., da Cunha, M.J., Schuch, C.P., et al., 2021. Movement smoothness in chronic post-stroke individuals walking in an outdoor environment—a cross-sectional study using IMU sensors. PLoS One. 16, e0250100

Gijbels, D., Lamers, I., Kerkhofs, L., et al., 2011. The Armeo Spring as training tool to improve upper limb functionality in multiple sclerosis: a pilot study. J. Neuroeng. Rehabil. 8, 1–8.

Goble, D.J., Cone, B.L., Fling, B.W., 2014. Using the Wii Fit as a tool for balance assessment and neurorehabilitation: the first half decade of "Wii-search". J. Neuroeng. Rehabil. 11, 1–9.

Grau-Pellicer, M., Lalanza, J., Jovell-Fernández, E., Capdevila, L., 2020. Impact of mHealth technology on adherence to healthy PA after stroke: a randomized study. Top. Stroke Rehabil. 27, 354–368.

Hassett, L., van den Berg, M., Lindley, R.I., et al., 2020. Digitally enabled aged care and neurological rehabilitation to enhance outcomes with Activity and MObility UsiNg Technology (AMOUNT) in Australia: a randomised controlled trial. PLoS Med. 17, e1003029.

Hesse, S., Uhlenbrock, D., 2000. A mechanized gait trainer for restoration of gait. J. Rehabil. Res. Devel. 37, 701–708.

Hinge Health., 2022. Hinge Health. Available at: https://www.hingehealth.com/. Accessed on 5 Dec 2022.

Hocoma., 2022. ArmeoSenso. Available at: https://www.hocoma.com/solutions/armeo-senso/. Accessed on 5 Dec 2022.

Høeg, E.R., Bruun-Pedersen, J.R., Cheary, S., et al., 2021a. Buddy biking: a user study on social collaboration in a virtual reality exergame for rehabilitation. Virt. Reality. 1–18.

Høeg, E.R., Povlsen, T.M., Bruun-Pedersen, J.R., et al., 2021b. System immersion in virtual reality-based rehabilitation of motor function in older adults: a systematic review and meta-analysis. Front. Virtual Real. 2, 30.

Hogan, N., 1987. Stable execution of contact tasks using impedance control. Proceedings. 1987 IEEE International Conference on Robotics and Automation, Raleigh, NC, USA. 4, 1047–1054.

Holden, M.K., 2005. Virtual environments for motor rehabilitation: review. Cyberpsychol. Behav. 8, 187–189.

Holmes, J.D., Jenkins, M.E., Johnson, A.M., et al., 2013. Validity of the Nintendo Wii® balance board for the assessment of standing balance in Parkinson's disease. Clin. Rehabil. 27, 361–366.

Hubbard, B., Pothier, D., Hughes, C., et al., 2012. A portable, low-cost system for posturography: a platform for longitudinal balance telemetry. J. Otolaryngol. Head Neck Surg. 41, S31.

InMotionVR., 2022. InMotionVR. Available at: https://inmotionvr.com/. Accessed on 5 Dec 2022.

Insafutdinov, E., Andriluka, M., Pishchulin, L., et al., 2017. ArtTrack: articulated multi-person tracking in the wild. Proceedings of the IEEE Conference on Computer Vision and Pattern Recognition. 2017, 1293–1301.

Insafutdinov, E., Pishchulin, L., Andres, B., et al., 2016. DeeperCut: a deeper, stronger, and faster multi-person pose estimation model. In: Leibe, B., Matas, J., Sebe, N., Welling, M. (Eds.), Computer Vision – ECCV 2016. ECCV 2016. Lecture Notes in Computer Science. Springer, Cham, pp. 9910.

Jezernik, S., Colombo, G., Keller, T., et al., 2003. Robotic orthosis lokomat: a rehabilitation and research tool. Neuromodulation. 6, 108–115.

Kaia Health., 2022. Kaia Health. Available at: https://kaiahealth.com/. Accessed on 5 Dec 2022.

Kalron, A., Frid, L., Fonkatz, I., et al., 2022. The design, development, and testing of a virtual reality device for upper limb training in people with multiple sclerosis: single-center feasibility study. JMIR Serious Games. 10, e36288.

Keshner, E.A., Weiss, P.T., Geifman, D., 2019. Tracking the evolution of virtual reality applications to rehabilitation as a field of study. J. Neuroeng. Rehabil. 16, 76.

Kim, J., Lee, G., Heimgartner, R., et al., 2019. Reducing the metabolic rate of walking and running with a versatile, portable exosuit. Science. 365, 668–672.

Kim, W.-S., Cho, S., Ku, J., et al., 2020. Clinical application of virtual reality for upper limb motor rehabilitation in stroke: review of technologies and clinical evidence. J. Clin. Med. 9, 3369.

Klamroth-Marganska, V., Blanco, J., Campen, K., et al., 2014. Three-dimensional, task-specific robot therapy of the arm after stroke: a multicentre, parallel-group randomised trial. Lancet Neurol. 13, 159–166.

Kleim, J.A.J., Theresa, A., 2008. Principles of experience-dependent neural plasticity: implications for rehabilitation after brain damage. J. Speech Lang. Hear. Res. 51, S225–239.

Krebs, H.I., Hogan, N., Aisen, M.L., Volpe, B.T., 1998. Robot-aided neurorehabilitation. IEEE Trans. Rehabil. Eng. 6, 75–87.

Królikowska, A., Maj, A., Dejnek, M., et al., 2023. Wrist motion assessment using Microsoft Azure Kinect DK: a reliability study in healthy individuals. Adv. Clin. Exp. Med. 32, 203–209.

Lage, G.M., Ugrinowitsch, H., Apolinário-Souza, T., et al., 2015. Repetition and variation in motor practice: a review of neural correlates. Neurosci. Biobehav. Rev. 57, 132–141.

Lang, C.E., Bland, M.D., Bailey, R.R., et al., 2013. Assessment of upper extremity impairment, function, and activity after stroke: foundations for clinical decision making. J. Hand Ther. 26, 104–115.

Lange, B., Flynn, S., Proffitt, R., et al., 2010. Development of an interactive game-based rehabilitation tool for dynamic balance training. Top. Stroke Rehabil. 17, 345–352.

Lange, B., Flynn, S., Rizzo, A., 2009. Initial usability assessment of off-the-shelf video, game consoles for clinical game-based motor rehabilitation. Phys. Ther. Rev. 14, 355–363.

Lange, B., Koenig, S., McConnell, E., et al., 2012. Interactive game-based rehabilitation using the Microsoft Kinect. IEEE Virtual Reality Workshops (VRW), Costa Mesa. CA, USA 2012, 171–172.

Langhorne, P., Bernhardt, J., Kwakkel, G., 2011. Stroke rehabilitation. Lancet. 377, 1693–1702.

Laver, K.E., Lange, B., George, S., et al., 2017. Virtual reality for stroke rehabilitation. Cochrane Database Syst. Rev. 11, CD008349

Lee, S.I., Adans-Dester, C.P., Grimaldi, M., et al., 2018. Enabling stroke rehabilitation in home and community settings: a wearable sensor-based approach for upper-limb motor training. IEEE J Trans. Eng. Health Med. 6, 1–11.

Leon, D., Cortes, M., Elder, J., et al., 2017. tDCS does not enhance the effects of robot-assisted gait training in patients with subacute stroke. Restor. Neurol. Neurosci. 35, 377–384.

Levac, D.E., Glegg, S.M., Sveistrup, H., et al., 2016. Promoting therapists' use of motor learning strategies within virtual reality-based stroke rehabilitation. PloS One. 11, e0168311

Levac, D.E., Huber, M.E., Sternad, D., 2019. Learning and transfer of complex motor skills in virtual reality: a perspective review. J. Neuroeng. Rehabil. 16, 1–15.

Levac, D.E., Miller, P.A., 2013. Integrating virtual reality video games into practice: clinicians' experiences. Physiother. Theory Pract. 29, 504–512.

Lynch, E.A., Jones, T.M., Simpson, D.B., et al., 2018. Activity monitors for increasing physical activity in adult stroke survivors. Cochrane Database Syst. Rev. 7, CD012543

Maceira-Elvira, P., Popa, T., Schmid, A.-C., Hummel, F.C., 2019. Wearable technology in stroke rehabilitation: towards improved diagnosis and treatment of upper-limb motor impairment. J. Neuroeng. Rehabil. 16, 1–18.

Maggio, M.G., Russo, M., Cuzzola, M.F., et al., 2019. Virtual reality in multiple sclerosis rehabilitation: a review on cognitive and motor outcomes. J. Clin. Neurosci. 65, 106–111.

Maier, M., Ballester, B.R., Verschure, P.F., 2019. Principles of neurorehabilitation after stroke based on motor learning and brain plasticity mechanisms. Front. Syst. Neurosci. 13, 74.

Makhataeva, Z., Varol, H.A., 2020. Augmented reality for robotics: a review. Robotics. 9, 21.

Makino, H., Hwang, E.J., Hedrick, N.G., Komiyama, T., 2016. Circuit mechanisms of sensorimotor learning. Neuron. 92, 705–721.

Marin-Pardo, O., Laine, C.M., Rennie, M., et al., 2020. A virtual reality muscle–computer interface for neurorehabilitation in chronic stroke: a pilot study. Sensors. 20, 3754.

Mathis, A., Mamidanna, P., Cury, K.M., et al., 2018. DeepLabCut: markerless pose estimation of user-defined body parts with deep learning. Nat. Neurosci. 21, 1281–1289.

MedBridge., 2022. MedBridge. Available at: https://www.medbridgeeducation.com/. Accessed on 5 Dec 2022.

Mehdizadeh, S., Nabavi, H., Sabo, A., et al., 2021. Concurrent validity of human pose tracking in video for measuring gait parameters in older adults: a preliminary analysis with multiple trackers, viewing angles, and walking directions. J. Neuroeng. Rehabil. 18, 1–16.

Merlo, A., Longhi, M., Giannotti, E., et al., 2013. Upper limb evaluation with robotic exoskeleton. Normative values for indices of accuracy, speed and smoothness. NeuroRehabilitation. 33, 523–530.

Merriam-Webster., (n.d.a). Augmented reality. Merriam-Webster. Available at: https://www.merriam-webster.com/dictionary/augmented%20reality. Accessed 9 December 2022.

Merriam-Webster., (n.d.b). Virtual reality. Merriam-Webster. Available at: https://www.merriam-webster.com/dictionary/virtual%20reality. Accessed 9 December 2022.

Miller, L.C., Dewald, J.P., 2012. Involuntary paretic wrist/finger flexion forces and EMG increase with shoulder abduction load in individuals with chronic stroke. Clin. Neurophysiol. 123, 1216–1225.

Mirelman, A., Bonato, P., Deutsch, J.E., 2009. Effects of training with a robot-virtual reality system compared with a robot alone on the gait of individuals after stroke. Stroke. 40, 169–174.

Mosadegh, B., Polygerinos, P., Keplinger, C., et al., 2014. Pneumatic networks for soft robotics that actuate rapidly. Adv. Funct. Mater. 24, 2163–2170.

Mousavi Hondori, H., Khademi, M., 2014. A review on technical and clinical impact of microsoft kinect on physical therapy and rehabilitation. J. Med. Eng. 2014.

Mubin, O., Alnajjar, F., Jishtu, N., et al., 2019. Exoskeletons with virtual reality, augmented reality, and gamification for stroke patients' rehabilitation: systematic review. JMIR Rehabil. Assist. Technol. 6, e12010.

Nam, K.Y., Kim, H.J., Kwon, B.S., et al., 2017. Robot-assisted gait training (Lokomat) improves walking function and activity in people with spinal cord injury: a systematic review. J. Neuroeng. Rehabil. 14, 1–13.

Nascimento, A.S., Fagundes, C.V., dos Santos Mendes, F.A., Leal, J.C., 2021. Effectiveness of virtual reality rehabilitation in persons with multiple sclerosis: a systematic review and meta-analysis of randomized controlled trials. Mult. Scler. Relat. Disord. 54, 103128.

Navarro-Lozano, F., Kiper, P., Carmona-Pérez, C., et al., 2022. Effects of non-immersive virtual reality and video games on walking speed in Parkinson disease: a systematic review and meta-analysis. J. Clin. Med. 11, 6610.

Nef, T., Mihelj, M., Riener, R., 2007. ARMin: a robot for patient-cooperative arm therapy. Med. Biol. Eng. Comput. 45, 887–900.

Nizamis, K., Athanasiou, A., Almpani, S., et al., 2021. Converging robotic technologies in targeted neural rehabilitation: a review of emerging solutions and challenges. Sensors. 21, 2084.

Nudo, R.J., Wise, B.M., SiFuentes, F., Milliken, G.W., 1996. Neural substrates for the effects of rehabilitative training on motor recovery after ischemic infarct. Science. 272, 1791–1794.

Palmas, F., Klinker, G., 2020. Defining extended reality training: a long-term definition for all industries. 2020 IEEE 20th International Conference on Advanced Learning Technologies (ICALT). 2020, 322–324.

Patel, S., Hughes, R., Hester, T., et al., 2010. A novel approach to monitor rehabilitation outcomes in stroke survivors using wearable technology. Proc. IEEE. 98, 450–461.

Patel, S., Park, H., Bonato, P., et al., 2012. A review of wearable sensors and systems with application in rehabilitation. J. Neuroeng. Rehabil. 9, 1–17.

Pelosin, E., Avanzino, L., Bove, M., et al., 2010. Action observation improves freezing of gait in patients with Parkinson's disease. Neurorehabil. Neural Repair. 24, 746–752.

Pelosin, E., Bove, M., Ruggeri, P., et al., 2013. Reduction of bradykinesia of finger movements by a single session of action observation in Parkinson disease. Neurorehabil. Neural Repair. 27, 552–560.

Pennati, G., Da, Re, C., Messineo, I., Bonaiuti, D., 2015. How could robotic training and botolinum toxin be combined in chronic post stroke upper limb spasticity? A pilot study. Eur. J. Phys. Rehabil. Med. 51, 381–387.

Penumbra., 2022. RealSystemVR. Available at: https://www.real-system.com/. Accessed on 5 Dec 2022.

Physiotech., 2022. Physiotech. Available at: https://physiotec.ca/ca/en/. Accessed on 5 Dec 2022.

Physitrack., 2022. Physitrack. Available at: https://www.physitrack.com/. Accessed on 5 Dec 2022.

Pietrusinski, M., Cajigas, I., Severini, G., et al., 2013. Robotic gait rehabilitation trainer. IEEE/ASME Trans. Mechatron. 19, 490–499.

Pohl, M., Werner, C., Holzgraefe, M., et al., 2007. Repetitive locomotor training and physiotherapy improve walking and basic activities of daily living after stroke: a single-blind, randomized multicentre trial (DEutsche GAngtrainerStudie, DEGAS). Clin. Rehabil. 21, 17–27.

Polygerinos, P., Wang, Z., Galloway, K.C., et al., 2015a. Soft robotic glove for combined assistance and at-home rehabilitation. Robot. Auton. Syst. 73, 135–143.

Polygerinos, P., Wang, Z., Overvelde, J.T., et al., 2015b. Modeling of soft fiber-reinforced bending actuators. IEEE Trans. Robot. 31, 778–789.

Real Time Rehab. Real Time Rehab. Available at: http://www.realtimerehab.com/. Accessed on 5 Dec 2022.

Ren, S., He, K., Girshick, R., Sun, J., 2015. Faster r-cnn: towards real-time object detection with region proposal networks. Adv. Neural Inform. Proc. Syst. 28.

Repnik, E., Puh, U., Goljar, N., et al., 2018. Using inertial measurement units and electromyography to quantify movement during action research arm test execution. Sensors. 18, 2767.

Rodgers, M.M., Alon, G., Pai, V.M., Conroy, R.S., 2019. Wearable technologies for active living and rehabilitation: current research challenges and future opportunities. J. Rehabil. Assist. Technol. Eng. 6, 2055668319839607

Rose, F.D., Brooks, B.M., Rizzo, A.A., 2005. Virtual reality in brain damage rehabilitation: review. Cyberpsychol. Behav. 8, 241–271.

Salarian, A., Horak, F.B., Zampieri, C., et al., 2010. iTUG, a sensitive and reliable measure of mobility. IEEE Trans. Neural Syst. Rehabil. Eng. 18, 303–310.

Schmidt, H., Werner, C., Bernhardt, R., et al., 2007. Gait rehabilitation machines based on programmable footplates. J. Neuroeng. Rehabil. 4, 1–7.

Schwerz de Lucena, D., Rowe, J., Chan, V., Reinkensmeyer, D.J., 2021. Magnetically counting hand movements: validation of a calibration-free algorithm and application to testing the threshold hypothesis of real-world hand use after stroke. Sensors. 21, 1502.

Seethapathi, N., Wang, S., Saluja, R., et al., 2019. Movement science needs different pose tracking algorithms. arXiv:1907.10226v1.

Sevcenko, K., Lindgren, I., 2022. The effects of virtual reality training in stroke and Parkinson's disease rehabilitation: a systematic review and a perspective on usability. Eur. Rev. Aging Phys. Act. 19, 4.

Shah, S.H.H., Karlsen, A.S.T., Solberg, M., Hameed, I.A., 2022. A social VR-based collaborative exergame for rehabilitation: codesign, development and user study. Virtual Real, 1–18.

Shen, J., Xiang, H., Luna, J., et al., 2020. Virtual reality-based executive function rehabilitation system for children with traumatic brain injury: design and usability study. JMIR Serious Games. 8, e16947.

Shin, S.Y., Hohl, K., Giffhorn, M., et al., 2022. Soft robotic exosuit augmented high intensity gait training on stroke survivors: a pilot study. J. Neuroeng. Rehabil. 19, 1–12.

Shishov, N., Melzer, I., Bar-Haim, S., 2017. Parameters and measures in assessment of motor learning in neurorehabilitation; a systematic review of the literature. Front. Hum. Neurosci. 11, 82.

Shumway-Cook, A., Woollacott, M., 2017. Motor Control: Translating Research into Clinical Practise, fifth edition Wolters Kluwer, Philadelphia.

Signal, N.E.J., McLaren, R., Rashid, U., et al., 2020. Haptic nudges increase affected upper limb movement during inpatient stroke rehabilitation: multiple-period randomized crossover study. JMIR mHealth uHealth. 8, e17036.

Stenum, J., Cherry-Allen, K.M., Pyles, C.O., et al., 2021. Applications of pose estimation in human health and performance across the lifespan. Sensors. 21, 7315.

Stenum, J., Rossi, C., Roemmich, R.T., 2021. Two-dimensional video-based analysis of human gait using pose estimation. PLoS Comput. Biol. 17, e1008935.

Straudi, S., Chew, E., Iahn, C., et al., 2015. Combining transcranial direct current stimulation and gravity-supported, computer-enhanced arm training in a chronic pediatric stroke survivor: a case report. Clin. Case Rep. Rev. 2, 301–306.

Sword Health., 2022. Sword Health. Available at: https://sword-health.com/. Accessed on 5 Dec 2022.

Takeda, I., Yamada, A., Onodera, H., 2021. Artificial intelligence-assisted motion capture for medical applications: a comparative study between markerless and passive marker motion capture. Comput. Methods Biomech. Biomed. Eng. 24, 864–873.

Taveggia, G., Borboni, A., Salvi, L., et al., 2016. Efficacy of robot-assisted rehabilitation for the functional recovery of the upper limb in post-stroke patients: a randomized controlled study. Eur. J. Phys. Rehabil. Med. 52, 767–773.

Toshev, A., Szegedy, C., 2014. DeepPose: human pose estimation via deep neural networks. 2014 IEEE Conference on Computer Vision and Pattern Recognition, Columbus, OH, USA, 2014, 1653–1660.

Tran, D.A., Pajaro-Blazquez, M., Daneault, J.-F., et al., 2016. Combining dopaminergic facilitation with robot-assisted upper limb therapy in stroke survivors: a focused review. Am. J. Phys. Med. Rehabil. 95, 459.

UINCARE., 2022. UINCARE. Available at: https://www.uincare.com/. Accessed on 5 Dec 2022.

Vaezipour, A., Aldridge, D., Koenig, S., et al., 2022. "It's really exciting to think where it could go": a mixed-method investigation of clinician acceptance, barriers and enablers of virtual reality technology in communication rehabilitation. Disabil. Rehabil. 44, 3946–3958.

Viswakumar, A., Rajagopalan, V., Ray, T., et al., 2021. Development of a robust, simple, and affordable human gait analysis system using bottom-up pose estimation with a smartphone camera. Front. Physiol. 12, 784865.

Voinescu, A., Sui, J., Stanton Fraser, D., 2021. Virtual reality in neurorehabilitation: an umbrella review of meta-analyses. J. Clin. Med. 10, 1478.

Volpe, B.T., Huerta, P.T., Zipse, J.L., et al., 2009. Robotic devices as therapeutic and diagnostic tools for stroke recovery. Arch. Neurol. 66, 1086–1090.

Wardani, R., Salsabila, S., Rahman, A.N., Rakhmatiar, R., 2021. Effectivity of nintendo wii as rehabilitation therapy in post stroke patients: a systematic review. MNJ Malang Neurol. J. 7, 56–59.

Webster, D., Celik, O., 2014. Systematic review of Kinect applications in elderly care and stroke rehabilitation. J. Neuroeng. Rehabil. 11, 1–24.

Webster, A., Poyade, M., Rooney, S., Paul, L., 2021. Upper limb rehabilitation interventions using virtual reality for people with multiple sclerosis: a systematic review. Mult. Scler. Relat. Disord. 47, 102610.

Wei, W.X., Fong, K.N., Chung, R.C., et al., 2018. "Remind-to-move" for promoting upper extremity recovery using wearable devices in subacute stroke: a multi-center randomized controlled study. IEEE Trans. Neural Syst. Rehabil. Eng. 27, 51–59.

Wellpepper., 2022. Wellpepper. Available at: https://www.well-pepper.com/. Accessed on 5 Dec 2022.

Whitford, M., Schearer, E., Rowlett, M., 2018. Effects of in home high dose accelerometer-based feedback on perceived and actual use in participants chronic post-stroke. Physiother. Theory Pract. 36, 799–809.

Widmer, M., Held, J.P.O., Wittmann, F., et al., 2022. Reward during arm training improves impairment and activity after stroke: a randomized controlled trial. Neurorehabilit. Neural Repair. 36, 140–150.

Wittmann, F., Held, J.P., Lambercy, O., et al., 2016. Self-directed arm therapy at home after stroke with a sensor-based virtual reality training system. J. Neuroeng. Rehabil. 13, 75.

WizeCare., 2022. WizeCare. Available at: https://wizecare.com/. Accessed on 5 Dec 2022.

Wu, X., Liu, H., Zhang, J., Chen, W., 2019. Virtual reality training system for upper limb rehabilitation. 2019 14th IEEE Conference on Industrial Electronics and Applications (ICIEA).

Wüest, S., Massé, F., Aminian, K., et al., 2016. Reliability and validity of the inertial sensor-based Timed "Up and Go" test in individuals affected by stroke. J. Rehabil. Res. Devel. 53, 599–610.

Wulf, G., Shea, C., Lewthwaite, R., 2010. Motor skill learning and performance: a review of influential factors. Med. Educ. 44, 75–84.

XRHealth., 2022. XRHealth. Available at: https://www.xr.health/. Accessed on 5 Dec 2022.

Yamato, T.P., Pompeu, J.E., Pompeu, S.M., Hassett, L., 2016. Virtual reality for stroke rehabilitation. Phys. Ther. 96, 1508–1513.

Yeh, S.W., Lin, L.F., Tam, K.W., et al., 2020. Efficacy of robot-assisted gait training in multiple sclerosis: a systematic review and meta-analysis. Mult. Scler. Relat. Disord. 41, 102034.

Yeo, E., Chau, B., Chi, B., et al., 2019. Virtual reality neurorehabilitation for mobility in spinal cord injury: a structured review. Innov. Clin. Neurosci. 16, 13–20.

You, S.H., Jang, S.H., Kim, Y.-H., et al., 2005. Virtual reality–induced cortical reorganization and associated locomotor recovery in chronic stroke: an experimenter-blind randomized study. Stroke. 36, 1166–1171.

Yu, L., Xiong, D., Guo, L., et al., 2016. A remote quantitative Fugl-Meyer assessment framework for stroke patients based on wearable sensor networks. Comput methods programs biomed. 128, 100–110.

Zanatta, F., Giardini, A., Pierobon, A., et al., 2022. A systematic review on the usability of robotic and virtual reality devices in neuromotor rehabilitation: patients' and healthcare professionals' perspective. BMC Health Serv. Res. 22, 523.

Zariffa, J., Kapadia, N., Kramer, J.L., et al., 2011. Relationship between clinical assessments of function and measurements from an upper-limb robotic rehabilitation device in cervical spinal cord injury. IEEE Trans. Neural Syst. Rehabil. Eng. 20, 341–350.

Zhang, L., Lin, F., Sun, L., Chen, C., 2022. Comparison of efficacy of Lokomat and wearable exoskeleton-assisted gait training in people with spinal cord injury: a systematic review and network meta-analysis. Front. Neurol. 13, 772660.

Zhu, Y., Lu, W., Gan, W., Hou, W., 2021. A contactless method to measure real-time finger motion using depth-based pose estimation. Comput. Biol. Med. 131, 104282.

Falls and Their Management

Dorit Kunkel and Digna de Kam

OUTLINE

Introduction, 545
Falls and Falling, 546
   Extent of the Problem, 546
   Causes of Falling, 547
   Consequences of Falling, 548
Assessing People at Risk of Falling, 548
   Interviewing Patients and Carers, 550
   Falls Diaries, 550
   Observing Fall-Related Activities, 551
     Video, 552
   Standard Tests and Outcome Measures, 552
Preventing Falls and Managing People Who Have
   Fallen, 553

The Person at Risk for Falling, 554
   Exercise and Other Training Programmes, 554
   Continued Physical Activity, 556
   Movement Strategies, 556
Physical Environment, 557
   Footwear and Orthotics, 557
   External Environment, 558
   Indoor Versus Outdoor Falls, 558
   Walking Aids, 559
Engagement With Fall Prevention, 559
Not Every Fall Is Preventable, 559
Multifactorial Approach to Fall Prevention, 560
Conclusion, 560

KEY POINTS

- When stability is challenged, we may fear falling, almost fall or actually fall.
- Do not underestimate their seriousness: falls can be calamitous, terrifying events.
- Elderly people and neurological patients are at high risk for falling.
- The consequences of falling are various and costly, from activity restriction to death.
- Falls are high on the agenda of those who fund and provide rehabilitation.
- The literature, common sense and thorough assessment will identify individuals at risk.

There are more than 400 interacting risk factors for falling; focus on modifiable risk factors.

INTRODUCTION

Falls are 'events which cause you to come to rest on the ground or other lower level unintentionally, not because of seizure, stroke/myocardial infarction or an overwhelming displacing force' (Tinetti et al 1988). Although this definition is commonly used, no universally accepted falls definition exists (Yoshida-Intern 2007), giving rise to different interpretations. For example, some health professionals focus on injury and other consequences, whereas older people tend to describe falls as a loss of balance (Zecevic et al 2006). When considering falls, it is important to try to talk to all involved to define and use an agreed definition. This chapter will explore the epidemiology of falls in relation to different neurological pathologies and risk factors followed by suggestions for falls assessment and treatments.

FALLS AND FALLING

Any situation that challenges our postural stability has the potential to: (a) instil within us (and those who care for us) a swiftly passing or enduring fear of falling, and/or (b) give rise to a 'near miss' (if a fall feels imminent but does not actually occur), and/or (c) result in a fall (which may have devastating consequences, including death).

Fear of falling tops the list of concerns for older people (Age UK 2019), and falls are high on the agenda of those who fund and provide healthcare. They are a major cause of disability and the leading cause of mortality because of injury in people older than 65 years (Tian et al 2013). One in six people in England were aged 65 years or older in 2011; this figure is forecast to increase to one in four by 2050 (Morgan 2021). The economic impact of falls among elderly people in the UK is considerable and increasing. An estimated 220,160 people were admitted to hospital after a fall from 2018 to 2019 (Public Health England 2022, Public Health Outcomes Framework 2022). Falls cost the National Health Service (NHS) more than £2 billion per year and account for more than 4 million bed days (Public Health England 2017, Royal College of Physicians 2013). People with neurological disorders are more vulnerable to falls than healthy young and older people, and they form the focus of this chapter. Other populations vulnerable to falls are beyond the scope of this chapter. These populations are likely to form part of the rehabilitation caseload and include:

People with dementia: At least 50% of people with dementia experience falls each year (Ansai et al 2019, Kröpelin et al 2013, Li and Harmer 2020,). In addition to the risk factors listed later, mobile people with dementia who have slow or unsteady gait and depressive symptoms tend to be at highest risk (Bansal et al 2016, Chantanachai et al 2021). Among people with dementia living in residential homes, fall frequency peaks in the late afternoon and evening, and this may be associated with 'sun downing syndrome'. Sun downing in people with dementia is linked with increased agitation, disorientation, confusion, anxiety, restlessness and wandering which suggests that increased awareness and careful supervision during this time may help to reduce falls (Bouwen et al 2008, Cipriani et al 2015).

People admitted or recently discharged from hospital: A hospital admission increases the risk for falls partially because of the unfamiliar surroundings but also because hospital admission is often associated with being acutely unwell or because of a deterioration in physical or mental well-being (National Institute for Health and Care Excellence [NICE] 2013, Stubbs et al 2014). Following consideration of the 'extent of the problem', the extensive literature to identify

patient groups at high risk for instability and falling has been outlined (see Causes of Falling on page 545).

To identify *an individual* at high risk for falling, be aware of the risk factors and use common sense. Haines et al (2009) showed that physiotherapists were highly accurate in predicting patient falls during rehabilitation when completing a comprehensive patient assessment (see Assessing People at Risk of Falling on page 546). There is no such thing as 'a faller': every patient who has fallen is an individual. Although an individual carries their risk factors for falling with them 24 hours a day, they only fall at particular moments. The path to preventing someone from falling (or, at least, falling again) stems from understanding their fall history in detail (see Preventing Falls and Managing People Who Have Fallen on page 551 and Multifactorial Approach to Fall Prevention on page 558); that is, the circumstances (Stack & Ashburn 1999) in which they fear falling, have nearly fallen or have actually fallen. It is important not to overlook near misses, which Skelton et al (2005) defined as 'a potential fall corrected'.

Extent of the Problem

Approximately one-third of community-dwelling people aged 65 and older fall annually, rising to 50% for those aged 80 and older (Public Health England 2022). Falling is also a problem for younger people living with a neurological condition, with an average 50% of those younger than 55 reporting at least one fall per year (Saverino et al 2014). People with neurological conditions, particularly people with stroke (see Chapter 7), multiple sclerosis (MS) (see Chapter 10), Parkinson's (see Chapter 11) or Huntington's disease (see Chapter 12) fall frequently and are at high risk for injuries and fractures (Gunn et al 2014, Schmid et al 2013, Wielinski et al 2005). Up to 65% of people with stroke fall in hospital (Batchelor et al 2012, Nyberg & Gustafson 1995, Teasell et al 2002). Between one-quarter and three-quarters of community-dwelling elderly people with chronic stroke fall over 6 months (Forster & Young 1995, Kerse et al 2008, Mackintosh et al 2006), and 50% report falls 1 year post-stroke (Ashburn et al 2008a, Schmid et al 2013). Among people with Parkinson's, approximately 60% fall and, of these, one-third fall repeatedly (Allen et al 2013, Amar et al 2015). Fall rates are similar among people with MS; approximately 56% experience falls and 37% experience repeated falls (Nilsagård et al 2015). Among those with Huntington's disease, 58% reported repeated falls in the previous 12 months (Busse et al 2009).

For someone with a neurological disorder, it takes less of a challenge to threaten postural stability than it does for someone with an intact system. In the model in Fig. 21.1, someone with good postural stability is likely to fall only

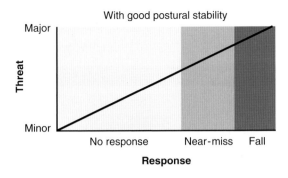

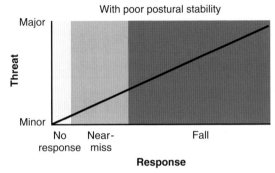

FIG. 21.1 Relation between postural threat and outcome for individuals with good and poor postural stability.

after a major challenge, a moderate threat may challenge their stability and register a near miss, and any lesser threat may not even cause a near miss. Healthy young and older individuals are often able to recover balance from a postural perturbation (Maki & McIlroy 1997) because they can adjust their balance in anticipation of potential balance disturbances (proactive balance) and can compensate quickly in response to unpredicted (reactive balance) postural disturbances (Shumway-Cook & Woollacott 2017). Conversely, someone with poor postural stability, such as people with stroke, Parkinson's or MS, may fall even when they experience minor balance threats. Even higher functional individuals with a neurological condition often have slowed, ineffective or absent reactive balance reactions (de Kam et al 2014, 2017a, Giulio et al 2016, Mansfield et al 2013, Massot et al 2019, Zadravec et al 2020). Because of the lack of these balance reactions, almost any threat to postural stability can result in a fall. As patients progress through rehabilitation, they may reacquire some of the skills to withstand moderate threats to balance (Jöbges et al 2004, Mansfield et al 2018, Protas et al 2005, Schinkel-Ivy et al 2020). Reactive balance training has shown potential to improve balance reactions even in people with chronic stroke (van Duijnhoven et al 2018).

Causes of Falling

The literature mentions more than 400 risk factors for falling ('Preventing Falls and Injuries in Older People' 1996). Grouped simply, some of the most frequently cited risk factors for falls are:

- *Nutritional status:* e.g., vitamin D or calcium deficiency
- *Environmental hazards:* e.g., loose carpets, poor lighting, poor footwear
- *Movement problems and lack of exercise:* e.g., muscle weakness, poor balance, gait disturbance, bone loss
- *Medication:* e.g., antidepressants, hypnotics, diuretics
- *Age and medical condition:* e.g., visual impairment, cognitive impairment, osteoarthritis

The three most predictive factors for falls that should be considered by clinicians assessing people at risk for falls both in community and extended-care settings are a history of previous falls, gait impairments and balance impairments (NICE 2013, Montero-Odasso et al 2022). Falls increase when multiple risk factors are present (Tinetti et al 1988).

Impairments such as muscle weakness, impaired cognition or attention, limited range of motion and activities of daily living (ADLs) ability, sensorimotor dysfunction, balance and mobility problems contribute to the large number of falls among people with stroke (Cho et al 2015, Hyndman & Ashburn 2002, 2003, Marigold & Misiaszek 2009, Tan & Tan 2016). Among people with Parkinson's, increased disease severity and duration of the disease, motor and cognitive impairments, slowness or freezing of gait, fear of falling, orthostatic hypotension, treatment with dopamine agonists and increased levodopa dosage contribute to recurrent falls (Allen et al 2013, Francois et al 2017, Pelicioni et al 2019).

Those with primary progressive MS who experience imbalance and cognitive dysfunction appear to be at greatest risk (Nilsagård et al 2015). Targets for physical intervention in those with Huntington's disease include gait bradykinesia, stride variability and chorea often leading to increased sway, cognitive decline and behavioural changes (Grimbergen et al 2008). Postural instability and unsteady gait are among the most common symptoms in people with neurological conditions, playing a part in many falls among these patients (Brozova et al 2011, Saverino et al 2014).

Encouragingly, many risk factors are amenable to intervention and will be the focus in this chapter. For example, van der Marck et al (2014) explored the fall risk factors that have been identified for people with Parkinson's and, through a consensus and expert panel review, recommended that assessments should focus mainly on 31 amenable risk factors. The final list included generic risk factors (highlighted earlier) but also disease-specific factors such as previous falls, disease severity, Parkinson's medication, slow mobility, shuffling and freezing of gait, stooped posture, axial rigidity, dyskinesias and cognitive impairment (van der Marck et al 2014). Similar lists exist for people with MS (Gianni et al 2014), stroke (Tan & Tan 2016) and Huntington's disease (Bachoud-Levi et al 2019).

Significantly, the *interaction* between risk factors is often more important than the risk factors themselves. As Berry and Miller (2008, p. 149) stated, 'falls result from an interaction between characteristics that increase an individual's propensity to fall and acute mediating risk factors that provide the opportunity to fall'. To reduce falls, therapists target potentially hazardous interactions by identifying the circumstances in which the patient falls and relating them to the pathology to determine the factors causing falls; these factors are likely to be disease and even patient specific. In many cases a multidisciplinary assessment will be necessary, drawing on the skills and expertise of those trained to assess factors ranging from balance and mobility to underlying medical conditions and the surrounding environment, and multidisciplinary intervention may follow (see A Multifactorial Approach to Fall Prevention section).

Consequences of Falling

The consequences of falling are wide ranging, interconnected and costly, and they may be devastating (Table 21.1).

KEY POINTS

- Take a thorough fall history before observing the patient move.
- Identify the circumstances surrounding previous falls and near misses.
- Interview the person who fell (or witnesses) and consider using a falls diary.
- Observe the person who fell performing fall-related activities in a functional way.
- Consider the careful use of a video recording.
- Complete a battery of appropriate tests and outcome measures.

ASSESSING PEOPLE AT RISK OF FALLING

A history of falls and balance and gait problems are among the most important risk factors for falling (Panel on Prevention of Falls in Older Persons 2011). Therefore

TABLE 21.1	Consequences of Falling
Fear of falling	Between 21% and 85% of older people express fall-related fear of falling which is correlated with psychological distress, reduced balance confidence and restriction of activity (Hadjistavropoulos et al 2011, Scheffer et al 2008, Terroso et al 2014).
	Factors that are associated with fear of falling include (Denkinger et al 2015):
	• Female gender
	• Using a walking aid
	• Poor physical function
	• Anxiety
	• History of falls
	A fear of falls can lead to (Lach & Parsons 2013):
	• Activity restriction
	• Increase risk for falls
	• Reduced quality of life
	• Depression
	• Potential fallers taking extra care
	An enduring fear can also negatively affect carers (Dow et al 2013).
	Fear, alongside other factors that restrict activity, should feature in fall prevention. Multifactorial interventions that include behavioural strategies to reduce avoidance behaviours and catastrophic thinking and include exercises may decrease some sources of fear during the intervention period (Huang et al 2016, Kumar et al 2016, Whipple et al. 2018).
Functional decline and increased dependence	Those who live alone, have poor self-rated health and are physically inactive are most at risk (Ek et al 2021) of functional decline and increased dependence. This can result in consequences ranging from people needing more support at home to requiring admission to long-term care facilities (Terroso et al 2014).

TABLE 21.1	Consequences of Falling—Cont'd
Injury	Fall descent, impact and bone strength are important determinants of whether a fall will result in a fracture (Berry & Miller 2008). Fractured femur is one of the most costly and debilitating consequences of falling (Terroso et al 2014). Cummings and Nevitt (1989) and Hwang et al (2011) summarised risk factors that increased the likelihood of a fall resulting in a hip fracture: • Fall direction/faller orientation (moving slowly, with little forwards momentum, a fall would result in direct application of impact energy to the femur) • Bone strength (several disorders can weaken the bone around the hip and increase the risk for fracture) • Depression (may be linked to medication use and slower reaction times) • Lack of protective response (grabbing something or stumbling might prevent a fall, change the faller's orientation or dissipate impact) • Local shock absorption (muscle or fat would be protective, whereas a hard landing surface would increase fracture risk) In a review of the literature, Moon and Sosnoff (2017) described landing strategies that reduce the load during a fall: • Squatting with flexed knees and hips during a backwards fall • Flexing elbows during a forwards fall • Rotating forwards or relaxing muscles during a sideways fall and stepping to reposition the foot in a more lateral position However, to date most studies explored safe landing strategies in younger people; few have explored the feasibility of retraining safe landing strategies in older people (Groen et al 2010).
Costly intervention	Injurious falls may require medical attention. Costs include: • Ambulance journey • Accident and emergency attendance • Hospital stay • Outpatient attendance • General practitioner consultations • Long-term care
Carer strain/injury	Dow et al (2013) highlighted that carer strain increased significantly after the first fall. Carers increased supervision, changed their daily routines in an attempt to be constantly vigilant and highlighted a lack of knowledge of available support services. Carers can be injured attempting to prevent falls and helping someone up after a fall: rehabilitation must not overlook them.
Death	Accidental injurious falls are the leading cause of death among elderly people (Royal College of Physicians 2013) with >5,000 older people dying in 2017 as a result of the fall (Age UK 2019). A long lie on after a fall has been reported in 30% of fallers and was linked to hospital admission, serious injury and the need for long-term care (Fleming & Brayne 2008).

further evaluation of fall risk factors is recommended if patients report a history of falls or difficulties with balance or gait. The first step for every fall assessment is to take a good fall history (with the patient in a safe, stable position) before performing a functional observation or a mobility test. This allows for choosing assessment tools suitable to the functional level of the patient. When, for example, a person who has fallen reports 'turning is fatal' or 'all falls are to do with turning' (Stack & Ashburn 1999), the therapist will be suitably alert to the risks inherent in asking that patient to perform a turn test. On the other hand, if a patient reports difficulties during walking under challenging circumstances, it is recommended to choose an assessment tool that mimics these circumstances. A final key aspect of a fall risk assessment is an evaluation of the home environment (Gillespie et al 2012), particularly for those individuals who spend most of their time indoors or those with a history of indoors falls. Taken together, the assessment of individuals at risk of falls consists of (1) a thorough history taking, (2) functional observation, (3) functional mobility testing and (4) evaluation of the home environment if indicated.

Interviewing Patients and Carers

Previous falls and near falls provide important information about a patient's fall risk profile (Kunkel et al 2011, Sanders et al 2015, Stack & Ashburn 1999). However, falls are not always well documented in patients' medical records; patients may not share the same ideas as healthcare professionals about what constitutes a fall (e.g., 'I didn't fall, I slipped'), nor may they always wish to disclose a fall (Amar et al 2015). It is imperative that therapists use all their interviewing skills to talk to patients about previous falls or near falls. The key to understanding what has happened (and thus being able to prevent a repetition) is being able to identify the circumstances in which the individual has fallen. Falls are distinct events that happen in a specific time and place and for a specific reason; although people with neurological conditions fall more frequently than people without, they do not fall continuously. An individual's risk factors for falling act on them *all day every day*, but people fall only occasionally, when they cannot preserve their postural stability as they move about their environment. Researchers have identified the most common circumstances in which people with stroke (Batchelor 2012, Goto et al 2019, Hyndman et al 2002, Mackintosh et al 2005, Schmid et al 2013, Weerdesteyn et al 2008), Parkinson's (Ashburn et al 2008b, Lamont et al 2017, Pelicioni 2019, Stack & Ashburn 1999, Stack & Roberts 2013) and MS (Gunn et al 2014, Mazumder et al 2014) fall. Limited information is available on falls among people with Huntington's disease (Grimbergen et al 2008, Kalkers et al 2016). Patients with neurological conditions are more likely than community-dwelling elderly persons to fall in or around their home (Batchelor et al 2012, Goto et al 2019, Gunn et al 2014, Hyndman et al 2002, Schmid et al 2013, Weerdesteyn 2008), where they spend most of their time. Outdoor falls are more common in patients who are less severely affected (Lamont et al 2017) and are therefore able to leave the house more regularly. Falls are often experienced during activities such as walking and turning transfers and ADLs (Ashburn et al 2008b, Batchelor et al 2012, Goto et al 2019, Hyndman et al 2002, Pelicioni et al 2019). Many people fall because of a trip, slip or loss of balance. In patients with Parkinson's, freezing of gait is an important cause of falls (Pelicioni et al 2019). Moreover, syncope and orthostatic hypotension should be considered as causes of falls because those

issues often require medical intervention (Fanciulli et al 2020, McDonald et al 2017).

In other words, the therapist must attempt to discover, through questioning and observation:
1. Where the patient fell;
2. What the patient was trying to do at the time: the 'fall-related activity';
3. What might have caused the patient to fall at that instant;
4. Whether the patient was able to break their fall in any way; and
5. What happened when and after the patient hit the floor.

Information on the circumstances and causes of falls can be obtained from the patient and those who may have witnessed the (near) fall. Unfortunately, in the case of most inpatient falls, the person documenting the fall did not see it happen. Hignett et al (2013) reported that staff witnessed only 8% of inpatient falls. Although a witness can easily record the location in which they found the faller, the time and evident injuries, they can only surmise what had happened (i.e., the fall-precipitating circumstances). This is reflected in the quality of the reports that staff can complete; in more than half of the sample of inpatient fall reports the record contained no information on the fall location, or the circumstances or risk factors that may have contributed (Hignett et al 2013).

Even the act of taking a detailed falls history may be a fall-preventive intervention, boosting insight and confidence. Elderly people who reflect on their falls and seek understanding are better able (than are their nonreflecting peers) to develop strategies to prevent future falls, face their fear of falling and remain active (Roe et al 2008). Self-reported impaired balance is a readily assessed risk factor for future fractures in elderly people (Wagner et al 2009). On completion of the interview, refer patients to other specialists if their input is necessary.

In addition to asking about past falls, it is also recommended to collect information about near misses and situations where the patient struggles to maintain balance. Those situations may lead to falls in the future or cause a fear of falling. Fear of falling is common in patients with neurological conditions (Kalkers et al 2016, Kalron et al 2017, Lindholm et al 2014, Schmid & Rittman 2009) and often leads to avoidance of activities. This results in deconditioning and thus further deterioration of balance and gait capacities (Lach & Parsons 2013, Schmid & Rittman 2009).

Falls Diaries

When information on falls and their circumstances is obtained retrospectively, patients may not be able to recall all their falls and fall circumstances. This is particularly the case for those who fall frequently (Antcliff et al 2022).

Hence a therapist can consider asking the patient to keep a falls diary when they are on the waiting list for physiotherapy or during active rehabilitation. The same questions that one might ask a patient directly can form the basis of a falls diary. The use of fall diaries is common in research studies on fall prevention interventions (Goodwin et al 2015, Mansfield 2018, Morris et al 2017, Sanders et al 2015). In addition, the European physiotherapy practice guideline on Parkinson's recommends the use of a falls diary (Keus et al 2014). On a calendar sheet patients mark any day on which they had a fall or a near miss. For each fall or near miss, information is obtained on (1) where the patient was, (2) what activity was performed and (3) the cause of the fall (see Table 21.2 for example falls diary use for injurious falls during turning; Ashburn et al 2008b).

For actual falls additional information is obtained on the consequences of the fall.

A falls diary can assist professionals with their assessments (and guide intervention) by:

1. Detailing the circumstances in which a patient is unstable; and
2. Illuminating the patient's level of insight; multiple 'don't know' or 'no idea' type responses may suggest that the patient lacks insight or interest or was not conscious.

Having someone who has fallen recently jot down the circumstances shortly after the incident may seem a promising way of recording the details before they fade from memory, but there is no guarantee. Diaries will not suit everyone. Interviews, reenactments and diaries all have strengths and weakness, but ultimately they all rely on the patient's perception.

Observing Fall-Related Activities

Now that the reader is clear about what type of activities cause the patient to fear falling or have previously caused near misses or actual falls, it is time to observe the patient attempting such activities.

- Embed the activities within representative 'real-life' activities, rather than asking the patient to perform isolated movements outside a functional context. For example, if a patient reports having fallen reaching, watch them reach for something from a high shelf and/ or a low cupboard rather than ask them to perform the Functional Reach Test (Duncan et al 1990).
- Functional tasks replicate more closely the type of challenge that meaningful action poses, whereas outcome measures are likely to impose certain limitations on the way patients move. Certain turn tests, for example, dictate where the subject should turn and in what direction; such a test will not reveal how subjects spontaneously turn when it is necessary to do so.
- Another advantage of observing functional tasks rather than relying only on standard tests is that the patient has something on which to focus other than the movement

TABLE 21.2 Examples of Injurious Falls During Turning That Require Health Service Input: An Example of Falls Diary Use (Ashburn et al 2008b)

Location	Activity/Cause	Landing	Injury	Getting Up	Intervention
Hotel	Turned too quickly	Right side	Fractured hand, bruises	Wife and son helped me	X-ray; surgery
Descending stairs	Twisted	On back	Fractured ribs, concussion		Husband called ambulance; 10 hours in hospital
Putting food in fridge	Turned	Very hard on back	Fractured ribs, bruises		Friends called ambulance; general practitioner called 2 days later
Sitting room	Turned too sharply	Left side	Hurt left shoulder	With help of chair	Called general practitioner; sent to accident and emergency
Shop	Turned quickly	Face-first	Cut face, nosebleed	Two ambulance men helped me	Ambulance
Kitchen	Turned quickly opening door	Heavily on side	Banged head, arm and shoulder	Crawled to lounge; used chair	Paramedics called

of interest. You could ask a patient who has fallen turning and reaching to perform the Timed Up and Go test (Podsiadlo & Richardson 1991) and the Functional Reach Test (Duncan et al 1990), or you could ask them to make a cup of tea (ideally in their own environment) while you observe them. The former will give you the time taken and distance reached. The latter will illuminate how the person moves during challenging tasks, whether they compensate and to what hazards they may be exposing themselves.

- Stack et al (2016) highlighted that extended in-home observation has several advantages over the one-off 'home visit'. Ticking off a checklist of theoretical challenges and hazards within a single session is likely to be unrepresentative, whereas 'assessing' someone descending the steps into her kitchen is unlikely to reflect how she does it when hurrying towards a saucepan that is boiling over. We recommend the assessor observes how the person uses their space, how they pace activities and how they manage tasks when their attention is on a goal, not on the task itself. Asking someone to walk you from their favourite chair to the top or bottom of their stairs is likely to provide opportunities to observe transfers, turns, walking and tackling steps naturally.

Video

In addition to traditional observation, using a video as a record of a patient assessment can be useful for feedback to the patient. Traditional handheld or static video cameras were most often used in the past (Stack et al 2016), but other mobile media such as smartphones and iPads provide a feasible alternative (Koh et al 2015). A video record allows repeated playback, which facilitates the rating, timing or step counting required by certain outcome measures. It also facilitates discussion with colleagues who may not have been able to attend a patient assessment in person. Always secure the permission of a patient to make, store and use a video record, and take all reasonable precautions not to record other patients' images or conversations inadvertently. Remember that a camera with a trailing power lead is a trip hazard, and that a handheld camera or holding an iPad prevents the therapist's hands from being free to catch a falling patient: be careful (Stack et al 2005). We recommend batteries and tripods or stable movable iPad stands (Koh et al 2015). Several wearable, sensor and other technologies for fall assessment and fall prevention have been documented, but the cost, availability and current evidence base do not yet support adoption into fall assessments in clinical practice (Chaudhuri et al 2014, Godfrey 2017).

Standard Tests and Outcome Measures

In assessing patients who have fallen, there is certainly a place for standardised measures. Armed with a detailed fall history and having observed the patient perform the culprit activities naturally, the therapist can progress to evaluating aspects of the patient's mobility and balance that:

1. May be contributing to their risk for falling, and
2. Will form the focus of intervention.

Although there has been considerable interest in developing screening tools to identify people at risk for falling, the results are contentious. Remembering the variety of risk factors for falling, it is apparent that predicting who will and who will not fall within a given time is no simple task (Oliver 2008, Oliver et al 2008). NICE (2013) does not recommend using fall prediction tools to attempt to predict an inpatient's risk for falling. Therefore we will not discuss the issue of population screening tools here but focus instead on the type of tools that will help a therapist track their patient's progress as their condition changes and/or they progress through rehabilitation.

Because balance deficits are among the most important risk factors for falling (Panel on Prevention of Falls in Older Persons 2011), we recommend a balance assessment tool as part of the fall risk assessment. A wide variety of balance assessment tools are available, which differ in the type and difficulty of the tasks included. Balance control tasks can roughly be divided in three main categories: steady-state balance control, proactive balance control and reactive balance control (Shumway-Cook & Woolacott 2017). Steady-state balance control involves maintaining balance under predictable and nonchanging circumstances. Examples of steady-state balance control tasks involve standing quietly or walking at a constant speed. Proactive balance control involves maintaining balance during voluntary movements with a predictable effect on postural stability. Examples of proactive balance control tasks are transfers or lifting objects. Moreover, proactive balance control is required when making adjustments to the gait pattern under dynamic and challenging circumstances (e.g., walking on an uneven surface or in a crowded environment). Neurological patients typically struggle with adjusting their gait to changes in the environment (unexpected obstacles, walking in crowds). This is particularly difficult when they must do so under time pressure (van Swigchem et al 2013), which may increase the risk of falls when walking outside. A last category of balance control is reactive balance, which involves restoring stability after a balance perturbation. Balance perturbations can result from either an external force (e.g., bumping into another person) or failing proactive balance control such as during turning or performing a transfer. When selecting a balance assessment tool, it is important to consider the type of tasks the patient experiences difficulties with and the level of functioning of the patient. For example, community-dwelling individuals need to control their balance under more challenging circumstances than patients residing mostly indoors. Table 21.3 illustrates examples of commonly used balance assessment tools in relation to the different categories of balance tasks.

Fig. 21.2 shows the relation between history taking, observation and standardised tests in the fall risk assessment.

PREVENTING FALLS AND MANAGING PEOPLE WHO HAVE FALLEN

After a comprehensive assessment, the therapist will be able to target the interactions between the individual and their environment that place them at risk for falling. For a patient with a condition (or other risk factor for falling)

that will be ongoing, the therapist must consider the challenges that person will face over 24 hours and address each one; the history of falls, near misses and fears will highlight

---

KEY POINTS

- Target the hazardous interactions between the individual and their environment.
- Exercise can reduce risk for falling and stimulate continued physical activity.
- Developing new movement strategies can make everyday activities safer.
- Appropriate footwear reduces the risk for falling.
- Modifying the environment reduces falls where hazards play a part.

TABLE 21.3 Balance Assessment Tools

Assessment Tool	Steady-State Balance	Proactive Balance	Dynamic Gait	Reactive Balance
Tinetti/POMA (Tinetti 1986)	X	X		X
Timed Up & Go test (Podsiadlo & Richardson 1991)		X		
Functional reach test (Duncan et al 1990)		X		
Berg Balance Scale (Berg et al 1992)	X	X		
Mini-BesTEST (Franchignoni et al. 2010)	X	X	X	X
Dynamic Gait Index (Shumway-Cook & Woollacott 1995)		X	X	
Functional Gait Assessment (Wrisley et al 2004)		X	X	
Push and release test (Jacobs et al 2006)				X

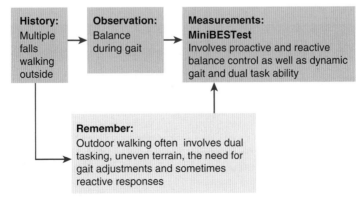

FIG. 21.2 Relation between history taking, observation and selection of measurement tools.

the priorities. Specifically, individuals with a mild to moderate fall risk may benefit from exercise alone, whereas more severely affected individuals more likely need a multifactorial approach (Gillespie et al 2012).

The Person at Risk for Falling

Exercise and Other Training Programmes

Physical activity (or exercise) is an important contributor to healthy ageing and fall prevention among elderly people and those with neurological conditions (Bauman et al 2016, Denissen et al 2019, Rose 2008, Sherrington et al 2019, World Health Organization 2010, Montero-Odasso et al 2022). Being physically active can:

- Delay or prevent the pathology and impairments that lead to disability and increased fall risk;
- Slow the progression of disease and system impairments;
- Restore function to a level that allows for more autonomy in the ADLs; and
- Reduce fear of falling as an important contributor to activity limitations.

Exercise interventions are effective in reducing fall risk in older individuals (Sherrington et al 2019) and in populations with stroke (Denissen et al 2019), mild Parkinson's (Canning et al 2015, O'Malley et al 2021, Seymour et al 2019), MS (Abou et al 2022) and Huntington's disease (Quinn et al 2020).

A meta-analysis of 108 trials in older individuals (with more than 23,000 participants) by Sherrington et al (2019) revealed that exercise reduced the rate of falling by 23%. Moreover, exercise programmes reduced the number of fallers by 15%. In particular, programmes with balance and functional exercises either with or without resistance exercises were effective in reducing fall rates and the number of fallers. Strength exercises may be a good addition to functional balance training because muscle strength contributes to postural control (MuehlBauer et al 2015). Thus strength training (as part of a multifactorial intervention) often shows a reduction in fall rates (Hill et al 2015, Ishigaki et al 2014). Although not all the example programmes outlined in Boxes 21.1–21.5 have been adequately tested in fully powered fall prevention trials, each one contains ideas for intervention that may suit specific patients.

In addition to older individuals, exercise interventions may also be effective to reduce fall risk in patients with neurological conditions. Specifically, a meta-analysis obtained in people with stroke (Denissen et al 2019) showed a 28% reduction in fall rate for interventions with an exercise component (8 studies, 765 participants). Although it was not possible to compare the effectiveness of different exercise interventions, most of the training programmes involved functional balance and/or gait exercises. Thus functional balance and gait training can be recommended

---

BOX 21.1   Example Programme 1: Individually Tailored Progressive Home-Based Exercise Programme for Parkinson's Patients (PDSAFE, Ashburn 2019, Goodwin 2015, Seymour 2019)

Patients were guided by a physiotherapist to target modifiable fall risk factors such as freezing of gait, balance and mobility problems and physical activity. The programme involved the following components:

- Task-oriented movement strategy training for improvement of freezing of gait and the performance of complex tasks involving fall-related activities.
- Progressive strengthening exercises for the lower limb.
- Progressive dynamic balance exercises at a moderate to hard intensity.

BOX 21.2   Example Programme 2: The FALLS Programme for People With Chronic Stroke (van Duijnhoven et al 2012)

The FALLS programme was adapted from the Nijmegen Falls Prevention programme, which successfully reduced fall rates in older individuals (Weerdesteyn et al 2006). The 5-week group programme consisted of the following elements:

- Obstacle course mimicking hazards from daily life such as uneven pavements, slopes, uneven surfaces, narrow passages and kneeling. The complexity of the obstacle course was increased using dual tasks.

- Fall training derived from martial arts techniques and involving forward, backward and sideways falling. Difficulty was gradually increased in terms of fall height.
- Walking exercises simulated walking in crowded environments. During the exercises, participants were challenged to change the speed and direction of walking. In addition, dual tasks were involved.

BOX 21.3   Example Programme 3: Example Programme for People With Multiple Sclerosis (Hogan et al 2014)

- Self-paced circuit strength and balance group exercise class 1 hour per week for 10 weeks
- Exercises included sit to stand, squatting, heel raises and stepping exercises (step-ups, side step and tandem stance)

- Each exercise had three difficulty levels depending on ability and was performed in sets of 12 (and progressed up to 3 sets of 12 if able)
- Included people with a confirmed diagnosis of multiple sclerosis with no relapse in the previous 12 weeks

BOX 21.4   Example Programme for People With Parkinson's (Morris et al 2011, 2015)

Two hour-long outpatient group exercise sessions once-weekly home exercises for 8 weeks
Included progressive resistance strength training:
- Exercises were progressed when exertion level dropped below the required level on the Modified Perceived Exertion scale (Foster et al 2001)
  - Exercises included sit to stand, trunk extension and rotation, step-ups, lateral pelvic hold/hitch, heel raises, toe standing, abdominal strengthening exercises in sitting
  - Completed in 1–2 sets with 8–15 repetitions (as able)
  - Therapists ensured safety, taught, progressed and corrected movements
  - Progression included changing the starting position, increasing weights or resistance (in 2% body weight increments) and increasing the number of repetitions

- Movement strategy training
  - Teaching and practicing individualised movement strategies: to use and incorporate cues, focus attention, break down complex movements and practice individual components of specific activities
  - Strategies for walking, turning, reaching, sit to stand, transfers and stepping tasks were included
  - Those with mild impairments practiced dual tasking; those with advanced disease were taught how to avoid dual tasking
- Community-dwelling people with confirmed diagnosis of idiopathic Parkinson's willing and able to attend an outpatient exercise programme

BOX 21.5   Example Programme 5: Toronto Perturbation-Based Balance Training in the Chronic Phase After Stroke (Mansfield et al 2018, Schinkel-Ivy et al. 2019).

Individual supervised training sessions aimed at improving reactive balance control. The programme consisted of two categories of balance perturbations:
- Internal perturbations were evoked using challenging agility tasks that were designed to cause a loss of balance (i.e., rapid stepping, kicking)

- External perturbations are caused by an external force (i.e., physiotherapist). The following external perturbations were used: lean-and-release, push/pull and trips during walking
Participants wore a safety harness during the training, and the intensity of the perturbations was progressive based on the performance of the individual.

to reduce the risk of falling after a stroke. For patients with Parkinson's, home exercise programmes involving strategy training, strength training and behavioural modification may reduce the risk of falls (Morris et al 2015). Positive effects on falls were mainly observed in individuals with milder disease severity but not in those who are more severely affected (Canning et al 2015, Seymour et al 2019). In addition, virtual reality treadmill training (Mirelman et al 2016) and tai chi (Gao et al 2014, Li et al 2012) may reduce the risk of falls in patients with Parkinson's.

The effect of physical therapy interventions on fall risk in persons with other neurological conditions is limited. Yet, the results of a recent meta-analysis in individuals with MS suggest that home-based exercise programmes may reduce fall risk in ambulatory patients (Abou et al 2022). Taken together, exercise interventions should be considered to reduce the risk of falls in both elderly persons and patients with neurological conditions.

Although direct evidence for the effect of exercise interventions on fall risk needs further study, it has been well-established that challenging and task-specific exercise interventions have a beneficial effect on key determinants of falls, such as balance, dynamic gait, strength functional mobility and balance confidence (Allen et al 2011, Canning et al 2015, Conradsson et al 2015, Goodwin et al 2008, Gunn et al 2015, Pollock et al 2014, Seymour et al 2019, Shen et al 2016, Smania 2010, Tang et al 2015, Tomlinson et al 2012, van Duijnhoven et al 2016, 2018, Veerbeek et al 2014).

Because the effects of balance training are task specific (Mansfield 2018), it is important to tailor the training intervention to the daily life activities of the individual patient and the observed deficits in balance control (steady-state, proactive control and/or reactive control; see Standardized Tests and Outcome Measures). For example, training of steady-state balance control may focus on maintaining a sitting or a standing position. Proactive balance training may consist of practicing functional tasks such as reaching, turning and making transfers. In addition, walking is a task in which patients struggle with proactive balance control, particularly if the gait pattern needs to be adjusted to a changing environment (e.g., uneven surfaces, stepping on the sidewalk, navigating through a crowded environment). It has been shown that training programmes focusing on gait adaptations (particularly under time pressure) can improve gait adaptability in people with stroke and Parkinson's (Mirelman 2011, van Ooijen 2015). Such training programmes are particularly useful for patients walking outside. A final aspect of balance control that needs to be considered is reactive balance training. It must be emphasised that the effect of conventional balance training on reactive control is limited (Kannan 2020, Mansfield 2018). Hence reactive balance training (perturbation-based balance training) needs to be considered in patients with reactive balance control deficits. Particularly reactive stepping in response to a balance perturbation is often challenging for older individuals and those with neurological conditions (de Kam et al 2014, 2017a, Gray et al 2019, Handelzalts et al 2019, Honeycutt et al 2016, Patel & Bhatt 2018, Peterson et al 2016a). Several studies have shown improved reactive stepping responses after perturbation-based training in patients with stroke, Parkinson's and MS (Dusane et al 2020, Peterson et al 2016b, Schinkel-Ivy et al 2019, 2020, van Duijnhoven et al 2018, van Liew et al 2021). Moreover, perturbation-based balance training may reduce fall risk (Mansfield et al 2015). Many perturbation-based training programmes require advanced lab equipment such as

moveable platforms or instrumented treadmills. However, a programme developed by Mansfield et al consists of therapist-induced perturbations and was shown to be effective in reactive stepping performance (Mansfield et al 2018, Schinkel-Ivy et al 2019). This programme is displayed in Box 21.5.

Continued Physical Activity

Although maintaining an active lifestyle is recommended for everyone, it is even more crucial for patients with neurological conditions. For those individuals, physical inactivity may lead to deterioration of strength, balance and gait capacity (Bhalsing et al 2018, Sandroff et al 2015), thereby increasing the risk of falls. On the other hand, functional mobility impairments and fear of falling resulting from neurological conditions often form a barrier for adopting an active lifestyle. Therefore fall-prevention programmes focusing on improving functional mobility and balance confidence (Abou et al 2021) may have the potential to stimulate continued involvement in physical activity (Laforest et al 2009). Keep in mind that different people are motivated in different ways towards exercise; patients will probably abandon boring home exercises quickly. Think about the various reasons you enjoy exercise (spending time alone or with other people, relaxing or competing, being outdoors or achieving obvious results), and think about finding ways for your patients to experience the same satisfaction (see also Chapter 20).

Movement Strategies

During rehabilitation, fall risk can be reduced by exercise programmes targeting the physical fall risk factors (Boxes 21.1–21.5) and by home evaluations and modifications to minimise environmental risk factors (see Physical Environment section on page 555). With these interventions, fall risk can be reduced but not eliminated, given that physical limitations may persist to some extent. The third strand to fall prevention for people at ongoing risk for falling is for them to learn to move through their world safely in light of the risk. For example, a patient struggling with a stand-to-sit transfer towards a chair may reduce the risk of falling by appropriately positioning themselves in front of the chair before transferring and using the handrails when performing the transfer. Such movement strategies are often used in the treatment of patients with Parkinson's but can also be useful for other populations. The patient and therapist work together to instigate new movement strategies, with the therapist drawing on their assessment and teaching skills:

Step 1: Extract the fall-related activities from an individual's fall history.

Step 2: Devise suitable movement strategies.

Step 3: Help the person at risk for falling to learn these strategies.

Deviations in posture and movement are common in individuals with neurological conditions. It is important to observe these deviations and consider whether they may hinder or benefit the patient. For example, a slight weight-bearing asymmetry towards the nonparetic side may facilitate reactive stepping towards the paretic side of stroke patients (de Kam et al 2017b). It may sometimes be necessary to promote compensations that improve patient safety (e.g., slow down, take several small steps). Strategies that may enhance stability during common fall-related activities in persons with Parkinson's based on findings by Stack & Ashburn (1999) and Ashburn et al (2008b) are listed in Table 21.4.

People with neurological conditions often struggle with the performance of dual tasks during balance and gait activities. Dual task training may improve the ability to cope with distraction, and it can enhance postural stability in older people and people with stroke (Zhou et al 2021), MS (Martino Cinnera et al 2021) and Parkinson's patients with mild to moderate impairment (de Freitas et al 2020). In more severely affected patients, dual tasking may not be trainable. For those individuals, management strategies may include attempts to avoid distractions while tackling challenging activities.

Physical Environment

Most falls in neurological patients occur during the day and at home, where they spend most of their time (Ashburn et al 2008b, Nilsagard et al 2015, Schmid et al 2013, Stack et al 2016, Stack & Roberts 2013). It is important to assess, understand and address the physical environment of patients who are experiencing falls to identify and target any potential environmental factors that may contribute to falls, particularly among repeat fallers (Letts et al 2010).

Footwear and Orthotics

Footwear is a bridge between the person and their environment. Inappropriate footwear and foot problems can influence balance and increase fall risk (Randolph et al 2017), but supportive footwear may improve stability (Kunkel et al 2017, Menz et al 2017a) by:

1. Altering feedback to the foot and ankle, and
2. Modifying friction at the shoe–floor interface (Menant et al 2008).

A study exploring footwear worn indoors and outdoors among people with stroke and Parkinson's reported that more than 30% of people with stroke and Parkinson's wore slippers indoors; many slipper wearers had experienced falls and reported foot problems (Bowen et al 2016). Furthermore, balance and gait performance in people's own indoor shoes (particularly in slippers) was significantly worse compared with balance performance in their usual outdoor shoes (Kunkel et al 2017). Evidence suggests that walking indoors barefoot, in slippers or in socks increases the risk for falls; wearing shoes with low enclosed heels, firm slip-resistant soles and Velcro fastening, on the other hand, may improve balance and could potentially reduce the risk for falls (Kunkel et al 2017, Menant et al 2008, Menz et al 2017).

However, despite these risks many people with neurological conditions continue to wear slipper-type shoes or generally unsupportive footwear indoors (Bowen et al 2016, Donovan-Hall et al 2020). For example, people with stroke typically favoured slippers indoors because they provide comfort and warmth, are easy to get on and off, and accommodate swollen feet (Donovan-Hall et al 2020).

TABLE 21.4	Strategies That May Enhance Stability During Common Fall-Related Activities
Fall-Related Activity	**Strategies That May Prevent Falls**
Turning	• Visualise and follow wide arcs, not tight turns. • One direction may be easier; turn that way when possible. • Slow down; pause between walking and turning.
Reaching	• Reach forwards, using visual guidance. • Reach with one hand while using the other for support. • Keep both feet planted firmly on the floor.
Transferring	• Remember that both sit to stand and stand to sit are challenging. • Pause between movements. • Use support.
Walking	• Use well-maintained aids if they help or keep a hand free. • Plan the route from A to B and focus.
Washing and dressing	• Sit down for stability, particularly when vision is obscured.

Assistive products such as orthotics are also often considered in rehabilitation for older people and people with neurological conditions. Their use can be beneficial to improve balance and gait, as well as reducing fear of falling, and may support people to increase their physical activity levels (Daryabor et al 2022, Tyson et al 2013, Wang et al 2019). However, most studies to date that explored the use of orthotics to reduce falls did not observe a reduction in falls (Nikamp et al 2019, Paton et al 2016, Wang et al 2019). For example, in one study the people with stroke who were provided with an ankle–foot orthosis early after stroke experienced significantly more falls compared with those who had not yet been provided with an orthosis (Nikamp et al 2019). The authors noted that most of the falls reported occurred when the stroke patients who had been provided with an orthosis undertook activities whilst not wearing the orthosis.

External Environment

Key hazards for people at risk for falling (Becker et al 2003, Pighills et al 2011) include:

- Poor lighting
- Chair and bed heights
- Floor surfaces and clutter
- Insufficient grab rails (toilets and bathrooms)
- Improperly used and maintained walking aids

Indoor Versus Outdoor Falls

Many falls by people with neurological conditions happen without the involvement of external and environmental hazards, for example, two-thirds of falls in people with stroke (Mackintosh et al 2005). However, environmental dimensions increase fall risk in this patient group, particularly during complex and dynamic situations such as walking outdoors (Lamont et al 2017, Saverino et al 2014). For example, the association of indoor trip hazards with falls was similar among people with stroke and matched controls, but the outdoor environment was associated with greater risk for falls in people with stroke (Wing et al 2017). This might be because of the increased impact of factors such as terrain and increased attentional demands when walking outdoors; both were the most common contributors to outdoor falls among people with Parkinson's (Lamont et al 2017).

Among the general population, people older than 75 years were more likely to fall indoors and those younger than 75 more often experienced falls outdoors (Bath & Morgan 1999). Analysis of indoor and outdoor falls revealed that indoor falls were more often associated with frailty, disability and inactivity, whereas outdoor falls occurred in more physically active people and were linked to compromised health status (Bath & Morgan 1999, Kelsey et al 2010). Outdoor falls by people with Parkinson's were often related to tripping and slipping, and indoor falls were linked to weakness, postural instability and vertigo (Gazibara et al 2016). In people with MS, higher physical activity levels in younger people with MS were linked to greater risk of falling, possibly because this group of people was undertaking more and higher risk (recreational, shopping) outdoor activities (Nilsagard et al 2015).

Current guidelines recommend that people who were hospitalised after a fall have a home hazard assessment (NICE 2013, Montero-Odasso et al 2022). Home hazard modifications can be beneficial (Carnemolla et al 2020, Keall et al 2015) and most effective when health professionals conduct the assessment (Gillespie et al 2012, Pighills et al 2011).

With a patient at high risk for falling, it may be helpful to sketch the layout of their home and mark on the sketch the environmental hazards and hazardous activities that are unavoidable (Fig. 21.3). This can already be started whilst patients are in hospital (Ueda et al 2017) and should include the pathways and entrance to the home and garden, and

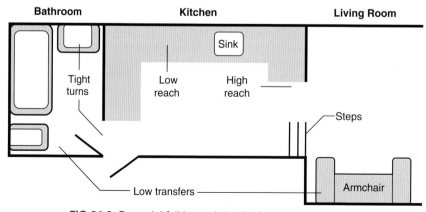

FIG 21.3 Potential fall hazards in the home environment.

walking routes from the bedroom to the bathroom, living room and kitchen. This exercise will identify the challenges to patients and therapists and may guide rehabilitation.

Walking Aids

Often assistive devices such as walking sticks or frames will be considered in the rehabilitation for patients who are unstable. Walking aids cannot be considered as fall-prevention strategies in themselves, but they can be a helpful tool to increase physical activity levels to prevent further deconditioning (Graafmans et al 2003, O'Hare et al 2013). The benefits of walking aids include improved balance by increasing the base of support area, reducing pain experienced during weight bearing, reduction in energy cost during walking, improved confidence and increased activity levels (Bateni et al 2005, Ijmker et al 2013). However, these benefits can be achieved only if walking aid selection is based on a person-centred assessment and aids are correctly adjusted and maintained (Bateni et al 2005, O'Hare et al 2013).

Keep in mind that walking aid use has been associated with 2- to 3-fold increased risk of falling (Deandrea et al 2010). Many factors may contribute to this, including incorrect use and the fact that walking aids are prescribed to those who are most frail and at risk of injuries (Costamagna et al 2017). In addition, up to 50% of patients abandon their devices soon after receiving them because they find them difficult or risky to use (Bateni et al 2005, Jimenez-Arberas & Ordonez-Fernandez 2021, Skymne et al 2012).

When considering footwear, orthotics and walking aids as part of rehabilitation, health professionals should aim to discuss individuals' needs and reasons for their current choices before considering options and alternatives together. Ideally prescription, selection and situational use of alternative footwear and assistive devices should be practiced with the patient to ensure that they are able to manage them correctly. Focus discussions on the potential benefits for balance rather than fall risk because positive framing was viewed as more acceptable to older people and people with stroke (Donovan-Hall et al 2020, Yardley at al. 2006).

Engagement With Fall Prevention

In practice, you will encounter some people who fall very frequently, accept that they will continue to fall and might not be willing to engage with fall prevention. Despite the evidence supporting fall-prevention interventions, adherence and uptake remain low (Robinson et al 2014). In Yardley et al's (2008) survey of people older than 54 years, home-based strength and balance training appeared more acceptable than classes, but neither option appeared in great demand: 36% said they would definitely train at home; only 23% would attend group sessions. A recent fall

was associated with a greater willingness to train at home and accept help with home hazards, and respondents from minority groups reported an increased likelihood to engage with fall-prevention interventions. In contrast, Nyman and Victor (2014) reported recruitment rates of 41% and acceptance (willing to participate but excluded) rates of 71% for falls intervention run in community settings, and higher recruitment (49%) and acceptance rates (89%) for falls intervention in institutional settings.

Several factors have been identified that help or hinder engagement with fall prevention (Aidemark & Askenäs 2018, Schnock et al 2019, Tzeng et al 2020).

Barriers to engagement include health problems, frailty, advancing age, lack of motivation, self-denial of risk, language and communication difficulties and lack of social or community support. In contrast, good self-reported health, younger age (which was linked to being fit and more inclined), high motivation, higher fall-prevention self-efficacy and not living alone were linked to better engagement with fall-prevention self-management activities. There is no one-size-fits-all approach to fall prevention. Ensuring that you have considered a faller's culture and lifestyle and the suitability and cultural appropriateness of the venue, as well as dates and times offered, can reduce some of the barriers of engagement (Dickinson et al 2011).

These findings highlight that often those most in need of intervention are often the hardest group to engage. Older people at risk for falling would like access to physiotherapists' professional knowledge, exchange information and be able to maintain their independence through shared decision making (Robinson et al 2014). However, they also reported that physiotherapists often displayed professional dominance to remain in control of the fall-prevention treatment programme. If therapists can move away from being the 'experts' and instead use their skills to promote self-management, uptake of fall prevention may improve. People are more likely to engage with fall-prevention activities if they are given the opportunity to express their needs, can choose activities that suit them best and are empowered to take control of their health (Age UK 2016). A focus on the positive messages about the potential benefits and enjoyment of exercises to help people to 'remain active' or 'stay steady' is preferrable to framing discussions about fall prevention just on instability and falls (Age UK 2012).

Not Every Fall Is Preventable

People with neurological conditions can often present with a high number and a high frequency of falls, and as a result have a high likelihood of experiencing injurious falls (Poss & Hirdes 2016). When a patient is clearly at risk for further and potentially injurious falls (e.g., a repeat faller with Parkinson's who has minimal saving reactions but remains mobile; see Chapter 11), therapists must raise the priorities of injury and death prevention over fall prevention. Expecting the patient to fall again, attention needs to turn to the landing and to what happens next. Could the environment be safer? Home modifications have been shown to be beneficial to reduce the likelihood of injurious falls (Keall et al 2015). Could the patient learn to get up from the floor alone? It has been shown that it is possible and safe to teach most people with stroke how to get off the floor independently after a fall (Hollands et al 2021). If the patient is unable to get up again alone, attention needs to turn to preventing a long lay, or at least minimising the consequences of one. How will the person who has fallen attract help? How will they stay warm, nourished and alive?

MULTIFACTORIAL APPROACH TO FALL PREVENTION

As discussed earlier, falling is a multifactorial problem with many potential risk factors. This suggests multifactorial risk assessment and intervention may be indicated (NICE 2013, Montero-Odasso et al 2022). Multifactorial interventions may reduce fall risk in community-dwelling elderly persons (Hopewell 2018, 2020), but the effect of such interventions on fall risk in care facilities is uncertain (Cameron 2018, Vlaeyen et al 2015). In addition, limited evidence for multifactorial fall-prevention programmes is available for people with stroke (Denissen et al 2019), MS (Hugos et al 2016) and Parkinson's (Owen et al 2019). Nevertheless, as a physical therapist it is important to consider the variety of fall risk factors a patient may present with and, if necessary, collaborate with other professionals in the diagnosis or treatment of fall risk.

Here, we present two examples of multifactorial programs for elderly people living in the community (Box 21.6) and in a care home setting (Box 21.7).

A variety of effective fall-prevention programmes for elderly people exist; Public Health England (2017) makes the following recommendations:
1. Identify people at risk for falls:
   - through a multifactorial multidisciplinary risk assessment.
2. Refer people at risk for falls:
   - to receive a tailored evidence-based fall-prevention programme.
3. Fall-intervention programmes should include:
   - highly challenging progressive strength and balance exercises,
   - medication and vision assessments,
   - home hazard assessments, and
   - bone-strengthening medicines.
4. Support older people to maintain activity levels and promote healthy ageing.
   - Offer information on or provide follow-up classes.

A few recent publications illustrate the scope of fall-prevention services (Table 21.5).

CONCLUSION

Fall prevention is a key area of healthcare. The extensive literature base is growing continuously and incorporates fall prevention in a wide range of settings. Taken as a whole, the literature shows that the coordination of multidisciplinary assessment and intervention is possible (but challenging) everywhere from the hospital emergency department to community care, both with cognitively intact and cognitively impaired patient groups.

BOX 21.6   Example 1: Multifactorial Interdisciplinary Intervention (Fairhall et al 2008, 2014)

Participant's general health status was assessed.
- Medication review
- Chronic disease and pain management
- Carer support

Intervention was tailored to each participant based on frailty characteristics (Fried et al 2001).
- Including weakness, slow walking speed, low physical activity level, unintentional weight loss, self-reported fatigue, depression and social isolation

Those presenting with weakness, slow walking speed and low physical activity levels received up to 10 home-based exercise sessions delivered by a physiotherapist over 12 months.

- Included targeted strength, balance and endurance exercises
- Mobility aid and equipment recommendations

Those presenting with unintentional weight loss received a clinical evaluation of nutritional intake.
- Included recommended home-delivered meals
- Prescription of high-energy, high-protein nutritional supplements

Those presenting with fatigue and depression
- Were referred to a psychiatrist or psychologist,
- Were given options to encourage social engagement and activity group participation, and
- Enabled telephone contact with volunteers.

BOX 21.7 Example 2: A Multifactorial Risk Factor Modification Programme (Dyer et al 2004)

Exercise Programme

- Experienced exercise assistants supported by a physiotherapist visited each home thrice weekly.
- Exercise sessions aimed to improve balance and gait, flexibility, strength and endurance.
- If possible, exercises were linked to tasks such as transfers, dressing and using walking aids.
- Group sessions (40 minutes) consisted of a warm up, a targeted circuit and a warm down. Sessions included dancing and games.
- Exercises were progressed as appropriate, using weights and thera-bands.
- Individual sessions were provided for residents with physical frailty and cognitive impairment.
- Participants were encouraged to carry out individual exercise outside of the visits.

Staff Education

All staff members were encouraged to be involved in the interventions, and each care home manager received written information.

Medical Reviews

Residents with suspected medical risk factors were examined, and recommendations were reported by letter to general practitioners (notably sedative and diuretic medication, polypharmacy, orthostatic hypotension and osteoporosis).

Environmental Modification

An occupational therapy assistant visited each home to assess risk factors on an individual basis and provided each home with a written report. Environmental health teams also visited the homes to carry out their routine assessments and to alert homes to any major risks.

Optician and Podiatry

A review from an optician was arranged for residents with a visual acuity of 6/12 or less, or if they had not seen an optician in the previous year. Podiatry was arranged for residents whose foot condition was of concern.

TABLE 21.5 Examples of Effective Fall-Prevention Services in Different Settings

In Hospital	Day Hospital	In the Community	In the Nursing Home
Individualised patient education programme staff training and feedback: consists of digital video and information booklet and individual physiotherapy sessions to facilitate self-efficacy with regards to patients 'knowing if they need help to get up and walk around', when to 'ask or wait for help' (Hill et al 2014)	Multidisciplinary 10-week exercise and education programme involving medical review, education, exercise (weekly gait, balance and lower limb strengthening, and tailored home exercises) and access to dietician, psychologist and podiatrist depending on the individual's risk factors (Leahy & Chan 2014)	Many effective programmes exist, e.g., Son et al (2016) compared tai chi and Otago – both were effective. Tai chi showed greater balance and gait velocity improvements, and Otago greater leg strength improvements	Jung et al (2014) summarised nursing home fall-prevention evidence into a three-step approach: (1) Identify previous fallers. If yes, commence comprehensive intervention. (2) If no, assess whether the patient has balance or gait problems, takes multiple medications or has dementia. (3) If no, review regularly. If yes, review medication, introduce exercise and reassess regularly.

Falls necessitate thorough investigation and a coordinated approach to intervention. As clinicians and services move away from trying to predict falls in a whole group of patients, more emphasis needs to be placed on identifying fall risk in an individual. To achieve this, clinicians are encouraged to take a thorough fall history to identify the circumstances surrounding previous falls and near misses, complete a battery of appropriate tests and outcome measures to identify an individual's disease-specific fall risk factors and observe the person who fell performing their fall-related activities in a functional way. Based on the interview and assessment outcomes, clinicians can target the hazardous interactions between the individual and their environment, use targeted exercises and stimulate continued physical activity, develop new movement strategies to make everyday activities safer and provide advice on appropriate footwear and environmental modification. When skilled practitioners and committed teams tackle falls by successfully involving people who have fallen in their care to make shared decisions, many falls are preventable, and the reduction of fear, injury and dependence is significant.

SELF-ASSESSMENT QUESTIONS

1. Which groups of people are at greatest risk for falling, and which disease-specific factors contribute to the increased fall risk?
2. What are the most frequently cited causes of falls?
3. What are the key points to remember when assessing falls?
4. When interviewing patients and carers about falls, what do therapists attempt to discover, through questioning and observation?
5. What are the key points to remember when managing people who have fallen?

REFERENCES

Abou, L., Alluri, A., Flifet, A., Du, Y., Rice, L.A., 2021. Effectiveness of physical therapy interventions in reducing fear of falling among individuals with neurologic diseases: a systematic review and meta-analysis. Arch. Phys. Med. Rehabil. 102, 132–154.

Abou, L., Qin, K., Alluri, A., Du, Y., Rice, L.A., 2022. The effectiveness of physical therapy interventions in reducing falls among people with multiple sclerosis: a systematic review and meta-analysis. J. Bodyw Mov. Ther. 29, 74–85.

Age, U.K., 2012. Don't mention the F-Word: advice to practitioners on communicating messages to older people. Available at: https://www.ageuk.org.uk/globalassets/age-uk/documents/reports-and-publications/reports-and-briefings/health--wellbeing/rb_2012_falls_prevention_dont_mention_the_f_word.pdf.

Age, U.K., 2016. Falls in older people: prevention. Available at: https://www.ageuk.org.uk/globalassets/age-uk/documents/reports-and-publications/consultation-responses-and-submissions/health--wellbeing/crs_aug16_falls_in_older_people_prevention.pdf.

Age, U.K., 2019. Falls in later life: a huge concern for older people. Available at: https://www.ageuk.org.uk/latest-press/articles/2019/may/falls-in-later-life-a-huge-concern-for-older-people/. Accessed on 24 June 2023.

Aidemark, J., Askenäs, L., 2018. Motivation for adopting fall prevention measures: a literature review searching for technology acceptance factors. Procedia. Comp. Sci. 138, 3–11.

Allen, N.E., Schwarzel, A.K., Canning, C.G., 2013. Recurrent falls in Parkinson's disease: a systematic review. Parkinson. Dis. 2013, 906274.

Allen, N.E., Sherrington, C., Paul, S.S., Canning, C.G., 2011. Balance and falls in Parkinson's disease: a meta-analysis of the effect of exercise and motor training. Mov. Disord. 26, 1605–1615.

Amar, K., Stack, E., Fitton, C., Ashburn, A., Roberts, H.C., 2015. Fall frequency, predicting falls and participating in falls research: similarities among people with PD with and without cognitive impairment. Parkinsonism. Relat. Disord. 21, 55–60.

Ansai, J.H., de Andrade, L.P., Masse, F.A.A., et al., 2019. Risk factors for falls in older adults with mild cognitive impairment and mild Alzheimer disease. J. Geriatr. Phys. Ther. 42, E116–E121.

Antcliff, S.R., Witchalls, J.B., Wallwork, S.B., Welvaert, M., Waddington, G.S., 2022. Daily surveillance of falls is feasible and reveals a high incidence of falls among older adults. Australas. J. Ageing. 41, e201–e205.

Ashburn, A., Hyndman, D., Pickering, R., Yardley, L., Harris, S., 2008a. Predicting people with stroke at risk of falls. Age. Ageing. 37, 270–276.

Ashburn, A., Stack, E., Ballinger, C., Fazakarley, L., Fitton, C., 2008b. The circumstances of falls among people with PD and the use of Falls Diaries to facilitate reporting. Disabil. Rehabil. 30, 1205–1212.

Ashburn, A., Pickering, R., McIntosh, E., et al., 2019. Exercise- and strategy-based physiotherapy-delivered intervention for preventing repeat falls in people with Parkinson's: the PDSAFE RCT. Health. Technol. Assess. 23, 1–150.

Bachoud-Lévi, A.C., Ferreira, J., Massart, R., et al., 2019. International guidelines for the treatment of Huntington's disease. Front. Neurol. 10, 710.

Bansal, S., Hirdes, J.P., Maxwell, C.J., Papaioannou, A., Giangregorio, L.M., 2016. Identifying fallers among home care clients with dementia and Parkinson's disease. Can. J. Aging. 35, 319–331.

Batchelor, F.A., Mackintosh, S.F., Said, C.M., Hill, K.D., 2012. Falls after stroke. Int. J. Stroke. 7, 482–490.

Bateni, H., Maki, B.E., 2005. Assistive devices for balance and mobility: benefits, demands, and adverse consequences. Arch. Phys. Med. Rehabil. 86, 134–145.

Bath, P.A., Morgan, K., 1999. Differential risk factor profiles for indoor and outdoor falls in older people living at home in Nottingham, UK. Eur. J. Epidemiol. 15, 65–73.

Bauman, A., Merom, D., Bull, F.C., Buchner, D.M., Singh, M.A., 2016. Updating the evidence for physical activity: summative reviews of the epidemiological evidence, prevalence, and interventions to promote 'active aging'. Gerontologist. 56 (Suppl. 2), S268–S280.

Becker, C., Kron, M., Lindemann, U., Sturm, E., Eichner, B., Walter-Jung, B., et al., 2003. Effectiveness of a multifaceted intervention on falls in nursing home residents. J. Am. Geriatr. Soc. 51, 306–313.

Berg, K.O., Wood-Dauphinee, S.L., Williams, J.I., Maki, B., 1992. Measuring balance in the elderly: validation of an instrument. Can J Public Health. 83 (Suppl 2), S7–11.

Berry, S.D., Miller, R.R., 2008. Falls: epidemiology, pathophysiology, and relationship to fracture. Curr. Osteoporos. Rep. 6, 149–154.

Bhalsing, K.S., Abbas, M.M., Tan, L.C., 2018. Role of physical activity in Parkinson's disease. Ann. Ind. Acad. Neurol. 21, 242.

Bouwen, A., Lepeleire, J.D., Buntinx, F., 2008. Rate of accidental falls in institutionalised older people with and without cognitive impairment halved as a result of a staff-oriented intervention. Age. Ageing. 37, 306–310.

Bowen, C., Ashburn, A., Cole M., et al., 2016. A survey exploring self-reported indoor and outdoor footwear habits, foot problems and fall status in people with stroke and Parkinson's. J. Foot. Ankle. Res. 9, 39.

Brozova, H., Stochl, J., Klempir, J., Kucharik, M., Ruzicka, E., Roth, J., 2011. A sensitivity comparison of clinical tests for postural instability in patients with Huntington's disease. Gait. Posture. 34, 245–247.

Busse, M.E., Wiles, C.M., Rosser, A.E., 2009. Mobility and falls in people with Huntington's disease. J. Neurol. Neurosurg. Psychiatry. 80, 88–90.

Carnemolla, P., Bridge, C., 2020. A scoping review of home modification interventions – Mapping the evidence base. Indoor. Built. Environ. 29, 299–310.

Cameron, I.D., Dyer, S.M., Panagoda, C.E., Murray, G.R., Hill, K.D., Cumming, R.G., Kerse, N., 2018. Interventions for preventing falls in older people in care facilities and hospitals. Cochrane. Database. Syst. Rev. 9, CD005465

Canning, C.G., Sherrington, C., Lord, S.R., et al., 2015. Exercise for falls prevention in Parkinson disease: a randomized controlled trial. Neurology. 84, 304–312.

Chantanachai, T., Sturnieks, D.L., Lord, S.R., Payne, N., Webster, L., Taylor, M.E., 2021. Risk factors for falls in older people with cognitive impairment living in the community: systematic review and meta-analysis. Ageing. Res. Rev. 71, 101452.

Chaudhuri, S., Thompson, H., Demiris, G., 2014. Fall detection devices and their use with older adults: a systematic review. J. Geriatr. Phys. Ther. 37, 178–196.

Cho, K., Yu, J., Rhee, H., 2015. Risk factors related to falling in stroke patients: a cross-sectional study. J. Phys. Ther. Sci. 27, 1751–1753.

Cipriani, G., Lucetti, C., Carlesi, C., Danti, S., Nuti, A., 2015. Sundown syndrome and dementia. Eur. Geriatr. Med. 6, 375–380.

Conradsson, D., Löfgren, N., Nero, H., et al., 2015. The effects of highly challenging balance training in elderly with Parkinson's disease: a randomized controlled trial. Neurorehabil. Neural. Repair. 29, 827–836.

Costamagna, E., Thies, S.B., Kenney, L.P., Howard, D., Liu, A., Ogden, D., 2017. A generalisable methodology for stability assessment of walking aid users. Med. Eng. Phys. 47, 167–175.

Cummings, S.R., Nevitt, M.C., 1989. A hypothesis: the causes of hip fractures. J. Gerontol. 44, M107–M111.

Daryabor, A., Yamamoto, S., Orendurff, M., Kobayashi, T., 2022. Effect of types of ankle-foot orthoses on energy expenditure metrics during walking in individuals with stroke: a systematic review. Disabil. Rehabil. 44, 166–176.

Deandrea, S., Lucenteforte, E., Bravi, F., Foschi, R., La Vecchia, C., Negri, E., 2010. Risk factors for falls in community-dwelling older people: a systematic review and meta-analysis. Epidemiology. 1, 658–668.

De Freitas, T.B., Leite, P.H.W., Doná, F., Pompeu, J.E., Swarowsky, A., Torriani-Pasin, C., 2020. The effects of dual task gait and balance training in Parkinson's disease: a systematic review. Physiother. Theory. Pract. 36, 1088–1096.

de Kam, D., Nonnekes, J., Nijhuis, L.B.O., Geurts, A.C., Bloem, B.R., Weerdesteyn, V., 2014. Dopaminergic medication does not improve stepping responses following backward and forward balance perturbations in patients with Parkinson's disease. J. Neurol. 261, 2330–2337.

de Kam, D., Roelofs, J.M.B., Bruijnes, A., et al., 2017a. The next step in understanding impaired reactive balance control in people with stroke: the role of defective early automatic postural responses. Neurorehabil. Neural. Repair. 31, 708–716.

de Kam, D., Kamphuis, J.F., Weerdesteyn, V., Geurts, A.C.H., 2017b. The effect of weight-bearing asymmetry on dynamic postural stability in people with chronic stroke. Gait. Posture. 53, 5–10.

Denissen, S., Staring, W., Kunkel, D., et al., 2019. Interventions for preventing falls in people after stroke. Cochrane. Database. Syst. Rev. 10, CD008728

Denkinger, M.D., Lukas, A.L., Nikolaus, T., Hauer, K., 2015. Factors associated with fear of falling and associated activity restriction in community-dwelling older adults: a systematic review. Am. J. Geriatr. Psychiatry. 23, 72–86.

Dickinson, A., Machen, I., Horton, K., Jain, D., Maddex, T., Cove, J., 2011. Fall prevention in the community: what older people say they need. Br. J. Community. Nurs. 16, 174–180.

Donovan-Hall, M., Robison, J., Cole, M., et al., 2020. The trouble with footwear following stroke: a qualitative study of the views and experience of people with stroke. Disabil. Rehabil. 42, 1107–1114.

Dow, B., Meyer, C., Morre, K.J., Hill, K.D., 2013. The impact of care recipient falls on caregivers. Aust. Health. Rev. 37, 152–157.

Duncan, P.W., Weiner, D.K., Chandler, J., Studenski, S., 1990. Functional reach: a new clinical measure of balance. J. Gerontol. 45, M192–M197.

Dusane, S., Bhatt, T., 2020. Mixed slip-trip perturbation training for improving reactive responses in people with chronic stroke. J. Neurophysiol. 124, 20–31.

Dyer, C., Taylor, G., Reed, M., Dyer, C.A., Robertson, D., Harrington, R., 2004. Falls prevention in residential care homes: a randomised controlled trial. Age. Ageing. 33, 596–602.

Ek, S., Rizzuto, D., Xu, W., Calderón-Larrañaga, A., Welmer, A.K., 2021. Predictors for functional decline after an injurious fall: a population-based cohort study. Aging. Clin. Exp. Res. 33, 2183–2190.

Fairhall, N., Aggar, C., Kurrle, S.E., Sherrington, C., Lord, S., Lockwood, K., et al., 2008. Frailty intervention trial (FIT). BMC Geriatr. 8, 27.

Fairhall, N., Sherrington, C., Lord, S.R., et al., 2014. Effect of a multifactorial, interdisciplinary intervention on risk factors for falls and fall rate in frail older people: a randomised controlled trial. Age. Ageing. 43, 616–622.

Fanciulli, A., Campese, N., Goebel, G., et al., 2020. Association of transient orthostatic hypotension with falls and syncope in patients with Parkinson disease. Neurology. 95, e2854–e2865.

Fleming, J., Brayne, C., 2008. Inability to get up after falling, subsequent time on floor, and summoning help: prospective cohort study in people over 90. BMJ. 337, a2227

Forster, A., Young, J., 1995. Incidence and consequences of falls due to stroke: a systematic inquiry. BMJ. 311, 83–86.

Foster, C., Florhaug, J.A., Franklin, J., et al., 2001. Monitoring exercise training during non-steady state exercise. J. Strength. Cond. Res. 15, 109–115.

Franchignoni, F., Horak, F., Godi, M., Nardone, A., Giordano, A., 2010. Using psychometric techniques to improve the Balance Evaluation Systems Test: the mini-BESTest. J. Rehabil. Med. 42, 323–331.

François, C., Biaggioni, I., Shibao, C., et al., 2017. Fall-related healthcare use and costs in neurogenic orthostatic hypotension with Parkinson's disease. J. Med. Econ. 20, 525–532.

Fried, L.P., Tangen, C.M., Walston, J., et al., 2001. Frailty in older adults: evidence for a phenotype. J. Gerontol. A. Biol. Sci. Med. Sci. 56, M146–M157.

Gao, Q., Leung, A., Yang, Y., et al., 2014. Effects of Tai Chi on balance and fall prevention in Parkinson's disease: a randomized controlled trial. Clin. Rehabil. 28, 748–753.

Gazibara, T., Kisic-Tepavcevic, D., Svetel, M., Tomic, A., Stankovic, I., Kostic, V.S., Pekmezovic, T., 2016. Indoor and outdoor falls in persons with Parkinson's disease after 1 year follow-up study: differences and consequences. Neurol. Sci. 37, 597–602.

Gianni, C., Prosperini, L., Jonsdottir, J., Cattaneo, D., 2014. A systematic review of factors associated with accidental falls in people with multiple sclerosis: a meta-analytic approach. Clin. Rehabil. 28, 704–716.

Gillespie, L.D., Robertson, M.C., Gillespie, W.J., et al., 2012. Interventions for preventing falls in older people living in the community. Cochrane. Database. Syst. Rev. 9

Giulio St, I.D., George, R.J., Kalliolia, E., Peters, A.L., Limousin, P., Day, B.L., 2016. Maintaining balance against force perturbations: impaired mechanisms unresponsive to levodopa in Parkinson's disease. J. Neurophysiol. 116, 493–502.

Godfrey, A., 2017. Wearables for independent living in older adults: gait and falls. Maturitas. 100, 16–26.

Goodwin, V.A., Richards, S.H., Taylor, R.S., Taylor, A.H., Campbell, J.L., 2008. The effectiveness of exercise interventions for people with Parkinson's disease: a systematic review and meta-analysis. Mov. Disord. 23, 631–640.

Goodwin, V.A., Pickering, R., Ballinger, C., et al., 2015. A multi-centre, randomised controlled trial of the effectiveness of PDSAFE to prevent falls among people with Parkinson's: study protocol. BMC Neurol. 15, 81.

Goto, Y., Otaka, Y., Suzuki, K., Inoue, S., Kondo, K., Shimizu, E., 2019. Incidence and circumstances of falls among community- dwelling ambulatory stroke survivors: a prospective study. Geriatr. Gerontol. Int. 19, 240–244.

Graafmans, W.C., Lips, P.T.A.M., Wijlhuizen, G.J., Pluijm, S.M., Bouter, L.M., 2003. Daily physical activity and the use of a walking aid in relation to falls in elderly people in a residential care setting. Z. Gerontol. Geriatr. 36, 23–28.

Gray, V.L., Yang, C.L., Fujimoto, M., McCombe Waller, S., Rogers, M.W., 2019. Stepping characteristics during externally induced lateral reactive and voluntary steps in chronic stroke. Gait. Posture. 71, 198–204.

Grimbergen, Y.A., Knol, M.J., Bloem, B.R., Kremer, B.P., Roos, R.A., Munneke, M., 2008. Falls and gait disturbances in Huntington's disease. Mov. Disord. 23, 970–976.

Groen, B.E., Smulders, E., de Kam, D., Duysens, J., Weerdesteyn, V., 2010. Martial arts fall training to prevent hip fractures in the elderly. Osteoporos. Int. 21, 215–221.

Gunn, H., Creanor, S., Haas, B., Marsden, J., Freeman, J., 2014. Frequency, characteristics and consequences of falls in multiple sclerosis: findings from a cohort study. Arch. Phys. Med. Rehabil. 95, 538–545.

Gunn, H., Markevics, S., Haas, B., Marsden, J., Freeman, J., 2015. Systematic review: the effectiveness of interventions to reduce falls and improve balance in adults with multiple sclerosis. Arch. Phys. Med. Rehabil. 96, 1898–1912.

Hadjistavropoulos, T., Delbaere, K., Fitzgerald, T.D., 2011. Reconceptualizing the role of fear of falling and balance confidence in fall risk. J. Aging. Health. 23, 3–23.

Haines, T., Kuys, S.S., Morrison, G., Clarke, J., Bew, P., 2009. Cost-effectiveness analysis of screening for risk of in-hospital falls using physiotherapist clinical judgement. Med. Care. 47, 448–456.

Handelzalts, S., Steinberg-Henn, F., Levy, S., Shani, G., Soroker, N., Melzer, I., 2019. Insufficient balance recovery following unannounced external perturbations in persons with stroke. Neurorehabil. Neural. Repair. 33, 730–739.

Hignett, S., Sands, G., Griffiths, P., 2013. In-patient falls: what can we learn from incident reports? Age. Ageing. 42, 527–531.

Hill, A.M., Waldron, N., Etherton-Beer, C., et al., 2014. A stepped-wedge cluster randomised controlled trial for evaluating rates of falls among inpatients in aged care rehabilitation units receiving tailored multimedia education in addition to usual care: a trial protocol. BMJ Open. 4, e004195

Hill, K.D., Hunter, S.W., Batchelor, F.A., Cavalheri, V., Burton, E., 2015. Individualized home-based exercise programs for older people to reduce falls and improve physical performance: a systematic review and meta-analysis. Maturitas. 82, 72–84.

Hogan, N., Kehoe, M., Larkin, A., Coote, S., 2014. The effect of community exercise interventions for people with MS who use bilateral support for gait. Mult. Scler. Int. 2014, 109142.

Hollands, L., Calitri, R., Warmoth, K., Shepherd, A., Allison, R., Dean, S., ReTrain Trial and team, 2021. Assessing the fidelity of the independently getting up off the floor (IGO) technique as part of the ReTrain pilot feasibility randomised controlled trial for stroke survivors. Disabil. Rehabil. 11, 1–10.

Honeycutt, C.F., Nevisipour, M., Grabiner, M.D., 2016. Characteristics and adaptive strategies linked with falls in stroke survivors from analysis of laboratory-induced falls. J. Biomech. 49, 3313–3319.

Hopewell, S., Adedire, O., Copsey, B.J., et al., 2018. Multifactorial and multiple component interventions for preventing falls in older people living in the community. Cochrane. Database. Syst. Rev. 7, CD012221

Hopewell, S., Copsey, B., Nicolson, P., Adedire, B., Boniface, G., Lamb, S., 2020. Multifactorial interventions for preventing falls in older people living in the community: a systematic review and meta-analysis of 41 trials and almost 20 000 participants. Br. J. Sports. Med. 54, 1340–1350.

Huang, T.T., Chung, M.L., Chen, F.R., Chin, Y.F., Wang, B.H., 2016. Evaluation of a combined cognitive behavioural and exercise intervention to manage fear of falling among elderly residents in nursing homes. Aging. Mental. Health. 20, 2–12.

Hugos, C.L., Frankel, D., Tompkins, S.A., Cameron, M., 2016. Community delivery of a comprehensive fall-prevention program in people with multiple sclerosis: a retrospective observational study. Int. J. MS. Care. 18, 42–48.

Hwang, H.F., Lee, H.D., Juan, H.H., Chen, C.Y., Lin, M.R., 2011. Fall mechanisms, bone strength, and hip fractures in elderly men and women in Taiwan. Osteoporos. Int. 22, 2385–2393.

Hyndman, D., Ashburn, A., 2003. People with stroke living in the community: attention deficits, balance, ADL ability and falls. Disabil. Rehabil. 25, 817–822.

Hyndman, D., Ashburn, A., Stack, E., 2002. Fall events among people with stroke living in the community: circumstances of falls and characteristics of fallers. Arch. Phys. Med. Rehabil. 83, 165–170.

Ijmker, T., Houdijk, H., Lamoth, C.J., et al., 2013. Effect of balance support on the energy cost of walking after stroke. Arch. Phys. Med. Rehabil. 94, 2255–2261.

Ishigaki, E.Y., Ramos, L.G., Carvalho, E.S., Lunardi, A.C., 2014. Effectiveness of muscle strengthening and description of protocols for preventing falls in the elderly: a systematic review. Braz. J. Phys. Ther. 18, 111–118.

Jacobs, J.V., Horak, F.B., Van Tran, K., Nutt, J.G., 2006. An alternative clinical postural stability test for patients with Parkinson's disease. J Neurol. 253, 1404–1413.

Jimenez-Arberas, E., Ordonez-Fernandez, F.F., 2021. Discontinuation or abandonment of mobility assistive technology among people with neurological conditions. Rev. Neurol. 72, 426–432.

Jöbges, M., Heuschkel, G., Pretzel, C., Illhardt, C., Renner, C., Hummelsheim, H., 2004. Repetitive training of compensatory steps: a therapeutic approach for postural instability in Parkinson's disease. J. Neurol. Neurosurg. Psychiatry. 75, 1682–1687.

Jung, D., Shin, S., Kim, H., 2014. A fall prevention guideline for older adults living in long-term care facilities. Int. Nursing. Rev. 61, 525–533.

Kalkers, K., Neyens, J.C.L., Wolterbeek, R., Halfens, R.J.G., Schols, J.M.G.A., Roos, R.A.C., 2016. Falls and fear of falling in nursing home residents with Huntington's disease. J. Nursing. Home. Res. Sci. 2, 83–89.

Kalron, A., Allali, G., 2017. Gait and cognitive impairments in multiple sclerosis: the specific contribution of falls and fear of falling. J. Neural. Trans. 124, 1407–1416.

Kannan, L., Vora, J., Varas-Diaz, G., Bhatt, T., Hughes, S., 2020. Does exercise-based conventional training improve reactive balance control among people with chronic stroke? Brain. Sci. 11, 2.

Keall, M.D., Pierse, N., Howden-Chapman, P., et al., 2015. Home modifications to reduce injuries from falls in the home injury prevention intervention (HIPI) study: a cluster-randomised controlled trial. Lancet. 385, 231–238.

Kelsey, J.L., Berry, S.D., Procter-Gray, E., et al., 2010. Indoor and outdoor falls in older adults are different: the maintenance of balance, independent living, intellect, and Zest in the Elderly of Boston Study. J. Am. Geriatr. Soc. 58, 2135–2141.

Kerse, N., Parag, V., Feigin, V.L., et al., 2008. Auckland Regional Community Stroke (ARCOS) Study Group. Falls after stroke. Stroke. 39, 1890–1893.

Keus, S.J.H., Munneke, M., Graziano, M., et al. 2014. European Physiotherapy Guideline for Parkinson's disease. KNGF/ ParkinsonNet, the Netherlands.

Koh, G.C., Yen, S.C., Tay, A., et al., 2015. Singapore Tele-technology Aided Rehabilitation in Stroke (STARS) trial: protocol of a randomized clinical trial on tele-rehabilitation for stroke patients. BMC Neurol. 15, 161.

Kröpelin, T.F., Neyens, J.C.L., Halfens, R.J.G., Kempen, G.I.J.M., Hamers, J.P.H., 2013. Fall determinants in older long-term care residents with dementia: a systematic review. Int. Psychogeriatr. 25, 549–563.

Kumar, A., Delbaere, K., Zijlstra, G.A., et al., 2016. Exercise for reducing fear of falling in older people living in the community: Cochrane systematic review and meta-analysis. Age. Ageing. 45, 345–352.

Kunkel, D., Burnett, M., Mamode, L., et al., 2017. The effects of wearing usual indoor and outdoor footwear on balance and gait performance in people with Parkinson's disease using clinical tests and instrumented movement analysis. Mov. Disord. 32 (Suppl. 2)

Kunkel, D., Pickering, R.M., Ashburn, A., 2011. Comparison of retrospective interviews and prospective diaries to facilitate fall reports among people with stroke. Age. Ageing. 40, 277–280.

Lach, H.W., Parsons, J.L., 2013. Impact of fear of falling in long term care: an integrative review. JAMA. 14, 573–577.

Laforest, S., Pelletier, A., Gauvin, L., et al., 2009. Impact of a community-based falls prevention program on maintenance of physical activity among older adults. J. Aging. Health. 21, 480–500.

Lamont, R.M., Morris, M.E., Hylton, H.B., McGinley, J.L., Brauer, S.G., 2017. Falls in people with Parkinson's disease: a prospective comparison of community and home-based falls. Gait. Posture. 55, 62–67.

Leahy, C., Chan, D.K., 2014. Day hospital fall prevention programme for elderly people to reduce re-presentation with fall. Asian. J. Gerontol. Geriatr. 9, 67–70.

Letts, L., Moreland, J., Richardson, J., et al., 2010. The physical environment as a fall risk factor in older adults: systematic review and meta-analysis of cross-sectional and cohort studies. Aust. Occup. Ther. J. 57, 51–64.

Li, F., Harmer, P., Fitzgerald, K., et al., 2012. Tai chi and postural stability in patients with Parkinson's disease. N. Engl. J. Med. 366, 511–519.

Li, F., Harmer, P., 2020. Prevalence of falls, physical performance, and dual-task cost while walking in older adults at high risk of falling with and without cognitive impairment. Clin. Intervent. Aging. 15, 945.

Lindholm, B., Hagell, P., Hansson, O., Nilsson, M.H., 2014. Factors associated with fear of falling in people with Parkinson's disease. BMC Neurol. 14 (1), 1–7.

Mackintosh, S.F.H., Hill, K., Dodd, K.J., Goldie, P., Culham, E., 2005. Falls and injury prevention should be part of every stroke rehabilitation plan. Clin. Rehabil. 19, 441–451.

Mackintosh, S.F., Hill, K.D., Dodd, K.J., Goldie, P.A., Culham, E.G., 2006. Balance score and a history of falls in hospital predict recurrent falls in the 6 months following stroke rehabilitation. Arch. Phys. Med. Rehabil. 87, 1583–1589.

Maki, B.E., McIlroy, W.E., 1997. The role of limb movements in maintaining upright stance: the 'change-in-support' strategy. Phys. Ther. 77, 488–507.

Mansfield, A., Inness, E.L., Wong, J.S., Fraser, J.E., Mcilroy, W.E., 2013. Is impaired control of reactive stepping related to falls during inpatient stroke rehabilitation? Neurorehabil. Neural. Repair. 27, 526–533.

Mansfield, A., Wong, J.S., Bryce, J., Knorr, S., Patterson, K.K., 2015. Does perturbation-based balance training prevent falls? Systematic review and meta-analysis of preliminary randomized controlled trials. Phys. Ther. 95, 700–709.

Mansfield, A., Aqui, A., Danells, C.J., et al., 2018. Does perturbation-based balance training prevent falls among individuals with chronic stroke? A randomised controlled trial. BMJ Open. 8, 021510.

Marigold, D.S., Misiaszek, J.E., 2009. Whole-body responses: neural control and implications for rehabilitation and fall prevention. Neuroscientist. 15, 36–46.

Martino Cinnera, A., Bisirri, A., Leone, E., Morone, G., Gaeta, A., 2021. Effect of dual-task training on balance in patients with multiple sclerosis: a systematic review and meta-analysis. Clin. Rehabil. 35, 1399–1412.

Massot, C., Simoneau-Buessinger, E., Agnani, O., Donze, C., Leteneur, S., 2019. Anticipatory postural adjustment during gait initiation in multiple sclerosis patients: a systematic review. Gait. Posture. 73, 180–188.

Mazumder, R., Murchison, C., Bourdette, D., Cameron, M., 2014. Falls in people with multiple sclerosis compared with falls in healthy controls. PloS One. 9, e107620

McDonald, C., Pearce, M., Kerr, S.R., Newton, J., 2017. A prospective study of the association between orthostatic hypotension and falls: definition matters. Age Ageing. 46, 439–445.

Menant, J.C., Steele, J.R., Menz, H.B., Munro, B.J., Lord, S.R., 2008. Optimizing footwear for older people at risk of falls. J. Rehabil. Res. Dev. 45, 1167–1181.

Menz, H.B., Auhl, M., Munteanu, S.E., 2017. Effects of indoor footwear on balance and gait patterns in community-dwelling older women. Gerontology. 63, 129–136.

Menz, H.B., Auhl, M., Munteanu, S.E., 2017a. Preliminary evaluation of prototype footwear and insoles to optimise balance and gait in older people. BMC Geriatr. 17, 1–8.

Mirelman, A., Maidan, I., Herman, T., Deutsch, J.E., Giladi, N., Hausdorff, J.M., 2011. Virtual reality for gait training: can it induce motor learning to enhance complex walking and reduce fall risk in patients with Parkinson's disease? J. Gerontol. A. Biol. Sci. Med. Sci. 66, 234–240.

Mirelman, A., Rochester, L., Maidan, I., et al., 2016. Addition of a non-immersive virtual reality component to treadmill training to reduce fall risk in older adults (V-TIME): a randomised controlled trial. Lancet. 388, 1170–1182.

Montero-Odasso, M., van der Velde, N., Martin, F.C., et al, 2022. World guidelines for falls prevention and management for older adults: a global initiative. Age Ageing. 51, 1–36.

Moon, Y., Sosnoff, J.J., 2017. Safe Landing strategies during a fall: systematic review and meta-analysis. Arch. Phys. Med. Rehabil. 98, 783–794.

Morgan, E., 2019. Living longer and old-age dependency—what does the future hold. Office for National Statistics., Available at: https://www.ons.gov.uk/peoplepopulationandcommunity/birthsdeathsandmarriages/ageing/articles/livinglongeranddoldagedependencywhatdoesthefuturehold/2019-06-24. Accessed on 24 June 2023.

Morris, M.E., Menz, H.B., McGinley, J.L., et al., 2011. Falls and mobility in Parkinson's disease: protocol for a randomised controlled clinical trial. BMC Neurol. 11, 93.

Morris, M.E., Menz, H.B., McGinley, J.L., et al., 2015. A randomized controlled trial to reduce falls in people with Parkinson's disease. Neurorehabil. Neural. Repair. 29, 777–785.

Morris, M.E., Taylor, N.F., Watts, 2017. A home program of strength training, movement strategy training and education did not prevent falls in people with Parkinson's disease: a randomised trial. J. Physiother. 63, 94–100.

Muehlbauer, T., Gollhofer, A., Granacher, U., 2015. Associations between measures of balance and lower-extremity muscle strength/power in healthy individuals across the lifespan: a systematic review and meta-analysis. Sports Med. 45, 1671–1692.

National Institute for Health and Care Excellence (NICE), 2013. Falls in older people: assessing risk and prevention. NICE guideline (CG161). www.nice.org.uk/guidance/cg161. Accessed on 24 June 2023.

Nikamp, C.D., Hobbelink, M.S., Van der Palen, J., Hermens, H.J., Rietman, J.S., Buurke, J.H., 2019. The effect of ankle-foot orthoses on fall/near fall incidence in patients with (sub-) acute stroke: A randomized controlled trial. PLoS One. 14 (3), 0213538.

Nilsagård, Y., Gunn, H., Freeman, J., et al., 2015. Falls in people with MS—an individual data meta-analysis from studies from

Australia, Sweden, United Kingdom and the United States. Mult. Scler. J. 21, 92–100.

Nyberg, L., Gustafson, Y., 1995. Patient falls in stroke rehabilitation. Stroke. 26, 838–842.

Nyman, S.R., Victor, C.R., 2014. Older people's participation and engagement in falls prevention interventions: comparing rates and settings. Eur. Geriatr. Med. 5, 18–20.

O'Hare, M.P., Pryde, S.J., Gracey, J.H., 2013. A systematic review of the evidence for the provision of walking frames for older people. Phys. Ther. Rev. 18, 11–23.

Oliver, D., 2008. Falls risk-prediction tools for hospital inpatients. Time to put them to bed? Age. Ageing. 37, 248–250.

Oliver, D., Papaioannou, A., Giangregorio, L., Thabane, L., Reizgys, K., Foster, G., 2008. A systematic review and meta-analysis of studies using the STRATIFY tool for prediction of falls in hospital patients: how well does it work? Age. Ageing. 37, 621–627.

O'Malley, N., Clifford, A.M., Conneely, M., Casey, B., Coote, S., 2021. Effectiveness of interventions to prevent falls for people with multiple sclerosis, Parkinson's disease and stroke: an umbrella review. BMC Neurol. 21, 1–31.

Owen, C.L., Ibrahim, K., Dennison, L., Roberts, H.C., 2019. Falls self-management interventions for people with Parkinson's disease: a systematic review. J. Parkinson. Dis. 9, 283–299.

Panel on Prevention of Falls in Older Persons, American Geriatrics Society and British Geriatrics Society, 2011. Summary of the updated American Geriatrics Society/British Geriatrics Society clinical practice guideline for prevention of falls in older persons. J. Am. Geriatr. Soc. 59, 148–157.

Patel, P.J., Bhatt, T., 2018. Fall risk during opposing stance perturbations among healthy adults and chronic stroke survivors. Exp. Brain. Res. 6, 619–628.

Paton, J., Hatton, A.L., Rome, K., Kent, B., 2016. Effects of foot and ankle devices on balance, gait and falls in adults with sensory perception loss: a systematic review. JBI Database. Syst. Rev. Implement. Rep. 14, 127.

Pelicioni, P.H.S., Menant, J.C., Latt, M.D., Lord, S.R., 2019. Falls in Parkinson's disease subtypes: risk factors, locations and circumstances. Int. J. Environ. Res. Public. Health. 16, 2216.

Peterson, D.S., Huisinga, J.M., Spain, R.I., Horak, F.B., 2016a. Characterization of compensatory stepping in people with multiple sclerosis. Arch. Phys. Med. Rehabil. 97, 513–521.

Peterson, D.S., Dijkstra, B.W., Horak, F.B., 2016b. Postural motor learning in people with Parkinson's disease. J. Neurol. 263, 1518–1529.

Pighills, A.C., Torgerson, D.J., Sheldon, T.A., Drummond, A.E., Bland, J.M., 2011. Environmental assessment and modification to prevent falls in older people. J. Am. Geriatr. Soc. 59, 26–33.

Podsiadlo, D., Richardson, S., 1991. The Timed "Up & Go": a test of basic functional mobility for frail elderly persons. J. Am. Geriatr. Soc. 39, 142–148.

Pollock, A., Baer, G., Campbell, P., et al., 2014. Physical rehabilitation approaches for the recovery of function and mobility following stroke. Cochrane. Database. Syst. Rev. 4

Preventing falls and injuries in older people, 1996. Effect. Healthcare. Bull. 2, 1–15.

Poss, J.W., Hirdes, J.P., 2016. Very frequent fallers and future fall injury: continuous risk among community-dwelling home care recipients. J. Aging. Health. 28, 587–599.

Protas, E.J., Mitchell, K., Williams, A., Qureshy, H., Caroline, K., Lai, E.C., 2005. Gait and step training to reduce falls in Parkinson's disease. NeuroRehabilitation. 20, 183–190.

Public Health England, 2017. Falls and fractures: consensus statement [PHE publications gateway number: 2016588]. 1–22. Available at: https://www.gov.uk/government/publications/falls-and-fractures-consensus-statement. Accessed on 24 June 2023.

Public Health England, 2022. Falls: applying all our health. Available at: https://www.gov.uk/government/publications/falls-applying-all-our-health/falls-applying-all-our-health. Accessed on 24 June 2023.

Public Health Outcomes Framework, 2022. Available at: https://www.gov.uk/government/statistics/public-health-outcomes-framework-november-2022-data-update. Accessed on 24 June 2023

Quinn, L., Kegelmeyer, D., Kloos, A., Rao, A.K., Busse, M., Fritz, N.E., 2020. Clinical recommendations to guide physical therapy practice for Huntington disease. Neurology. 94, 217–228.

Randolph, S., Dalal, R.A., Asumu, E., Colbert, V., Isom, A.T., Mayfield, S.R., 2017. The effect of inappropriate footwear on gait and falls in older adults: a literature review. J. Natl. Soc. Allied. Health. 14 (1).

Robinson, L., Newton, J.L., Jones, D., Dawson, P., 2014. Self-management and adherence with exercise-based falls prevention programmes: a qualitative study to explore the views and experiences of older people and physiotherapists. Disabil. Rehabil. 36, 379–386.

Roe, B., Howell, F., Riniotis, K., Beech, R., Crome, P., Ong, B.N., 2008. Older people's experience of falls: understanding, interpretation and autonomy. J. Adv. Nurs. 63, 586–596.

Rose, D.J., 2008. Preventing falls among older adults: no 'one size suits all' intervention strategy. J. Rehabil. Res. Dev. 45, 1153–1166.

Royal College of Physicians, 2013. Falling standards, broken promises: Report of the National Audit of Falls and Bone Health. Available at: https://www.rcplondon.ac.uk/projects/outputs/falling-standards-broken-promises-report-national-audit-falls-and-bone-health. Accessed on 24 June 2023.

Sanders, K.M., Stuart, A.L., Scott, D., Kotowicz, M.A., Nicholson, G.C., 2015. Validity of 12-month falls recall in community-dwelling older women participating in a clinical trial. Int. J. Endocrinol. 2015, 210527.

Sandroff, B.M., Klaren, R.E., Motl, R.W., 2015. Relationships among physical inactivity, deconditioning, and walking impairment in persons with multiple sclerosis. J. Neurol. Phys. Ther. 39, 103–110.

Saverino, A., Moriarty, A., Playford, D., 2014. The risk of falling in young adults with neurological conditions: a systematic review. Disabil. Rehabil. 36, 963–977.

Scheffer, A.C., Schuurmans, M.J., Van Dijk, N., Van Der Hooft, T., De Rooij, S.E., 2008. Fear of falling: measurement strategy, prevalence, risk factors and consequences among older persons. Age. Ageing. 37, 19–24.

Schinkel-Ivy, A., Huntley, A.H., Aqui, A., Mansfield, A., 2019. Does perturbation-based balance training improve control of reactive stepping in individuals with chronic stroke? J. Stroke. Cerebrovasc. Dis. 28, 935–943.

Schinkel-Ivy, A., Huntley, A.H., Danells, C.J., Inness, E.L., Mansfield, A., 2020. Improvements in balance reaction impairments following reactive balance training in individuals with sub-acute stroke: a prospective cohort study with historical control. Top. Stroke. Rehabil. 27, 262–271.

Schmid, A.A., Rittman, M., 2009. Consequences of poststroke falls: activity limitation, increased dependence, and the development of fear of falling. Am. J. Occup. Ther. 63, 310–316.

Schmid, A.A., Yaggi, H.K., Burrus, N., et al., 2013. Circumstances and consequences of falls among people with chronic stroke. J. Rehabil. Res. Dev. 50, 1277–1286.

Schnock, K.O., Howard, E.P., Dykes, P.C., 2019. Fall prevention self-management among older adults: a systematic review. Am. J. Prev. Med. 56, 747–755.

Seymour, K.C., Pickering, R., Rochester, L., et al., 2019. Multicentre, randomised controlled trial of PDSAFE, a physiotherapist-delivered fall prevention programme for people with Parkinson's. J. Neurol. Neurosurg. Psychiatry. 90, 774–782.

Shen, X., Wong-Yu, I.S., Mak, M.K., 2016. Effects of exercise on falls, balance, and gait ability in Parkinson's disease: a meta-analysis. Neurorehabil. Neural. Repair. 30, 512–527.

Sherrington, C., Fairhall, N.J., Wallbank, G.K., et al., 2019. Exercise for preventing falls in older people living in the community. Cochrane Database Syst Rev. 1, CD012424

Shumway-Cook, A., Woollacott, M., 1995. Motor Control Theory and Applications. Williams and Wilkins, Baltimore. 323–324.

Shumway-Cook, A., Woollacott, M.H., 2017. Normal Postural Control. Motor Control: Translating Research into Clinical Practice. Wolters Kluwer, Philadelphia.153–182.

Skelton, D., Dinan, S., Campbell, M., Rutherford, O., 2005. Tailored group exercise (Falls Management Exercise – FaME) reduces falls in community-dwelling older frequent fallers (an RCT). Age. Ageing. 34, 636–639.

Skymne, C., Dahlin-Ivanoff, S., Claesson, L., Eklund, K., 2012. Getting used to assistive devices: ambivalent experiences by frail elderly persons. Scand. J. Occup. Ther. 19, 194–203.

Smania, N., Corato, E., Tinazzi, M., et al., 2010. Effect of balance training on postural instability in patients with idiopathic Parkinson's disease. Neurorehabil. Neural. Repair. 24, 826–834.

Son, N.K., Ryu, Y.U., Jeong, H.W., Jang, Y.H., Kim, H.D., 2016. Comparison of 2 different exercise approaches: tai chi versus Otago, in community-dwelling older women. J. Geriatr. Phys. Ther. 39, 51–57.

Stack, E., Ashburn, A., 1999. Fall-events described by people with PD: implications for clinical interviewing and the research agenda. Physiother. Res. Int. 4, 190–200.

Stack, E., Ashburn, A., Jupp, K., 2005. Postural instability during reaching tasks in Parkinson's disease. Physiother. Res. Int. 10, 146–153.

Stack, E., King, R., Janko, B., et al., 2016. Could in-home sensors surpass human observation of people with Parkinson's at high risk of falling? An ethnographic study. Bio. Med. Res. Int. 2016, 3703745.

Stack, E., Roberts, H., 2013. Slow down and concentrate: time for a paradigm shift in fall prevention among people with Parkinson's disease? Parkinson. Dis. 2013, 704237.

Stubbs, B., Binnekade, T., Eggermont, L., Sepehry, A.A., Patchay, S., Schofield, P., 2014. Pain and the risk for fall in community-dwelling older adults: systematic review and meta-analysis. Arch. Phys. Med. Rehabil. 95, 175–187.

Tan, K.M., Tan, M.P., 2016. Stroke and falls – clash of the two titans in geriatrics. Geriatrics. 1, 31.

Tang, A., Tao, A., Soh, M., et al., 2015. The effect of interventions on balance self-efficacy in the stroke population: a systematic review and meta-analysis. Clin. Rehabil. 29, 1168–1177.

Teasell, R., McRae, M., Foley, N., Bhardwaj, A., 2002. The incidence and consequences of falls in stroke patients during inpatient rehabilitation: factors associated with high risk. Arch. Phys. Med. Rehabil. 83, 329–333.

Terroso, M., Rosa, N., Margues, A.T., Simoes, R., 2014. Physical consequences of falls in the elderly: a literature review. Eur. Rev. Aging. Phys. Act. 11, 51–59.

Tian, Y., Thompson, J., Buck, D., Sonola, L., 2013. Exploring the System-Wide Costs of Falls in Older People in Torbay. The King's Fund, London.

Tinetti, M.E., 1986. Performance-oriented assessment of mobility problems in elderly patients. J. Am. Geriatr. Soc. 34, 119–126.

Tinetti, M.E., Speechley, M., Ginter, S.F., 1988. Risk factors for falls among elderly persons living in the community. N. Engl. J. Med. 319, 1701–1707.

Tomlinson, C.L., Patel, S., Meek, C., et al., 2012. Physiotherapy intervention in Parkinson's disease: systematic review and meta-analysis. BMJ. 345, e5004.

Tyson, S.F., Sadeghi-Demneh, E., Nester, C.J., 2013. A systematic review and meta-analysis of the effect of an ankle-foot orthosis on gait biomechanics after stroke. Clin. Rehabil. 27, 879–891.

Tzeng, H.M., Okpalauwaekwe, U., Lyons, E.J., 2020. Barriers and facilitators to older adults participating in fall-prevention strategies after transitioning home from acute hospitalization: a scoping review. Clin. Intervent. Aging. 15, 971.

Ueda, T., Higuchi, Y., Imaoka, M., Todo, E., Kitagawa, T., Ando, S., 2017. Tailored education program using home floor plans for falls prevention in discharged older patients: a pilot randomized controlled trial. Arch. Gerontol. Geriatr. 71, 9–13.

van der Marck, M.A., Klok, M.P.C., Okun, M., Giladi, N., Munneke, M., 2014. Bloem BR on behalf of the NPF Falls Task Force. Consensus-based clinical practice recommendations for the examination and management of falls in patients with Parkinson's disease. Parkinsonism. Relat. Disord. 20, 360–369.

van Duijnhoven, H.J., De Kam, D., Hellebrand, W., Smulders, E., Geurts, A.C., Weerdesteyn, V., 2012. Development and process evaluation of a 5-week exercise program to prevent falls in people after stroke: the FALLS program. Stroke. Res. Treat. 2012, 407693.

van Duijnhoven, H.J., Heeren, A., Peters, M.A., Veerbeek, J.M., Kwakkel, G., Geurts, A.C., Weerdesteyn, V., 2016. Effects of exercise therapy on balance capacity in chronic stroke: systematic review and meta-analysis. Stroke. 47, 2603–2610.

van Duijnhoven, H.J.R., Roelofs, J.M.B., den Boer, J.J., et al., 2018. Perturbation-based balance training to improve step quality in the chronic phase after stroke: a proof-of-concept study. Front. Neurol. 9, 980.

Van Liew, C., Monaghan, A.S., Dibble, L.E., Foreman, K.B., MacKinnon, D.P., Peterson, D.S., 2021. Perturbation practice in multiple sclerosis: assessing generalization from support surface translations to tether-release tasks. Mult. Scler. Relat. Disord. 56, 103218.

van Ooijen, M.W., Heeren, A., Smulders, K., et al., 2015. Improved gait adjustments after gait adaptability training are associated with reduced attentional demands in persons with stroke. Exp. Brain. Res. 233, 1007–1018.

van Swigchem, R., van Duijnhoven, H.J., den Boer, J., Geurts, A.C., Weerdesteyn, V., 2013. Deficits in motor response to avoid sudden obstacles during gait in functional walkers post-stroke. Neurorehabil. Neural. Repair. 27, 230–239.

Veerbeek, J.M., van Wegen, E., van Peppen, R., et al., 2014. What is the evidence for physical therapy poststroke? A systematic review and meta-analysis. PloS One. 9, e87987.

Vlaeyen, E., Coussement, J., Leysens, G., et al., 2015. Characteristics and effectiveness of fall prevention programs in nursing homes: a systematic review and meta-analysis of randomized controlled trials. J. Am. Geriatr. Soc. 63, 211–221.

Wagner, H., Melhus, H., Gedeborg, R., Pedersen, N.L., Michaelsson, K., 2009. Simply ask them about their balance – future fracture risk in a nationwide cohort study of twins. Am. J. Epidemiol. 169, 143–149.

Wang, C., Goel, R., Rahemi, H., Zhang, Q., Lepow, B., Najafi, B., 2019. Effectiveness of daily use of bilateral custom-made ankle-foot orthoses on balance, fear of falling, and physical activity in older adults: a randomized controlled trial. Gerontology. 65, 299–307.

Weerdesteyn, V., de Niet, M., van Duijnhoven, H.J., Geurts, A.C., 2008. Falls in individuals with stroke. J. Rehabil. Res. Dev. 45, 1195–1213.

Weerdesteyn, V., Rijken, H., Geurts, A.C., Smits-Engelsman, B.C., Mulder, T., Duysens, J., 2006. A five-week exercise program can reduce falls and improve obstacle avoidance in the elderly. Gerontology. 52, 131–141.

Whipple, M.O., Hamel, A.V., Talley, K.M., 2018. Fear of falling among community-dwelling older adults: a scoping review to identify effective evidence-based interventions. Geriatr. Nurs. 39, 170–177.

Wielinski, C.L., Erickson-Davis, C., Wichmann, R., Walde-Douglas, M., Parashos, S.A., 2005. Falls and injuries resulting from falls among patients with Parkinson's disease and other parkinsonian syndromes. Mov. Disord. 20, 410–415.

Wing, J.J., Burke, J.F., Clarke, P.J., Feng, C., Skolarus, L.E., 2017. The role of the environment in falls among stroke survivors. Arch. Gerontol. Geriatr. 72, 1–5.

World Health Organization, 2010. Global recommendations on physical activity for health. World Health Organization, Geneva.

Wrisley, D.M., Marchetti, G.F., Kuharsky, D.K., Whitney, S.L., 2004. Reliability, internal consistency, and validity of data obtained with the functional gait assessment. Phys. Ther. 84, 906–918.

Yardley, L., Donovan-Hall, M., Francis, K., Todd, C., 2006. Older people's views of advice about falls prevention: a qualitative study. Health Educ. Res. 21, 508–517.

Yardley, L., Kirby, S., Ben-Shlomo, Y., Gilbert, R., Whitehead, S., Todd, C., 2008. How likely are older people to take up different falls prevention activities? Prevent. Med. 47, 554–558.

Yoshida-Intern, S., 2007. A global report on falls prevention epidemiology of falls. World Health Organization, Geneva.

Zadravec, M., Olenšek, A., Rudolf, M., Bizovičar, N., Goljar, N., Matjačić, Z., 2020. Assessment of dynamic balancing responses following perturbations during slow walking in relation to clinical outcome measures for high-functioning post-stroke subjects. J. Neuroeng. Rehabil. 17, 85.

Zecevic, A.A., et al., 2006. Defining a fall and reasons for falling: comparisons among the views of seniors, health care providers, and the research literature. Gerontologist. 46, 367–376.

Zhou, Q., Yang, H., Zhou, Q., Pan, H., 2021. Effects of cognitive motor dual-task training on stroke patients: a RCT-based meta-analysis. J. Clin. Neurosci. 92, 175–182.

Physical Activity and Exercise in Neurological Rehabilitation

Helen Dawes

OUTLINE

Neurological Conditions, 571
Physical Activity, 572
  Exercise, 573
  Fitness, 573
  Physical Activity, Exercise and Fitness in Long-Term Neurological Conditions, 573
  Considerations for Prescribing Neurological Conditions, 574
    Stage and Severity of Disease, 574
    Condition Progression, 574
    Neurological Symptoms, 574
    Likelihood of Secondary Conditions, 574
    Exercise Response and Recovery, 574
Assessment and Monitoring of Exercise, 575
  Safety, 575
  International Classification of Function Model and Exercise, Physical Activity and Fitness, 575
  Assessment of Key Body Functioning Fitness Components, 575

Assessment and Monitoring of Health, 576
  Monitoring Symptoms, 576
  Monitoring Participation, Health and Well-being, 576
Monitoring Exercise and Physical Activity Levels, 576
  Wider Assessment, 577
Exercise Prescription, 577
  Exercise Prescription Setting, 577
  Exercise Prescription Content, 577
Limit to Capacity, 577
Exercise Response and Recovery, 577
  Frequency, 577
  Intensity, 578
  Timing, 578
  Type, 578
Reducing Sedentary Time, 578
Barriers and Facilitators, 578
Changing Behaviour, 578
Conclusion, 580
Summary of Exercise Prescription Guidance, 580

NEUROLOGICAL CONDITIONS

Neurological disorders are diseases of the central and peripheral nervous systems: the brain, spinal cord, cranial nerves, peripheral nerves, nerve roots, autonomic nervous system, neuromuscular junction and muscles (World Health Organization [WHO] 2015). More than 3 million people in the UK and 1 billion worldwide, according to the WHO, are affected by neurological disorders which affect their mobility and participation in physical activities (WHO 2015). Considering a single condition, more than 6 million people die because of stroke each year, with more than 80% of these deaths taking place in low- and middle-income countries. The more common disorders include epilepsy, Alzheimer's disease and other dementias, cerebrovascular diseases including stroke, migraine and other headache disorders, multiple sclerosis, Parkinson's, Huntington's disease, neuroinfections, brain tumours, traumatic disorders of the nervous system caused by head trauma and neurological disorders as a result of malnutrition (WHO 2015). A number of rare disorders and infections also cause neurological disorders. These include bacterial (i.e., *Mycobacterial tuberculosis, Neisseria meningitides*), viral (i.e., HIV, enteroviruses, West Nile virus, Zika), fungal (i.e., *Cryptococcus, Aspergillus*) and parasitical (i.e., malaria, Chagas) infections that can affect the nervous system (WHO 2015).

Neurological conditions have a great human, societal and economic cost because of the complexity of the systems they affect. Clinicians need a detailed awareness of the basic structure and function of the neuromuscular system and pathological processes. Several excellent textbooks, including *Neurology: An Illustrated Colour Text*, can be consulted to inform practice (Fuller 2010). Conditions affecting the nervous system can be categorised into areas affected, including the brain, spinal cord, nerve roots, plexus and peripheral nerves, or broad pathological processes involving (Fuller 2010) systemic pathology (metabolic, toxic, nutritional, immunological or endocrine disorders), intrinsic pathology (metabolic, infectious, neoplastic, degenerative, paroxysmal, immunological and genetic disorders), vascular pathology *and* extrinsic pathology (Fuller 2010). Typical symptoms include headaches, memory disturbance, balance issues, blackouts, change in taste or smell, visual problems, difficulty with speech or swallowing, weakness or altered sensation or tingling (Fuller 2010). Underlying pathology and symptoms will be considered in the context of exercise assessment and prescription for long-term neurological conditions.

People with conditions report wanting to be active and gain associated health and well-being benefits, and that they would like to be able to be active in their locality using local resources. Importantly, across conditions physical activity (PA) levels remain low: approximately one-third of healthy control subjects of the same age (whether measured by activity monitors or questionnaires) with activity levels reducing as the disease progresses (Collett et al 2017a, 2017b, Reider et al 2017). This low activity may reflect the complexity of symptoms associated with these conditions. The evidence supports the importance of achieving an active lifestyle as early as possible after diagnosis and using an approach that adapts to the progressing needs of the individual. UK PA-promoting schemes including exercise referral schemes encourage PA in sedentary and clinical populations but have not been developed for people with neurological conditions. It is therefore unsurprising that activity levels are low, despite individuals expressing a desire to be active and comply with government PA advice.

The UK Department of Health (DOH) supported the development of the PA support system for people with long-term neurological conditions (LTNCs) to safely exercise using community fitness resources and fitness providers supported by a National Health Service (NHS) clinician (physiotherapist) (Elsworth et al 2011, Winward 2011, Winward & Dawes 2010). National Occupational Standards have been written and Accredited Exercise Professionals Courses implemented across the UK and globally to support professionals working with these conditions. More recently Moving Medicine (https://movingmedicine.ac.uk/) has developed conversations for healthcare professionals to use in practice to support people with some neurological conditions to be more active.

PHYSICAL ACTIVITY

The benefits of regular PA are now well documented in healthy and chronic disease populations. The WHO defines PA as any body movement produced by the skeletal muscles to perform tasks which result in energy expenditure (WHO 2017). Current recommendations from the UK DOH advocate daily activity in bouts of 10 minutes or more, with 150 minutes of moderate activity per week or 75 minutes of vigorous activity and minimisation of sedentary behaviour (WHO 2017). PA includes any activity which uses energy, including sporting, exercise, occupational, household chores, gardening, active transport and recreational activities (WHO 2017). Current advice also supports the importance of strong muscles and more vigorous activities for health, particularly when involving the large gluteal and quadriceps leg muscles, both for maintaining physical functioning and for health and preventing or delaying onset of long-term conditions such as diabetes (WHO 2017).

Maintaining PA is known to benefit physical and cognitive health and well-being with benefits including reducing the risk for hypertension, maintaining bone health, improving mood and controlling weight (Department of Health and Social Care 2019, WHO 2017). A lack of PA is a significant risk factor for noncommunicable diseases such as stroke, diabetes and cancer. However, less and less PA is occurring in adults and children worldwide (Department of Health and Social Care 2019). Globally, 23% of adults and 81% of school-going adolescents are not active enough (WHO 2010). Of particular note is the impact of PA on energy balance and weight control which is associated with numerous diseases and conditions. We know that women and girls are less active than men and boys. The Covid-19 pandemic has had a negative impact on the physical activity levels of people with neurological diseases, and this change was related to the worsening of disease symptoms and psychosocial factors.

In 2010 the chief medical officer in the UK highlighted that PA was a 'wonder drug' in his annual report; however, 2000 years ago Plato commented on the beneficial effects of being active on the body and mind: *'Lack of activity destroys the good condition of every human being, while movement and methodical physical exercise save it and preserve it'*. These thoughts were more recently reflected by Edward Stanley, Earl of Derby (1826-93) and British statesman, in his The Conduct of Life address at Liverpool College on 20 December 1873: *'Those who don't make time for exercise now will have to make time for ill health later'*. The recent evidence supports both physical and cognitive benefits of an active lifestyle, although the optimal timing of PA interventions through the life course or its optimal content is not yet known. Indeed for neurological conditions, whilst we know that for all conditions PA is beneficial, the optimal and minimal content, delivery and timing and mode of delivery are not clear.

Exercise

Exercise is PA which involves planned, structured and repetitive movements with the aim to maintain or improve physical fitness (American College of Sports Medicine [ACSM] 2017).

Fitness

Fitness includes a set of attributes relating to the ability to perform PA and is composed of skills-related, health-related and physiological components (ACSM 2017). Physical fitness, according to the ACSM (2017), consists of fitness components. Fitness components should typically include cardiorespiratory endurance, body composition, muscular strength and endurance, flexibility, agility, balance, coordination, power, speed and reaction time.

Physical Activity, Exercise and Fitness in Long-Term Neurological Conditions

The required dose of PA for health and well-being is high and perhaps daunting for some people affected by a neurological condition. Consideration should be given for the health condition and stage of the disease and the age of the individual in the context of the person's environment and personal factors (WHO 2001). It is important to consider PA epidemiology health trajectories which support that; although recommendations are for achieving levels of 150 minutes of moderate activity or 75 minutes of

vigorous activity per week, increasing activity by as little as 30 minutes of moderate PA a week is health promoting, particularly for those performing less than the 150 minutes of activity, and consider the importance of both PA and reducing sedentary time (Fig. 22.1) (Ekelund et al 2016, Powell et al 2011, Rafferty et al 2017).

Several systems (including those affecting movement) continence, cognition and mood, may be affected by neurological pathology, which can result in a range of possible symptomatic presentations and progressions. Some conditions are progressive (such as Parkinson's and motor neurone disease), some have a sudden onset and variable levels of recovery (such as a stroke or transient ischaemic attack) and others may relapse and remit at any time point over several years (e.g., multiple sclerosis). The type and level of impairment of body function will affect the choice of activity and its delivery, and needs to be considered to enable safe, effective and sympathetic exercise prescription. For successful exercise participation, health and fitness professionals may need to consider the underlying pathology alongside possible symptoms and adapt exercises appropriately whatever the chosen exercise modality or setting. Day-to-day performance in people with neurological conditions may be more variable than that observed in healthy individuals. Condition-specific pathology affecting physical, cognitive, social and emotional factors, as well as medication and its timing in relation to exercise sessions, may also affect ability to exercise on a given day.

Importantly, people with neurological conditions universally report wishing to achieve an active lifestyle and how being active following personalised activities helps them to focus on positive aspects of disability (Elsworth et al

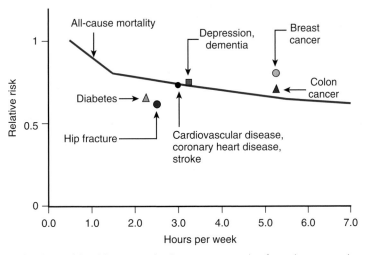

FIG. 22.1 Risk of selected health events by hours per week of moderate to vigorous physical activity (Powell et al 2011).

2009a, 2009b). Positive benefits of being active reported by people with long-term neurological conditions include social aspects and enhancing feelings of 'normality' (Elsworth et al 2009a, 2009b).

Considerations for Prescribing Neurological Conditions

Exercise prescription has become more popular over recent years and is now a common component of rehabilitation programmes. In part this has been because of increasing evidence of benefit for all for specific neurological conditions, and in part because of earlier diagnosis in most of these conditions. People with a range of long-term neurological conditions are no different than the general population, with participation in a range of physical activities having demonstrated benefits at International Classification of Function (ICF) levels of body function, activity and participation (Dawes 2008).

Measurement tools should consider physical functioning directly affected by the condition, alongside a focus on exercise as an intervention for prevention of secondary conditions and health and well-being benefits. There is still limited evidence as to the effect of participation in regular exercise on long-term general health and well-being within an individual's daily life, mainly because of a paucity of trials. There is a wealth of evidence of the impact of PA on cardiovascular, neurological, metabolic, immune, respiratory and musculoskeletal systems and an indication that long-term effects of exercise in neurological conditions may also exert effects by reducing disease activity.

So what is different in prescribing PA and exercise for neurological conditions? There are various aspects of the presentation that make prescription more complex.

Stage and Severity of Disease

The severity of the disease activity and level of disability will vary through the course of the condition and between individuals. The disease stage will affect the selected content and delivery of exercise.

Condition Progression

Health conditions may have different forms of presentation:
- Deteriorating disorder (slow/fast) – amyotrophic lateral sclerosis
- Relapse and remit – multiple sclerosis
- Recovery/motor recovery – traumatic brain injury

Neurological Symptoms

Health conditions may have a number of symptoms:
- Ataxia
- Spasticity
- Apraxia
- Weakness

- Variability
- Fatigue
- Altered movement skill and cost of moving – neural and muscular
- Sensory
- Behavioural
- Autonomic dysfunction
- Cognitive
- Emotional

Likelihood of Secondary Conditions

The likelihood of comorbidities is extremely high (ACSM 2017) with one-third of adults living with at least one condition (WHO 2015). In an audit of 28 participants with long-term neurological conditions attending an exercise class in Cornwall, the concurrent comorbidities included epilepsy (2), osteoporosis (3), asthma (3), heart disease (2), arthritis (6), cancer (2) and stroke and brain injury (2). This should be factored into training programmes.

Exercise Response and Recovery

Exercise response and recovery may be altered compared with healthy age-matched individuals in the following systems:
- Neuromuscular system
- Cardiovascular system
- Autonomic system
- Metabolic system

When training people with neurological conditions, it may be wise to consider and monitor these different systems during exercise and to be aware of possible challenges for patients. Affected symptoms may include an altered metabolic functioning with reduced aerobic and anaerobic metabolism in people with Huntington's disease or Parkinson's affecting response and recovery from exercise (Dawes et al 2015, Foteini Mavrommati et al 2017, Steventon et al 2015). The underpinning mechanism is not clearly understood, but possible factors include abnormalities in bioenergetic functioning (Foteini Mavrommati et al 2017, Steventon et al 2015). Alternatively, individuals may present with an altered autonomic control such as observed temperature control challenges in people with multiple sclerosis or orthostatic hypotension during or after exercise in people with Parkinson's (Foteini Mavrommati et al 2017, Hansen et al 2015, Kobal et al 2014). Again potential mechanisms are complex with possible primary and secondary involvement of motor, sensory and autonomic structures. Importantly, individuals may be slower to respond to exercise stress (Feltham et al 2013) and take longer to recover (Dawes et al 2014), and this should be factored into exercise programmes (Collett et al 2017a, 2017b, Dawes et al 2014). Variability in how people feel from day to day is higher than in the general

Impairments

Cognitive
Emotional
Behavioural
Neurological
Cardiovascular
Respiratory
Metabolic
Musculo-skeletal

Impact on mobility → Detraining

FIG. 22.2 Logic flow of the effect of impairments on mobility and detraining.

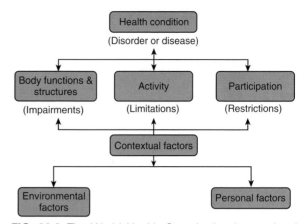

FIG. 22.3 The World Health Organization International Classification of function model of body structures, functions, activity and participation.

population, and again this should be factored into prescription with some flexibility in when to push harder and perform more vigorous intensity exercise and when not to. The impaired body functioning can lead to reduced PA and increased sedentary time (Fig. 22.2).

Detraining will occur in neuromuscular, autonomic, metabolic and cardiorespiratory systems affecting all components of fitness, including muscle strength, speed and power, balance, coordination, flexibility and cardiovascular endurance. This can lead to a downwards spiral, and it is important to remember to consider regular activity that addresses each of these components in people with long-term neurological conditions.

ASSESSMENT AND MONITORING OF EXERCISE

Safety

The patient's safety should be the first consideration for exercise prescription, both for the safety of the delivery mechanism and the exercise content. All individuals should follow the industry standard ACSM guidelines for exercise testing and prescription for long-term condition safety guidelines that incorporate the Physical Activity Readiness Questionnaire, which measures key cardiac, respiratory and musculoskeletal risk factors and then clearly outlines whether a potential client can immediately start or requires further investigation before participation (Shephard 2015). In addition to these basic safety considerations, there are further considerations for people with long-term neurological conditions. It may be wise to take a detailed prescribed medication and medical history to ensure that clients are started when on a stable medical regime and to allow all symptoms, such as orthostatic intolerance, to be considered in adapting exercises for prescribing. It is also important to determine cognitive impairment affecting independent safe participation (e.g., dementia), history of additional neurological

conditions, unstable psychiatric disease and other metabolic comorbidities. However, it is important to iterate that exercise is rarely contraindicated; rather,prescription should be modified to allow safe engagement.

International Classification of Function Model and Exercise, Physical Activity and Fitness

When monitoring the impact of an exercise prescription in a person with neurological conditions, consideration should be given for the ICF WHO model of classification which allows for measurement of changes in body functioning to be assessed in the context of a pathway to their impact on participatory activities and allows for changes in the health condition of the individual and other contextual influences such as personal social or environmental factors (Fig. 22.3) (Khan & Pallant 2007, Mayo et al 2004, Ptyushkin et al 2010). In addition, when prescribing behavioural interventions an important consideration is the logical flow of prescription on behavioural change, so care should be taken to measure compliance with the intervention as well as the desired impact. This will enable adaptation of exercise as appropriate and an understanding of what is working and what is not.

Assessment of Key Body Functioning Fitness Components

Measurement of the key fitness components of endurance, strength, speed, power, balance, agility and flexibility linked to the body functioning of the ICF model should be considered, and measures may take the form of surrogate markers such as the 6-minute walk, sit-to-stand and standing balance tests (http://www.rehabmeasures.org/default.aspx) or could be determined from changes in performance on exercise activities included in the programme, such as an increase in the work volume in a strengthening regime or distance achieved on a bike or in a swimming pool.

Assessment and Monitoring of Health

General health measures such as blood pressure, weight, height, grip strength and mobility should be monitored as general health markers.

Monitoring Symptoms

After prescribing exercise, the professional should monitor a patient's symptoms to either ensure that they do not get worse or to determine whether the intervention is helping. Some areas of typical interest may be fatigue, cognition and mood. Appropriate measures may be found at the AbilityLab website (http://www.rehabmeasures.org/default.aspx).

Monitoring Participation, Health and Well-being

Health-related Quality of Life Euroqol-5D-5L, well-being Short Form 36 and participation WHO disability assessment schedule (WODAS) could be monitored to show the impact of the exercise prescription (http://www.rehabmeasures.org/default.aspx).

The MOVES tool is an available resource which compares groups or populations of participants engaging in a sport or PA with the same group as if they had not taken part in that activity. It estimates the reduction in risk of key diseases from increased PA and assigns an economic value to the resulting health improvements. The tool may be a useful resource for professionals to support their case for prescription if considering the sustainability of services (https://www.sportengland.org/our-work/partnering-local-government/tools-directory/moves-tool/).

Monitoring Exercise and Physical Activity Levels

When measuring PA, there is a Sport England–validated single-item PA measure (achieving/not achieving 30 minutes of PA per week). This tool offers a quick way to quantify activity and also to categorise people as sedentary (<30 minutes of activity a week) or active (achieving 30 minutes activity a week). Further sensitivity can be achieved using measures such as the International Physical Activity Questionnaire (physical activity) (Craig et al 2003). Implementation and delivery of the intervention should be considered if remotely prescribing, along with the perceptions and experiences of the client. Any issues may be easily rectifiable and enable participation. Diaries can be used as a self-report method to determine adherence and fidelity of an exercise intervention. PA and exercise occur within social, work, transport and home domains, and it is important to consider all of these.

In healthy populations most PA is undertaken socially or as a means of transport (WHO 2010), but for populations with neurological conditions most PA would appear to occur in the home, particularly for individuals with more severe disease (Martin Ginis et al 2016). A further consideration is that models of exercise prescription and monitoring developed for healthy individuals, such as heart rate estimates, metabolic equivalents or pedometer step counts, may not be accurate, particularly for individuals with more severely affected movement or changed metabolic, respiratory and cardiovascular functioning. Typically, these measures will underestimate the effort or energy cost of an activity in people with neurological conditions, with the discrepancy greater for those more severely affected (Dawes et al 2004, Sandroff et al 2014).

Monitoring should attempt to consider the components of the prescription: what mode or type of activity and then how frequently, intensively and for how long the activity is performed. Technological measurement tools, such as accelerometer devices including off-the-shelf systems, can be used in neurological populations. They record activity counts and heart rate. Several systems exist which have been validated to monitor sitting and activity intensity in those with neurological conditions, but these systems are often expensive and not suitable for routine clinical practice, and off-the-shelf systems developed to measure activity in the general population may not be totally reliable or accurate. However, some wrist-worn systems are usually accurate enough, if recording average activity over 10 or more minutes, and are stable in their level of accuracy and thus are useful if used to look for relative change in an individual's activity levels over time. Their validity in more severely affected individuals is often lower, but several still can be useful tools for monitoring the effectiveness of interventions within individuals. Heart rate may give an indication of activity intensity, but reduced capacity and possible effect of medications should be considered (ACSM 2017).

It is extremely useful to monitor exertional symptoms (Borg et al 1987, Dawes et al 2005). Our perception of exertional symptoms is what limits and dictates how hard we believe we can exercise and for how long (Kinsman & Weiser 1975). Although reporting may be less sensitive and more variable than in healthy populations, particularly if used to direct the intensity of performing exercises, it is important to consider how hard an exercise session feels for an individual and how fatigued the individual is after exercise because both have been shown to coincide with how hard people work and the time it takes to recover for neurological populations, including those with multiple sclerosis, Parkinson's and Huntington's disease (Collett et al 2017a, 2017b, Dawes et al 2014). There are numerous scales, but the one most commonly used by exercise practitioners is the category ratio scale developed by Borg, which provides interindividual and intraindividual comparisons (Borg 1998). The category ratio CR-10 scale, which rates from 0 to 10, has been used to safely and effectively prescribe both aerobic and strength exercises for people with a range of neurological conditions (Busse et al 2014, Dawes et al 2014, Elsworth et al 2011, Quinn et al 2016).

Wider Assessment

When prescribing, it may be sensible to consider the wider effect of the exercise on service use, work, and family and carers.

Exercise Prescription

When prescribing exercise for persons with long-term conditions, the trainer should be both promoting PA for health and well-being and also giving a specific rehabilitation and maintenance exercise programme. There are several areas to consider, including the content, delivery and setting for exercise interventions, which are outlined in the following subsections.

Exercise Prescription Setting

People with long-term conditions will need to exercise in their locality but still require safe and appropriate exercise venues. Overwhelming evidence supports the need to enjoy an activity for individuals to adhere longer term. Considering available resources and the stage of each condition, exercise prescription may be carried out in several possible environments, including the individual's home or local community environment (health walks, park, shopping mall), voluntary sector provision from charities (neurological alliance, specific charities) or public providers including NHS organisations, primary care, neurological specialisms (clinical links), community physiotherapy team and rehabilitation services, County Council providers and exercise referral, that is, GoActive or private providers and funders such as Virgin or other centres. The complexity of provision, which varies in different geographies both between and within countries, is confusing for all, and support to navigate and take advantage of local initiatives and to participate in activities of choice is a critical area.

Exercise Prescription Content

The core principles of training apply: frequency, intensity, type and timing (FITT). However, there may be a need to adapt training considering an individual's condition, symptoms, medication, diet, medical history, disease severity, comorbidities, age, gender, capacity, mobility and baseline fitness level in all components of fitness (ACSM 2017). An altered response and recovery from exercise may direct exercise prescription (Collett et al 2017a, 2017b, Dawes et al 2014).

Limit to Capacity

When measuring exercise, most individuals with neurological conditions will tend to have a reduced exercise capacity, approximately one-third lower than sedentary matched healthy control subjects (Buckley et al 2008), although this depends on disease severity. Individuals will be less active for less time, in general approximately one-third as active at lower intensities (mostly in light or moderate intensity), will have reduced exercise capacity, lower strength dependent on muscle group and be less able to elevate heart rate to the same levels because of less movement and motor ability (Buckley et al 2008). This should be considered in exercise prescription.

Exercise Response and Recovery

Most individuals with neurological conditions will have a normal linear submaximal exercise (Collett et al 2017a, 2017b, Dawes et al 2014, 2015, Foteini Mavrommati et al 2017, Steventon et al 2015) response of cardiovascular, respiratory and aerobic/anaerobic metabolic systems to exercise, although there may be differences in some or all of these systems, which should be considered when prescribing and monitored if symptoms presenting themselves indicate (Collett et al 2017a, 2017b, Dawes et al 2014, 2015, Feltham et al 2013, Foteini Mavrommati et al 2017, Hansen et al 2015, Kobal et al 2014).

Frequency

There is good evidence that those with neurological conditions align to the ACSM (2017) and WHO (2010) guidelines for exercise testing and prescription for the general population. Most individuals will benefit from an exercise dose of 5 or more days of 30 minutes of activity a week. Several studies have shown across a range of neurological conditions that functional, health and well-being benefits can be achieved with a single session of exercise a week as a minimum for those who are starting from an inactive base (Busse et al 2013, Collett et al 2011, 2016, Rafferty et al 2017). More has been shown to be better, but again numerous studies demonstrate that most individuals will achieve a single session of exercise a week, whereas fewer achieve twice-weekly sessions and very few the government guidance (Busse et al 2013, Collett et al 2011, 2016, Rafferty et al 2017). However, when considering cognitive benefits, it appears that more frequent exercise may be required (Demnitz et al 2016, Kalron et al 2015, Thomas et al 2016).

Intensity

Again there is good evidence for benefits from achieving the exercise intensities suggested by ACSM (2017) guidelines for exercise testing and prescription for the general population. They suggest a dose that meets 150 minutes of moderate or 75 minutes of vigorous PA or a combination may improve functioning, health and well-being; an example of moderate-intensity PA is brisk walking (heart rate 60%–70% of maximum) and vigorous-intensity PA is running (heart rate 71%–85% of maximum). There is emerging evidence to suggest a case for higher intensity for training cardiovascular and neuromuscular systems. To date, evidence for cognitive changes is in individuals who perform 40 minutes of moderate to vigorous PA at least three times a week (ACSM 2017, WHO 2010).

Timing

There is also good evidence for following suggested timings by the WHO and ACSM aiming to achieve sessions of at least 10 minutes and ideally sessions lasting for 30 minutes or more for physical functioning, health and well-being, and 40 minutes or more for cognitive functioning (ACSM 2017, WHO 2010). Evidence is emerging that timing during the day should be considered.

Type

Adherence to all physical activities is greater when exercise is either essential or enjoyable. Prescriptions should attempt to tap into essential physical activities such as cleaning, active transport or gardening and to make other activities as enjoyable as possible. There is no evidence that any type of activity is better for health, well-being or cognitive functioning, although the mode of activity may affect transfer of physical functioning; that is, walking will improve walking more than cycling.

Reducing Sedentary Time

There is increasing evidence that not only should individuals increase PA but also they should reduce sedentary time to benefit health and well-being. Exercise prescriptions should take this into consideration, and individuals should be encouraged to break sitting time whenever possible. Several possible approaches may include memory aids such as texting, using smartphone or watch applications, simple diary completion or the use of off-the-shelf commercially available activity systems.

Barriers and Facilitators

On a daily basis, people with neurological conditions have to tackle social and environmental factors, including suitable transport, access and facilities and negative attitudes of people in fitness and community centres (their beliefs about risk and benefit), and they may rely on a high level of family support to be able to participate (Martin Ginis et al 2016, Rimmer et al 2004). People with neurological conditions express a desire to be able to participate in a range of activities, including those that are not just gym based, and in a range of environments. Factors that affect ongoing PA participation integration into peoples' lives are multiple and complex, and this is true for people with neurological conditions. Long-term engagement in PA may require both a medical and a social model, using community facilities and also using medical support as required, possibly from a self-management system. Clinicians should be aware that people with neurological conditions may be motivated to be active by several factors that reflect those observed in the healthy population, such as weight control, body image and social factors. These factors should be considered in behaviour change approaches.

Changing Behaviour

Inactivity and increased time spent in sedentary activities are a problem worldwide. Several strategies have been introduced to increase activity with limited impact. A historical and evolutionary view of human activity levels may be helpful when considering how to change behaviour considering modern lifestyles. Historically, we have been active either out of necessity or for play. This may be helpful to consider when planning interventions. People with neurological conditions report numerous barriers and facilitators to achieving a physically active lifestyle which are true for all of us. Several barriers affecting engagement reported by people with long-term neurological conditions can be categorised under societal, economic and physical factors (Martin Ginis et al 2016). These include issues of access to activities such as travel, cost, time and disability access, and knowledge issues such as lack of knowledge of a condition and exercise for each condition and general lack of awareness of condition symptoms, which may limit participation or cause embarrassment (Martin Ginis et al 2016). In addition, it is important to consider motivators to achieving a physically active lifestyle. Data from those with long-term conditions support that people are not just motivated by health factors but rather by factors that motivate us all, such as body image, weight management, strength gains, fun and enjoyment, fitness, stress relieving, socialising and meeting people (Elsworth et al 2009a, 2009b, Martin Ginis et al 2016).

Changing people's behaviour is an important aim for policy-makers, healthcare providers, educators, researchers and others, but the task is challenging and all of the necessary resources are rarely available. Even when we know what we are trying to achieve, we may lack the time, the multidisciplinary team, access to the people whose behaviour needs to change, understanding of behaviour change theories, or knowledge and skills relevant to changing behaviour. Several theories relate to behaviour change. A well-used model is behaviour change theory (Bandura 1997, Hagger et al 2002), which supports the need to consider giving people the ability, confidence and motivation to change. However, changing behaviour is complex, with hundreds of possible models describing components of behaviour changes such as motivational, socioeconomic and public health theories. A theoretical framework to support PA that incorporates numerous models is the behaviour change wheel (BCW) model (http://www.behaviourchangewheel.com). The BCW was developed from 19 such frameworks of behaviour change theories identified in a systematic literature review (Fig. 22.4) (WHO 2015). The model places behaviour change theories under three main areas of Capability, Opportunity and Motivation, which are all required

to change behaviour (COM-B) (Barker et al 2016). The prescribing exercise practitioner needs to consider and address each of the three areas if they wish to change behaviour. They need to ensure that the individual is capable of performing the activity, has the opportunity to perform the activity and finally has the motivation. For example, if a person wants to swim, the exercise practitioner needs to support the individual to attend a suitably adapted pool (opportunity), make sure the individual is capable of using the facilities or performing the activity, and finally the practitioner needs to consider how best to motivate an individual.

The NICE guideline standards of care for people with neurological conditions state that patients should be actively involved in setting their own goals. A recent review supports this strategy for use in exercise and therapeutic exercise (Room et al 2017). Interventions used to improve exercise adherence in older people and to evaluate the behavioural theories underpinning the interventions

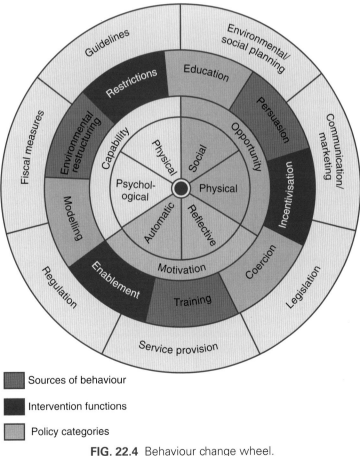

FIG. 22.4 Behaviour change wheel.

reviewed were classified into categories according to the Behaviour Change taxonomy: shaping knowledge, feedback and monitoring, social support, comparison of outcomes, identity, and goals and planning. Only four studies used behavioural approaches within their study, including social learning theory, socioemotional selectivity theory, cognitive behavioural therapy and self-efficacy. Interventions included in the feedback and monitoring category showed positive outcomes and promise (Room et al 2017). Novel technologies may help support such approaches in individuals.

CONCLUSION

There are several key messages for professionals working with patients with neurological conditions. When considering engaging with PA for health benefits, it is important to consider what, how often, how frequently and how hard.

- PA benefits brain and body health and well-being for those with neurological conditions.
- Participation in PA is associated with low risk and unlikely to do harm.
- The optimal or most effective setting, mode and format for delivery for health and wellbeing has not been established, and activity should be encouraged in all settings.
- The optimal or most effective content and dose of PA for health and well-being has not been established, but current guidance indicates that optimal levels may be in line with government guidance for the population.
- The optimal or most effective timing and PA content for health and well-being for people at different stages of neurological conditions is not established.
- The minimal dose of exercise for health benefits may be as low as an increase of 30 minutes a week, with more activity being better.
- Individualised exercise prescription and ongoing monitoring should be undertaken.

Participation in PA brings health and well-being benefits to people with neurological conditions. However, activity remains lower than for the rest of the population, and governments may need to enforce policies and strategies that positively support activity for people with conditions and disabilities alongside those introduced for healthy populations to make a step change in this area. In summary the possible benefits of being active are substantial, and people with neurological disease should be encouraged to increase their activity levels to achieve the benefits of an active lifestyle.

SUMMARY OF EXERCISE PRESCRIPTION GUIDANCE

Prescription should be biopsychosocial and individualised, and consider an individual's goals, views, pathology, history, symptoms and social and environmental factors.

Mode	Selection of activities that are enjoyable.
Delivery	Consider all possible delivery options including home and community, and that support (formal/informal) may enable participation. Consider group or individual approaches.
Frequency	Exercise at least once a week but aim to achieve WHO guidance of five sessions of moderate to vigorous physical activity and two strength and flexibility sessions.
Intensity	Activity should be moderate or vigorous.
Timing	Promote increases of 10 minutes or more; aim for 30 minutes in a session for physical and 40 minutes for cognitive health at least once a week, but more may be better.
Type	There should be a selection of activities to train; fitness components aim for training of cardiovascular fitness, strength, balance and flexibility.
Monitoring	Exercise should be monitored and progressed.

SELF-ASSESSMENT QUESTIONS

1. What exercise dose is optimal for those with neurological conditions?
2. Which fitness components should be trained (cardiovascular fitness, flexibility, balance, coordination and skill, muscle strength, speed and power or muscle endurance)?
3. For best uptake of exercise and successful implementation into peoples' lives, where and how should exercise be undertaken?
4. How should exercise intensity, duration, frequency and type be measured in neurological populations?

REFERENCES

American College of Sports Medicine (ACSM), 2017. ACSM's Guidelines for Exercise Testing and Prescription Guidelines for Graded Exercise Testing and Training, 10th ed. Lippincott Williams and Wilkins, Philadelphia.

Bandura, A., 1997. Self-Efficacy: the Exercise of Control. WH Freeman and Company, New York.

Barker, F., Atkins, L., de Lusignan, S., 2016. Applying the COM-B behaviour model and behaviour change wheel to develop an intervention to improve hearing-aid use in adult auditory rehabilitation. Int. J. Audiol. 55 (Suppl. 3), S90–S98.

Borg, G., 1998. Borg's Perceived Exertion and Pain Scales. Human Kinetics, Champaign, IL.

Borg, G., Hassmen, P., Lagerstrom, M., 1987. Perceived exertion related to heart rate and blood lactate during arm and leg exercise. Eur. J. Appl. Physiol. 65, 679–685.

Buckley, E.L., 2008. Exercise physiology in special populations: advances in sport and exercise science. In: Spurway, N. (Ed.), Advances in Sport and Exercise Science. Elsevier, Oxford.

Busse, M., Quinn, L., Dawes, H., et al., 2014. Supporting physical activity engagement in people with Huntington's disease (ENGAGE-HD): study protocol for a randomized controlled feasibility trial. Trials. 15, 487.

Busse, M., Quinn, L., Debono, K., et al., 2013. A randomized feasibility study of a 12-week community-based exercise program for people with Huntington's disease. J. Neurol. Phys. Ther. 37, 149–158.

Collett, J., Dawes, H., Meaney, A., et al., 2011. Exercise for multiple sclerosis: a single-blind randomized trial comparing three exercise intensities. Mult. Scler. 17, 594–603.

Collett, J., Franssen, M., Meaney, A., et al., 2017a. Phase II randomised controlled trial of a 6-month self-managed community exercise programme for people with Parkinson's disease. J. Neurol. Neurosurg. Psychiatry. 88, 204–211.

Collett, J., Meaney, A., Howells, K., et al., 2017b. Acute recovery froxm exercise in people with multiple sclerosis: an exploratory study on the effect of exercise intensities. Disabil. Rehabil. 39, 551–558.

Craig, C.L., Marshall, A.L., Sjöström, M., et al., 2003. International physical activity questionnaire: 12-country reliability and validity. Med. Sci. Sports Exerc. 35, 1381–1395.

Dawes, H., 2008. The role of exercise in rehabilitation. Clin. Rehabil. 22, 867–870.

Dawes, H., Collett, J., Debono, K., et al., 2015. Exercise testing and training in people with Huntington's disease. Clin. Rehabil. 29, 196–206.

Dawes, H., Collett, J., Meaney, A., et al., 2014. Delayed recovery of leg fatigue symptoms following a maximal exercise session in people with multiple sclerosis. Neurorehabil. Neural Repair. 28, 139–148.

Dawes, H., Collett, J., Ramsbottom, R., et al., 2004. Measuring oxygen cost during level walking in individuals with acquired brain injury in the clinical setting. J. Sports Sci. Med. 3, 76–82.

Dawes, H.N., Barker, K.L., Cockburn, J., et al., 2005. Borg's rating of perceived exertion scales: do the verbal anchors mean the same for different clinical groups? Arch. Phys. Med. Rehabil. 86, 912–916.

Demnitz, N., Esser, P., Dawes, H., et al., 2016. A systematic review and meta-analysis of cross-sectional studies examining the relationship between mobility and cognition in healthy older adults. Gait Posture. 50, 164–174.

Department of Health and Social Care, 2019. UK Chief Medical Officers' Physical Activity Guidelines. Available at: https://assets.publishing.service.gov.uk/government/uploads/system/uploads/attachment_data/file/832868/uk-chief-medical-officers-physical-activity-guidelines.pdf.Accessed on 27 July 2023.

Ekelund, U., Steene-Johannessen, J., Brown, W.J., et al., 2016. Does physical activity attenuate, or even eliminate, the detrimental association of sitting time with mortality? A harmonised meta-analysis of data from more than 1 million men and women. Lancet. 388, 1302–1310.

Elsworth, C., Dawes, H., Sackley, C., et al., 2009a. A study of perceived facilitators to physical activity in neurological conditions. Int. J. Ther. Rehabil. 16, 17–24.

Elsworth, C., Winward, C., Sackley, C., et al., 2011. Supported community exercise in people with long-term neurological conditions: a phase II randomized controlled trial. Clin. Rehabil. 25, 588–598.

Elsworth, C.H.D., Sackley, C., Soundy, A., et al., 2009b. Perceived facilitators to physical activity in individuals with progressive neurological conditions; a focus group and questionnaire study. Int. J. Ther. Rehabil. 16, 17–24.

Feltham, M.G., Collett, J., Izadi, H., et al., 2013. Cardiovascular adaptation in people with multiple sclerosis following a twelve week exercise programme suggest deconditioning rather than autonomic dysfunction caused by the disease. Results from a randomized controlled trial. Eur. J. Phys. Rehabil. Med. 49, 765–774.

Foteini Mavrommati, J.C., Franssen, M., Meaney, A., et al., 2017. Exercise response in Parkinson's disease: insights from a cross-sectional comparison with sedentary controls and a per-protocol analysis of a randomised controlled trial. BMJ Open 7, e017194.

Fuller, G., Manford, M., 2010. Neurology: an Illustrated Colour Text, second ed. Elsevier Health Sciences, Oxford.148.

Hagger, M.S., Chatzisarantis, N.L., Biddle, S.J., 2002. The influence of autonomous and controlling motives on physical activity intentions within the Theory of Planned Behaviour. Br. J. Health Psychol. 7, 283–297.

Hansen, D., Wens, I., Keytsman, C., et al., 2015. Is long-term exercise intervention effective to improve cardiac autonomic control during exercise in subjects with multiple sclerosis? A randomized controlled trial. Eur. J. Physiol. Rehabil. Med. 51, 223–231.

Kalron, A., Zeilig, G., 2015. Efficacy of exercise intervention programs on cognition in people suffering from multiple sclerosis, stroke and Parkinson's disease: a systematic review and meta-analysis of current evidence. NeuroRehabilitation. 37, 273–289.

Khan, F., Pallant, J.F., 2007. Use of the International Classification of Functioning, Disability and Health (ICF) to identify preliminary comprehensive and brief core sets for multiple sclerosis. Disabil. Rehabil. 29, 205–213.

Kinsman, R.A., Weiser, P.C., 1975. Subjective symptomatology during work and fatigue. In: Simonson, E., Weiser, P.C. (Eds.), Psychological Aspects and Physiological Correlates of Work and Fatigue. Charles C Thomas, Springfield, IL, pp. 336–405.

Kobal, J., Melik, Z., Cankar, K., Strucl, M., 2014. Cognitive and autonomic dysfunction in presymptomatic and early Huntington's disease. J. Neurol. 261, 1119–1125.

Martin Ginis, K.A., Ma, J.K., Latimer-Cheung, A.E., Rimmer, J.H., 2016. A systematic review of review articles addressing factors related to physical activity participation among children and adults with physical disabilities. Health Psychol. Rev. 10, 478–494.

Mayo, N.E., Poissant, L., Ahmed, S., et al., 2004. Incorporating the International Classification of Functioning, Disability, and Health (ICF) into an electronic health record to create indicators of function: proof of concept using the SF-12. J. Am. Med. Inform. Assoc. 11, 514–522.

Powell, K.E., Paluch, A.E., Blair, S.N., 2011. Physical activity for health: What kind? How much? How intense? On top of what? Ann. Rev. Public Health. 32, 349–365.

Ptyushkin, P., Vidmar, G., Burger, H., Marincek, C., 2010. Use of the International Classification of Functioning, Disability and Health (ICF) in patients with traumatic brain injury. Brain Inj. 24, 1519–1527.

Quinn, L., Trubey, R., Gobat, N., et al., 2016. Development and delivery of a physical activity intervention for people with Huntington disease: facilitating translation to clinical practice. J. Neurol. Phys. Ther. 40, 71–80.

Rafferty, M.R., Schmidt, P.N., Luo, S.T., et al., 2017. Regular exercise, quality of life, and mobility in Parkinson's disease: a longitudinal analysis of National Parkinson Foundation Quality Improvement Initiative Data. J. Parkinsons Dis. 7, 193–202.

Reider, N., Salter, A.R., Cutter, G.R., et al., 2017. Potentially modifiable factors associated with physical activity in individuals with multiple sclerosis. Res. Nurs. Health. 40, 143–152.

Rimmer, J.H., Riley, B., Wang, E., et al., 2004. Physical activity participation among persons with disabilities: barriers and facilitators. Am. J. Prevent. Med. 26, 419–425.

Room, J., Hannink, E., Dawes, H., Barker, K., 2017. What interventions are used to improve exercise adherence in older people? And what behavioral theories are they based on? A systematic review. BMJ Open. 7, e019221.

Sandroff, B.M., Motl, R.W., Pilutti, L.A., et al., 2014. Accuracy of StepWatch and ActiGraph accelerometers for measuring steps taken among persons with multiple sclerosis. PLoS One. 9, e93511.

Shephard, R.J., 2015. Qualified fitness and exercise as professionals and exercise prescription: evolution of the PAR-Q and Canadian Aerobic Fitness Test. J. Phys. Act. Health. 12, 454–461.

Steventon, J.J.C., Furby, H., Ralph, J., et al., 2015. Exercise-induced metabolic and cardiorespiratory abnormalities in Huntington's disease. Mov. Disord. 29, 196–206.

Thomas, A.G., Dennis, A., Rawlings, N.B., et al., 2016. Multimodal characterization of rapid anterior hippocampal volume increase associated with aerobic exercise. Neuroimage. 131, 162–170.

Winward, C., 2011. Supporting community-based exercise in long-term neurological conditions: experience from the Long-term Individual Fitness Enablement (LIFE) project. Clin. Rehabil. 25, 579–587.

Winward, C., Dawes, E.H., 2010. Physical Activity for Neurological Conditions. Oxford Brookes University, Oxford.

World Health Organization (WHO), 2001. International Classification of Functioning, Disability, and Health (ICF). WHO, Geneva.

World Health Organization (WHO), 2010. Global Recommendations on Physical Activity for Health. WHO, Geneva.

World Health Organization (WHO), 2015. Neurological Disorders: Public Health Challenges World, Health Organisation. What Are Neurological Disorders? Available at: http://www.who.int/features/qa/55/en/. Accessed June 2017.

World Health Organization (WHO), 2017. Global Strategy on Diet. Physical Activity Health. Available at: http://www.who.int/mediacentre/factsheets/fs385/en/.

Pain Management

Mark I. Johnson and Chih-Chung Chen

OUTLINE

Introduction, 583
    Contemporary Views About Pain, 585
    Patient Experience of Pain, 585
    Types of Pain, 585
Anatomy and Pathophysiology, 586
Signs and Symptoms and Clinical Presentation, 587
    Musculoskeletal Pain, 587
    Neuropathic Pain, 588
    Peripheral Neuropathic Pain,, 588
    Central Neuropathic Pain, 588
Epidemiology of Pain Associated with Neurological
    Conditions, 589
    Progressive Neurological Conditions, 589
    Multiple Sclerosis, 589
    Parkinson's, 589
    Huntington's Disease, 589
    Amyotrophic Lateral Sclerosis: Motor Neurone
        Disease, 589
    Other Neurological Diseases, 590
    Acute Neurological Conditions, 590
    Stroke, 590
    Traumatic Brain Injuries, 590
    Spinal Cord Injuries,, 590
Diagnosis, Assessment and Prognosis, 591
    Subjective Assessment, 591
    Red and Yellow Flags, 592
    Factors That Influence the Reliability of Subjective
        Pain Report, 592

    Objective Assessment, 593
Principles of Pain Management, 593
    Pharmacological Management of Pain, 593
    Surgical Management of Pain, 596
    Rehabilitation, 596
    Physical Activity and Exercise, 596
    Manual Therapy, 596
    Splinting, Casting and Bracing, 597
    Electrophysical Techniques, 597
    Electrotherapy, 597
    Psychological Approaches, 599
    Self-Management, 599
Pain Treatment Selection, Goal Setting and Outcome
    Monitoring, 600
    Initiating Treatment, 600
    Setting Treatment Goals, 600
    Evaluating Response to Treatment, 600
    Strategies to Improve Treatment Effect, 601
    Impact of Covid-19, 601
Conclusions, 602
Case Studies, 602
    Case 1: Diabetic Neuropathic Pain, 602
    History, 602
    Medications, 602
    Case 2: Phantom Limb Pain, 603
    History, 603
    Medications, 603

INTRODUCTION

Pain is a global health problem, with the prevalence of persistent (chronic) pain estimated to be one in five adults and expected to rise with an ageing population (Goldberg & McGee 2011, Vos et al 2020). The treatment and management of pain is financially expensive in terms of health service delivery and time lost from work, and socially expensive in terms of suffering and impaired quality of life resulting from disability, depressive mood and social isolation (Gaskin & Richard 2012, Pitcher et al 2019). Annual costs attributable

TABLE 23.1	Mean Prevalence of Pain in Adults With Neurological Conditions
Condition	**Prevalence of Pain**
Progressive Neurological Condition	
Multiple sclerosis	• 63% (95% CI: 55%–70%) (Foley et al 2013) • 50%–86% (in review by Borsook 2012)
Parkinson's	• 67.6% (range: 40%–85%) (Broen et al 2012) • 40%–60% (in review by Borsook 2012)
Huntington's disease	• 41% (95% CI: 36%–46%) (Sprenger et al 2019)
Motor neurone disease	• 60%, with 41.5% reporting limb/shoulder pain (Hurwitz et al 2021) • Range: 19%–85% (in review by de Tommaso et al 2016)
Guillain–Barré syndrome	• 89%, 38% after 1 year (in review by Borsook 2012)
Alzheimer's disease	• 57% (in review by Borsook 2012) • 38%–75% (in review by de Tommaso et al 2016)
Other	• Muscular dystrophy (MD): chronic pain 68% (95% CI: 52%–82%) in facioscapulohumeral MD, 65% (95% CI: 51%–77%) in myotonic dystrophy, 62% (95% CI: 50%–73%) in Becker/Duchenne MD and 60% (95% CI: 48%–73%) in limb/girdle MD (Huang et al 2021) • Frequency: 50% of adolescents have chronic pain with spinal muscular atrophy and Duchenne and Becker MDs (Lager & Kroksmark 2015)
Nervous System Damage	
Poststroke	• 29.56% (Paolucci et al 2016a) • Central poststroke neuropathic pain: any location 11% (95% CI: 7%–18%) but >50% in subgroups; at stroke 26% (95% CI: 18%–35%), within 1 month 31% (95% CI: 22%–42%), within 1 year 41% (95% CI: 33.9%–49.0%) (Liampas et al 2020)
Traumatic brain injury	• 49.8%–53.2% had chronic pain (Nampiaparampil 2008)
Spinal cord injury	• 61% ± 20% (mean ± SD) pain (van Gorp et al 2015) • 53% neuropathic pain (Burke et al 2017) • 68% (95% CI: 63%–73%) chronic pain, neuropathic pain, 58% (95% CI: 49%–68%), musculoskeletal pain 56% (95%: CI 41%–70%), visceral pain 20% (95% CI: 11%–29%) (Hunt et al 2021)
Syringomyelia	• 37% (in review by Borsook 2012)
Diabetic neuropathy	• 63% (in review by Borsook 2012)

Adapted from Borsook (2012).

to total healthcare and lower worker productivity associated with pain are greater than those for heart disease, cancer and diabetes. The International Association for the Study of Pain (IASP) declared the management of pain is a human right (Brennan et al 2019), and the International Classification for Diseases, 11th revision (ICD-11) recognises chronic primary pain is a disease entity in its own right (World Health Organization [WHO] 2019).

Pain is integral to neurological disease, and there is a high prevalence of pain associated with neurological conditions (see Table 23.1). Pain is not as visible as functional impairment, and traditionally treatment tends to focus on cure, slowing disease progression and improving functional outcome often at the expense of pain management. Until recently, guidelines for the treatment of specific neurological conditions gave little consideration to pain, leaving decisions to the clinicians alone.

The spatial and temporal characteristics of bodily pain are often dynamic, resulting from a complex interplay of sensory, emotional and cognitive processes that are malleable and influenced by social, psychological and biological factors, that is, 'everything matters for pain and its management'. The origin of pain associated with specific neurological conditions is often varied and may occur as a direct consequence of disease or trauma on the nervous system or as an indirect consequence of the effects of the neurological condition on neural and nonneural structures. Consequently, pain associated with neurological conditions is complex. A detailed investigation of 176 home-living patients with Parkinson's found that 83% of patients reported having pain, with 29% having more than one type of pain. Musculoskeletal pain was the most common, reported by 70% of patients, and peripheral neuropathic pain (20%) and central neuropathic pain (10%) were present in a minority of patients (Beiske et al 2009). Only 34% of patients were receiving analgesic medication, suggesting a need for better assessment and management of pain. This chapter outlines the science and management of pain in neurological conditions, including multiple sclerosis (MS), Parkinson's, motor neurone disease, stroke, traumatic brain injury (TBI) and spinal cord injury (SCI).

Contemporary Views About Pain

The IASP defines pain as 'An unpleasant sensory and emotional experience associated with, or resembling that associated with, actual or potential tissue damage' (IASP 2022, Raja et al 2020). Pain serves to protect an organism from threats t o the integrity of tissue rather than as an indicator of tissue status, that is, 'pain is a protector not a monitor'. Pain is an inferred perceptual experience and should be distinguished from nociception, which is a neural process of encoding noxious stimuli (i.e., pain and nociception are different phenomena). Nociception may lead to a variety of physiological consequences including autonomic (e.g., fight-flight-fright) or behavioural (e.g., withdrawal reflex or complex nocifensive behaviour) responses that may occur in the absence of pain sensation. Thus pain cannot, and should not, be inferred solely from activity in sensory neurones or solely from pathological findings. Pain is always a psychological state that is influenced to varying degrees by social, psychological and biological factors including social context, environment, genetics, sex, anthropometrics, previous medical history and perhaps, but not always, the presence of tissue damage.

The traditional approach to manage pain has been to identify and treat (fix) damaged and diseased tissue that is believed to be causing the pain. In some circumstances this can save a person's life. For example, sudden-onset abdominal and lower back pain may indicate a perforated ulcer or an abdominal aortic aneurysm, sudden-onset chest pain may indicate myocardial infarction and sudden-onset headache with numbness and loss of balance may indicate a stroke. In these instances, pain is a clear warning sign that tissue damage is occurring, and that treatments that target the cause of the pain (i.e., curative) are not only necessary but may also be lifesaving.

However, the link between pain and tissue damage can be tenuous. Examples include:
- Pain that is much more severe than expected from tissue damage (e.g., when a sliver of metal embeds beneath a fingernail);
- Pain that is much less severe than expected from tissue damage (e.g., when seriously injured soldiers do not feel pain [battlefield analgesia]);

- Pain that is absent despite a life-threatening disease (e.g., cancerous tumours); and
- Pain that persists despite detectable pathology (e.g., mechanical low-back pain).

Clinicians should accept that pain may not always be a reliable sign of tissue status, and treating damaged and diseased tissue does not always alleviate pain.

Persistent pain that lasts beyond the time of normal healing and/or has been present for more than 3–6 months (i.e., longstanding, persistent or chronic pain) may no longer serve an adaptive 'protective' role. The WHO recognises this and has categorised chronic pain as (1) secondary to pathology associated with cancer, surgery or physical trauma, the nervous system, headache or the orofacial region, viscera and musculoskeletal system, and (2) distinct from traditional pathology-based diagnoses (i.e., chronic primary pain) (WHO 2019).

Patient Experience of Pain

Pain is a subjective phenomenon with no objective means of measurement. Pain is always a personal experience learned through experiences related to injury and harm in early life. Pain is expressed to others via verbal description or pain-related gestures and behaviours; an inability to communicate does not negate the possibility that a human or a nonhuman animal experiences pain. Hence expression of pain may vary markedly between individuals. If an individual reports their subjective experience in the same way as pain caused by tissue damage, it should be accepted as pain, even if it is not possible to find pathology or a cause. Pain is what the person says it is (McCaffery & Pasero 1999). By attending to the status of their body rather than fighting it, some patients are able to live meaningful lives with pain by focusing less on diagnosis and cure, becoming the expert and making informed choices, telling others about pain and redefining relationships. Being skilled at actively listening and comprehending the language used by people in the stories they tell (narratives) about their pain experience is critical to diagnosing the impact of pain on the person's life (Fishman 2012, Johnson & Hudson 2016).

Types of Pain

Pain is often categorised according to duration of pain (i.e., acute and chronic) or pathophysiology (i.e., nociceptive, neuropathic and nociplastic). Often clinical service is dichotomised as acute pain and chronic pain. Acute pain serves to (1) warn of bodily threat by instigating avoidance and/or escape behaviours, and (2) aid recovery of damaged tissue, making body parts sensitive to stimuli that might cause further harm. The relationship between pain and tissue damage often weakens as pain persists and may even completely break down, with changes in the central nervous system perpetuating pain despite minimal peripheral input. In these circumstances, the biological significance of persistent pain becomes less clear.

In the general population risk factors associated with the development of chronic pain include previous history of pain, psychological distress, lack of physical activity, long-term exposure to manual labour and dissatisfaction with work (MacFarlane et al 1999). Risk factors after surgery include inadequate treatment of acute pain, severe acute pain, emotional stress and the presence of neuropathic pain (Kehlet et al 2006).

The terms acute and chronic pain do not reflect physiological mechanisms, and Loeser (2019) argues that mechanistic descriptors are more relevant because there are no specific changes in psychophysiological processes occurring at 3- or 6-month timepoints. The most common mechanistic descriptors of pain used in clinical practice are nociceptive, neuropathic and nociplastic pain.

Nociceptive pain is associated with activation of nociceptors by a noxious stimulus that is damaging or threatens damage to healthy tissues as occurs during traumatic injury and burns, and chemical stimuli arising from inflammation or ischaemia. Neuropathic pain is associated with a lesion or disease of the somatosensory nervous system. Neuropathic pain is not a diagnosis but a clinical description, sometimes referred to as *neuropathic pain syndrome*. Nociplastic pain is associated with pain arising from altered nociception without clear evidence of actual or threatened tissue damage (Kosek et al 2016). Different drugs are used to manage pain of predominantly nociceptive and neuropathic origin.

A disturbance of the function of a nerve is termed a *neuropathy*, with a mononeuropathy affecting one nerve, a mononeuropathy multiplex affecting several nerves and a polyneuropathy affecting several diffuse and bilateral nerves. Patients often describe peripheral neuropathies as sharp, throbbing, freezing or burning pain with numbness, prickling or tingling in the extremities. If motor nerves are affected, there may be weakness or paralysis, and if autonomic nerves are affected, there may be disturbances in sweating, heat and cold sensation, blood pressure, bowel, bladder or digestive function. Central neuropathic pain may be caused by stroke, brain injury, MS or SCI, and is more widespread and diffuse than peripheral neuropathic pain. Pain adjuvant drugs are used to alleviate neuropathic pain and include antidepressants, anticonvulsants and membrane stabilisers.

KEY POINTS

The prevalence of pain in neurological conditions is higher than previously believed and neurological pain affects all aspects of an individual's life, including work, hobbies, self-esteem, relationships, mood and sleep quality. Practitioners need to be skilled at deciding when pain indicates sinister pathology and when it does not. Pain is usually accompanied by an increased sensitivity of the nervous system resulting in amplification of signals related to tissue damage.

ANATOMY AND PATHOPHYSIOLOGY

Classically, physiological processes involved in producing the perceptual experience of pain have been described using a 'bottom-up' stimulus-organism-response model. This model is overly simplistic and inadvertently implies that pain is an inevitable consequence of activity in the nociceptive system driven by tissue damage. Contemporary neuroscience suggests that pain emerges to reduce threat and preserve coherent behaviour according to situational context ('pain as a protector'). This is achieved via patterns of impulses within multiple widely distributed brain neural networks that are genetically determined and modified by sensory experience. Pain emerges via a process of perceptual inference based on snippets of multisensory input resulting in localisation of sensory events, including pain, within bodily parts (Tabor et al 2017). The characteristics of sensory experiences are malleable and are updated by the brain according to social, psychological and biological context. In fact, perceptual inference may generate paradoxical sensory experiences such as pain in the absence of tissue damage (Fisher et al 1995) and serious tissue damage with an absence of pain (Beecher 1946). This is achieved in part by altering the sensitivity (excitability) of the nociceptive transmission system via facilitatory and inhibitory processes operating via top-down (central neural pathways) and bottom-up (peripheral pathways) processes ('gating' mechanisms).

A working knowledge of the physiology of the nociceptive system aids understanding of the consequence of neural lesions on nociceptive processing and the mechanism of action of pharmacological and nonpharmacological pain-relieving treatments (Fig. 23.1). Johnson has described both bottom-up (Johnson 2014, Chapter 2) and top-down processing (Johnson 2019) in the nociceptive system.

Lesions that affect sensory, motor and autonomic fibres often result in hypersensitive central nociceptive cells, abnormal inputs to central nociceptive cells, reflex muscle spasm, ectopic impulse generation, loss of large-diameter afferent inhibition, sympathetic hyperactivity and persistent activity in descending facilitatory pathways. All of these amplify nociceptive input to higher centres of the brain with the potential to increase pain.

Injury of peripheral nerves instigates degeneration of the axon distal to the site of damage (Wallerian degeneration). Lesions to peripheral nerves, distal to the cell body (e.g., peripheral neuropathies), cause distal branches of the nerve fibre to degenerate initially followed by a period of regeneration. Axonal sprouts develop and attempt to reinnervate their peripheral target (axon path finding, axon guidance). If axonal sprouts fail to find their target, a clump of regenerating neuronal sprouts forms (neuroma). There may be spontaneous nerve activity (ectopic firing) at the neuroma (primary site) or at the dorsal root ganglion

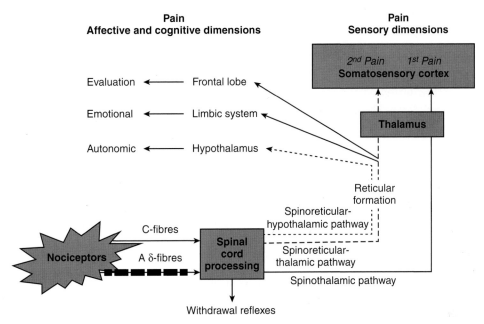

FIG. 23.1 Overview of the basic elements of the nociceptive system.

(secondary site) generating pain in the absence of stimuli. Pressure applied to neuroma may produce excessive pain because of lowered thresholds of excitation at the neuroma. Lesions proximal to the cell body (e.g., brachial plexus avulsion) diminish afferent input to central nociceptive cells, which become spontaneously hyperactive.

Injury to the central nervous system can be devastating because this is where neural centres for physiological processes are located. Peripheral input converges in the central nervous system, so damage may affect widespread areas of the body, as seen in tetraplegia associated with cervical damage and hemiplegia associated with stroke. Damage to the central nervous system results in central sensitisation, loss of descending inhibitory (and possibly facilitatory) pathways and neuroinflammation caused by glial cell activation. Glial cell activation also causes hyperarousal of the sympathetic nervous system and the hypothalamic-pituitary complex. Glial cell dysfunction is a cause of central neuropathic pain (Gosselin et al 2010, Yanguas-Casas et al 2014).

Reorganisation of neuronal circuitry (central neuroplasticity) occurs with persistent input from nociceptors and/or after nerve damage and has a major role in the development of chronic pain (Pelletier et al 2015, Seifert & Maihofner 2011). Nerve damage causes changes in afferent input to the 'neuromatrix' that subserves body sensation and pain, which in turn causes reorganisation of neural circuitry, creating delocalised, unusual and exaggerated pain (Melzack 2005). Rehabilitation techniques that target neuroplastic changes in somatosensory and motor cortices

resulting from tissue damage are likely to be beneficial (Pelletier et al 2015).

SIGNS AND SYMPTOMS AND CLINICAL PRESENTATION

Pain presents as a multidimensional experience encompassing sensory, emotional, cognitive, social, environmental and spiritual elements of a person's life. Although neurological conditions affect the nervous system, neuropathic pain is less common than musculoskeletal pain.

Musculoskeletal Pain

Musculoskeletal pain may present as a primary or secondary consequence of the neurological condition or as a comorbidity such as osteoarthritis. Musculoskeletal pain arises from involvement of nociceptors in bones, muscles, ligaments, tendons, fasciae and blood vessels, and often presents as less well-defined deep somatic pain that may be referred and may have nerve involvement.

Muscle pain may present as a dull, aching, poorly localised pain which may worsen on activity. For example, individuals with myasthenia gravis may experience painful, aching muscles (myalgia) during or after physical activity. Individuals with mitochondrial disease may experience myalgia, neuropathy, abdominal pain, chest pain, headaches and Raynaud's-like pain in hands and feet. Joint and capsule pain may result from a variety of causes including inflammatory (e.g., rheumatoid arthritis) and noninflammatory (osteoarthritis) conditions. Joint pain is more localised than muscle pain and may be dull or sharp, present at rest and provoked by movement of the joint. The pain may arise from a variety of soft tissues around the joint including tendons, ligaments and bursa. Tendon pain (e.g., tendinitis and tendon injuries), ligament pain (e.g., sprains) and bursa pain (e.g., bursitis and overuse injury) often present as a sharp, movement-evoked pain when the affected structure is stretched or compressed. It may be alleviated on rest. Bone pain commonly results from injury, infection or tumour and is often more intense than joint pain; the pain is described as dull, deep and penetrating, and may vary between localised and diffuse.

Pain from muscle spasticity (increased abnormal muscle tone) resulting from damage to the upper motor neurone in the central nervous system may hinder movement and generate long-lasting pain and reduced functional activity. A systematic review by Milinis et al (2015) found that spasticity was associated with poorer health status, and that it contributed to multiple factors including pain, bladder problems, fatigue and sleep. Failure to manage these factors has negative effects on quality of life. If untreated, permanent shortening of a muscle will occur, causing a muscular contracture deformity where it becomes impossible to move joints and muscles.

Painful muscle spasms are transient and generally short lasting, and may occur as painful night cramps. A wide variety of causes have been suggested for painful muscle spasms including a protective response to an injury, reduced blood flow muscle, dehydration and depletion of electrolytes. In functional movement disorders where there is abnormal movement or positioning, patients may experience painful muscle spasms, contractures and fixed postures that are hard to overcome. Muscle relaxants and physiotherapy are first-line treatment for muscle spasticity. Medications used for muscle spasms include cyclobenzaprine and baclofen coupled with exercise, stretching, massage and acupuncture.

Neuropathic Pain

Neuropathic pain arises from a variety of aetiologies. There may be uncertainty as to the nature and location of the lesion, especially in nonspecialist clinical settings. Neuropathic pain may be constant or intermittent, spontaneous or evoked. The onset and offset of neuropathic pain may be predictable or unpredictable. It may be paroxysmal with a sudden rise in the intensity of pain (e.g., shooting, spasmlike). Adjectives used to describe neuropathic pain include tingling, pins and needles, electric shocklike, numb, prickling, itching, burning, shooting, stabbing and lancinating. Concurrent symptoms may include allodynia, hyperalgesia, anaesthesia dolorosa, and sensory gain or loss. Patients may report bizarre sensations that they find very distressing. Patients may become frustrated at trying

to convey the legitimacy of condition, especially if the precipitating injury was trivial. People with neuropathic pain experience poorer physical and mental health than people with other forms of pain, even when adjusted for pain intensity (Finnerup et al 2021).

Peripheral Neuropathic Pain

Peripheral neuropathic pain usually has an anatomical distribution related to the affected nerve(s) and may be provoked by mechanical stimulus of the nerve. Common conditions with peripheral neuropathic pain as a symptom include nerve root damage (radiculopathy), painful diabetic neuropathy, neuropathic pains from tumours, virus postherpetic neuralgia, trigeminal neuralgia and postsurgical chronic neuropathic pain. The symptoms associated with radiculopathy include radicular pain, anaesthesia, paraesthesia, hypoesthesia, and weakness and reduced motor control radiating to body parts served by the nerve. Radiculopathy is one of the sources of referred pain from the spine. Radicular pain could arise from nonnerve root structures such as pain referred from visceral or somatic tissues (discs, ligaments, muscles and tendons). Peripheral neuropathy may present as a sharp, throbbing, freezing or burning pain with numbness, prickling or tingling that has a gradual onset in the extremities spreading into the legs and arms. There may be severe touch allodynia. If motor nerves are affected, there may be weakness or paralysis, ataxia and falling. If autonomic nerves are affected, there may be altered sweating, intolerance to heat and alterations in cardiovascular, bowel, bladder or digestive function.

Central Neuropathic Pain

Central neuropathic pain often presents as more widespread and diffuse than peripheral neuropathic pain, and patients may have difficulty locating the pain. Central

> ## KEY POINTS
>
> Bodily pain emerges from activity in widely distributed brain networks through a process of perceptual inference based on extracts of multisensory input. Pain alerts a person to potential threat to preserve coherent behaviour according to situational context ('pain as a protector').
>
> Musculoskeletal pain and neuropathic pain are common in neurological conditions. Peripheral neuropathic pain usually has an anatomical distribution related to the affected nerve(s), whereas central neuropathic pain is more widespread and diffuse. Rehabilitation techniques targeting neuroplastic changes in somatosensory and motor cortices are likely to be beneficial.

neuropathic pain may arise from any level in the central nervous system and should have a somatopically plausible distribution to the lesion. Common conditions that present with central neuropathic pain include progressive neurological conditions such as MS, Parkinson's, Huntington's disease and motor neurone disease, and insults to the central nervous system after stroke, TBI and SCI.

EPIDEMIOLOGY OF PAIN ASSOCIATED WITH NEUROLOGICAL CONDITIONS

Pain in those with neurological conditions is common (see Table 23.1). Cragg et al (2018) assessed self-reports of chronic pain for 16 neurological conditions using data from a cross-sectional national survey in Canada and estimated overall prevalence to be 36% (95% confidence interval [CI]: 31%–42%) with greater odds of chronic pain for people with spinal cord trauma.

Progressive Neurological Conditions

Pain in progressive neurological conditions may be caused by the disease or result from the consequences of disease on the body, such as protective responses by the musculoskeletal system or concurrent health condition including infections, and the side effect of drugs.

Multiple Sclerosis

Pain is very common with MS and is often varied in its presentation. Foley et al (2013) estimated the 95% CI for prevalence of different types of pain as follows: headache (33%–52%), neuropathic extremity pain (7%–53%), back pain (13%–28%), painful spasms (8.5%–23%), Lhermitte's sign (10%–25%) and trigeminal neuralgia (2%–6%). Pain is generally caused by nerve and muscle damage and/or dysfunction. A systematic review of 38 studies that used magnetic resonance imaging (MRI) found that the location of demyelinating lesions was associated with neuropathic pain syndromes such as headache and facial pain (Seixas et al 2014). Patients may report a burning, aching, tightness in the chest and abdomen caused by muscle stiffness or spasms, known as the 'MS girdle' or 'MS hug'. Central neuropathic pain results from damage to myelinated nerves in the central nervous system causing ectopic impulses in damaged nociceptive fibres and a loss of pain modulation because of damage to descending inhibitory pathways. This may present as partial numbness, paraesthesia, sharp pain and electrical 'buzzing' and shocklike dysesthesia in the back and limbs by movement of the neck (i.e., Lhermitte's sign). Trigeminal neuralgia can occur as an initial symptom of MS. Musculoskeletal pain is common and usually secondary to problems with mobility, balance and posture from fatigue, muscle weakness and spasticity, causing stresses and strains on joints, ligaments or muscles.

Parkinson's

Pain is a major complaint in Parkinson's but often remains underdiagnosed and inadequately managed, although pain scales specific for Parkinson's are available (Skogar & Lokk 2016). Its onset may be very early in the condition and is reported to be the most bothersome symptom (Young Blood et al 2016). Musculoskeletal pain presenting in the neck, upper back and extremities is common and accounts for 40%–90% of reported pain. Musculoskeletal pain is associated with persistent tremor, muscle rigidity and dystonia with twisting, cramping or posturing of the painful body part. Musculoskeletal injuries caused by falls presenting as fractures, sprains and bruises are also common. Neuropathic pain appears to be less common. Central neuropathic pain may present in Parkinson's unprovoked and in unusual locations such as the face, mouth, genitalia, pelvis, anus or abdomen. Neuropathic pain associated with akathisia and inner restlessness may also present. Evidence suggests that dysfunction in dopaminergic centres regulating the autonomic functions and inhibitory modulation of pain inputs may be contributing to central neuropathic pain in Parkinson's. L-dopa may transiently alleviate pain, and individuals in the levodopa 'on' state report less pain than those in the 'off' state.

Huntington's Disease

Huntington's disease primarily affects the basal ganglia and the thalamus, and these structures are known to be involved in sensorimotor integration and pain processing. The mean prevalence of pain in Huntington's disease is estimated to be 41% (95% CI: 36%–46%), which is comparable with other neurodegenerative diseases, although pain interference with daily activities was lower than that observed in the general population (Sprenger et al 2019). A large worldwide cohort study found that the prevalence of pain interference increased up to 42% in the middle stage of Huntington's disease, whereas the prevalence of painful conditions and analgesic use decreased as Huntington's disease progresses (Sprenger et al 2021). Pain may be underreported and undertreated because patients with Huntington's disease have impairments in negative emotion recognition and empathy for pain (Baez et al 2015). Patients with Huntington's disease may experience pain from comorbidities such as diabetes and are at risk for painful diabetic neuropathy.

Amyotrophic Lateral Sclerosis: Motor Neurone Disease

Motor neurone disease is the most common neurodegenerative disorder of the motor system in adults with upper and lower motor neurones affected. Pain and sensory disturbance may not be a common feature in the initial phase, helping to distinguish motor neurone disease from radiculopathies. The prevalence of pain over the course of the disease is estimated to be 60% (95% CI: 50%–69%) and commonly located in the upper limbs and shoulders (Hurwitz et al 2021). Most patients have limb-onset disease manifesting as weakness in the hand (grip), shoulder, and ankle or hip with associated muscle cramps. As the disease becomes more advanced, limbs become weaker and spasticity develops. Musculoskeletal pain may result from mechanical stress on joints from muscle weakness, spasticity and muscle cramps. Neuropathic pain occurs in a small proportion of patients, and pain may also arise from constipation, oedema related to reduced activity, pressure sores caused by immobility and episodes of excessive yawning causing jaw pain.

Other Neurological Diseases

Rarer neurological diseases also affect the musculoskeletal system, causing spasticity, contractions and spasms. It is likely that pain is underestimated, or underdetected and undertreated. The prevalence of chronic pain in muscular dystrophies is estimated to be greater than 60%, with the lumbar spine, shoulders and legs the most frequent sites (Huang et al 2021). Spinal muscular atrophy is a neuromuscular, degenerative disease characterised by loss of alpha motor neurone function in the spinal cord resulting in progressive muscle weakness, atrophy and paralysis that is greater in the legs than in the arms, and eventually affecting respiration and swallowing dysphagia. Muscle weakness and limited mobility may lead to contractures and deformity of the spine with resultant pain. Spinocerebellar ataxia disorders are a group of neurodegenerative disorders characterised by ataxia and oculomotor disturbances, cognitive deficits and dysfunction of pyramidal and extrapyramidal systems. Reports on the frequency of pain vary from 19% to 64% of patients, although a systematic review found pain to be reported in only 1 of 30 patients with spinocerebellar ataxia (Rossi et al 2014).

Acute Neurological Conditions

Damage to the central nervous system occurs after a stroke or from traumatic injury with pain being common.

Stroke

Stroke damages specific structures of the brain. Paolucci et al (2016a) evaluated 443 stroke patients and estimated mean overall prevalence rate of pain to be 29.6%, with 14.1% reporting pain in the poststroke acute stage, 42.7% in the subacute stage and 31.9% in the chronic stage. Many different types of pain may present after a stroke, including musculoskeletal pain and central poststroke pain (central pain syndrome) on the affected side of the body. Musculoskeletal pain from spasticity with painful spasms on the affected (weaker) side of the body affects more than 30% of stroke patients. Shoulder pain is also common and may present as severe stiffness and pain on movement (i.e., capsulitis, 'frozen shoulder') because of damage and inflammation in the capsule, muscle and ligaments. Weakness in the muscles that hold the shoulder joint in place may lead to partial dislocation of the upper arm bone and shoulder blade (i.e., shoulder subluxation), which may also contribute to shoulder pain (i.e., poststroke complex regional pain syndrome). Stroke patients may experience a painfully swollen paralysed hand, which may develop as a result of oedema because of the lack of movement, especially if the hand is hanging downwards. Repositioning the hand and using oedema gloves may help.

Central poststroke neuropathic pain often presents as severe, spontaneous 'icy' burning pain or throbbing, shooting-like pain sometimes accompanied with paraesthesia and numbness contralateral to the site of the stroke. Mechanical and thermal allodynia may be present causing pain on movement or from a change in temperature. Prevalence at any location is 11% (95% CI: 7%–18%) and greater than 50% in subgroups of patients with medullary or thalamic strokes (Liampas et al 2020). At stroke onset, central poststroke neuropathic pain occurs in 26% (95% CI: 18%–35%) of patients, rising to 41% (95% CI: 33.9%–49.0%) in the first year.

Traumatic Brain Injuries

Chronic pain is a common consequence after TBI with the prevalence of chronic pain estimated to be 49.8%–53.2% (95% CI) and independent of posttraumatic stress disorder and depression (Nampiaparampil 2008). Prevalence of headache was 55.5%–60.2%, and the frequency of low-back pain was 46%, extremity pain 39% and complex regional pain syndrome 12%. Pain may be caused by injury to brain tissue, an indirect consequence of the injury such as deep venous thrombosis, or unrelated to the injury. Most pain involves the musculoskeletal system presenting as spasticity, muscle spasms, joint contractures, tendinitis and painful postural abnormalities, although neuropathic pain and autonomic symptoms may also be present. TBIs require early pain management by a multidisciplinary team and integrated into existing treatment strategies (Gironda et al 2009). Analgesic medication, rehabilitation and psychological techniques have been used with success to alleviate pain (Moshourab et al 2015).

Spinal Cord Injuries

SCI includes traumatic and nontraumatic aetiology and cauda equina lesions. The International Spinal Cord Injury

Pain classification system categorises nociceptive pain as musculoskeletal (e.g., spasm-related pain), visceral (e.g., constipation pain) or other (e.g., pressure sore pain), and neuropathic pain as SCI-related pain (e.g., cauda equina lesion), at-level SCI pain (e.g., spinal cord lesion) or below-level SCI pain (e.g., postthoracotomy pain) (Bryce et al 2012). Approximately half of patients experience musculoskeletal pain in acute and chronic phases with extremity and back pain related to ossification and muscle spasms and contractures present (Michailidou et al 2014). Between 40% and 50% of individuals experience neuropathic pain within the first year. The prevalence of chronic pain is estimated to be 68% (95% CI: 63%–73%), 58% (95% CI: 49%–68%) for neuropathic pain, 56% (95% CI: 41%–70%) for musculoskeletal pain and 20% (95% CI: 11%–29%) for visceral pain (Hunt et al 2021). Mechanisms contributing to SCI neuropathic pain are multiple and complex, with sensory loss and central neuropathic pain typically present below the level of the injury within weeks. Segmental pain associated with mechanical and/or thermal allodynia and hyperalgesia may also occur around the border between normal sensation and loss of sensation. Visceral pain is often related to constipation.

A systematic review of 19 studies provided evidence that multicomponent treatments targeting mood disturbance and fostering community connections were important in the management of pain associated with SCI (Tran et al 2016). Treatment of pain related to SCI is challenging because pain is often accompanied by alterations in autonomic, metabolic and biochemical processes (Saulino & Averna 2016). Management of musculoskeletal pain, neuropathic pain and visceral pain follows conventional approaches previously described and is aligned to National Institute of Health and Care Excellence (NICE) guidelines for SCI (NICE 2016). A systematic review of the effectiveness of 22 physiotherapy interventions concluded that four interventions were effective: fitness, hand and wheelchair training and transcutaneous electrical nerve stimulation (TENS) (Harvey et al 2016).

KEY POINTS

Pain presents as a subjective personal experience including sensory, emotional and cognitive dimensions that are influenced by social, environmental and spiritual factors. Clinically neuropathic pain is observed less commonly than musculoskeletal pain. People with neuropathic pain often experience poorer physical and mental health than people with other pains. Neuropathic pain arises from a variety of aetiologies. A comprehensive assessment of pain is necessary when exploring the pain in patients with progressive as well as acute neurological conditions.

DIAGNOSIS, ASSESSMENT AND PROGNOSIS

A wide range of healthcare professionals may be involved in diagnosis, assessment and rehabilitation for pain including occupational therapists, physical therapists, physicians, nurses and chiropractic, osteopathic and massage therapists. A holistic approach to the management of pain is necessary for optimal care. A comprehensive biopsychosocial assessment should be undertaken. This should include assessment of sensory, affective, cognitive, physiological and behavioural aspects of the pain and screening for the development of chronicity and/or factors that prevent progress of recovery from chronic pain, disability and poor quality of daily life. Curricula on pain for physical therapy include guidance on pain assessment (Slater et al 2017). The Italian Consensus Conference on Pain in Neurorehabilitation has defined criteria for assessing and treating pain associated with neurological conditions (Bartolo et al 2016, Paolucci et al 2016b). The primary focus of the consultation is to establish the pain problem, help patients understand what might be causing the pain and to assist in the relief of pain and improvement of physical and cognitive functioning. Pain diagnosis is far from an exact science, and labels given to pain conditions often cut across categories and may be of little value. For example, diagnosis based on location of pain (e.g., low-back pain, shoulder pain, knee pain) may be of limited use other than identifying where to target a treatment. Diagnosis based on probable cause informs clinical decision making going forwards, and the possibility of treating injuries or disease. The assessment of an episode of pain needs to establish the following:

- Is there a sinister pathology (red flags)? Does this require specialist referral?
- Is there a clearly identifiable medical, neurological or surgical cause of pain that can be treated? Does this require specialist referral?
- Are there factors that prevent progress of recovery from chronic pain, disability and quality of life (yellow flags)? Does this require specialist referral?
- Are there biopsychosocial drivers of pain to inform an appropriate rehabilitation treatment algorithm?

Subjective Assessment

Subjective assessment, the self-report of pain, is an accepted standard rather than a gold standard, and objective measures of physical performance and physiological/autonomic responses may be useful. The consultation should include a discussion about pain in relation to the presenting condition, history of the presenting condition, past medical history, treatment history and social history. The description of pain may provide a 'rough' indication to structures that may drive pain, although this is by no means

TABLE 23.2 Potential Damaged Tissues and Pain Description

Potential Tissues Involved	Description of Pain
Cutaneous, superficial tissue	Well-defined localised
Deeper tissue (such as bone, muscle, ligament, tendon, fasciae, blood vessels)	Less well-defined pain
Muscle involvement	Dull, aching (poorly localised, may worsen on activity)
Vascular involvement	Throbbing, aching, diffuse
Connective tissue involvement	Localised and affected more by movement
Bone involvement	Dull, deep and nagging (localised and diffuse)
Neural involvement	Sharp, shooting, burning, freezing, pins and needles, tingling, numbing
Autonomic neural involvement	Burning, freezing, pressure-like, stinging, pallor, heat intolerance, hypohidrosis
Visceral	Sickening, squeezing, tightness, bloating
	Diffuse, difficult to locate, referred to superficial structures

TABLE 23.3 Red and Yellow Flags

Red Flags	Yellow Flags
• Thoracic pain • Fever/unexplained weight loss • Bladder or bowel dysfunction • History of carcinoma • Ill health or presence of other medical illness • Progressive neurological deficit • Disturbed gait, saddle anaesthesia • Age of onset <20 years or >55 years	• Negative attitude that pain is harmful or potentially severely disabling • Fear avoidance behaviour/reduced activity levels • Expectation that passive, rather than active, treatment will be beneficial • Tendency to depression, low morale and social withdrawal • Social or financial problems

Red flags for serious pathology and yellow flags for psychosocial factors that cloud assessment and treatment and negatively affect outcome (Samanta et al 2003).

Red and Yellow Flags

A careful history of the present condition is necessary, including medical history, family history and social history to help screening for red flags. Red flags were originally developed as an aid to think about sinister pathology in acute low back such as cancer, infection or fracture and are used in conjunction with other information to refer patients for further investigation (Table 23.3).

Factors That Influence the Reliability of Subjective Pain Report

A person's mental map of themselves and their world is often conveyed in the stories the patient tells (narratives) about their pain experience. An individual's underlying thinking, reflected in the language that the patient uses, affects their final experience of pain. Individuals rarely communicate their experiences as they actually happened, but tend to generalise, delete and distort the information through cognitive biases, and this can influence a person's sense of self. Sometimes thoughts, attitudes and behaviours can prevent individuals from achieving their desired goals in a process of 'self-sabotage' (Johnson & Hudson 2016). If a practitioner understands an individual's experience and the context within which it is situated, the patient is more likely to establish what pain means to that individual.

an exact science (Table 23.2). The evaluation should document pain severity and its effect on daily activities (sleep, fatigue, mobility), possible cause of pain, whether the condition has deteriorated or improved, what exacerbates and relieves pain, physical or psychological problems and concurrent medications. A variety of clinical tools are available to assist the assessment and documentation of an individual's description of pain severity or intensity (i.e., visual analogue scales, numerical rating scales and categorical scales), pain quality (i.e., McGill Pain Questionnaire), pain distribution (site, depth and expanse; i.e., Body Chart), pain impact (i.e., Brief Pain Inventory, Short-Form health survey [SF-36]), pain beliefs (i.e., pain catastrophising scale, fear-avoidance beliefs, survey of pain attitudes) and pain coping (i.e., pain-coping strategies questionnaire, pain self-efficacy questionnaire). The selection of which tools are appropriate to use varies between clinics and practitioners.

Objective Assessment

Objective information can be gathered through systematic investigation of the patient's symptoms.

Observation and palpation are used to identify gross trauma and anatomical anomalies that may be contributing to symptoms. Observation of standing, walking, sitting, fidgeting and repositioning may provide insights into the bothersomeness and effect of pain on activities of daily living. Palpation of anatomical landmarks is used to detect the anatomical abnormalities, range of motion and quality of movement, and may be used to assess structures contributing to movement and pressure-evoked pain. Likewise, passive and active movements that increase or reduce pain provide useful information about potential contributing factors and can aid rehabilitation strategies and advice about how to improve activities of daily living including exercise.

Clinical tests may be crucial for assessing the presence of sinister pathology. Confirmatory tests may include blood tests for inflammatory biomarkers (e.g., rheumatoid arthritis), X-ray scans and computerised tomography scans for bone fractures, ultrasonography for muscular or tendon damage and MRI for soft tissue damage including nerve compression or infiltration. Nerve conduction tests and somatosensory-evoked potentials and biopsies can be used to evaluate large- and small-fibre neuropathies. The rationale for undertaking clinical tests should be carefully considered because it may be costly, harmful to the patient and produce irrelevant information. Thus practitioners are discouraged from routinely referring patients for diagnostic imaging unless the result is likely to change management.

> ### KEY POINTS
> A comprehensive biopsychosocial assessment of pain should be undertaken to establish the pain problem. The assessment should include screening for factors that worsen the functional activity, quality of life and social participation to assist in the relief of pain and improvement of physical and cognitive functioning. Pain diagnosis based on probable causes informs clinical decision making for the possibility of treating injuries or disease. However, the pathophysiology of pain is often multifactorial.

PRINCIPLES OF PAIN MANAGEMENT

Early pain management is critical to reduce the likelihood of acute pain becoming chronic. Undertreating pain for fear of masking important pathological symptoms or incurring side effects is dangerous because pain has harmful physiological effects, including increased blood pressure, changes in blood gases, delayed gastric emptying, urinary retention and increased secretion of cortisol. Referral to a specialist pain service for comprehensive assessment and multimodal management may be appropriate if the case is overly complex and/or there has been deterioration in the patient's underlying health condition.

Effective pain management strategies take a patient-centred, biopsychosocial approach tailored to the individual to relieve pain and improve physiological functioning associated with activities of daily living, role functioning associated with jobs and hobbies, and emotional, cognitive and social functioning to improve quality of life. As a general rule, the focus shifts from a biopsychosocial approach to manage acute pain to a social-psycho-bio approach to manage chronic pain (Fig. 23.2). The concerns and expectations of the patient should be at the core of a pain treatment plan with a clear explanation why a particular treatment is offered, possible adverse effects and coping strategies for pain.

Open and consistent communication between the multidisciplinary team and patient will build trust and is critical for patients embarking on a rehabilitation programme. Optimal strategies include practitioners working with the patient to cocreate an explanatory model for pain and to codesign a personalised treatment and care plan. Empowerment of patients and caregivers to self-manage pain is the cornerstone of effective treatment. Document the patient's expectations about pain prognosis and treatment outcome, and engage in a dialogue about factors that may hinder treatment success such as treatments that interfere with daily functions. Perform regular reviews to evaluate and monitor treatment outcome and support the patient becoming competent in self-management of their pain.

Pharmacological Management of Pain

A working knowledge of the principles of prescribing and likely adverse events related to the different classes of drugs used in pain management is pivotal in managing and advising any pain patient, even if the therapist is not a prescriber (Table 23.4). Patients may have been prescribed pharmacological treatment before they arrive at clinic and will seek advice from their therapist. Educating the patient about their pain often involves discussions about the benefits and possible adverse effects of the drugs, and the importance of dose titration and adherence to the regime.

Medication may act to resolve the damage or disease causing the pain or interact with the nociceptive system to relieve the experience of pain (i.e., analgesic medication). Analgesic and adjuvant medication remains mainstay treatment for acute and chronic pain and is particularly

• Acute Pain = Bio Psycho Social

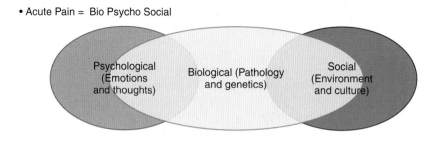

• Chronic Pain [Syndrome] = Social Psycho Bio

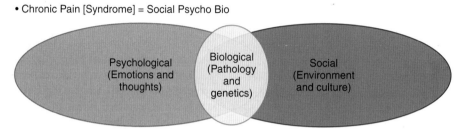

FIG. 23.2 Shifting emphasis in the biopsychosocial model of acute and chronic pain. Biological components often drive acute pain, and a biomedical approach to treat the cause of the pain (e.g., the injury or disease) is often appropriate with medication as first-line treatment and nonpharmacological treatments as adjuncts. However, treatment must also focus on psychosocial factors that may hinder recovery because inadequate management of individuals with acute pain is a risk factor for the development of chronic pain. It is critical that patients are provided with pain education, empowerment to self-manage their pain and early access to care to prevent acute pain becoming chronic. Psychosocial components often dominate persistent pain, so a psychosocial approach to rehabilitation and pain management is likely to be more successful. Involvement of multidisciplinary teams is critical.

useful for pain of recent onset, including acute exacerbations. Pain adjuvants are drugs whose primary use was not originally pain, but they may be helpful for pain management in certain circumstances. Analgesic and adjuvant medications are associated with side effects, tolerance and dependence, and should be given for short periods because patients may become habitually dependent on drugs. Drug choice depends on diagnosis, practice guidelines and care pathways recommended by professional bodies such as the NICE.

For nonneuropathic pain, analgesic medication is usually prescribed using a stepwise approach often guided by the WHO analgesic ladder, which was initially developed for cancer pain but is now used for noncancer pain as well (Leung 2012). The principles of prescribing using the WHO analgesic ladder are to start with mild analgesics and increase dose or switch to more powerful analgesics if pain is not adequately managed. Paracetamol or nonsteroidal antiinflammatory drugs such as diclofenac and ibuprofen

are indicated for mild to moderate pain; weak opioid drugs, including codeine, hydrocodone and tramadol, are indicated for moderate pain; and strong opioids, including morphine, oxycodone and hydromorphone, are used for moderate to severe pain. Muscle relaxants are for spasticity and muscle spasms, and steroid injections are used for inflamed areas such as the shoulder.

Open-ended, indiscriminate long-term prescribing of opioids has resulted in opioid abuse and death, leading to concern about the use of opioids. Opioids are indicated to relieve short-lived intensely painful events and at the end of life. For acute pain, opioids may be less effective than medicines with other different mechanisms of action, so opioids are often used in combination with paracetamol, nonsteroidal antiinflammatory drugs and local anaesthetics; they should not be used beyond the expected period of tissue healing, and a clear strategy for tapering opioid dose should be in place. For end-of-life-care, especially for cancer pain, optimal treatment is opioids combined

TABLE 23.4 Main Analgesic Agents and Pain Adjuvants

Drug Class	Examples	Indications
Analgesic Medication		
Simple, nonopioid nonsteroidal antiinflammatory drugs	Diclofenac, ibuprofen	Mild to moderate pain including musculoskeletal conditions
Simple, nonopioid analgesics	Paracetamol	Mild to moderate pain including musculoskeletal conditions
Opioid	Codeine, hydrocodone, morphine, oxycodone, hydromorphone, buprenorphine, tramadol[a]	Moderate to severe pain, particularly of visceral origin
Compound medications (simple nonopioid analgesic with an opioid)	Co-codamol (codeine/paracetamol), co-codaprin (codeine/aspirin), co-dydramol (dihydrocodeine/paracetamol)	Moderate pain
Corticosteroids	Local – dexamethasone, hydrocortisone acetate Systemic – prednisolone	Inflammatory pain (rheumatoid arthritis or compression neuropathy)[b]
Local anaesthetics	Lignocaine, bupivacaine, lidocaine	Local pain[b]
Pain Adjuvant Medication		
Muscle relaxants	Baclofen, cyclobenzaprine, botulinum toxin (Botox), diazepam (also anxiolytic)	Musculoskeletal pain, spasticity
Antidepressants	Tricyclic antidepressants (amitriptyline, nortriptyline) Serotonin and/or norepinephrine reuptake inhibitors (venlafaxine, duloxetine)	Neuropathic pain, migraine, fibromyalgia, rheumatoid arthritis
Antiepileptics	Gabapentin, pregabalin, carbamazepine	Neuropathic pain
Capsaicin	Zacin (topical cream), Axsain (topical cream), Qutenza (patch)	Neuropathic pain, osteoarthritis
Cannabinoids	Nabilone	Neuropathic pain, fibromyalgia, multiple sclerosis
Ketamine (anaesthetic)	Ketalar	Neuropathic pain, postoperative pain, cancer pain
Antianxiety and sedatives	Zopiclone, lorazepam, temazepam	Pain-related anxiety and sleep disturbance

[a]Acts as a weak opioid receptor agonist and a serotonin-noradrenaline reuptake inhibitor.
[b]As for interventional procedure – joint injection, spinal injection, sympathetic block, myofascial block.

with other drug and nondrug treatments because of variability in the benefit–harm profile between patients. There should be caution when considering opioids for long-term pain because of the development of tolerance, dependence and neuroadaptations that reduce efficacy and safety, so patients must be carefully selected and monitored.

For neuropathic pain, prescribers follow NICE guidelines that recommend amitriptyline, duloxetine, gabapentin or pregabalin as initial treatment. Capsaicin cream may be recommended for people with localised neuropathic pain who cannot tolerate oral treatments. Combination therapy using smaller doses of individual drugs combined with other drugs is commonly prescribed for neuropathic pain to reduce tolerability.

Routes of administration are predominantly oral (systemic), although transdermal (topical cream, transdermal patch), sublingual and various methods of injection or infusion including intradermal, subcutaneous, intramuscular, intravenous, intraarticular, intraperitoneal, intrathecal and epidural are used in certain circumstances. Injections and infiltration of drugs (e.g., anaesthetic or antiinflammatory medications) in or around the painful sites are used when patients cannot tolerate systemic medication or oral routes of administration cannot be tolerated.

Surgical Management of Pain

Surgery may be used to treat the cause of pain. For example, surgery may be used to lengthen tendons as a last resort for severe contractures or to remove structures that are compressing nerves and contributing to neuropathic pain. Examples of surgical techniques include lumbar microdiscectomy for a herniated lumbar disc or microvascular decompression for trigeminal neuralgia. Stereotactic radiosurgery is not surgery in the true sense because it is a noninvasive lesion technique. Stereotactic radiosurgery delivers a high dose of radiation precisely to a target area to manage brain tumours, blood vessel problems, neurological problems (e.g., Parkinson's) and neuropathic pain such as trigeminal neuralgia. Surgery may provide an immediate reduction in pain but at the expense of surgical morbidity and procedural risk, which is generally low but can be serious. Complications associated with neurolesion techniques include interference with somatosensory, motor and autonomic functioning.

Invasive neuromodulation techniques using surgically implanted devices may be used to manage symptoms of intractable pain and include implantable drug delivery systems and invasive electrical stimulation techniques. Implantable drug delivery systems involve subcutaneous implantation of a pump filled with drug(s) that is connected to a catheter that administers the drug(s) into the cerebrospinal fluid (i.e., intrathecal). Opioids coadministered with other drugs that act synergistically and reduce opiate side effects are often used for intrathecal drug delivery for chronic pain. Catheter complications include catheter obstruction, dislodgement and migration, and side effects associated with medication.

Rehabilitation

Strategies and interventions to enable and support recovery or adjustment to live as full and active lives as possible requires open and consistent communication between the multidisciplinary team and the patient, family and carers. Building trust is necessary before the patient undertakes any treatment or rehabilitation programme. When handling the patient, the therapist should facilitate them rather than support using limited 'hands-on'.

Physical Activity and Exercise

Graded physical activity, exercise and movement is the foundation of pain management. Guidelines for the use of exercise prescription for the management of neuropathic and musculoskeletal pain in, for instance, Parkinson's, are available (Allen et al 2015). Physical activity and exercise relieve chronic musculoskeletal pain and especially osteoarthritis (Juhl et al 2014, Tanaka et al 2013, Uthman et al 2013) and neck, shoulder and back pain (Gomes-Neto et al

2017, Saragiotto et al 2016). There are fewer systematic reviews on chronic neuropathic pain, although evidence supports the use of exercise for peripheral neuropathy (Davies et al 2015, Streckmann et al 2014). The main barriers to the use of physical activity and exercise to manage pain associated with neurological conditions are functional disability, tiredness and fatigue. For individuals with MS, the main barriers were being too tired, functional impairment and a lack of time (Asano et al 2013). In addition, the physical condition of the individual and the presence of movement-evoked pain needs to be considered to determine an appropriate type, intensity and dosage of exercises.

Manual Therapy

Techniques that are used to reduce spasticity and muscle spasms are likely to alleviate musculoskeletal pain. Physiotherapy rehabilitation using manual therapy techniques is beneficial for the management of MS (Campbell et al 2016), Parkinson's (Yitayeh & Teshome 2016), Alzheimer's disease (Zhu et al 2015), motor neurone disease (Morris et al 2006), cerebral palsy (Franki et al 2012), stroke (Pollock et al 2014), TBI (Bland et al 2011) and SCI (Harvey et al 2016).

Soft tissue therapy involves assessment, evaluation and treatment of soft tissues including ligaments, muscles, tendons and fascia to manage pain and neuromusculoskeletal dysfunction. A range of practitioners are licensed to administer soft tissue therapy including physiotherapists and massage therapists who assess posture, range of motion and biomechanics to aid selection of manual therapy techniques to facilitate flexibility and mobility. Soft tissue mobilisation, joint mobilisation and nerve mobilisation techniques are commonly used to manage pain associated with neurological conditions. Soft tissue techniques use rhythmic stretching and the application of firm, direct pressure to tissue to stretch tight fascial structures and reduce muscle tension. Soft tissue mobilisation is used to relax muscles, break down myofascial adhesions such as scar tissue and move tissue fluids.

Myofascial techniques promote flexibility and mobility of connective tissue by targeting muscle and fascial tissue and mobilising fibrous adhesions. Trigger point techniques are used to 'deactivate' or 'release' the taut band of muscle to reduce the hyperirritability of the trigger point.

Massage includes a range of techniques, with Swedish massage being the most commonly used and consisting of effleurage (sliding or gliding), petrissage (kneading), tapotement (rhythmic tapping), friction (cross fibre or with the fibres) and vibration/shaking. Massage of the hands and feet can be particularly useful to reduce stress and relax patients and can be administered by caregivers. Systematic reviews suggest that massage may reduce pain and associated symptoms, and that patients with neurological conditions like it for MS (Salarvand et al 2021), movement disorders (Angelopoulou et al 2020), dementia (Margenfeld et al 2019) and stroke (Cabanas-Valdés 2021), although evidence is inconclusive for motor neurone disease (Blatzheim 2009), cerebral palsy (Guchan Topu & Tomac 2020) and SCI (Fattal et al 2009).

Mobilisation of joints is used to improve range of motion and pain relief by slow velocity (i.e., speed) and increasing amplitude (i.e., distance of movement) movement of the joint using high-velocity, low-amplitude thrusting and muscle energy techniques. Nerve mobilisation involves movement of neural tissues and their surrounding tissues by gentle stretching (i.e., neural stretching) to relieve nerve-related chronic musculoskeletal pain. A systematic review found neural mobilisation to be superior to minimal intervention to alleviate pain and reduce disability associated with nerve-related chronic musculoskeletal pain, although there was insufficient evidence to judge whether neural mobilisation was superior to other interventions (Su & Lim 2016).

Splinting, Casting and Bracing

Splinting, casting, and bracing are used to immobilise and stabilise structures such as joints, and to reduce workload and hold a structure in place to prevent further injury of soft tissue. Splinting, casting and bracing may also help stretch muscles that are limiting range of motion and are sometimes used to prevent contractures from forming by preventing an abnormal position, although this may be uncomfortable to the patient. Orthotics may be used to limit mobility, to promote the underworking loading and to increase realignment of posture. A systematic review of 21 studies of people with neuromuscular disease and central nervous system conditions including poststroke and SCI found only limited evidence on the effectiveness of orthotics for knee stability for pain, falls and trips (Su & Lim 2016).

Electrophysical Techniques

A variety of electrophysical techniques are recommended in physiotherapy guidelines to relieve pain and to promote recovery of injury or function as a standalone treatment or combined with other techniques, including physical activity and exercises (stretching or strengthening), manual therapies (massage or mobilisation) or splinting or bracing. Electrophysical agents introduce thermal (thermotherapy, cryotherapy), mechanical (ultrasound, acupuncture) or electromagnetic (electricity, light, low-level laser) energy into the body. A detailed critique of electrophysical agents can be found in the book *Electrophysical Agents: Evidence-Based Practice* (Watson & Nasbaum 2020).

Electrotherapy

Invasive Electrical Techniques. Invasive electrical techniques include percutaneous electrical nerve stimulation, spinal cord stimulation, deep brain stimulation and motor cortex stimulation. Percutaneous electrical nerve stimulation is the least invasive of the techniques and delivers mild currents to nerves by inserting needles underneath the skin. NICE (2013) recommends use of percutaneous electrical nerve stimulation for refractory neuropathic pain. Spinal cord stimulation involves implantation of electrodes into the epidural space to target the dorsal columns and is recommended by NICE to manage adults with pain of neuropathic origin who continue to experience severe chronic pain for at least 6 months and who are resistant to medical management including complex regional pain syndrome and pain associated with peripheral vascular disease (NICE 2008, Simpson et al 2009). Deep brain stimulation involves implantation of electrodes into the thalamus, periaqueductal/periventricular grey or cingulate gyrus, and is often used to manage severely intractably central poststroke pain and facial pains. Motor cortex stimulation involves implantation of electrodes into the motor cortex to manage central poststroke pain and also for refractory facial pain. Shortwave, microwave, and therapeutic ultrasound diathermy are contraindicated when a patient has an implanted electrical stimulator because of the risk for heat-induced neurological damage at electrode contact points. Likewise, MRI has the potential to interfere with electrodes, resulting in heating to surrounding tissue damage.

Noninvasive Electrical Brain Stimulation Techniques. Noninvasive electrical stimulation of the brain includes repetitive transcranial magnetic stimulation and transcranial direct current stimulation, and these techniques are increasingly being used for the management of chronic pain because they are safe and easy to administer. When used to relieve pain, noninvasive electrical brain stimulation is usually applied to the primary motor cortex or dorsolateral prefrontal cortex. The European Federation of Neurological Societies guidelines on neurostimulation for neuropathic pain concluded that there was weak evidence to support the use of repetitive transcranial magnetic stimulation or transcranial direct current stimulation for neuropathic pain and fibromyalgia, and inconclusive evidence for SCI pain (Cruccu et al 2016).

The European Chapter of the International Federation of Clinical Neurophysiology has developed evidence-based guidelines on the use of transcranial direct current stimulation after an evaluation of research that found that there was possible efficacy for anodal transcranial direct current stimulation of the contralateral primary motor cortex for chronic lower limb neuropathic pain secondary to spinal cord lesion (Lefaucheur et al 2016). A systematic review of five studies provided evidence that transcranial direct current stimulation reduced neuropathic pain associated with SCI (Mehta et al 2015).

Transcutaneous Electrical Nerve Stimulation. The purpose of TENS is to stimulate peripheral nerves using pulsed electrical currents generated by a portable battery-powered device and delivered across the intact surface of the skin via self-adhering electrodes for symptomatic relief of pain. TENS is available without prescription and is inexpensive and safe compared with medication and can be self-administered by the patient following instruction from a healthcare practitioner. Contraindications include patients who also have implantable devices, and precautions include pregnancy, epilepsy and active malignancy (Houghton et al 2010). A large systematic review and meta-analysis found moderate-certainty evidence that TENS relieves pain, suggesting that TENS is a useful adjunct to core treatment (Johnson et al 2022).

Acupuncture. Acupuncture involves inserting fine needles at selected points in the body to stimulate underlying nerve and muscle tissue to inhibit nociceptive input and influence autonomic nervous system activity. More powerful acupuncture stimulation may be achieved by 'twirling' inserted needles or by passing mild currents through pairs of needles using a portable electrical stimulator (i.e., electroacupuncture). An appraisal of acupuncture for neurological conditions by Grant (2016) suggests that acupuncture is beneficial for musculoskeletal pain, including spasticity, but is less effective for neuropathic pain. Systematic reviews provide tentative evidence that acupuncture is efficacious for MS (Campbell et al 2016, Khodaie et al 2022), Parkinson's (Lee & Lim 2017), Alzheimer's disease (Huang et al 2019, Zhou et al 2015) and SCI (He et al 2022, Ma et al 2015).

Therapeutic Ultrasound. In neurological diseases, therapeutic ultrasound can be used to induce focused lesions, clear protein aggregates, facilitate drug uptake and modulate neuronal function, and these effects may indirectly reduce pain (Leinenga et al 2016). There is a lack of studies evaluating the efficacy of therapeutic ultrasound on pain associated with neurological conditions. Sánchez et al (2017) evaluated the effect of therapeutic ultrasound on nodules in MS and found that reductions in pain and redness associated with nodules in MS were greater when therapeutic ultrasound was added to conventional gel prescribed for cellulite and nodules. Evidence on the efficacy of therapeutic ultrasound to manage musculoskeletal pain is inconsistent.

Thermal Therapies. Warmth therapies (thermotherapy) and cold therapies (cryotherapy) are used to produce comfort, relaxation and analgesia. Thermal therapies may be delivered 'moist' as immersion in a bath or a damp towel, or 'dry' using wraps or electric pads. Heat dilates blood vessels, improving perfusion and delivery of oxygen and nutrients to target tissue, and can aid stretching of muscle and connective tissue which may reduce spasticity and increase flexibility. In contrast, cold therapy constricts blood vessels, reducing perfusion and delivery of inflammatory mediators to target tissue. Ice massage may be used to create numbness in a painful area of injury without burning the skin. Often alternating heat with cold therapy is most beneficial. Precautions should be taken to prevent hot or cold burning of the skin. There is a lack of good-quality research on the effectiveness of simple thermal therapies on pain outcomes, and especially their use in pain associated with neurological conditions.

Low-Level Laser Therapy. Treatment using irradiation with light amplification by stimulated emission of radiation (LASER) of low-output power intensity, when the effects are not caused by heat, is termed low-level laser therapy. The outcome of low-level laser therapy is dose dependent. In general, laser treatment is administered daily for acute conditions and less frequently (e.g., a few times a week) for chronic inflammatory conditions. To date, few studies have investigated the effect of low-level laser therapy on pain associated with neurological conditions, although studies using animal models have found that low-level laser therapy may reduce disease progression in MS (Goncalves et al 2016) and Alzheimer's disease (Lu et al 2016). A meta-analysis of four human studies concluded that there was weak evidence that low-level laser therapy reduced neuropathic pain (de Andrade et al 2016).

Visual Feedback, Motor Imagery and Body Illusions. Over the previous decade, interest has arisen in the use of visual feedback, motor imagery and body illusions to reduce pain, improve function and normalise sensations of dysmorphic body parts, where individuals cannot easily locate their body parts in space (Boesch et al 2016, Moseley et al 2008, Wittkopf & Johnson 2016). Mirror visual feedback is used in rehabilitation settings to manage pain and dysfunction associated with cortical and subcortical reorganisation, especially when body image has been affected, such as limbs being perceived as large, swollen, heavy or stuck in one position (e.g., posttrauma, complex regional pain syndrome and phantom limb pain) or small and withered (e.g., osteoarthritic hands) (Gilpin et al 2015, Moseley 2007, O'Connell et al 2013).

Motor imagery techniques have been used in a variety of neurological conditions including neurodegenerative disease, stroke and SCI, and involve mentally rehearsing movements of affected body parts without actually moving, such as imagining picking up and drinking a cup of water. The process involves visualising the movement in the mind's eye (visual motor imagery) and imagining the feeling of the movement (kinaesthetic motor imagery) (Dickstein & Deutsch 2007). Evidence from systematic reviews for alleviation of chronic pain (Bowering et al 2013) and limb pain (Harris & Hebert 2015, Thieme et al 2016) by mental imagery is promising but not conclusive.

Psychological Approaches

Often people with chronic pain struggle to manage their mental health, which in turn affects their 'physical' pain. Chronic pain is known to affect a person's identity and narrative of themselves.

Patients should be empowered with strategies to promote healthier lifestyles and reduce fear and anxiety about the consequences of their pain. Increasing confidence by reducing fear and anxiety, reducing dramatisation (catastrophising) of pain and creating new social contexts reduce pain and improve quality of life.

Various psychological approaches are used alongside other treatments to alter an individual's beliefs, attitudes and behaviours about their pain and to provide individuals with effective coping strategies, including taking an active role in self-management of their pain. Psychological approaches include cognitive behavioural therapy (CBT) that includes reconceptualisation of pain as a problem to solve and coping skills training; behavioural interventions that include altering pain-relevant communication and behavioural activation via contingency management; and self-regulatory treatments such as biofeedback, hypnosis and relaxation training such as mindfulness (Simpson et al 2014), progressive muscle relaxation and autogenic training. Recently, attention has focused on the use of resilience-based positive activity interventions (Hassett & Finan 2016, Sturgeon & Zautra 2016).

A patient-centred approach is used in all cases to modify maladaptive cognitions and behaviours so that the experience of living with pain is improved (Dixon et al 2007, Hoffman et al 2007, Pike et al 2016). CBT techniques delivered over a series of sessions are the foundation of most practice and aim to develop adaptive cognitive and behavioural pain coping skills, including restructuring of maladaptive cognitions, appropriate goal setting, stress management through relaxation, breathing and visual imagery, sleep hygiene, activity pacing to prevent relapse and effective use of social reinforcement. Barriers to success include limited availability of psychological therapies in service provision because of prohibitive costs.

A report following the Italian Consensus Conference on Pain in Neurorehabilitation concluded that psychological treatments are proven to be the most valuable component of a multidisciplinary approach to manage pain associated with neurological conditions, but there was still a need to determine which psychological therapies should be matched with specific pathologies for neurorehabilitation teams (Castelnuovo et al 2016). They provided a summary table of evidence and recommendations for the use of psychological therapies in neurological conditions.

Self-Management

Self-management is a patient-centred intervention that provides individuals with knowledge and skill to improve behaviours required for day-to-day management of chronic conditions (i.e., pain) by promoting self-efficiency to take action dealing with their pain to enhance quality of life. It is currently believed to expand the effects from physical or biomedical treatments with cost-effectiveness (Boyers et al 2013). In the literature, 'self-management' means that the patient is an active participant in a treatment (Lorig & Holman 2003).

Types of psychological interventions often used in the self-management of chronic pain include the Stanford model, used to deal with physical, emotional and social consequences of pain; acceptance and commitment therapy, used to change the fear-of-pain behaviours to meaningful activities; and CBT, used to develop a preexisting intervention of self-management (Mann et al 2013). The therapy originally proceeds through a series of stages that emphasise reconceptualisation of pain as manageable by self-control, which is followed by skills acquisition and practice that promote behavioural change and maintenance of the change. The therapy is currently modified for helping patients to identify the relationships between their thoughts and emotions, and aims to restructure pain-avoidance beliefs and behaviours to change daily lifestyle by self-regulatory skills on a biopsychosocial model.

Current evidence suggests that patients with TBI favour the delivery of self-management via the internet (Jones et al 2016). In people with peripheral nerve injury, a questionnaire has been developed to reflect key reported outcomes for neuropathic pain treatment, and its baseline and follow-up versions could assess the change in self-management over time (Wiklund et al 2013). Two SCI studies (n = 99) reported that the important components in self-management were exercise (54%), nutrition (52%) and pain management (44%) (Munce et al 2014), and perceived importance and self-efficacy influenced the motivation (Molton et al 2008). Future research is urged to develop self-management which could be modified over time as the participant's needs changed.

An MS study reported that perceived importance and self-efficacy beliefs on behaviours of change were mediated or partially mediated by readiness to engage in those behaviours (Kratz et al 2011). Recently, a pamphlet-based intervention (n = 30) of physical activity was found to improve stages of change placement and social support (Plow et al 2014). This study also found pain as one of the common barriers to engage in a physical activity programme, whereas pamphlets, phone calls and action planning were motivators. However, a self-management intervention (n = 84) with self-monitoring using electronic personal health records did not augment MS centre-based care compared with usual care (n = 83) (Miller et al 2011). A tailored programme with web-based delivery and therapist telephone support may be optimal (Harrison et al 2017). A recent study found that a combined CBT and acceptance and commitment therapy programme in self-management for MS pain improved the severity and the impact of pain (Harrison et al 2017). However, the reduction was not observed in those with more complex comorbidities.

KEY POINTS

The principles of pain management are to make long-standing pain tolerable to improve physical, role, emotional, cognitive and social functionality. A biopsychosocial model of care is adopted where pain is considered an illness rather than a disease. Multiprofessional involvement in treating pain associated with neurological conditions combines a progressive approach to pharmacological treatment as part of neurorehabilitation. Surgery may be necessary to treat underlying pathology and offered through specialist services. Electrophysical and psychological therapies may be offered through a rehabilitation service as standalone treatment or as adjuncts to medication. Electrophysical and psychological therapies are generally safer than medication and can be used to reduce medication and concurrent side effects. The principles of pain management are the same irrespective of whether the pain is of primary or secondary origin, although consideration needs to be given to potential interactions between treatments for the primary condition and secondary symptoms.

PAIN TREATMENT SELECTION, GOAL SETTING AND OUTCOME MONITORING

Initiating Treatment

There are no robust indicators to predict whether a new patient will respond for most pain treatments, so patients need to be followed up carefully. An individual is not suitable for a specific treatment if the treatment is contraindicated, the patient refuses to use the treatment, does not

understand the principles of the treatment and, if appropriate, is unable to self-administer unless a caregiver takes on the responsibility to do so. A serious adverse event and/or worsening pain may prompt treatment withdrawal. A careful assessment of reported lack of treatment response should be undertaken before deciding treatment failure. Patients should be screened for suitability of self-administered treatments and time taken to familiarise the patient with the treatment, explain how the treatment should be administered and, importantly, to evaluate competence to self-administer and, if possible, initial response in the clinic. Expert patients can be valuable to support new patients. Set treatment goals as measurable functional outcomes that can monitor progress and can be verified with quantifiable changes in behaviour and quality of life.

Setting Treatment Goals

It is important to negotiate the objectives of treatment and to manage the patient's expectation of outcome, especially if the patient needs to commit to self-administering treatment regularly. A written treatment agreement with the patient reduces misunderstanding and includes the patient in collaborative decision making and treatment delivery, reinforcing an internal focus of control and engagement in treatment outcome. It may act as a motivational reminder to the patient about the treatment regime. Reducing pain by 20% may be significant with respect to regaining function, but primary outcomes should not be framed as reductions in pain sensation or 'feeling better' because pain severity is amorphous and like trying to hit a moving target. Achieving zero pain is usually unrealistic unless there are strong reasons to believe that pain pathology will completely resolve. Treatment outcome should be framed as SMART (specific, measurable, achievable, realistic and time-bound) functional goals that can monitor progress and can be verified with quantifiable changes in behaviour and quality of life. Patients should have a strong sense of ownership of treatment objectives through honest, transparent, realistic dialogue. A verification protocol may be useful to monitor progress of treatment objectives and shows the patient the seriousness of agreement of functional goals. Evidence of achievement of goals can be communicated to friends and family using social media to sustain motivation to self-manage the painful condition (Fishman 2012).

Evaluating Response to Treatment

Nonresponse of a treatment to relieve pain during an initial consultation should not be taken as treatment failure because time may be required to optimise outcome. Likewise, success of a treatment during the initial consultation should not be taken as long-term treatment success because optimism can fuel positive expectation which declines over time. Undertake a careful assessment of what a patient means if the patient claims that they are not responding to a treatment and compare this with their expectation of what a satisfactory treatment response would consist of. Establish whether the patient has previously experienced a beneficial response. Disentangle pain severity and pain bothersomeness. Temporarily withdrawing treatments may help a patient to evaluate the situation. Initial enthusiasm for a new treatment often wanes, so you may need to revisit patient expectation of outcome. If the patient is genuinely experiencing no physiological, psychological or social benefit, then a different treatment approach may be necessary.

Research to determine the efficacy of rehabilitation programmes for managing pain in neurological conditions is challenging because of the variety of treatments and techniques used. An assessment of the status of tissues including musculoskeletal, nerve and blood supply is necessary to evaluate potential hazards associated with using a particular technique that may lead to an increased risk for complications. In general, spasticity is managed either by a therapist or caregiver by regular (daily) passive stretching and movement of joints to reduce risk for contractures. Advice, education and training about correct positioning of limbs and how to undertake movements of daily activities without causing strain on joints is crucial to protect affected tissues. Evidence for the value of foam supports, pillows, arm slings and cuffs or straps is equivocal.

Strategies to Improve Treatment Effect

Empowering patients to self-manage pain is critical for individuals with chronic pain because regularly bringing patients to clinic for supervised passive treatments generates an external locus of control and dependency on the practitioner. Strategies to empower patients to self-manage pain are challenging to implement within an operational healthcare model that dictates attending short consultations at clinics to receive treatments. The problem is further compounded with pain associated with neurological conditions because individuals often have complex functional and social life challenges that are difficult to resolve. The number and variety of books, charities and online resources to support individuals live well with pain using self-management techniques and strategies has increased in recent years and can be found via a simple internet search.

Approaches to 'soothe pain' and changing how a painful area 'feels' such as manual therapy (massage), physical activity, thermal stimulation, neuromodulation and analgesic medication should be given priority. Likewise, empowering patients to integrate activities that create positive sensory experiences, such as hydrotherapy, mindfulness, yoga

or Pilates, can markedly improve quality of life. Soaking in a warm bath, pleasantly stroking body parts that are sore and listening to soothing music, temporarily supporting a body part with a sling, or investing in inexpensive over-the-counter aids such as TENS, thermal gels or wraps are all simple techniques that alleviate pain, anxiety and stress. These sensory techniques should be used to make the painful area feel safe, protected, stabilised and should not provoke moderate to severe pain. Light stroking will not be appropriate in the presence of touch allodynia, yet deep rubbing or thermal therapy may be pleasant.

> ### KEY POINTS
>
> Current research to determine the efficacy of rehabilitation programmes for managing pain in neurological conditions is challenging. These pain management options are considered if they are not contraindicated. The patient's motivation and familiarisation of the treatment principle and protocol are critical. It is important to meet the treatment objectives with the patient's expectation of outcome. Reduction of 20% of pain intensity may be significant with respect to regaining function. SMART functional goals are set to monitor quantifiable changes in behaviour and quality of life. Empowering patients to integrate activities that create positive sensory experiences can markedly improve quality of life.

Impact of Covid-19

Coronavirus disease 2019 (Covid-19), caused by SARS-CoV-2 (i.e., severe acute respiratory syndrome coronavirus 2), affects pain in several ways. Covid-19 infection is associated with a variety of types of pain and neurological signs and symptoms reflecting damage to different body systems (Weng et al 2021). Headache and nonspecific musculoskeletal pain (low back, neck and widespread) may be a symptom of infection (Abdullahi et al 2020). More than 35% of Covid-19 patients develop neurological problems (e.g., viral encephalitis, ischaemic stroke, haemorrhagic stroke and Guillain–Barré syndromes) which can be life-threatening. Covid-19 patients may experience concomitant pain as a result of these neurological conditions (e.g., peripheral neuralgia to poststroke pain syndrome) and long-lasting symptoms (long Covid) that are similar to chronic fatigue syndrome and functional neurological disorder (Wildwing & Holt 2021). SARS-CoV-2 can invade the nervous system, and neurological involvement is associated with more severe infection.

A higher incidence of Covid-19 is observed in populations with existing pain burden, amplifying risk factors for pain morbidity and mortality. For example, pain medication can compromise the immune system causing immunosuppression (steroids and opioids) or increase risk of respiratory depression (opioids) or mask Covid-19-related fever (nonsteroidal antiinflammatory drugs). Potential risk factors for the development of chronic pain after Covid-19 include acute pain, being at high-risk of Covid-19, admission to intensive care, neurological insult, mental health burden and rehabilitation challenges (Kemp et al 2020).

Redistribution of healthcare services during the pandemic resulted in interruptions of pain services. Undertreatment of acute pain increased the risk of patients developing chronic pain, disability and psychological ill health. Interruptions to chronic pain services compromised support for biopsychosocial and self-management of pain, resulting in passive coping strategies that were magnified further by the negative psychological impact of social isolation during 'lockdown'. Decisions about who, when and how in-person consultations were undertaken were made on a case-by-case decision, informed by guidelines for risk mitigation of patients and healthcare providers accessing pain services (Emerick et al 2020, Puntillo et al 2020).

Often services adopted remote assessment and treatment of pain using telehealth approaches, via electronic information and telecommunication technologies to triage urgency of in-person visits, diagnose and evaluate patients, plan and deliver treatments (e.g., prescriptive drugs), and support biopsychosocial management of pain and emotional distress associated with pain and/or the pandemic (Eccleston et al 2020). Low-cost mobile health technologies using smartphones, tablets or laptops were used to scheduled visits, undertake consultations and share messages, information and images between patients and healthcare professionals. Generic web-based systems were adapted for pain services such as the Collaborative Health Outcome Information Registry (https://choir.stanford.edu) and PAIN OUT (http://pain-out.med.uni-jena.de).

Evidence is growing for the effectiveness of telemedicine for chronic pain including online delivery of psychological therapies and self-management programmes integrating healthy lifestyles and active strategies of coping for pain, disability, depression and anxiety (Slattery et al 2019). Poor access to technologies used in remote care and privacy protection and data security remain concerns of telemedicine (Perez et al 2021).

CONCLUSIONS

Pain associated with neurological conditions is common, and clinical guidelines for the treatment of neurological conditions acknowledge the need for pain management. When assessing individuals with pain, practitioners need to be skilled at deciding when pain indicates sinister pathology and when it does not. Clinical red flags help in this process. In a rehabilitation setting, the goal of pain management is to make long-standing pain tolerable to improve physical, role, emotional, cognitive and social functionality. A patient-centred biopsychosocial model of care is adopted where multidisciplinary treatments are used often combining pharmacological and nonpharmacological treatments including surgical, psychological and electrophysical techniques. There is a bewildering variety of nonpharmacological interventions used by therapists in rehabilitation settings, including manual therapy, physical activity and exercise, splinting, casting and bracing, electrical stimulation techniques, acupuncture, therapeutic ultrasound, thermal therapies, low-level laser therapy, visual feedback, motor imagery and body illusions. There is growing evidence of benefit from many of these interventions, although there are no robust indicators to predict whether a patient will respond. Hence treatment selection is based on the core principles of rehabilitation to make pain tolerable to improve physical, emotional, cognitive and social functionality through a process of negotiation with the patient. This is achieved using care plans that manage expectations of outcome through a process of cocreation and empower the patient with self-management techniques and resources (e.g., Ravindran 2021, https://my.livewellwithpain.co.uk).

CASE STUDIES

Case 1: Diabetic Neuropathic Pain
History

The patient was a 73-year-old unmarried woman with painful diabetic neuropathy, cerebrovascular accident and cardiovascular disorders including ventricular arrhythmias, hypertension and angina pectoris for more than 3 years (Somers & Somers 1999). The patient was admitted to hospital because of atrial fibrillation. Her stay at the hospital was extended after the patient fell from bed and fractured her right lateral malleolus 5 days after admission. Her right leg was casted below the knee, and the patient was transferred to a rehabilitation hospital 4 days after the fall.

Medications

The patient was taking Procan for ventricular arrhythmias, Lopressor for hypertension and Isordil for angina pectoris. The patient had a right cerebrovascular accident and was taking Ticlid to prevent a second infarct. The patient self-administered Humulin N insulin for type 1 diabetes. Because of her painful diabetic neuropathy in the left lower extremity, the patient applied Zostrix cream at home to control the pain, but the patient described this treatment as ineffective (Table 23.5).

TABLE 23.5 Case Example of Diabetic Neuropathic Pain

Findings	Problem List	Goals	Treatment Plan	Progress in Therapy
• Stocking and glove paraesthesia • Severe burning pain in LE • Focal aching pain in right ankle (fracture) • 4/5 MMT on right LE and 2/5 to 3/5 MMT on left LE • Cannot sleep • Unable to clean or go shopping	• Sensation loss • Neuropathic and musculoskeletal pains • Muscle weakness • Poor quality sleep • Reduction of social participation	• Prevent injury • Reduce pain • Increase muscle strength • Return to normal sleep pattern • Return to 80% of household activities in 2 months	• Education for safety on daily care • Medication and TENS for pain control and sleep quality • Muscle strengthening exercise and functional training • Assess the need for assistive devices	Week 1: therapeutic exercise and functional training (2/day; 6 days/week). Pain remained relatively constant Week 2: treatments were added as follows: (1) oral medications for neuropathic pain; (2) TENS self-administered as required and continued as home treatment after discharge Weeks 2–4: the intensity of pain was reduced from 7.4 to 4.6 cm (2.8-cm change) on VAS after TENS. The patient slept through the night for the first time in years Week 4 (discharge): the distribution of pain was reduced to two small areas; the intensity of pain was reduced to zero on the VAS after TENS

LE, Lower extremity; *MMT*, manual muscle testing; *TENS*, transcutaneous electrical nerve stimulation; *VAS*, visual analogue scale.
Adapted from Somers & Somers (1999).

Case 2: Phantom Limb Pain

History

A 24-year-old male nonsmoker with no medications and no substance misuse had a history of motorcycle collision leading to a chest wall avulsion and partial amputation of the left arm (Wilcher et al 2011). The patient received 10 weeks of acute care in a surgical medical unit to repair the chest wall and internal organs. After surgical repair, the patient was transferred to the acute rehabilitation unit where phantom limb pain became his major issue (Table 23.6).

The patient described the pain as cramping and aching, becoming searing and burning on the missing left limb as if his missing hand was clenched in a fist formation. The pain often occurred at random intervals during the day from 15 minutes to up to 90 minutes. The patient rated the pain as between 8 and 10 cm on a 10-cm visual analogue scale. At this point, the pain clinic was consulted for possible nerve block, which was deemed not appropriate. Hence a series of aggressive pain management methods was administrated.

Medications

The patient was taking naproxen (250 mg TID), tramadol (50 mg QID), extended-release morphine (150 mg BID) and hydrocodone/acetaminophen (5/500 mg q4h) as needed for pain control. The patient also received two lidocaine patches every 24 hours, and gabapentin (400 mg QID). TENS was also used. The patient's blood pressure, which was affected by severe pain, was treated by clonidine (0.4 mg BID), metoprolol (125 mg BID) and lisinopril (20 mg QD).

TABLE 23.6	Case Example of Phantom Limb Pain				

Findings	Problem List	Goals	Treatment Plan	Progress in Therapy
• Severe pain with cramping, aching, searing, burning sensations on the missing limb	• Phantom limb pains	• Reduce pain	• Medication • TENS • Mirror visual feedback therapy	Week 2: The patient rated the pain as 8–10 out of 10 cm on a VAS and took the medications and TENS as previously described. Week 4: The patient performed these practices of mirror therapy (15 min/time and no less than twice daily) with his mother clapping her hands in synchrony to give him hearing hand clapping (auditory feedback). All pain medications except gabapentin were gradually discontinued. Gabapentin was decreased from four to three times a day. His blood pressure decreased after 2 days of mirror therapy. The patient rated his maximal pain as 6 out of 10 cm on a VAS. Week 5 (discharge): The patient was discharged home with continuation of outpatient mirror and auditory feedback therapy.

TENS, Transcutaneous electrical nerve stimulation; *VAS*, visual analogue scale.

SELF-ASSESSMENT QUESTIONS

1. What is pain? Explain the different ways that pain can be classified.
2. Describe the basic elements of the nociceptive system, and explain how functioning of the nociceptive system may be affected by injury to the central nervous system.
3. What are the key elements involved in assessing the biopsychosocial aspects of pain associated with neurological conditions?
4. Explain how to make pain management effective.
5. What should clinical professionals consider when managing pain in a patient with a neurological condition in relation to treatment selection, goal setting and monitoring outcome? Please explain.

REFERENCES

Abdullahi, A., Candan, S.A., Abba, M.A., et al., 2020. Neurological and musculoskeletal features of COVID-19: a systematic review and meta-analysis. Front. Neurol. 11, 687.

Allen, N.E., Moloney, N., Van Vliet, V., Canning, C.G., 2015. The rationale for exercise in the management of pain in Parkinson's disease. J. Parkinsons Dis. 5, 229–239.

Angelopoulou, E., Anagnostouli, M., Chrousos, G.P., Bougea, A., 2020. Massage therapy as a complementary treatment for Parkinson's disease: a systematic literature review. Complement. Ther. Med. 49, 102340.

Asano, M., Duquette, P., Andersen, R., et al., 2013. Exercise barriers and preferences among women and men with multiple sclerosis. Disabil. Rehabil. 35, 353–361.

Baez, S., Herrera, E., Gershanik, O., et al., 2015. Impairments in negative emotion recognition and empathy for pain in Huntington's disease families. Neuropsychologia. 68, 158–167.

Bartolo, M., Chiò, A., Ferrari, S., Italian Consensus Conference on Pain in Neurorehabilitation (ICCPN), 2016. Assessing and treating pain in movement disorders, amyotrophic lateral sclerosis, severe acquired brain injury, disorders of consciousness, dementia, oncology and neuroinfectivology. Evidence and recommendations from the Italian Consensus Conference on Pain in Neurorehabilitation. Eur. J. Phys. Rehabil. Med. 52, 841–854.

Beecher, H.K., 1946. Pain in men wounded in battle. Bull. U.S. Army Med. Dep. 5, 445–454.

Beiske, A.G., Loge, J.H., Ronningen, A., Svensson, E., 2009. Pain in Parkinson's disease: prevalence and characteristics. Pain. 141, 173–177.

Bland, D.C., Zampieri, C., Damiano, D.L., 2011. Effectiveness of physical therapy for improving gait and balance in individuals with traumatic brain injury: a systematic review. Brain Inj. 25, 664–679.

Blatzheim, K., 2009. Interdisciplinary palliative care, including massage, in treatment of amyotrophic lateral sclerosis. J. Body Mov. Ther. 13, 328–335.

Boesch, E., Bellan, V., Moseley, G.L., Stanton, T.R., 2016. The effect of bodily illusions on clinical pain: a systematic review and meta-analysis. Pain. 157, 516–529.

Borsook, D., 2012. Neurological diseases and pain. Brain. 135, 320–344.

Bowering, K.J., O'Connell, N.E., Tabor, A., et al., 2013. The effects of graded motor imagery and its components on chronic pain: a systematic review and meta-analysis. J. Pain. 14, 3–13.

Boyers, D., McNamee, P., Clarke, A., et al., 2013. Cost-effectiveness of self-management methods for the treatment of chronic pain in an aging adult population: a systematic review of the literature. Clin. J. Pain. 29, 366–375.

Brennan, F., Lohman, D., Gwyther, L., 2019. Access to pain management as a human right. Am. J. Public Health. 109, 61–65.

Broen, M.P., Braaksma, M.M., Patijn, J., Weber, W.E., 2012. Prevalence of pain in Parkinson's disease: a systematic review using the modified QUADAS tool. Mov. Disord. 27, 480–484.

Bryce, T.N., Biering-Sorensen, F., Finnerup, N.B., et al., 2012. International spinal cord injury pain classification: part I. Background and description. March 6–7, 2009. Spinal Cord. 50, 413–417.

Burke, D., Fullen, B.M., Stokes, D., Lennon, O., 2017. Neuropathic pain prevalence following spinal cord injury: a systematic review and meta-analysis. Eur. J. Pain. 21, 29–44.

Cabanas-Valdés, R., Calvo-Sanz, J., Serra-Llobet, P., et al., 2021. The effectiveness of massage therapy for improving sequelae in post-stroke survivors. A systematic review and meta-analysis. Int. J. Environ. Res. Public Health. 18, 4424.

Campbell, E., Coulter, E.H., Mattison, P.G., et al., 2016. Physiotherapy rehabilitation for people with progressive multiple sclerosis: a systematic review. Arch. Phys. Med. Rehabil. 97, 141–151. e3

Castelnuovo, G., Giusti, E.M., Manzoni, G.M., et al., 2016. Psychological considerations in the assessment and treatment of pain in neurorehabilitation and psychological factors predictive of therapeutic response: evidence and recommendations from the Italian consensus conference on pain in neurorehabilitation. Front. Psychol. 7, 468.

Cragg, J.J., Warner, F.M., Shupler, M.S., et al., 2018. Prevalence of chronic pain among individuals with neurological conditions. Health Rep. 21, 11–16.

Cruccu, G., Garcia-Larrea, L., Hansson, P., et al., 2016. EAN guidelines on central neurostimulation therapy in chronic pain conditions. Eur. J. Neurol. 23, 1489–1499.

Davies, B., Cramp, F., Gauntlett-Gilbert, J., et al., 2015. The role of physical activity and psychological coping strategies in the management of painful diabetic neuropathy – a systematic review of the literature. Physiotherapy. 101, 319–326.

de Andrade, A.L., Bossini, P.S., Parizotto, N.A., 2016. Use of low level laser therapy to control neuropathic pain: a systematic review. J. Photochem. Photobiol. 164, 36–42.

de Tommaso, M., Arendt-Nielsen, L., Defrin, R., et al., 2016. Pain in neurodegenerative disease: current knowledge and future perspectives. Behav. Neurol. 2016, 7576292.

Dickstein, R., Deutsch, J.E., 2007. Motor imagery in physical therapist practice. Phys. Ther. 87, 942–953.

Dixon, K.E., Keefe, F.J., Scipio, C.D., et al., 2007. Psychological interventions for arthritis pain management in adults: a meta-analysis. Health Psychol. 26, 241–250.

Eccleston, C., Blyth, F.M., Dear, B.F., et al., 2020. Managing patients with chronic pain during the COVID-19 outbreak: considerations for the rapid introduction of remotely supported (eHealth) pain management services. Pain. 161, 889–893.

Emerick, T., Alter, B., Jarquin, S., et al., 2020. Telemedicine for chronic pain in the COVID-19 era and beyond. Pain Med. 21, 1743–1748.

Fattal, C., Kong, A.S.D., Gilbert, C., et al., 2009. What is the efficacy of physical therapeutics for treating neuropathic pain in spinal cord injury patients? Ann. Phys. Rehabil. Med. 52, 149–166.

Finnerup, N.B., Kuner, R., Jensen, T.S., 2021. Neuropathic pain: from mechanisms to treatment. Physiol. Rev. 101, 259–301.

Fisher, J.P., Hassan, D.T., O'Connor, N., 1995. Minerva. BMJ. 310, 70.

Fishman, S.M., 2012. Listening to Pain. A Clinician's Guide to Improving Pain Management Through Better Communication. Oxford University Press, Oxford.

Foley, P.L., Vesterinen, H.M., Laird, B.J., et al., 2013. Prevalence and natural history of pain in adults with multiple sclerosis: systematic review and meta-analysis. Pain. 154, 632–642.

Franki, I., Desloovere, K., De Cat, J., et al., 2012. The evidence-base for basic physical therapy techniques targeting lower limb function in children with cerebral palsy: a systematic review using the International Classification of Functioning, Disability and Health as a conceptual framework. J. Rehabil. Med. 44, 385–395.

Gaskin, D., Richard, P., 2012. The economic costs of pain in the United States. J. Pain. 13, 715–724.

Gilpin, H.R., Moseley, G.L., Stanton, T.R., Newport, R., 2015. Evidence for distorted mental representation of the hand in osteoarthritis. Rheumatology (Oxford). 54, 678–682.

Gironda, R.J., Clark, M.E., Ruff, R.L., et al., 2009. Traumatic brain injury, polytrauma, and pain: challenges and treatment strategies for the polytrauma rehabilitation. Rehabil. Psychol. 54, 247–258.

Goldberg, D., McGee, S., 2011. Pain as a global public health priority. BMC Public Health. 11, 770.

Gomes-Neto, M., Lopes, J.M., Conceicao, C.S., et al., 2017. Stabilization exercise compared to general exercises or manual therapy for the management of low back pain: a systematic review and meta-analysis. Phys. Ther. Sport. 23, 136–142.

Goncalves, E.D., Souza, P.S., Lieberknecht, V., et al., 2016. Low-level laser therapy ameliorates disease progression in a mouse model of multiple sclerosis. Autoimmunity. 49, 132–142.

Gosselin, R.D., Suter, M.R., Ji, R.R., Decosterd, I., 2010. Glial cells and chronic pain. Neuroscientist. 16, 519–531.

Grant, D.J., 2016. Acupuncture for neurological conditions. In: Filshie, J., White, A., Cummings, M. (Eds.), Medical Acupuncture: A Western Scientific Approach, 2nd ed. Elsevier, Edinburgh.

Güçhan Topcu, Z., Tomaç, H., 2020. The effectiveness of massage for children with cerebral palsy: a systematic review. Adv. Mind Body Med. 34, 4–13.

Harris, J.E., Hebert, A., 2015. Utilization of motor imagery in upper limb rehabilitation: a systematic scoping review. Clin. Rehabil. 29, 1092–1107.

Harrison, A.M., McCracken, L.M., Jones, K., et al., 2017. Using mixed methods case-series evaluation in the development of a guided self-management hybrid CBT and ACT intervention for multiple sclerosis pain. Disabil. Rehabil. 39, 1785–1798.

Harvey, L.A., Glinsky, J.V., Bowden, J.L., 2016. The effectiveness of 22 commonly administered physiotherapy interventions for people with spinal cord injury: a systematic review. Spinal Cord. 54, 914–923.

Hassett, A.L., Finan, P.H., 2016. The role of resilience in the clinical management of chronic pain. Curr. Pain Headache Rep. 20, 39.

He, K., Hu, R., Huang, Y., et al., 2022. Effects of acupuncture on neuropathic pain induced by spinal cord injury: a systematic review and meta-analysis. Evid. Based Complement. Alternat. Med. 2022, 6297484.

Hoffman, B.M., Papas, R.K., Chatkoff, D.K., Kerns, R.D., 2007. Meta-analysis of psychological interventions for chronic low back pain. Health Psychol. 26, 1–9.

Houghton, P., Nussbaum, E., Hoens, A., 2010. Electrophysical agents. Contraindications and precautions: an evidence-based approach to clinical decision making in physical therapy. Physiother. Can. 62, 5–80.

Huang, M., Magni, N., Rice, D., 2021. The prevalence, characteristics and impact of chronic pain in people with muscular dystrophies: a systematic review and meta-analysis. J. Pain. 22, 1343–1359.

Huang, Q., Luo, D., Chen, L., et al., 2019. Effectiveness of acupuncture for Alzheimer's disease: an updated systematic review and meta-analysis. Curr. Med. Sci. 39, 500–511.

Hunt, C., Moman, R., Peterson, A., et al., 2021. Prevalence of chronic pain after spinal cord injury: a systematic review and meta-analysis. Reg. Anesth. Pain Med. 46, 328–336.

Hurwitz, N., Radakovic, R., Boyce, E., Peryer, G., 2021. Prevalence of pain in amyotrophic lateral sclerosis: a systematic review and meta-analysis. Amyotroph. Lateral Scler. Frontotemporal Degener. 22, 7–8.

IASP Task Force on Taxonomy, 2022. IASP Taxonomy. IASP Press., Available at: https://www.iasp-pain.org/resources/terminology/. Accessed on 14 June 2023.

Johnson, M., 2014. Transcutaneous Electrical Nerve Stimulation (TENS). Research to Support Clinical Practice. Oxford University Press, Oxford, UK.

Johnson, M.I., 2019. The landscape of chronic pain: broader perspectives. Medicina (Kaunas). 55, 182.

Johnson, M.I., Hudson, M., 2016. Generalizing, deleting and distorting information about the experience and communication of chronic pain. Pain Manag. 6, 411–414.

Johnson, M.I., Paley, C., Jones, G., et al., 2022. Efficacy and safety of transcutaneous electrical nerve stimulation (TENS) for acute and chronic pain in adults: a systematic review and meta-analysis of 381 studies (The Meta-TENS Study). BMJOpen. 12, e051073.

Jones, T.M., Dean, C.M., Dear, B.F., et al., 2016. An internet survey of the characteristics and physical activity of community-dwelling Australian adults with acquired brain injury: exploring interest in an internet-delivered self-management program focused on physical activity. Disabil. Health J. 9, 54–63.

Juhl, C., Christensen, R., Roos, E.M., et al., 2014. Impact of exercise type and dose on pain and disability in knee osteoarthritis: a systematic review and meta-regression analysis of randomized controlled trials. Arthr. Rheumatol. 66, 622–636.

Kehlet, H., Jensen, T.S., Woolf, C.J., 2006. Persistent postsurgical pain: risk factors and prevention. Lancet. 367, 1618–1625.

Kemp, H.I., Corner, E., Colvin, L.A., 2020. Chronic pain after COVID-19: implications for rehabilitation. Br. J. Anaesth. 125, 436–440.

Khodaie, F., Abbasi, N., Kazemi Motlagh, A.H., et al., 2022. Acupuncture for multiple sclerosis: a literature review. Mult. Scler. Relat. Disord. 60, 103715.

Kosek, E., Cohen, M., Baron, R., et al., 2016. Do we need a third mechanistic descriptor for chronic pain states? Pain. 157, 1382–1386.

Kratz, A.L., Molton, I.R., Jensen, M.P., et al., 2011. Further evaluation of the Motivational Model of Pain Self-Management: coping with chronic pain in multiple sclerosis. Ann. Behav. Med. 41, 391–400.

Lager, C., Kroksmark, A.K., 2015. Pain in adolescents with spinal muscular atrophy and Duchenne and Becker muscular dystrophy. Eur. J. Paediatr. Neurol. 19, 537–546.

Lee, S.H., Lim, S., 2017. Clinical effectiveness of acupuncture on Parkinson disease: a PRISMA-compliant systematic review and meta-analysis. Medicine (Baltimore). 96, e5836.

Lefaucheur, J.P., Antal, A., Ayache, S.S., et al., 2016. Evidence-based guidelines on the therapeutic use of transcranial direct current stimulation (tDCS). Clin. Neurophysiol. 128, 56–92.

Leinenga, G., Langton, C., Nisbet, R., Gotz, J., 2016. Ultrasound treatment of neurological diseases – current and emerging applications. Nat. Rev. Neurol. 12, 161–174.

Leung, L., 2012. From ladder to platform: a new concept for pain management. J. Prim. Health Care. 4, 254–258.

Liampas, A., Velidakis, N., Georgiou, T., et al., 2020. Prevalence and management challenges in central post-stroke neuropathic pain: a systematic review and meta-analysis. Adv. Ther. 37, 3278–3291.

Loeser, J.D., 2019. A new way of thinking about pain. Pain Manag. 9, 5–7.

Lorig, K.R., Holman, H., 2003. Self-management education: history, definition, outcomes, and mechanisms. Ann. Behav. Med. 26, 1–7.

Lu, Y., Wang, R., Dong, Y., et al., 2016. Low-level laser therapy for beta amyloid toxicity in rat hippocampus. Neurobiol. Aging. 49, 165–182.

Ma, R.J., Liu, X., Clark, J., et al., 2015. The impact of acupuncture on neurological recovery in spinal cord injury: a systematic review and meta-analysis. J. Neurotrauma. 32, 1943–1957.

MacFarlane, G.J., Thomas, E., Croft, P.R., et al., 1999. Predictors of early improvement in low back pain amongst consulters to general practice: the influence of pre-morbid and episode-related factors. Pain. 80, 113–119.

Mann, E.G., Lefort, S., Vandenkerkhof, E.G., 2013. Self-management interventions for chronic pain. Pain Manag. 3, 211–222.

Margenfeld, F., Klocke, C., Joos, S., 2019. Manual massage for persons living with dementia: a systematic review and meta-analysis. Int. J. Nurs. Stud. 96, 132–142.

McCaffery, M., Pasero, C., 1999. Pain: A Clinical Manual, second ed. C.V. Mosby, St. Louis.

Mehta, S., McIntyre, A., Guy, S., et al., 2015. Effectiveness of transcranial direct current stimulation for the management of neuropathic pain after spinal cord injury: a meta-analysis. Spinal Cord. 53, 780–785.

Melzack, R., 2005. Evolution of the neuromatrix theory of pain. The Prithvi Raj Lecture: presented at the Third World Congress of World Institute of Pain, Barcelona 2004. Pain. Pract. 5, 85–94.

Michailidou, C., Marston, L., De Souza, L.H., Sutherland, I., 2014. A systematic review of the prevalence of musculoskel-etal pain, back and low back pain in people with spinal cord injury. Disabil. Rehabil. 36, 705–715.

Milinis, K., Young, C.A., Trajectories of Outcome in Neurological Conditions (TONiC) study., 2015. Systematic review of the influence of spasticity on quality of life in adults with chronic neurological conditions. Disabil. Rehabil. 38, 1431–1441.

Miller, D.M., Moore, S.M., Fox, R.J., et al., 2011. Web-based self-management for patients with multiple sclerosis: a practical, randomized trial. Telemed. J. E. Health. 17, 5–13.

Molton, I.R., Jensen, M.P., Nielson, W., et al., 2008. A preliminary evaluation of the motivational model of pain self-manage-ment in persons with spinal cord injury-related pain. J. Pain. 9, 606–612.

Morris, M.E., Perry, A., Bilney, B., et al., 2006. Outcomes of physical therapy, speech pathology, and occupational therapy for people with motor neuron disease: a systematic review. Neurorehabil. Neural Repair. 20, 424–434.

Moseley, G.L., 2007. Using visual illusion to reduce at-level neu-ropathic pain in paraplegia. Pain. 130, 294–298.

Moseley, G.L., Gallace, A., Spence, C., 2008. Is mirror therapy all it is cracked up to be? Current evidence and future directions. Pain. 138, 7–10.

Moshourab, R.A., Schafer, M., Al-Chaer, E.D., 2015. Chronic pain in neurotrauma: implications on spinal cord and traumatic brain injury. In: Kobeissy, F.H. (Ed.), Brain Neurotrauma: Molecular, Neuropsychological, and Rehabilitation Aspects. CRC Press/Taylor & Francis, Boca Raton (FL).

Munce, S.E., Fehlings, M.G., Straus, S.E., et al., 2014. Views of people with traumatic spinal cord injury about the compo-nents of self-management programs and program delivery: a Canadian pilot study. BMC Neurol. 14, 209.

Nampiaparampil, D.E., 2008. Prevalence of chronic pain after traumatic brain injury: a systematic review. JAMA. 300, 711–719.

National Institute for Health and Care Excellence (NICE), 2008. Spinal cord stimulation for chronic pain of neuropathic or ischaemic origin [Technology appraisal guidance, TA159]. NICE, London, Available at: https://www.nice.org.uk/guid-ance/ta159. Accessed on 14 June 2023..

National Institute for Health and Care Excellence (NICE), 2013. Percutaneous electrical nerve stimulation for refractory neu-ropathic pain [Interventional procedures guidance, IPG450]. NICE, London, Available at: https://www.nice.org.uk/guid-ance/ipg450. Accessed on 14 June 2023.

National Institute for Health and Care Excellence (NICE), 2016. Spinal injury: assessment and initial management [NICE guideline, NG41]. NICE, London, Available at: https://www.nice.org.uk/guidance/ng41. Accessed on 14 June 2023.

O'Connell, N.E., Wand, B.M., McAuley, J., et al., 2013. Interventions for treating pain and disability in adults with complex regional pain syndrome. Cochrane Database Syst. Rev. 4, CD009416.

Paolucci, S., Iosa, M., Toni, D., Neuropathic Pain Special Interest Group of the Italian Neurological Society, 2016. Prevalence and time course of post-stroke pain: a multicenter prospective hospital-based study. Pain Med. 17, 924–930.

Paolucci, S., Martinuzzi, A., Scivoletto, G., Italian Consensus Conference on Pain in Neurorehabilitation (ICCPN)., 2016. Assessing and treating pain associated with stroke, multiple sclerosis, cerebral palsy, spinal cord injury and spasticity. Evidence and recommendations from the Italian Consensus conference on Pain in Neurorehabilitation. Eur. J. Phys. Rehabil. Med. 52, 827–840.

Pelletier, R., Higgins, J., Bourbonnais, D., 2015. Is neuroplas-ticity in the central nervous system the missing link to our understanding of chronic musculoskeletal disorders? BMC Musculoskelet. Disord. 16, 25.

Perez, J., Niburski, K., Stoopler, M., Ingelmo, P., 2021. Telehealth and chronic pain management from rapid adaptation to long-term implementation in pain medicine: a narrative review. Pain Rep. 6, e912.

Pike, A., Hearn, L., de, C., Williams, A.C., 2016. Effectiveness of psychological interventions for chronic pain on health care use and work absence: systematic review and meta-analysis. Pain. 157, 777–785.

Pitcher, M.H., Von Korff, M., Bushnell, M.C., Porter, L., 2019. Prevalence and profile of high-impact chronic pain in the United States. J. Pain. 20, 146–160.

Plow, M., Bethoux, F., Mai, K., Marcus, B., 2014. A formative evaluation of customized pamphlets to promote physical activity and symptom self-management in women with mul-tiple sclerosis. Health Educ. Res. 29, 883–896.

Pollock, A., Baer, G., Campbell, P., et al., 2014. Physical rehabili-tation approaches for the recovery of function and mobility following stroke. Cochrane Database Syst. Rev. 4, CD001920.

Puntillo, F., Giglio, M., Brienza, N., et al., 2020. Impact of COVID-19 pandemic on chronic pain management: look-ing for the best way to deliver care. Best Pract. Res. Clin. Anaesthesiol. 34, 529–537.

Raja, S.N., Carr, D.B., Cohen, M., et al., 2020. The revised International Association for the Study of Pain definition of pain: concepts, challenges, and compromises. Pain. 161, 1976–1982.

Ravindran, D., 2021. The pain-free mindset. Vermilion Publishing, London, UK.

Rossi, M., Perez-Lloret, S., Doldan, L., et al., 2014. Autosomal dominant cerebellar ataxias: a systematic review of clinical features. Eur. J. Neurol. 21, 607–615.

Salarvand, S., Heidari, M.E., Farahi, K., et al., 2021. Effectiveness of massage therapy on fatigue and pain in patients with multiple sclerosis: a systematic review and meta-analysis. Mult. Scler. J. Exp. Transl. Clin. 7 20552173211022779

Samanta, J., Kendall, J., Samanta, A., 2003. 10-minute consultation: chronic low back pain. BMJ. 326, 535.

Sánchez, A.G., Andrade, E.L., Marsal, J.V., et al., 2017. A study to evaluate the effect of ultrasound treatment on nodules in multiple sclerosis patients. Int. J. Neurosci. 127, 404–411.

Saragiotto, B.T., Maher, C.G., Yamato, T.P., et al., 2016. Motor control exercise for nonspecific low back pain: a Cochrane Review. Spine. 41, 1284–1295.

Saulino, M., Averna, J.F., 2016. Evaluation and management of SCI-associated pain. Curr. Pain Headache Rep. 20, 53.

Seifert, F., Maihofner, C., 2011. Functional and structural imaging of pain-induced neuroplasticity. Curr. Opin. Anaesthesiol. 24, 515–523.

Seixas, D., Foley, P., Palace, J., et al., 2014. Pain in multiple sclerosis: a systematic review of neuroimaging studies. Neuroimage Clin. 5, 322–331.

Simpson, E.L., Duenas, A., Holmes, M.W., et al., 2009. Spinal cord stimulation for chronic pain of neuropathic or ischaemic origin: systematic review and economic evaluation. Health Technol. Assess. 13, 1–154. iii, ix–x

Simpson, R., Booth, J., Lawrence, M., et al., 2014. Mindfulness based interventions in multiple sclerosis – a systematic review. BMC Neurol. 14, 15.

Skogar, O., Lokk, J., 2016. Pain management in patients with Parkinson's disease: challenges and solutions. J. Multidiscip. Healthc. 9, 469–479.

Slater, H., Sluka, K., Derlund, S., et al., 2017. IASP Curriculum Outline on Pain for Physical Therapy. IASP Press., Available at: http://www.iasp-pain.org/Education/CurriculumDetail.aspx?ItemNumber=2055. Accessed on 14 June 2023.

Slattery, B.W., Haugh, S., O'Connor, L., et al., 2019. An evaluation of the effectiveness of the modalities used to deliver electronic health interventions for chronic pain: systematic review with network meta-analysis. J. Med. Internet Res. 21, e11086.

Somers, D.L., Somers, M.F., 1999. Treatment of neuropathic pain in a patient with diabetic neuropathy using transcutaneous electrical nerve stimulation applied to the skin of the lumbar region. Phys. Ther. 79, 767–775.

Sprenger, G.P., Roos, R.A.C., van Zwet, E., et al., 2021. The prevalence of pain in Huntington's disease in a large worldwide cohort. Parkinsonism Relat. Disord. 89, 73–78.

Sprenger, G.P., van der Zwaan, K.F., Roos, R.A.C., Achterberg, W.P., 2019. The prevalence and the burden of pain in patients with Huntington's disease. Pain. 160, 773–783.

Streckmann, F., Zopf, E.M., Lehmann, H.C., et al., 2014. Exercise intervention studies in patients with peripheral neuropathy: a systematic review. Sports Med. 44, 1289–1304.

Sturgeon, J.A., Zautra, A.J., 2016. Social pain and physical pain: shared paths to resilience. Pain Manag. 6, 63–74.

Su, Y., Lim, E.C., 2016. Does evidence support the use of neural tissue management to reduce pain and disability in nerve-related chronic musculoskeletal pain? A systematic review with meta-analysis. Clin. J. Pain. 32, 991–1004.

Tabor, A., Thacker, M.A., Moseley, G.L., Körding, K.P., 2017. Pain: a statistical account. PLoS Comput. Biol. 13, e1005142.

Tanaka, R., Ozawa, J., Kito, N., Moriyama, H., 2013. Efficacy of strengthening or aerobic exercise on pain relief in people with knee osteoarthritis: a systematic review and meta-analysis of randomized controlled trials. Clin. Rehabil. 27, 1059–1071.

Thieme, H., Morkisch, N., Rietz, C., et al., 2016. The efficacy of movement representation techniques for treatment of limb pain – a systematic review and meta-analysis. J. Pain. 17, 167–180.

Tran, J., Dorstyn, D.S., Burke, A.L., 2016. Psychosocial aspects of spinal cord injury pain: a meta-analysis. Spinal Cord. 54, 640–648.

Uthman, O.A., van der Windt, D.A., Jordan, J.L., et al., 2013. Exercise for lower limb osteoarthritis: systematic review incorporating trial sequential analysis and network meta-analysis. BMJ. 347, f5555.

van Gorp, S., Kessels, A.G., Joosten, E.A., et al., 2015. Pain prevalence and its determinants after spinal cord injury: a systematic review. Eur. J. Pain. 19, 5–14.

Vos, T., Diseases and Injuries Collaborators., 2020. Global burden of 369 diseases and injuries in 204 countries and territories, 1990–2019: a systematic analysis for the Global Burden of Disease Study 2019. Lancet. 396, 1204–1222.

Watson, T., Nasbaum, E.L., 2020. Electrophysical Agents: Evidence-Based Practice, 13th edition Elsevier, Edinburgh.

Weng, L.M., Su, X., Wang, X.Q., 2021. Pain symptoms in patients with coronavirus disease (COVID-19): a literature review. J. Pain Res. 14, 147–159.

Wiklund, I., Holmstrom, S., Stoker, M., et al., 2013. Are treatment benefits in neuropathic pain reflected in the Self Assessment of Treatment questionnaire? Health Qual. Life Outcomes. 11, 8.

Wilcher, D.G., Chernev, I., Yan, K., 2011. Combined mirror visual and auditory feedback therapy for upper limb phantom pain: a case report. J. Med. Case Rep. 5, 41.

Wildwing, T., Holt, N., 2021. The neurological symptoms of COVID-19: a systematic overview of systematic reviews, comparison with other neurological conditions and implications for healthcare services. Ther. Adv. Chronic Dis. 12 2040622320976979

Wittkopf, P.G., Johnson, M.I., 2016. Managing pain by visually distorting the size of painful body parts: is there any therapeutic value? Pain Manag. 6, 201–204.

World Health Organization, 2019. International Statistical Classification of Diseases and Related Health Problems, 11th edition.

Yanguas-Casas, N., Barreda-Manso, M.A., Nieto-Sampedro, M., Romero-Ramirez, L., 2014. Tauroursodeoxycholic acid reduces glial cell activation in an animal model of acute neuroinflammation. J. Neuroinflamm. 11, 50.

Yitayeh, A., Teshome, A., 2016. The effectiveness of physiotherapy treatment on balance dysfunction and postural instability in persons with Parkinson's disease: a systematic review and meta-analysis. BMC Sports Sci. Med. Rehabil. 8, 17.

Young Blood, M.R., Ferro, M.M., Munhoz, R.P., et al., 2016. Classification and characteristics of pain associated with Parkinson's disease. Parkinsons Dis. 2016, 6067132.

Zhou, J., Peng, W., Xu, M., et al., 2015. The effectiveness and safety of acupuncture for patients with Alzheimer disease: a systematic review and meta-analysis of randomized controlled trials. Medicine (Baltimore). 94, e933.

Zhu, X.C., Yu, Y., Wang, H.F., et al., 2015. Physiotherapy intervention in Alzheimer's disease: systematic review and meta-analysis. J. Alzheimer Dis. 44, 163–174.

Clinical Neuropsychology in Rehabilitation

F. Colin Wilson

OUTLINE

Introduction, 611
Neuropsychological Assessment, 612
    Cognitive Functions, 612
    Assessment of Emotional and Behavioural
        Adjustment, 613
    Affective and Mediating Factors, 614
    Assessment of Outcomes and Quality of Life, 614
Neuropsychological Interventions, 615
    Cognitive Interventions, 615
    Behavioural Interventions, 615
    Psychotherapy: Staff, Team and Organisational Support
        and Research, 616
Neuropsychological Consequences of Neurological
**   Disorders, 616**
    Age of Acquisition and Neuroplasticity, 616
    Focal Versus Diffuse, 617

Acute Versus Chronic, 617
Progressive Versus Static, 617
Site and Lateralisation, 617
Traumatic Brain Injury, 617
Stroke, 618
Hypoxic Brain Injury, 618
Covid-19, 619
Degenerative Conditions, 621
Spinal Injuries, 621
Neuropsychological Disorders of Movement, 621
Apraxia, 621
Neglect, 622
Functional Disorders, 622
Process of Rehabilitation, 622
Conclusion, 622
    Psychological Adjustment, 623

INTRODUCTION

The field of postqualification applied psychology that is concerned with the assessment, rehabilitation and management of people with neurological disorders is known as *clinical neuropsychology*. In essence, clinical neuropsychologists use a scientific and analytical approach to understand the brain and neurocognitive/neurobehavioural functioning in clinical contexts. Within the United Kingdom, most neuropsychologists initially qualify as clinical psychologists before developing a more in-depth knowledge base, postqualification clinical experience and practice within the context of a competency-based framework, which promotes professional standards of practice (British Psychological Society 2012). By way of contrast,

Hokkanen et al (2019) noted that up to one-third of European countries have no training model in place for clinical neuropsychology. Notwithstanding, benchmarking of standards and competencies across Europe are being developed (Hokkanen et al 2020). In general, clinical neuropsychologists aim to identify and interpret disorders of cognitive function such as memory, language, learning, and thinking and reasoning; this also includes perceptual (integration of information from the environment), emotional and behavioural disorders arising from neuropathology. The rehabilitation team needs to have an understanding of these disorders to screen patients for cognitive perceptual dysfunction as well as neurobehavioural difficulties and address these deficits as part of their planned intervention.

Early work from a behavioural neurology approach demonstrated value in terms of the fractionation of cognitive and affective functions arising from neurological insult. Clinical neuropsychology developed rapidly in the context of worldwide conflicts (World Wars I and II) which fostered the study of injured service personnel and the impact of often focal (open) brain insults on cognitive functioning. Much of this work helped to establish the fractionated anatomy of neurocognitive functions. In neurorehabilitation, it is important to appreciate the distinction between focal injuries such as stroke and diffuse insults such as traumatic brain injury (TBI); diffuse injuries are associated with widespread tearing and shearing of neuronal connections. The effects of these acquired injuries can affect cognitive functioning, mood, motivation and engagement in rehabilitation. Although it is conceded that many functions depend on highly localised and specialised areas, other cognitive domains may be dependent on a wide area network of interconnected anatomical structures. In everyday practice, most clinical neuropsychologists generally adopt the working assumption that many neurofunctions are localised to regions of the cortex but are also often heavily interdependent on other affected or preserved cerebral tissue. It is beyond the scope of this chapter to address this issue in depth. Over the past 50 years neurorehabilitation has increasingly become an active area of clinical neuropsychology practice and applied research activity. Before that point, practitioners generally working within the context of neurosciences would have had a primarily diagnosis and assessment role; with the exception of a few notable clinicians such as A. R. Luria, H.-L. Teuber and Oliver Zangwill, the area of rehabilitation was relatively neglected. The emergence of neuroimaging from the 1980's onwards provided impetus to clinical neuropsychologists to move beyond the realms of assessment into a more practice-based role including rehabilitative approaches, within which tailored assessment provided the theoretical scaffolding which when combined with experimental case study methodology enables the planning and evaluation of practical rehabilitation approaches. In essence, cognitive neuropsychology concentrates upon the single case or case-series approach and seeks to explain psychological deficits in terms of the components of cognitive information-processing models. Cognitive neuropsychological analysis has been very influential in developing our understanding of both normal and abnormal cognitive psychological functions within the brain. Today clinical neuropsychologists are involved in acute, postacute and community-based neurorehabilitation involving patients in disorders of consciousness (DOC) through to those with concussion or mild TBI resuming a former work role or alternative prevocational or educational opportunities.

NEUROPSYCHOLOGICAL ASSESSMENT

Clinical neuropsychological management and/or treatment involves detailed tailored assessment before planning tailored interventions. Neuropsychological assessment should be understood as the essential precursor to the planning and implementation of rehabilitation. It is a description in psychological terms of the client's current state with respect to the clinical problems the neuropsychologist or rehabilitation team is actively seeking to address. This assessment aims to provide a concise overview into the processes which are no longer functioning normally, as well as a sound rationale upon which a planned intervention is based. Subsequent reassessments allow progress to be monitored and interventions to be adjusted, according to the client's current state.

Practitioners continue to draw from three historical positions in everyday practice. The first position would commonly draw on the work of A. R. Luria (see Christensen 1974) and is based upon behavioural neurology. As such, this approach uses relatively simple tasks, selected from a wide variety of available tests which are easily completed by most normal adults. Accordingly, any particular task failure is arguably a pathological sign, and the pattern of these structural observations facilitates a psychological description to be established.

The second historical position emanating from North America is a psychometric battery-based approach articulated in measures such as Halstead–Reitan and Luria Nebraska Neuropsychological Test Batteries, as well as the Wechsler suite of tests. In this approach, a standardised extensive test battery is administered, and the resulting descriptions of patient deficits arise out of a psychometric analysis of test scores relative to age-based norms.

The third position which is dominant within the UK and Europe is the normative person-centred approach which draws on specific tests, associated wherever possible with adequate normative data, as well as ecological validity, to investigate clinical hypotheses about the patient's strengths as well as areas of deficits or decrement. In practice, many neuropsychologists will use a mixture of these approaches depending on the patient's presentation, time, available resources and reliable data from other sources to develop a robust working formulation and plan treatment.

Cognitive Functions

Commonly, neuropsychological assessment concentrates upon cognitive functions such as perception, attention and concentration, learning and memory, language, thinking and reasoning. At least in the past because of the extensive variety of tests available to the neuropsychologist, most such tests present test materials in a controlled way and thereby yield reliable scores relative to appropriate norms. It is nevertheless still the case that such test norms may be more or less adequate for the clinical population under consideration, and some may have questionable test–retest reliability, content, or indeed more importantly in a rehabilitation context, ecological validity. Clearly, test use required even more careful thought within the context of the global Covid-19 pandemic. Before the pandemic, teleneuropsychology had been somewhat limited in use and scope. However, in the wake of Covid-19, various practice guidelines (Bunnage et al 2020, Kitaigorodsky et al 2021) have provided a framework for both assessment and therapy. It is worth noting that most tests have not actively explored issues of performance validity as part of their development (Bigler 2012, DeRight & Jorgensen 2015), which has implications for normative samples and clinical populations under consideration. The interested reader is referred to such seminal textbooks as by Goldstein and McNeil (2012), Lezak et al (2012) and in particular Strauss et al (2006), which provide a detailed description of some commonly used tests (Table 24.1).

Assessment of Emotional and Behavioural Adjustment

After acquired brain injury (ABI), patients in general are at increased risk for development of a range of emotional and behavioural disorders. Emotional disturbance with a mixture of reactive anxiety and depression is particularly common and can influence patient engagement with therapy and rehabilitation outcome unless addressed. Bipolar disorders, mania, obsessive-compulsive disorder and psychotic episodes unless presenting before the ABI are rare (circa 1%–2%; Brown 2012) and require referral to and consultation with neuropsychiatry.

Individuals with emerging insight of their acquired physical, communicative and cognitive deficits are probably more at risk for depression particularly over time.

TABLE 24.1 Commonly Used Tests in Clinical Practice

Cognitive Domain	Test Purpose	Test
Premorbid functioning	Established level of functioning before illness	Educational attainments Occupational status Tests of word recognition or single word reading
Processing speed	Reduced information processing	Psychomotor tasks, simple reaction time tests
Overall intellectual functioning	Establish baseline current cognitive functioning	Measures such as Wechsler Adult Intelligence Scale, Raven's Matrices
Language	Level of receptive understanding and expression	Verbal comprehension, object to word matching, command following, object naming, verbal fluency
Memory	Establish level of memory deficit, ability to learn	Tests of immediate recall, recognition, capacity to learn and retain new verbal or visual information
Attention	Capacity to attend, manage distractions, divide and sustain attention	Attend to instructions, attend to sound in presence of distraction, vigilance tasks
Perception	Visuoperceptual and visuospatial functions	Object and face recognition Hand–eye coordination Spatial location and orientation
Executive functioning	Detect cognitive impairments in terms of self-organisation, planning, problem solving and independent reasoning	Simple step-by-step problem solving, strategic planning tasks, planning and organising an event, complex problem solving, managing to complete multiple errands in a set time

The reader is referred to Strauss et al (2006), who provide a much more comprehensive overview and critique of tests in common clinical practice.

Those surviving TBI also have an increased risk for suicide, which remains fairly constant over time after injury (1%, at least three times the standard mortality rate; Fleminger et al 2003), which may be associated with ongoing alcohol/drug abuse. Table 24.2 provides an overview of frequently occurring emotional and behavioural difficulties within the first year after TBI, stroke and hypoxic/anoxic injury [for more details, see Brown (2012)].

Historically, behavioural assessment depends on observational recording to identify the antecedent triggers of the target *problematic* behaviour repertoire, as well as an analysis of the consequences of the behaviour for the individual and/or others. Such observations furnish an understanding of causative and maintenance factors which can inform the design of behavioural programme(s), intrinsic to effective team management of patients; examples of such approaches are provided by Wilson et al (2003a), as well as McMillan and Wood (2017). In addition, those interested in applying behavioural approaches should consider the value and clinical appropriateness of methods in common use among people with intellectual disability, particularly positive behaviour support approaches (British Psychological Society 2018).

Affective and Mediating Factors

Beyond assessment of cognition and behaviour, clinical neuropsychologists commonly evaluate the patient's adjustment to disability, affective states, coping mechanisms, forensic history, insight and awareness, motivation, trauma history as well as premorbid background as part of a comprehensive assessment. This component of assessment maybe elicited via structured clinical interview, interview with family or significant other, and/or the use of standard questionnaires and rating scales. This element of clinical assessment draws heavily from other branches of applied psychology and mental health approaches. However, without such information, any rehabilitative approach is likely to be either ill-informed or in extreme cases clinically inappropriate.

Assessment of Outcomes and Quality of Life

Few can be oblivious to the current theme of establishing the clinical and cost-effectiveness of rehabilitation services delivered whilst still ensuring quality provision. Within neuropsychological rehabilitation, a variety of measures such as the Barthel index (Wade 1992), Functional Independence Measure–Functional Assessment Measure (Cook et al 1994) and Rehabilitation Complexity Scale

TABLE 24.2	**Common Emotional-Behavioural Difficulties After Acquired Brain Injury (Brown 2012)**
Traumatic brain injury	• Apathy (46%) • Depression (20%–40%) • Anxiety (10%–25%) • Pain (>50%): headaches, spasticity, contractures, heterotopic ossification, complex regional pain syndromes • Reduced anger control, posttraumatic stress disorder (19%–26%) • Reduced community involvement • Reduced relationship satisfaction and quality • Inability to return to work or previous enjoyed leisure pursuits • Severe behavioural disorders (verbal, physical and sexual disinhibition, aggression)
Stroke	• Apathy (57%) • Depression (20%–40%) • Anxiety (30%) • Pain (spasticity, contractures, complex regional pain syndromes)
Hypoxia/anoxia	• Apathy (79%) • Depression • Anxiety • Agitation • Reduced anger control • Affective dysregulation (inability to control internal emotional state) • Egocentric or childish behaviour • Poor psychosocial and vocational reintegration • Severe behavioural disorders (lack of initiation, disinhibition, loss of judgement)

(Turner-Strokes et al 2007) have been used in the planning and evaluation of patient-centred rehabilitation. However, none of the available scales is adequate to assess the status of those in DOC, and there is a relative dearth of good measures of the specific outcome of psychological interventions. Notwithstanding, robust evidence of the clinical and cost-effectiveness of neurorehabilitation is available (Oddy & da Silva Ramos 2013, Turner-Stokes et al 2016).

NEUROPSYCHOLOGICAL INTERVENTIONS

Management strategies include cognitive and behavioural interventions, as well as various forms of psychotherapy. Most approaches rely at least to some degree on an individual's capacity to attend, form new memories and have a degree of insight/awareness of the deficits/decrements under active management. Some tentative suggestions in relation to how therapists can minimise the effect of these deficits on therapy activity are provided in Box 24.1, which outlines guiding principles to consider in assessment and when planning intervention(s) particularly in acute and postacute settings.

BOX 24.1   Guiding Cognitive Principles for Rehabilitation (Wilson 2009)

1. Establish nature, site and extent of acquired brain injury.
2. Assess level of responsiveness/orientation to current environment.
3. Assess patient understanding of their current problems/deficits (awareness).
4. Alter environment (minimise noise, distractions) and promote active attention to therapy activity, which may require using a set number of repetitions.
5. Tailor therapy to maximise patient understanding of therapy demands within the interdisciplinary team working context.
6. Implement errorless learning [Wilson (2004) provides details about learning without errors] as part of holistic therapy practice and ward-based activity.
7. Use SMART goals (specific, measurable, achievable, realistic and timed goals; Cott & Finch 1990) in therapy to minimise patient confusion and anxiety.
8. Provide concise feedback to patient and family to promote positive engagement (consider the use of agreed tangible rewards to reinforce engagement; e.g., watching a chosen favourite DVD after physiotherapy).
9. Facilitate multiple opportunities for practice across functional contexts (skill generalisation) from therapy to ward to home setting.

Cognitive Interventions

Cognitive interventions aim to reduce the effect of deficits in the areas of memory, learning, perception, language, and thinking and reasoning. How this is achieved depends in part upon the model of recovery that is adopted but, in general, requires a fundamental level of some basis for new learning and/or the development of strategies which circumvent the disrupted components within the cognitive system.

Besides the explicit teaching of new strategies, appropriately structured training may be used; this is often based upon errorless learning which has been shown to be most effective after ABI. Aids to performance, which may be either external (such as diaries to aid memory) or internal (mnemonics), may also be successfully used. These interventions are more fully developed than others in some areas such as attention, memory and executive dysfunction, but the basic principles can be applied in any area of cognitive function. The reader is referred to Cicerone et al (2019), who provides an up-to-date meta-analytical literature review.

Behavioural Interventions

Behavioural interventions have become less common. However, such tailored interventions may be appropriate to address the remediation of aberrant behaviours and in situations where an individual's residual cognitive function is significantly impaired. Behavioural interventions are founded upon psychological learning theory. Behaviours that are desirable or prosocial (in a rehabilitation context) can therefore be increased by ensuring that they are positively reinforced (good outcome), whereas undesirable negative behaviours are not reinforced. Although theoretically negative reinforcement (punishment) might be used to reduce the frequency of a behaviour in clinical practice, such an approach should be considered in only extreme circumstances such as significant life-threatening behaviour. In practice, the lack of positive reinforcement delivered consistently is often sufficient in itself for the unwanted/negative behaviour to reduce.

Behavioural problems can directly interfere with therapy engagement and compliance, such as kicking directed towards staff, biting or indirectly reduced participation resulting from use of verbal aggression or use of inappropriate/disinhibited language throughout therapy. Nonetheless, often behaviour problems can be relatively easily addressed in the context of good interdisciplinary team (IDT) working including regular communication between neurorehabilitation team members, as well as the patient and their family. In addition, it is important that all interdisciplinary staff can commence and complete structured behavioural observation(s) records with antecedent (A), behaviour (B) and consequence (C) sections at the very least [see Table 24.3; Wilson et al (2003b, p. 46), McMillan and Wood (2017)].

Such recording methods permit patient–staff and/ or patient–family interactions to be reviewed and possible behavioural/environmental triggers to be identified. Without these, it is difficult to reliably identify reductions or escalations in aberrant behaviour patterns or to establish whether a planned behavioural management plan is effective.

Although behavioural approaches may be considered somewhat simplistic, that is not necessarily the case, and indeed many are both effective and sophisticated. A detailed description of such approaches is adequately outlined by McMillan and Wood (2017). Undoubtedly, within the rehabilitative context, behavioural approaches do place significant demands on staff resources and must be applied on a consistent basis and often over a prolonged period. The patient-related benefits to the rehabilitation team in being able to provide meaningful rehabilitation within a structured and effective behavioural protocol outweigh the necessary time given to training. For this reason, behavioural approaches are less commonly used outside specialist facilities. However, their role in postacute settings where someone is exhibiting significant levels of challenging behaviour affecting their engagement in rehabilitation should be actively considered as part of a positive behaviour support management plan.

Psychotherapy: Staff, Team and Organisational Support and Research

Psychologists in neuropsychological practice are also involved in a variety of more general clinical psychological issues. Among these is the provision of psychotherapy or counselling, which may follow one of a large variety of models and is often eclectic, addressing issues of personal loss, life changes and adjustment to disability. The psychotherapeutic techniques appropriate to neuropsychological disability are relatively underdeveloped and are associated with several specific problems, such as cognitive limitations and disorders of insight and awareness.

In light of their formative training and knowledge of social relations, as well as organisational processes, psychologists are often in a position to provide practical support to the construction, as well as ongoing 'healthy' functioning of rehabilitation teams. Bateman et al (2002) provide evidence of one approach delivered in the context of multidisciplinary teams. Staff stressors are often high in the neurorehabilitation setting, and the health and welfare of staff is important; not only as an end in itself but also because it has consequences for the care of patients, as well as critical interactions with families and carers, many of whom are in highly distressed states or enduring complex grief.

NEUROPSYCHOLOGICAL CONSEQUENCES OF NEUROLOGICAL DISORDERS

The consequences and detailed management of specific neuropsychological problems cannot be discussed in any detail within this chapter, notwithstanding Gurd et al (2010) and Goldstein & McNeil (2012) provide the reader with a detailed account. The neuropsychological consequences of neurological insult depend on several factors, not all of which are determined by the neurological aetiology (Box 24.2).

Age of Acquisition and Neuroplasticity

The age at which a lesion is acquired can also powerfully influence outcome. Previously, it was argued that the

TABLE 24.3	Sample ABC Behavioural Record			
Date/Time	A (Antecedents)	B (Behaviour)	C (Consequences)	Possible Options
May 4, 2022 8:30 a.m.	Two staff were with J helping him to get washed and dressed before breakfast	J started shouting at S (nurse) and then attempted to hit L (physio) as we were standing him from his wheelchair	I told J to 'stop shouting' and helped J to return to sitting in his wheelchair	Discuss with other team members regarding alternatives Inform J about care task and how he can be involved Ignore shouting Temporarily withdraw and return to J when he is calmer Establish reward for J when he does not shout or is not attempting to hit out at staff

developing brain's 'plasticity' could actively support an alternative brain region to assume cognitive functions previously destined to be located within the lesion area. This hypothesis has not been supported in all contexts, particularly where critical structures have been entirely ablated. In addition, neuroplasticity has been found to extend well beyond childhood and adolescence (DeFlna et al 2009, Hoffman & Harrison 2009). In this context, the role of neurogenesis in individual patient outcomes has become increasingly recognised. From a theoretical perspective, Robertson and Murre (1999) critically posited a key role for Hebbian learning, that is, the relative strengthening of neuronal connections and structured guided recovery where a particular cognitive domain is at least partly spared after brain insult.

Focal Versus Diffuse

Focal circumscribed lesions result in quite different effects from lesions which diffusely affect the cerebral cortex. Specific neuropsychological deficits of cognitive function are generally associated with relatively focal lesions (after trauma, cerebral tumour or neurosurgical resection). By way of contrast, diffuse lesions (after infections, generalised degeneration or severe TBI) tend to affect level of consciousness, processing speed, attention, motivation and initiation and affect, rather than specific neurocognitive functions.

Acute Versus Chronic

Acute lesions have greater effects than chronic lesions. After the acute lesion acquisition, there is likely to be widespread disruption of neurocognitive functions, together with changes in the level of consciousness, confusion and loss of orientation. Amnesia is common in the acute period, and the duration of posttraumatic amnesia before the restoration of continuous memory remains a good clinical indicator of injury severity even in the absence of clinical imaging findings. In the context of TBI, most improvements in neurocognitive functioning occur within the first 6–12 months with further improvements occurring over the next few years (Lezak et al 2012, Ponsford 1995).

Progressive Versus Static

Cerebral lesions (tumour growth or degenerative condition) that develop over time are likely to exert a greater deleterious impact than lesions that are static after a period of acute trauma. The former requires the cerebral cortex to continue to adapt and recompensate for structural changes.

Within progressive lesions, those that develop more rapidly generally cause more marked cognitive disruption than those which develop more slowly. This effect is seen most clearly in the case of tumours, where slow-growing tumours such as meningiomas have much less effect than more rapidly growing tumours such as gliomas. Historically, clinicians have observed that meningiomas can grow to a considerable size before they cause sufficient interference with cognitive function to come to neurosurgical attention, whereas among more aggressive tumours, a smaller but rapid multiplying lesion can give rise to notable cognitive and neurobehavioural consequences. By way of contrast, for those with benign acoustic neuromas, managed by stereotactic radiosurgery, the cognitive and quality of life outcomes are not necessarily bleak. Although subjective cognitive complaints can be linked with lower reported quality of life (Brownlee et al 2022).

Site and Lateralisation

The site is obviously of relevance in the case of a focal lesion and will determine the neuropsychological consequences within the principle of relative localisation. Lateralisation, whether the lesion is primarily located in the left or right hemisphere of the cerebral cortex, is also of relevance because the cognitive functions assumed by the two hemispheres are known to differ. There is a large and growing body of literature on cerebral lateralisation which is beyond the scope of this chapter. The clearest example of lateralisation is that of speech, which is exclusively located in the left hemisphere of about 95% of right-handed individuals (Kolb & Whishaw 2003).

An overview of neuropsychological deficits related to common conditions is presented in the next section. It is not possible to describe the management of neuropsychological problems in each condition. The reader is referred to Greenwood et al (2003), who address cognitive and behavioural problems arising in the context of neurological rehabilitation for common conditions.

Traumatic Brain Injury

TBI is the most frequent worldwide cause of injury-related disability (Hyder et al 2007), affecting about 50 million people per annum with annual global cost of circa 400 billion US dollars (Maas et al 2017). In high-income economies, falls among the elderly population are an increasing cause. Although overall, TBI affects young males, mostly as a result of road traffic accidents or assaults, more than any other group, and effective holistic intervention(s) can result in favourable outcomes. Head injuries range from very mild to very severe and profound, with dramatic differences in the neurobehavioural sequelae up to and including those in DOC. The lesions associated with head injury are generally focal or multifocal and static. Essentially, acceleration–deceleration closed head injuries may result in widespread and diffuse lesions across the cortex. In particular, even apparently very mild head injuries associated with a brief period of concussion may sometimes have significant cognitive and emotional consequences in terms of anxiety, depression, changes in personality and subtle disorders of processing speed, attention and memory, with consequent effects upon occupational role performance, social activity and personal relationships (see Table 24.4 for common neuropsychological symptoms after TBI). Helpfully, Silverberg et al (2020) provide a recent synthesis of practice guidelines for the management of concussion and mild TBI.

Stroke

Stroke illness occurs more commonly in older adults. The effects of strokes and other cerebrovascular accidents will depend on the area and proportion of the arterial distribution which is damaged or disrupted, ranging from the whole territory of one of the main cerebral arteries, which

is a substantial proportion of the cortex, down to relatively discrete focal lesions associated with a distal portion of one of these arteries. Wilson (2009) provides an overview of the functional and neuropsychological consequences of stroke which depend primarily on the area of cortex affected. However, the clinical presentation can be complicated by the occurrence of further, perhaps minor, strokes that prevent the psychological condition from being stable and by associated arterial disease, which may result in restricted blood supply to the entire cortex (see Table 24.5 for common neuropsychological symptoms poststroke).

Hypoxic Brain Injury

After hypoxic/anoxic injury which can occur in association with TBI or separately after cardiac/respiratory arrest or carbon monoxide poisoning, the pattern of cognitive deficits is dependent on the nature and duration of the period of loss or reduction of cerebral blood supply. The neuropathology associated with hypoxic/anoxic injury is often widespread involving the basal ganglia, thalamus, white matter projections and diffuse cortical areas (Anderson & Arciniegas 2010). Acquired deficits can include ataxia, extrapyramidal symptoms, 'mental slowness', memory problems, a combination of memory and executive difficulties, dysarthria, dyspraxia, naming difficulties, impaired

---

TABLE 24.4 Common Symptoms After Traumatic Brain Injury (Wilson 2009)

Postconcussional Symptoms	Mild-to-Moderate TBI (GCS: mild = 13–15; moderate = 9–12)	Severe TBI (GCS < 8 for 6+ hours)
• Dizziness & vestibular disturbance • Persistent headaches • Reduced stamina • Fatigue/sleep disturbance • Noise/light sensitivity • Blurred/double vision • Tinnitus • Slowed thinking • Reduced concentration • Poor memory	• Impaired speed of processing (thinking speed) • Poor divided attention • Poor memory • Reduced 'frustrative' tolerance • Low mood (depression) • Marked anxiety • Posttraumatic stress disorder	• Reduced speed of thought/information processing • Overall decline in intellectual functioning • Difficulties with word finding and sentence construction • Impaired divided attention and marked distractibility • Limited concentration • Poor memory and new learning ability • Reduced independent planning, problem solving and reasoning • Reduced or total lack of initiation • Poor self-regulation (verbal, physical or sexual disinhibition) • Mood swings, irritability • Limited insight or awareness of their acquired neurological deficits

Severity levels are from Campbell (2004, p. 106).
GCS, Glasgow Coma Scale; *TBI*, traumatic brain injury.

visual recognition including agnosia (inability to recognise objects) and prosopagnosia (inability to recognise faces), as well as altered attentional control. A recent systematic literature review by Brownlee et al (2020) provides a useful overview of commonly observed cognitive deficits after hypoxia. Critically, as Hopkins et al (2005) have argued that it is loss of tissue volume rather than aetiology per se which dictates the extent of cognitive deficits.

Covid-19

In late 2019 a new virus was recognised, namely SARS-CoV-19 (Covid-19), which can affect multiple organs including the central nervous system. Covid-19 follows on from previous respiratory viral infections such as SARS (in 2002) and MERS (in 2012) which have been associated with known neurological symptoms and cognitive dysfunction. Initially the robustness of studies involving Covid-19 patients varied widely. Over time, strong evidence of brain-related changes after Covid-19 infection has become clear. Indeed, Douaud et al (2022) in a longitudinal UK Biobank study identified changes in those who tested positive for Covid-19 in the orbitofrontal cortex, parahippocampal gyrus, primary olfactory cortex and global brain size relative to available pre-illness imaging. With regard

TABLE 24.5	Common Cognitive and Behavioural Deficits After Stroke (Wilson 2009)		
Arterial Lesion	**Observed Deficits**	**Assessment**	**Rehabilitation Strategies**
ACA	Severe hemiplegia sensory loss (affected lower limb)	Neurological examination Somatosensory examination	Limb care and positioning Facilitated movement repetitive training
ACA damage to supplementary motor area	Poor initiation/control of voluntary movement Limited speech Ideomotor apraxia (disorder of skilled voluntary movements)	Ability to follow verbal or gestural commands Assess ability to demonstrate actions on request	Errorless learning (hand-overhand facilitation to shape series of movement(s) in sequence
ACA mesial/orbital frontal areas	Personality change Apathy Marked disinhibition	Use patient and family interviews and self-report measures	Information to family members and staff Structure environment to minimise opportunities for disinhibited behaviour
Anterior communicating artery aneurysms	Acute/chronic confusion Impaired memory and new learning Confabulation (includes events or details in conversation which have not occurred)	Orientation Ability to recall new information Safety awareness Route finding	Supervision Provide environmental cues Structure activity Minimise risks for wandering, e.g., alarms/sensor switches
MCA	Contralesional hemiplegia Visual field loss Global dysphasia (DOM) Unilateral neglect (disorder of visuospatial awareness usually NON-DOM)	Visual fields testing Tests for neglect and sustained attention (concentration)	Establish level of comprehension and awareness Promote use of neglected side via visual/auditory cues, positioning of therapy tasks, use of prism lenses
Superior MCA	Upper limb and facial paresis Poor expression Poor speech prosody (deficit in rate of speech) Ideomotor apraxia (DOM) Unilateral neglect (NON-DOM)	Ability to copy movements via instruction or gesture Personal and extrapersonal neglect tests (Comb-Razor Test, Line Cancellation, Star Cancellation, etc.)	Repetitive practice Intensive SLT programme involving shaping of speech sounds Affected limb activation

(Continued)

TABLE 24.5   Common Cognitive and Behavioural Deficits After Stroke (Wilson 2009)—Cont'd

Arterial Lesion	Observed Deficits	Assessment	Rehabilitation Strategies
Inferior MCA	Homonymous hemianopia (deficit of nasal and temporal visual field on same side of hemiplegia) Receptive understanding Dysgraphia (problems with writing) Dyscalculia (DOM problems with numbers) Unilateral neglect Anosognosia (lack of awareness of illness) Constructional and dressing dyspraxia Agitation (NON-DOM)	Visual fields testing Pen and paper neglect tests Interview and self-report measures to establish level of awareness/insight Copying gestures, use of objects Interview – identify possible sources of agitation	Advice to visually scan into affected visual field Establish mode of communication Establish 'real-life' use of memory via errorless learning Use compensatory aids Visual scanning training and limb activation Directive feedback to patient and family Provide opportunities to learn and adapt to acquired deficits Frequent practice using shaping of affected limb Commence ABC behavioural records
PCA	Cortical blindness (total or partial loss of vision with intact pupil response to light) Confusion Impaired memory Poor shape, size and colour perception Ability to perceive moving but not static objects	Visual fields testing Orientation Ability to recall new information Visuospatial/ visuoperceptual assessments such as Cortical Vision Screening Test (CORVIST; James et al 2001), the Visual Object and Space Perception Battery (VOSPB; Warrington & James 1991)	Establish level of visual field deficit and patient awareness Consistently orientate to task/ activity Organise environment to minimise real-life perceptual difficulties
PCA (DOM)	Alexia without agraphia (impaired ability to read but not write) Visual agnosia (impaired ability to identify objects)	Pencil and paper tasks of writing and reading prose Able to identify and use common and uncommon objects	Consider talking books Consider use of visual markers or anchors placed on commonly used objects Provide opportunities to learn and adapt to acquired deficits
PCA (NON-DOM)	Unilateral neglect Constructional dyspraxia Agitation/confusion	Visual fields testing Pen and paper neglect tests Tests for dyspraxia	Establish level of visual field deficit and patient awareness Consistently orientate to task/ activity Organise environment to minimise real-life perceptual difficulties

ABC, Antecedents, behaviours, consequences; *ACA*, anterior cerebral artery; *DOM*, dominant; *MCA*, middle cerebral artery; *NON DOM*, nondominant; *PCA*, posterior cerebral artery; *SLT*, speech and language therapist.

to the cognitive sequelae of Covid-19, Rogers et al (2021) in a meta-analysis of 147 studies noted common symptom complaints including anosmia, weakness, dysgeusia, fatigue, depression, headache, anxiety and altered mental status. Principal cognitive complaints included 'brain fog', impaired memory and attention. Although not definitive, the need for long-term monitoring and follow-up for those presenting with long Covid-19 symptoms in keeping with past outbreaks is clearly indicated. At this time, the long-term health, well-being, economic and societal impact of this worldwide pandemic remain evident and ongoing.

Degenerative Conditions

Interest in the degenerative conditions from a neuropsychological perspective has grown in recent years. In addition to dementia of the Alzheimer's type, which is clearly associated with deficits of cognitive function of a progressive nature, there are several other degenerative conditions which occur in adult life. Over the past 30 years, the neuropsychological consequences are increasingly better understood. Multiple sclerosis (MS), Parkinson's, Huntington's disease and motor neurone disease, sometimes referred to collectively as the 'subcortical dementias', are all associated with cognitive, affective and neurobehavioural deficits in a significant proportion of those with the disease, and almost all of those whose disease progresses to an advanced stage suffer neurocognitive and emotional sequelae. Disorders of memory, attention and affect are common as primary consequences of the disease in this group, and there are naturally significant psychological disturbances associated with being a sufferer of one of these diseases. Ferreira (2010) provides a detailed description of cognitive deficits in MS, and Mitolo et al (2015) review the literature with regard to evidence-based cognitive remediation in people with MS.

Spinal Injuries

Spinal cord injury clearly differs from other neurological conditions in that the patient has suffered a disabling condition, but all neural systems supporting psychological functions are intact. However, this working assumption does not hold for persons after significant polytrauma. In practice, the main issue after spinal cord injury is one of adjustment, both in terms of the primary impairment dependent on the level of spinal cord lesion and the secondary consequences of acquired functional restrictions that follow from the disability. Among the primary disabilities are loss of mobility and other functional capacities (especially if the upper limbs are affected), together with loss of bladder and bowel control, and, most importantly for psychological health, sexual function may also be affected. Depression is common after spinal injury, and the facilitation of insight and adjustment to the disability is a primary task for the psychologist working as an integral part of the rehabilitation team.

Neuropsychological Disorders of Movement

Memory for motor acts, and in particular motor skills, has been shown to be distinct from memory for semantic or episodic information. It is noteworthy that even patients with a dense global amnesia may retain the ability to perform previously learned motor skills. This capacity to acquire new motor skills may be less impaired than their ability to learn new semantic information or recall recent events. Although disorders of motor memory and motor skills are much less well researched than other aspects of memory, it is worth noting that even a serious impairment of memory will not necessarily prevent the learning of new motor tasks. Notwithstanding, it is now well established that selective damage to such structures as the cerebellum, commonly linked with coordination and movement, can give rise to cognitive and affective complaints (Balsters et al 2013, Schmahmann & Sherman 1998).

Apraxia

Apraxia refers to disorders of voluntary movement in the absence of sensory loss, paresis or motor weakness, which is commonly observed when the patient is asked to respond to a command or to produce an action outside its normal context. It is therefore probably the intentional aspects of the task that are the root of the problem. A distinction is often drawn between ideomotor and ideational apraxia. Ideomotor apraxia is a disorder affecting the ability to produce simple gestures either on command or by imitation, while the ability to perform more complex tasks may be largely intact; that is, the patient knows what to do but not how to do it. By contrast, ideational apraxia refers to the inability to perform actions that require a well-ordered sequence of elements. Although this is an important distinction in the literature, there remains debate about the absolute distinction between these two conditions. Both conditions are primarily associated with lesions in the posterior cortical regions, especially the parietal lobe, and in the dominant usually left hemisphere. Typically for both conditions, relevant behaviour(s) may be performed without difficulty in everyday life relative to when conscious attention is directed to the task. Dressing apraxia has been regarded as an independent form of apraxia, but there is some reason to believe that it is only the difficulty of this particular task which involves the integration of body elements with external space, and complex personal movements in relation to highly plastic objects that make it appear a distinct entity. Constructional apraxia is, however, a distinct type and involves a deficit in the spatial aspects of a task in relation to individual motor movements. The problem appears to lie in the integration of visuospatial information and voluntary motor acts, and may be apparent in drawing or in the construction of three-dimensional models. The disorder is also associated with lesions of the parietal cortex, and some have argued that it may take a different form depending on whether the right hemisphere affecting visuospatial perception or the left hemisphere affecting motor execution is damaged.

Neglect

Unilateral visual neglect, or unilateral hemi-inattention, has attracted considerable research interest in recent decades. It affects at least 30% of stroke patients in the acute setting (Hammerbeck et al 2019). Patients with this disorder essentially act as if one side of space, commonly their left side after right frontoparietal lesion(s), does not exist or is not internally attend to. This disorder can occur in the absence of any visual field defect. In extreme cases the patient may eat food on only the right half of their plate, dress the right side of their body and attend to right-sided visual events. It can occur in relation to imagined scenes as to real stimuli. There is still considerable debate about whether the problem is one of disordered internal representations or one of attentional deficit. It seems clear, however, that patients have some semantic access to the information appearing in the neglected space, but this information does not enter consciousness or direct behaviour. Longley et al (2021) provide a recent Cochrane review of nonpharmacological rehabilitation approaches to neglect which indicates a limited evidence base for a range of interventions in terms of persistent improvements in activities of daily living as well as neglect assessment measures.

Functional Disorders

No account of the management of physical and cognitive disorders in neurorehabilitation can overlook the not insignificant proportion of patients who present with a range of physical symptoms unexplained by organic pathology (see Chapter 16 for a more detailed overview). It is now well established that approximately one-third of neurology outpatients have symptom complaints, including gait disturbance, weakness and sensory disturbance, cognitive complaints that are not explained by organic disease profiles (Carson et al 2011). Moreover, Carson et al (2011) in a large cohort study showed that patients presenting with such symptoms relative to those with medically explained neurological symptoms had poorer physical health statuses, elevated levels of distress and were more likely to be unemployed and/or in receipt of disability benefits. Within the United Kingdom, the term commonly adopted to denote such physical symptoms is *functional motor disorders* (FMDs). It is known that most physiotherapists in

UK clinical practice see and treat such patients (Edwards et al 2012). Nielsen et al (2015) have developed multidisciplinary consensus recommendations which seek to frame the delivery of physiotherapy and psychological support to such patients, and special interest groups for clinicians and researchers have been formed. Currently, most treatment approaches draw on a biopsychosocial framework. Nielsen et al (2015) provide an overview of a wide range of biopsychosocial variables which may contribute to patient presentation. Treating therapists and clinicians should be aware of the range of possible contributing proximal and distal psychosocial factors which may influence patient engagement and outcome. At present, therapy intervention including information giving and psychoeducation, recruitment and demonstration of normal movement capacity, and movement retraining including overt or covert distraction may be delivered either before or in conjunction with tailored psychotherapy. Regrettably, to date there are a limited number of high-quality studies involving patients with FMDs, although Nielsen et al (2013) in a systematic review did identify some promising findings for physiotherapy input. Notwithstanding, additional larger well-designed treatment trials involving IDT input are required.

PROCESS OF REHABILITATION

Neuropsychologists generally work within an IDT, particularly in rehabilitation settings. They should contribute to the team not only by their support but also by effectively playing the appropriate multidisciplinary role within the team. Observation of the patient and the IDT in the rehabilitation and care environment, to inform best practice and treatment strategies, is essential in the effective provision of care. This affords opportunity for ongoing discussion, learning, support and evaluation of patient, IDT and carer interactions, which is a key component of tailored rehabilitation of patients with complex neurodisability. A psychologist who is based within an expert and committed IDT will respect the particular contributions made by other team members. They will come to realise that it is only by the collaborative efforts of the disciplines within the team that the optimal outcome will be achieved for the patient, and that the patient will have the best chance of a good psychological adjustment to their condition and obtain the best quality of life that is possible.

CONCLUSION

Factors that influence psychological management that need to be considered include the cognitive ability and psychological adjustment of the patient and a collaborative team approach.

An important determinant of the psychological effects of neurological injury or disease is the cognitive status of the individual. Besides specific cognitive deficits, which may limit both psychological and functional adjustment to the disease, more general factors, such as attentional capacity, motivation, premorbid views and beliefs, as well as the capacity for learning and the acquisition of skills, will all contribute to the eventual outcome.

Premorbid intellectual capacity will also be a factor; it is known that the best protective factor against dementia in advanced age is to be more intelligent as an adult, and the same principle applies to all neuropsychological deficits. The more you have, the less you will be affected by a given proportional loss, and the more you have left with which to compensate. Nevertheless, those who functioned at a high intellectual level with a mentally demanding occupation before illness may also be more acutely aware of relatively subtle deficits in their ability, and this may have a disproportionate effect upon their capacity to pursue a previous occupation.

Relatively intact cognitive abilities may contribute to the ability to benefit from rehabilitation interventions, and to gain insight and consequent adjustment to the disability, although in some severely affected individuals the lack of insight and memory for what has been lost may result in an unawareness which is in some respects protective against overwhelming psychological distress, even if it cannot be regarded as psychologically healthy.

Psychological Adjustment

In summary, good long-term psychological adjustment depends on:

- Satisfactory (or at least some) insight into the events and psychological changes that have occurred and at least some intrapersonal capacity for acceptance of these changes;
- An appropriate adjustment of the perception of self;
- A capacity to modify beliefs and personal goals;
- The acquisition of appropriate strategies to compensate as far as is possible for any residual handicap or acquired cognitive deficit/decrement; and
- Organising the rehabilitation environment to optimise engagement and patient-relevant outcome.

It implies not only psychological adjustment but also the reestablishment of personal, family and social relationships, both intimate and more distant. It may also involve occupational adjustment and redefinition of personal roles in all of these contexts. This is something that the psychologist must understand and have the skills to facilitate within a variety of adapted therapeutic approaches. In addition, it should also be recognised that not all of those who acquire neurological diseases had perfect psychological adjustment

before the index injury occurred; occasionally, the personality of a patient, as perceived by those close to them, has actually been improved by the condition. Not everyone who is neurologically intact is in good psychological health, and the goal of returning the client to this state may be confounded by circumstances unrelated to the primary neurological insult.

SELF-ASSESSMENT QUESTIONS

1. What are the most common types of emotional disturbance observed after ABI?
2. What is the evidence base for cognitive interventions?
3. Outline aetiological factors which contribute to neuropsychological disability.
4. What are the key deficits after right middle cerebral artery stroke, and what assessments are commonly used?
5. What are the common deficits arising after hypoxic brain injury?
6. What cognitive factors are implicated in disorders of movement?
7. What key factors affect psychological adjustment after brain injury?

ACKNOWLEDGEMENTS

The author is grateful to Laura Wheatley-Smith, Lead Clinical Physiotherapist, Regional Acquired Brain Injury Unit (RABIU), Belfast HSC Trust for her careful review of an earlier version of this chapter.

REFERENCES

Anderson, C.A., Arciniegas, D.B., 2010. Cognitive sequelae of hypoxic-ischemic brain injury: a review. NeuroRehabilitation. 26, 47–63.

Balsters, J.H., Whelan, C.D., Robertson, I.H., Ramnani, N., 2013. Cerebellum and cognition: evidence for the encoding of higher order rules. Cereb. Cortex 23, 1433–1443.

Bateman, W., Wilson, F.C., Bingham, D., 2002. Team effectiveness – development of an audit tool. J. Manag. Dev 21, 215–226.

Bigler, E.D., 2012. Symptom validity testing, effort and neuropsychological assessment. J. Int. Neuropsychol. Soc 18, 632–642.

British Psychological Society, 2012. Competency framework for the UK Clinical Neuropsychology profession. Leicester (UK), BPS Division of Neuropsychology.

British Psychological Society, 2018. Positive Behaviour Support. Leicester (UK), BPS Division of Clinical Psychology.

Brown, R., 2012. Psychological and psychiatric aspects of brain disorder: nature, assessment and implications for clinical neuropsychology. In: Goldstein, L.H., McNeil, J.E. (Eds.), Clinical Neuropsychology: A Practical Guide to Assessment and Management for Clinicians. Wiley Blackwell, Chichester, pp. 87–104.

Brownlee, N.N.M., Wilson, F.C., Curran, D.B., Lyttle, N., McCann, J.P., 2020. Neurocognitive outcomes in adults following cerebral hypoxia: a systematic literature review. NeuroRehabilitation. 47, 83–97.

Brownlee, N., Wilson, F.C., Curran, D.B., Wright, G., Flannery, T., Caldwell, S.B., 2022. Cognitive and psychosocial outcomes following stereotactic radiosurgery for acoustic neuroma. NeuroRehabilitation. 50, 151–159.

Bunnage, M., Evans, J.J., Wright, I., et al., 2020. Guidelines to colleagues on the use of tele-neuropsychology. British Psychological Society: Division of Neuropsychology Professional Standards Unit.

Campbell, M., 2004. Acquired brain injury: trauma and pathology. In: Stokes, M. (Ed.), Physical management in neurological rehabilitation, 2nd ed. Elsevier, London, pp. 103–124.

Carson, A., Stone, J., Hibberd, C., Murray, G., Duncan, R., Coleman, R., 2011. Disability, distress and unemployment in neurology outpatients with symptoms unexplained by organic disease. J. Neurol. Neurosurg. Psychiatry. 82, 810–813.

Christensen, A.L., 1974. Luria's Neuropsychological Investigation. Munksgaard, Copenhagen.

Cicerone, K.D., Goldin, Y., Ganci, K., Rosenbaum, A., Wethe, J.V., Langenbahn, D.M., 2019. Evidence-based cognitive rehabilitation: systematic review of the literature from 2009 through 2014. Arch. Phys. Med. Rehabil. 100, 1515–1533.

Cook, L., Smith, D.S., Truman, G., 1994. Using Functional Independence Measure profiles as an index of outcome in the rehabilitation of brain-injured patients. Arch. Phys. Med. Rehabil. 75, 390–393.

Cott, C., Finch, E., 1990. Goal setting in physical therapy practice. Physiother. Can. 43, 19–22.

DeFlna, P., Fellus, J., Polito, M.Z., Thompson, J.W., Moser, R.S., DeLuca, J., 2009. The new neuroscience frontier: promoting neuroplasticity and brain repair in traumatic brain injury. Cogn. Neuropsychologist. 23, 1391–1399.

DeRight, J., Jorgensen, R.S., 2015. I just want my research credit: frequency of suboptimal effort in a non-clinical healthy undergraduate sample. Cogn. Neuropsychologist. 29, 101–117.

Douaud, G., Lee, S., Alfaro-Almargo, F., Arthofer, C., Wang, C., et al., 2022. SARS-CoV-2 is associated with changes in brain structure in UK Biobank. Nature. 604, 697–707.

Edwards, M.J., Stone, J., Nielsen, G., 2012. Physiotherapists and patients with functional (psychogenic) motor symptoms: a survey of attitudes and interest. J. Neurol. Neurosurg. Psychiatry. 83, 655–658.

Ferreira, M.L.B., 2010. Cognitive deficits in multiple sclerosis. Arq. Neuropsiquiatr. 68, 632–641.

Fleminger, S., Oliver, D.L., Williams, W.H., Evans, J., 2003. The neuropsychiatry of depression after brain injury. In: Williams, W.H., Evans, J.J. (Eds.), Biopsychosocial Approaches in Neurorehabilitation. Psychology Press, Hove, pp. 65–87.

Goldstein, L.H., McNeil, J.E., 2012. Clinical Neuropsychology: A Practical Guide to Assessment and Management, 2nd ed. Wiley Blackwell, Chichester.

Greenwood, R., et al., 2003. In: Greenwood, R., Barnes, M.P., McMillan, T.M. (Eds.), Handbook of Neurological Rehabilitation. Psychology Press, London.

Gurd, J., Kischka, U., Marshall, J., 2010. The Handbook of Clinical Neuropsychology, 2nd ed. Oxford University Press, Oxford.

Hammerbeck, U., Gittins, M., Vail, A., Paley, L., Tyson, S.F., Bowen, A., 2019. Spatial neglect in stroke: identification, disease process and association with outcome during inpatient rehabilitation. Brain. Sci. 9, 1–10.

Hoffman, S.W., Harrison, C., 2009. The interaction between psychological health and traumatic brain injury: a neuroscience perspective. Cogn Neuropsychologist. 23, 1400–1415.

Hokkanen, L., Lettner, S., Barbosa, F., et al., 2019. Training models and status of clinical neuropsychologists in Europe: results of a survey of 30 countries. Clin. Neuropsychol. 33, 32–56.

Hokkanen, L., Barbosa, F., Ponchel, A., et al., 2020. Clinical neuropsychology as a specialist profession in European health care: developing a benchmark for training standards and competencies using the Europsy model? Front. Psychol. 11, 559134.

Hopkins, R., Tate, D., Bigler, E., 2005. Anoxic versus traumatic brain injury: amount of tissue loss, not etiology, alters cognitive and emotional function. Neuropsychology. 19, 233–242.

Hyder, A.A., Wunderlich, C.A., Puvanachandra, P., Gururaj, G., Kobusingye, O.C., 2007. The impact of traumatic brain injury: a global perspective. Neurorehabilitation. 22, 341–353.

James, M., Plant, G.T., Warrington, E.K., 2001. Cortical Vision Screening Test. Thames Valley Test Company, Bury St. Edmunds (UK).

Kitaigorodsky, M., Loewenstein, D., Curiel Cid, R., Crocco, E., Gorman, K., Gonzalez-Jimenez, C., 2021. A teleneuropsychology protocol for the cognitive assessment of older adults during COVID-19. Front. Psychol. 12, 651136.

Kolb, B., Whishaw, I.Q., 2003. Fundamentals of Human Neuropsychology, 5th ed. WH Freeman and Co, New York.

Lezak, M.D., Howieson, D.B., Bigler, E.D., Loring, D.W., 2012. Neuropsychological Assessment, 5th ed. Oxford University Press, New York.

Longley, V., Hazelton, C., Heal, C., et al., 2021. Non-pharmacological interventions for spatial neglect or inattention following stroke and other non-progressive brain injury. Cochrane. Database. Syst. Rev. 7, CD003586

Maas, A.I.R., Menon, D.K., Adelson, P.D., et al., 2017. Traumatic brain injury: integrated approaches to improve prevention, clinical care, and research. Lancet. Neurol. 16, 987–1048.

McMillan, T.M., Wood, R.L.I., 2017. Neurobehavioural Disability and Social Handicap Following Traumatic Brain Injury, 2nd ed. Taylor & Francis, London.

Mitolo, M., Venneri, A., Wilkinson, I.D., Sharrack, B., 2015. Cognitive rehabilitation in multiple sclerosis: a systematic review. J. Neurol. Sci. 354, 1–9.

Nielsen, G., Stone, J., Edwards, M.J., 2013. Physiotherapy for functional (psychogenic) motor symptoms: a systematic review. J. Psychosom. Res. 75, 93–102.

Nielsen, G., Stone, J., Matthews, A., Brown, M., Sparkes, C., Farmer, R., 2015. Physiotherapy for functional motor disorders: a consensus recommendation. J. Neurol. Neurosurg. Psychiatry. 86, 1113–1119.

Oddy, M., Ramos, S., da Silva, 2013. The clinical and cost-benefits of investing in neurobehavioural rehabilitation: a multi-centre study. Brain. Inj. 27, 1500–1507.

Ponsford, J., 1995. Traumatic Brain Injury; Rehabilitation for Everyday Adaptive Living. Psychology Press, Hove.

Robertson, I.H., Murre, J.M.P., 1999. Rehabilitation of brain damage: brain plasticity and principle of guided recovery. Psychol. Bull. 125, 544–575.

Rogers, J.P., Watson, C.J., Badenoch, J., et al., 2021. Neurology and neuropsychiatry of COVID-19: a systematic review and meta-analysis of the early literature reveals frequent CNS manifestations and key emerging narratives. J. Neurol. Neurosurg. Psychiatry. 92, 932–941.

Schmahmann, J.D., Sherman, J.C., 1998. The cerebellar cognitive affective syndrome. Brain. 121, 561–579.

Silverberg, N.D., Iaccarino, M.A., Panenka, W.J., et al., 2020. Management of concussion and mild traumatic brain injury: a synthesis of practice guidelines. Arch. Phys. Med. Rehabil. 101, 382–393.

Strauss, E.A., Sherman, E.M.S., Spreen, O., 2006. A Compendium of Neuropsychological Tests: Administration, Norms and Commentary, 3rd ed. Oxford University Press, New York.

Turner-Stokes, L., Disler, R., Williams, H., 2007. The rehabilitation complexity scale: a simple, practical tool to identify 'complex specialised' services in neurological rehabilitation. Clin. Med. 7, 593–599.

Turner-Stokes, L., Williams, H., Bill, A., Bassett, P., Sephton, K., 2016. Cost-efficiency of specialist inpatient rehabilitation for working aged adults with complex neurological disabilities: a multi-centre cohort analysis of a national clinical data set. BMJ Open. 6, e010238.

Wade, D.T., 1992. The Barthel ADL Index: Guidelines. In: Wade, D.T. (Ed.), Measurement in Neurological Rehabilitation. Oxford University Press, Oxford, pp. 177–178.

Warrington, E.K., James, M., 1991. The Visual Object and Space Perception Battery. Thames Valley Test Company, Bury St Edmunds.

Wilson, B.A., 2004. Management and remediation of memory problems in brain-injured adults. In: Baddeley, A.D., Kopelman, M.D., Wilson, B.A. (Eds.), The Essential Handbook of Memory Disorders for Clinicians. John Wiley & Sons, Chichester, pp. 199–226.

Wilson, F.C., 2009. Cognitive perceptual considerations. In: Lennon, S., Stokes, M. (Eds.), Pocketbook of Neurological Physiotherapy. Churchill Livingstone, London.

Wilson, B.A., Herbert, C.M., Shiel, A., 2003a. Behavioural Approaches in Neuropsychological Rehabilitation – Optimising Rehabilitation Procedures. Taylor & Francis, East Sussex.

Wilson, F.C., Harpur, J., Watson, T., Morrow, J.I., 2003b. Adult survivors of severe cerebral hypoxia – case series survey and comparative analysis. Neurorehabilitation. 18, 291–298.

25

Selected Topics in Physical Management for Neurological Conditions

Liesbet De Baets, Stephen Ashford, Hannes Devos, Abiodun E. Akinwuntan, Joseph Buttell, Camilla Erwee, Alexandra Henson, Prue Morgan, and Carlee Holmes

OUTLINE

Introduction, 628
Musculoskeletal Integration in Neurological Upper Limb Approach — Movement And Muscle Activation of the Shoulder Complex After Stroke: A Musculoskeletal View on Poststroke Shoulder Assessment and Rehabilitation, 628
Evaluation of the Shoulder Complex From a Musculoskeletal Viewpoint, 629
Normal Kinematics of the Shoulder Complex, 629
Shoulder Kinematics After Stroke, 629
Normal Muscle Timing at the Shoulder Complex, 630
Muscle Timing at the Shoulder Complex After Stroke, 631
Clinical Scapular Protocol, 631
Musculoskeletal Management of Shoulder Complex Dysfunctions After Stroke, 635
Motor Control Training, 635
Neuroplasticity and Timing of Motor Control Training in Individuals With Stroke, 635
Illustration by Means of a Case Presentation, 636
Summary, 636
Spasticity: When and How to Treat the Clinical Problem in Neurological Rehabilitation, 637
Upper Motor Neurone Syndrome, 637
Spasticity, 638
Principles of Management, 639
Clinical Case Illustration, 639
Physical and Pharmacological Treatment, 639
Clinical Case Illustration, 640
Evaluation of Outcome, 641
Clinical Case Illustration, 643
Summary, 643

On the Road With Multiple Sclerosis – Challenges in Screening, Assessment and Training of Driving, 643
Driving as an Important Instrumental Activity of Daily Living, 643
Aspects of the Driving Evaluation Process, 644
Fitness-to-Drive Legislation, 644
Screening, 645
Assessment, 645
Intervention, 646
Case Presentation, 647
Consultation, 647
Screening, 647
Assessment, 647
Interpretation of Driving Evaluation Results, 649
Driving Training Programme, 649
Posttraining Assessment, 649
Summary, 649
Physical Management of People with Prolonged Disorder of Consciousness – Disability Management, Ethics and Legal Frameworks, 649
Introduction, 649
What Is a Disorder of Consciousness?, 650
How Is Rehabilitation Different for People in PDOC?, 650
Legal and Ethical Considerations, 651
Management from the Acute Setting to the Community, 651
Acute Phase, 651
Rehabilitation Phase, 652
Transition of Care – Community Phase, 652
Case Study – Sarah, 653

Stimulation and Responsiveness, 653
  Oral Care, 653
    Postural Management, 654
    Swallowing, 654
    Nutrition, 654
    Outcomes, 654
    Summary, 654
Adults With Cerebral Palsy, 654
  Introduction, 654
  Classification Systems, 655
  Childhood Management, 655

Transition From Paediatric to Adult Health
    Services, 657
  Age-Related Health Issues in Adults With CP, 657
Case Study, 659
  Assessment of Kellie's Neuromuscular and Postural
    Status, 659
  Measures of Posture, 659
  Measures of Spasticity, Pain and Skin Integrity, 659
  Management Strategies, 662
  Case Summary, 662
  Summary, 662

INTRODUCTION

Patients with neurological conditions are frequently considered complex cases because of the diversity of symptoms with which they present. Throughout this book, general physical management principles have been presented in detail for a wide variety of neurological pathologies. This chapter will focus on five additional topics, with a theoretical background section and case study presentation, implementing theoretical constructs into clinical care. Firstly, the neurological upper limb approach from a musculoskeletal perspective will be discussed because therapists with a focus on neurorehabilitation tend to neglect integrating different physical management domains into the clinical care of a patient. This section describes a musculoskeletal approach for a common clinical phenomenon: poststroke shoulder pain. Secondly, spasticity and spasticity management are revisited because, although not necessarily neglected in clinical practice, the topic is not universally addressed in the same manner despite the evidence base in this area of practice. The multidisciplinary approach required is highlighted and presented as part of an overall management strategy and treatment selection process. Thirdly, the concept of driving with neurological conditions is covered, highlighting the need for, again, a multidisciplinary approach in what is for most of us a common, basic activity of daily living. As one can imagine, the decision for a patient to refrain from driving has life-changing consequences, but this part presents a driving evaluation process and rehabilitation perspective to consider driving as a regular part of the physical management for neurological conditions. Fourthly, the physical management for people with prolonged disorders of consciousness will be discussed because this is a group of patients requiring a specific approach compared with more regularly seen patients in rehabilitation wards and private practices. Attention will also be given to the important ethical guidelines and legislation. Finally, we present a relatively new domain in neurological management: adults with cerebral palsy. Individuals

with developmental disabilities such as cerebral palsy experience unique challenges associated with lifelong neuromuscular dysfunction. Although once considered exclusively a 'paediatric' condition, many people living with cerebral palsy are adults. This section describes potential impairments and activity limitations to consider in a comprehensive lifespan assessment and management of the adult with cerebral palsy to enhance participation outcomes.

MUSCULOSKELETAL INTEGRATION IN NEUROLOGICAL UPPER LIMB APPROACH — MOVEMENT AND MUSCLE ACTIVATION OF THE SHOULDER COMPLEX AFTER STROKE: A MUSCULOSKELETAL VIEW ON POSTSTROKE SHOULDER ASSESSMENT AND REHABILITATION

Liesbet De Baets

A proper and pain-free shoulder function is important for accurate performance of daily activities and contributes to daily life autonomy and quality of life. At the level of the shoulder complex, poststroke motor impairments such as muscle weakness, increased muscle tone, pathological muscle synergies and altered temporal muscle activity may specifically hamper scapulohumeral control (Frontera et al 1997, McComas et al 1973), that is, the adaptation of scapular position and movement according to the humeral position. This altered scapular control might impede optimal upper limb function (De Baets et al 2016a, 2016b).

Most pathologies or functional impairments around the shoulder do not originate from bony disorders but rather from soft tissue disturbances. These exist in the form of inflexibility, like tightness in muscles or capsular structures around the shoulder girdle or intrinsic muscle pathology within the subacromial space (e.g., supraspinatus tendinopathy) (Kibler et al 2012). Accurate assessment of scapular movements and key scapulothoracic and scapulohumeral musculature (m. trapezius, m. serratus anterior, rotator cuff) and their relation to upper extremity function is crucial to gain a deeper understanding of pathologies and impairments of the shoulder in individuals with stroke. These insights are considered the foundation to design or optimise treatment strategies for enhancing shoulder and upper limb function in individuals with stroke.

Evaluation of the Shoulder Complex From a Musculoskeletal Viewpoint

Currently available clinical measurement scales for stroke are typically limited to a global upper limb assessment (Baker et al 2011). However, a painful poststroke shoulder can be attributable to painful underlying musculoskeletal structures, which should be specifically assessed. It is accepted that abnormal joint torques caused by spastic muscles induce abnormal joint forces, leading to pain within the musculoskeletal system. Abnormal joint alignment, movement patterns and muscle activation patterns of the shoulder complex through mechanisms including muscle weakness and loss of voluntary motor control might additionally induce pain in musculoskeletal structures. Earlier mentioned changes negatively influence the stability of the shoulder complex and can thereby contribute to the development of musculoskeletal shoulder pain conditions (e.g., tendinopathy of the rotator cuff, subluxation of the humeral head, adhesive capsulitis).

Normal Kinematics of the Shoulder Complex

In the evaluation of movement patterns of the shoulder complex, specific attention should be paid towards movements occurring at the scapulothoracic and glenohumeral joint. To interpret the observed movements, knowledge of normal movement patterns as described later is essential.

Movement at the scapulothoracic joint results from the combination of movement in the sternoclavicular and acromioclavicular joints. Scapulothoracic lateral rotation at full arm elevation is the combination of clavicular elevation in the sternoclavicular joint and lateral rotation of the scapula in the acromioclavicular joint (Ludewig et al 2009). Scapulothoracic posterior tilting is predominantly a tilting movement in the acromioclavicular joint, with only little contribution from retraction in the sternoclavicular joint (Ludewig et al 2009, Sahara et al 2006). Late in the elevation range, the clavicula also rotates posteriorly because of a tensioned coracoclavicular ligament, which furthermore contributes to the posterior tilting of the scapula in the scapulothoracic joint (Ludewig et al 2004). No consensus is reached in literature on scapulothoracic protraction or retraction during arm elevation. Scapulothoracic protraction/retraction is furthermore minimal before 100° of arm elevation (Ludewig et al 2009, McClure et al 2001) (Fig. 25.1).

In the glenohumeral joint, abduction/adduction, forwards flexion/extension and internal/external rotation are the three degrees of freedom. During arm elevation, the humerus rotates externally (Ludewig et al 2009) (see Fig. 25.1).

Angular positions of the clavicula and scapula at resting posture, with the arm at the side, have also been described. In the sternoclavicular joint, retraction, elevation and very little posterior rotation are reported. In the acromioclavicular, as well as scapulothoracic, joint the scapular resting posture is in protraction, lateral rotation and anterior tilt (Ludewig et al 2009).

Although an agreement on the direction of movement during arm elevation is reached for most joints of the shoulder complex, large variations in absolute degrees or in normal ranges of movement have been reported. These variations are attributable to differences in population samples, addition of external load and the individual's movement variability.

Shoulder Kinematics After Stroke

Given that poststroke impairments such as muscle weakness, spasticity, and/or loss of voluntary motor control adversely affect the normal position and movement of the shoulder complex, this will inadvertently affect scapular kinematics in individuals with stroke.

Niessen et al (2008) have reported increased scapulothoracic lateral rotation at the hemiplegic side in individuals with stroke with shoulder pain compared with controls, during both active and passive abduction and forwards flexion. Compared with individuals with stroke without shoulder pain, this increased scapulothoracic lateral rotation was found only during passive abduction (Niessen et al 2008). In contrast, Hardwick and Lang (2011a) found that those individuals with stroke with more shoulder pain had less scapulothoracic scapular lateral rotation during scapular plane elevation. These authors also reported a significant decreased scapulothoracic lateral rotation in individuals with stroke without shoulder pain compared with control subjects during a person-assisted forwards flexion task (Hardwick & Lang 2011b). Robertson et al (2012) showed less scapulothoracic protraction in individuals with stroke without shoulder pain compared with controls during various reaching tasks. Finally, in individuals with stroke with a low proximal arm function, increased lateral rotation at higher passive arm elevation angles was observed compared with in healthy individuals and individuals with stroke with a moderate to high arm function (De Baets et al 2016a). Individuals with stroke with a moderate proximal arm function without shoulder pain also showed increased lateral rotation, as well as scapular malpositioning and dyskinesia, and less active humeral elevation compared with high-functioning individuals with stroke and healthy control subjects (De Baets et al 2016a). In a high arm forwards flexion, less posterior tilting and more lateral rotation were

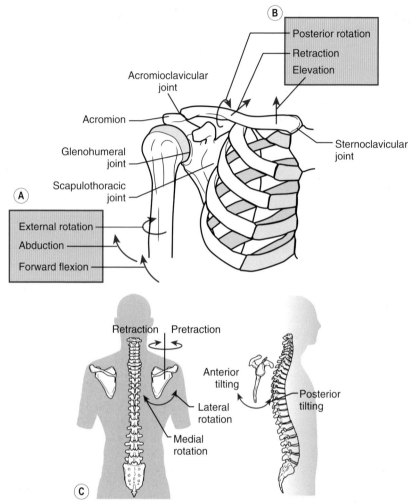

FIG. 25.1 Kinematics of the glenohumeral (A), sternoclavicular (B) and acromioclavicular (C) joints.

observed in individuals with stroke with a high proximal arm function without pain (De Baets et al 2016b).

None of the earlier mentioned studies linked the alterations in movement of the shoulder complex to changes in muscle activation patterns. However, given that the coordinated movement of the scapula relative to the thorax (i.e., scapulothoracic movement) and the scapular movement relative to the humerus (i.e., scapulohumeral rhythm) rely on the proper functioning of scapulothoracic and glenohumeral muscles (Inman et al 1996, Kibler & McMullen 2003, Kibler et al 2013), these are important to assess poststroke.

Normal Muscle Timing at the Shoulder Complex

Scapulothoracic muscles are the main contributors to correct scapulothoracic movement patterns, whereas glenohumeral muscles, such as the rotator cuff, provide the dynamic stability at the level of the glenohumeral joint. Large humerothoracic and glenohumeral muscles like pectoralis major, latissimus dorsi and deltoid subsequently provide the actual arm movement. A change in scapulothoracic, glenohumeral or humerothoracic muscle coordination can induce alterations in scapulothoracic and glenohumeral movement patterns. Deficient movement is characterised by an asynchronous pattern of muscle activation or termination. Specifically for the shoulder complex, early activation of the scapular stabilisers and a correct temporal sequence of scapular musculature in relation to prime mover activity and actual arm movement at the glenohumeral joint are essential for proper scapular position and coordinated scapulohumeral motion (Kibler 1998, Magarey & Jones 2003).

A very important scapulothoracic stabiliser is the serratus anterior muscle. The main function of the serratus anterior is to stabilise the scapula on the thorax and to furthermore work in a force couple together with upper and lower trapezius to laterally rotate the scapula. Regarding upper trapezius activity, some research suggests a link between increased upper trapezius activity and shoulder pathology (Cools et al 2014, Struyf et al 2014a), whereas others want to train upper trapezius as part of the lateral scapular rotation force couple in patients with shoulder pain (Mottram et al 2009, Pizzari et al 2014).

In persons with glenohumeral instability, Jaggi et al (2012) suggested that increased activation of pectoralis major played a role in both anterior and posterior glenohumeral instability, and that increased activation of pectoralis major played a role in anterior instability (Jaggi et al 2012). From increased pectoralis major and pectoralis major activity, it is known that they contribute to increased glenohumeral internal rotation and scapulothoracic protraction movement.

Only very recently, research focused towards more deeply lying scapulothoracic musculature, like rhomboid major, pectoralis minor and levator scapulae, which are also considered important for scapulothoracic movement but from which it is believed that they are prone to tightness and adaptive shortening, and cause muscle imbalances (Castelein et al 2015, 2016a, 2016b, 2016c, Quesnele 2011). Levator scapulae are a scapular elevator and retract the scapula together with the rhomboid major. Levator scapulae and rhomboid major additionally medially rotate the scapula (Escamilla et al 2009). As such, normal scapular lateral rotation can be hampered by shortened or hyperactive levator scapulae and rhomboid major (Behrsin & Maguire 1986). Pectoralis minor is a synergist of serratus anterior, and both contribute to the protraction of the scapula. Furthermore, pectoralis minor is responsible for anterior tilting and scapula depression and internal rotation (Oatis 2004) and might as such hinder correct posterior tilting and external rotation (Borstad & Ludewig 2005). Recent research indicated increased pectoralis minor activity in persons with subacromial impingement syndrome during arm elevation (Castelein et al 2016a). Increased muscle activity might result in adaptive shortening of the muscle, leading to an aberrant scapulothoracic position and movement. A shortened pectoralis major is already associated with abnormal scapular positioning, increased anterior tilting and internal scapular rotation (Borstad 2008, Tate et al 2012). These kinematic alterations lengthen scapular stabilisers such as lower and middle trapezius, and thereby negatively influence their stabilising function (Kibler et al 2013, McClure et al 2012, Tate et al 2012). As such, these alterations are known to lead to glenohumeral joint disorders and subacromial shoulder pain (Borstad 2008, Struyf et al 2014b, Tate et al 2012).

Muscle Timing at the Shoulder Complex After Stroke

Scapular muscle recruitment patterns in individuals after stroke with a high proximal upper limb function, but without shoulder pain, indicated early and prolonged infraspinatus activity during a high arm forwards flexion compared with controls and compared with individuals with stroke with a high proximal arm function with shoulder pain (De Baets et al 2014, 2016b). Individuals with stroke with a high proximal arm function with shoulder pain showed later activity of lower trapezius compared with high functioning individuals with stroke without shoulder pain. Serratus anterior was furthermore earlier inactive compared with control subjects and high functioning individuals with stroke without shoulder pain (De Baets et al 2014). Finally, in individuals with stroke with a moderate to high proximal arm function without shoulder pain, delayed activation and early inactivation of serratus anterior, early lower trapezius activation and late infraspinatus inactivation were reported during a low arm forwards flexion compared with healthy control subjects. In a high arm forwards flexion, less posterior tilting and more lateral rotation were observed (De Baets et al 2016b).

Clinical Scapular Protocol

A clinical scapular protocol (ClinScap) was introduced in individuals after stroke (De Baets et al 2016a). This protocol consists of five tests, with several subtests (Figs. 25.2 and 25.3), and assesses key elements of upper limb shoulder girdle poststroke.

Test 1: Observation of tilting and winging. While seated upright in a chair with lower back support, the presence (score 1) or absence (score 0) of scapular tilting and winging is scored by observing the participant's scapular position on the thorax. This scoring is done during rest (both arms alongside the body, thumbs pointing forwards) and during active unloaded forwards flexion. Individuals with stroke are instructed to move bilaterally at a rate of 3 seconds up towards their maximal forwards flexion and 3 seconds down towards the rest position. Observation is done from a dorsal and lateral position. Presence of tilting or winging indicates a prominence of the inferior tip of the scapula dorsally (tilting) or prominence of the medial scapular border (winging). Palpation is used to verify anatomical landmarks. A total score is calculated for observation at rest and for observation during movement. Score 0 indicates no presence of tilting or winging, score 1 the presence of tilting or winging, and score 2 the presence of both tilting and winging.

Test 2: Shoulder girdle position. Three different measures are used to evaluate the participant's shoulder girdle position. Acromial index (AI): This index is assessed with the patient lying supine, the arms relaxed alongside the body with the palms placed on the table. The patient is instructed

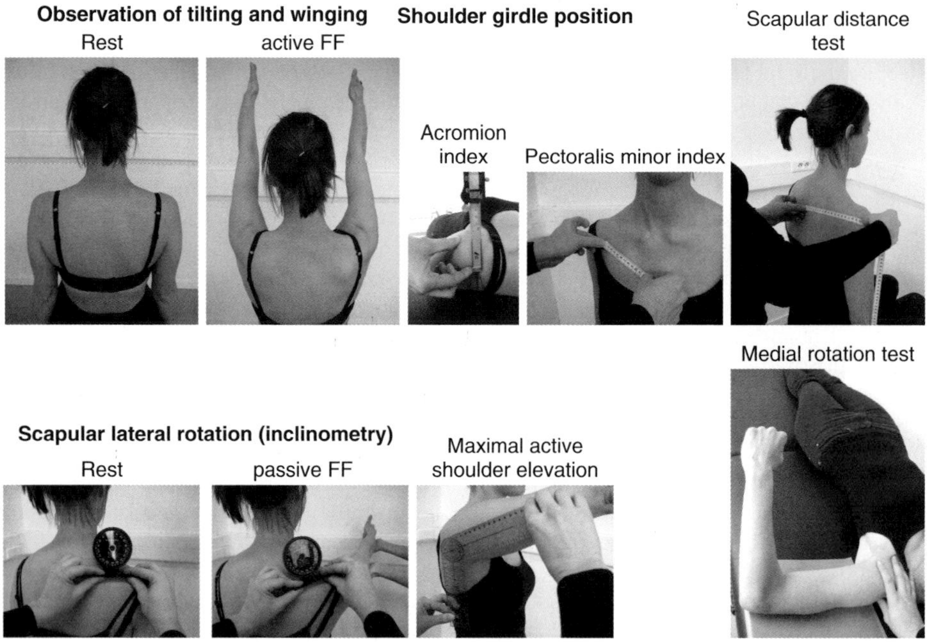

FIG. 25.2 Clinical scapular protocol. *FF,* Forwards flexion.

to stay relaxed during the measurement. In this position the acromial angle is palpated and the vertical distance between this angle and the table (cm) is measured with a sliding carpenter. This distance is divided by the subject height (cm) and defined as the AI (no unit).

Pectoralis minor index (PMI): This index is assessed with the patient seated upright in a chair with lower back support and the arms relaxed alongside the body. The resting length of the pectoralis minor muscle is assessed by measuring the length (measurement tape) between the inferior medial tip of the coracoids process and the caudal edge of rib four (at its attachment to the sternum). Both reference points are first palpated and marked using a pen. Participants are instructed to exhale during the palpation, marking and measurement itself. The PMI (no unit) is defined as the pectoralis minor resting length (cm) divided by the subject height (cm).

Scapular distance test (SDT): This test assesses the position of the scapula on the trunk in an upright-seated position with lower back support with the arms relaxed alongside of the body. The SDT (no unit) is calculated by dividing the distance between the acromial angle and the spinous process of T3 (cm) by the distance between the acromial angle and the scapular trigonum (cm). Anatomical landmarks are first palpated and marked using a pen, and distances are subsequently measured with flexible measurement tape.

Test 3: Scapular lateral rotation. Scapular lateral rotation is assessed with an inclinometer (Plurimeter-V gravity inclinometer, Dr Rippstein, Switzerland) while patients are seated upright on a chair with lower back support. The inclinometer is held manually on the scapular spine by the skilled physiotherapist while an assisting physiotherapist passively elevates the participant's arm in the sagittal plane (forwards flexion). The amount of lateral rotation (degrees) is read from the inclinometer at rest (arm alongside the body) and at 45°, 90° and 135° of passive forwards flexion (determined by goniometry). The elbow is extended, and the thumb pointed upwards during task performance.

Test 4: Maximal active humeral elevation. While seated upright with lower back support, the maximal range of active humerothoracic elevation in the sagittal plane (forwards flexion) is read from a goniometer (degrees). Patients are instructed to extend the elbow and to keep the thumb pointing upwards during movement.

Test 5: Medial rotation test. This test assesses scapular dynamic control while participants lay supine with the upper arm passively supported by a wedge in 90° of humerothoracic scapular plane elevation (30° anterior to the frontal plane) and the elbow flexed. While actively performing a movement towards glenohumeral internal rotation (i.e., moving the forearm towards the table), the patient is instructed to keep the scapula still. Meanwhile, the assessor palpates the anterior humeral head and the coracoid

CLINICAL SCAPULAR PROTOCOL

Name: ....

Date: ....

TEST 1

Observation of tilting and winging

Rest   active FF

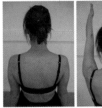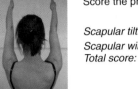

Score the presence (score 1) or absence (score 0) of scapular tilting and winging

Scapular tilting: *0/1*
Scapular winging: *0/1*
Total score: *0/1/2*

TEST 2

Shoulder girdle position

Acromion index

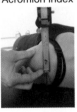

Measure the distance between the acromial angle and the table, and divide this by the subject's height

Acromial length: ... cm
Acromial index (acromial length/subject's height): ...

Pectoralis minor index

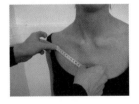

Measure the distance between the coracoid process and the insertion of the 4th rib on the sternum, and divide this by the subject's height.

Pectoralis minor length: ... cm
Pectoralis minor index (Pectoralis minor length/subject's height): ...

Scapular distance test

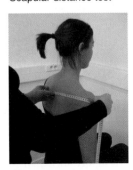

Divide the distance between the acromial angle and the spinous process of T3 (cm) by the distance between the acromial angle and the scapular trigonum (cm).

Distance acromial angle and the spinous process of T3: ... cm
Distance acromial angle and the scapular trigonum: ... cm

Scapular distance: ...

Ⓐ

FIG. 25.3 Scoring sheet for clinical scapular protocol.

TEST 3

Scapular lateral rotation (inclinometry)

Rest   passive FF

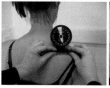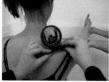

Read the degree of scapular lateral rotation from the inclinometer at rest and during passive arm elevation.

Degree of lateral rotation at rest: ... degrees
Degree of lateral rotation at 30 degrees of forward flexion: ... degrees
Degree of lateral rotation at 60 degrees of forward flexion: ... degrees
Degree of lateral rotation at 90 degrees of forward flexion: ... degrees
Degree of lateral rotation at 120 degrees of forward flexion: ... degrees

TEST 4

Maximal active
shoulder elevation

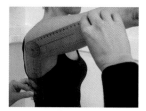

Read the degree of humeral elevation from the inclinometer at maximal active arm elevation.

Degree of humeral elevation: ... degrees

TEST 5

Medial rotation test

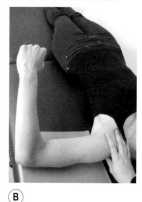

Judges the amount of anterior humeral translation and scapular movement during glenohumeral internal rotation.

Anterior humeral translation: 0/1
Scapular movement: 0/1
Total score: 0/1/2

(B)

FIG. 25.3, cont'd

process and judges the amount of anterior humeral translation and scapular movement. Aberrant dynamic control indicates excessive anterior humeral translation (more than 4 mm, judged by palpation) or scapular movement (more than 6 mm, judged by palpation in the direction of anterior tilt, downwards rotation or scapular elevation) before 60° of internal glenohumeral rotation. A total score of 0 indicates correct humeral translation and scapular movement, a score of 1 means aberrant humeral translation or aberrant scapular movement, and a score of 2 indicates aberrant humeral translation and aberrant scapular movement.

Scapular malpositioning and dyskinesia are linked to, for example, delayed lower trapezius activation or decreased serratus anterior activity. This might induce scapular winging (protraction), increased anterior tilting or reduced lateral rotation. Also, static measures like the acromial distance, scapular distance, PMI and observation at rest can be performed to assess shoulder girdle position and scapular positioning at rest (De Baets et al 2016a). Inflexibility or shortening of soft tissue structures has been suggested as a possible contributor to shoulder disorders. For example, stiffness of pectoralis minor can induce increased scapular anterior tilt and protraction because of its pull on the coracoid (Borstad & Ludewig 2005). Many authors have suggested that such an altered scapular position is associated with a reduction of the subacromial space (Seitz et al

2011, Solem-Bertoft et al 1993), and that it leads to muscle imbalances and adaptive shortening of postural muscles and other soft tissue, for example, posterior shoulder structures (Laudner et al 2010). Inflexibility of posterior shoulder structures in return is associated with glenohumeral internal rotation deficits, which is related to a more anteriorly tilted scapular position (Borich et al 2006). As such, a vicious circle of inflexibility, leading to scapular malposition and further inflexibility, is created.

Musculoskeletal Management of Shoulder Complex Dysfunctions After Stroke

It is well accepted that movement control depends on the contribution of active, passive and control systems. Within this interpretation, ideal control relies on the appropriate passive support (i.e., proper flexibility of passive structures) combined with proper muscle control (i.e., correct timing characteristics of, e.g., lower trapezius and serratus anterior) that is coordinated by the nervous system. Conversely, changes in any of these systems can lead to less than optimal control. This has formed the basis of a range of passive (manual therapy and muscle stretching) and active (motor control retraining) rehabilitation techniques that aim to restore control and reduce disability and/or pain. However, the implementation of this musculoskeletal model into clinical stroke rehabilitation is not straightforward given the complexity and heterogeneity in clinical presentation of the poststroke individual. This emphasises the application of individualised therapy planning, rather than a one-size-fits-all rehabilitation model.

Motor Control Training

Motor control has been broadly defined as the combination of neurophysiological and biomechanical mechanisms that contribute to movement control (Littlewood et al 2013). Various brain areas are involved in motor control, including cortical (primary somatosensory cortex, posterior parietal cortex, primary motor cortex, supplementary motor area, premotor cortex, prefrontal cortex) and subcortical structures (basal ganglia), the brainstem (vestibular nuclei, reticular formation), as well as the cerebellum, and spinal networks. Any of these areas might be affected because of stroke, and thus affect motor control, which causes the sensorimotor impairments that underlie the development and persistence of dysfunction and pain. Motor control alterations can be either, neither or both cause and consequence of movement dysfunctions or pain, and thereby initiate a vicious circle of pathology leading to pain, which negatively influences motor control in turn. Sensorimotor adaptations after stroke are, for example: (1) redistribution of activity within and between muscles, both augmented

or compromised (i.e., earlier activity in lower trapezius or delayed serratus anterior activity in individuals with stroke without shoulder pain, respectively); and (2) changes in mechanical features including posture and movement (i.e., increased scapular lateral rotation and decreased scapular posterior tilting in individuals with stroke without shoulder pain).

In general, motor control training aims to optimise muscle activation patterns and proprioception, and to improve posture, joint alignment and movement patterns. When translated to the shoulder complex in individuals with stroke, this involves training of not only the upper limb but also the core of the body (Kibler et al 2006) and the trunk (Saeys et al 2012). Postural anticipatory adaptations, core and proximal trunk stability, correct scapulothoracic setting and control of glenohumeral external rotators (infraspinatus, posterior deltoid) and triceps brachii are prerequisites to efficiently take the hand forwards and perform a proper reach (Aimola et al 2011, Barker et al 2009, Kisiel-Sajewicz et al 2011).

Neuroplasticity and Timing of Motor Control Training in Individuals With Stroke

Cortical neuroplasticity can be defined as a morphological or functional change in neuronal properties, such as strength of internal connections, altered representational patterns or reorganisation of neuronal territories (Calford 2002, Sanes & Donoghue 2000), and aims to complete or almost complete recovery in the long run. In individuals with stroke, neuroplastic changes underlie the patients' functional recovery. As such, therapy focused on the restorative potential of the brain and neural structures constitutes an important part of neurological rehabilitation poststroke (Nowak 2008, Oujamaa et al 2009).

Neuroplasticity occurs mainly in the acute and subacute stage after stroke (Kreisel et al 2007, Vahedi et al 2007), and patients will benefit most from targeted neurorehabilitation in these early stages (Cumming et al 2011, Hubbard et al 2015). Although it is assumed that spontaneous recovery slows down after a few weeks and reaches a plateau after several months, an exact limit for recovery potential has never been established (Demain et al 2006). In contrast, it has been shown that adapted neurorehabilitation leads to functional gains and reorganisation of brain activity even in chronic stroke patients (Carey et al 2002). This suggests that the complete potential of neuroplasticity and the associated recovery is often not yet fully exploited.

In healthy individuals, novel motor skill training, and not repetition of general exercise, is associated with improvement in task performance and increase in representation of the trained muscle in the primary motor cortex (Karni et al 1995). Given the evidence that novel motor skill training is associated with rapid changes in cortical excitability and cortical reorganisation, this type of training is also considered relevant for individuals with stroke. Motor control exercises for the trunk and scapulothoracic and glenohumeral joints can be regarded as such novel motor skill training and should thus, as soon as possible, be added to the rehabilitation protocol. As such, a novel skill stimulus is given early after stroke towards the injured side of the brain, enhancing the likelihood for neuroplastic advantageous changes.

Illustration by Means of a Case Presentation

DN, a 48 year-old man, had a first unilateral stroke, located subcortically in the left posterior limb of the internal capsule. Three months after stroke onset, anterolateral shoulder pain occurred. Results of a clinical shoulder assessment were scapular dyskinesia at rest and during movement (as scored by visual observation), pain during active shoulder movement (arm elevation, humeral internal rotation), restriction in glenohumeral internal rotation (passive shoulder examination), positive impingement tests (Neer test, Jobe test) (Hughes 2011, Jobe & Jobe 1983), positive scapular assistance test (pain is related to scapular position/movement) (Rabin et al 2006) and positive test for scapular control (kinetic medial rotation test) (Morrissey et al 2008). Ultrasound examination revealed a supraspinatus tendinopathy.

DN was evaluated by means of three-dimensional scapulothoracic movement analysis and a clinical examination. The clinical examination consisted of the ClinScap (De Baets et al 2016b), the VAS pain scale during active movement, the Fugl-Meyer test (Platz et al 2005), the Action Research Arm Test (ARAT) (Platz et al 2005) and the Motor Activity Log (MAL) (Uswatte et al 2005). All assessments were performed before and at 6 weeks after a scapula-focused rehabilitation protocol.

The aim of the scapula-focused rehabilitation protocol was to normalise the scapulothoracic movement pattern and scapulohumeral rhythm. The programme consisted of 30 minutes of physical therapy, three times per week, for 6 weeks. This physical therapy was in addition to the regular physical therapy and focused on the scapulothoracic and glenohumeral joint solely.

The content of the rehabilitation was twofold. The first focus was towards optimisation of the passive glenohumeral joint range of motion by means of manual therapy techniques (i.e., passive translations in the dorsal and caudal direction of the glenohumeral joint capsule). Also, passive and active stretches were applied, especially to posteroinferior shoulder structures by means of the sleeper stretch and the cross-arm stretch (McClure et al 2007). Shortened muscles such as pectoralis minor and teres major were addressed by means of manual stretch and manual techniques.

The second focus was on motor control exercises to correct alignment and coordination, which involved: (1) learning optimal scapular orientation at rest and then controlling optimal orientation during active arm movements; (2) muscle-specific exercises for the middle and lower trapezius, serratus anterior and rotator cuff. The motor control exercises were performed according to Worsley et al (2013). DN's scapulothoracic position was optimised, initially by using visual (observation) and tactile (palpation) feedback to improve the alignment of the scapula and clavicle. The following guidelines were used: the acromion should be higher than the superior medial border of the scapula, the scapular spine should be 15–25° rotated in the frontal plane, the scapular medial border and inferior angle should be tight against the rib cage and the clavicle should have a slight posterior rotation in the frontal plane (Mottram 1997, Wegner et al 2010). DN was then taught to actively reproduce this scapular and clavicular 'setting' using auditory feedback (from therapist) and tactile feedback by palpation (Comerford & Mottram 2012). Once the scapular setting was controlled, DN was asked to control the scapular setting during reaching tasks with a maximal humeral elevation of 90° in the frontal, sagittal and scapular planes, executed at a slow, controlled pace and repeated until the movement could not be controlled anymore (on average 10 repetitions). Once DN had regained sufficient control of scapular orientation during arm movements, muscle-specific motor control exercises were introduced (after 4–6 weeks). These exercises required DN to initiate and maintain the optimal scapular orientation whilst he performed specific exercises for the lower and middle trapezius, serratus anterior and infraspinatus (Cools et al 2007). Side-lying external rotation, side-lying forwards flexion, prone horizontal abduction with external rotation and prone extension were performed to optimise the intramuscular trapezius muscle balance. Serratus anterior was targeted by means of protraction exercises in supine. Infraspinatus was exercised by means of external rotation exercises.

After 6 weeks, the pattern of anterior-posterior tilting and protraction-retraction was evolved towards the mean of a healthy control population. The lateral rotation was already increased initially and even increased further after therapy. Probably, more emphasis towards the improvement in range of motion by means of scapular mobilisations in the inferior, posterior direction, together with stretches of these structures, must be incorporated. In Tables 25.1 and 25.2 the results of, respectively, the ClinScap and the Fugl-Meyer, ARAT and MAL can be found for both measurement sessions.

Summary

In this section we provided an overview of essential knowledge on normal shoulder complex kinematics and muscle function, and on shoulder girdle movement patterns and muscle function observed in individuals after stroke with and without shoulder pain. This knowledge is essential to keep in mind when evaluating the upper extremity of an

TABLE 25.1 Results of the Scapular-Focused Treatment on the Clinical Scapular Protocol

	Before Treatment	After 6 Weeks of Treatment
Scapular dyskinesia at rest	2	1
Acromial index	4.69	3.87
Pectoralis minor index	5.53	6.15
Scapular distance	1.45	1.23
Inclinometry – rest	2° of lateral rotation	2° of lateral rotation
Inclinometry – passive forwards flexion 120°	48° of lateral rotation	58° of lateral rotation
Maximal humerothoracic elevation	85°	120°
Medial rotation test	2	2

TABLE 25.2 Results of the Scapular-Focused Treatment on Pain, Fugl-Meyer, Action Research Arm Test and Motor Activity Log

	Before Treatment	After 6 Weeks of Treatment
Visual analogue scale pain scale during active movement (max 10)		
During arm elevation	5	2
During internal rotation	3	2
Fugl-Meyer test		
Upper limb motor part (max 66)	51	57
Proximal arm part Fugl-Meyer (max 36)	24	28
Action Research Arm Test (max 57)	41	53
Motor Activity Log (max 5)		
Amount scale	5	5
How well scale	2.2	4.4

individual with stroke, with or without shoulder pain. The ClinScap is an easy-to-use battery of tests to objectively investigate different aspects of shoulder complex kinematics in clinical practice. Regarding shoulder complex rehabilitation, principles of motor control training and neuroplasticity are essential to include in the upper extremity treatment plan of an individual after stroke.

SPASTICITY: WHEN AND HOW TO TREAT THE CLINICAL PROBLEM IN NEUROLOGICAL REHABILITATION

Stephen Ashford

Neurological damage, for example, as a result of stroke, trauma or degeneration to the brain or spinal cord, typically leads to paralysis or weakness, which may be partial or complete. In the early stages, the affected limbs are often flaccid (low-toned paresis), but muscle tone may increase and may result from the development of muscle overactivity or 'spasticity'. Spasticity will often have unwanted effects, such as

pain, and result in secondary problems, such as muscle stiffness and contracture (Intercollegiate Stroke Working Party 2016, Martin et al 2014). Even if return of active movement occurs, spasticity may still interfere with the fine motor coordination required for highly skilled tasks.

Spasticity is characterised by disordered sensorimotor control, presenting as intermittent or sustained involuntary activation of muscles. Spasticity as a clinical problem has been seen in 38%–42% of patients after stroke (Sommerfeld et al 2011, Urban et al 2010), 13% of patients after traumatic brain injury and 41%–66% of people with multiple sclerosis (MS) (Martin et al 2014), depending on the time of assessment after injury or onset. It may cause additional unwanted effects such as pain, deformity and impaired function (Burke et al 1988). The implications of paresis and spasticity for people with neurological damage are summarised with examples in Table 25.3.

Upper Motor Neurone Syndrome

The group of motor impairments resulting from damage to the central nervous system are termed the *upper motor neurone*

TABLE 25.3   Problems Experienced by People With Neurological Damage

International Classification of Function, Disability and Health (ICF) Domain	Problems Experienced
Impairment to body structure and function	Paralysis Spasticity Contracture Pain
Limitation of Activity Passive Active	Difficulty with caring: • maintaining hygiene • cutting fingernails • dressing Unable to use the limb for active tasks: • mobility, transfers and walking • lifting, carrying • reaching • manipulating objects • activities of daily living
Restriction of participation	Loss of employment Inability to engage in leisure activities

TABLE 25.4   Positive and Negative Features of the Upper Motor Neurone Syndrome

Positive Features	Negative Features
Spasticity	Muscle weakness
Spastic dystonia	Loss of dexterity
Increased tendon reflexes	Fatigability
Clonus	
Cocontraction	
Spasms	
Associated reactions	

syndrome (UMNS) (Stevenson & Jarrett 2006, Thompson et al 2005). The UMNS is divided into positive and negative features (Pandyan et al 2005, Thompson et al 2005). Positive features are those characterised by muscle overactivity including spasticity, and negative features are noted by underactivity, primarily weakness, as shown in Table 25.4.

Spasticity

Spasticity presents in a variety of ways depending on the size, location and age of the lesion (Burke et al 1988). Spasticity was defined by Lance in 1980 as 'a motor disorder, characterised by a velocity-dependent increase in tonic stretch reflexes (muscle tone) with exaggerated tendon jerks, resulting from hyperexcitability of the stretch reflex as one component of the UMNS' (Lance 1980, p. 5). However, the SPASM consortium, a European thematic network tasked to develop standardised measures of spasticity (Pandyan et al 2005), has proposed a broader definition: 'disordered sensory-motor control, resulting from an upper motor neurone lesion, presenting as intermittent or sustained involuntary activation of muscles'. This broader definition incorporates the positive features of the UMNS but still excludes the negative features and biomechanical changes to muscle and associated structures. The authors argue that, in so doing, it is more clinically relevant.

If spasticity is not managed effectively, affected muscles adopt a shortened position with corresponding contribution to abnormal limb and trunk posture (Barnes 2003). This may result in soft tissue shortening and biomechanical changes in the contracted muscles. Resistance to passive movement in muscle (after neurological insult) may be caused by spasticity, thixotropy or contracture (Vattanaslip et al 2000). Thixotropy is stiffness in muscle, which is dependent on the history of the limb movement (Vattanaslip et al 2000). If muscle is not moved, there is a tendency for it to become stiffer and therefore more resistant to movement. If movement is not undertaken for long periods, contracture will also develop. Contracture represents physical shortening of the muscle and other soft tissues around the joint (e.g., joint capsule), with loss of passive range of movement, which is irrespective of thixotropy or spasticity (Vattanaslip et al 2000). However, contracture may also cause some stiffness towards the end of range of movement. Prevention of contracture and minimisation of thixotropy are therefore important in management of an immobile limb. In addition, spasticity may also be painful for two reasons. First, the overactivity (contraction) of the muscle itself can be painful (similar to 'cramp') because of the strength and duration of contraction (Stevenson & Jarrett 2006). Second, the resulting malalignment can cause pain by adversely stressing interconnecting muscle tissue and joint structures (Thompson et al 2005). Both the positive features of the UMNS and biomechanical changes seen in the clinical presentation will contribute to resistance to passive stretch, which is important to consider in clinical examination and treatment, as discussed further in the next section.

Principles of Management

Clinical management should address spasticity when it is causing pain or harm to the patient's care provision or function or when risk for further deterioration exists, but it should not treat spasticity indiscriminately without the possibility of meaningful benefit (Barnes 2003, Bhakta 2000, Intercollegiate Stroke Working Party 2016, Thompson et al 2005, Williams et al 2020). For example, the implication of spasticity in the hand may be leading to contracture in the long finger flexors. The resulting difficulty in cleaning the palm of the hand may lead to maceration of skin tissue in the palm. Risk for secondary contracture and damage to the skin would warrant intervention to prevent this, and management of spasticity is indicated. In contrast, if spasticity is present as a symptom without other adverse effects, then intervention is not warranted.

At a clinical level, treatment will often be concerned with management of spasticity and other features of the UMNS, such as spastic dystonia, cocontraction and associated reactions (Intercollegiate Stroke Working Party 2016, Stevenson & Jarrett 2006). Spasticity may present a significant clinical problem in terms of limiting function at the level of activity performance by the individual, otherwise known as 'active function' (Intercollegiate Stroke Working Party 2016, Sheean 2001). Alternatively, it may affect carrying out care tasks by a caregiver or by the person themself to a paretic limb, otherwise known as 'passive function' (Intercollegiate Stroke Working Party 2016, Sheean 2001). The combined intervention package will also address other issues, such as joint range of movement relevant to passive or active function improvements, and task retraining relevant to active function improvements (Thompson et al 2005). In some patients who have active function goals, the negative UMN feature of weakness will be the main issue addressed by both task training and specific strengthening (Thompson et al 2005).

Spasticity may be focal (localised to a specific anatomical area affecting one or two muscle groups), regional (affecting the whole limb, e.g., arm) or generalised (affecting the whole body) (Bergfeldt et al 2006, Royal College of Physicians et al 2018). The approach to management has often included passive stretch, which was to both maintain structural length of muscle and inhibit expression of spasticity through an inhibitory effect on the stretch reflex

(Thompson et al 2005). However, although inhibition of the stretch reflex may reduce spasticity for a short period, different strategies are needed for longer-term management.

Clinical Case Illustration

Julia, a 44-year-old woman with no significant medical history, suffered a traumatic brain injury after a mountain bike accident in the Brecon Beacons area of Wales in the UK. She was undertaking a steep descent, lost control of her bike and collided with a fence post at the side of the track.

On initial meeting, Julia explained that her right arm had been getting 'tighter', with pain in her shoulder and in the area of her upper arm. The discomfort had worsened over the past 1–2 months, and there was also now some 'tightness' in her right leg. She reported increasing difficulty with getting comfortable in bed and in her wheelchair because of the knee flexion spasticity.

On examination, she had full range extension at her right knee and minus 20° extension at her right elbow. A velocity-dependent 'catch' indicative of spasticity was evident at both elbow and knee (Lance 1980) but was more significant at her elbow when evaluated against a clinical measure of spasticity (Modified Ashworth Scale [MAS] 3 out of 4) (Brashear et al 2002, Pandyan et al 1999). Identifying a velocity-dependent element in muscle extensibility is helpful for differential diagnosis between spasticity and established contracture or muscle stiffness. Although both spasticity and contracture require management, only spasticity will respond to focal (e.g., botulinum toxin-A [BoNT-A]) or systemic antispasmodic medications (e.g., baclofen). It is therefore important to identify spasticity before initiating spasticity medication. It can be difficult clinically to differentiate between spasticity and contracture, and use of electromyogram is valuable in these circumstances to confirm clinical findings.

Physical and Pharmacological Treatment

The evidence for physical interventions to manage contracture and muscle shortening is limited. The aim of such intervention is to counteract the dominant posture, which may lead to muscle and soft tissue shortening if unchecked (College of Occupational Therapists & Association of Chartered Physiotherapists in Neurology 2015). Passive movement, active movement or interventions such as splinting or casting can achieve muscle stretch. The advantage of splinting or casting is that they produce stretch of a longer duration than manual passive movement alone (College of Occupational Therapists & Association of Chartered Physiotherapists in Neurology 2015, Lai et al 2009, Stevenson & Jarrett 2006).

However, current reviews have not supported splinting and casting applications in the upper limb for maintaining muscle length particularly in the acute period immediately after insult (Katalinic et al 2010, Tyson & Kent 2010). The primary sources of evidence in the reviews were patients with a paretic limb, the majority of whom would not normally be considered for splinting intervention particularly acutely. The lack of difference between the intervention and control groups is therefore not as surprising as it first seems. In addition, an acknowledged weakness of several included studies was that patients often did not receive the intended splinting dosage (Lannin & Herbert 2003, Lannin et al 2007). Most trials reviewed in both of these systematic reviews were examining patients in the more acute phase after stroke, and therefore differences are possible (although not proven) in patients in a more chronic state with appropriate methods and dosage. The effectiveness, methods and dosage required with physical interventions of this type are yet to be adequately identified, and future work may contribute to views on effectiveness (College of Occupational Therapists & Association of Chartered Physiotherapists in Neurology 2015).

In many studies of BoNT intervention for focal spasticity, physical interventions have not been included or described, and the focus for evaluation has been on reduction in spasticity rather than functional or meaningful outcome for the individual. Some studies have attempted to evaluate the influence of physical interventions, however. Giovannelli and colleagues (2007) demonstrated in a single-blind randomised controlled trial of patients with MS that patients who received physiotherapy in combination with BoNT had a significantly greater reduction in spasticity measured on the MAS than those receiving BoNT alone. Unfortunately, the study did not evaluate functional outcome. In addition, the specific physical interventions used in this study were not described, and other limitations included small sample size, incomplete blinding and measurement bias.

Other studies have attempted to explore specific physical interventions used in combination with BoNT. Hesse and colleagues (1998) conducted a small, randomised, double-blind, placebo-controlled trial investigating BoNT in combination with functional electrical stimulation (FES). Four groups were compared: BoNT, FES, BoNT + FES and no intervention. Spasticity was measured using the MAS. They also measured limb position and difficulties encountered by the patient or carer in performing care tasks (passive function) such as cleaning the palm, cutting fingernails and putting the affected arm through a sleeve. Improvements were most prominent for spasticity reduction in the group who received combined BoNT and FES. Of the functional tasks, only 'cleaning the palm of the hand' showed significant improvement, which occurred in both the BoNT + FES and the FES-only groups. These results suggest that specific physical intervention such as FES may

have a role in combination with BoNT, but also that FES in some cases may be an effective management alone to improve passive function in some patients.

Physical interventions may be sufficient to inhibit the development of contracture in muscle and soft tissue in some cases of limb spasticity (Lai et al 2009, Stevenson & Jarrett 2006), although this is yet to be clearly demonstrated by research studies (College of Occupational Therapists and Association of Chartered Physiotherapists in Neurology 2015, Katalinic et al 2010, Tyson & Kent 2010). However, in patients with moderate to severe spasticity pharmacological treatment may be needed to support an effective management programme (Stevenson & Jarrett 2006). Systemic medications to decrease spasticity are available such as baclofen and tizanidine, two of the more commonly used medications. In some individuals these medications are poorly tolerated, and it is necessary to evaluate the potential benefits and side effects before commencing and during treatment. Medications are often used in combination with physical interventions, with the selection of agents depending on the severity and distribution of spasticity (generalised or focal), and whether the spasticity produces any benefit to the patient (e.g., enabling standing due to leg extensor spasticity). For focal spasticity the pharmacological intervention of choice is intramuscular BoNT injection (Royal College of Physicians 2002, 2009, 2018); see the BEST study (Ward et al 2014), the ULIS II study (Turner-Stokes et al 2013) and the ULIS III study (Turner-Stokes et al 2021).

BoNT is a neurotoxin which acts by blocking transmission presynaptically at the neuromuscular junction (Barnes 2003, Dressler et al 2005). The toxin is produced by *Clostridium botulinum*, and strains of the bacterium have been identified as producing seven distinct toxins labelled A–G (Hambleton & Moore 1995). Toxin A is the serotype that has been developed into a therapeutic agent and widely applied in clinical practice and research (Elia et al 2009, Royal College of Physicians et al 2018). Other serotypes have also been developed for use, and BoNT-B is available but less frequently applied in management of spasticity because of its shorter duration of action (Brashear et al 2004, Davis & Barnes 2000).

Clinical Case Illustration

Because Julia had spasticity affecting both her right arm and leg, baclofen was considered as a generalised spasticity agent for management. However, baclofen crosses the blood–brain barrier and can cause sedation, fatigue, dizziness, lowering of seizure threshold and cognitive dysfunction. The proposed dosage after titrating was 15 mg three times daily. Because of the relatively short half-life of baclofen (3.5 hours), it was recommended that the medication be taken in the morning, midday and evening to maintain concentration in the body and produce the required clinical effect.

Julia was also thought to potentially benefit from injection of BoNT-A for her arm spasticity according to the goals of treatment. In particular, spasticity was making putting her arm through a garment sleeve difficult, and there was believed to be a significant risk to loss of further joint range at the elbow. Further assessment was carried out physically and using needle electromyogram to assist in localising the relevant muscle groups and confirm the presence of active muscle spasticity. Spasticity was confirmed in right biceps brachii, brachialis and brachioradialis, and these muscles were injected with BoNT-A. Intervention and baseline measures were documented for spasticity (MAS), goal setting (Goal Attainment Scaling [GAS]) and function (Arm Activity Measure and Leg Activity Measure); see Table 25.5 for further details.

Julia was also provided with a specialised wheelchair with a pommel integrated in the pressure-relieving cushion, allowing optimal positioning of her legs. She had a positioning programme in bed, which included positioning of her legs to keep her knees apart and her legs generally

extended. In her arm she had some return of active movement control and was given an exercise programme to encourage arm and hand extension and function. When not using her arm, she supported it in sitting with an arm support in her wheelchair, which comfortably prevented internal rotation of her arm at the shoulder and encouraged elbow extension.

Fig. 25.4 summarises the overall management strategy and treatment selection process for spasticity management and is a progression of the model from the Royal College of Physicians guideline document (Royal College of Physicians et al 2009).

Evaluation of Outcome

Specific evaluation of spasticity is commonly undertaken using clinician-reported measures such as the MAS or the Tardieu Scale. These methods have limitations because of challenges with both validity and reliability. The MAS in particular conflates resistance to passive stretch with spasticity, when spasticity is only one factor that affects resistance. Both scales when tested also have limited interrater reliability. Quantification of resistance to passive stretch using force measurement and evaluation of associated

TABLE 25.5   Measures of Outcome Applied After Spasticity Treatment

Measure/Evaluation Method	Description	Baseline (Before Intervention)	Outcome (After Intervention)
GAS (Ashford & Turner-Stokes 2006)	A method of evaluating the extent to which a patient's individual goals are achieved in the course of intervention. An overall total ('T') score of 50.0 indicates achievement of goals as predicted	GAS total 36.4	GAS total 50.0
Modified Ashworth Scale (Brashear et al 2002)	Clinical measure of spasticity (resistance to passive stretch) which forms a single-item scale from 0 (no increase in muscle tone) to 4 (affected part rigid in flexion or extension), with an additional point at +1 (slight increase in muscle tone...)	Elbow 3	Elbow 1
Arm Activity measure (Ashford et al 2013a, 2013b, 2014)	A patient or carer-rated 20-item measure of difficulty in passive and active arm function	Active 46 Passive 22	Active 42 Passive 8
Leg Activity measure (Ashford et al 2016)	Patient or carer-rated 33-item measure of difficulty in passive and active arm function, as well as spasticity-related quality of life (symptoms and participatory impact)	Active 43 Passive 13 Impact 16	Active 38 Passive 6 Impact 12

GAS, Goal Attainment Scaling.

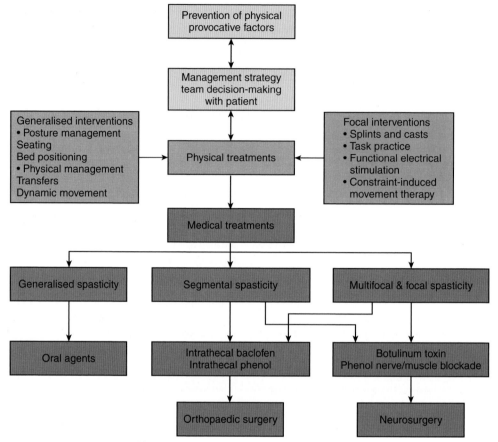

FIG. 25.4 Management of spasticity in adults.

muscle activity using electromyogram have been demonstrated. These methods have limitations for application in daily clinical practice because of the time and equipment required. However, these assessments are becoming more clinically accessible, and may be more practical for use in the future.

GAS is increasingly used as a method to plan treatment and evaluate outcome for limb spasticity (Ashford & Turner-Stokes 2006, 2009, Sutherland et al 2021, Turner-Stokes et al 2010). Goals for treatment of spasticity are widely diverse, depending on the individual aspirations and priorities of the patient and/or their family. They may be directed at reducing impairment to body systems (e.g., preventing contractures and deformity), improving activities (such as personal care) or use of the limb for participatory activities (such as work, hobbies, recreation, etc.). In other words, goals may be directed at achieving change at any level of the World Health Organization *International Classification of Function, Disability and Health*, but most commonly at activity for both passive and active function.

GAS has now been used as the primary outcome measure in three large multicentre trials of focal spasticity intervention in the upper limb: the BEST study (Ward et al 2014) and the ULIS II and III studies (Turner-Stokes et al 2013, 2021). Through these studies GAS demonstrated clinically important change in outcome for people with limb spasticity after intervention. Goal setting is only one element of treatment planning and outcome evaluation. In addition to detailed goal setting and attainment, it is also key to quantify improvements against relevant standardised measures, and the Arm Activity and Leg Activity measures have been developed for this purpose (Ashford et al 2013a, 2013b, 2014, 2016). These measures enable not only evaluation of goal attainment but also quantification of goal improvements against a recognised, patient-reported measure of functional change.

Clinical Case Illustration

The combined interventions incorporating both physical and pharmacological treatments resulted in Julia's specific treatment goals being met. The overall GAS total ('T') score indicated the achievement of all goals as planned at the start of treatment. Improvements included improved ease of upper body dressing by carers and improvements in the ease of her positioning and tolerance in her wheelchair. Her ability to transfer with assistance and an aid also improved. Standardised measures reflected these improvements with a reduction in patient-reported Arm Activity measure passive function score from 22 before treatment to 8 after (Ashford et al 2013a, 2013b), indicating reduced care difficulty at a clinically meaningful level. Reduction in spasticity as measured by the MAS changed after treatment from 3 to 1 for elbow flexors (Brashear et al 2002), indicating reduction in resistance to passive stretch because of spasticity. See Table 25.5 for a summary of the measures and the changes seen in this case.

Summary

The importance of a management plan developed in conjunction with the patient, carers and multidisciplinary team (MDT) should be emphasised in addressing exacerbating factors for spasticity and physical as well as pharmacological methods for management. In most cases of clinical spasticity, it is envisaged that it will be necessary to make recommendations about physical management before pharmacological interventions or in combination with them. The benefits of coordinated interdisciplinary work in spasticity management, encompassing elements of physical management, supplemented by pharmacological interventions, are key to providing optimal spasticity control for patients and facilitating their rehabilitation or management.

ON THE ROAD WITH MULTIPLE SCLEROSIS – CHALLENGES IN SCREENING, ASSESSMENT AND TRAINING OF DRIVING

Hannes Devos and Abiodun E. Akinwuntan

For many individuals with MS, driving a car symbolises mobility, independence, freedom and self-esteem. Making fitness-to-drive recommendations for drivers with MS is particularly challenging because of the relatively young onset of the disease, the unpredictable progression of the disease and the heterogeneity of symptoms depending on the site and extent of the damage in the central nervous system.

In most countries, assessment of fitness-to-drive is a multidisciplinary approach, where the issue of driving continuation, restriction or cessation is discussed with the physician, psychologist, occupational therapist, physical therapist and occasionally the social worker. An accurate fitness-to-drive decision warrants each member of the MDT to be knowledgeable about the characteristics of the disease (see Chapter 10); the legal, ethical and deontological boundaries of fitness to drive; the most accurate screening and assessment tools; and finally, the opportunities for driving training. Each of these aspects will be described later using a schematic overview of a driving evaluation process (Fig. 25.5). This schematic overview is by no means ideal, yet it may be used as a practice guideline for fitness-to-drive referral. Afterwards, a case will be presented using the same schematic diagram.

Driving as an Important Instrumental Activity of Daily Living

Driving a car is one of the most important modes of transportation, especially in Western industrialised countries. Driving is a highly overlearned, yet complex instrumental activity of daily living that requires intact visual, sensory, motor and cognitive skills to respond timely and appropriately to a constantly changing, dynamic and challenging environment (Akinwuntan et al 2012b). Some authors claim that about 90% of all the information used while driving is visual (Sivak 1996). Indeed, drivers need to scan from side to side to check for blind spots, oncoming vehicles when merging and potential hazards approaching in the periphery. Additionally, drivers need to be able to scan vertically for signs and traffic lights, and monitor the rearview mirror, dashboard and other operational instruments in the vehicle. An optimum amount of visual field needs to be accessible to the driver to be able to respond quickly and accurately to traffic cues, physical landscape and unexpected hazards whilst maintaining the complex task of driving. Visual acuity, contrast sensitivity, glare recovery and eye coordination are other visual sensory skills that are paramount for safe driving. Accurate information of these visual stimuli will inform the driver to make appropriate decisions in traffic. In addition, drivers need sufficient strength, coordination, muscle tone, coordination and range of motion to operate the steering wheel and pedals. MS may potentially affect all these functions.

For many individuals with MS, driving a car is very important to maintain independence in life, work and hobbies (Neven et al 2013). The ability to drive is frequently affected by the multiple complications experienced with MS. Drivers with MS are 3.4 times more likely to be treated in the emergency department for motor vehicle crashes (MVCs) compared with age- and sex-matched controls (Lings 2002). Individuals with MS who exhibit cognitive symptoms are particularly at risk for MVCs (Schultheis et al 2002). To some extent, drivers with MS are aware of

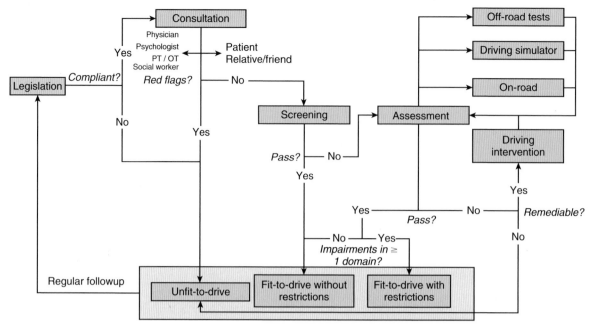

FIG. 25.5 Framework for driving evaluation and intervention in multiple sclerosis based on best practice and evidence. *OT*, Occupational therapy; *PT*, physical therapy.

the potential implications of the disease (Schultheis et al 2009). Drivers with moderate to severe MS tend to change their driving patterns by reducing the number of trips and relying more on the input of passengers (Neven et al 2013). Fatigue and daytime sleepiness, two important symptoms of MS, may affect driving habits and driving performance (Chipchase et al 2003, Devos et al 2021).

Aspects of the Driving Evaluation Process

Fitness-to-Drive Legislation

Minimum medical requirements for fitness-to-drive have been established in many countries to mitigate the number of MVCs as a result of medical conditions. However, such standards are often not based on evidence and do not particularly pertain to drivers with MS (Devos et al 2012). Almost all states in the United States and most driver licensing agencies in many countries of the world have minimum criteria for visual acuity and visual field requirements for driving. Drivers with MS must comply with these visual requirements to be considered fit to drive (see Fig. 25.5).

When an individual with MS meets all the legislative criteria, a medical fitness-to-drive recommendation will be required by a healthcare professional. In most countries, physicians have the ultimate responsibility to determine fitness to drive. However, physicians often struggle to make

such a decision by themselves. The vague legislation criteria, perceived risk of liability suits, fear of compromising the patient–doctor relationship, lack of time and limited knowledge of the evidence-based screening and assessment tools often see physicians requesting the input of other healthcare experts in making a decision (Devos et al 2012). This team will discuss the issue of driving resumption with the candidate driver and, if applicable, get proxy information on driving risks from family and friends (see Fig. 25.5).

When serious red flags are observed during the consultation, such as anosognosia, neglect, unstable disease status, less than 1 month after exacerbation, epilepsy and others, patients should be advised to refrain from driving until those symptoms have resolved. If no such red flags are noticed, physicians may be comfortable issuing a fitness-to-drive recommendation (see Fig. 25.5).

Overall, physicians are accurate in making such fitness-to-drive recommendations. In a relatively large study including 218 active drivers with MS, Ranchet et al (2015) compared the reliability between the physician's rating of fitness to drive with the recommendation by a specialised on-road driving assessor. Both physicians and experts agreed on 191 (88%) of the cases. Yet physicians were more likely to overestimate the true driving capabilities compared with the on-road assessor's judgement. Therefore, screening tools have been developed to assist healthcare professionals in determining who should require a more detailed assessment.

Screening

The goal of a clinical screening tool is to determine any functional deficits that might hinder safe driving. These screening tools are relatively inexpensive and can be easily administered during the consultation routine of the healthcare professional. A failed performance on the screening battery warrants a more detailed assessment at a specialised driving centre (see Fig. 25.5). Although most screening tools lack face validity, some have shown moderate accuracy in predicting fitness to drive. Current evidence available in the literature suggests that the Stroke Drivers Screening Assessment (SDSA) is most accurate in predicting fitness to drive in MS patients (Krasniuk et al 2019). The SDSA was originally developed in the United Kingdom to screen for driving impairments after stroke (Nouri & Lincoln 1993), but it has also been used successfully for drivers with MS in the United Kingdom (Lincoln & Radford 2008) and the United States (Akinwuntan et al 2012a). The SDSA comprises four tests: dot cancellation, directions, compass and road sign recognition (Fig. 25.6). The performance on each of the tests is entered into a discriminant equation to predict the person's likelihood of passing an on-road assessment (Akinwuntan et al 2012a), Lincoln & Radford 2008). These algorithms have been developed to rule out anyone with serious concerns with

driving. The equations are therefore conservative in issuing a passing performance. Individuals with MS who perform poorly on the screening should proceed to a more detailed assessment of fitness to drive, which is usually conducted at a specialised driving assessment centre. These assessments may be free of charge, reimbursed by insurance or an out-of-pocket expense.

Assessment

An elaborate assessment of driving will include off-road tests, driving simulator tests or on-road tests (see Fig. 25.5). The off-road tests will provide a detailed assessment of visual, motor and cognitive functions because these functions are known to affect driving with MS (Akinwuntan et al 2013).

Visual functions that are traditionally assessed include binocular acuity, colour perception, glare recovery, eye movement coordination, depth perception and contrast sensitivity (Fig. 25.7). Binocular acuity correlates significantly with performance on the road (Devos et al 2016, Ranchet et al 2015). Motor and functional tests typically comprise range of motion, manual muscle testing, nine-hole peg test and disease severity status [indexed by the Expanded Disability Status Scale (Kurtzke 1983) and Barthel index (Mahoney & Barthel 1965)]. There are a myriad of cognitive tests used for fitness-to-drive assessment in MS patients. Among those, the Useful Field of View (UFOV®) (Fig. 25.8) test is a preferred computerised cognitive test to measure the effect of MS on speed of processing, divided attention and selective attention (Akinwuntan et al 2013, Badenes et al 2014, Krasniuk et al 2019, Shawaryn et al 2002). The combined score of the UFOV® test produces

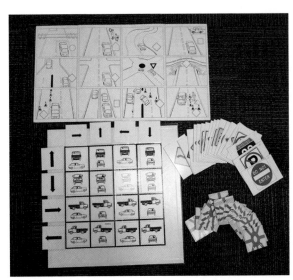

FIG. 25.6 Directions, compass and road sign recognition subtests of the US version of the stroke drivers screening assessment.

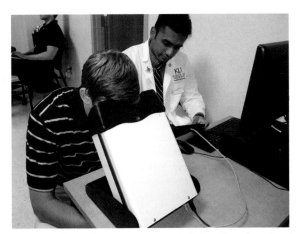

FIG. 25.7 Health professional administering the visual assessment battery.

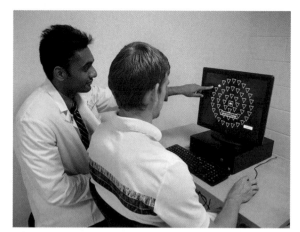

FIG. 25.8 Health professional explaining the selective attention subtest of the Useful Field of View®.

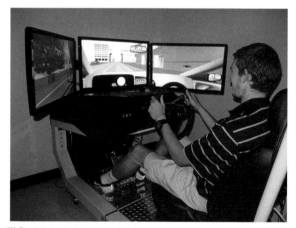

FIG. 25.9 Example of an Interactive Driving Simulator (STI*SIM* Drive®) for assessment and training of driving.

a score ranging from 1 (very low) to 5 (very high) risk for future car crashes.

Driving simulators, especially the recent versions (Fig. 25.9), with interactive driving scenarios, immersive fidelity, and data specification and reduction capabilities offer a wide range of opportunities to assess several levels of driving skill (Krasniuk et al 2022). Unlike off-road tests, driving simulators have the capability to evaluate the integrated visual, motor and cognitive functions in a safe, standardised and reliable environment that approximates real-world driving. The driving simulator can also be used to get clients familiarised with any car modifications such as spinner knob, left-sided accelerator pedal or hand controls that may be needed to be successful during

an on-road test. However, the evidence supporting use of driving simulators for assessment and training of driving for MS patients is limited (Krasniuk et al 2022).

Finally, certified on-road assessors or driving rehabilitation specialists will administer a standardised on-road route in a car that is adapted with dual controls to ensure safety (Akinwuntan et al 2013, Classen et al 2016, Devos et al 2016, Krasniuk et al 2017). The driver's practical fitness to drive will be assessed, including the amount of weaving, checking mirrors and blind spots, maintaining appropriate gap distance, obeying traffic rules, merging lanes, adapting speed, turning left and right and navigating roundabouts.

Individuals with MS who successfully complete the assessment battery with no major impairments in any of the visual, motor or cognitive functions should be allowed to continue driving with no restrictions (see Fig. 25.5). Still, regular follow-up is indicated, especially after a relapse. If there are minor to moderate impairments in one or more domains, appropriate restrictions can be imposed. Although the type and number of restrictions vary greatly between countries, common restrictions include not driving on highways, not driving at night and not driving in unfamiliar areas. However, if the symptoms are too severe and not remediable with training, driving cessation should be advised. Such decisions sometimes evoke anxiety, anger, disbelief and/or distress. It is important to recognise these sentiments by listening to the patient and exploring transportation alternatives. In some countries, professional and volunteer support groups are available to assist individuals with limited transportation options (Akinwuntan & Devos 2015).

Finally, driving intervention programmes might be indicated for remediable problems (see Fig. 25.5). These driving interventions can focus on car adaptations (e.g., extra or larger mirrors, spinner knobs, hand controls), compensation (e.g., driving slower, planning ahead of time, leaving more gap distance), remediation (e.g., training of road sign recognition, anticipatory braking, speed control, lane positioning, merging) or a combination of those intervention strategies.

Intervention

Intervention programmes to improve on-road driving in MS patients are still in their infancy. Although there are some anecdotal reports of improved driving performance after training, only one pilot study has empirically tested the potential benefits of an intervention programme geared to improve driving-related skills in MS patients (Akinwuntan et al 2014). A total of 36 active drivers with relapsing-remitting MS underwent 5 hours of training in a wide field-of-view driving simulator. The driving simulator was a full-sized sedan with all mechanical parts and could be adapted with modifications such as hand controls, spinner knob and left-side accelerator pedal. The training sessions were customised to the participants' performance during the on-road driving test at pretraining.

Four of the seven participants with failing performance at pretraining passed the road test after completion of training. The training group improved on colour perception, speed of processing and visual scanning. They also reported less fatigue after training. However, more well-conducted studies are needed to convincingly establish the usefulness of driving simulators as meaningful training tools to improve fitness to drive in MS patients.

Participants who successfully complete the intervention programme should be recommended to retake the assessment to determine their fitness to drive (see Fig. 25.5).

Case Presentation

Eva, a 44-year-old woman diagnosed with relapsing-remitting MS 4 years ago, was referred by her MS neurologist for a comprehensive driving evaluation. She expressed to her neurologist that she noted decreased attention behind the wheel. Her spouse confirmed that Eva had drifted off the road a few times and tended not to keep to the posted speed limits, especially in city traffic or while driving on highways.

Eva currently has a part-time job as an administrative assistant at a local hospital. She walks independently but uses a cane for outdoor activities, especially in the mornings when she feels tired. She has a valid driver's license, 26 years of driving experience and drove about 12,000 miles in the previous year. She uses her car daily for commuting and small errands. She reports a daily mileage of 10 miles. She had incurred one speeding violation but no crash in the past 5 years. Eva wants to be cleared to continue driving.

Using the same framework presented in Fig. 25.5, Eva's request for a driving evaluation will be addressed in the following subsections.

Consultation

The MS neurologist acquired information on Eva's disease duration and the type of MS. This information is detailed in the case description. Eva scored 2 on the Expanded Disability Status Scale, indicating minimal disability. Eva reported no significant comorbidities that could be considered detrimental to safe driving. Eva's last exacerbation was about 20 months ago. She did not take any medication. After the interview with Eva and her spouse, the MS neurologist decided to prescribe a fitness-to-drive assessment.

Screening

The US version of the SDSA was administered (Fig. 25.6 and Table 25.6). Based on her performance on the SDSA, Eva

was predicted to fail the on-road assessment (Akinwuntan et al 2012a). Her results on the SDSA warranted a more detailed assessment of fitness to drive.

Assessment

The off-road assessment included tests of motor function, vision and cognition (see Table 25.6). The motor and functional assessments included the manual muscle test of key upper and lower extremity muscles (Kendall et al 1993), range of motion of key upper and lower extremity joints (Gajdosik & Bohannon 1987), Barthel index (Mahoney & Barthel 1965) and Expanded Disability Status Scale (Kurtzke 1983). Eva did not have any significant limitations in range of motion or strength. Her muscles in the lower extremities, especially the quadriceps and foot extensor muscles, were submaximal (4 out of 5). Five points were deducted from the maximum score of the Barthel index because she was using a cane when she came in for the assessment.

Her visual functions were administered using the Keystone vision screener (see Fig. 25.7). Assessment of binocular acuity and horizontal field of view was essential to meet the legal criteria of the State of Georgia in the United States, where Eva obtained her driver's license. She passed the binocular visual field test (20/30) and the horizontal field-of-view test (170°). She passed the contrast sensitivity test but failed the colour perception, eye coordination, depth perception, and glare recovery tests.

The cognitive battery consisted of the Mini-Mental State Examination (Folstein et al 1975), Trail Making Tests parts A and B (Reitan 1986), Rey-Osterrieth Complex Figure (Rey 1941) and the Useful Field of View (UFOV®) test (Ball et al 1990). Her results are shown in Table 25.6.

Before the simulator test, Eva completed the simulator sickness questionnaire (Kennedy et al 1993) and was determined not to be prone to simulator adaptation syndrome, a potential side effect of driving simulation that can cause nausea. She first got acquainted with the driving simulator setup by driving a 3.5-mile scenario with very light traffic. After familiarisation, Eva proceeded to drive through a 9.5-mile evaluation scenario that simulated daily life driving on residential, urban and interstate roads. She committed eight traffic violations (speeding tickets) and two crashes. She hit a pedestrian and she did not see a vehicle suddenly pulling out from the curb (see Table 25.6). Finally, her reaction time was assessed driving a 1.5-mile scenario with the instructions to bring the car to a stop when a red stop sign suddenly appeared in the centre of the screen. Her brake response time (see Table 25.6) was similar to age-matched norms (394 ± 45 ms) (Akinwuntan et al 2009). After completion of the simulated drive, the simulator sickness

TABLE 25.6   Results of the Clinical Assessment

Tests	First Visit (Pretraining)	Posttraining
Legal Criteria[a]		
Binocular acuity	Pass (>20/60)	N/A
Horizontal visual field	Pass (>140°)	N/A
Screening: Stroke Drivers Screening Assessment		
Dot cancellation time (s)	685	573
Dot cancellation errors	14	3
Dot cancellation false positives	0	1
Directions, /32	32	32
Compass, /32	20	28
Road sign recognition	5	7
Assessment		
Off-road		
Motor and Functional Tests		
Range of motion, limits		
Neck	Within normal limit	Within normal limit
Right upper extremity	Within normal limit	Within normal limit
Left upper extremity	Within normal limit	Within normal limit
Right lower extremity	Within normal limit	Within normal limit
Left lower extremity	Within normal limit	Within normal limit
Manual muscle testing, /5		
Neck	5	5
Right upper extremity	5	5
Left upper extremity	5	5
Right lower extremity	4	4
Left lower extremity	4	4
Barthel index, /100	95	100
Expanded Disability Status Scale, /12	2	2
Vision Tests		
Binocular acuity	20/30	N/A
Field of view (horizontal)	170	N/A
Contrast sensitivity	Pass	N/A
Colour perception	Fail	N/A
Eye coordination	Fail	N/A
Depth perception	Fail	N/A
Glare recovery	Fail	N/A
Cognitive Tests		
Mini-Mental State Examination, /30	28	28
Trail Making Test A (s)	47	44
Trail Making Test B (s)	211	138
Rey-Osterrieth Complex Figure, /36	35	36
UFOV processing speed (ms)	80.2	213.4
UFOV divided attention (ms)	313.5	213.4
UFOV selective attention (ms)	313.5	366.8

TABLE 25.6	Results of the Clinical Assessment—Cont'd	
Tests	**First Visit (Pretraining)**	**Posttraining**
Driving simulator		
Crashes	2	0
Tickets	8	2
Brake response time (ms)	394	309
On-road assessment, /50	44	46

[a]According to the licensing requirements of the State of Georgia. Please check your own legal criteria.
N/A, Not applicable; *UFOV®*, Useful Field of View.

questionnaire was administered again to confirm that Eva did not show any symptoms of simulator adaptation syndrome.

The road test was conducted by an independent on-road assessor. Performed on a standardised traffic route, the on-road driving performance of Eva was scored on a 50-point scale. She scored 44 of 50 maximum points. A minimum of 45 points is required for a passing performance, hence she was judged as failing the practical road test.

Interpretation of Driving Evaluation Results

Eva was in a mild stage of MS and was actively driving at the time of testing. Binocular acuity and visual field met the legal standard for fitness to drive. The outcome of the screening battery and the off-road driving assessment revealed difficulties with other visual sensory functions and difficulties with speed of processing, attention and reasoning skills. Her results on the driving simulator assessment confirmed the test results of the cognitive assessment. These impairments may have affected her fitness to drive. Eva was therefore scheduled for an on-road assessment. She scored one point below the cutoff value for passing.

Driving Training Programme

Eva's borderline performance in the cognitive, simulator and on-road tests made her an ideal candidate for driving simulator training. Eva underwent 5 hours of driving training. Her training focused on lane positioning on straight and curvy roads, speed adaptations, hazard perception and divided attention, following a previously described protocol (Akinwuntan et al 2014).

Posttraining Assessment

After training Eva was rescheduled for a posttraining assessment (see Table 25.6). She improved on all cognitive, simulator and on-road tests, except for the speed of processing subtest of the UFOV® test. Her results on the posttraining assessment were reassuring enough for the driving assessor to render a recommendation of fit to drive with restrictions. These restrictions included not driving at

night (because of poor glare recovery), not driving on highways (because of difficulties with speed of processing) and driving only in a familiar area (15 miles around the home address). Eva was encouraged to retake the assessment within 1 year or sooner if she experienced any exacerbation of symptoms. A copy of the fitness-to-drive recommendation was sent to the referring neurologist to assist in making the final determination of fitness to drive.

Summary

Drivers with MS rely heavily on a car for daily life activities. Several procedures are in place to prolong safe driving for patients with MS. A framework for fitness to drive, including legislation, screening, assessment and intervention, may assist healthcare professionals in this difficult decision-making process. A multidisciplinary approach, in which members of the team provide a recommendation of fitness to drive based on their expertise, is the right course of action.

PHYSICAL MANAGEMENT OF PEOPLE WITH PROLONGED DISORDER OF CONSCIOUSNESS – DISABILITY MANAGEMENT, ETHICS AND LEGAL FRAMEWORKS

Joseph Buttell, Camilla Erwee, Alexandra Henson

Introduction

This subsection introduces physical management for people with disorders of consciousness (DOC). In the United Kingdom there was a 10% increase in the number of head injury admissions between 2005 and 2019 (Headway.org). In addition, improvements in acute health systems and medical/surgical treatments enable higher survival rates Caplan et al 2015. This inevitably results in more survivors with catastrophic cognitive and physical disabilities needing appropriate skilled management at every point in the pathway from hyperacute to community settings. Despite the demand for specialist intervention, this is a group whose prevalence is unclear, with UK estimates ranging from 12,000 to 50,000 people (Houses of Parliament, PN489).

Ethics and the legal framework around clinical decision-making are constantly being revised in response to emerging understanding and detection of consciousness itself in this group. The legal and clinical guidance presented here outlines the current situation in England and Wales, and thus maybe different in other regions and countries. We advise readers and practitioners to familiarise themselves with respective guidelines and regulations.

We start by outlining the diagnosis and prognostic expectations for this caseload and the key relevant ethical and legal context. Then we focus on physical management approaches in acute, rehabilitation and long-term settings as part of multidisciplinary intervention and care.

This subsection addresses people in DOC after sudden-onset acquired brain injury (ABI) such as cerebrovascular accident, trauma and hypoxia, as opposed to those in terminal disorders of consciousness following chronic illness (TDOC). In TDOC, advance discussion about treatment choices ahead of this point will guide treatment (NHS Improving Quality 2018).

What Is a Disorder of Consciousness?

Persistent disorder of consciousness (PDOC) comprises presentations between unconsciousness and consistent awareness lasting beyond 4 weeks, diagnosed by an expert PDOC physician (Royal College of Physicians 2020). The diagnosis is distinct from coma, which presents as prolonged deep sleep, and locked-in syndrome, where the person is conscious and often cognitively intact but brainstem damage causes widespread or total paralysis. With PDOC, people are awake at times and reflexively responsive to stimuli (e.g., withdrawing from pain) but exhibit at best limited and inconsistent conscious awareness. They are dependent for care beyond somatic function (e.g., nutrition, continence care, pressure relief). The diagnosis comprises a continuum from a state where the individual evinces no cortical responses ('vegetative' state [VS]) to indications of 'islands' of awareness of self and/or the environment (minimally conscious state [MCS]). Prevalence of VS to MCS in the UK is estimated to be 1:3 (Houses of Parliament, PN489). Worldwide the incidence is largely unknown because of differences in diagnostic criteria, reporting and assessments used (Giacino et al 2018). In 2018, a comprehensive review by Wade (2018) estimated the prevalence to be 2–5 per 100,000 with an incidence of 2.6 per 100,000. Many people with PDOC will live for years beyond the initial injury, some for decades, and national guidance recommends annual expert medical review (Royal College of Physicians 2020). Life expectancy

is influenced by health and age before injury, comorbidities and severity and nature of brain injury.

Although a few patients in PDOC make significant gains after diagnosis, many remain stable for extended periods or for the rest of their lives. Prognostication in relation to recovery of consciousness and meaningful function is difficult at the single patient level, but typically the longer the duration of PDOC, the less likely there is to be subsequent change and it will be smaller in scale. Increase in awareness is best predicted by trajectory of responsiveness in early stages postinjury (Shiel et al 2000, Turner-Stokes et al 2015).

For this caseload where ability to self-advocate is lost and the family's understanding is often reliant on the professionals, it is vital for the MDT to include family from the outset in care and information gathering, and to collaborate closely throughout. Integrating observations and sharing analysis supports understanding, inclusion and joint decision-making with the family as part of the team. It is a detailed, iterative process elucidating reflexive from cortical responses at the edges of consciousness. Behaviour indicating responsiveness is most likely to emerge first with family if it does occur, so joint sessions and analysis are essential.

How Is Rehabilitation Different for People in PDOC?

For much of the ABI caseload, the MDT are focused on restitution of function and independence which is often prognostically unlikely or limited for this group. In addition, the long-term sequelae of being dependent for basic care, immobile, incontinent and largely uncommunicative can lead to severe, painful and possibly life-limiting conditions.

MDT goals for these individuals are therefore centred around:

- Providing the best opportunity for level of consciousness to be enabled and assessed;
- Management of physical needs to reduce or prevent secondary complications such as aspiration, pain, contractures and pressure sores;
- Facilitation of family participation, understanding, adjustment and decision-making; and
- Treatment planning and decision-making in line with the patient's best interests.

The whole team collaborates in creating conditions to support the patient to respond or evidence their awareness, and to monitor for behaviour indicating this. Since a landmark study in 2006 discovering cortical responsiveness in people clinically diagnosed as being in VS via highly sensitive serial functional magnetic resonance imaging (fMRI) testing (Owen et al 2006), there has been extensive global research exploring the prevalence and extent of this cognitive motor dissociation, and into ways to verify it in the clinical setting (Cruse et al 2011). Despite evidence of 'covert awareness' in up to 17% of persistent VS cases in research (Owen et al 2006), clinical services do not have access to the requisite level of imaging and rely on exacting serial behavioural observations over time to establish an individual's level of responsiveness.

Standardised tools are used to objectively log and analyse the patient's behaviours, classify them in relation to level of responsiveness and note triggering stimuli to construct a robust clinical hypothesis over time. National guidelines recommend using two different measures concurrently (for recommendations, see National Guideline by Royal College of Physicians 2020). It is important that assessments are completed in a range of conditions. Physical activity is likely to be most stimulating, so it is key to involve family and MDT members in physiotherapy sessions to optimise motivation. Awareness may be evidenced by repeated lower-level responses (e.g., turning towards familiar people, brief visual focus or tracking) or by rare or single high-level responses such as appropriate laughter or smiling, following commands or appropriate speech within context (Royal College of Physicians 2020).

Legal and Ethical Considerations

Legally, clinicians in England and Wales work within the context of the Mental Capacity Act, which establishes people's rights to decline treatment and how capacity to make decisions is assessed (Mental Capacity Act 2005). When the individual cannot choose for themselves, universal in the PDOC caseload, decisions must be made 'in their best interests' by the person responsible for actioning the intervention in question, having consulted with their family, friends and MDT.

The growing understanding that people in PDOC can be stabilised long-term in this highly dependent and potentially physically or psychologically painful state has focused increasing ethical and legal query on the assumption that sustaining life is justified (England and Wales Court of Protection 2021, Graham 2019, Kitsinger 2021). Teams are challenged to adapt their perspective, and whilst starting from a strong presumption that life-saving treatment is in a person's best interests, this should be tested against evidence of the individual's beliefs, wishes and values. Overall the onus is on the team to demonstrate thorough consideration of rationales for prolonging life rather than halting treatment (British Medical Association 2018).

Management from the Acute Setting to the Community

Acute Phase

Physiotherapists' role in acute management of people in PDOC focuses primarily on the respiratory and musculoskeletal systems to support medical stabilisation. Many PDOC patients have protracted weaning from mechanical ventilation (Fan et al 2015). Failure to protect the airway successfully due to compromised cough and swallow strength or reflexes can cause aspiration pneumonia. Many patients require a tracheostomy to become successfully independent of assisted ventilation (Bellon et al 2022, Melotte et al 2022). MDT weaning in neurologically impaired adults has been shown to take longer than single-disciplinary models but is more successful in avoiding airway reinsertion and readmissions to intensive care units (ITUs) (Garrubba et al 2009). Physiotherapists, speech language therapists (SLTs), nurses and anaesthetists collaborate on safe weaning, incorporating positioning with oral hygiene, saliva management, reflux management and respiratory hygiene.

Oral hygiene often requires MDT input for this population. Oral access is often complicated by emergence of hypersensitivity and protective bite reflex. These are understood to be triggered by repeated noxious stimulation from suction, long-term endotracheal tubes and oral discomfort from difficulties delivering mouth care in the early stages combined with downregulated conscious processing of stimuli. Physiotherapists can contribute to structured desensitisation and stimulation programmes to reduce and prevent the development of this problem alongside SLTs. Research evidence for specific therapy approaches remains poor but have been described (Konradi 2015).

Within the MDT, physiotherapists direct 24-hour postural management with both disability management and restorative goals. Disability management aims include minimising muscle length and joint changes (and subsequent pain), reducing aspiration risk and optimising functional positioning for graded stimulation in collaboration with occupational therapists and nurses to maintain skin health. This will include side lying in bed on both sides, supine, sitting (including specialist wheelchairs), splinting for vulnerable joints and therapeutic standing. Limbs may need to be handled to assess for the presence of spasticity, low tone, joints vulnerable to subluxation, high tone from adaptive shortening and to improve comfort during position changes or donning splints. The physiotherapist identifies needs and triggers interventions when unhelpful changes are occurring (e.g., spasticity). Although patients in VS are unlikely to experience pain, for those in MCS this cannot be ruled out and pain is likely to be perceived.

The aim in the acute phase is to begin developing a 24-hour pattern of management that prevents secondary complications; anticipates needs; minimises pain, distress and carer burden; and maximises the person's potential to move on from an acute setting while establishing a baseline. Clear communication with family education about the condition and pathway should be introduced, and they should be supported to monitor and record the patient's behaviours. The physiotherapist will contribute to MDT referral of patients to appropriate onward services and long-term case management if available.

Rehabilitation Phase

During rehabilitation, physiotherapists focus on establishing a comprehensive 24-hour physical management plan to stimulate awareness, offer functional stimulation through movement and positioning, and monitor for evidence of change in behaviour. This includes continuous assessment of the effectiveness of selected interventions (joint ranges, carer burden, skin integrity) alongside objective observations of behaviours and responsiveness during structured stimulation therapy. Although direct evidence for stimulation programmes remains lacking (Cheng et al 2018, Lombardy et al 2002), they form the basis for clinical MDT diagnosis and intervention. The physiotherapist may take the lead in specific stimulating activities such as therapeutic standing, usually via equipment such as a tilt table. Tilt tables allow staff to bring a patient towards an upright position safely. Standing and upright postures have begun to be investigated for their potential to increase patient's responsiveness, purportedly via the reticular activating system (Moriki 2013). Therapeutic standing allows for weight bearing through the feet and loading of the lower limb muscles. Within the context of a comprehensive 24-hour postural management and medical treatment plan, this may reduce loss of muscle length and contracture formation (Bohannon & Green 2021). Physiotherapists work with occupational therapy and nursing colleagues to identify the most appropriate way to achieve static postures to facilitate function, as well as to minimise secondary complications caused by immobility or pressure areas. This typically includes bed positioning such as side lying, sitting up in bed and sleep systems; seating including adapted wheelchairs; trialling of splints and pressure-relieving equipment.

Physiotherapists will typically be involved in assessing and handling joints, and they have a key role in identifying tone changes consistent with spasticity and disorders of the musculoskeletal system. With PDOC patients, therapists should be vigilant for signs of heterotopic ossification (Bargellesi et al 2017), a posttrauma pathology resulting in formation of painful bony deposits in muscles. Responses that may indicate pain or distress during movement should be assessed, and physiotherapists can provide valuable insight to the wider team regarding the use or weaning of pain relief and tone-modifying medications which may also

have sedating effects. The use of BoNT injections and other tone-modifying treatments should be instigated within the context of thorough assessment by specialised team members. Physiotherapists contribute to these assessments and increasingly deliver injections as their knowledge and skills allow them to select appropriate muscle targets, goals and outcome measures. Goals for management of focal spasticity using BoNT injection can be classified as enabling passive care such as reducing adductor spasticity to allow for the placement of a hoist sling, or active function, such as enabling standing through reducing spastic plantar flexion (Royal College of Physicians 2018).

Reducing dependence on artificial airways is another key rehabilitation goal for PDOC patients because tracheostomies require skilled management to maintain a healthy patent airway and are vulnerable to problems in the long-term including tracheal injury, infection and accidental decannulation. Tracheostomies are surgical devices and need changing at regular intervals. Relying on a tracheostomy tube with an inflated cuff represents a risk in an unconscious patient because of the risk of asphyxiation if it becomes blocked. Accidental occlusion or 'blocking off' of the tube is a rare but life-threatening circumstance requiring 24-hour monitoring. Therefore rehabilitation effort is well invested in facilitating independence from an artificial airway, and the physiotherapist contributes to this objective through respiratory assessment and treatment for respiratory hygiene and increasing cough effectiveness and lung volumes to maximise potential for successful weaning.

Engagement with the family is essential for stimulation activities to be meaningful and relevant to the patient. Family can use time with the patient to stretch the therapeutic opportunities available and provide family with an active role, bringing them into the team and aligning their observations with those of the MDT. This can allow for rapport building and a collaborative space where advance planning based on an understanding of the patient's values can guide long-term decision-making. Medicolegal frameworks exist to support staff and families with the difficult decisions regarding escalation of care, ceiling of treatment and treatment withdrawal. These frameworks should be discussed with families within the rehabilitation period and form part of the carer guidelines and handover to a long-term care setting.

Transition of Care – Community Phase

Community care for people in PDOC in the United Kingdom but also elsewhere is typically provided in specialised care homes with skilled and experienced staff maintaining the 24-hour care plan established during rehabilitation. Patients may have a period of community physiotherapy provision during transition, or the patient may be transferred to a care setting with a physiotherapist in the team. Prevention of physical deterioration is the primary goal, through long-term review and maintenance of the therapeutic physical routine. This aims to prevent pain and difficulty in meeting care needs because of spasticity or contracture, and the loss of joint range. It will also facilitate access to different positions, preventing avoidable conditions such as contractures or pressure wounds. Long-term management will include training for staff when needed. Change in spasticity may require referral and the provision or sourcing of splints and devices to best suit the patient as appropriate. The secondary role is to support the long-term monitoring of PDOC and observe for behaviours that might suggest a change in conscious level which would require consideration of a repeat rehabilitation admission. In the United Kingdom, guidelines (Royal College of Physicians 2020) recommend quarterly review by a physiotherapist for the first year followed by annual review thereafter to ensure physical management is optimised and appropriate referrals are made should the presentation have changed.

CASE STUDY – SARAH

Sarah was a 27-year-old woman living with her parents and studying pharmacy full time. She swam four times a week and volunteered for the local homeless shelter. Sarah had type 1 diabetes mellitus since childhood and self-administered insulin. One morning, she was found unconscious in bed by her father after a hypoglycaemic episode (BM 1.3 mmol/L) of unknown duration. She had gone to bed as normal the night before and was otherwise fit and healthy.

Upon hospital admission, initial computerised tomography brain scans showed no change. There was no recovery of consciousness with correction of blood glucose, and she remained intubated in the ITU. Two days later, a repeat scan reported diffuse cerebral oedema and Sarah underwent urgent bifrontal decompressive craniectomy. Three weeks into Sarah's admission she continued to require intensive chest physiotherapy to manage secretions and had a tracheotomy. Later, a percutaneous endoscopic gastrostomy tube was placed, and she was diagnosed as being in PDOC. After 6 weeks in ITU she moved to the ward where the tracheostomy was weaned. Sarah transferred to a specialist neurorehabilitation unit 4 months after her brain injury.

Rehabilitation focused on multidisciplinary assessment of her awareness and long-term disability management. Sarah had myoclonic jerks in her right leg, extensor patterning of limbs and was fully dependent on the assistance of two people for all activities. She had severe dysphagia, creating high risk of aspirating her secretions, and was

dependent on chest physio and repeated Yankauer suctioning to manage secretions.

In rehabilitation, long-term goals formulated by the patient or family direct meaningful person-centred intervention and will often extend beyond the admission (Evans 2012). The centrality of the individual and their family is acknowledged by using their own wording. Short-term goals are devised to work towards these headline aims in achievable, measurable and realistic steps within the admission. Outcomes from the achievement or nonachievement of these short-term targets are used to describe the rehabilitation trajectory.

Sarah's long-term goals:
- To be able to squeeze my family's hands
- To keep my mouth clean
- To keep my limbs moving fully
- To explore whether I can eat safely

STIMULATION AND RESPONSIVENESS

Assessing Sarah's level of consciousness was central in her programme, for her family and to inform her rehabilitation, care plan and discharge planning. Her behaviours were noted and classified using the Sensory Modality Assessment and Rehabilitation Technique (Gill-Thwaites et al 1997), Wessex Head Injury Matrix (Shiel et al 2000) and Coma Recovery Scale–Revised (Giacino et al 2014). Sarah demonstrated a limited range of inconsistent behaviours during tactile, auditory and olfactory stimulation with family and with therapists. The behaviours seen were all reflexive or spontaneous movement, many being myoclonic jerks of her leg. Sarah was concluded to be in persistent VS, and education and support were provided for her family.

The MDT created a timetable providing opportunities for structured tactile, auditory and olfactory activities as more behaviours were observed during assessment in these modalities. The programme included 30 minutes of activity at a time spaced through the day, providing one type of stimuli at a time to avoid fatigue and overstimulation. Activities included gentle massage on her left hand, exposing to preferred aromatherapy scents and playing her favourite music with either team members or family with their consent. Sarah's responses were observed and noted.

Oral Care

On admission Sarah presented with oral hypersensitivity and reemergence of bite reflex, with concurrent trismus. The team devised an MDT approach incorporating postural management and desensitisation to enable comfortable and effective regular oral hygiene. For Sarah, this included positioning in supported side lying with wedges and pillows to reduce the risk of aspiration and minimise distress during graded desensitisation before cleaning her teeth and tongue. She also received BoNT to her masseter muscles to allow mouth opening.

Postural Management

Sarah presented with axial muscle weakness requiring support to maintain head position and to maintain a sitting position. Recurrent coughing caused by pooled secretions necessitated frequent repositioning. Furthermore, Sarah had repeated jerks of her right lower limb related to cortical myoclonus, disturbing her postural alignment in bed and in the chair over time. Her posture and positioning were optimised through provision of a tilt-in-space wheelchair including contoured occipital head support, a two-point pelvic strap and a four-point chest harness. The chair was set with a seat angle of 30° to facilitate a tilted position to maintain a stable, upright position and an additional 10° of recline to minimise the alterations to her head position when coughing, and to maintain her pelvis at the back of the chair when she experienced a myoclonic jerk in her right leg. She was able to sit for 4 hours at a time without repositioning.

Sarah had retained passive range of movement (ROM) in her upper limbs, despite evidence of hyperreflexia in her right wrist and finger flexors, and elbow extensors. She had hyperreflexia in her left pronators, elbow flexors and extensors. Throughout the admission, comfort and range was assessed through a daily ROM programme. Larger joints were gently mobilised through full range during personal care, during position changes and when hoisting to a chair. The joints of her hands were reviewed daily. Sarah's upper limb ROM was consistently monitored and maintained with a 24-hour postural management plan. Lower limb ROM was maintained through overnight bilateral ankle splints and 20-minute spans of therapeutic standing at 70° on the tilt table which was found to be adequate to maintain ankle range. No focal or global medical spasticity treatment was indicated.

Swallowing

Sarah was offered small amounts of pureed food after therapeutic desensitisation and stimulation by therapists and family with training and guidance. Because of her lack of swallow response this was not pursued.

Upon discharge, Sarah had reduced frequency and increased efficacy of cough and swallowing; however, she continued to benefit from assistance in managing secretions through provision of suctioning, saline nebulisers and frequent oral care.

Nutrition

Initially, Sarah presented with severe fluctuations in blood glucose levels creating a risk of further hyperglycaemic or hypoglycaemic injury. Coordinated liaison between the medical, diabetes and dietetics teams successfully devised a consistent plan to control her blood sugar within acceptable levels.

Outcomes

Sarah's rehabilitation improved her symptom management and considerably reduced her care needs because her management became predictable, despite minimal change in her level of impairment or functional ability. She moved to a local brain injury specialist placement with 24-hour care and maintenance therapy. Upon transfer, her family and team were provided with comprehensive postural management and care guidelines to optimise her stability and well-being. The medical team also provided handover for her brittle diabetic management, reducing the risk of future hypoglycaemic events. Maxillofacial review was set up to monitor the trismus to maintain oral hygiene and reduce the risk of aspiration pneumonia. Ceiling of care and resuscitation status were discussed and agreed with the family and care setting. Behaviours consistent with emergence into MCS were described. Planned neurology followup and neuronavigator allocation were arranged.

Summary

In conclusion, this is a complex caseload in which the clinical team must use highly specialist skills and close multidisciplinary working to achieve the best outcomes. It requires a demanding paradigm shift for clinicians, from working towards independence to minimising disability and providing support for the patient and family in line with their values. Ultimately, the profound nature of the change to consciousness for these people affects identity itself and challenges the basis on which we consider the rationale for treatment, and our roles as professionals.

ADULTS WITH CEREBRAL PALSY

Prue Elizabeth Morgan and Carlee Holmes

Introduction

Cerebral palsy (CP) is the most common cause of disability in childhood, with current estimated worldwide incidence of 2.0 per 1,000 births in well-resourced countries (Australian Cerebral Palsy Register Group 2018). It arises from nonprogressive interference, lesion or abnormality within the developing foetal or infant brain resulting in motor and postural dysfunction and other nonmotor impairments such as disorders of sensation, perception, cognition and behaviour (Smithers-Sheedy et al 2016). In addition, comorbidities such as intellectual disability, respiratory disorders and epilepsy may occur (Galea et al

2019). Among individuals with CP the severity of the disability ranges from minimal (independent in all activities) through to severe (requiring full assistance for daily tasks). The condition complexity is increased by co-occurrence of associated impairments, with greater severity of motor impairment associated with greater likelihood of associated impairments (Galea et al 2019). As a result of varying combinations of motor and nonmotor impairments, people with CP may experience difficulty with activities such as walking, balance, upper limb function and communication, resulting in participation restrictions.

Although CP is described as a nonprogressive disorder, resultant neuromuscular physical impairments may change over the lifespan, particularly in those with more severe CP. Occurrence of joint dysfunction, contractures, weakness, fatigue, pain, falls and mental health disorders develop over time and are prevalent in many, affecting quality of life (Morgan et al 2014). For example, 30%–40% of ambulant adults with CP report mobility decline (Morgan & McGinley 2013), experience six times more falls than adults without CP (Ryan et al 2020) and up to 70% experience daily pain (van der Slot et al 2021). Further, adults with CP are twice as likely to be diagnosed with a psychiatric disorder than the general population (McMorris et al 2021). Despite this, because of improvements in neonatal care and early intervention, life expectancy for many with CP approaches that of the general population, with reduction in life expectancy associated with more severe forms of CP and significant comorbidities (Blair et al 2019). Although in the past decade there have been significant improvements in early diagnosis, prevention and treatment, with a reduction in the frequency of nonambulant forms of CP and associated comorbidities (Novak et al 2020), around 75% of people with CP are adults and continue to need lifelong care.

Classification Systems

The motor impairments of CP are classified into four main subtypes – spastic, dyskinetic, ataxic and hypotonic – of which spasticity is the predominant motor type (86%) (Smithers-Sheedy et al 2016). A proportion may present with more than one motor type, for example, exhibiting spasticity with dystonia. The distribution of the motor impairments may also vary, resulting in either unilateral (hemiplegia) or bilateral (diplegia, quadriplegia) distribution. Spastic diplegia is the predominant motor subtype (Australian Cerebral Palsy Register Group 2018).

Given the heterogeneity of the condition, a range of validated measurement tools have been developed to describe the functional status of individuals with CP. The Gross Motor Function Classification System (GMFCS) – Expanded and Revised (Palisano et al 2008) (Fig. 25.10)

allows determination of gross motor function from Level I (demonstrates independent gait, some difficulties with balance and coordination) through to Level V (no independent mobility, transported in wheelchair, limited ability to control posture and limbs). Sixty-two percent of children in the most recent registry report are described as functioning at GMFCS Level I or II (Australian Cerebral Palsy Register Group 2018). Although the GMFCS is not validated for use in adults, GMFCS level at age 12 is a reasonable predictor of adult mobility status, particularly at milder and more severe levels (McCormick et al 2007).

Validated tools to classify upper limb function (the Manual Ability Classification system [MAC]) (Eliasson et al 2006) and communication function (Communication Function Classification System [CFCS]) (Hidecker et al 2011) have similarly been developed and use a 5-level scoring system (Level I, relatively independent; Level V, require considerable support). Knowing a person's performance using these tools can assist families, educators and health professionals understand areas of an individual's strengths, and where additional support may be needed. It can also assist in tailoring specific healthcare needs over the lifespan. For example, a child's GMFCS level may determine frequency of hip radiograph recommendations for hip surveillance purposes (Wynter et al 2015).

Childhood Management

There is considerable high-quality evidence to support a range of motor interventions to enhance outcomes in children with CP. Novak and colleagues (2020) have succinctly summarised effective training-based interventions suitable for use in childhood such as bimanual training, constraint induced movement therapy (CIMT), treadmill training and goal-directed training that may be implemented. Effective strategies when practiced at high intensity result in experience-dependent plasticity (Novak et al 2020). Strategies for the management of abnormal tone and contracture have also been evaluated, with recommendations regarding the use of casting, BoNT or combination therapies made (Novak et al 2020).

Management algorithms, diagnostic matrices, care pathways and clinical guidelines have been developed to assist in the management of issues presenting in people with CP, for example, hip surveillance programmes (Wynter et al 2015), single-event multilevel surgery (SEMLS), osteoporosis (Whitney et al 2021), scoliosis risk scores (Pettersson et al 2020), musculoskeletal management algorithms (Cerebral Palsy Follow Up Program 2022) and exercise and physical activity recommendations (Verschuren et al 2016). However, application of these guidelines to individuals with the most complex CP can be challenging, particularly adults who may not be able

GMFCS E & R between 12th and 18th birthday: Descriptors and illustrations

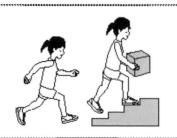
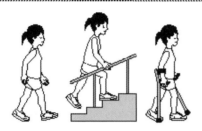

GMFCS Level I

Youth walk at home, school, outdoors and in the community. Youth are able to climb curbs and stairs without physical assistance or a railing. They perform gross motor skills such as running and jumping but speed, balance and coordination are limited.

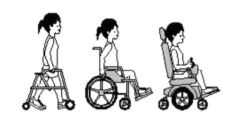

GMFCS Level II

Youth walk in most settings but environmental factors and personal choice influence mobility choices. At school or work they may require a hand held mobility device for safety and climb stairs holding onto a railing. Outdoors and in the community youth may use wheeled mobility when traveling long distances.

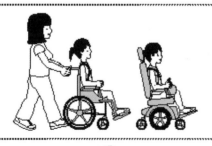

GMFCS Level III

Youth are capable of walking using a hand-held mobility device. Youth may climb stairs holding onto a railing with supervision or assistance. At school they may self-propel a manual wheelchair or use powered mobility. Outdoors and in the community youth are transported in a wheelchair or use powered mobility.

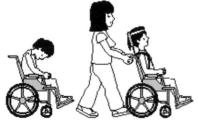

GMFCS Level IV

Youth use wheeled mobility in most settings. Physical assistance of 1-2 people is required for transfers. Indoors, youth may walk short distances with physical assistance, use wheeled mobility or a body support walker when positioned. They may operate a powered chair, otherwise are transported in a manual wheelchair.

GMFCS Level V

Youth are transported in a manual wheelchair in all settings. Youth are limited in their ability to maintain antigravity head and trunk postures and control leg and arm movements. Self-mobility is severely limited, even with the use of assistive technology.

FIG 25.10 Gross Motor Function Classification System – Expanded and Revised illustrated descriptors. (Illustrations: Graham, Reid and Harvey, RCH, Melbourne; Descriptors: Palisano et al 2008. Reprinted with permission.)

to access surveillance equipment or resources (Holmes et al 2020). The research upon which these guidelines are developed is typically focused on children with CP, and on management of single impairments, resulting in difficulty when searching for effective treatments for adults with complex needs to enhance participation outcomes. Evidence to support interventions in adults is only recently emerging, with recognition of the need for individualised evidence-based lifespan care. Finally, optimal management of those with complex CP ideally is delivered by a skilled specialist MDT, which may not always be accessible or available.

Transition From Paediatric to Adult Health Services

Transition is most widely defined as the purposeful, planned movement of adolescents and young adults with chronic physical and medical conditions from child-centred to adult-orientated healthcare systems (Rosen et al 2003). The current situation in well-resourced countries involves the transition of children with CP from paediatric to adult healthcare services at approximately 18 years of age. However, the occurrence of transition at a predetermined chronological age rather than at a developmental age may place vulnerable young adults, such as those with complex CP, into adult healthcare facilities that do not have the expertise, time or resources to adequately meet their needs (Li et al 2020). Some of these reported barriers experienced by those both undergoing and providing transition services are summarised in Table 25.7 below.

Guidelines to establishing successful transition processes have been published (Stewart 2009) based on research evidence alongside input from an expert panel consisting of young people with disabilities, researchers, clinicians, community members, parents and families. These guidelines stress essential elements of collaboration, capacity building at all levels, the involvement of community facilitators, readily accessible information and resources and a standardised educational strategy (Stewart 2009).

Age-Related Health Issues in Adults With CP

Preventative healthcare requires prioritisation for adults with complex CP who are at high risk for the development of cardiometabolic disease and early mortality, premature sarcopenia and functional deterioration (Peterson et al 2013). Secondary impairments are most common in the more severely affected individuals, with the effects of ageing and functional decline occurring earlier in adults with CP than the general population (Haak et al 2009). This may be related to earlier development of osteoporosis and arthritis, poor nutrition, sedentary lifestyles and fatigue (Haak et al 2009, Peterson et al 2013), setting up an ongoing cycle of progression and decline.

Respiratory disease accounts for most premature deaths in all people with CP, accounting for a 14-fold increased risk of death in adults with CP compared with their nondisabled peers (Gibson et al 2021, Ryan 2019). This vulnerable and often medically fragile population of adults with CP may experience increased hospital admissions (Gill et al 2021), crisis care and emergency department admissions and increased mortality (Ryan 2019). Hence neither paediatric CP knowledge nor knowledge gleaned from those without disability can necessarily be applied to the adult CP population who require specific guidelines for best practice healthcare throughout adulthood.

TABLE 25.7 Barriers Experienced in the Transition to Adult Healthcare (Collis et al 2008, Joly 2015, Young et al 2009)	
Barriers to Transition	
Patient and family perspectives	**Service provider perspectives**
Lack of communication between paediatric and adult healthcare providers	Lack of dedicated transition clinics
Lack of specialist knowledge	Lack of dedicated staff (medical and allied health)
Lack of care coordination (i.e., paediatrician equivalent)	Limited specific resources (equipment, space, time)
Inappropriate facilities and equipment	Limited funding
Discontinuity in care	Inadequate collaboration between paediatric and adult healthcare providers
Difficulty adjusting to adult healthcare	Limited infrastructure
Lack of access	
Feelings of loss, abandonment and uncertainty	

Adults with complex CP may present for management of several potentially interrelated issues often requiring an MDT approach:

- **Low bone density and fracture risk:** The risk of fracture (any cause) is 6.4% in adults with CP compared with 2.7% in the general population, occurring at an earlier age in adults with CP and progressing throughout the lifespan as mobility and weight bearing decline and the risk of osteoporosis increases (Whitney et al 2019). Effective management requires screening for, and addressing, risk factors such as weight-bearing status and mobility, falls history, body weight and nutrition, medication use that may negatively affect bone health and a history of low-impact fractures (Bromham et al 2019).

- **Contracture development:** The incidence of contractures in adults with CP is high with 14%–100% experiencing hip contractures and 32%–87% experiencing knee contractures (Holmes et al 2018). Such musculoskeletal issues are progressive and adversely affect many aspects of care and function inclusive of mobility, seating and pressure care. Effective management in those with more severe CP requires a global focus on postural strategies and supports to minimise contracture progression and associated pressure injury development.

- **Mobility and balance dysfunction:** A decline in mobility and balance and resultant falls is common in adults with CP occurring up to 40 years earlier than in the general population (Morgan & McGinley 2013). Up to 58% of adults with CP experience a decline in mobility with a greater deterioration experienced by those with bilateral CP, higher levels of fatigue and in individuals with an initial poorer gait function (Morgan & McGinley 2013). Higher levels of pain and perceptions of balance dysfunction are also associated with an earlier decline in mobility (Gjesdal et al 2020, Opheim et al 2009). The reported incidence of falls varies, with some studies reporting it to be as high as 75% in adults with CP (Morgan & McGinley 2013), which poses a significant risk of adverse consequences including fear, functional decline and ultimately increased morbidity and mortality. Improvements can be achieved with targeted physiotherapy interventions inclusive of strategies to enhance walking confidence, reduce falls risk and pain and fatigue (Morgan & McGinley 2013).

- **Physical inactivity:** Adults with CP are at a greater risk of preventable cardiometabolic disease and progressive functional limitations as a result of reduced physical activity (Verschuren et al 2016). Across all ages and levels of motor function, young people with cerebral palsy participated in 13%–53% less habitual physical activity than their peers (Carlon et al 2013). Increasing physical activity through participation in community gymnasium programmes can not only improve physical health-related outcomes but also mental health outcomes as demonstrated in a student-mentored weekly community gymnasium-based exercise programme (Shields et al 2019).

- **Pain:** The prevalence of pain in adults with CP is reported to be as high as 89% with a range of contributing factors inclusive of sensory and autonomic dysfunction, abnormal neuromotor function, clinical procedures and therapy (van der Slot et al 2021). Commonly reported sites of pain for adults with CP (all GMFCS levels) include neck and back (66%), legs (76%) and arms (38%) (van der Slot et al 2021). For adults with disorders of cognition and communication, reporting and localisation of pain are challenging, with greater risk of pain neglect and undermanagement (McDowell et al 2017) and potential negative impacts on resultant quality of life and function (van der Slot et al 2021).

- **Spasticity:** Spasticity is the most common motor disorder in individuals with CP, affecting up to 86.5% (Smithers-Sheedy et al 2016). Spasticity is poorly understood in adults with CP (Smith et al 2021), leading to underdiagnosis and treatment, and is a likely contributing factor to pain, joint deformity and contracture, pressure injury risk, decreased motor control and function. Spasticity management may consider a combination of interventions including medications such as BoNT and oral and intrathecal baclofen (Tosi et al 2009). Although conservative interventions have been well established in children (Novak et al 2020), a strong evidence base for spasticity management is lacking for adults with CP (Smith et al 2021). Complicating the assessment and management of spasticity in this population is the potential to develop new comorbidities such as stroke and myelopathy (Smith et al 2021).

- **Fatigue:** Fatigue affects 18%–39% of adults with CP (Brunton 2018) and is reported more frequently in adults more severe disability (GMFCS III–V) (van Gorp et al 2021). Correlations exist between pain, fatigue and mental health, highlighting the need for CP-specific assessments and interventions to address the adverse implications for quality of life, independence and function (Brunton 2018, van Gorp et al 2021).

- **Mental health disorders:** Mental health issues in adults with CP are prevalent, with approximately 1 in 3 adults with CP suffering from a psychiatric disorder which may present as a psychotic illness or an anxiety or mood disorder (Eres et al 2021). Assessment and treatment may be more complicated because of communication disorders, lack of specific psychosocial language available on Augmentative and Alternative Communication

(AAC) systems, proxy reporting and lack of CP-specific assessment tools (Whitney et al 2019). Common problems experienced by those with CP such as pain, fatigue and medication side effects may further exacerbate mental health issues (Whitney et al 2019).

CASE STUDY

Kellie is a 43-year-old woman with CP functioning at GMFCS level V. She is dependent for all aspects of her care inclusive of mobility, transfers, position changes, hygiene and nutrition. Kellie is nonverbal and because of decreased motor control, including inconsistent eye gaze, use of AAC is challenging. Kellie lives at home with her elderly parents and is supported through the National Disability Insurance Scheme (NDIS) for disability-related supports. The NDIS is a publicly funded insurance scheme providing eligible Australians, with permanent and significant disability, access to funding for specialist disability supports (National Disability Insurance Agency 2020). Kellie enjoys water activities including visits to the pool and disability-accessible beaches. Social interaction with her peers, family and the local community is an important participation goal for Kellie.

Kellie's transition to adult healthcare was complicated by the number of concurrent medical specialists she required (neurology, respiratory, gastroenterology, endocrinology, orthopaedics and radiology) and her rural location. Kellie travels up to 4 hours for specialist appointments at the public tertiary hospital because of limited access to a suitable facility closer to home. Although she engages with community-based allied health services, access to ongoing specialist allied health is also difficult because of limited rural resources and retention of a skilled workforce.

Kellie presents to the tertiary hospital for review of her increasing postural asymmetry and associated pain and pressure injury risk. Because of her inability to independently change position, the adoption of prolonged static asymmetrical postures remains a risk for ongoing progression and secondary associated complications (Fig. 25.11). Her increasing pain and pressure injury risk had meant that she was no longer able to tolerate sitting in her wheelchair to enable transport to her weekly community pool activity and participate in the associated social activities.

The interrelationship between Kellie's impairments, activity limitations and participation restrictions are illustrated using the ICF classification (World Health Organisation 2022) in Fig. 25.12.

Given Kellie's extremely limited function and medical fragility, the focus of assessment was on her neuromuscular and postural status.

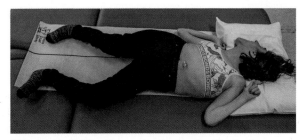

FIG 25.11 Kellie: Postural asymmetry illustrating presence of windswept hips, chest asymmetry and limb contractures. (Reproduced with permission.)

Assessment of Kellie's Neuromuscular and Postural Status

A comprehensive assessment of Kellie's neuromuscular and postural status used a variety of assessment tools. Her assessment results are provided in Table 25.8.

To note, the feasibility of obtaining standardised positioning for spinal/pelvic radiographs is compromised for Kellie because of her established contractures, cognitive challenges and spasticity (Fig. 25.13).

Measures of Posture

The Goldsmith Indices of Body Symmetry (GIofBS) (Fig. 25.14), using an impairment focus, was used to provide a clinical three-dimensional measure of her chest shape and symmetry and hip and pelvic mobility inclusive of a measure of wind sweeping (external rotation/abduction of one hip and internal rotation/adduction of the contralateral hip). Kellie's results suggest considerable asymmetry resulting in a fixed windswept posture towards the left.

The GIofBS was supplemented with the Posture and Postural Ability Scale (PPAS) (Rodby-Bousquet et al 2014), an activity-based framework, which enables description of Kellie's postural ability in supine, prone, sitting and standing, noting relationships between body parts, weight bearing and symmetry. Postural ability is described using a 7-point scale ranging from Level 1, unplaceable in an aligned posture, to Level 7, able to move in and out of a position (Rodby-Bousquet et al 2014). Kellie's results suggest asymmetry and considerable difficulty in being placed in an aligned posture in any position.

Measures of Spasticity, Pain and Skin Integrity

Kellie is at high risk for pressure injuries based on her low weight, incontinence, diet, inability to independently move and postural asymmetries causing the potential for uneven weight bearing through bony prominences.

The commonly used spasticity measures – the Tardieu scale (Gracies et al 2010) and the Modified Ashworth Scale (Bohannon & Smith 1987) – have limited use for Kellie in

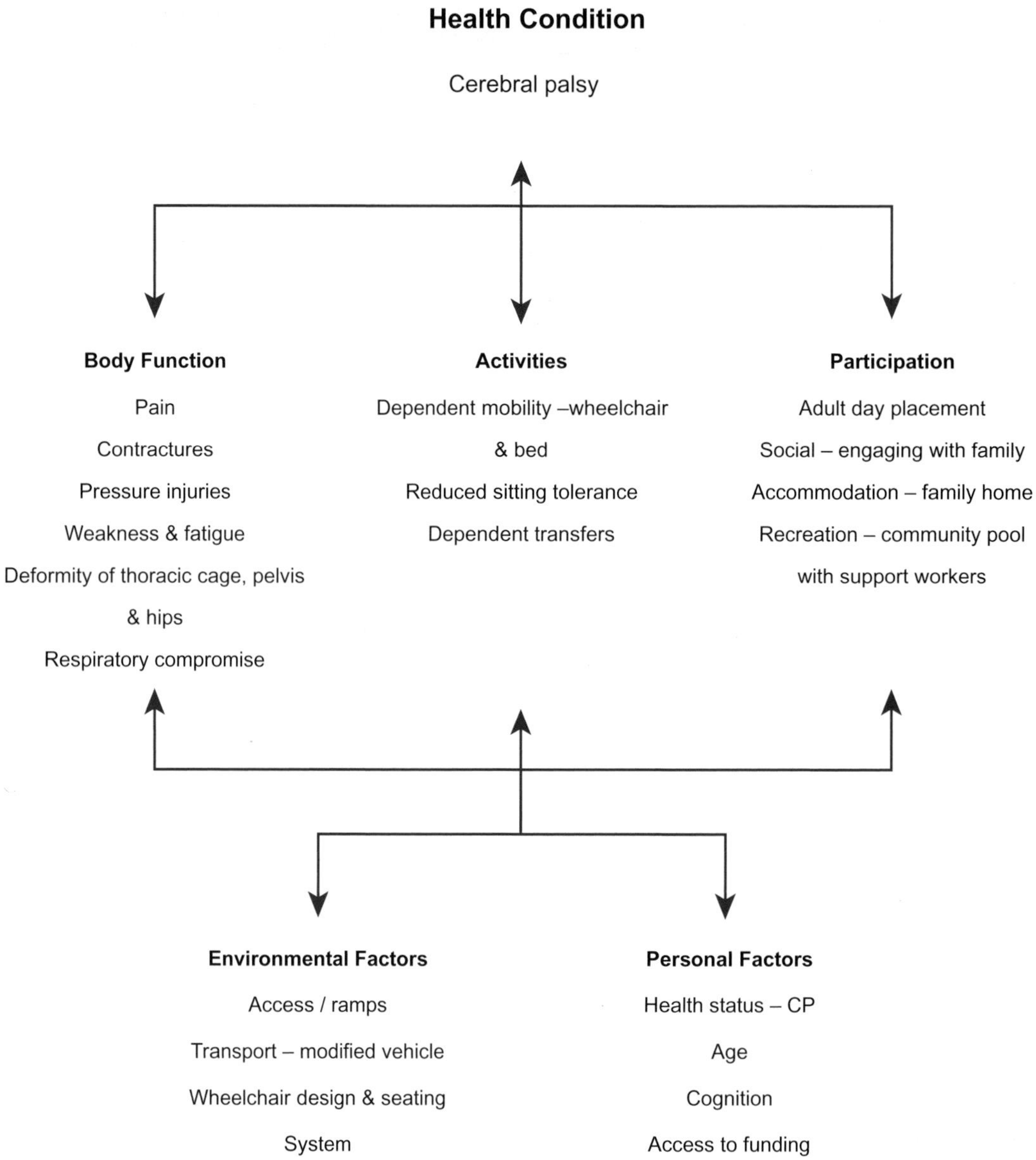

Health Condition

Cerebral palsy

Body Function

Pain

Contractures

Pressure injuries

Weakness & fatigue

Deformity of thoracic cage, pelvis

& hips

Respiratory compromise

Activities

Dependent mobility –wheelchair

& bed

Reduced sitting tolerance

Dependent transfers

Participation

Adult day placement

Social – engaging with family

Accommodation – family home

Recreation – community pool

with support workers

Environmental Factors

Access / ramps

Transport – modified vehicle

Wheelchair design & seating

System

Personal Factors

Health status – CP

Age

Cognition

Access to funding

FIG 25.12 Modified ICF diagram illustrating Kellie's function across ICF domains.

the presence of such significant fixed postural asymmetry and the presence of contractures, prior tendon transfers and pain. Hence the GAS was used to measure treatment efficacy (Turner-Stokes et al 2013), supplemented with goniometric measures of key joints. For example, a goal identified using the GAS for Kellie was 'One carer is able to access, clean and dry her palm preventing skin redness and breakdown'. Given Kellie's difficulties with communication, pain was optimally measured using the Non-Communicating Adult Pain Checklist (NCAPC), an 18-item scale describing six subdimensions of pain behaviour (vocal reaction, emotional reaction, facial expression, body language, protective reaction and physiological reaction) (Lotan et al 2009, 2010). Results using the NCAPC, Tardieu scale and goniometer findings suggest fixed contractures in hips and knees and high levels of pain (before spasticity management).

TABLE 25.8   Assessment Results

	Kellie's Results	Interpretation
Radiographs		
Hip migration (%)	Right: 100% Left: unable to measure – extreme hip external rotation and abduction	>30% = abnormal or 'at risk'[a] 100% = complete dislocation
Cobb angle (spine)	43°	Scoliosis defined as Cobb angle ≥10°[b]Corrective surgery considered at >30°
Pelvic obliquity	29°	0° = level pelvis in frontal plane
Range of motion		
Hip flexion	Right: 30°–50 ° Left: 30°–60°	Asymmetrical limited hip flexion requiring accommodation in seating
Knee flexion	Right: 15°–110° Left: 30°–70°	Asymmetrical limited knee ROM requiring accommodation in seating
Ankle plantarflexion	Right: 30° PF Left: 15° PF	Fixed plantar flexion contractures
Elbow flexion	Right: 100°–130° Left: 85°–130°	Asymmetrical limited elbow ROM
Noncommunicating Adult Pain Checklist[c]		
Prespasticity management	21 of 54 (postmanagement: 7 of 54)	≥10 of 54 indicative of high pain level
Goldsmith Indices of Body Symmetry[d]		**Control data**[d]
Chest depth width ratio	0.62	Control data (0.52–0.75); lower value indicative of a flattened chest shape
Chest left right ratio	0.88	Control data: (0.00–0.27); 0 indicative of symmetry between right and left sides
Combined hip external rotation/abduction	Right: 14° Left: 64°	Control data: Right: 35–65°; Left: 42–69°
Windswept Index	37	Control data: (0–14; 0 = symmetry between right and left sides
Posture and Postural Ability Scale[e]		
Level of postural ability in supine, prone, sitting and standing	Level 1	Unplaceable in an aligned posture
Quality of posture in supine, prone, sitting and standing	Frontal plane: 0/6 Sagittal plane: 0/6	Relates to ability to achieve symmetry of head, trunk, pelvis, limbs and even weight distribution

[a]Wynter et al 2011,
[b]Saito et al 1998,
[c]Lotan et al 2010,
[d]Holmes et al 2020,
[e]Rodby-Bousquet et al 2014.
PF, Plantarflexion; *ROM*, range of movement.

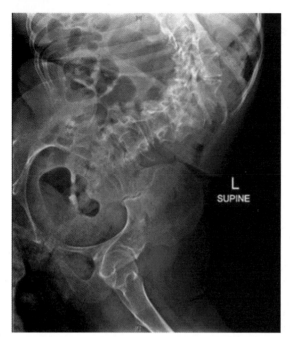

FIG 25.13 Kellie: Radiograph of spine and left hip. (Reproduced with permission.)

Management Strategies

The proposed strategies and interventions to comprehensively manage a range of Kellie's impairments and activity limitations linked to assessment tools are summarised in Table 25.9 and illustrated in Fig. 25.15. Although largely impairment-focused, once these were addressed, Kellie could tolerate sitting in her wheelchair for extended periods free from pain and pressure injury risks. This enabled achievement of her participation goals of attending the pool weekly and engaging in social events in her local rural community of which she is a well-known and valued member.

Case Summary

Kellie's complex CP increases her risk of ongoing deterioration in her health status, such as decline in respiratory function, skin integrity, movement and posture as she ages. Through a comprehensive management programme administered by an MDT, Kellie's postural status was stabilised through the use of customised seating and bed supports, and spasticity management. As a result of these interventions Kellie's pain and the pressure injury on her ear resolved. She was able to spend more time in her tilt-in-space chair to attend the pool and the social activities she enjoys with her peers, family and local community. The interrelationship between Kellie's impairments, activity limitations and participation restrictions support the need for access to a skilled MDT to optimise her ongoing care.

Summary

Adults ageing with developmental disabilities, such as CP, need lifespan care to minimise adverse neuromuscular consequences and enhance participation outcomes. Evidence suggests those with complex CP are particularly at risk for developing high-risk comorbidities including cardiorespiratory, neurological and musculoskeletal disorders. There is a clear need for improved awareness and screening alongside the development of services and clinicians equipped to address the complexities of lifespan healthcare in adults with CP.

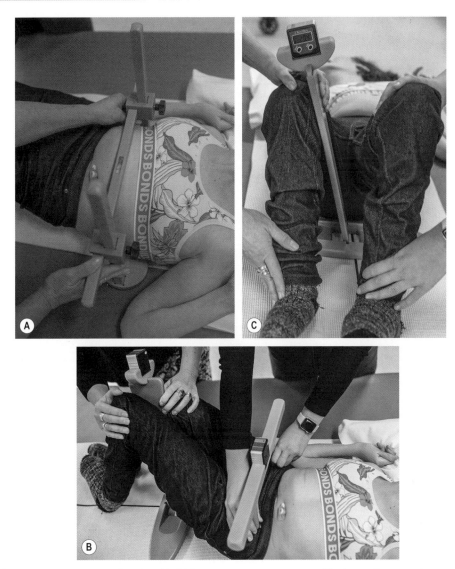

FIG 25.14 Kellie undergoing the GIofBS measurement process: (A) chest shape and symmetry, (B) pelvic mobility, (C) hip mobility. (Reproduced with permission.)

TABLE 25.9   Measurement Tools and Proposed Strategy/Intervention

Issue	Measurement Tool	Strategy/Intervention
Spasticity	GAS[1] Goniometer Modified Tardieu Scale[2] Skin integrity checks	Oral medications including baclofen, dantrium and gabapentin Botulinum toxin to wrist and elbow flexors, splinting and ROM exercises Sciatic and femoral nerve blocks to reduce hip and knee extension and improve wheelchair positioning and comfort
Contractures and Postural asymmetry	GIofBS[3] Radiographs PPAS[4] MAT[5]	Custom moulded wheelchair, and commode to accommodate asymmetrical limited hip flexion, pelvic obliquity, thoracic deformity, limb contractures, maintain skin integrity, facilitate respiration, vision, comfort, engagement and participation Customised hoist sling to accommodate asymmetrical limited hip flexion Bed positioning equipment (Fig. 6)
Pain	NCAPC[6]	Spasticity management Assistive technology and positioning equipment (Fig. 6) Pressure care Gastrointestinal care (bowel regime)
Lack of independent movement	PPAS[4]	24-hour postural management plan utilising time spent in wheelchair (tilt in space), bed positioning, commode and splinting
Pressure injuries	Skin integrity checks	Silk pillow case for R ear pressure injury ROHO mattress insert for trunk/pelvis & heels. Assistive technology (custom moulded seating and bed positioning equipment) Spasticity management

[1]Turner-Stokes et al., 2013;
[2]Gracies et al., 2010;
[3]Holmes et al., 2020;
[4]Rodby-Bousquet et al., 2014;
[5]State Spinal Cord Injury Service, 2021;
[6]Lotan et al., 2009.

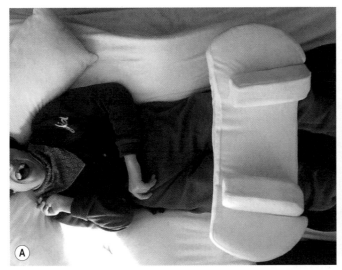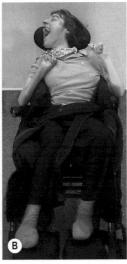

FIG 25.15 Kellie supported in bed (A) using assistive technology products and in her wheelchair, (B) with a custom moulded seating system to accommodate her fixed postural asymmetries (pelvic obliquity, asymmetrical limited hip flexion and scoliosis).

SELF-ASSESSMENT QUESTIONS

1. What are normal movement directions of the scapulothoracic joint during arm elevation? How can this movement in the scapulothoracic joint be explained?
2. Which clinical tests exist to assess shoulder girdle position? How should you interpret the outcome of these tests?
3. What are the two core elements for treatment and management of severe spasticity?
4. When might you consider treatment of spasticity with botulinum toxin?
5. What is the difference between screening and assessment for fitness to drive?
6. What are the main steps of a fitness-to-drive referral process?
7. What are some common age-related health issues that arise in adults with cerebral palsy?
8. What assessment tools might you use to enable a comprehensive assessment of the posture and associated impairments of an adult with severe cerebral palsy?

REFERENCES

Aimola, E., Santello, M., La Grua, G., Casabona, A., 2011. Anticipatory postural adjustments in reach-to-grasp: effect of object mass predictability. Neurosci. Lett. 502, 84–88.

Akinwuntan, A.E., Devos, H., 2015. Decisions about driving for persons with neurodegenerative conditions. Arch. Phys. Med. Rehabil. 96, 767–768.

Akinwuntan, A.E., Devos, H., Kumar, V., et al., 2014. Improvement of driving skills in persons with relapsing-remitting multiple sclerosis: a pilot study. Arch. Phys. Med. Rehabil. 95, 531–537.

Akinwuntan, A.E., Devos, H., Stepleman, L., et al., 2013. Predictors of driving in individuals with relapsing-remitting multiple sclerosis. Mult. Scler. J. 19, 344–350.

Akinwuntan, A.E., O'Connor, C., McGonegal, E., et al., 2012a. Prediction of driving ability in people with relapsing-remitting multiple sclerosis using the stroke driver screening assessment. Int. J. MS Care. 14, 65–70.

Akinwuntan, A.E., Tank, R., Vaughn, L., et al., 2009. Normative values for driving simulation parameters: a pilot study. Paper presented at the Proceedings of the Fifth International Driving Symposium on Human Factors in Driver Assessment. Training, and Vehicle Design, Big Sky, Montana.

Akinwuntan, A.E., Wachtel, J., Rosen, P.N., 2012b. Driving simulation for evaluation and rehabilitation of driving after stroke. J. Stroke Cerebrovasc. Dis. 21, 478–486.

Ashford, S., Jackson, D., Mahaffey, P., et al., 2016. Conceptualisation and development of the Leg Activity measure (LegA) for patient and carer reported assessment of activity (function) in the paretic leg in people with acquired brain injury. Physiother. Res. Int. 22, e1660.

Ashford, S., Slade, M., Nair, A., Turner-Stokes, L., 2014. Arm Activity measure (ArmA) application for recording functional gain following focal spasticity treatment. Int. J. Ther. Rehabil. 21, 10–17.

Ashford, S., Slade, M., Turner-Stokes, L., 2013a. Conceptualisation and development of the Arm Activity measure (ArmA) for assessment of activity in the hemiparetic arm. Disabil. Rehabil. 18, 1513–1518.

Ashford, S., Slade, M., Turner-Stokes, L., 2013b. Initial psychometric evaluation of the Arm Activity measure (ArmA): a measure of activity in the hemiparetic arm. Clin. Rehabil. 27, 728–740.

Ashford, S., Turner-Stokes, L., 2006. Goal attainment for spasticity management using botulinum toxin. Physiother. Res. Int. 11, 24–34.

Ashford, S., Turner-Stokes, L., 2009. Management of shoulder and proximal upper limb spasticity using botulinum toxin and concurrent therapy interventions: a preliminary analysis of goals and outcomes. Disabil. Rehabil. 31, 220–226.

Australian Cerebral Palsy Register Group., 2018. Report of the Australian Cerebral Palsy Register. Birth years 1995-2012. Available at: https://cpregister.com/wp-content/uploads/2019/02/Report-of-the-Australian-Cerebral-Palsy-Register-Birth-Years-1995-2012.pdf. Accessed on 19 July 2023.

Badenes, D., Garolera, M., Casas, L., et al., 2014. Driving competences and neuropsychological factors associated to driving counselling in multiple sclerosis. J. Int. Neuropsychol. Soc. 20, 555–565.

Baker, K., Cano, S.J., Playford, E.D., 2011. Outcome measurement in stroke: a scale selection strategy. Stroke. 42, 1787–1794.

Ball, K.K., Roenker, D.L., Bruni, J.R., 1990. Developmental Changes in Attention and Visual Search Through Adulthood. Elsevier, Amsterdam.

Bargellesi, S., et al., 2017. Occurrence and predictive factors of heterotopic ossification in severe acquired brain injured patients during rehabilitation stay: cross-sectional survey. Clin. Rehabil. 32, 255–262.

Barker, R.N., Brauer, S., Carson, R., 2009. Training-induced changes in the pattern of triceps to biceps activation during reaching tasks after chronic and severe stroke. Exp. Brain. Res. 196, 483–496.

Barnes, M., 2003. Botulinum toxin – mechanisms of action and clinical use in spasticity. J. Rehabil. Med. 9, 1650–1677.

Behrsin, J.F., Maguire, K., 1986. Levator scapulae action during shoulder movement: a possible mechanism for shoulder pain of cervical origin. Aust. J. Physiother. 32, 101–106.

Bellon, P.A., Bosso, M.J., Echegaray, J.E.C., et al., 2022. Tracheostomy decannulation and disorders of consciousness evolution. Respir. Care. 67, 209–215.

Bergfeldt, U., Borg, K., Kullander, K., Julin, P., 2006. Focal spasticity therapy with botulinum toxin: effects on function, activities of daily living and pain in 100 adult patients. J. Rehabil. Med. 38, 166–171.

Bhakta, B.B., 2000. Management of spasticity in stroke. Br. Med. Bull. 56, 476–485.

Blair, E., Langdon, K., McIntyre, S., et al., 2019. Survival and mortality in cerebral palsy: observations to the sixth decade from a data linkage study of a total population register and National Death Index. BMC Neurol. 19, 1–11.

Bohannon, R.W., Green, M.D., 2021. Neurologic and musculoskeletal effects of tilt-table standing on adults: a systematic review. J. Phys. Ther. Sci. 33, 700–706.

Bohannon, R.W., Smith, M.B., 1987. Interrater reliability of a modified Ashworth scale of muscle spasticity. Phys. Ther. 67, 206–207.

Borich, M.R., Bright, J.M., Lorello, D.J., et al., 2006. Scapular angular positioning at end range internal rotation in cases of glenohumeral internal rotation deficit. J. Orthopaed. Sports Phys. Ther. 36, 926–934.

Borstad, J.D., 2008. Measurement of pectoralis minor muscle length: validation and clinical application. J. Orthopaed. Sports Phys. Ther. 38, 169–174.

Borstad, J.D., Ludewig, P.M., 2005. The effect of long versus short pectoralis minor resting length on scapular kinematics in healthy individuals. J. Orthopaed. Sports Phys. Ther. 35, 227–238.

Brashear, A., McAfee, A.L., Kuhn, E.R., Fyffe, J., 2004. Botulinum toxin type B in upper-limb post-stroke spasticity: a double-blind, placebo-controlled trial. Arch. Phys. Med. Rehabil. 85, 705–709.

Brashear, A., Zafonte, R., Corcoran, M., et al., 2002. Inter- and intrarater reliability of the Ashworth Scale and the Disability Assessment Scale in patients with upper-limb post-stroke spasticity. Arch. Phys. Med. Rehabil. 83, 1349–1354.

British Medical Association., 2018. Clinically Assisted Nutrition and Hydration (CANH) and Adults Who Lack the Capacity to Consent, guidance for decision making in England and Wales. Available at: https://www.bma.org.uk/media/1161/bma-clinically-assisted-nutrition-hydration-canh-full-guidance.pdf Accessed on 19 July 2023.

Bromham, N., Dworzynski, K., Eunson, P., et al., 2019. Cerebral palsy in adults: summary of NICE guidance. BMJ. 364, l806.

Brunton, L.K., 2018. Descriptive report of the impact of fatigue and current management strategies in cerebral palsy. Pediatr. Phys. Ther. 30, 135–141.

Burke, W., Wesolowski, M., Guth, M., 1988. Comprehensive head injury rehabilitation: an outcome evaluation. Brain Inj. 2, 313–322.

Calford, M.B., 2002. Mechanisms for acute changes in sensory maps. Adv. Exp. Med. Biol. 508, 451–460.

Carey, J.R., Kimberley, T.J., Lewis, S.M., et al., 2002. Analysis of fMRI and finger tracking training in subjects with chronic stroke. Brain. 125 (Pt 4), 773–788.

Caplan, H., Cox, C., 2019. Resuscitation strategies for traumatic brain injury. Current Surgery Reports. 7, 1–14.

Carlon, S.L., Taylor, N.F., Dodd, K.J., Shields, N., 2013. Differences in habitual physical activity levels of young people with cerebral palsy and their typically developing peers: a systematic review. Disabil. Rehabil. 35, 647–655.

Castelein, B., Cagnie, B., Parlevliet, T., et al., 2015. Optimal normalization tests for muscle activation of the levator scapulae, pectoralis minor, and rhomboid major: an electromyography study using maximum voluntary isometric contractions. Arch. Phys. Med. Rehabil. 96, 1820–1827.

Castelein, B., Cagnie, B., Parlevliet, T., Cools, A., 2016a. Scapulothoracic muscle activity during elevation exercises measured with surface and fine wire EMG: a comparative study between patients with subacromial impingement syndrome and healthy controls. Man. Ther. 23, 33–39.

Castelein, B., Cagnie, B., Parlevliet, T., Cools, A., 2016b. Serratus anterior or pectoralis minor: which muscle has the upper hand during protraction exercises? Man. Ther. 22, 158–164.

Castelein, B., Cagnie, B., Parlevliet, T., Cools, A., 2016c. Superficial and deep scapulothoracic muscle electromyographic activity during elevation exercises in the scapular plane. J. Orthopaed. Sports Phys. Ther. 46, 184–193.

Cerebral Palsy Follow Up Program., 2022. Manual for CPUP adult assessment form. Avsailable at: https://cpup.se/in-english/manuals-and-evaluation-forms/. Accessed on19 July 2023.

Cheng, L., Cortese, D., Monti, M.M., et al., 2018. Do sensory stimulation programs have an impact on consciousness recovery? Front Neurol. 9, 826.

Classen, S., Krasniuk, S., Knott, M., et al., 2016. Interrater reliability of Western University's on-road assessment. Can. J. Occup. Ther. 83, 317–325.

College of Occupational Therapists and Association of Chartered Physiotherapists in Neurology, 2015. Splinting for the Prevention and Correction of Contractures in Adults with Neurological Dysfunction Practice Guideline for Occupational Therapists and Physiotherapists. College of Occupataional Therapists, London.

Collis, F., Finger, E., Okerstrom, E., Owens, K., 2008. Review of transition of young adult clinics. Final report–Attachment, 6.

Comerford, M.J., Mottram, S., 2012. Kinetic Control: The Management of Uncontrolled Movement. Elsevier, Chatswood.

Cools, A.M., Dewitte, V., Lanszweert, F., et al., 2007. Rehabilitation of scapular muscle balance: which exercises to prescribe? Am. J. Sports Med. 35, 1744–1751.

Cools, A.M., Struyf, F., De Mey, K., et al., 2014. Rehabilitation of scapular dyskinesis: from the office worker to the elite overhead athlete. Br. J. Sports Med. 48, 692–697.

Cumming, T.B., Thrift, A.G., Collier, J.M., et al., 2011. Very early mobilization after stroke fast-tracks return to walking: further results from the phase II AVERT randomized controlled trial. Stroke. 42, 153–158.

Chipchase, S.Y., Lincoln, N.B., Radford, K.A., 2003. A survey of the effects of fatigue on driving in people with multiple sclerosis. Disabil. Rehabil. 25, 712–721.

Cruse, D., Chennu, S., Chatelle, C., et al., 2011. Bedside detection of awareness in the vegetative state: a cohort study. Lancet. 378, 2088–2094.

Davis, E.C., Barnes, M., 2000. Botulinum toxin and spasticity. J. Neurol. Neurosurg. Psychiatry. 69, 143–149.

De Baets, L., Jaspers, E., Janssens, L., Van Deun, S., 2014. Characteristics of neuromuscular control of the scapula after stroke: a first exploration. Front. Hum. Sci. 8, 933.

De Baets, L., Jaspers, E., Van Deun, S., 2016a. Scapulohumeral control after stroke: a preliminary study of the test-retest reliability and discriminative validity of a clinical scapular protocol (ClinScaP). NeuroRehabilitation. 38, 359–370.

De Baets, L., Van Deun, S., Monari, D., Jaspers, E., 2016b. Three-dimensional kinematics of the scapula and trunk, and associated scapular muscle timing in individuals with stroke. Hum. Mov. Sci 48, 82–90.

Demain, S., Wiles, R., Roberts, L., McPherson, K., 2006. Recovery plateau following stroke: fact or fiction? Disabil. Rehabil. 28, 815–821.

Devos, H., Akinwuntan, A.E., Gelinas, I., et al., 2012. Shifting up a gear: considerations on assessment and rehabilitation of driving in people with neurological conditions. An extended editorial. Physiother. Res. Int. 17, 125–131.

Devos, H., Alissa, N., Lynch, S., et al., 2021. Real-time assessment of daytime sleepiness in drivers with multiple sclerosis. Mult. Scler. Relat. Disord. 47, 102607.

Devos, H., Ranchet, M., Backus, D., et al., 2016. Determinants of on-road driving in multiple sclerosis. Arch. Phys. Med. Rehabil. 98, 1332–1338.

Dressler, D., Saberi, F.A., Barbosa, E.R., 2005. Botulinum toxin – mechanisms of action. Arqu. Neuropsi. 63, 180–185.

England and Wales Court of Protection Decisions, North West London Clinical Commissioning Group v GU EWCOP 59 (11 November 2021). Available at: https://www.bailii.org/ew/cases/EWCOP/2021/59.html Accessed on 5 July 2023.

Elia, A.E., Filippini, G., Calandrella, D., Albanese, A., 2009. Botulinum neurotoxins for post-stroke spasticity in adults: a systematic review. Mov. Disord. 24, 801–812.

Eliasson, A.C., Krumlinde-Sundholm, L., Rosblad, B., et al., 2006. The Manual Ability Classification System (MACS) for children with cerebral palsy: scale development and evidence of validity and reliability. Devel. Med. Child Neurol. 48, 549–554.

Escamilla, R.F., Yamashiro, K., Paulos, L., Andrews, J.R., 2009. Shoulder muscle activity and function in common shoulder rehabilitation exercises. Sports Med. 39, 663–685.

Eres, R., Reddihough, D., Coghill, D., 2021. Addressing mental health problems in Australians with cerebral palsy: a need for specialist mental health services. Adv. Mental Health., 1–4.

Evans, J.J., 2012. Goal setting during rehabilitation early and late after acquired brain injury. Curr. Opin. Neurol. 25, 651–655.

Fan, L., Su, Y., Elmadhoun, O.A., et al., 2015. Protocol-directed weaning from mechanical ventilation in neurological patients: a randomised controlled trial and subgroup analyses based on consciousness. Neurol. Res. 37, 1006–1014.

Folstein, M.F., Folstein, S.E., McHugh, P.R., 1975. Mini-mental state'. A practical method for grading the cognitive state of patients for the clinician. J. Psychiatr. Res. 12, 189–198.

Frontera, W.R., Grimby, L., Larsson, L., 1997. Firing rate of the lower motoneuron and contractile properties of its muscle fibers after upper motoneuron lesion in man. Muscle Nerve 20, 938–947.

Gajdosik, R.L., Bohannon, R.W., 1987. Clinical measurement of range of motion. Review of goniometry emphasizing reliability and validity. Phys. Ther. 67, 1867–1872.

Galea, C., McIntyre, S., Smithers-Sheedy, H., et al., 2019. Cerebral palsy trends in Australia (1995–2009): a population-based observational study. Devel. Med. Child Neurol. 61, 186–193.

Graham, M., Wallace, E., Doherty, C., et al., 2019. From awareness to prognosis: ethical implications of uncovering hidden awareness in behaviorally nonresponsive patients. Cambridge Q. Healthcare Ethics. 28, 616–631.

Garrubba, M., Turner, T., Grieveson, C., 2009. Multidisciplinary care for tracheostomy patients: a systematic review. Crit. Care. 13, R177.

Giacino, J.T., Fins, J.J., Laureys, S., Schiff, N.D., 2014. Disorders of consciousness after acquired brain injury: the state of the science. Nat. Rev. Neurol. 10, 99–114.

Giacino, J.T., Katz, D.I., Schiff, N.D., et al., 2018. Comprehensive systematic review update summary: Disorders of consciousness: Report of the Guideline Development, Dissemination, and Implementation Subcommittee of the American Academy of Neurology; the American Congress of Rehabilitation Medicine; and the National Institute on Disability, Independent Living, and Rehabilitation Research. Neurology. 91, 461–470.

Gibson, N., Blackmore, A.M., Chang, A.B., et al., 2021. Prevention and management of respiratory disease in young people with cerebral palsy: consensus statement. Devel. Med. Child Neurol. 63, 172–182.

Gill-Thwaites, H., 1997. The Sensory Modality Assessment Rehabilitation Technique – a tool for assessment and treatment of patients with severe brain injury in a vegetative state. Brain Inj. 11, 723–734.

Gill, J., Morgan, P., Enticott, J., 2021. Emergency department usage by adults with cerebral palsy: a retrospective cohort study. Emerg. Med. Australas. 34, 169–175.

Giovannelli, M., Borriello, G., Castri, P., et al., 2007. Early physiotherapy after injection of botulinum toxin increases the beneficial effects on spasticity in patients with multiple sclerosis. Clin. Rehabil. 21, 331–337.

Gjesdal, B.E., Jahnsen, R., Morgan, P., et al., 2020. Walking through life with cerebral palsy: reflections on daily walking by adults with cerebral palsy. Int. J. Qual. Stud. Health Wellbeing. 15, 1746577.

Gracies, J.M., Burke, K., Clegg, N.J., et al., 2010. Reliability of the Tardieu Scale for assessing spasticity in children with cerebral palsy. Arch Phys Med Rehabil. 91, 421–428.

Graham, M., 2019. Can they feel? The capacity for pain and pleasure in patients with cognitive motor dissociation. Neuroethics. 12, 153–169.

Haak, P., Lenski, M., Hidecker, M.J., et al., 2009. Cerebral palsy and aging. Devel. Med. Child Neurol. 51 (Suppl 4), 16–23.

Hambleton, P., Moore, A.P., 1995. Botulinum neurotoxins: origin, structure, molecular actions and antibodies. In: Moore, A.P. (Ed.), Handbook of Botulinum Toxin Treatment. Blackwell Science, Oxford, pp. 16–27.

Hardwick, D.D., Lang, C.E., 2011a. Scapula and humeral movement patterns and their relationship with pain: a preliminary investigation. Int. J. Ther. Rehabil. 18, 210–220.

Hardwick, D.D., Lang, C.E., 2011b. Scapular and humeral movement patterns of people with stroke during range-of-motion exercises. J. Neurol. Phys. Ther. 35, 18–25.

Hesse, S., Reiter, F., Konrad, M., Jahnke, M.T., 1998. Botulinum toxin type A and short-term electrical stimulation in the treatment of upper limb flexor spasticity after stroke: a randomised, double-blind placebo-controlled study. Clin. Rehabil. 12, 381–388.

Hidecker, M.J., Paneth, N., Rosenbaum, P.L., et al., 2011. Developing and validating the Communication Function Classification System for individuals with cerebral palsy. Devel. Med. Child Neurol. 53, 704–710.

Holmes, C., Brock, K., Morgan, P., 2018. Postural asymmetry in non-ambulant adults with cerebral palsy: a scoping review. Disabil. Rehabil., 1–10.

Holmes, C., Fredrickson, E., Brock, K., Morgan, P., 2020. The intra- and inter-rater reliability of the Goldsmith indices of body symmetry in nonambulant adults with cerebral palsy. Disabil. Rehabil. 43, 2640–2646.

Hubbard, I.J., Carey, L.M., Budd, T.W., et al., 2015. A randomized controlled trial of the effect of early upper-limb training on stroke recovery and brain activation. Neurorehabil. Neural Repair. 29, 703–713.

Hughes, P., 2011. The Neer sign and Hawkins-Kennedy test for shoulder impingement. J. Physiother. 57, 260.

Inman, V.T., Saunders, J.B., Abbott, L.C., 1996. Observations of the function of the shoulder joint. 1944. Clin. Orthopaed. Relat. Res. 330, 3–12.

Intercollegiate Stroke Working Party, 2016. National Clinical Guideline for Stroke, fifth ed. Royal College of Physicians, London, UK.

Jaggi, A., Noorani, A., Malone, A., et al., 2012. Muscle activation patterns in patients with recurrent shoulder instability. Int. J. Shoulder Res. 6, 101–107.

Jobe, F.W., Jobe, C.M., 1983. Painful athletic injuries of the shoulder. Clin. Orthopaed. Relat. Res. 173, 117–124.

Joly, E., 2015. Transition to adulthood for young people with medical complexity: an integrative literature review. J. Pediatr. Nurs. 30, e91–e103.

Karni, A., Meyer, G., Jezzard, P., et al., 1995. Functional MRI evidence for adult motor cortex plasticity during motor skill learning. Nature. 377, 155–158.

Katalinic, O.M., Harvey, L.A., Herbert, R.D., et al., 2010. Stretch for the treatment and prevention of contractures. Cochrane Database Syst. Rev. 9, 1–29.

Kendall, F.P., McCreary, E.K., Provance, P.G., 1993. Muscles: Testing and Function. Williams & Wilkins, Baltimore.

Kennedy, R.S., Lane, N.E., Berbaum, K. S., & Lilienthal, M.G., 1993. Simulator sickness questionnaire: An enhanced method for quantifying simulator sickness. Int J Aviation Psychol. 3, 203–220.

Kibler, W.B., 1998. The role of the scapula in athletic shoulder function. Am. J. Sports Med. 26, 325–337.

Kibler, W.B., McMullen, J., 2003. Scapular dyskinesis and its relation to shoulder pain. JAMA. 11, 142–151.

Kibler, W.B., Press, J., Sciascia, A., 2006. The role of core stability in athletic function. Sports Med. 36, 189–198.

Kibler, W.B., Sciascia, A., Wilkes, T., 2012. Scapular dyskinesis and its relation to shoulder injury. JAMA. 20, 364–372.

Kibler, W.B., Ludewig, P.M., McClure, P.W., et al., 2013. Clinical implications of scapular dyskinesis in shoulder injury: the 2013 consensus statement from the 'Scapular Summit'. Br. J. Sports Med. 47, 877–885.

Kisiel-Sajewicz, K., Fang, Y., Hrovat, K., et al., 2011. Weakening of synergist muscle coupling during reaching movement in stroke patients. Neurorehabil. Neural Repair. 25, 359–368.

Kitsinger, J., 2021. Life-Sustaining Treatment Contrary to His Best Interests: Lessons from a Supplementary Hearing. Open Justice, Court of Justice Protection Project, July 2021 Available at: https://openjusticecourtofprotection. org/2021/07/30/life-sustaining-treatment-contrary-to-his-best-interests-lessons-from-a-supplementary-hearing/ Accessed on 5 July 2023.

Konradi, J., Lerch, A., Cataldo, M., Kerz, T., 2015. Direct effects of Facio-Oral Tract Therapy® on swallowing frequency of non-tracheotomised patients with acute neurogenic dysphagia. SAGE Open Med. 3, 2050312115578958.

Krasniuk, S., Classen, S., Morrow, S.A., et al., 2017. Driving errors that predict on-road outcomes in adults with multiple sclerosis. OTJR (Thorofare NJ). 1539449217708554.

Krasniuk, S., Classen, S., Morrow, S.A., et al., 2019. Clinical determinants of fitness to drive in persons with multiple sclerosis: systematic review. Arch. Phys. Med Rehabil. 100 1534–155

Krasniuk, S., Knott, M., Bagajati, R., et al., 2022. Utilizing driving simulators for persons with multiple sclerosis: a scoping review. Transport. Res. Part F. 85, 103–118.

Kreisel, S.H., Hennerici, M.G., Bazner, H., 2007. Pathophysiology of stroke rehabilitation: the natural course of clinical recovery, use-dependent plasticity and rehabilitative outcome. Cerebrovasc. Dis. 23, 243–255.

Kurtzke, J.F., 1983. Rating neurologic impairment in multiple sclerosis: an expanded disability status scale (EDSS). Neurology. 33, 1444–1452.

Lai, J., Francisco, G., Willis, F., 2009. Dynamic splinting after treatment with botulinum toxin type-A: a randomized controlled pilot study. Adv. Ther. 26, 241–248.

Lance, J.W., 1980. Symposium synopsis. In: Feldman, R.G., Young, R.R., Koella, W.P. (Eds.), Spasticity: Disordered Motor Control. Yearbook Medical Publishers, Chicago, pp. 465–494.

Lannin, N., Cusick, A., McCluskey, A., Herbert, R.D., 2007. Effects of splinting on wrist contracture after stroke; a randomised controlled trial. Stroke. 38, 111–116.

Lannin, N., Herbert, R.D., 2003. Is hand splinting effective for adults following stroke? A systematic review and methodological critique of published research. Clin. Rehabil. 17, 807–816.

Laudner, K.G., Moline, M.T., Meister, K., 2010. The relationship between forward scapular posture and posterior shoulder tightness among baseball players. Am. J. Sports Med. 38, 2106–2112.

Li, L., Bird, M., Carter, N., et al., 2020. Experiences of youth with medical complexity and their families during the transition to adulthood. J Transition Med. 2, 1.

Lincoln, N.B., Radford, K.A., 2008. Cognitive abilities as predictors of safety to drive in people with multiple sclerosis. Mult. Scler. 14, 123–128.

Lings, S., 2002. Driving accident frequency increased in patients with multiple sclerosis. Acta Neurol. Scand. 105, 169–173.

Littlewood, C., Malliaras, P., Bateman, M., et al., 2013. The central nervous system – an additional consideration in 'rotator cuff tendinopathy' and a potential basis for understanding response to loaded therapeutic exercise. Man. Ther. 18, 468–472.

Lombardi, F., Taricco, M., De Tanti, A., et al., 2002. Sensory stimulation for brain injured individuals in coma or vegetative state. Cochrane Database Syst. Rev. 2, CD001427.

Lotan, M., Moe-Nilssen, R., Ljunggren, A.E., Strand, L.I., 2009. Reliability of the Non-Communicating Adult Pain Checklist (NCAPC), assessed by different groups of health workers. Res. Dev. Disabil. 30, 735–745.

Lotan, M., Moe-Nilssen, R., Ljunggren, A.E., Strand, L.I., 2010. Measurement properties of the Non-Communicating Adult Pain Checklist (NCAPC): a pain scale for adults with Intellectual and Developmental Disabilities, scored in a clinical setting. Res. Dev. Disabil. 31, 367–375.

Ludewig, P.M., Behrens, S.A., Meyer, S.M., et al., 2004. Three-dimensional clavicular motion during arm elevation: reliability and descriptive data. J. Orthopaed. Sports Phys. Ther. 34, 140–149.

Ludewig, P.M., Phadke, V., Braman, J.P., et al., 2009. Motion of the shoulder complex during multiplanar humeral elevation. J. Bone Joint Surg. 91, 378–389.

Magarey, M.E., Jones, M.A., 2003. Dynamic evaluation and early management of altered motor control around the shoulder complex. Man. Ther. 8, 195–206.

Mahoney, F.I., Barthel, D.W., 1965. Functional evaluation: the Barthel Index. Md. State Med. J. 14, 61–65.

Martin, A., Abogunrin, S., Kurth, H., Dinet, J., 2014. Epidemiological, humanistic and economic burden of illness of lower limb spasticity in adults: a systematic review. Neuropsychiatry Dis. Treat. 10, 111–122.

McClure, P., Balaicuis, J., Heiland, D., et al., 2007. A randomized controlled comparison of stretching procedures for posterior shoulder tightness. J. Orthopaed. Sports Phys. Med. 37, 108–114.

McClure, P., Greenberg, E., Kareha, S., 2012. Evaluation and management of scapular dysfunction. Sports Med. Arthrosc. Rev. 20, 39–48.

McClure, P.W., Michener, L.A., Sennett, B.J., Karduna, A.R., 2001. Direct 3-dimensional measurement of scapular kinematics during dynamic movements in vivo. J. Shoulder Elbow Surg. 10, 269–277.

McComas, A.J., Sica, R.E., Upton, A.R., Aguilera, N., 1973. Functional changes in motoneurones of hemiparetic patients. J. Neurol. Neurosurg. Psychiatry. 36, 183–193.

McCormick, A., Brien, M., Plourde, J., et al., 2007. Stability of the Gross Motor Function Classification System in adults with cerebral palsy. Devel. Med. Child Neurol. 49, 265–269.

McDowell, B.C., Duffy, Lundy, C., 2017. Pain report and musculoskeletal impairment in young people with severe forms of cerebral palsy: a population-based series. Res. Dev. Disabil. 60, 277–284.

McMorris, C.A., Lake, J., Dobranowski, K., et al., 2021. Psychiatric disorders in adults with cerebral palsy. Res. Devel. Disabil 111, 103859.

Mélotte, E., Maudoux, A., Panda, R., et al., 2022. Links between swallowing and consciousness: a narrative review. Dysphagia.

Morgan, P., McGinley, J., 2013. Falls, fear of falling and falls risk in adults with cerebral palsy: a pilot observational study. Eur. J. Physiother. 15, 93–100.

Morgan, P., Soh, S., McGinley, J., 2014. Health-related quality of life of ambulant adults with cerebral palsy and its association with falls and mobility decline: a preliminary cross sectional study. Health Qual. Life Outcomes. 12, 132.

Moriki, T., Nakamura, T., Kojima, D., et al., 2013. Sitting position improves consciousness level in patients with cerebral disorders. Open J. Ther. Rehabil. 1, 1–3.

Morrissey, D., Morrissey, M.C., Driver, W., et al., 2008. Manual landmark identification and tracking during the medial rotation test of the shoulder: an accuracy study using three-dimensional ultrasound and motion analysis measures. Man. Ther. 13, 529–535.

Mottram, S.L., 1997. Dynamic stability of the scapula. Man. Ther. 2, 123–131.

Mottram, S.L., Woledge, R.C., Morrissey, D., 2009. Motion analysis study of a scapular orientation exercise and subjects' ability to learn the exercise. Man. Ther. 14, 13–18.

National Disability Insurance Agency., 2020. National Disability Insurance Scheme. Available at: https://www.ndis.gov.au/. Accessed on 5 July 2023.

Neven, A., Janssens, D., Alders, G., et al., 2013. Documenting outdoor activity and travel behaviour in persons with neurological conditions using travel diaries and GPS tracking technology: a pilot study in multiple sclerosis. Disabil. Rehabil. 35, 1718–1725.

NHS., 2018. Improving quality capacity, care planning and advance care planning in life limiting illness – A Guide for Health and Social Care Staff. Available at: https://www.england.nhs.uk/improvement-hub/wp-content/uploads/sites/44/2017/11/ACP_Booklet_2014.pdf. Accessed on 5 July 2023.

Niessen, M., Janssen, T., Meskers, C., et al., 2008. Kinematics of the contralateral and ipsilateral shoulder: a possible relationship with post-stroke shoulder pain. J. Rehabil. Med. 40, 482–486.

Nouri, F.M., Lincoln, N.B., 1993. Predicting driving performance after stroke. BMJ. 307, 482–483.

Novak, I., Morgan, C., Fahey, M., et al., 2020. State of the evidence traffic lights 2019: systematic review of interventions for preventing and treating children with cerebral palsy. Curr. Neurol. Neurosci. Rep. 20, 3.

Nowak, D.A., 2008. The impact of stroke on the performance of grasping: usefulness of kinetic and kinematic motion analysis. Neurosci. Biobehav. Rev. 32, 1439–1450.

Oatis, 2004. Kinesiology: The Mechanics and Pathomechanics of Human Movement. Lippincott Williams & Wilkins.

Opheim, A., Jahnsen, R., Olsson, E., Stanghelle, J.K., 2009. Walking function, pain, and fatigue in adults with cerebral palsy: a 7-year follow-up study. Devel. Med. Child Neurol. 51, 381–388.

Oujamaa, L., Relave, I., Froger, J., et al., 2009. Rehabilitation of arm function after stroke. Literature review. Ann. Phys. Rehabil. Med. 52, 269–293.

Owen, A.M., Coleman, M., Boly, M., et al., 2006. Detecting awareness in the vegetative state. Science. 313, 1402.

Palisano, R.J., Rosenbaum, P., Bartlett, D., Livingston, M.H., 2008. Content validity of the expanded and revised Gross Motor Function Classification System. Devel. Med. Child Neurol. 50, 744–750.

Pandyan, A.D., Gregoric, M., Barnes, M.P., et al., 2005. Spasticity: clinical perceptions, neurological realities and meaningful measurement. Disabil. Rehabil. 27, 2–6.

Pandyan, A.D., Price, C.I.M., Curless, R.H., 1999. A review of the properties and limitations of the Ashworth and modified Ashworth Scales. Clin. Rehabil. 13, 373–383.

Peterson, M., Gordon, P., Hurvitz, E., 2013. Chronic disease risk among adults with cerebral palsy: the role of premature sarcopoenia, obesity and sedentary behaviour. Obesity Rev.

Pettersson, K., Wagner, P., Rodby-Bousquet, E., 2020. Development of a risk score for scoliosis in children with cerebral palsy. Acta Orthop. 91, 203–208.

Pizzari, T., Wickham, J., Balster, S., et al., 2014. Modifying a shrug exercise can facilitate the upward rotator muscles of the scapula. Clin. Biomech. 29, 201–205.

Platz, T., Pinkowski, C., van Wijck, F., et al., 2005. Reliability and validity of arm function assessment with standardized guidelines for the Fugl-Meyer Test, Action Research Arm Test and Box and Block Test: a multicentre study. Clin. Rehabil. 19, 404–411.

Quesnele, D.C.J., 2011. The assessment and treatment of muscular imbalance. Man. Ther. 16, e4.

Rabin, A., Irrgang, J.J., Fitzgerald, G.K., Eubanks, A., 2006. The intertester reliability of the Scapular Assistance Test. J. Orthopaed. Sports Phys. Ther. 36, 653–660.

Ranchet, M., Akinwuntan, A.E., Tant, M., et al., 2015. Agreement between physician recommendation and fitness-to-drive decision in multiple sclerosis. Arch. Phys. Med. Rehabil. 96, 1840–1844.

Reitan, R.M., 1986. Trail Making Test Manual for Administration and Scoring. Reitan Neuropsychology Laboratory, Tucson, AZ.

Rey, A., 1941. L'examen psychologique dans les cas d'encéphalopathie traumatique. Arch. Psychol. 28, 215–285.

Robertson, J.V., Roche, N., Roby-Brami, A., 2012. Influence of the side of brain damage on postural upper-limb control including the scapula in stroke patients. Exp. Brain Res. 218, 141–155.

Rodby-Bousquet, E., Agustsson, A., Jonsdottir, G., et al., 2014. Interrater reliability and construct validity of the Posture and Postural Ability Scale in adults with cerebral palsy in supine, prone, sitting and standing positions. Clin. Rehabil. 28, 82–90.

Rosen, D.S., Blum, R.W., Britto, M., et al., 2003. Transition to adult health care for adolescents and young adults with chronic conditions: position paper of the Society for Adolescent Medicine. J. Adolesc. Health. 33, 309–311.

Royal College of Physicians, British Society of Rehabilitation Medicine, The Chartered Society of Physiotherapy, Association of Chartered Physiotherapists Interested in Neurology and the Royal College of Occupational Therapists.,

2018. Spasticity in adults: management using botulinum toxin. National guidelines. London: RCP, 2018.

Royal College of Physicians., 2020. Prolonged Disorders of Consciousness Following Sudden Onset Brain Injury, National Clinical Guidelines. Available at: https://bit.ly/38rdU5q. Accessed on 5 July 2023.

Ryan, J., Cameron, M., Liverani, S., et al., 2020. Incidence of falls among adults with cerebral palsy: a cohort study using primary care data. Devel. Med. Child Neurol. 62, 477–482.

Ryan, J.M., Peterson, M.D., Ryan, N., et al., 2019. Mortality due to cardiovascular disease, respiratory disease, and cancer in adults with cerebral palsy. Devel. Med. Child Neurol. 61, 924–928.

Saeys, W., Vereeck, L., Truijen, S., et al., 2012. Randomized controlled trial of truncal exercises early after stroke to improve balance and mobility. Neurorehabil. Neural Repair. 26, 231–238.

Sahara, W., Sugamoto, K., Murai, M., et al., 2006. 3D kinematic analysis of the acromioclavicular joint during arm abduction using vertically open MRI. J. Orthopaeds. Res. 24, 1823–1831.

Saito, N., Ebara, S., Ohotsuka, K., et al., 1998. Natural history of scoliosis in spastic cerebral palsy. Lancet. 351, 1687–1692.

Sanes, J.N., Donoghue, J.P., 2000. Plasticity and primary motor cortex. Ann. Rev. Neurosci. 23, 393–415.

Schultheis, M.T., Garay, E., Millis, S.R., Deluca, J., 2002. Motor vehicle crashes and violations among drivers with multiple sclerosis. Arch. Phys. Med. Rehabil. 83, 1175–1178.

Schultheis, M.T., Weisser, V., Manning, K., et al., 2009. Driving behaviors among community-dwelling persons with multiple sclerosis. Arch. Phys. Med. Rehabil. 90, 975–981.

Seitz, A.L., McClure, P.W., Finucane, S., et al., 2011. Mechanisms of rotator cuff tendinopathy: intrinsic, extrinsic, or both? Clin. Biomech. 26, 1–12.

Shawaryn, M.A., Schultheis, M.T., Garay, E., Deluca, J., 2002. Assessing functional status: exploring the relationship between the multiple sclerosis functional composite and driving. Arch. Phys. Med. Rehabil. 83, 1123–1129.

Sheean, G.L., 2001. Botulinum treatment of spasticity: Why is it difficult to show a functional benefit? Trauma Rehabil. 14, 771–776.

Shiel, A., Horn, S.A., Wilson, B.A., et al., 2000. The Wessex Head Injury Matrix (WHIM) main scale: a preliminary report on a scale to assess and monitor patient recovery after severe head injury. Clin. Rehabil. 14, 408–416.

Shiel, A., Wilson, B., McLellan, D.L., et al., 2000. Wessex Head Injury Matrix (WHIM) – Manual. Harcourt Assessment, London.

Shields, N., van den Bos, R., Buhlert-Smith, K., et al., 2019. A community-based exercise program to increase participation in physical activities among youth with disability: a feasibility study. Disabil. Rehabil. 41, 1152–1159.

Sivak, M., 1996. The information that drivers use: is it indeed 90% visual? Perception. 25, 1081–1089.

Smith, S.E., Gannotti, M., Hurvitz, E.A., et al., 2021. Adults with cerebral palsy require ongoing neurologic care: a systematic review. Ann. Neurol. 89, 860–871.

Smithers-Sheedy, H., McIntyre, S., Gibson, C., et al., 2016. A special supplement: findings from the Australian Cerebral Palsy Register, birth years 1993 to 2006. Dev. Med. Child Neurol. 58 (Suppl. 2), 5–10.

Solem-Bertoft, E., Thuomas, K.A., Westerberg, C.E., 1993. The influence of scapular retraction and protraction on the width of the subacromial space. An MRI study. Clin. Orthopaed. Relat. Res. 296, 99–103.

Sommerfeld, D.K., Johansson, H., Jonsson, A.-L., et al., 2011. Rivermead mobility index can be used to predict length of stay for elderly persons, 5 days after stroke onset. J. Geriatr. Phys. Ther. 34, 64–71.

State Spinal Cord Injury Service., 2021. Spinal Seating Professional Development Program. Available at: https://aci.health.nsw.gov.au/networks/spinal-cord-injury/spinal-seating. Accessed on 5 July 2023.

Stevenson, V.L., Jarrett, L., 2006. Spasticity Management – A Practical Multidisciplinary Guide. Informa Healthcare, London.

Stewart, D., 2009. Transition to adult services for young people with disabilities: current evidence to guide future research. Dev. Med. Child Neurol. 51 (Suppl. 4), 169–173.

Struyf, F., Cagnie, B., Cools, A., et al., 2014a. Scapulothoracic muscle activity and recruitment timing in patients with shoulder impingement symptoms and glenohumeral instability. J. Electromyol. Kinesiol. 24, 277–284.

Struyf, F., Meeus, M., Fransen, E., et al., 2014b. Interrater and intrarater reliability of the pectoralis minor muscle length measurement in subjects with and without shoulder impingement symptoms. Man. Ther. 19, 294–298.

Sutherland, E., Hill, B., Singer, B., et al., 2021. Clinical trial adherence to focal muscle spasticity guidelines: a systematic review. Arch. Phys. Med. Rehabil. 102, e112.

Tate, A., Turner, G.N., Knab, S.E., et al., 2012. Risk factors associated with shoulder pain and disability across the lifespan of competitive swimmers. J. Athl. Train. 47, 149–158.

The Mental Capacity Act., 2005. Available at: https://www.legislation.gov.uk/ukpga/2005/9/contents. Accessed on 5 July 2023.

Thompson, A., Jarrett, L., Lockley, L., et al., 2005. Clinical management of spasticity. J. Neurol. Neurosurg. Psychiatry. 76, 459–463.

Tosi, L.L., Maher, N., Moore, D.W., et al., 2009. Adults with cerebral palsy: a workshop to define the challenges of treating and preventing secondary musculoskeletal and neuromuscular complications in this rapidly growing population. Dev. Med. Child Neurol. 51 (Suppl. 4), 2–11.

Turner-Stokes, L., Baguley, I., De Graaff, S., et al., 2010. Goal attainment scaling in the evaluation of treatment of upper limb spasticity with botulinum toxin: a secondary analysis from a double-blind placebo-controlled randomised clinical trial. J. Rehabil. Med. 42, 81–89.

Turner-Stokes, L., Bassett, P., Rose, H., et al., 2015. Serial measurement of Wessex Head Injury Matrix in the diagnosis of patients in vegetative and minimally conscious states: a cohort analysis. BMJ Open. 5, e006051.

Turner-Stokes, L., Fheodoroff, K., Jacinto, J., Maisonobe, P., 2013. Results from the Upper Limb International Spasticity Study-II (ULIS-II): a large, international, prospective cohort study investigating practice and goal attainment following treatment with botulinum toxin A in real-life clinical management. BMJ Open. 3, e002771.

Turner-Stokes, L., Jacinto, J., Fheodoroff, K., et al., 2021. Assessing the effectiveness of upper-limb spasticity management using a structured approach to goal-setting and outcome measurement: First cycle results from the Upper Limb International Spasticity-III study. J. Rehabil. Med. 53.

Tyson, S.F., Kent, R.M., 2010. Orthotic devices after stroke and other nonprogressive brain lesions. Stroke. 1, 1–3.

Urban, P., Wolf, T., Uebele, M., et al., 2010. Occurrence and clinical predictors of spasticity after ischemic stroke. Stroke. 41, 2016–2020.

Uswatte, G., Taub, E., Morris, D., et al., 2005. Reliability and validity of the upper-extremity Motor Activity Log-14 for measuring real-world arm use. Stroke. 36, 2493–2496.

Vahedi, K., Hofmeijer, J., Juettler, E., et al., 2007. Early decompressive surgery in malignant infarction of the middle cerebral artery: a pooled analysis of three randomised controlled trials. Lancet Neurol. 6, 215–222.

van der Slot, W.M.A., Benner, J.L., Brunton, L., et al., 2021. Pain in adults with cerebral palsy: A systematic review and meta-analysis of individual participant data. Ann. Phys. Rehabil. Med. 64, 101359.

van Gorp, M., Dallmeijer, A.J., van Wely, L., et al., 2021. Pain, fatigue, depressive symptoms and sleep disturbance in young adults with cerebral palsy. Disabil. Rehabil. 43, 2164–2171.

Vattanaslip, W., Ada, L., Crosbie, J., 2000. Contribution of thixotropy, spasticity and contracture to ankle stiffness after stroke. J. Neurol. Neurosurg. Psychiatry. 69, 34–39.

Vegetative and Minimally Conscious States, 2015. Houses of Parliament POSTNOTE. PN489.

Verschuren, O., Peterson, M.D., Balemans, A.C., et al., 2016. Exercise and physical activity recommendations for people with cerebral palsy. Devel. Med. Child Neurol. 58, 798–808.

Wade, D.T., 2018. How many patients in a prolonged disorder of consciousness might need a best interests meeting about starting or continuing gastrostomy feeding? Clin. Rehabil. 32, 1551–1564.

Ward, A.B., Wissel, J., Borg, J., et al., 2014. Functional goal achievement in post-stroke spasticity patients: the BOTOX®

Economic Spasticity Trial (BEST) BEST Study Group. J. Rehabil. Med. 46, 504–513.

Wegner, S., Jull, G., O'Leary, S., Johnston, V., 2010. The effect of a scapular postural correction strategy on trapezius activity in patients with neck pain. Man. Ther. 15, 562–566.

Whitney, D., Alford, A., Devlin, M., et al., 2019. Adults with cerebral palsy have higher prevalence of fracture compared with adults without cerebral palsy independent of osteoporosis and cardiometabolic diseases. J. Bone Miner. Res. 34, 1240–1247.

Whitney, D., Hurvitz, E., Caird, M., 2021. Critical periods of bone health across the lifespan for individuals with cerebral palsy: informing clinical guidelines for fracture prevention and monitoring. Bone. 150, 116009.

Whitney, D., Warschausky, S., Ng, S., et al., 2019. Prevalence of mental health disorders among adults with cerebral palsy: a cross-sectional analysis. Ann. Intern. Med. 171, 328–333.

Williams, G., Singer, B., Ashford, S., et al., 2020. A synthesis and appraisal of clinical practice guidelines, consensus statements and Cochrane systematic reviews for the management of focal spasticity in adults and children. Disabil. Rehabil. 44, 509–519.

World Health Organisation., 2022. International Classification of Functioning, Disability and Health (ICF). Available at: https://www.who.int/standards/classifications/international-classification-of-functioning-disability-and-health. Accessed on 5 July 2023.

Worsley, P., Warner, M., Mottram, S., et al., 2013. Motor control retraining exercises for shoulder impingement: effects on function, muscle activation, and biomechanics in young adults. J. Shoulder Elbow Surg. 22, e11–e19.

Wynter, M., Gibson, N., Kentish, M., et al., 2011. The consensus statement on hip surveillance for children with cerebral palsy: Australian standards of care. J. Pediatr. Rehabil. Med. 4, 183–195.

Wynter, M., Gibson, N., Willoughby, K., et al., 2015. Australian hip surveillance guidelines for children with cerebral palsy: 5-year review. Devel. Med. Child Neurol. 57, 808–820.

Young, N.L., Barden, W.S., Mills, W.A., et al., 2009. Transition to adult-oriented health care: perspectives of youth and adults with complex physical disabilities. Phys. Occup. Ther. Pediatr. 29, 345–361.

Answers to Self-Assessment Questions

CHAPTER 1

1. • The rehabilitation process comprises four main steps: assessment, goal setting, intervention planning and outcome measurement.
   • The ICF provides a common terminology understood by team members, the patient and the patient's family. The ICF enables the team to describe all aspects of disability including contextual factors across all four steps of the rehabilitation process.
   • An ICF-based rehabilitation plan can facilitate team working and clinical reasoning.
   • Refer to Lexell and Brogardh (2015) for an example of a rehabilitation plan based on the ICF.

2. • Have written protocols and pathways which help remove organisational and professional barriers.
   • Have specialist training and knowledge.
   • Agree on a consistent approach for clinical problems.
   • Share treatment sessions.
   • Understand the thinking and beliefs of different disciplines.
   • Have an information provision strategy with consistent messages and access to further information when required.
   • Refer to Clarke and Forster (2015) for further reading.

3. • Fast access to reliable healthcare evidence
   • Effective treatment by trusted professionals
   • Continuity of care and smooth transitions
   • Involvement of and support for family and carers
   • Clear and comprehensive information, and support for self-care
   • Involvement and shared decision making with respect for patient preferences
   • Emotional support, empathy and respect
   • Attention to both physical and environmental needs
   Refer to the Pickering Institute (http://www.pickering.org).

4. The three principles are: enhance the learner's expectation, enhance the learner's autonomy and provide an external focus of attention for the learner. For a sit-to-stand task example:
   • Enhance learner's expectation. The therapist might choose three chair heights that are sufficiently high so the patient can achieve standing with minimal to no assistance from the therapist; the therapist will provide verbal encouragement by stating that the patient will be able to stand up from these higher heights; and after the patient performs a trial well the therapist will acknowledge that trial verbally.
   • Enhance learner's autonomy. Encourage the patient to make choices. The therapist might tell the patient that they will practice the task a total number of times and allow the patient to order the practice sequence.
   • External focus of attention. The therapist is telling the patient to 'push into the floor' to achieve the extension to enhance the momentum transfer into the extension phase of the transfer. If the flexion phase is to be accentuated, then the therapist instructs the patient to 'bring your nose forward past your feet'.

5. Therapists make predictions at all points of care for their patient: during acute hospitalisation, rehabilitation stays and home/outpatient departments. Depending on the prediction information for a specific diagnosis, this information is useful in discharge planning and to encourage through interventions the elicitation of these predictors. It is also useful to determine the intervention strategies used to encourage the positively predicted functional recovery.

6. Primary prevention seeks to prevent the onset of disease through healthy living. It is achieved by health education and lifestyle and behavioural changes. Secondary prevention aims to stop or slow disease progression and prevent complications through early diagnosis and adequate treatment. Tertiary prevention is focused on reducing impairments and activity restrictions. By encouraging an active lifestyle through proper nutrition and following the American College of Sports Medicine guidelines for exercise, individuals may be able to primarily prevent hypertension or diabetes mellitus or

manage them sufficiently (secondary prevention) so they do not escalate to a stroke. If that occurred, then the therapist would be called in for tertiary prevention.

CHAPTER 2

1. Clinical reasoning is defined as the sum of the thinking and decision-making processes, within which the therapist interacts with significant others to agree on goals and health management strategies. The American Physical Therapy Association (2020) defines clinical reasoning as an ability to organise, synthesise, integrate and apply sound clinical rationale for patient management.

2. There is a lack of consensus on essential components of clinical reasoning (Elven & Dean 2017). This chapter identifies five primary components of clinical reasoning: assessment, interpretation, treatment planning, intervention and reassessment (+ outcomes).

3. This acronym relates to the main aims of therapy: recovery, adaptation, maintenance and prevention. See also Fig. 2.3.

4. The ICF Framework is provided in Fig. 2.2. This framework provides a comprehensive and detailed list to identify issues that relate to people's lives. It helps formulate a working plan based on individual goals and includes input from multiple health professionals.
   Case Study 1

5. Low mood and low motivation may affect her ability to engage in therapy. As a person who smokes this may affect her cardiovascular fitness and endurance during therapy. Premorbidly she attended the gym three times per week so has a reasonable fitness level and some understanding of the need to exercise.

6. You would need to consider her goals and that you are on a path to reach them; it may be that she does not reach her goal of walking her dog by discharge or may be performing this task in a different way. An example of this may be in a wheelchair and she may be walking her dog with her husband holding the leash. She would also need to be independent with bed mobility lie to sit or stand and transfer or complete these tasks with the aid of her husband. She lives in a two-storey home with nine stairs; if she cannot manage these safely it may be she lives upstairs or downstairs temporarily or has a stair lift installed.
   Case Study 2

7. In the first sessions in particular, low exercise self-efficacy scores indicated that home exercises were not likely to be completed, especially with low confidence after two falls, a busy home with children at home schooling during Covid lockdown and with multiple sclerosis-related fatigue. Balance exercises chosen were less challenging

and were demonstrated to be performed successfully within the session. These exercises were easier to complete and fit into a busy daily routine. Despite being easier to perform, the importance of performing these exercises regularly was reinforced.

8. Gait biomechanics – ankle push-off and knee flexion and toe clearance.
   Exertion levels – between 'light' and 'somewhat hard' to allow for doses to be replicated at the gym with the exercise physiologist, without detrimental experiences of fatigue after the session.
   Confidence – the chosen speed had a rhythm and exertion level that Mrs M preferred.

CHAPTER 3

1. Fatigue experienced by people with neurological conditions such as multiple sclerosis (MS) or stroke can have a negative impact on many aspects of a person's life, such as mobility and cognitive function, with subsequent impact on issues such as employment. It is therefore this impact of the overwhelming fatigue that distinguishes it from fatigue experienced in the healthy population.

2. MS is a chronic, inflammatory, demyelinating disease of the central nervous system. It is not uncommon for inflammatory lesions to occur in the cerebellum or brainstem which can lead to postural and/or limb ataxia. Additional lesions to the ascending sensory pathways in the spinal cord or brainstem can also lead to additional overlay of sensory ataxia. This mixed presentation can vary but may affect the type of rehabilitation strategies used.

3. Several preliminary clinical research studies indicate that vestibular rehabilitation can be useful for people with MS, stroke, traumatic brain injury (including concussion) and vestibular migraine.

4. Many older methods that use hands-on neuromuscular facilitation provide extra sensory information to guide, resist, block, perturbate and provide guidance and feedback to enable more active movement and control in patients with sensory loss. It is hoped that in coming years robotics may also provide this kind of sensory information with movement. Early research suggests vibration and textured insoles may also be a novel idea to improve balance. Sensory-based priming provided by electrical stimulation, vibration or even motor imagery/action observation such as mirror therapy may also enhance sensory awareness and motor planning. Aligning discriminatory sensory touch with movement, attention and perceptual learning provides the bases of more recent neuroscience-based approaches that show improvement in sensory tasks after brain injury.

5. Ankle plantar flexors, shoulder internal rotators and wrist/finger flexors are often at risk of contracture because of a combination of a prolonged shortened resting position, weakness and increased tone. Contracture can lead to secondary complications such as joint and ligament changes, pain and pressure areas.

CHAPTER 4

Walking

1. Propulsion, postural control and adaptation
2. Stance phase: initial contact, loading response, midstance, terminal stance, preswing (push-off); swing phase: initial swing, mid-swing, terminal swing
3. Up to 50% of everyday tasks are composed of turning steps (Glaister et al 2007); walking assessment should therefore include questions about how patients experience turning in their home and everyday life situations, and you should observe turning in both directions, as well as negotiation of turns through thresholds and turning in confined places like toilets or kitchens.
4. With reference to Table 3 in Bohannon and Williams Andrews (2011): (a) 1.34 m/s; (b) 1.24 m/s

Sit to Stand

1. 60 times a day
2. Flexion momentum, momentum transfer, extension, stabilisation
3. 75° dorsiflexion
4. Foot position, seat height, arm rests, age, strength, balance, range of movement, body weight, vision, sensation, pain, psychological status

Rolling and Getting Out of Bed

1. 5.3 s (SD 2.9 s), range 2.3–17.3 s
2. Record the start position and instructions (e.g., sit up over the edge of the bed or stand up; self-paced or as fast as possible), observe and record the movement of each key component (i.e., head and trunk, far upper limb, near upper limb, lower limbs), and time the manoeuvre over several trials.
3. Answers may include nocturnal hypokinesia, early morning akinesia, tremor, dystonia, light-headedness, dizziness, weakness, slow turning speed, reduced range in the turn or reduced axial acceleration.

Reach and Grasp

1. Object location and identification, postural control, transport phase (acceleration/deceleration), manipulation
2. (a) Size, weight, shape, texture and fragility of the object, location of the object, and the goal/task; (b) the goal/task

3. (a) At the start of the transport phase; (b) at the end of acceleration, between 50% and 60% of the transport phase
4. The role of vision in reach and grasp is object location and monitoring changes in location, size and orientation of the object. Visual fixation on the object stops before the critical period for final hand shape and is redirected to subsequent landmarks required for action with the grasped object. Guidance from visual and tactile receptors provides feed-forwards information to control fingertip forces and grasp kinematics during manipulation.

Posture and Balance

1. Posture is the relative alignment of body segments and the overall position of joints to balance these segments against gravity. The process through which this balance is obtained (either statically or dynamically) is known as balance. Balance describes both sensory and motor control.
2. The vestibular, proprioceptive and visual systems all contribute to balance control. All appear to be processed within the cerebellum and brainstem nuclei. The value placed on each sensory input in determining a motor response is referred to as *sensory weighting*. The cortex can also determine how sensory inputs are perceived to effect a motor response.
3. The triceps surae (soleus and gastrocnemius muscles) on the posterior aspect of the ankles principally control standing body sway when no additional perturbations are incurred. These act in a ballistic fashion to prevent a forwards fall of an individual. This is known as the *ballistic bias theory* (Loram et al 2005a).
4. A person with ataxia typically features postural tremor, affecting standing balance and entropy of standing. They have increased instability (multidirectional body sway) often associated with frequent falls and an adopted widened stance. When responding to balance perturbations, motor responses are often increased in magnitude and an 'overresponse' is observed.

CHAPTER 5

1. There are four types of data: nominal, ordinal, interval and ratio. Nominal tools consist of two or more categories but without order (i.e., one is not better than the other); an example is gender. Ordinal tools consist of two or more categories with an order between the categories, but the difference between categories is not equal; an example is the Berg Balance Scale or the Hoehn and Yahr scale for people with Parkinson's. Interval tools consist of two or more categories with order and with

equal differences between categories, but a score of zero is not an absence of the construct evaluated; an example is the Brunel Balance Assessment. Ratio tools have two or more categories with order, equal difference between categories and an absolute zero value; an example is gait speed from a 10-metre walk test or distance reached from a functional reach.

2. (a) False. It is interrater reliability. Test-retest reliability refers to stability of scores when repeated on different occasions.

  (b) False. Pearson correlation coefficients should not be used for examining reliability because systematic differences between assessments can be unnoticed, leading to a very high or perfect correlation when in fact there is lack of agreement between the assessments. Because results from a 10-metre walk test provide ratio data, an intraclass correlation coefficient with Bland–Altman analysis should be used for investigating reliability.

3. There are two types of predictive validity: linear and logistic regression. The outcome variable to be predicted in a linear regression model is a continuous (interval or ratio) variable. In a logistic regression model the outcome variable is a dichotomous or binary variable, that is, consisting of two categories. The strength of the prediction model in a linear regression is determined by the R^2 value (explained variance), expressed as a percentage with a higher percentage representing a better prediction model. For a logistic regression model, the strength of the prediction can be interpreted by the reported sensitivity, specificity and positive and negative predicted values.

4. When considering two assessments, either by one therapist on two different occasions or by two therapists on one occasion, there is always a degree of error between both assessments, irrespective of whether ordinal scales, functional performance or instrumented measures are used. Hence it is crucial to determine the measurement error of a measurement tool which is crucial to interpret whether the difference between two measurements is caused by error, or when the difference is greater than the measurement error, a true change in performance. Of course, a change in performance does not mean that the difference is also clinically relevant. Therefore the minimal clinically important difference (MCID) can be calculated. If a change in performance is greater than the MCID, the change in performance is also clinically relevant. It is important to understand the measurement error and MCID of a measurement tool to interpret a change in score. A change needs to be greater than the error and MCID to be able to say that the patient's performance/ability has changed. A change below the error

is merely because of natural variability in the testing protocol.

5. There is not a right or wrong answer to this question because it all depends on the context in which you work. This question is to prompt you to reflect on how measurement tools may benefit your practice and how they could be implemented. However, reports of the impact of implementing measurement indicate that they can improve communication with colleagues and patients; enhance the effectiveness of assessment, goal setting and monitoring progress; and speed clinical decision making and planning. One of the most frequently reported barriers to using measurement tools is a lack of know-how – which to choose, why to choose them and how to use them. The recommendations with links to instruction manuals in Table 5.1 and the online resources provide this know-how.

CHAPTER 6

1. Find out about the context of a person's life outside of the health system and before injury or illness (i.e., at work, home, school). Find out about their preferences and values. Involve the person in decisions around the selection of goals. Involve there family in these discussions. Use language that the person can understand. Actively listen; do not just talk. Provide information about prognosis and the expected level of difficulty for specific goals, but allow people to choose goals that may be challenging or highly ambitious. Use goal setting to drive the selection of therapeutic interventions and rehabilitation plans. Do not set goals that just reflect what interventions you, as a clinician, want to provide. Involve the person in the evaluation of their progress towards goals and the success of the rehabilitation programme.

2. Family members can be a good source of information about a person's life outside of the health system and before injury or illness. They can represent the views of people who are not able to fully participate in goal setting because of severe communication or cognitive impairments. They can advocate for the preferences and values of people with illnesses or injuries. Family members are often going to be the people involved in supporting someone after the person leaves hospital or the health service, so having them involved in decision making about the objectives of rehabilitation is valuable. Sometimes it can be challenging to involve family members when health professionals believe that this might affect or conflict with the therapeutic relationship they have with their clients/patients. For instance, it can be difficult when family members appear to have different

ideas about the goals of rehabilitation from the apparent preferences of clients/patients or expectations of the health professionals. However, it is usually better to involve family members in goal setting than to avoid their involvement because involving family members helps identify any such differences in opinion early so that these differences can at least be openly discussed and addressed.

3. Approaches to goal setting ought to be adapted to the different contexts in which they are used. People have different social, motivational, psychological and information needs at different stages of their recovery after stroke. In the acute stages of a first-time stroke, people know very little about stroke or what to expect. They need hope and encouragement to make the most of rehabilitation opportunities, and they benefit from strong leadership provided by knowledgeable health professionals regarding early plans for rehabilitation. As people gain more information about rehabilitation and stroke recovery, and as they learn what stroke means in the context of their own lives, they should be encouraged to take more control over decision making around the objectives of rehabilitation. Approaches to goal setting ought to be modified to accommodate these and other changing needs over time as a person recovers from stroke. Ultimately, people after stroke ought to be encouraged to act as their own rehabilitation professionals so that they can continue to set objectives and develop their own strategies to work towards them after the rehabilitation professionals are no longer involved.

4. Goal Attainment Scaling (GAS) goals are considered time consuming to develop, although this criticism has been addressed in part by the introduction of a GAS-Light approach. GAS T-scores are questionable because the calculation for T-scores requires GAS data to be interval, where each step on the scale is equivalent (like centimetre increments on a ruler), when this is unlikely to be the case. GAS T-scores can be avoided, however, by just reporting raw GAS scores and analysing them with nonparametric methods. More problematic is the question of what GAS scores actually measure. Changes in scores on measures of goal attainment reflect two things: firstly, change in a person's health, functioning or well-being from a baseline state; and secondly, the expectations of the person or people setting the goals. This means that it is possible for one person to do worse in terms of their rehabilitation outcomes but score better than another person if the expectations for the first person were initially lower. If health professionals are 100% accurate with their predictions regarding what outcomes patients will achieve, then all patients should always achieve a GAS score of 0 (the expected outcome).

For this reason, GAS scores cannot distinguish between substandard therapy oriented towards easily achievable goals and extremely high standards of therapy with very ambitious goals. Even if a rehabilitation team improves the quality of its service delivery, its average GAS score ought to remain at a steady 0. GAS scores therefore cannot be used to meaningfully benchmark performance between two rehabilitation services or within one rehabilitation service over time.

CHAPTER 7

1. A stroke is a disorder of the blood supply in the brain. There are two types of stroke: an ischaemic stroke where the blood vessel is blocked, and a haemorrhagic stroke where because of a ruptured blood vessel, blood leaks into the brain. In an ischaemic stroke, the blocked blood vessel prohibits the provision of blood to the area of the brain after the blockage. In the case of a haemorrhagic stroke, there is also a reduced blood supply to a region of the brain. The loss of body functions after stroke is caused by the deprived blood supply to regions of the brain responsible for the respective body function.

2. Please refer to Fig. 7.1 where the list can be found.

3. This is false. Literature has established independent predictors of upper limb outcome based on parameters collected early after stroke. The presence of shoulder abduction and finger extension measured within 72 hours poststroke is a valid predictor of regaining some dexterity at 6 months after stroke.

4. Please refer to Fig. 7.3 and compare your recovery pattern with the depicted pattern. The core physical treatment focus in the different phases would be as follows:
   - Hyperacute phase: early mobilisation
   - Early and later rehabilitation phase: restoring impairments to regain activities by focusing on task-oriented practice and rehabilitation interventions to improve (extended) activities of daily living (ADLs) and social interaction
   - Chronic phase: environmental adaptations and services at home, focusing on maintaining physical condition and monitoring quality of life

5. Currently, there are no evidence-based interventions for optimising motor function in patients with a paralysis of the paretic upper and lower limb. In these patients, monitoring of return of some volitional movement should be made regularly during the first 6 months after stroke. As long as there is no voluntary movement in the affected limbs, the treatment will normally be task oriented, with the focus on optimising mobility such as sitting and transferring and using a wheelchair

independently, optimising ADLs and social interaction, arranging home adaptations, and enhancing physical condition and quality of life.

CHAPTER 8

1. The most severe grading of traumatic brain injury (TBI) (based on grading of length of coma).
2. An extremely severe brain injury (the most severe grading) based on length of posttraumatic amnesia (PTA).
3. The Glasgow Coma Scale (GCS) and PTA scores indicate a high chance of a poor outcome. A 'poor' outcome is typically determined by factors such as
   - the need for long-term care;
   - requires assistance for self-care;
   - inability to work, study, drive or play sports; and
   - limited mobility (i.e., difficulty walking) and may require assistive devices.
4. Penny has significant spasticity and hypertonicity which may lead to further loss of range of motion (ROM) and restrict her ability to regain function. A tilt-table is a great option to stretch tight calves. However, even if it is performed twice daily for 30 minutes, that still leaves 23 hours a day for the calf muscles to become contracted. Resting or night splints have the advantage that they can be worn for extended periods, but they are dependent on being firmly donned and the straps used to secure them may cause pressure areas. Further, any splints worn overnight may disrupt sleep and contribute to further fatigue and difficulty engaging in therapy, but resting splints may be taken on/off for therapy. Serial casts also provide a sustained stretch, but they cannot be taken off for therapy. Because Penny's problems with ROM have a neurological basis (i.e., spasticity and hypertonicity), botulinum toxin (BoNT) or baclofen may be an option. Higher levels of baclofen contribute to fatigue in many patients and may not be tolerable. BoNT is effective for reducing spasticity, which may allow other measures (tilt-tabling, casting, splinting) to be more effective or better tolerated.
5. Penny has severe quadriparesis and spasticity and is involved in an intensive daily physiotherapy program. She is likely to have many 'aches and pains' that will need to be monitored, as delayed-onset muscle soreness is common in any intensive rehabilitation programme. However, because there was no initial injury identified in Penny's left hip, and the loss of ROM is associated with an 'ache', this pain needs to be closely monitored. If it does not resolve in days (as would be expected with delayed-onset muscle soreness), a bone scan may be required to confirm or exclude heterotrophic ossification.

6. All families have roles such as mother, father, sister, girlfriend and so on. These roles vary widely from family to family. When a person with a brain injury returns home from hospital, these roles may change and this change is often a source of significant stress. It is reasonably normal for couples to delegate jobs such as cooking and cleaning. Noninjured family members and significant others may have to pick up jobs that the person with a TBI can no longer perform. They may also have to assist with showering, dressing and other self-care tasks, as well as assisting with a home exercise programme of stretching and strengthening exercises. This is a time of enormous adjustment for all family members, and the change in family dynamics may cause conflict. It is most important that the patient and the family are well supported through this time by a multidisciplinary team, and that physiotherapists are aware of the burden and implications that their home exercise programme may have on an already stressed family.
7. The effect of any physiotherapy or medical intervention should be monitored and evaluated. In relation to mobility and walking after insertion of a baclofen pump or orthopaedic surgery, a range of standardised outcome measures should be used. With respect to physical impairment, the key domains to assess are ROM (goniometry), strength (handheld dynamometry) and balance (Berg Balance Scale). When an intervention is applied to target spasticity or muscle hypertonicity, such as a baclofen pump, then the Modified Tardieu and Modified Ashworth scales should be used. With respect to mobility and walking, the measure of performance needs to be aligned with the person's goals. In this case, it is reasonable to consider a Timed Up and Go, 10-metre walk test (+/−) gait aid, 6-minute walk test or the Functional Ambulation Categories.

CHAPTER 9

1. International Standards for Neurological Classification of Spinal Cord Injury (INSCSCI) assessment tool. Identifies impairments to inform neurological level of injury and can give indication of prognosis postinjury. Helps to evaluate the potential for recovery during initial phases of rehabilitation.
2. Use of a spirometer to assess forced vital capacity (FVC) and peak flow meter to assess peak cough flow. Elective ventilation would be considered with an FVC of ≤1.0 L.
3. Abdominal muscles are innervated from T6 to T12. Spinal cord injury (SCI) lesions in the thoracic and cervical cord will impair a patient's ability to cough effectively to varying degrees.

4. All body systems controlled by the nervous system below the level of the lesion are affected. These are the musculoskeletal, sensory, cardiovascular, respiratory, urinogenital and gastrointestinal systems.

5. Yes, they develop neuropathic pain resulting from trauma to peripheral nerve structures and because of central cord sensitisation.

6. Appropriate wheelchair size for the individual, postural support to provide optimum trunk stability and enable effective pushing technique, appropriate pressure-relieving cushion that also optimises stability.

CHAPTER 10

1. Multiple sclerosis (MS) is an inflammatory demyelinating polyneuropathy affecting the central nervous system. Both inflammatory and neurodegenerative processes contribute to the presentation and disease course, which is highly variable between individuals and over time (see Fig. 10.1 for a summary).

2. The different types of MS and their management approaches are:
   (a) MS has relapsing and progressive subtypes, with most patients presenting with relapsing MS at the outset.
   (b) At all stages, the principles of comprehensive patient-centred care are key, as is comprehensive assessment and discussion with the patient, their family and any caregivers about their priorities.
   (c) Main approaches include health promotion and prevention, restorative and ameliorative interventions. Evaluate common key issues at each stage of the clinical course (see Table 10.5).

3. Use recommended outcome measures which reflect the patient's problems and goals (see Outcome Measures box). Ensure that your selected measure(s) reflect outcomes across the ICF classification framework.

4. The approaches available to help manage ataxia in MS patients are:
   (a) Approaches include restorative approaches (such as exercise strategies), compensatory strategies (such as provision of aids and adaptations) and medication. Surgical options may be considered for some.
   (b) Refer to appropriate best practice guidelines, such as those provided by Ataxia UK.

5. (a) Consider if and how cognitive problems may affect the processing of information you provide and the accuracy of patient recall. Consider the patient's ability to engage effectively and safely with therapeutic interventions, including home programmes.
   (b) Sensitively discuss how cognitive issues (if any) may affect daily life, and refer to a psychologist where appropriate.
   (c) Use simple strategies to assist memory, such as providing a written summary of any verbal advice and information given.

6. (a) People should consider making changes that support a brain healthy lifestyle and minimise risks for developing comorbidities. Lifestyle changes are achievable at all stages of the disease. Tailored education and ongoing support are essential.
   (b) There is now evidence that both cardiovascular and resistance exercises are safe, effective and feasible in people across the disease course.
   (c) Physical activity advice should include careful consideration of pacing, progression and maintaining motivation.
   (d) Use the available evidence-based guidelines (see Sedentary Behaviour, Weakness and Deconditioning section).

7. Comorbidities can affect both the primary disease course and overall health, as well as possibly affect the effectiveness of disease-modifying therapies (see Health Promotion, Lifestyle Modifications and Comorbidities section).

8. (a) A range of primary and secondary factors affect MS fatigue (see Fatigue section).
   (b) Management approaches include rehabilitation and behavioural approaches such as graduated physical activity and pacing. Medications can be useful for some people.

9. (a) Clear guidance about how to access local services should be available; this may include self-referral systems.
   (b) People should request a review when existing symptoms change or new symptoms occur which affect function.
   (c) Emphasise the importance of early contact, particularly when people are at risk for secondary complications (e.g., pressure sores, contractures).

10. (a) There are a wide range of different options that you may offer your patient (face-to-face, telephone, videoconferencing). Consider the right place, right person, right time approach to meet the individual's needs.
    (b) Key considerations for remotely delivered reviews include safety, digital literacy and ability to achieve the required goals of the intervention.

11. There is a wealth of information available, but it is important for people to access relevant resources

and to undertake a questioning approach to the information they glean. Third sector organisations can be a helpful and high-quality source of information, ongoing support and advice. Approved health apps are being used increasingly to support self-management.

CHAPTER 11

1. Physiotherapy aims to optimise function and independence, thus improving or maintaining a person's quality of life. When communicating with people with Parkinson's and their family, it is important to develop a trusting relationship and truthful approach that explores the incurable and neurodegenerative nature of the condition. Information and education should be provided using language that emphasises positive options for management, giving people time to understand the condition and recognise they could manage the condition with support. The cause of Parkinson's is not always known but has been linked to environmental/toxic factors or genetic mutations. This means the course of the condition differs greatly between individuals. Encourage the person to both seek and share experiences with others who have Parkinson's, as well as use information from expert professionals to help understand and deal with symptoms individual to them. The use of the Preassessment Information Form (PIF) will help develop the conversation.

2. Diagnosis is mainly based on expert clinical observation and assessment. The criteria for diagnosis can now include the presence of dementia and attempts to identify Parkinson's early, even when: (a) in an asymptomatic preclinical stage; (b) in a prodromal stage of emerging motor and nonmotor symptoms, which may be experienced years before motor symptoms are expressed; and (c) clinical Parkinson's.

    Clinical Parkinson's remains defined by dopamine-responsive motor features of bradykinesia (slowness with reduced movement amplitude that must be present), plus rigidity (stiffness) or rest tremor or both, which are initially unilateral.

3. Symptomatic control is the way Parkinson's is managed at present, with the prescription of exercise playing an increasingly important role. The complexity of motor and nonmotor presentation requires encouragement in activity and social participation to optimise the person's potential from diagnosis throughout the condition. Management is best achieved through involvement of a multidisciplinary team with expertise in the condition, and referral to services that encourage the social aspect of management.

4. People with Parkinson's should be referred for assessment soon after diagnosis and to a therapist with experience in Parkinson's.

5. Assessment is based on evidence, which demonstrates effectiveness in physiotherapy techniques for improving physical capacity, transfers, manual activities, balance, gait, respiratory function and pain management. The approach should combine the knowledge of the therapist and perspective of the individual seeking treatment to set realistic goals.

6. Interventions for people with Parkinson's fall broadly into three categories:
    * Exercise (related to conditioning)
    * Practice (related to motor learning and performance)
    * Movement strategy training

CHAPTER 12

Huntington's Disease

1. Executive dysfunction could affect the ability to remember instructions and may require approaches such as reinforcement with written information and regular prompts; apathy would affect the engagement in self-management programmes and means that treatments should be relevant to the person and tasks and be goal oriented; and behavioural symptoms (e.g., irritability) could affect carer burden and compliance with treatment.

2. Consider graded exercise programmes which are goal oriented and involve peers with the disease when possible to aid motivation and the development of support networks. As the condition shows a progression of motor and cognitive symptoms over time, consider implementing environmental strategies to reduce falls risk and teaching strategies to avoid falls (e.g., fast turns) and to get up off the floor early in the disease course when motor and cognitive learning would be less affected.

3. The genetic diagnosis of Huntington's disease (HD) can be determined before symptom onset (premanifest stage). In the premanifest/early stage of manifest HD, focus should be on targeting strength, mobility and aerobic capacity to minimise long-term disability.

4. Although large-scale randomised controlled trials are not available, there is evidence from small-scale trials and case studies that exercise programmes, exergaming, multidisciplinary interventions and breathing exercises may lead to a maintenance of functional independence and improvements at an impairment level (e.g., increased pulmonary function).

5. (a) Executive dysfunction can affect task switching. Therefore self-management programmes should have clear instructions to allow switching between

activities. Consider engaging carers in facilitating interventions at home.

(b) Apathy and associated depression can affect the motivation to produce goal-directed behaviour. Interventions should therefore be task oriented, goal oriented and relevant to the person, and incorporated into everyday activities to aid compliance and engagement.

(c) Irritability can result in loss of temper. Working with patient and carers to understand potential fears and sources of frustration around the disease and its progression can help structure the intervention so that trigger factors are avoided. Consider safety when working alone (e.g., in the community).

Hereditary Ataxia

1. The cognitive affective syndrome includes reduced executive function, impaired spatial cognition and linguistic difficulties. This could affect the planning of daily routines and engagement in management programmes, understanding of verbal instructions, as well as difficulties in remembering diagrams.

2. Large-scale randomised controlled trials do not exist, but there is evidence that intensive training (3–13 hours/week for at least 4 weeks) can lead to improvements in balance and mobility. Exergaming is interactive, so it can aid with motivation and provide feedback about performance.

3. People with cerebellar dysfunction can show impairments in smooth pursuit and saccadic eye movements, as well as nystagmus. There can be a mild reduction in vestibulo-ocular reflex gain. Impairments in oculomotor control will make foveation of targets difficult and thus reduce visual acuity and the accuracy of reaching movements, as well as accurate foot placement while walking.

4. Reducing the mouse cursor speed; adding viscous resistance to the mouse; increasing double click time (i.e., the time between clicks to activate/open a function).

5. Before hydrotherapy and aerobic capacity, symptoms of cardiomyopathy should be screened by a cardiologist. The intensity of training may need to be reduced and/or gradually increased whilst monitoring symptoms (e.g., dyspnoea, thoracic pain and dizziness).

Henoch-Schonlein Purpura (HSP)

1. Symptoms mainly affect the legs. Muscle weakness particularly distally results in foot drop and reduced push-off and swing phase initiation. Spasticity and increased passive stiffness in muscles can affect fast movements (e.g., knee flexion during preswing and swing phase). Corticospinal tract degeneration may mean that synergies of movement under subcortical control (e.g., reticulospinal activity) may develop.

2. Weakness (arising from myopathy), weakness and sensory loss affecting balance (caused by neuropathy), ataxia (associated with cerebellar degeneration), dementia (associated with thinning of the corpus callosum).

3. Functional electrical stimulation (FES) can be used to help with foot drop bilaterally by stimulating the common peroneal nerve. However, setting up times can be long for people with HSP. Case studies have looked at FES targeting proximal muscle groups and aiding proximal stability while walking. In type II HSP, peripheral neuropathy would mean that stimulating the peripheral nerve would not be effective.

4. People with rare hereditary conditions often report a lack of local understanding of the condition and expertise in the condition amongst doctors and allied health professionals alike. Because of the lack of clinical trials there is often a poor evidence base for intervention, and evidence from similar but more common conditions (e.g., multiple sclerosis, Parkinson's) may need to be used. Access to specialist centres for people in rural areas may result in long travel times that can be tiring and costly for patients and carers.

CHAPTER 13

1. b. Amyotrophic lateral sclerosis (ALS)
2. a. Riluzole
3. b. Affects the bladder and bowel in the early stage of the condition
4. a. Distal limb weakness
   b. History of trips and falls
5. a. Hobbies – physical activity/football
   d. Occupational history – industrial engineer
6. c. C9ORF72
7. a. Education on preventing the cycle of deconditioning
   b. Considering and managing fatigue
   c. Advice on suitable aerobic and resistance exercise programmes
   d. Balancing the intensity and type of exercise
8. e. All of the above
9. d. Eye test
10. a. 160 L/min
11. c. Confusion

CHAPTER 14

1. Acute or chronic; acquired or inherited; axonal or demyelinating
2. Axonal transport
3. Spasticity

4. False. There is little evidence of a mechanism of overwork weakness in polyneuropathy, and there is no evidence of deterioration in exercise trials in polyneuropathies.

5. Redistribution of pressure under the foot, realignment and correction of foot deformities, reduction of foot drop, stabilisation of the ankle joint, and increasing sensory feedback to the foot and/or ankle.

CHAPTER 15

1. Assess jaw tightness with a Willis bite gauge. Improvements in range can come with stretches best done with a specific jaw jack which allows a carer to apply stretch pressure without overstretching. Gains can also be measured using ability to manage items such as a sandwich or burger now fits.

2. In addition to skeletal muscle, limb girdle muscular dystrophy (LGMD) can affect respiratory and cardiac systems.

3. Involvement of cardiac system, respiratory system, muscle fatigue, balance and cognitive impairments which may affect carryover.

4. Mitochondrial disease is an 'umbrella' term covering many different types of mitochondrial disorders with a wide variety of symptoms. It is sometimes helpful to find out the genotype, levels of heteroplasmy and whether they have a recognised phenotype with typical symptoms. If a formal exercise test has been performed this can be very helpful in guiding exercise prescription.

5. Primary muscle atrophy is caused by the primary pathology owing to either denervation or direct degeneration of the muscle tissue. There is fatty infiltration and fibrosis of the muscle tissue that can be observed on magnetic resonance imaging (MRI) as fatty streaking. Secondary muscle atrophy is caused by disuse and deconditioning. There is volume loss of the muscle observable on MRI. Secondary muscle atrophy can be reversed with targeted exercise.

CHAPTER 16

1. A clinically useful way to conceptualise functional motor disorder (FMD) is to consider predisposing factors, precipitating factors and perpetuating factors. Each factor may be biological, psychological or social in nature. Although many clinicians consider psychological factors to be central to the aetiology of FMD, others consider psychological issues to be risk factors, rather than directly causative. From a biological point of view, self-focused attention can be considered as a mechanism that drives functional symptoms.

2. FMD can be considered as an abnormal learnt pattern of movement that is driven by self-focused attention and erroneous illness beliefs/expectations. Physical rehabilitation can address FMD by retraining movement with redirection of attention and addressing unhelpful illness beliefs and expectations about movement.

3. • Create an expectation of improvement.
   • Promote open and consistent communication between the multidisciplinary team and patient.
   • Involve family and carers in treatment.
   • Limit passive treatment. When handling the patient is required, facilitate rather than support.
   • Encourage early weight bearing.
   • Foster independence and self-management.
   • Use goal-directed rehabilitation focusing on function and automatic movement (e.g., walking) rather than the impairment (e.g., weakness) and specific muscle strengthening exercises.
   • Minimise reinforcement of maladaptive movement patterns and postures.
   • Avoid use of adaptive equipment and mobility aids, although these are not always contraindicated, particularly in patients who have completed rehabilitation without improvement.
   • Avoid use of splints and devices that immobilise joints.
   • Recognise and challenge unhelpful thoughts and behaviours.

4. Key members of the multidisciplinary team include:
   • Neurologist
   • Psychiatrist
   • Psychologist
   • Physiotherapist
   • Occupational therapist
   • Speech and language therapist
   • Specialist nurses
   Other professionals who may have a role in rehabilitation of patients with FMD include social workers, exercise professionals, art therapists and rehabilitation assistants.

5. Mobility aids and environmental adaptations have the potential to limit rehabilitation progress. Mobility aids may hinder return to normal (automatic) movement patterns, increase self-focus (and therefore exacerbate the functional symptoms) and be a cause of secondary pain and abnormal movement. There are situations when it is appropriate to support a patient with adaptive equipment, for example, if they have completed treatment and require a mobility aid for independent mobilisation. Immobilisation of joints in casts has been associated with triggering and exacerbating fixed functional dystonia (with

complex regional pain syndrome features) and therefore should be avoided.

CHAPTER 17

1. Vestibular neuritis is thought to be as a result of a virus (maybe the herpes simplex virus) activated in the vestibular nerve and results in nerve damage and hair cell loss. Please refer to Table 17.1 where the list of body functions that can be affected is found.
2. Vestibular compensation is the means by which the central nervous system recalibrates the asymmetrical input to the vestibular nuclei which occurs as a result of hair cell loss or vestibular nerve damage. In humans, when hair cells die, they do not regenerate so the pathology may not recover but the patient does. The cerebellum plays a crucial role in vestibular rehabilitation. A patient may fail to compensate after a vestibular lesion if the lesion is too great, if it is fluctuating or if the central nervous system is abnormal.
3. Please refer to Table 17.2 for a list of common peripheral and central vestibular disorders.
4. Nystagmus is a rhythmical oscillation of the eyes. In peripheral vestibular nystagmus, it has a fast phase and a slow phase. It is named by the direction of the fast phase. With right unilateral vestibular loss, a left beating nystagmus is observed (i.e., the eyes slowly drift to the right). This is because the right side is inactive and therefore the left side is relatively more active and thus drives a vestibular ocular reflex to the right. The central nervous system corrects this drift with a fast eye movement (or phase) to the left.
5. BPPV stands for *benign paroxysmal positional vertigo*. The main symptoms are vertigo that is short lived and associated with a head-dependent position. Most commonly the patient reports vertigo when lying down into bed, turning in bed or getting up. Nausea, vomiting and anxiety frequently accompany the spells.

   The posterior semicircular canal is most commonly affected, and one effective treatment is Epley's manoeuvre.

CHAPTER 18

1. Close observation of mean arterial blood pressure (MAP) and intracranial pressure (ICP) is essential. Any decline in MAP, increase in ICP, or a combination of both will have a detrimental effect on cerebral perfusion pressure (CPP), leading to the risk for cerebral hypoxia and further ischaemic damage (MAP − ICP = CPP). Normal values are CPP 70–100 mmHg, ICP <10 mmHg.
2. Peak cough flow needs to be greater than 270 mL. When below this level, consider using active cycle of breathing

techniques (ACBT), airway clearance, breath stacking, lung volume recruitment (LVR) bags and provision of mechanical in-exsufflation (MI:E); refer to speech and language therapist (SLT) as part of the chest management programme.
3. The respiratory control centres (RCCs) control breathing through activation and modulation of the muscles that drive respiration. Neurones within the medulla trigger inspiration, providing signals to the phrenic and intercostal nerves. The pneumotaxic centre determines the frequency of respiration, whereas the apneustic centre controls the intensity of breathing.

CHAPTER 19

1. It has been described as a person's ability to manage their symptoms, treatment, physical and psychosocial consequences, and lifestyle changes inherent in living with a chronic condition. Self-management support means supporting the person to develop their self-management skills, resourcefulness and self-confidence, to ultimately live in an optimum way with their condition. It is important to be clear that self-management does not mean patient adherence to a prescribed self-exercise programme or just education. Neither does it mean leaving the patient to 'manage by themselves'.
2. A self-management programme might include elements of patient education or information provision but goes much further and facilitates behaviour change. Behaviour change is achieved through different means, for example, drawing on psychological theories such as Social Cognitive Theory (SCT).
3. Self-efficacy is a person's belief in their own capability to bring about a change in a specific behaviour. In other words, it is a person's self-confidence in their ability to do or change something. The four sources of self-efficacy are mastery experiences, vicarious experiences, verbal persuasion and physiological feedback.
4. Active listening; getting to know the patient's story and them as a person, not a condition; helping people reflect on the skills they already have and can use to self-manage. Working in a self-management model also requires a commitment to partnership working and shared decision making, and recognition that professionals do not hold all the answers.
5. Self-management programmes can be delivered in groups, or one to one, by professionals, lay leaders or a combination of both. It is widely accepted that programmes work best when participants can tailor content to their own situation and needs. Didactic approaches such as information giving are least effective in changing behaviour.

CHAPTER 20

1. A range of interactive technologies could have been chosen to achieve the therapy goals for this client to improve upper limb function and increase independence with mobility. This client is attending outpatient hospital sessions with the therapist. (1) The ArmeoSenseo (Hocoma) can be used to improve upper limb function because the system includes tracking devices on the wrist and arm to provide more specific tracking and feedback on performance than the Nintendo Wii. Additional arm weight support can be added to the system to provide additional assistance during training. (2) The Lokomat (Hocoma) may be used to target mobility through gait training. The Lokomat offers options for the clinician to modify body weight support, velocity and active assistance. This would provide more specific gait training for the client than the Nintendo Wii. The clinician may use visual feedback through a mirror in front of the client or adding game-based activities controlled through the client's gait activity. (3) A virtual reality (VR) headset system such as REALSystem VR, XRHealth or InMotionVR may be suitable to use with this client. The clinician could choose appropriate games that target upper limb movement, weight shift in standing, or pregait activities. These systems may provide more rehabilitation-specific activities and more options for the clinician to adjust the level of challenge than the Nintendo Wii.

2. Video games designed for entertainment can provide opportunities and motivation for repetitive practice. (1) In the rehabilitation setting, the quality of the movements is important. Some commercially available video games can encourage players to perform movements that are not suitable in rehabilitation (e.g., too fast, too challenging) and can cause compensatory movements. (2) The scores provided in commercially available video games do not record meaningful information for tracking player/client progress. Scores do not often represent the quality of movement of the player. (3) The type, amount and content of feedback provided in commercially available video game systems can be perceived as negative and discouraging by some people. Feedback is not designed to be clinically appropriate and may not provide the player/client with enough information to modify performance.

3. Technology:
   - What does the technology add to clinical practice?
   - What is the amount and type of equipment required?
   - Where will the equipment be stored?
   - Where will the equipment be set up, for example, in the clinic or home?
   - Who will have access to the equipment?
   - Who will provide technical support and troubleshooting?

   Game/activity content:
   - Does the game/activity meet the intended goal of the therapy sessions (assessment, support, intervention)?
   - Does the game/activity meet the intended core challenge of the therapy (balance, memory, dual tasking, physical interaction, cognitive interaction)?
   - Does the game/activity suit the time that the intervention is anticipated to be used (e.g., in one session, multiple sessions)?
   - Is there flexibility of the game/activity to be used within sessions, and does the game/activity allow for continuity across sessions if needed?
   - Can the game/activity be tailored to meet the needs of the client and/or goals of the therapy?
   - How quickly does the level of challenge change? Does the level of challenge change once a certain criterion is met, or does the level of challenge change after a certain period?

   Client needs:
   - Does the client have any physical impairments that would prevent them from using the mouse, touchscreen, controller or physical tracking?
   - Does the client have cognitive impairments in which VR interventions with multiple simultaneous commands and complex controls could be too challenging?
   - Does the client have visual impairments?
   - Does the client have auditory impairments?
   - Does the client have speech/language impairments?
   - Do the goals of the game/activity match the therapeutic goals of the client?
   - Is there a tutorial that is suitable to explain the game/activity to the client? Or are different instructions required?
   - Is the feedback (audio/visual/haptic) provided appropriate for this client?
   - Is the scoring provided appropriate for this client?
   - Are the game/activity interactions helpful or harmful to the client's rehabilitation?
   - Can the tasks be customised for my client? If not, can I do something with the environment and setup to customise?
   - Is this level of challenge appropriate for my patient and our rehabilitation goals?
   - Can the game/activity be used independently by this client, or is supervision/assistance required?

4. There is great potential for the integration of interactive technology hardware with customised software

developed specifically for rehabilitation. Limitations of current research include:

- Small sample sizes.
- Variations in the intensity and duration of the intervention.
- Variations in the content (software) and level of interaction/interactivity of the intervention.
- Differences in outcome measures used.
- Heterogeneity of the participant populations.
- Limited information about the characteristics of the interventions that support the use of these interactive technologies.

CHAPTER 21

1. Elderly people and neurological patients are at high risk for falling.

   Most common risk factors in people with neurological conditions are postural instability and unsteady gait. Disease-specific risk factors in people with stroke include muscle weakness, impaired cognition or attention, limited range of motion and activities of daily living ability, sensorimotor dysfunction, and balance and mobility problems.

   In people with Parkinson's, explore disease severity and duration of the disease, motor and cognitive impairments, freezing of gait, fear of falling and medication (treatment with dopamine agonists and increased levodopa dosage).

   In people with multiple sclerosis (MS) explore the type of MS (those with primary progressive MS are at greatest risk), imbalance and cognitive dysfunction.

   In people with Huntington's disease, explore gait bradykinesia, stride variability and chorea, increased sway, cognitive decline and behavioural changes.

2.
   - Nutritional status (e.g., vitamin D or calcium deficiency)
   - Environmental hazards (e.g., loose carpets, poor lighting, poor footwear)
   - Movement problems and lack of exercise (e.g., muscle weakness, poor balance, gait disturbance, bone loss)
   - Medication (e.g., antidepressants, hypnotics, diuretics)
   - Age and medical condition (e.g., visual impairment, cognitive impairment, osteoarthritis)

3.
   - Take a thorough fall history before observing the patient move.
   - Identify the circumstances surrounding previous falls and near misses.
   - Interview the person who fell (or witnesses) and consider using a falls diary.

- Observe the person who fell performing their fall-related activities in a functional way.
- Consider the careful use of a video camera.
- Complete a battery of appropriate tests and outcome measures.

4. The key to understanding what has happened is to identify the circumstances in which the individual has fallen. Therapists must attempt to discover, through questioning and observation:
   - Where the patient fell,
   - What the patient was trying to do at the time: the 'fall-related activity',
   - What might have caused the patient to fall at that instant,
   - Whether the patient was able to break their fall in any way, and
   - What happened when and after the patient hit the floor.

5.
   - Target the hazardous interactions between the individual and their environment.
   - Exercise can reduce risk for falling and stimulate continued physical activity.
   - Developing new movement strategies can make everyday activities safer.
   - Appropriate footwear reduces the risk for falling.
   - Modifying the environment reduces falls where hazards play a part.
   - Not everyone is interested in falls prevention, and some falls are unavoidable.

CHAPTER 22

1. Standard guidance regarding the effective dose: moderate or vigorous physical activity for 30 minutes five times per week, strength/power twice a week and flexibility twice a week. Set goals for functioning, health and well-being. This will vary depending on the individual, disease severity, age, etc. There is no clear guidance regarding safe or optimal dose for all conditions, and this may vary on an individual basis. Current advice is individualised prescription with monitoring and adaptation as required.

2. All components are to be integrated with consideration to guidance. This is moderate or vigorous physical activity for 30 minutes five times per week, strength/power twice a week and flexibility twice a week.

3. In locality, including community settings, and individualised prescription for long-term engagement. Consider body functioning alongside personal and environmental context.

4. Intensity: self-report methods using questionnaires or diaries (validated questionnaires include International

Physical Activity Questionnaire [IPAQ], Global Physical Activity Questionnaire [GPAQ] and Physical Activity Score for the Elderly [PASE]) or objective measures such as accelerometers and pedometers; accuracy will depend on level of mobility impairment.

Duration: self-report methods using questionnaires or diaries (validated questionnaires include IPAQ, GPAQ and PASE) or objective measures such as accelerometers and pedometers.

Frequency: self-report methods using questionnaires or diaries (validated questionnaires include IPAQ, GPAQ and PASE) or objective measures such as accelerometers and pedometers; the latter may underestimate but tends to be reliable within individuals.

Type: self-report methods using questionnaires or diaries (validated questionnaires include IPAQ, GPAQ and PASE).

CHAPTER 23

1. Pain is described as 'an unpleasant sensory and emotional experience associated with, or resembling that associated with, actual or potential tissue damage', as defined by the International Association for the Study of Pain (IASP). The two common ways to categorise pain are according to duration of pain (i.e., acute and chronic) and pathophysiology (i.e., nociceptive and neuropathic). The common classification used in clinical practice and service delivery is acute and chronic. Often the intensity and duration of acute pain are related to severity and extent of tissue damage, and this serves to protect the body from the threat of further harm. The relationship between chronic pain and tissue damage may be weak, and pain may persist because of a dysfunction of the nociceptive system (i.e., pain may be persisting beyond the expected time for healing and be present in the absence of observable pathology). Nociceptive pain is caused by activation of nociceptors by a noxious stimulus from damaging or threatening tissues. Neuropathic pain arises from a lesion or disease of the somatosensory nervous system. Distinguishing between nociceptive and neuropathic pain is necessary in the selection of analgesic medication.

2. Please refer to Fig. 23.1 for the basic elements of the nociceptive system. Damage to the central nervous system may result in a variety of changes that affect somatosensory processing including central sensitisation, loss of descending pain inhibitory (and possibly facilitatory) pathways and neuroinflammation characterised by glial cell activation leading to hyperarousal of the sympathetic nervous system and the hypothalamic-pituitary complex. Glial cell dysfunction, such as persistent activation after spinal cord injury (SCI), contributes to neuronal hyperexcitability and central neuropathic pain. Reorganisation of neuronal circuitry (central neuroplasticity) occurs with persistent input from nociceptors and/or after nerve damage and has a major role in the development and maintenance of chronic pain. Nerve damage causes changes in afferent input to the 'neuromatrix' that subserves body sensation and pain, which in turn causes reorganisation of neural circuitry creating delocalised, unusual, and exaggerated pain.

3. A comprehensive biopsychosocial assessment should evaluate sensory, affective, cognitive, physiological, and behavioural aspects of a person's lived experience of pain and screen for risk factors for the development of chronicity or prevention of recovery. The focus of the consultation is to establish the nature of the person's pain and how it affects their health, well-being and daily living, and to cocreate an explanation of what is causing the pain and how best to manage the pain to facilitate physical and cognitive functioning. Pain diagnosis is far from an exact science, and labels given to pain conditions often cut across categories and may be of little value. For example, diagnosis based on location of pain (e.g., low back pain, shoulder pain, knee pain) may be of limited value other than identifying where to target a treatment. Diagnosis based on probable cause informs clinical decision making going forward and the possibility of treating injuries or disease.

4. Effective pain management strategies are person-centred (i.e., treating the person and the pain) and use a biopsychosocial approach that is tailored to the individual. Goals include relieving (soothing) pain and improving activities of daily living, role functioning (e.g., jobs and hobbies), and emotional, cognitive and social functioning associated with quality of life. As a general rule the focus shifts from a bio-psycho-social approach to manage acute pain to a social-psycho-bio approach to manage chronic pain (Fig. 23.2). The concerns and expectations of the patient should be at the core of a pain treatment plan with a clear explanation why a particular treatment is offered, possible adverse effects and coping strategies for pain. Open and consistent communication between the multidisciplinary team and patient will build trust and is critical for patients embarking on a rehabilitation programme. Empowerment of patients and caregivers to self-manage pain is the cornerstone of effective treatment. Document the patient's expectations about pain prognosis and treatment outcome, and engage in a dialogue about factors

that may hinder treatment success such as treatments that interfere with daily functions. Conduct regular reviews to evaluate, monitor treatment outcome and support the patient becoming competent in self-management of their pain.

5. Managing pain in neurological conditions is challenging. Check for contraindications and consider the following: match treatment objectives with the patient's expectation of outcome; ensure patient motivation and familiarisation of the principles and protocols of treatment offered; set SMART functional goals to monitor quantifiable changes in behaviour and quality of life. Remember to empower patients to integrate activities that create positive sensory experiences which can markedly improve quality of life. Please refer to the section Pain Treatment Selection, Goal Setting and Outcome Monitoring for further detail.

CHAPTER 24

1. The list of common as well as less common types of emotional difficulties is detailed in Table 24.2. Respondents should mention at least depression, anxiety and pain as a minimum.

2. There is a growing evidence base to support cognitive rehabilitation in persons after traumatic brain injury (TBI) and stroke. Respondents should refer to capacity for new learning and key literature such as Cicerone et al (2011).

3. Core factors contributing to neuropsychological disability are provided in Box 24.2. In particular, clinicians should actively consider whether the injury is focal or diffuse, acute or chronic, static or evolving and what is the scope for spontaneous change, neurogenesis or practice-based therapy.

4. The main deficits after middle cerebral artery stroke or aneurysm are outlined in Table 24.5.

5. Common deficits arising after hypoxic brain injury are outlined in the text (see Hypoxic Brain Injury section). Respondents at a minimum should cite ataxia, memory and/or executive deficits.

6. Current understanding of motor skills learning is less well researched than other aspects of memory functioning. Notwithstanding, studies have clearly identified that cognitive and affective deficits can arise after discrete damage to the cerebellum.

7. Some key factors for psychological adjustment are insight, ability to adopt compensatory or other strategies, as well as capacity to modify personal objectives in the face of neurological injury or illness.

CHAPTER 25

1. During arm elevation, the scapulothoracic joint moves towards lateral rotation and posterior tilt. Both scapulothoracic protraction and retraction can occur during arm elevation, depending on the movement plane. Scapulothoracic movement is a combination of movement in the acromioclavicular and sternoclavicular joints.

2. Three tests are described to assess shoulder girdle position at rest. The acromion index assesses the distance from the acromion to the table in lying position, and the scapular distance measures the distance of the scapula relative to the spine. A more protracted posture of the shoulder girdle results in a higher acromion index and a higher scapular distance. The pectoralis minor index also assesses the degree of protraction of the shoulder complex. A smaller index means a more protracted posture.

3. The two core elements for treatment and management of severe spasticity are physical and pharmacological intervention delivered through a coordinated treatment plan.

4. Treatment of spasticity with botulinum toxin should be considered if the spasticity is focal (i.e., localised to a smaller number of muscles affecting one region) and there is a clear goal (rationale) for treatment.

5. Screening refers to identifying any functional deficits that may potentially hinder safe driving. Screening tools can be used by any healthcare professional because they are relatively inexpensive, accurate and do not take much time. An assessment of fitness to drive is a detailed evaluation of visual, motor and cognitive functions through paper-and-pencil testing, computerised tests, simulator tests or on-road driving tests. This assessment is usually conducted by a healthcare professional specialised in determining fitness to drive for individuals with medical conditions.

6. Please refer to Fig. 25.5.

7. Some of the common age-related issues arising in adults with cerebral palsy are (1) low bone density and heightened fracture risk, (2) contracture development, (3) mobility and balance dysfunction, (4) cardiometabolic disease and progressive functional limitations, (5) pain, (6) fatigue, (7) spasticity and (8) mental health disorders.

8. Assessment tools enabling a comprehensive assessment of an adult with severe cerebral palsy may include radiographs (pelvis and spine), range of motion of the upper and lower limbs (goniometry), pain (Non-Communicating Adult Pain Checklist), posture (Goldsmith Indices of Body Symmetry, Posture and Postural Ability Scale), skin integrity, spasticity (Modified Tardieu) and patient-focused goals (Goal Attainment Scale).

Abbreviations

6MWT	6-minute walk test		CBT	cognitive behavioural therapy
α-syn	alpha-synuclein		CCT	circuit class training
A&E	Accidents & Emergency		CDSP	Chronic Disease Self-management Programme
ABI	acquired brain injury		CI	confidence interval
ACA	anterior cerebral artery		CIDP	chronic inflammatory demyelinating polyradiculoneuropathy
ACBT	active cycle of breathing technique		CIMT	constraint-induced movement therapy
AD	autonomic dysreflexia		CK	serum creatine kinase
ADCA	autosomal dominant cerebellar ataxia		ClinScap	clinical scapular protocol
ADHD	attention deficit hyperactivity disorder		CMAP	compound muscle action potential
ADL	activities of daily living		CMT1	Charcot–Marie–Tooth disease type 1
AFO	ankle–foot orthosis		CMT2	Charcot–Marie–Tooth disease type 2
AI	acromial index		CNS	central nervous system
AIDP	acute inflammatory demyelinating polyradiculoneuropathy		CO_2	carbon dioxide
AIS	ASIA Impairment Scale		CoM	centre of mass
ALS	amyotrophic lateral sclerosis		CoP	centre of pressure
ALSAQ-40	ALS Assessment Questionnaire 40		COPM	Canadian Occupational Performance Measure
ALSFRS	Amyotrophic Lateral Sclerosis Functional Rating Scale		CP	cerebral palsy
			CPG	central pattern generator
ALSFRS-R	Amyotrophic Lateral Sclerosis Functional Rating Scale–Revised		CPP	cerebral perfusion pressure
			CRPS	complex regional pain syndrome
ALSSQOL	ALS-specific QOL instrument		CSF	cerebrospinal fluid
AMAN	acute motor axonal neuropathy		CVA	cerebrovascular accident
AMSAN	acute motor sensory axonal neuropathy		DADL	domestic activities of daily living
AP	anteroposterior		DAI	diffuse axonal injury
app	mobile application		DBS	deep brain stimulation
APPDE	Association of Physiotherapists in Parkinson's Disease Europe		DIP	distal interphalangeal joint
			DMD	Duchenne muscular dystrophy
ARAT	Action Research Arm Test		DMT	disease-modifying therapy
ASIA	American Spinal Injuries Association		DN	diabetic neuropathy
BAT	bilateral arm training		DSM 5	*Diagnostic Statistical Manual of Mental Disorders, Fifth Edition*
BCW	behaviour change wheel			
BMD	Becker muscular dystrophy		DVT	deep venous thrombosis
BoNT-A	botulinum toxin A		EBP	evidence-based practice
BoNT-B	botulinum toxin B		ECG	electrocardiogram
BP	blood pressure		EDH	extradural haematoma
BPPV	benign paroxysmal positional vertigo		EDMD	Emery Dreifuss muscular dystrophy
BWSTT	body weight–supported treadmill training		EEG	electroencephalogram
CAD	cough assist device		EHDN	European Huntington's Disease Network
CBD	corticobasal disease		EMG	electromyogram; electromyography

EMG-NMS	electromyography-triggered neuromuscular electrostimulation	IVIg	intravenous immunoglobulin
		KAFO	knee–ankle–foot orthoses
EPDA	European Parkinson's Disease Association	KNGF	Royal Dutch Society for Physical Therapy
FAC	Functional Ambulation Category	LBD	Lewy body dementia
FES	functional electrical stimulation	L-dopa	L-3,4-dihydroxyphenylalanine
FFD	fixed functional dystonia	LE	lower extremity
FIM	Functional Independence Measure	LGMD	limb girdle muscular dystrophy
FMD	functional motor disorder	LGMD2A;	limb girdle muscular dystrophy type 2A or type
fMND	familial motor neurone disease	LGMD2I	2I
fMRI	functional magnetic resonance imaging	LiFE	Lifestyle Integration Functional Exercise
FOG	freezing of gait	LMN	lower motor neurone
FRDA	Friedreich's ataxia	LMNAD	LMNA dystrophy (LMNA gene creates Lamin A and C proteins)
FSHD	facioscapulohumeral muscular dystrophy		
FTD	frontotemporal dementia	LOC	level of consciousness
FTSST	five times sit to stand test	LOFA	late-onset FRDA
FVC	forced vital capacity	LV	left ventricular
GAS	Goal Attainment Scaling	LVR	lung volume recruitment
GBS	Guillain–Barré syndrome	MAC	manual assisted cough
GCS	Glasgow Coma Scale	MAL	Motor Activity Log
GOAT	Galveston Orientation and Amnesia Test	MAP	mean arterial pressure
GP	general practitioner	MAS	Modified Ashworth Scale
GRADE	Grading of Recommendations Assessment, Development and Evaluation	MASCIP	Multidisciplinary Association of Spinal Cord Injury Professionals
GRF	ground reaction force	MCA	middle cerebral artery
HD	Huntington's disease	MCID	minimal clinically important difference
HD-FAC	Huntington's Disease–Functional Ambulation Category	MCS	minimally conscious state
		MDC	minimal detectable change
HDU	high dependency unit	MDS	Movement Disorder Society
HH	homonymous hemianopia	MDT	multidisciplinary team
HMAS	Hammersmith Motor Ability Scale	MHI	manual hyperinflation
HMD	head-mounted display	mHtt	mutation causing Huntington's disease
HO	heterotopic ossification	MI:E	mechanical insufflation and exsufflation
HPD	Hallpike–Dix	MIC	maximal insufflation capacity
HR	heart rate	MMT	manual muscle testing
HSP	hereditary spastic paraparesis	MND	motor neurone disease
Htt	huntingtin protein	MNDA	Motor Neurone Disease Association
IASP	International Association of the Study of Pain	MPAI	Mayo-Portland Adaptability Inventory
IBM	inclusion body myositis	MRC	Medical Research Council
ICARS	International Classification of Ataxia Rating Scale	MRI	magnetic resonance imaging
ICC	intraclass correlation coefficient	MS	multiple sclerosis
ICD-11	*International Classification of Disease*, version 11	MSA	multiple system atrophy
ICF	*International Classification of Functioning, Disability and Health*	MTPJ	metatarsal phalangeal joint
		MVC	motor vehicle crash
ICP	intracranial pressure	Na$^+$	sodium ion
IDT	interdisciplinary team	NES	nonepileptic seizures
IPD	idiopathic Parkinson's disease	NHS	National Health Service
IPPB	intermittent positive pressure breathing	NICE	National Institute for Health and Care Excellence
ISCoS	International Spinal Cord Injury Society	NIHSS	National Institutes of Health Stroke Scale
ISNCSCI	International Standard Neurological Classification of Spinal Cord Injury	NIV	noninvasive ventilation
		NMS	neuromuscular electrostimulation
ITB	intrathecal baclofen	NSAA	North Star Ambulatory Assessment
IVF	in vitro fertilisation	OCSP	Oxford Community Stroke Project

ODI	onset to diagnosis interval	SDSA	Stroke Drivers Screening Assessment
OLS	one-leg stance	SDT	scapular distance test
OT	occupational therapy	SEM	standard error of measurement
PA	physical activity	SF12	Short Form 12
$PaCO_2$	partial pressure of carbon dioxide	SF36	Short Form 36
PADL	personal activities of daily living	SLT	speech and language therapist
PaO_2	partial pressure of oxygen	SMA	spinal muscular atrophy
PCA	posterior cerebral artery	SMART	specific, measurable, achievable/ambitious, relevant, timed
PCF	peak cough flow		
PD	Parkinson's disease	sMND	sporadic motor neurone disease
PDOC	prolonged disorders of consciousness	SNAP	sensory nerve action potential
PDQ-39	Parkinson's Disease Questionaire of 39 questions	SNIP	sniff nasal inspiratory pressure
		SOM	standardised outcome measure
PE	plasma exchange	SpO_2	oxygen saturation
PEEP	peak end-expiratory pressure	SPRS	Spastic Paraplegia Rating Scale
PEG	percutaneous endoscopic gastrostomy	SRM	standardised response mean
PGD	preimplantation genetic diagnosis	STN	subthalamic nucleus
PIP	proximal interphalangeal joint	STS	sit to stand
PMI	pectoralis minor index	STT	speed-dependent treadmill training
PMP22	peripheral myelin protein 22 gene	SUTC	Stroke Unit Trialists Collaboration
PPPD	persistent postural perceptual dizziness	TA	tendo-Achilles
PREP	Predicting REcovery Potential for the hand and arm	TACI	total anterior circulation infarct
		TB	transfer board
PSCC	posterior semicircular canal	TBI	traumatic brain injury
PSP	progressive supranuclear palsy	TENS	transcutaneous electrical nerve stimulation
PTA	posttraumatic amnesia	TIA	transient ischaemic attack
QOL	quality of life	TIS	Trunk Impairment Scale
RAMP	Recovery, Adaptation, Maintenance and Prevention	TOAST	Trial of Org 10172 in Acute Stroke Treatment
		TUG	Timed Up and Go test
RBD	rapid eye movement sleep behavioural disorder	UE	upper extremity
		UFOV*	Useful Field of View
RCC	respiratory control centre	UMN	upper motor neurone
RCT	randomised controlled trial	UMNS	upper motor neurone syndrome
REM	rapid eye movement	UN	unilateral neglect
RHS	Revised Hammersmith Scale	UPDRS	Unified Parkinson's Disease Rating Scale
RMW	respiratory muscle weakness		
ROC	receiver operating characteristic curves	UTI	urinary tract infection
ROM	range of motion	VAS	visual analogue scale
RTI	respiratory tract infection	VC	vital capacity
RT-UL	robot-assisted therapy for the upper limb	VFB	ventilator-free breathing
RYR1	ryanodine receptor 1	VOR	vestibular ocular reflex
SARA	Scale for the Assessment and Rating of Ataxia	VR	virtual reality
		VSR	vestibulospinal reflex
SCA	spinocerebellar ataxia	WHO	World Health Organization
SCAT5	Sport Concussion Assessment Tool version 5	WOB	work of breathing
SCC	semicircular canal	WPT	World Physiotherapy
SCI	spinal cord injury		
SCT	social cognitive theory		
SDH	subdural haematoma		

INDEX

Note: Page numbers followed by *f* indicate figures; *t*, tables; *b*, boxes.

A

Abdominal binders, SCI rehabilitation, 207
ABR. *See* Activity-based rehabilitation
Academy of Neurologic Physical
　　Therapy Outcome Measures
　　Recommendations (EDGE), 39*t*
Acceleration, in transport and
　　manipulation phases, 90*t*
Acceptance and commitment therapy, for
　　pain, 597
Acetyl choline (ACh), 383–384
Acquired neuromuscular diseases, 386
Acquired neuropathies, 358–363
　　acute rehabilitation of, 370
Acromial index (AI), 627, 633*f*
Acromioclavicular joint, kinematics of,
　　627, 630*f*
ACSM. *See* American College of Sports
　　Medicine
Action
　　change and, 501*b*
　　in transport and manipulation phases,
　　　90*t*
Action-observation, in skill acquisition, 17
Action Research Arm Test (ARAT), 530–
　　531, 628
Active function, 630
Active inference, 416–417
Activity-based rehabilitation (ABR), 214
Activity limitations, measurement tools
　　and, 115, 115*t*–117*t*
Activity of daily living (ADL)
　　driving, 643–644
　　independence, stroke and, 158–159, 159*b*
Acupuncture, for pain, 598
Acute neurological conditions, for pain,
　　590–591
Acute phase, of stroke, 154–156
Acute respiratory failure, management of,
　　483
Adaptability, for neurorehabilitation, 518
Adaptation
　　in balance, 95
　　exercises, for vestibular disorders, 455*f*
　　therapists in, 12–13
　　in walking, 72*t*
Adaptive Test for Neuromuscular Disorders
　　(ATEND), 405

Adenosine triphosphate (ATP), 401
ADL. *See* Activity of daily living
Adult DMD North Star Network (ANSN),
　　389–390
Aerobic exercise
　　for MND, 342–343, 342*t*
　　in neural plasticity, 11
Aerosol-generating procedure (AGP), 474
AFOs. *See* Ankle-foot orthoses
Age of onset/acquisition
　　clinical neuropsychology and, 616–617
　　Parkinson's and, 266
　　in sit to stand, 83*t*, 84*t*–85*t*
AGP. *See* Aerosol-generating procedure
AI. *See* Acromial index
AICA. *See* Anterior inferior cerebellar
　　artery
Airway clearance techniques, in respiratory
　　management, 479–481, 483*f*
Akinesia, 60, 61*t*
Akinwuntan, Abiodun E., 635–636
Alpha-synuclein (α-syn), in Parkinson's,
　　267
ALS. *See* Amyotrophic lateral sclerosis
ALS Assessment Questionnaire 40
　　(ALSAQ-40), 337
ALS-CBS. *See* ALS Cognitive Behavioural
　　Screen
ALS Cognitive Behavioural Screen (ALS-
　　CBS), 337
ALS Depression Inventory 12, 337
ALS Functional Rating Scale (ALSFRS),
　　336–337
ALS Prognostic Index, 337
ALS-specific QOL instrument (ALSSQOL),
　　337
ALSAQ-40. *See* ALS Assessment
　　Questionnaire 40
Amantadine, in MS, 253–254
American College of Sports Medicine
　　(ACSM), 17
Amitriptyline, for neuropathic pain, 361
Amnesia, posttraumatic, in traumatic brain
　　injury, 180, 180*t*
Amyotrophic lateral sclerosis (ALS), 327,
　　329. *See also* Motor neurone disease
　　bulbar-onset, 329
　　pain and, 589–590
Analgesic ladder, WHO, 591

Analgesic medication, for pain, 591, 595*t*
Angular velocity, 439
Ankle-foot orthoses (AFOs)
　　facioscapulohumeral muscular
　　　dystrophy, 394
　　for MND, 341
Anosognosia, 62–63
ANSN. *See* Adult DMD North Star
　　Network
Anterior cord syndrome, 200–203, 206*t*
Anterior horn cell, respiratory function in,
　　486, 487*t*
Anterior inferior cerebellar artery (AICA),
　　444
Anterior posterior instability, in sit to
　　stand, 85*t*–86*t*
Anticholinergic therapy, Parkinson's, 270
Anticipatory postural adjustments
　　balance and, 95
　　during sit to stand, 83*t*
Antiepileptic drugs, pain management in
　　MS, 242
Antispasticity medication, for hereditary
　　paresis, 311
Anxiety
　　in MS, 252
　　self-management and, 500
APPDE. *See* Association of Physiotherapists
　　in Parkinson's Europe
Apraxia, 60
　　clinical neuropsychology and, 621–622
　　constructional, 622
　　defined, 622
　　dressing, 622
　　ideational, 622
　　ideomotor, 622
Aquatic therapy, SCI and, 214, 215*f*
AR. *See* Augmented reality
ARAT. *See* Action Research Arm Test
Arm Activity measure, 632, 641*t*
Arm, paretic, electrostimulation of, 168
Arm position, in sit to stand, 85*t*–86*t*
Arm rest, in sit to stand, 84*t*–85*t*
Arm training, bilateral, after stroke, 167
Armeo Power, 527*f*
ArmeoSenso system, 522, 523*f*
Arterial blood gases, in respiratory
　　assessment, 478, 478*b*
Arthritis Self-Management Programme, 506

Ashford, Stephen, 637
Assessment, in clinical reasoning, 4
Assistive devices, in MND, 341
Association of Physiotherapists in Parkinson's Europe (APPDE), 274
Associative stage, of motor learning, 518
Asymmetrical foot placement, in sit to stand, 85t–86t
Ataxia
   hereditary, 303–309
      anatomy, pathophysiology and clinical presentation of, 303–305, 304f
      autosomal dominant cerebellar ataxias of, 303
      autosomal recessive ataxias of, 303
      diagnosis and genetic testing for, 305
      epidemiology and genetics of, 303
      medical management for, 305–307
      physiotherapy assessment in, 307–308
      time course and corresponding management for, 308
      treatment selection and secondary complications/special problems in, 308–309, 310f
   measurement tools for, 115t–117t
   in MS, 247
   posture and balance in, 97–99, 100t–101t
Atelectasis
   common techniques for, 490t
   SCI and, 208
ATEND. See Adaptive Test for Neuromuscular Disorders
ATP. See Adenosine triphosphate
Atrophy, skeletal muscle tissue, 385
Attention, functional motor disorders and, 416–417
Attentional focus, in skill acquisition, 13–15
Audiology screening, for vestibular disorders, 446
Augmented reality (AR), for neurorehabilitation, 517, 520
Automatic stage, of motor learning, 518
Autonomic dysfunction, SCI and, 210
Autonomic dysreflexia, SCI and, 210, 211t
Autosomal dominant cerebellar ataxias, 303–305, 304f
Autosomal recessive ataxias, 303
Avatars, 519, 525f
Axonal damage, polyneuropathies, 355
Axonal degeneration, of HSP, 310–311
Axonal neuropathies, 355, 357b
Axonal sprouts, 585

B

B-IPQ. See Brief Illness Perception Questionnaire

Baclofen
   for hypertonicity, 185
   for spasticity, 185
   in MS, 242
Balance, 91–102
   assessment, 452t
      in Nintendo Wii Fi, 521–522
   clinical foci of, 97–102, 100t–101t
   defined, 438
   in hereditary ataxias, 309
   home exercise prescription, of clinical reasoning, 48
   impairment, measurement tools for, 115t–117t
   interventions, for polyneuropathies, 371–372
   measurement tools for, 115t–117t
   movement analysis strategies to quantify, 96–97, 97f, 98t–99t
   reeducation for, 454–456
   of SCI, 212
   sensorimotor control of, 93–95
      essential motor components in, 94–95
      essential sensory components in, 94
   in sit to stand, 84t–85t
   training, after stroke, 161t–162t, 163
      after traumatic brain injury, 184
      interventions for, 187–188
Balance assessment tools, falls and, 552–553, 553t
BARS. See Brief Ataxia Rating Scale
Barthel Index, 117, 615
Basal ganglia
   Huntington's disease and, 295, 296f
   Parkinson's and, 267
BBT. See Box and Block Test
BCTs. See Behaviour change techniques
BCW. See Behaviour change wheel
Bed mobility, of SCI, 212
Behaviour change, in neurological rehabilitation, 22–25
Behaviour change techniques (BCTs), 22–23
Behaviour change wheel (BCW), 23, 24f, 577, 579f
Behavioural adjustment, assessment of, 613–614, 614t
Behavioural interventions, in clinical neuropsychology, 615–616
Behavioural neurology, 612
Benign paroxysmal positional vertigo, 442
   case study for, 461–462
   Hallpike-Dix manoeuvre and, 442–443
   horizontal canal, 456–457, 458f
   management of, 456, 457f
Berg Balance Scale, 122, 452t
   for functional motor disorders, 424t
Biceps femoris, during sit to stand, 83t

Bilateral arm training, after stroke, 167
Bilateral vestibular hypofunction, 443
   treatment of, 456
Bimanual training, 651
Biopsychosocial model, in neurological rehabilitation, 3
Bladder
   of SCI, 211
   symptoms, in MS, 251–252
Bland-Altman plot, 120, 120f
Body illusions, for pain, 598–599
Body sway, 96
Body weight, in sit to stand, 84t–85t
Body weight-supported treadmill training, after stroke, 164
Bone pain, 585, 588b
BoNT-A, for spasticity, 185–186
'Bottom-up' methods, in hypertonus, 56
Botulinum toxin-A, for spasticity, 185–186
Botulinum toxin, intramuscular, spasticity management in MS, 242
Bow hunter's syndrome, 444–445
Bowel symptoms, in MS, 251–252
Bowels, of SCI, 211
Box and Block Test (BBT), 118, 530–531
Bracing, for pain, 597
Bradykinesia, 60, 61t
   execution of, with bed mobility, in Parkinson's, 88t
   in Parkinson's, 269
   with walking in Parkinson's, 79t–80t
Brain injury, traumatic, 177–192
   assessment of, 182–185, 184t, 190b
      abnormal tone in, 183, 183t
      balance and vestibular function in, 184
      concurrent musculoskeletal injuries in, 185
      disorders of movement in, 184
      function in, 185
      muscle and joint range of motion in, 184, 184t
      muscle paresis in, 184
      pain in, 185
   case presentation of, 190–192, 191t–192t, 192f, 193t
   clinical presentation of, 181–182, 182t
   Covid-19 pandemic, 189–190
   diagnosis of, 179–180
      coma in, 179t, 180
      posttraumatic amnesia in, 180, 180t
   epidemiology of, 178
   interventions for, 186–189
      for balance and vestibular function, 187–188
      for concurrent musculoskeletal injuries, 188
      for disorders of movement, 187

Brain injury, traumatic (*Continued*)
  for function, 189
  for hypertonicity and spasticity, 186–187
  for muscle and joint range of motion, 188, 188f
  for muscle paresis, 187
  other considerations for, 189
  for pain, 188–189
  medical management of, 180–181, 180b, 181t
  intracranial pressure in, 180–181
  multidisciplinary care in, 181, 181b
  pathophysiology of, 178–179, 178t
    associated injuries, 179
    primary brain injury, 178–179
    secondary brain injury, 179
  prognosis/time course for, 185–186
Breaking news, SCI and, 204
Breath stacking, for MND, 345
Breathing
  central nervous control of, 474
  SCI management of, 208
Brief Ataxia Rating Scale (BARS), 307–308
Brief Illness Perception Questionnaire (B-IPQ), for functional motor disorders, 424t
Brown-Séquard syndrome, 200–203, 206t
Brunel Balance Assessment, 122
Bursa pain, 585
Buttell, Joseph, 649

C

C90RF72 mutations, 328
Cadence, in gait cycle, 74t
Caloric/oculomotor testing, for vestibular disorders, 446
Cannabis, for MS, 247
Cardiac symptoms, of Friedreich's ataxia, 306
Cardiomyopathy, of neuromuscular disorders, 395–397
Cardiovascular dysfunction, of SCI, 210–211
Cardiovascular fitness, SCI and, 220
Carer strain/injury, falls and, 548t–549t
Carers, interviewing, falls and, 550
Case presentation, of traumatic brain injury, 190–192, 191t–192t, 192f, 193t
Case study, on stroke, 169–170, 170t, 171t
Casting
  for pain, 597
  of traumatic brain injury, 180
Categorical data, 119
Cauda equina syndrome, 198, 200–203, 206t

Cave Automatic Virtual Environment (CAVE) system, 520
CBT. *See* Cognitive behavioural therapy
CD. *See* Cervical dizziness
CDSP. *See* Chronic Disease Self-management Programme
Ceiling effect, in measurement tool, 122
Central conditions, respiratory function in, 484, 486t
Central cord syndromes, SCI, 200–203, 206t
Central nervous system
  control of breathing in, 474, 475f
  damage to, pain and, 585
Central neuropathic pain, 583, 588–589
  multiple sclerosis and, 586
  Parkinson's and, 586
  stroke and, 587
Central neuroplasticity, 585
Central vestibular disorders, 61–62, 441, 442t, 443–445
Cerebellar ataxia, 58–59, 59t
Cerebellar cognitive affective syndrome, 304
Cerebellum, vestibular compensation and, 450–452
Cerebral palsy (CP), for neurological conditions
  age-related health issues, 657–659
    contracture development, 628
    fatigue, 628
    low bone density and fracture risk, 627
    mental health disorders, 628
    mobility and balance dysfunction, 628
    pain, 628
    physical inactivity, 628
    spasticity, 628
  childhood management, 655–657
  classification systems, 655
  definition, 654–655
  paediatric to adult health services, 657, 657t
Cerebrospinal fluid (CSF), MS diagnosis, 237
Cervical dizziness (CD), 445
Cervicogenic dizziness. *See* Cervical dizziness
CFCS. *See* Communication Function Classification System
CFS. *See* Chronic fatigue syndrome
Change, stages of, 501b
Charcot, Jean-Martin, 328
Charcot-Marie-Tooth disease, 357t, 363–366
  disease course and prognosis of, 366
  medical management of, 365–366
  presentation of, 363–365, 364f, 365f

Charcot-Marie-Tooth disease (*Continued*)
  type 1, 361
  type 1A, 361, 364f
  type 2, 361
Chest infections, of neuromuscular disorders, 397–398
Chest radiographs, in respiratory assessment, 478
Children, SCI and, 222
Choking, MND and, 340
Chronic demyelinating polyradiculoneuropathy, 357t, 361–362
Chronic Disease Self-management Programme (CDSP), 503–504
Chronic fatigue, 55
Chronic fatigue syndrome (CFS), 55
Chronic phase, of stroke, 157, 157f, 158b
Chronic stroke, exercise for, 554b
CIMT. *See* Constraint-induced movement therapy
Circle of Willis, 152
Circuit class training, after stroke, 164–165
Circulation, SCI management of, 203
Classic tremor, 59
Clinical Global Impression (CGI) Scale, for functional motor disorders, 424t
Clinical neuropsychology, 611–623
  acute *versus* chronic lesions in, 617
  age of acquisition and, 616–617
  apraxia and, 621–622
  assessment, 612–615
    affective factors in, 614
    cognitive functions in, 612–613, 613t
    emotional and behavioural adjustment, 613–614, 614t
    mediating factors in, 614
    outcomes and quality of life, 614–615
  Covid-19 in, 619–621
  degenerative conditions and, 621
  focal *versus* diffuse lesions in, 617
  functional disorders and, 622
  history of, 612
  hypoxic brain injury and, 618–619
  interventions, 615–616, 615b
    behavioural, 615–616, 616t
    cognitive, 615
    psychotherapy in, 616
  lateralisation and, 617
  lesion site and, 617
  neglect and, 622
  neurological diseases in, neuropsychological consequences of, 616–622, 617b
  neuropsychological disorders of movement in, 621
  progressive *versus* static lesions in, 617

Clinical neuropsychology (*Continued*)
  psychological adjustment in, 623
  rehabilitation in, process of, 622
  spinal injuries and, 621
  stroke and, 618, 619*t*–620*t*
  traumatic brain injury and, 617–618, 618*t*
Clinical reasoning (CR), neurological physiotherapy
  assessment and treatment principles, 33–50
  clinical case, 39–50
  collaborative goal setting, 36
  components, 34–39, 35*f*
    assessment, 34–35, 35*t*
    interpretation, 35–36
    intervention, 38–39
    reassessment, 39
    treatment planning, 36–38
  considerations, 42*f*
  definition, 33
  evidence for, 34
  framework for, 34
  hypotheticodeductive reasoning strategy, 33
  interventions, 49
  prognosis, 36
  reassessment, 48–49
  reflection, 38–39, 46–49
Clinical reasoning approach, in neurological conditions, 3–4, 53
Clinical reasoning form (CRF), 37, 43*t*–46*t*, 47*t*–48*t*
Clinical scapular protocol (ClinScap), 631–635, 632*f*
  maximal active humeral elevation, 632
  medial rotation test, 632–635
  observation of tilting and winging, 631
  scapular-focused treatment, 637*t*
  scapular lateral rotation, 632, 632*f*
  scoring sheet, 633*f*
  shoulder girdle position, 631–632
Clinical Test of Sensory Interaction in Balance (CTSIB), 448–450, 452*t*
Clinical utility, 124
ClinScap. *See* Clinical scapular protocol
Clonazepam, spasticity management in MS, 242
Coenzyme Q10
  of Friedreich's ataxia, 306–307
Cognitive behavioural therapy (CBT)
  in MS, 249–250
  for pain, 596
Cognitive dysfunction, 62–63
Cognitive functions, in clinical neuropsychology, 612–613, 613*t*
Cognitive impairment, in MS, 252

Cognitive interventions, in clinical neuropsychology, 615
Cognitive stage, of motor learning, 518
Cogwheel rigidity, 269
Cold therapy, for pain, 598
Collaboration, self-management and, 502
Collapsing weakness, in functional motor disorders, 419*t*
Coma
  definition of, 182*t*
  in traumatic brain injury, 179*t*, 180
Coma Recovery Scale-Revised, 650
Communication Function Classification System (CFCS), 651
Community, self-management and, 499
Comorbidities, in functional motor disorders, 426–429
Compartmentalisation, functional motor disorders and, 415–416
Compensation, balance and, 95
Compensatory movements, 521
Compression stockings, SCI rehabilitation, 210–211
Conceptual framework
  CR in neurological physiotherapy, 34
  importance of, 3–4
Concurrent validity, 122
Consciousness, disorders of, 180, 182*t*
Constraint-induced movement therapy (CIMT), 16, 529–530, 651
  after stroke, 166–167
Construct validity, of measurement tools, 121–122
Contemplation, change and, 501*b*
Content validity, of measurement tools, 121
Continued physical activity, for falls, 556
Continuous data, 120
Contracture
  development, 390
  in impairments, 64
  measurement tools for, 115*t*–117*t*
  in MS, 252
  neurological impairments, 64
  spasticity and, 629–630
Contraversive pushing, 62
Coordination
  disorders of, 58–60
  measurement tools for, 115*t*–117*t*
Cortical neuroplasticity, 628
Corticosteroids
  for chronic demyelinating polyradiculoneuropathy, 361–362
  for MS management, 239
Cough
  MND and, 344
  SCI respiratory management, 208

Cough Assist, 345–346, 346*f*
Cough assist machines, 486
Cough augmentation techniques, MND and, 344–345, 345*f*
Counselling, genetics of, Huntington's disease, 295
Covid-19
  clinical neuropsychology and, 619–621
CP. *See* Cerebral palsy
CR. *See* Clinical reasoning
Cramps, MND and, 333
Craniotomy, for haemorrhagic stroke, 153
CRF. *See* Clinical reasoning form
Criterion-related validity, of measurement tools, 122–123
Crutches, for MND, 341
CSF. *See* Cerebrospinal fluid
CTSIB. *See* Clinical Test of Sensory Interaction in Balance
Customised software, in neurorehabilitation, 525–527

D

DAI. *See* Diffuse axonal injury
Dantrolene, for spasticity management in MS, 242
DASH. *See* Disabilities of the Arm, Shoulder and Hand
De Baets, Liesbet, 627
Death, falls and, 548*t*–549*t*
Deceleration, in transport and manipulation phases, 90*t*
Decision making, in self-management, 507–508, 511*f*
Deconditioning
  in impairments, 64–65
  in MS, 246
Deficient movement, 628
Degenerative conditions, clinical neuropsychology and, 621
Dementia, falls and, 546
Demyelination
  acute, 359*f*
  chronic, 364*f*
  of MS, 236
  in neuropathy, 355, 357*b*
Dependence, falls and, 548*t*–549*t*
Depression
  MND and, 337
  in MS, 252
Dermatomyositis (DM), 387
Detachment, functional motor disorders and, 415–416
Devos, Hannes, 635–636
Dexterity
  loss of, 59–60

Dexterity (*Continued*)
   measurement tools for, 115*t*–117*t*
   stroke and, 158–159, 159*b*
DGC. *See* Dystrophin-glycoprotein complex
Diabetic neuropathic pain, case study for, 602–603, 603*t*
Diabetic neuropathy, 357*t*, 362–363
Diaries, falls, 550–551, 551*t*
Diazepam, spasticity management in MS, 242
Difficulty turning
   execution of, with bed mobility, in Parkinson's, 88*t*
   with walking in Parkinson's, 79*t*–80*t*
Diffuse axonal injury (DAI), 178
Disabilities of the Arm, Shoulder and Hand (DASH), for functional motor disorders, 424*t*
Discharge planning, SCI and, 222–223
Discriminant validity, 122–123
Disease-modifying therapies (DMTs), in MS management
   active disease, 239
   challenges, 239
Disease specific interventions, in self-management, 504*t*
Disorders of consciousness (DOC), neurological conditions, 649–654
   definition, 650
   legal and ethical considerations, 651–653
      acute phase, 651–652
      rehabilitation phase, 652
      transition of care, community phase, 652–653
   persistent disorder of consciousness (PDOC), 650–651
Dissociation, in functional motor disorders, 415–416
Dissociative seizures (DSs), in functional motor disorders. *See* Nonepileptic seizures
Distractibility, in functional motor disorders, 419*t*
Disuse atrophy, 341–342
Dizziness, 438
   causes of, 445–446
   persistent postural perceptual, 445
DM. *See* Dermatomyositis
DMD. *See* Duchenne muscular dystrophy
DMTs. *See* Disease-modifying therapies
DOC. *See* Disorders of consciousness
Dopamine agonists, Parkinson's therapy, 270
Dopamine, for Parkinson's, 267–268
Dopaminergic systems, 13–15
Double support, in gait cycle, 74*t*
Dressing, falls and, 557*t*
Drift without pronation test, in functional motor disorders, 419*t*

Driving, multiple sclerosis and
   as activity of daily living, 643–644
   assessment of, 645–649, 645*f*, 646*f*, 648*t*–649*t*
   case presentation of, 647–649, 648*t*–649*t*
   challenges in, 643–649
   consultation for, 647
   evaluation process for, aspects of, 644–647, 644*f*
   fitness-to-drive legislation and, 644–645, 644*f*
   interpretation of, 649
   intervention for, 646–647
   posttraining assessment for, 649
   screening for, 645, 645*f*, 647
   training programme for, 649
Driving simulators, 638, 646*f*
Duchenne muscular dystrophy (DMD)
   assessment and outcome measures, 389–390
   childhood-onset, 388
   cognitive, 389
   disease course and prognosis, 389
   extramuscular systems, 388
   joints measured in adults, 390, 392*t*
   medical management, 390–392
   outcome measures, 389, 391*t*
   physical management, 392–393
   presentation, 388–389
   respiratory assessment, 392*t*
   stages of progression, 389*t*
   stages of pulmonary and respiratory decline, 388, 390*t*
Duloxetine, for neuropathic pain, 361
Dynamic Gait Index Long and Short Form, 452*t*
Dynamic visual acuity, 448
Dysaesthesia, 63
   diabetic neuropathy and, 361
Dysarthria, 59
   MND and, 339–340
   of MS, 247
Dysautonomia, 445–446
Dysdiadochokinesia, 59
Dyskinesias, 58
Dyslipidaemia, in diabetic neuropathy, 359
Dysmetria, 59
Dysphagia, MND and, 340
Dyspraxia, 60
Dyssynergia, 59
Dystonia, 57–58, 58*t*
   in ataxia, 305
   functional, in functional motor disorders, 420
   in hereditary ataxias, 305
Dystrophin-glycoprotein complex (DGC), 385*f*

E

Early acute management, of SCI, 203–207, 204*b*
   facilitation of range, length and movement, 205–207
   mobilisation, 207
   physical management, 204–205
   prognosis, 204
ECC. *See* Excitation contraction coupling
Edinburgh Cognitive and Behavioural ALS Screen, 337
Education, in functional motor disorders, 425
Egan Klassifikation Scale (EK2), 394
Electrical stimulation techniques, for pain
   invasive, 597
   noninvasive, of brain, 597–598
Electromyography (EMG), in sit to stand, 82
Electrostimulation
   of paretic arm and hand, 168
   of paretic lower limb, 165
Electrotherapy, for pain, 597–599
EMG. *See* Electromyography
Emotional lability, MND and, 333–334
Endolymphatic sac decompression, 447
Engagement, in neurological rehabilitation, 22
Environment, in sitting/getting out of bed, 87*t*
EPDA. *See* European Parkinson's Disease Association
EQ-5D-5L, for functional motor disorders, 424*t*
Erectile dysfunction, SCI and, 211
Erwee, Camilla, 643
ESE. *See* Exercise self-efficacy
European Chapter of the International Federation of Clinical Neurophysiology, 593–594
European Guideline, of Parkinson physiotherapy, 274
European Parkinson's Disease Association (EPDA), 271
Evoked potentials, MS diagnosis of, 237–238
Excitation contraction coupling (ECC), 383–384
Exercise, 573
   adaptation, 455*f*
   assessment and monitoring of, 575–580
   for falls, 554–556, 554*b*, 555*b*
   frequency of, 577
   gaze stability, 454
   habituation, 454
   intensity of, 578
   International Classification of Function model and, 575, 575*f*

Exercise (*Continued*)
  limit to capacity in, 577
  in MND, 341–342, 342*t*, 343*f*
  for pain, 596
  of Parkinson's physiotherapy, 279–281,
    282*f*
  for polyneuropathy, 370–371, 375–376
  prescription, 577
  response and recovery, 577–578
  safety, 575
  visual desensitisation, 454
Exercise prescription, in neurological
    rehabilitation, 17–18
Exercise self-efficacy (ESE), 46–48
Exergaming, 309
Exoskeletons, SCI and, 219, 219*b*, 219*f*
Expectation, functional motor disorders
    and, 416–417
Experiences
  mastery, 501
  vicarious, 501
Expert Patient Programme, 503–504
Extended reality (XR), 517, 520
Extension, in sit to stand, 81*t*
External environment, falls and, 558, 558*f*

F

Facilitation movement, of SCI, 214–216
Facioscapulohumeral muscular dystrophy
    (FSHD)
  assessment and outcome measures, 393
  autosomal dominant disease, 393
  disease course and prognosis, 393
  DUX4 protein, 393
  medical management, 393
  physical management, 393–394
  presentation, 393
Falls, 545–562, 545*b*
  activities related to, observation of,
    551–552
  assessment of, 548–553, 548*b*
  balance assessment tools, 552–553, 553*t*
  causes of, 547–548
  consequences of, 548, 548*t*–549*t*
  diaries, 550–551, 551*t*
  exercise for, 554–556, 554*b*, 555*b*
  extent of problem of, 546–547
  functional motor disorders and, 429
  history, 548–550
  management of, 553–560, 553*b*
  measurement tools for, 115*t*–117*t*
  in MS, 244–246
  multifactorial approach for, 560, 560*b*,
    561*b*, 561*t*
  Parkinson's, 269
  patient groups, 546

Falls (*Continued*)
  postural stability and, 546–547, 547*f*
  postural threat and outcome, 547*f*
  prevention of, 553–560, 553*b*
    engagement with, 559
    movement strategies for, 554*b*, 555*b*,
      556–557, 557*t*
    in physical environment, 557–559, 558*f*
  risk for, 554–557
  tests and outcome measures in, 552–553,
    553*f*
Family, involvement in goal setting, 133–134
FAS. *See* Functional Ability Scale
Fatigue, 55–56
  in Charcot-Marie-Tooth disease, 362
  in chronic demyelinating
      polyradiculoneuropathy, 358
  in functional motor disorders, 426
  in Guillain-Barré syndrome, 357
  measurement tools for, 115*t*–117*t*
  in MND, 340
  in MS, 248–250, 253–254
  in polyneuropathies, 374
    management of, 372, 376
Fear
  of falling, 548*t*–549*t*
  self-management and, 500
Feedback
  in motor learning, 14*t*–15*t*, 519
  in skill acquisition, 16
  in Social Cognitive Theory, 501
FES. *See* Functional electrical stimulation
Festination, with walking in Parkinson's,
    79*t*–80*t*
FitMi, 522
Fitness, 573
Fitness-to-drive legislation, 644–645, 644*f*
FITT principle. *See* Frequency, intensity,
    time, type principle
Fixed functional dystonia, in functional
    motor disorders, 420, 420*f*,
    427*t*–428*t*
Flexion momentum, in sit to stand, 81*t*
Floor effect, in measurement tool, 122
FMA-UE. *See* Fugl-Meyer Assessment
    Upper Extremity
FNDs. *See* Functional neurological
    disorders
FOG. *See* Freezing of gait
Fogg Behaviour Model, 25*f*
Follow-up, SCI and, 223
Foot flat, in gait cycle, 74*t*
Foot position, in sit to stand, 84*t*–85*t*
Foot Posture Index, 363
Footwear, falls and, 557–558
Forced vital capacity (FVC), 388, 405
  in spinal cord injury, 208, 208*t*

Forward Reach test, 118
Four Square Step Test, 452*t*
Freezing of gait (FOG), 60
  with walking in Parkinson's, 79*t*–80*t*
Frequency, intensity, time, type (FITT)
    principle, 17
Friedreich's ataxia, 305, 314*t*–315*t*
  pharmacological management of,
    306–307
FSHD. *See* Facioscapulohumeral muscular
    dystrophy
Fugl-Meyer Assessment Upper Extremity
    (FMA-UE), 522, 530–531
Fugl-Meyer test, 628
Function, in traumatic brain injury, 185
  interventions for, 189
Functional Ability Scale (FAS), 530–531
Functional decline, falls and, 548*t*–549*t*
Functional disorders, clinical
    neuropsychology and, 622
Functional dystonia, in functional motor
    disorders, 420
Functional electrical stimulation (FES),
    220*f*, 631–632
  SCI and, 215, 216*f*
Functional Gait Assessment, 452*t*
Functional Independence Measure, 336
Functional Independence Measure-
    Functional Assessment Measure,
    615
Functional jerks, in functional motor
    disorders, 419–420, 427*t*–428*t*
Functional Mobility Scale, for functional
    motor disorders, 424*t*
Functional motor disorders, 413–431
  adaptive aids for, 429
  biopsychosocial formulation for, 417–
    418, 417*t*
  case study in, 430–431, 431*t*
  clinical presentation of, 418–421
    fixed functional dystonia as, 420, 420*f*
    functional dystonia as, 420
    functional gait disorder as, 419
    functional jerks as, 419–420
    functional tremor as, 419
    functional weakness as, 418–419, 419*t*
    mixed movement disorder as, 420
    nonepileptic seizures as, 421
    persistent postural-perceptual
      dizziness as, 420
  concluding treatment of, 429–430
  diagnosis of, 418, 419*t*
  epidemiology of, 415, 415*b*
  historical perspective of, 414–415
  medications for, 429
  multidisciplinary team for, 421–422
  pathophysiology of, 415–418, 416*b*, 417*t*

Functional motor disorders (*Continued*)
  physiotherapy interventions of, 423–426
    considerations for, 426–429
    education as, 425
    intensity, duration and setting of, 429
    movement retraining as, 425–426, 427t–428t
    persistent pain and fatigue in, 426
    self-management as, 426
  prognosis of, 418
  rehabilitation of
    assessment for, 423
    before commencing, 422–423
    outcome measures of, 423
    physical, 423
Functional movement disorders, 60–61
Functional movement re-education, in neurological rehabilitation, 12–13
Functional neurological disorders (FNDs), 60–61
Functional neurological symptoms, 414
Functional performance tests, 118
Functional reach test, 452t
FVC. *See* Forced vital capacity

G

Gabapentin
  for neuropathic pain, 361
  spasticity management in MS, 242
Gait, assessment, for polyneuropathies, 363, 374
Gait cycle, in walking, 72, 73f, 74t
Gait disorder, functional, in functional motor disorders, 419, 427t–428t
Gait impairment, 77
Gait training
  robotic systems, 528, 528f
  SCI and, 218–220
  after stroke, 161t–162t, 163–164
  robot-assisted, 164
Game-based rehabilitation, 517, 520
Gamification, for neurorehabilitation, 517
Garner, Jill, 39–46
GAS. *See* Goal Attainment Scaling
Gaze-evoked nystagmus, 449t, 461
Gaze stability exercises, 454
General fatigue, 55
Generalisability, in motor learning, 14t–15t
Generic interventions, in self-management, 504t
Genetic factors, of MS, 235–236
Genetic neuromuscular disorders, 386
Gentamicin, for Ménière's disease, 447
GEO, robotic systems, 528, 528f
GFRs. *See* Ground reaction forces

GIofBS. *See* Goldsmith Indices of Body Symmetry
Give-way weakness, in functional motor disorders, 419t
Glasgow Coma Score, of traumatic brain injury, 179t
Glenohumeral instability, 628
Glenohumeral joint, kinematics of, 627, 630f
Globus pallidus, in Parkinson's, 267
GMFCS. *See* Gross Motor Function Classification System
Goal Attainment Scaling (GAS), 141–144, 142t
  for spasticity, 632, 641t
Goal-directed training, 651
Goal documentation, 132–133
Goal selection, 131–132
Goal setting
  definition of, 130
  self-management and, 502, 503t
  in stroke rehabilitation, 129–145
    case study example of interprofessional rehabilitation goals, 133t
    changing needs from acute care to community life, 134–141, 135f
    definitions and assumptions in, 130–131
    goal achievement as outcome measure, 141–144, 142t, 143f
    key points for, 140b–141b
    pragmatic person-centred, 131–134
    questions for gathering useful information for goal selection, 131b
    questions to address in goal statement, 132
Goldsmith Indices of Body Symmetry (GIofBS), 654, 663f
Google Cardboard, 525
Google Daydream, 525
Grasp, 83–91
  clinical focus on, for people with stroke, 91, 92t–93t
  essential components of, 87, 89t
  kinematics of, 87–88, 90t
  measurement tools for, 115t–117t
  muscle activity of, 89–91, 91f
Grip, measurement tools for, 115t–117t
Gross Motor Function Classification System (GMFCS), 651, 656f
Ground reaction forces (GFRs), 77, 78f
Group-based interventions, in self-management, 504t
Guillain-Barré syndrome, 357t, 358–361, 359f
  disease course and prognosis of, 360–361, 360f

Guillain-Barré syndrome (*Continued*)
  medical management of, 359–360
  presentation of, 359
Gut microbiota, of Parkinson's, 267

H

Habit formation, in behaviour change, 23–25
Habituation exercises, 454
Habituation, vestibular compensation and, 453
HADS. *See* Hospital Anxiety and Depression Scale
Haemorrhagic stroke, 152
Haemothorax, SCI, 207
Hair cells, 439
Hallpike-Dix (HPD) manoeuvre, 442–443, 443f, 449t
Hand, paretic, electrostimulation of, 168
HAQ. *See* Health Assessment Questionnaire
Head-mounted displays (HMDs), 520
Health, assessment and monitoring of, 576
Health Assessment Questionnaire (HAQ), 388
Health promotion
  of MS management, 243
  in neurological rehabilitation, 18
Healthcare services, redistribution of, 599
Healthy habits, in behaviour change, 24b
Heat sensitivity, of MS, 251
Heel-off, in gait cycle, 74t
Heel rise, in gait cycle, 74t
Heel strike, in gait cycle, 74t
Hemianopia, 62
Hemifacial muscle overactivity, in functional motor disorders, 419t
Hemiplegic stroke, posture and balance in, 99, 100t–101t
Henson, Alexandra, 643
Hereditary ataxias, 303–309
  anatomy, pathophysiology and clinical presentation of, 303–305, 304f
  autosomal dominant cerebellar ataxias of, 303
  autosomal recessive ataxias of, 303
  diagnosis and genetic testing for, 305
  epidemiology and genetics of, 303
  medical management for, 305–307
  physiotherapy assessment in, 307–308
  time course and corresponding management for, 308
  treatment selection and secondary complications/special problems in, 308–309, 310f
Hereditary neuropathies, 363–366

Hereditary spastic paresis, 309–313, 315t–316t
  anatomy, pathophysiology and clinical presentation of, 310–311
  diagnosis of, 311
  epidemiology and genetics of, 309–310
  medical management for, 311
  physiotherapy assessment for, 311–312
  time course and corresponding management for, 312
  treatment selection, secondary complications and special problems in, 312–313
Heterotropic ossification, of SCI, 222
HH. See Homonymous hemianopia
Hierarchy, 122
Hip abductor sign, in functional motor disorders, 419t
Hip and knee extensors, during sit to stand, 83t
History taking, of Parkinson's physiotherapy, 275–276, 277f
HMDs. See Head-mounted displays
Holmes, Carlee, 650
Home-based rehabilitation technologies, 520–527
  interventions, 521
  sensor-based systems, 521–523, 523f
  video analysis, 523–525
  VR headsets, 525–527, 526f
Home visit, falls and, 552
Homonymous hemianopia (HH), 62
Hoover's sign, in functional motor disorders, 418, 419t
Hope, in neurological rehabilitation, 8–9, 21–22, 22b
Horizontal roll test, 449t
Hospital admission, falls and, 546
Hospital Anxiety and Depression Scale (HADS), for functional motor disorders, 424t
HTC Vive, 525, 526f
Huntingtin, Huntington's disease, 294
Huntington's disease, 294–303, 315t–316t
  anatomy and pathophysiology of, 295
    basal ganglia and, 295, 296f
  behavioural symptoms of, 296
  clinical presentation of, 295–296
  counselling, genetics of, 295
  epidemiology of, 294
  genetics of, 294–295
  medical management of, 296–300
    physiotherapy assessment and prognosis of, 297–298, 299t, 300f
    standard care for, 297
    time course and corresponding physiotherapy management, 298–300

Huntington's disease (Continued)
  movement deficits in, 296–297, 296f
  natural history of, 295
  pain and, 589
  patient/client management of, 300f
  physiotherapy screening for, 299t
  prevalence of, 294
  treatment-based classification for, 301t–302t
  treatment selection and secondary complications/special problems in, 300–303
  Unified Huntington's Disease Rating Scale, 297
Hybrid exoskeletons, benefits of, 219
Hydrotherapy
  of SCI rehabilitation, 214
  traumatic brain injury for, 186, 190
Hyperacute phase, of stroke, 154–156
Hypertonicity, after traumatic brain injury, 183
  interventions for, 186–187
Hypertonus, 56–57
Hypothetical neurobiological model, for functional motor disorders, 416–417
Hypotheticodeductive reasoning strategy, 33
Hypotonus, 57
Hypoxic brain injury, clinical neuropsychology and, 618–619

I

IAM. See Internal acoustic meatus
IASP. See International Association for the Study of Pain
IBM. See Inclusion body myositis
IBMFRS. See Inclusion Body Myositis Functional Rating Scale
ICARS. See International Classification of Ataxia Rating Scale
ICCs. See Intraclass correlation coefficients
Ice gait, walking on, in functional motor disorders, 419t
ICF. See International Classification of Functioning, Disability and Health
ICF-based problem list, 35–36, 36f
Idebenone, of Friedreich's ataxia, 306–307
Idiopathic inflammatory myopathies (IIMs)
  acquired diseases, 387
  assessment and outcome measures, 388
  disease course and prognosis, 387
  medical management, 388
  physical management, 388
  presentation, 387

Idiopathic Parkinson's disease (IPD), 266
If-then plans, definition of, 139
IIMs. See Idiopathic inflammatory myopathies
Iliopsoas muscle, during sit to stand, 83t
IMACS. See International Myositis Assessment and Clinical Studies
Immobility, MND and, 339
Immune-mediated necrotising myopathy (IMNM), 387
Impaired balance, of MS, 245
Impairments, 6, 53–65
  coordination disorders, 58–60
  fatigue, 55–56
  measurement tools and, 114–115
  motor planning disorders, 60–61
  muscle tone disorders, 56–58
  in neurological practice, 54, 54t
  secondary complications in, 64–65
    contracture, 64
    deconditioning, 64–65
    learned non-use, 65
    physical inactivity, 64–65
  sensory disorders, 63–64
  vestibular disorders, 61–62
  visuospatial disorders, 62–63
  weakness, 54–55
Impedance control, 527
Inclinometer, 632, 633f
Inclusion body myositis (IBM), 387
Inclusion Body Myositis Functional Rating Scale (IBMFRS), 388
Incomplete syndromes, of SCI, 200–203, 204f, 205f, 206t
Inconsistency, in functional motor disorders, 419t
Individually Tailored Progressive Home-Based Exercise Programme, 554b
Indoor versus outdoor, falls and, 558–559
Inertial measurement units, 535b
Inflammatory neuropathies, 355
Inherited neurological conditions, 294–318
  case study in, 314–318
    classification of, 316
    condition overview, 314–316, 315t–316t, 317t
    examination in, 316–318
    intervention in, 318
    outcomes of, 318
    prognosis of, 318
  hereditary ataxias, 303–309
    anatomy, pathophysiology and clinical presentation of, 303–305, 304f
    autosomal dominant cerebellar ataxias of, 303
    autosomal recessive ataxias of, 303
    diagnosis and genetic testing for, 305

Inherited neurological conditions
    (*Continued*)
  epidemiology and genetics of, 303
  medical management for, 305–307
  physiotherapy assessment in, 307–308
  time course and corresponding
      management for, 308
  treatment selection and secondary
      complications/special problems in,
      308–309, 310*f*
  hereditary spastic paresis, 309–313,
      315*t*–316*t*
    anatomy, pathophysiology and clinical
        presentation of, 310–311
    diagnosis of, 311
    epidemiology and genetics of, 309–310
    medical management for, 311
    physiotherapy assessment for, 311–312
    time course and corresponding
        management for, 312
    treatment selection, secondary
        complications and special problems
        in, 312–313
  Huntington's disease, 294–303,
      315*t*–316*t*
    anatomy and pathophysiology of, 295
    behavioural symptoms of, 296
    clinical presentation of, 295–296
    counselling, genetics of, 295
    epidemiology of, 294
    genetics of, 294–295
    medical management of, 296–300
    movement deficits in, 296–297, 296*f*
    natural history of, 295
    patient/client management of, 300*f*
    physiotherapy screening for, 299*t*
    prevalence of, 294
    treatment-based classification for,
        301*t*–302*t*
    treatment selection and secondary
        complications/special problems in,
        300–303
    Unified Huntington's Disease Rating
        Scale, 297
    nonpharmacological treatment for,
        315*t*–316*t*
Initial contact, 76
  in gait cycle, 74*t*
Initial swing, in gait cycle, 74*t*
Injury, falls and, 548*t*–549*t*
Instructions, in sitting/getting out of
    bed, 87*t*
Instrumental activity of daily living,
    643–644
Intention tremor, 59, 60*t*
Interactive driving simulators, 638, 646*f*
Interactive gaming technologies, 537

Interactive technologies, 518–520, 519*b*,
    537*b*
  ambulation function, 535
  applications, 517
  clinical setting, 535
  development of, 517–518
  extended reality, 520
  game-based tasks, 518–519
  home-based rehabilitation, 520–521
  interventions, 535
  motor behaviours, 518
  spinal cord injury, 535
  video gaming systems, 521
Interactive video gaming, after stroke,
    167–168
Interdisciplinary team, after stroke, 153
Intermittent positive-pressure breathing
    (IPPB), SCI, 209
Internal acoustic meatus (IAM), 444
Internal consistency, 121
Internal validity, 122
International Association for the Study of
    Pain (IASP), 583
International Classification of Ataxia
    Rating Scale (ICARS), 307–308
International Classification of Functioning,
    Disability and Health (ICF)
  in neurological rehabilitation, 6–7, 6*f*
  Parkinson's history-taking, 274
International GBS Outcome Study, 357
International Myositis Assessment and
    Clinical Studies (IMACS), 388
International Spinal Cord Injury Pain
    classification system, 588
International Standard Neurological
    Classification of Spinal Cord Injury
    (ISNCSCI), 200*f*
Interval data, assessing reliability for,
    120–121, 120*f*
Interval tool, 118
Interventions
  falls and, 548*t*–549*t*
  therapists in, 12–13
Interview
  falls and, 550
  motivational, 502
Intracerebral haemorrhage, definition of, 152
Intraclass correlation coefficients (ICCs),
    120
Intracranial haemorrhage, definition of, 152
Intracranial pressure, in traumatic brain
    injury, 180–181
Intrathecal baclofen (ITB), 311
Intravenous immunoglobulin
  for chronic demyelinating
      polyradiculoneuropathy, 361–362
  for Guillain-Barré syndrome, 359–360

Intrinsic motivation, in skill acquisition,
    13–15
Involuntary muscle spasms, 58
IPD. *See* Idiopathic Parkinson's disease
IPPB. *See* Intermittent positive-pressure
    breathing
Ischaemic stroke, 152–154, 154*t*
ISNCSCI. *See* International Standard
    Neurological Classification of
    Spinal Cord Injury
Isoniazid, for MS, 247
ITB. *See* Intrathecal baclofen

J

Joint contractures
  in MS, 252
  in neuromuscular disorders, 405
Joint mobilisation, for pain, 593
Joint range measurement, 394

K

κ coefficients, 119
KAFOs. *See* Knee-ankle-foot orthoses
Kinematics
  of reach and grasp, 87–88, 90*t*
  of walking, 72–77, 75*f*, 76*f*
Kinetics, walking, 77
Knee-ankle-foot orthoses (KAFOs), 388
Knowledge of performance (KP), in
    feedback, 16
Knowledge of results (KR), in feedback, 16
Knowledge, self-management and, 502–503
KP. *See* Knowledge of performance
KR. *See* Knowledge of results

L

L-3,4-dihydroxyphenylalanine (L-DOPA),
    Parkinson's therapy, 270
Labyrinthitis, 441–442
Language therapy, for functional motor
    disorders, 421
Laser therapy, for pain, 598
Lateralisation, clinical neuropsychology
    and, 617
Lateropulsion, 62
Layperson leaders, in self-management, 504*t*
LBD. *See* Lewy body dementia
Lead leg, in gait cycle, 74*t*
Leap Motion, 524
Learned non-use, of hemiparetic
    extremity, 65
Leg Activity measure, 632, 641*t*
Leigh syndrome, 401

Leprosy, acquired neuropathies and, 355
Lesion site, clinical neuropsychology and, 617
Levator scapulae, muscle timing and, 628
Levodopa, for Parkinson's therapy, 270
Lewy body dementia (LBD), in Parkinson's, 267
LGMD. *See* Limb girdle muscular dystrophy
Lidocaine, for dysaesthesia, 361
Life Thread Model, 498–499
Lifestyle modifications, of MS management, 243
Lifting, SCI, 217–218
Ligament pain, 585
Likert scales, 117
Limb girdle muscular dystrophy (LGMD)
   assessment and outcome measures, 394
   case studies, 406
   disease course and prognosis, 394, 396*f*
   inheritance patterns, 394
   medical management, 394–395
   physical management, 395
   subtypes, 394, 396*t*
Limb weakness, in functional motor disorders, 418
   lower, 427*t*–428*t*
   upper, 427*t*–428*t*
Listening, in self-management, 507
LMNs. *See* Lower motor neurones
LOA. *See* Loss of ambulation
Loading response, 76
   in gait cycle, 74*t*
'Locked in' syndrome, 182*t*
Locomotor recovery, from stroke, 161*t*–162*t*, 163–169
   balance training for, 163
   bilateral arm training, 167
   circuit class training for, 164–165
   constraint-induced movement therapy, 166–167
   electrostimulation of paretic arm and hand, 168
   electrostimulation of paretic lower limb, 165
   gait training for, 163–164
   robot-assisted therapy, upper limb, 168
   therapy delivery, 168–169
   upper limb recovery, 165, 165*t*–166*t*
   virtual reality, interactive video gaming, 167–168
Lokomat, robotic systems, 528, 528*f*
Long Covid self-management, 508–510
Lorig, Kate, 498
Loss of ambulation (LOA), 390–392
Low-level laser therapy, for pain, 598

Lower limb peripheral sensory neuropathies, 63
Lower limb proprioceptive loss, 63
Lower limb recovery, from stroke, 161*t*–162*t*, 163–169
   balance training for, 163
   bilateral arm training, 167
   circuit class training for, 164–165
   constraint-induced movement therapy, 166–167
   electrostimulation of paretic arm and hand, 168
   electrostimulation of paretic lower limb, 165
   gait training for, 163–164
   robot-assisted therapy, upper limb, 168
   therapy delivery, 168–169
   upper limb recovery, 165, 165*t*–166*t*
   virtual reality, interactive video gaming, 167–168
Lower motor neurone weakness, 55
Lower motor neurones (LMNs) syndrome, 55, 327
Lumbar paraspinals, during sit to stand, 83*t*
Lumbar puncture, MS diagnosis of, 237
Lung function
   progression, 388
   in respiratory assessment, 474–477, 477*f*

M

MAC. *See* Manual assisted coughing
Machado-Joseph disease, 303
Magnetic resonance imaging (MRI)
   MS diagnosis of, 237
   neuromuscular disorders, 385
   for vestibular disorders, 446
Maintenance, change and, 501*b*
Maintenance rehabilitation, of MS management, 243–244
MAL. *See* Motor Activity Log
Manual Ability Classification system (MAC), 651
Manual assisted coughing (MAC), MND and, 345
Manual cough, in respiratory management, 482
Manual muscle testing (MMT), 388
Manual therapy, for pain, 596–597
MAP. *See* Myositis Activities Profile
MAS. *See* Modified Ashworth Scale
Massage, for pain, 593
Mastery experiences, in Social Cognitive Theory, 501
Maximal active humeral elevation test, 632
Maximal expiratory pressure (MEP), 476–477

Maximal inspiratory pressure (MIP), 476–477
Maximal insufflation capacity (MIC), 344–345
   in respiratory management, 481–482, 481*b*
McLoughlin, James, 46–50
mCTSIB. *See* Modified Clinical Test of the Sensory Interaction of Balance
MD. *See* Mitochondrial diseases
ME. *See* Myalgic encephalomyelitis
Measurement tools, 113–125
   activity limitations in, 115, 115*t*–117*t*
   applied measurement science in, 124–125
   impairments and, 114–115
   psychometric properties of, 119–124
      reliability as, 119–121
      responsiveness as, 123–124
      validity as, 121–123
   types of, 115*t*–117*t*, 117–119
Mechanical insufflation and exsufflation device, 345–346, 346*f*
   in respiratory management, 480*f*, 482
Medial rotation test, 632–635
Medical Research Council (MRC) score, 363
MELAS. *See* Mitochondrial encephalomyopathy, lactic acidosis and strokelike episodes
Ménière's disease, 443
   medical and surgical management of, 447
Mental practice, in motor learning, 14*t*–15*t*, 17
MEP. *See* Maximal expiratory pressure
MI. *See* Motivational interviewing
MIC. *See* Maximal insufflation capacity
Microsoft Azure Kinect, 524
Microsoft Kinect, 524, 524*f*
Microsoft Xbox with Kinect sensor, 524
Mid-stance, 76
   in gait cycle, 74*t*
Mid-swing, in gait cycle, 74*t*
Migraine, vestibular, 443–444
Mindset, in neurological rehabilitation, 19–22
Mini-Balance Evaluation Systems Test, 452*t*
Minimally conscious state, definition of, 182*t*
Ministroke, definition of, 151
MIP. *See* Maximal inspiratory pressure
MIT Manus, 527, 527*f*
Mitochondrial diseases (MD)
   assessment and outcome measures, 402–405
   cell, 401–402, 404*f*

Mitochondrial diseases (MD) (*Continued*)
 disease course and prognosis, 402
 exercise, 404, 404*t*
 maternal inheritance, 401, 402*f*
 medical management, 402–403
 organelles, 401
 physical management, 403–405
 presentation, 401–402, 403*f*
 subtypes, 401
Mitochondrial encephalomyopathy, lactic acidosis and strokelike episodes (MELAS), 401
Mitofusin 2, 361
Mixed movement disorder, in functional motor disorders, 420
MMT. *See* Manual muscle testing
MNDA. *See* Motor Neurone Disease Association
Mobile dystonia, 58
Mobility
 functional, SCI rehabilitation, 217–218
 in hereditary ataxias, 309
 measurement tools for, 115*t*–117*t*
Modelling
 in motor learning, 14*t*–15*t*
 in skill acquisition, 17
Modified Ashworth Scale (MAS), 632, 641*t*
Modified Clinical Test of the Sensory Interaction of Balance (mCTSIB), 451*f*
Modified Epley's manoeuvre, for benign paroxysmal positional vertigo, 457*f*
Momentum transfer, in sit to stand, 81*t*
Monoplegic gait, dragging, in functional motor disorders, 419*t*
Monroe Kellie doctrine, 489*f*
Morgan, Prue Elizabeth, 650
Mortality, in Parkinson's, 266
Motion sensitivity, 454
Motion Sensitivity Quotient, 454
Motion tracking techniques, for neurorehabilitation, 523–524
Motivation, in neurological rehabilitation, 20, 21*f*
Motivational interviewing (MI), 21, 502
Motor Activity Log (MAL), 628
Motor control, in neurological rehabilitation, 11–12
 variables for, 14*t*–15*t*
Motor control training, 635
 neuroplasticity and timing of, 635–636
Motor fatigue, 55–56
Motor imagery, for pain, 598–599
Motor learning, 518
 in neurological rehabilitation, 13–17, 14*t*–15*t*

Motor neurone disease, 327–349
 anatomy of, 328
 assessment of, 334–338, 335*t*, 336*t*
 bulbar-onset, 333
 case study on, 348–349, 349*t*–350*t*
 clinical phenotypes of, 329
 clinical presentation of, 333–334
 diagnosis of, 329–330, 330*b*, 331*f*
 disease-specific measures for, 336–337
 environmental factors of, 329
 epidemiology of, 327–328
 exercise for, 341–342, 342*t*, 343*f*
 genetic factors for, 328
 geographical factors of, 329, 329*b*
 management of, 338–339
 medical management for, 330–333
 pain and, 589–590
 pathophysiology of, 328
 prognosis of, 337–338, 338*t*
 respiratory issues in, 344–347, 345*f*, 346*f*
 secondary complications of, 339–347, 340*t*
 signs of, 333–334
 symptoms of, 333–334
 time course of, 338–339
 treatment selection for, 339–347
  assistive devices and orthoses for, 341
  exercise for, 341–342, 342*t*, 343*f*
  wheelchair as, 343–344
Motor Neurone Disease Association (MNDA), red flag diagnosis tool, 330, 331*f*
Motor planning, disorders of, 60–61
'Motor proteins', 355
Motor vehicle crashes (MVCs), 636
Movement
 deficits, Huntington's disease and, 296–297, 296*f*
 disorders, in traumatic brain injury, 184
  interventions for, 187
 neuropsychological disorders of, clinical neuropsychology and, 621
 observation and analysis of, 71–102
  posture and balance in, 91–102
  reach and grasp in, 83–91
  rolling and getting out of bed in, 82–83
  sit to stand in, 77–82
  in sitting/getting out of bed, 87*t*
  walking in, 71–77, 72*t*
 patterns, execution of, with bed mobility, in Parkinson's, 88*t*
 retraining, for functional motor disorders, 425–426, 427*t*–428*t*
 strategies, for falls, 554*b*, 555*b*, 556–557, 557*t*
 therapy, constraint-induced, after stroke, 166–167

MOVES tool, 574
MRC score. *See* Medical Research Council score
MRI. *See* Magnetic resonance imaging
MS. *See* Multiple sclerosis
MSA. *See* Multiple system atrophy
Multifactorial approach, for falls, 560, 560*b*, 561*b*, 561*t*
Multiple sclerosis (MS), 235–253
 case study of, 253
 classification of, 238–239, 238*f*
 client in standing frame, 236*f*
 clinical and MRI activity, 249*f*
 clinical neuropsychology and, 622
 clinical presentation of, 237
  visual symptoms, 237
 diagnosis of, 237–238
 driving and, 643–649
  as activity of daily living, 643–644
  assessment, 645–649, 648*t*–649*t*
  case presentation of, 647–649, 648*t*–649*t*
  challenges in, 643–649
  consultation for, 647
  evaluation process for, aspects of, 644–647, 644*f*
  fitness-to-drive legislation and, 644–645
  interpretation, 649
  intervention for, 646–647
  posttraining assessment, 649
  screening for, 645, 647
  training programme, 649
 epidemiology of, 235–236
 exercise for, 555*b*
 fatigue, 248–250
 history of complaint, 253–257
 initial outpatient physiotherapy session of, 254, 255*tb0010*
 intensity, supervised practice for, 245*f*
 interventions of, 244–252, 256*t*
  anxiety, 252
  ataxia, 247
  bladder, 251–252
  bowel, 251–252
  cognitive impairment, 252
  depression, 252
  fatigue, 248–250
  heat sensitivity, 251
  impaired mobility, balance and falls, 244–246
  pain, 250
  respiratory dysfunction of, 251
  sedentary behaviour, weakness and deconditioning, 246
  spasticity, 244*f*, 247–248
  upper limb impairment, 246–247

Multiple sclerosis (MS) (*Continued*)
   vestibulopathy, 250–251
   key assessment findings of, 254, 254*t*
   medical management of, 239–244
     challenges associated with disease-modifying therapies, 239
     disease-modifying therapies in active disease, 239
     health and social care team, 240–241
     physiotherapy assessment, 241–242, 242*t*
     prognosis, 239–240
     sign and symptoms, 240, 240*f*, 241*t*
     time course and management, 242–244
   medication, 253–254
   pain and, 589
   pathology of, 236
   pathophysiology of, 236–237
     demyelination, 236
     plaques, 236
   problem list, goals and plan, 255*t*
   progress review at 3 months, 255
   secondary complications of, 252–253
     contractures, 252
     pressure ulcers, 252–253
   Self-Efficacy Scale, 507*b*
   spasticity of, 244*f*, 247–248
   time course and management of, 242–244
     health promotion, lifestyle modifications and comorbidities of, 243
     maintenance rehabilitation of, 243–244
     restorative rehabilitation of, 243
     service delivery of, 244
   treatment plan of, 254
Multiple system atrophy (MSA), in Parkinson's, 267
Muscle action, during sit to stand, 82, 82*f*, 83*t*
Muscle activity
   of reach and grasp, 89–91, 91*f*
   walking kinematics and, 72–77, 74*t*, 79*t*
Muscle biopsy, for MND, 330
Muscle disorders, respiratory function in, 487, 488*t*
Muscle pain, 585
Muscle paresis, after traumatic brain injury, 184
   interventions for, 187
Muscle spasms, 585
Muscle spasticity
   measurement tools for, 115*t*–117*t*
   pain from, 585
Muscle strength
   and aerobic exercise, 375
   assessment of, for polyneuropathies, 363, 373
   impairments, 373, 374*t*

Muscle strength (*Continued*)
   measurement
     tools for, 115*t*–117*t*
     respiratory issues, 344
Muscle tone
   disorders of, 56–58
   measurement tools for, 115*t*–117*t*
   in traumatic brain injury, 183, 183*t*
Muscle training, respiratory, 483
Muscle wasting, in Charcot-Marie-Tooth disease, 363–365, 364*f*, 365*f*
Muscle weakness
   measurement tools for, 115*t*–117*t*
   MND and, 333, 339
   pain and, 587
Muscular atrophy, progressive, 329
Muscular dystrophies, 386
   Duchenne, 388–393. *See also* Duchenne muscular dystrophy
   facioscapulohumeral, 393–394. *See also* Facioscapulohumeral muscular dystrophy
   limb girdle, 394–395. *See also* Limb girdle muscular dystrophy
Muscular dystrophies, pain and, 587
Musculoskeletal injuries, concurrent, in traumatic brain injury, 185
   interventions for, 188
Musculoskeletal pain, 587–588, 588*b*
   in MS, 250
   spinal cord injuries and, 590–591
MusicGlove system, 522, 523*f*
MVCs. *See* Motor vehicle crashes
Myalgic encephalomyelitis (ME), 55
Myasthenia gravis, 487, 488*t*
Myelin
   of MS, 236–237
   of polyneuropathies, 355
Myoclonus, in functional motor disorders, 419–420, 427*t*–428*t*
Myositis Activities Profile (MAP), 388
Myotonic dystrophy type 1
   assessment and outcome measures, 397–398, 399*t*
   disease course and prognosis, 395–397
   gene codes, 395
   medical management, 398
   multisystem involvement, 395
   phenotypical characteristics, 395, 398*t*
   physical management, 398–399

N

National Disability Insurance Scheme (NDIS), 653
National Health Service (NHS), Parkinson's (PD), 272

National Institute for Health and Clinical Excellence (NICE), MS physical therapy guidelines of, 240–241
National Insurance Disability Scheme, 46
NCAPC. *See* Non-Communicating Adult Pain Checklist
NDIS. *See* National Disability Insurance Scheme
Negative predictive value, 123
Neglect, clinical neuropsychology and, 622
Nerve, anatomy and physiology of, 356
Nerve conduction studies, for MND, 330
NESs. *See* Nonepileptic seizures
Neural plasticity, 38
   in neurological rehabilitation, 10–11, 10*b*
Neuritis, peripheral vestibular, case studies for, 460–461
Neurological conditions
   acute, 590–591
   adults with cerebral palsy, 654–665
   case study, 653–654, 659–662
     assessment, neuromuscular and postural status, 659, 661*t*
     assistive technology products, 665*f*
     custom moulded seating system, 665*f*
     ICF domains, 653, 660*f*
     management strategies, 662, 664*t*
     measures of posture, 659
     measures of spasticity, pain and skin integrity, 659–660
     postural asymmetry, 653, 659*f*
     spine and left hip, 662*f*
   clinical reasoning approach in, 3–4
   disorders of consciousness, disability management, ethics and legal frameworks, 649–654
   inherited, 294–318
     case study in, 314–318
     hereditary ataxias, 303–309
     hereditary spastic paresis, 309–313, 315*t*–316*t*
     Huntington's disease, 294–303, 315*t*–316*t*
     nonpharmacological treatment for, 315*t*–316*t*
   multiple sclerosis, 643–649
   pain associated with, epidemiology of, 584*t*, 589–591
   physical management in, 4, 628–665
   poststroke shoulder assessment and rehabilitation, 628–637
   spasticity, 637–643
   stimulation and responsiveness, 653
     nutrition, 654
     oral care, 653–654
     outcomes, 654
     postural management, 654

Neurological conditions (*Continued*)
  swallowing, 654
Neurological disability, self-management and
  approach to, 503–505
  evidence base for, 503–507
  understanding responses to, 499–502
Neurological disorders, 571–572
  exercise and, 573
  falls and, 546–547
  fitness and, 573
  of MS, 235
  physical activity and, 572–575, 573*f*
Neurological impairments, 53, 54*t*
  clinical reasoning in, 53
  coordination, disorders of, 58–60
  fatigue as, 55–56
  motor planning, disorders of, 60–61
  muscle tone, disorders of, 56–58
  secondary complications in, 64–65
    contracture as, 64
    deconditioning as, 64–65
    learned non-use as, 65
    physical inactivity as, 64–65
  sensory disorders as, 63–64
  vestibular disorders as, 61–62
  visuospatial disorders as, 62–63
  weakness as, 54–55
Neurological physiotherapy
  clinical reasoning in, 33–50
  measurement tools for, 115*t*–117*t*
Neurological rehabilitation
  conceptual framework, 34
  definition of, 3
  guiding principles in, 3–25, 5*f*
    behaviour change in, 22–25
    exercise prescription, 17–18
    functional movement re-education
      in, 12–13
    health promotion in, 18
    ICF in, 6–7, 6*f*
    mindset in, 19–22
    motor control in, 11–12
    neural plasticity in, 10–11, 10*b*
    person-centred care in, 7–9, 8*b*, 9*t*
    prediction in, 10
    prognosis in, 9–10
    self-management (self-efficacy) in, 19,
      19*f*, 19*t*
    skill acquisition/motor learning in,
      13–17, 14*t*–15*t*
    team work in, 7
  physical activity in, 571–580
    barriers in, 578
    changing behaviour in, 578–580, 579*f*
    exercise in, 573
    facilitators of, 578
    fitness in, 573

Neurological rehabilitation (*Continued*)
    frequency of, 577
    intensity of, 578
    in long-term neurological conditions,
      573–574, 573*f*
    reducing sedentary time in, 578
    timing of, 578
    type of, 578
  theoretical framework in, 5–25, 5*f*
Neurological upper limb approach,
    musculoskeletal integration in,
    628–637
Neurology, for functional motor disorders,
    421
Neuromas, acoustic, neurological disorders
    of, 618
Neuromuscular disorders (NMDs)
  acquired, 386
  anatomy and physiology, 383–385
  anterior horn cell diseases, 383
  assessment, 387
  case studies, 405–406
  genetic, 386
  muscle structure and function, 385, 386*f*
  physical management and rehabilitation,
    387
  types
    idiopathic inflammatory myopathies,
      387–388
    mitochondrial diseases, 401–405
    muscular dystrophies, 388–395
    myotonic dystrophy type 1, 395–399
    spinal muscular atrophy, 399–401
Neuromuscular junction, respiratory
    function in, 487, 488*t*
Neuronal circuitry, reorganisation of, 585
Neurone, 355, 356*f*
Neuronitis, 441–442
Neuropathic pain, 583, 588–589, 588*b*
  central, 583, 588–589
    multiple sclerosis and, 586
    Parkinson's and, 586
    stroke and, 587
  diabetic, case study for, 602–603, 603*t*
  diabetic neuropathy and, 361
  in MS, 250
  peripheral, 588
Neuropathic pain syndrome, 583
Neuropathy, 583
  acquired, 358–363
    chronic demyelinating
      polyradiculoneuropathy, 357*t*,
      361–362
    Guillain-Barré syndrome, 357*t*, 358–
      361, 359*f*, 360*f*
  axonal, 355, 357*b*
  diabetic, 357*t*, 362–363

Neuropathy (*Continued*)
  hereditary, 363–366
  respiratory function in, 487, 487*t*
Neuroplasticity, in individuals with stroke
    and, 635–636
Neurorehabilitation, 517–538
  case history in, 537–538
  definition of, 517
  evidence, 535
  role of, 518–519, 519*b*
  self-management and, 501
  tips for choosing, 536–537, 537*b*
    activity/task/game, 536–537
    client considerations in, 537
    resources for clinicians, 536
    technology, 536
  types of, 519–535
    home-based rehabilitation, 521–527
    robot-assisted motor training, 527–
      530, 527*f*, 528*f*, 530*f*
    wearable technology, field assessments
      and interventions, 530–535, 535*b*
Neurotherapists, in hypertonus, 56
NHS. *See* National Health Service
NICE. *See* National Institute for Health and
    Clinical Excellence
Nintendo Wii, 521, 522*f*, 537
Nintendo Wii Fit, 521–522, 522*f*, 524
NMDs. *See* Neuromuscular disorders
Nociceptive pain, 583
  in MS, 250
Nominal data, with two scoring categories,
    assessing reliability for, 119
Nominal tool, 117
Non-Communicating Adult Pain Checklist
    (NCAPC), 654
Nondopaminergic cell dysfunction,
    Parkinson's, 268
Nonepileptic seizures (NESs), in functional
    motor disorders, 429
  physiotherapy for, 429
Noninvasive ventilation, for MND, 336*t*,
    346–347
Normative person-centred approach, in
    clinical neuropsychology, 614
North Star Ambulatory Assessment
    (NSAA), 391*t*
North Star Assessment for Limb Girdle
    Type Muscular Dystrophies
    (NSAD), 394
NSAA. *See* North Star Ambulatory
    Assessment
Nutrition, for neurological conditions, 654
Nystagmus, 442*b*
  benign paroxysmal positional vertigo
    and, 442–443
  spontaneous, 449*t*

O

Object contact, in transport and manipulation phases, 90t

Object location, in transport and manipulation phases, 90t

Objective assessment, of pain, 593

Occupational therapy, for functional motor disorders, 421

Oculomotor, balance and, 94

Oedema, measurement tools for, 115t–117t

One-leg stance test, 452t

One-to-one interventions, in self-management, 504t

Ongoing postural adjustments, during sit to stand, 83t

Optimal Theory of Motor Learning, 13

Optokinetic stimulation, 454

Ordinal data, assessing reliability for, 119–120

Ordinal tools, 117

Orthoses
  for MND, 341
  SCI and, 219b

Orthostatic blood pressure, 445–446

Orthostatic hypotension, 445–446

Orthotic management, 394
  in ataxia, 305–306
  for polyneuropathies, 372

Orthotics, falls and, 557–558

Oscillopsia, 443

Oswestry standing frame, 218f

Otoconia, 439

Otoliths, 439

Outcome measures, 113–114
  in DMD, 389, 553t
  in falls, 552–553, 553f
  of functional motor disorders, 423, 424t
  in spinal cord injury, 213t–214t

Overall Neuropathy Limitation scale, 363

Overground walking, after stroke, 163

Overlapping impairments, 54

Overnight pulse oximetry, 405

Overwork damage, 341–342

Oxford Community Stroke Project classification, for ischaemic strokes, 153–154, 154t

P

Pain, 63–64
  acute, 583
  anatomy and pathophysiology of, 586–587, 587f
  assessment of, 591–593
  in Charcot-Marie-Tooth disease, 362
  chronic, 583

Pain (*Continued*)
  clinical presentation of, 587–589
  contemporary views on, 585
  definition of, 583
  diagnosis of, 591–593
  in functional motor disorders, 426
  management of, 583–604
    electrophysical techniques for, 597–599
    pharmacological, 593–595, 595t
    principles of, 593–600, 594f, 600b
    psychological approaches to, 599–600
    surgical, 596
  measurement tools for, 115t–117t
  MND and, 339
  in MS, 250
  musculoskeletal, 587–588
    in MS, 250
  with neurological conditions, epidemiology of, 584t, 589–591
  neuropathic, 583, 588–589, 588b
    in MS, 250
  nociceptive, 583
  objective assessment of, 593
  origin of, 583
  outcome monitoring for, 600–602
  patient experience of, 585
  phantom limb, 603–604, 604t
  in polyneuropathies, 374
    management of, 372
  potential damaged tissues and, 592t
  prognosis for, 591–593
  progressive neurological conditions and, 589–590
  rehabilitation, 596–597
  in SCI, 212
  signs and symptoms of, 587–589
  subjective assessment of, 591–593
    red and yellow flags for, 592, 592t
    reliability of, factors influencing, 592
  in traumatic brain injury, 185
    interventions for, 188–189
  treatment for
    Covid-19 impact, 601–602
    effect of, strategies to improve, 601
    evaluating response to, 600–601
    initiating, 600
    selection of, 600–602
    setting goals, 600
  types of, 585–586

Pain adjuvants, 591, 595t

Paraesthesia, 63

Paraplegia, 198

Paraspinals, during sit to stand, 83t

Parkinson, James, 266

Parkinsonism, 266

Parkinson's (PD), 265–288
  aetiology of, 266–267, 266b
  age of onset, 266
  case study of, 284b–288b
  clinical features of, 269
  definition of, 265
  epidemiology of, 266–267, 266b
  exercise for, 555b
  getting out of bed for people with, 83, 88t
  idiopathic, 266
  incidence of, 266
  medical management of, 268–271
    clinical presentation of, 268–270
    diagnosis of, 268–270
    pharmacological, 270
    research, newer technologies, 271
    surgical, 270–271, 271b
  model for collaborative, 272f
  mortality in, 266
  neuroanatomy of, 267–268, 268b
  pain and, 589
  pathophysiology of, 267, 268b
  physical activity and, 571
  physiotherapy management of, 274–284
    choosing treatment of, 276–284, 284b
    exercise, 279–281, 282f
    framework intervention for, 274, 275b
    goal setting of, 276–284, 284b
    history taking, 275–276, 277f, 286
    movement strategies training, 282–284
    physical assessment, 276, 279b, 286–287
    physical examination, 278f
    practice of, 281–282
    referral to, 274–275, 275t
    treatment goals, 280f, 287–288
  posture and balance in, 99, 100t–101t
  team management of, 271–274
    time course from diagnosis and communication, 272–273, 273b, 273t, 274f
  walking for people with, 77, 79t–80t

Parkinson's UK exercise framework, 281, 282f

Participation, in ICF, 6–7

Passive function, 630

Passive movements, physical management and, 214

Patent airway, maintenance of, 479–481

Patient activation, 506

Patient Activation Measure, 506

Patient-centred care, Picker principles of, 7–8, 8b

Patient groups, in falls, 546

Patient-reported outcome measures (PROMs), 394

PD. *See* Parkinson's

PDOC. *See* Persistent disorder of consciousness

Peak cough flow, 405
    in respiratory assessment, 477–478, 477b
Pectoralis minor index (PMI), 627, 633f
Pectoralis minor muscle, 627
Peer support, self-management and, 499
Perceived fatigue, 55
    in MS, 248
Performance fatigability, in MS, 248
Performance of Upper Limb (PUL), 393
Performance of Upper Limb 2.0 (PUL 2.0), 391t
Peripheral neuropathic pain, 588
Peripheral vestibular disorders, 61
Peripheral vestibular neuritis, case studies for, 460–461
Peripheral vestibular system, 439–440, 439f
    disorders of, 441–443
Persistent disorder of consciousness (PDOC), 643, 650–651
Persistent postural perceptual dizziness (PPPD), 445
    in functional motor disorders, 420
    medical and surgical management of, 447
Person-centred care
    concept of, 6–7
    in neurological rehabilitation, 7–9, 8b, 9t
Person-centred goal setting, pragmatic, in stroke rehabilitation, 131–134
    family involvement in, 133–134
    goal documentation, 132–133
    goal selection, 131–132
    measurement in, 134
Persuasion, verbal, 501
Perturbation-based balance training, 556
Pes cavus, in Charcot-Marie-Tooth disease, 362
Phantom limb pain, 603–604, 604t
Phenothiazines, vestibular rehabilitation and, 446–447
Physical activity, 572–575
    barriers in, 578
    changing behaviour in, 578–580, 579f
    condition progression, 574
    exercise in, 573–574
    exercise response/ recovery, 574–575, 575f
    facilitators of, 578
    for falls, 554
    fitness in, 573–574
    frequency of, 577
    intensity of, 578
    likelihood of secondary conditions, 574
    in long-term neurological conditions, 573–574, 573f
    neurological symptoms in, 574
    for pain, 596
    for polyneuropathy, 370–371

Physical activity (Continued)
    reducing sedentary time in, 578
    stage/severity of disease and, 574
    timing of, 578
    type of, 578
Physical assessment, of functional motor disorders, 423
Physical capacity, Parkinson's diagnosis, 276
Physical examination, for Parkinson's physiotherapy, 278f
Physical inactivity, in impairments, 64–65
Physical management, SCI and, 204–205, 212–221
Physical rehabilitation, of functional motor disorders, 422
Physical therapy, in lower motor neurone weakness, 55
Physiotherapy assessment, of clinical reasoning, 40t–41t
Pickering principles, of patient-centred care, 7–8, 8b
Plantarflexors, during sit to stand, 83t
Plasma exchange, for Guillain-Barré syndrome, 359–360
Plasticity, SCI and, 199
PM. See Polymyositis
PMI. See Pectoralis minor index
Pneumothorax, SCI and, 207
Poliomyelitis, 386
Polymyositis (PM), 387
Polyneuropathy, 355–376
    acquired, 358–363
    anatomy of, 356
    assessment of, 366–369, 368t
    case study on, 372–376
        balance, 375
        hand splints and equipment, 376
        management of fatigue in, 376
        management of upper limb function in, 375–376
        muscle strength and aerobic exercise in, 375
        observation of activities on, 373–374
        orthotic prescription for, 374–375
        physiotherapy options for, 374
        presenting impairments in, 373, 373f
        range of movement, 375
        self-management, 376
    causes of, 356–358
    physical management and rehabilitation for, 369–372
        acute, 370
        long-term, 370–372
    physiology of, 356
    treatment of, 369t
    types of, 357t, 358–366

Polyradiculoneuropathy, chronic demyelinating, 357t, 361–362
Pose estimation, for neurorehabilitation, 523
Positional tests, 449t
Positioning, SCI rehabilitation of, 217b
Positive emotion, Engagement, Relationships, Meaning and Accomplishment (PERMA) theory, 20
Positive predictive value, 123
Posterior cord syndrome, 200–203
Posterior spinal fusion, for scoliosis, 305–306
Poststroke fatigue, 55
Poststroke shoulder pain. See also Shoulder complex
    case presentation, 636
    evaluation, 629–635
Posttraumatic amnesia
    definition of, 182t
    in traumatic brain injury, 180, 180t
Postural adjustments, balance and, 95
Postural control
    of reach and grasp, 89t
    in walking, 72t
Postural deformity, after SCI, 221, 221b
Postural instability, in Parkinson's, 269
Postural orthostatic tachycardia syndrome (POTS), 445–446
Posture, 91–102
    clinical foci of, 97–102, 100t–101t
    measurement tools for, 115t–117t
    movement analysis strategies to quantify, 95–96, 96t
Posture and Postural Ability Scale (PPAS), 654
Posturography, 452t
    for vestibular disorders, 446
POTS. See Postural orthostatic tachycardia syndrome
Power-assisted wheeling systems, 218
PPMS. See Primary progressive MS
PPPD. See Persistent postural perceptual dizziness
Practice
    amount of, in skill acquisition, 16
    definition of, 518
    in motor learning, 14t–15t
Pragmatic person-centred goal setting, in stroke rehabilitation, 131–134
    family involvement in, 133–134
    goal documentation, 132–133
    goal selection, 131–132
    measurement in, 134
'Preassessment Information Form', 275
Precontemplation, change and, 501b
'Prediagnosis' stage, of Parkinson's, 273

Prediction, in neurological rehabilitation, 10
Predictive validity, 123
Pregabalin
　for neuropathic pain, 361
　spasticity management in MS, 242
Preparation, change and, 501*b*
Preparatory phase, of sit to stand, 81*t*
Presbystasis, 443
Presbyvestibulopathy, 443
Pressure ulcers, in MS, 252–253
Preswing (push-off), in gait cycle, 74*t*
Primary gain, in functional motor
　disorders, 415
Primary lateral sclerosis, 329
Primary progressive MS (PPMS), 239
Problem-solving, self-management and, 502
Professional leaders, in self-management,
　504*t*
Prognosis, in neurological rehabilitation,
　9–10
Progressive muscular atrophy, 329
Progressive neurological conditions,
　589–590
PROMs. *See* Patient-reported outcome
　measures
Proprioceptive system, 94
Propulsion, in walking, 72*t*
Protein misfolding, MND and, 328
Pseudobulbar affect, 333–334
Psychiatry, for functional motor
　disorders, 421
Psychogenic Movement Disorders Rating
　Scale, for functional motor
　disorders, 424*t*
Psychological status, in sit to stand, 84*t*–85*t*
Psychological therapy, for functional motor
　disorders, 421
Psychometric battery-based approach, to
　clinical neuropsychology, 613–614
Psychotherapy, 616
PUL. *See* Performance of upper limb
PUL 2.0. *See* Performance of Upper
　Limb 2.0
Push-off, in gait cycle, 74*t*
Pusher syndrome, 62
Pyridoxine, for MS, 247

Q

QRCs. *See* Quick Reference Cards
Quadriceps muscle, during sit to stand, 83*t*
Quality of life, assessment of, clinical
　neuropsychology and, 614–615
Quick Reference Cards (QRCs), of
　Parkinson's therapy, 277*f*, 278*f*,
　280*f*, 286
Quiet stance, balance and, 94–95

R

Radicava ORS, for MND, 333
Radiculopathy, 585
RAMP acronym, in neurological
　physiotherapy, 12
Range of motion, in traumatic brain injury,
　184, 184*t*
　interventions for, 188, 188*f*
Range of movement
　loss of, after SCI, 221, 221*b*
　measurement tools for, 115*t*–117*t*
　in sit to stand, 84*t*–85*t*
Rasch-built Overall Disability Scale, for
　inflammatory neuropathy, 363
Ratio data, assessing reliability for, 120–
　121, 120*f*
Ratio measurement tool, 118
Reach, 83–91
　clinical focus on, for people with stroke,
　91, 92*t*–93*t*
　essential components of, 87, 89*t*
　kinematics of, 87–88, 90*t*
　muscle activity of, 89–91, 91*f*
Reaching
　falls and, 557*t*
　measurement tools for, 115*t*–117*t*
Recovery, from stroke
　lower limb and locomotor, 161*t*–162*t*,
　163–169
　　balance training for, 163
　　bilateral arm training, 167
　　circuit class training for, 164–165
　　constraint-induced movement
　　therapy, 166–167
　　electrostimulation of paretic arm and
　　hand, 168
　　electrostimulation of paretic lower
　　limb, 165
　　gait training for, 163–164
　　robot-assisted therapy, upper limb,
　　168
　　therapy delivery, 168–169
　　upper limb recovery, 165, 165*t*–166*t*
　　virtual reality, interactive video
　　gaming, 167–168
Rectus abdominis, during sit to stand, 83*t*
Reduced arm swing, with walking in
　Parkinson's, 79*t*–80*t*
Reduced bone density, after SCI, 221
Redundancy, 122
Reflection, of clinical reasoning, 38–39
Reflexive autonomous individuals, 498
Reflexology, for functional motor
　disorders, 422
Rehabilitation
　definition of, 3

Rehabilitation (*Continued*)
　neurological, physical activity in.
　　See Neurological rehabilitation,
　　physical activity in
　stroke, goal setting in, 129–145
　　case study example of
　　interprofessional rehabilitation
　　goals, 133*t*
　　changing needs from acute care to
　　community life, 134–141, 135*f*
　　definitions and assumptions in,
　　130–131
　　goal achievement as outcome
　　measure, 141–144, 142*t*, 143*f*
　　key points for, 140*b*–141*b*
　　pragmatic person-centred, 131–134
　　questions for gathering useful
　　information for goal selection, 131*b*
　　questions to address in goal statement,
　　132
'Rehabilitation 2030
　A Call for Action', 7
Rehabilitation Complexity Scale, 615
Rehabilitation goal, definition of, 130
Rehabilitation phase
　for neurological conditions, 652
　in stroke, 7
Rehabilitation process, carer on, 9*t*
Reintegration, SCI and, 222
Relapsing-remitting MS (RRMS), 238
Reliability, in measurement tools, 119–121
Repetitions, definition of, 160
Resilience, in neurological rehabilitation,
　21–22, 22*b*
Resistance exercise, for MND, 342–343, 342*t*
Resource utilisation, self-management and,
　502
Respiration
　common problems in neurological
　　conditions that affect, 474*b*
　red flags regarding, 476*b*
Respiratory assessment, 474–479, 476*b*
　arterial blood gases in, 478, 478*b*
　chest radiographs in, 478
　lung function in, 474–477, 477*f*
　for MND, 335–336, 336*t*
　peak cough flow in, 477–478, 477*b*
　for polyneuropathies, 363
　respiratory pattern in, 478
　respiratory reserve in, 478–479, 478*f*,
　479*b*
Respiratory dysfunction, in MS, 251
Respiratory failure, MND and, 335–336
Respiratory impairments, in MND, 339,
　340*t*
Respiratory management, 473–492
　assessment in, 474–479, 476*b*

Respiratory management (*Continued*)
  arterial blood gases in, 478, 478*b*
  chest radiographs in, 478
  lung function in, 474–477, 477*f*
  peak cough flow in, 477–478, 477*b*
  respiratory pattern in, 478
  respiratory reserve in, 478–479, 478*f*, 479*b*
  central nervous control of breathing in, 474, 475*f*
  Covid-19, 209–210
  early mobilisation in, 479, 480*f*
  function in neurological conditions, 484–488
    anterior horn cell conditions, 486, 487*t*
    central conditions, 484, 486*t*
    muscle conditions, 487, 488*t*
    neuromuscular junction, 487, 488*t*
    neuropathy, 487, 487*t*
    spinal cord injury and disease, 484–486, 486*t*
    subarachnoid haemorrhage, 484
  long-term, 210
  of traumatic brain injury, 488–492, 488*t*, 489*f*, 489*t*, 490*f*, 490*t*, 491*t*
  treatment and, 479–484
    acute respiratory failure in, 483
    manual cough in, 482
    maximal insufflation capacity in, 481–482, 481*b*
    mechanical insufflation and exsufflation in, 480*f*, 482
    muscle training in, 483
    other considerations in, 482–483, 482*b*
    patent airway maintenance in, 479–481
    tracheostomy in, 483–484, 485*f*
    weaning in, 483–484
Respiratory pattern, in respiratory assessment, 478
Respiratory reserve, in respiratory assessment, 478–479, 478*f*, 479*b*
Responsiveness, in measurement tools, 123–124
Resting tremor, 59
Restoration, Adaptation, Maintenance and Prevention (RAMP), 34
  definition, 37
  treatment planning for, 37, 37*f*
Restorative rehabilitation, of MS management, 243
Revised Hammersmith Scale (RHS), 401
Revised upper limb module (RULM), 401, 405
Rhomboid major muscle, muscle timing and, 628
RHS. *See* Revised Hammersmith Scale

Rigidity, of joint, in Parkinson's, 269
Rising phase, of sit to stand, 81*t*
Rivermead Mobility Index, 117
RNA processing, defects in, MND and, 328
Robot-assisted gait training, after stroke, 164
Robot-assisted motor training, for neurorehabilitation, 527–530
Robot-assisted therapy, after stroke, 168
Robotic systems, for neurorehabilitation
  augment gait, soft, 529, 530*f*
  definition, 529
  gait training, 528, 528*f*
  impedance control, 527
  upper limb motor training, 527, 527*f*
Rollator frames, for MND, 341
Rolling and getting out of bed, 82–83, 87*t*
  for people with Parkinson's, 83, 88*t*
Romberg test, 452*t*
Rotational vertebral artery syndrome, 444–445
RRMS. *See* Relapsing-remitting MS
RULM. *See* Revised upper limb module

S

S-FMDRS. *See* Simplified Functional Movement Disorders Rating Scale
Saccades, 449*t*
Saliva, excessive, MND and, 340
Samsung Gear VR, 525, 526*f*
SARA. *See* Scale for the assessment and rating of ataxia
SARAH system. *See* Semi-Automated Rehabilitation at the Home system
Sarcomere, 383–385, 384*f*
SCA. *See* Spinocerebellar ataxia
Scale for the assessment and rating of ataxia (SARA), 307–308, 310*f*
Scapular distance test (SDT), 627–628, 633*f*
Scapular lateral rotation
  clinical scapular protocol for, 632, 632*f*
  kinematics after stroke, 627
  muscle timing for, 628
Scapulothoracic joint, kinematics of, 627
Scapulothoracic posterior tilting, 627
SCAT5. *See* Sport Concussion Assessment Tool version 5
SCC. *See* Semicircular canal
SCI. *See* Spinal cord injury
Scoliosis, in ataxia, 305–306
SDSA. *See* Stroke Drivers Screening Assessment
SDT. *See* Scapular distance test
Seat height, in sit to stand, 84*t*–85*t*
Secondary gain, in functional motor disorders, 415

Secondary problems, for vestibular rehabilitation, 457–459
Secondary progressive MS (SPMS), 238–239
Sedentary behaviour, in MS, 246
Seizures, 402
Self-efficacy, 500–501
  in neurological rehabilitation, 19
Self-management, 495–512, 510*b*
  definition of, 497–499
  education, 497
  factors influencing, 500*t*
  for functional motor disorders, 426
  long Covid, 508–510
  measurement of, 506–507, 507*b*
  for neurological disability
    approach to, 503–505
    evidence base for, 503–507
    understanding responses to, 499–502
  in neurological rehabilitation, 19, 19*f*, 19*t*
  for pain, 599–600
  for polyneuropathy, 370
  programmes, 499–503
    components of, 502–503, 502*f*, 503*t*
    self-efficacy in, 500–501
    Social Cognitive Theory in, 500–501
    Stress Coping Model in, 501–502
    Transtheoretical Model of Behaviour Change in, 501*b*, 502
  research, issues in, 505
  strengths and limitations of, 504*t*
  stroke and, 505–506
  supporting, 507–510, 511*f*
Self-Management Behaviours scale, 506, 507*b*
Self-manager, 508
Self-reported self-efficacy scale, 506
SEM. *See* Standard error of measurement
Semi-Automated Rehabilitation at the Home (SARAH) system, 524
Semicircular canal (SCC), 439, 440*f*
Sensation, in sit to stand, 84*t*–85*t*
Sensitivity, 123
Sensor-based systems, for neurorehabilitation, 521–523, 523*f*
Sensorimotor control, of balance, 93–95
  essential motor components in, 94–95
  essential sensory components in, 94
Sensory ataxia, 59
Sensory changes, after SCI, 212
Sensory disorders, 63–64
Sensory disturbance, midline splitting of, in functional motor disorders, 418
Sensory integration, balance and, 94
Sensory loss, 63
  in Charcot-Marie-Tooth disease, 362
  in diabetic neuropathy, 360

Sensory Modality Assessment and Rehabilitation Technique, 650
Sensory substitution, vestibular compensation and, 452–453
Serial casting, for range of motion improvement, 187
Serratus anterior muscle, muscle timing and, 628
Service delivery, of MS management, 244
Sexual dysfunction, SCI and, 211
Shirley Ryan AbilityLab online Rehabilitation Measures Database, 124
Shoulder complex
    evaluation of, 629–635
    kinematics of, 629, 630f
    muscle timing at, 630–631
    after stroke
        clinical scapular protocol, 631–635, 632f
        kinematics, 629–630
        motor control training for, 635–636
        muscle timing at, 631
        musculoskeletal management of, 635–636
        neuroplasticity and timing, 635–636
Shoulder girdle position, in clinical scapular protocol, 631–632, 632f
Shoulder pain
    SCI rehabilitation and, 221
    stroke and, 587
Shoulder subluxation, measurement tools for, 115t–117t
Shuffling steps, with walking in Parkinson's, 79t–80t
Sialorrhea, MND and, 340
'Silent' lesions, of MS, 237
Simplified Functional Movement Disorders Rating Scale (S-FMDRS), for functional motor disorders, 424t
Single support, in gait cycle, 74t
Sit to stand (STS), 77–82
    clinical focus on, for people following stroke, 82, 85t–86t
    contextual factors influencing, 82, 84t–85t
    muscle action during, 82, 82f, 83t
    typical phases of, 78, 80f, 81t
Sitting balance, SCI, 212, 217–218, 225t–226t
Situational Characteristics Questionnaire, 454
Sjogren's disease, 386
Skill acquisition, in neurological rehabilitation, 13–17, 14t–15t
Skull vibration-induced nystagmus testing (SVINT), 446
SLEs. See Strokelike episodes

Slow STS performance, in sit to stand, 85t–86t
SMA. See Spinal muscular atrophy
SMART acronym, 132–133
    in team goals, 7
    treatment goal setting, 598
Smartphones, in neurorehabilitation, 525, 526f
Smooth pursuit, 449t
Sniff nasal inspiratory pressure (SNIP), 337, 475–476
SNIP. See Sniff nasal inspiratory pressure
SOC. See Standards of care
Social Cognitive Theory, 500–501
Social isolation, self-management and, 499
Soft foam collar, for MND, 341
Soft tissue therapy, for pain, 593
Spastic dystonia, 57
Spastic Paraplegia Rating Scale (SPRS), 312
Spastic paresis, hereditary, 309–313, 315t–316t
    anatomy, pathophysiology and clinical presentation of, 310–311
    diagnosis of, 311
    epidemiology and genetics of, 309–310
    medical management for, 311
    physiotherapy assessment for, 311–312
    time course and corresponding management for, 312
    treatment selection, secondary complications and special problems in, 312–313
Spasticity, 56, 637–643
    in ataxia, 305
    definition, 638–639
    evaluation of outcome for, 641–643, 641t
    management, principles of, 639, 642f
    measures of pain and skin integrity, 659–660
    in MS, 244f, 247–248
    physical and pharmacological treatment, 639–641
    problems experienced by people, 638t
    SCI and, 212
    after traumatic brain injury, 182
        interventions for, 186–187
    UMNS, 637–638, 638t
Specificity, 123
    of training, in motor learning, 14t–15t
Speech therapy, for functional motor disorders, 421
Speed-dependent treadmill training, after stroke, 163–164
Spinal cord injury (SCI), 198–228
    aetiology of, 198–199, 198t, 199f
    anterior cord syndrome, 200–203, 206t
    ASIA impairment scale, 199

Spinal cord injury (SCI) (Continued)
    assessment of, 212, 213t
    autonomic dysreflexia, 210
    Brown-Séquard syndrome, 200–203, 206t
    case study of, 223–228, 227f, 228f
    classification of, 199
    clinical neuropsychology and, 622
    clinical presentation of, 210–212
        pain, 212
        spasticity, 212
    definition of, 198
    diagnosis of, 199
    discharge planning of, 222–223
    early acute management of, 203–207, 204b
        facilitation of range, length and movement, 205–207
        mobilisation, 207
        physical management, 204–205
        prognosis, 204
    epidemiology of, 198
    functional outcomes after, 202t–203t
    heterotropic ossification, 222
    incomplete syndromes of, 200–203, 204f, 205f, 206t
    initial management plan of, 224t
    interactive technologies, 535
    lifelong care of, 222–223
    paediatric considerations of, 222
    pain and, 590–591
    pathological changes after, 199t
    pathophysiology of, 199
    physical management of, 204–205, 212–221
        aquatic therapy, 214, 215f
        cardiovascular fitness, 220
        facilitation movement, 214–216
        functional mobility, 217–218
        gait training, 218–220
        modalities, 220–221
        seating, 216–217, 217t
        splinting, 216, 216f, 217b
        standing, 218, 218f
        strength training, 214, 214b
    prognosis of, 200, 201b, 203t
    progress with rehabilitation of, 223
    rehabilitation, aims of, 212
    reintegration, 222
    respiratory assessment, 207–208, 207t
        long-term, 210
    respiratory function in, 484–486, 486t
    respiratory treatment of, 208–210
        precautions in, 205b, 208b
    special considerations of, 221–222
    updated problem list, goals and treatment plan during rehabilitation phase of, 225t–226t

Spinal muscular atrophy (SMA)
  assessment and outcome measures, 401
  autosomal recessive condition, 399
  case studies, 405–406
  disease course and prognosis, 400–401
  medical management, 401
  pain and, 587
  physical management, 401
  presentation, 399, 400t
Spinal shock, SCI and, 210
Spinocerebellar ataxia (SCA), 304f
Spinocerebellar ataxia disorders, pain
    and, 587
Splinting
  for pain, 597
  SCI and, 216, 216f, 217b
Splints, for range of motion improvement,
    187
SPMS. See Secondary progressive MS
Spontaneous nystagmus, 449t
Sport Concussion Assessment Tool version
    5 (SCAT5), for traumatic brain
    injury, 177
Sport-related concussions, TBI and, 177
SPRS. See Spastic Paraplegia Rating Scale
Sputum retention, common techniques
    for, 490t
Stabilisation, in sit to stand, 81t
Stability, falls and, 557t
Standard error of measurement (SEM), in
    reliability analysis, 119
Standard tests, for falls, 552–553, 553f
Standards of care (SOC), 389
Standing programme, SCI, 212–214
Stanford model, of self-management, 597
Step length, in gait cycle, 74t
Stereotactic radiosurgery, for pain, 591
Sternoclavicular joint, kinematics of, 627,
    630f
Sternomastoid test, in functional motor
    disorders, 419t
Strength, in sit to stand, 84t–85t
Strength training
  for muscle paresis, 186
  SCI and, 214, 214b
Strengthening, SCI, 214, 214b
Stress Coping Model, 501–502
Stretching exercises, for MND, 342–343
Striatum, Parkinson's and, 267
Stride length, in gait cycle, 74t
Stride width, in gait cycle, 74t
Stroke, 151–170
  assessment of, 154–159, 156b
    acute phase, 154–156
    in chronic phase, 157, 157f, 158b
    in hyperacute phase, 154–156
    interventions for, 159–163

Stroke (Continued)
    prognosis and time course in, 157–
      159, 158f, 159b
    subacute phase, 156–157
  case study on, 169–170, 170t, 171t
  clinical neuropsychology, 618,
    619t–620t
  clinical presentation of, 153–154, 154t,
    155f
  definition of, 151
  diagnosis of, 152
  epidemiology of, 152
  general therapy principles of, 160–163,
    161t–162t, 165t–166t
  haemorrhagic, 152
  interdisciplinary team for, 153
  interventions, 159–163
    general therapy principles, 160–163
  ischaemic, 152–154, 154t
  lower limb and locomotor recovery
      from, 161t–162t, 163–169
    balance training for, 163
    bilateral arm training, 167
    circuit class training for, 164–165
    constraint-induced movement
      therapy, 166–167
    electrostimulation of paretic arm and
      hand, 168
    electrostimulation of paretic lower
      limb, 165
    gait training for, 163–164
    robot-assisted therapy, upper limb,
      168
    therapy delivery, 168–169
    upper limb recovery, 165, 165t–166t
    virtual reality, interactive video
      gaming, 167–168
  medical management of, 152–153
  pain and, 590
  pathophysiology of, 152
  reach and grasp in, 91, 92t–93t
  self-management and, 505–506
  setting for, 153
  shoulder complex
    clinical scapular protocol, 631–635,
      632f
    kinematics, 629–630
    motor control training for, 635–636
    muscle timing at, 631
    musculoskeletal management of,
      635–636
    neuroplasticity and timing, 635–636
  sit to stand following, 82, 85t–86t
  therapy delivery of, 168–169
  vestibular system, 444
Stroke Drivers Screening Assessment
    (SDSA), 637, 645f

Stroke rehabilitation, goal setting in,
    129–145
  case study example of interprofessional
    rehabilitation goals, 133t
  changing needs from acute care to
      community life, 134–141, 135f
    acute rehabilitation, 134–136
    community-based late subacute
      rehabilitation, 138–139
    hospital-based early subacute
      rehabilitation, 136–138
    ongoing life after stroke, 139–141
  definitions and assumptions in, 130–131
    activities to enhance goal pursuit,
      130–131
    rehabilitation goals and goal setting,
      130
  goal achievement as outcome measure,
      141–144
    appeal of, 141
    Goal Attainment Scaling in, 141–144,
      142t
    problems with, 142–144, 143f
  key points for, 140b–141b
  pragmatic person-centred, 131–134
    family involvement in, 133–134
    goal documentation, 132–133
    goal selection, 131–132
    measurement in, 134
  questions for gathering useful
      information for goal selection, 131b
  questions to address in goal statement,
      132
Stroke Self-Efficacy Questionnaire, 506,
    507b
Stroke-specific databases: evidence-based
    review of stroke rehabilitation, 39t,
    124
Strokelike episodes (SLEs), 402–403
STS. See Sit to stand
Subacute phase, of stroke, 156–157
Subarachnoid haemorrhage, respiratory
    function in, 484
Subjective assessment
  of functional motor disorders, 423
  of pain, 591–593
  of SCI, 213t
Substantia nigra, Parkinson's and, 267
Subthalamic nucleus, Parkinson's, 267
Suction, SCI respiratory treatment, 209
Sun downing syndrome, 546
Supraspinatus tendinopathy, 627–628
Surgical management, of ataxia, 306
SVINT. See Skull vibration-induced
    nystagmus testing
Sway balance, 95
Swimming, aquatic therapy, 214, 215f

Swing phase, 76–77
Syringomyelia, of SCI, 222
Syrinx, of SCI, 222

T

Tandem Romberg test, 452t
Tandem walking, 452t
TANS. See Transition Assessment North Star Worksheet
Tardive dyskinesias, 58
Task, in sitting/getting out of bed, 87t
Task practice issues, in skill acquisition, 15
Task-specific practice, in hypertonus, 56–57
Task-specific training, in functional and neural plasticity, 10–11
TBI. See Traumatic brain injury
TDOC. See Terminal disorders of consciousness
Team goal setting, in neurological rehabilitation, 7
Team work, in neurological rehabilitation, 7
Technical skills, in self-management, 498
Telerehabilitation, therapy delivery, 162
10-m timed walk, for functional motor disorders, 424t
Tendon pain, 585
Tenodesis series, 215f
Terminal contact, in gait cycle, 74t
Terminal disorders of consciousness (TDOC), 643
Terminal stance, 76
    in gait cycle, 74t
Terminal swing, in gait cycle, 74t
Tetraplegia, definition of, 198
The Academy of Neurological Physical Therapy outcome measures recommendations section of the American Physical Therapy Association, 124
The Shaking Palsy, 266
Theoretical framework
    importance of, 4–5
    in neurological rehabilitation, 5–25, 5f
Theory, in clinical reasoning, 4
Therapeutic alliance, in neurological rehabilitation, 20
Thermal therapies, for pain, 598
Thermoregulation dysfunction, SCI and, 211
Thixotropy, for neurological conditions, 629–630
Thrombectomy, for stroke, 153
Thrombolysis, for stroke, 152–153
Tibialis anterior, during sit to stand, 83t

Tilt-tables, for range of motion improvement, 187
Tilting, in clinical scapular protocol, 631, 632f
Timed function tests, 390
Timing, in sitting/getting out of bed, 87t
Tinetti's Balance Performance Assessment, 452t
TIS. See Trunk Impairment Scale
Tissue viability, SCI of, 221–222
Tizanidine (Zanaflex), spasticity management in MS, 242
TOAST (Trial of Org 10172 in Acute Stroke Treatment) classification, of stroke, 152
Toe-off, in gait cycle, 74t
Toronto Perturbation-Based Balance Training, 555b
Tracheostomy
    for MND, 347
    in respiratory management, 483–484, 485f
Trail leg, in gait cycle, 74t
Transcutaneous electrical nerve stimulation, for pain, 598
Transfer of training, in motor learning, 14t–15t
Transferring, falls and, 557t
Transient ischaemic attack, definition of, 151
Transition Assessment North Star Worksheet (TANS), 391t
Transition, for neurological conditions, 657, 657t
Transition of care, community phase, 652–653
Transtheoretical Model of Behaviour Change, 501b, 502
Traumatic brain injury (TBI), 177–192
    assessment of, 182–185, 184t, 190b
        abnormal tone in, 183, 183t
        balance and vestibular function in, 184
        concurrent musculoskeletal injuries in, 185
        disorders of movement in, 184
        function in, 185
        muscle and joint range of motion in, 184, 184t
        muscle paresis in, 184
        pain in, 185
    case presentation of, 190–192, 191t–192t, 192f, 193t
    clinical neuropsychology and, 617–618, 618t
    clinical presentation of, 181–182, 182t
    Covid-19 pandemic, 189–190

Traumatic brain injury (TBI) (Continued)
    diagnosis of, 179–180
        coma in, 179t, 180
        posttraumatic amnesia in, 180, 180t
    epidemiology of, 178
    interventions for, 186–189
        for balance and vestibular function, 187–188
        for concurrent musculoskeletal injuries, 188
        for disorders of movement, 187
        for function, 189
        for hypertonicity and spasticity, 186–187
        for muscle and joint range of motion, 188, 188f
        for muscle paresis, 187
        other considerations for, 189
        for pain, 188–189
    medical management of, 180–181, 180b, 181t
        intracranial pressure in, 180–181
        multidisciplinary care in, 181, 181b
    pain and, 590
    pathophysiology of, 178–179, 178t
        associated injuries, 179
        primary brain injury, 178–179
        secondary brain injury, 179
    prognosis/time course for, 185–186
    respiratory management of, 488–492, 488t, 489f, 489t, 490f, 490t, 491t
    vestibular system, 444
Treadmill assessment, of clinical reasoning, 49
Treadmill deweighting gantry, 220f
Treadmill training, 651
    after stroke
        body weight-supported, 164
        speed-dependent, 163–164
Treatment planning, of clinical reasoning
    development of, 37–38
    implementation, 38
    RAMP, aims of, 37, 37f
Tremor, 59
    entrainment, in functional motor disorders, 419t
    functional, in functional motor disorders, 419, 427t–428t
    in Parkinson's, 269
Trigeminal neuralgia, multiple sclerosis and, 586
Trigger point techniques, for pain, 593
Trunk Impairment Scale (TIS), 121–123
Trunk muscles, during sit to stand, 83t
Tubular visual field, in functional motor disorders, 418
Turning, falls and, 557t

U

UFOV®. *See* Useful Field of View
Ultrasound, therapeutic, for pain, 598
UMNS. *See* Upper motor neurone syndrome
UMNs. *See* Upper motor neurones
Uncertainty, self-management and, 500
Uni-dimensionality, 121
Unilateral spatial neglect, 62
University of South Australia, International Centre for Allied Health Evidence, 39t
Upper limb
    for neurological conditions, 628–637
    positioning, SCI rehabilitation, 216
Upper limb activity, measurement tools for, 115t–117t
Upper limb function, in hereditary ataxias, 308
Upper limb impairment, in MS, 246–247
Upper limb motor practice, 532–534, 534f
Upper limb recovery, from stroke, 165, 165t–166t
Upper limb rehabilitation, 527, 527f
Upper limb rigidity, execution of, with bed mobility, in Parkinson's, 88t
Upper motor neurone syndrome (UMNS), 54, 637–638, 638t
Upper motor neurones (UMNs), 327
    degeneration, in MND, 333
    weakness, 54–55
Useful Field of View (UFOV®), 646f

V

Validity, in measurement tools, 121–123
Variable practice, in skill acquisition, 16–17
VAS. *See* Visual analogue scale
Vascular vertigo (VV), 444
Vegetative state, definition of, 182t
Velocity-dependent hypertonus, 56
Velocity, in gait cycle, 74t
VEMPs. *See* Vestibular evoked myogenic potentials
Ventilator-free breathing (VFB), 209
Ventilatory support, weaning from, 209–210
Verbal persuasion, in Social Cognitive Theory, 501
Vertebral artery compression syndrome, 444–445
Vertigo, 438
Vestibular agnosia, 444
Vestibular compensation, 450–452, 453b
    in MS, 250–251
Vestibular disorders, 61–62
    assessment of, 447–450, 448t
        functional ability in, 448, 451f, 452t

Vestibular disorders (*Continued*)
        outcome measures in, 448–450, 451f
        physical impairments in, 448, 449t, 450f
    central, 441, 442t, 443–445
    classification of, 441, 442t
    diagnosis of, 446
    epidemiology of, 438
    interventions for, 453–459
    medical and surgical management of, 446–447
    pathophysiology, 441
    peripheral, 441–443
    prognosis of, 450–453
    signs and symptoms of, 438t
    treatment plan and goals for, 453t
Vestibular evoked myogenic potentials (VEMPs), 446
Vestibular function, after traumatic brain injury, 184
    interventions for, 187–188
Vestibular hypofunction, bilateral, 443
Vestibular migraine (VM), 443–444
Vestibular nerve, 440
Vestibular neurectomy, for Ménière's disease, 447
Vestibular neuritis, 441–442
Vestibular nuclei, 440
Vestibular ocular motor screening, 452t
Vestibular ocular reflex (VOR), 440–441, 441f, 449t
Vestibular paresis, 441–442
Vestibular paroxysmia (VP), 445
Vestibular rehabilitation, 438–462
    case studies for, 460–462
    interventions in, 453–459
        for balance and gait reeducation, 454–456
        benign paroxysmal positional vertigo, management of, 456, 457f
        gaze stability exercises, 454
        habituation exercises, 454
        horizontal canal benign paroxysmal positional vertigo, 456–457, 458f
        secondary problems, 457–459
        visual desensitisation exercises, 454
    multidisciplinary team in, 459
    patient groups, 453t
    remote and digital, 459
    specialist centres and support groups in, 459–460
    support groups, 460
    useful resources for, 460
Vestibular rehabilitation therapy (VRT), 420
Vestibular schwannoma (VS), 444
    medical and surgical management of, 447
Vestibular sedatives, 446–447

Vestibular system, 94
    anatomy and physiology of, 438–440, 439f, 440f
    Covid-19, 459
    peripheral, 439–440, 439f
Vestibulopathy, in MS, 250–251
Vestibulospinal reflex (VSR), 440–441
VFB. *See* Ventilator-free breathing
vHIT. *See* Video head impulse test
Vicarious experience, in Social Cognitive Theory, 501
ViD. *See* Visually induced dizziness
Video analysis, for neurorehabilitation, 523–525
Video gaming, interactive, after stroke, 167–168
Video head impulse test (vHIT), 443, 446
Video, in assessment of falls, 552
Virtual reality (VR)
    for neurorehabilitation, 517, 520
    video gaming, after stroke, 167–168
Virtual rehabilitation, 517, 520, 535
Vision
    balance and, 94
    in sit to stand, 84t–85t
Visual analogue scale (VAS), 388
Visual assessment battery, 637–638, 645f
Visual desensitisation exercises, 454
Visual feedback, for pain, 598–599
Visual Vertigo Analogue Scale, 454
Visually induced dizziness (ViD), 454
Visuomotor integration, 529
Visuospatial disorders, 62–63
Vital capacity, critical values of, 477b
Vitamin B_{12} deficiency, polyneuropathy and, 355
Vitamin D, in MS, 253–254
VM. *See* Vestibular migraine
VOR. *See* Vestibular ocular reflex
VORx1 exercises, 454
VORx2 exercises, 454
VP. *See* Vestibular paroxysmia
VR. *See* Virtual reality
VR headsets, in neurorehabilitation, 525–527, 526f
VRT. *See* Vestibular rehabilitation therapy
VS. *See* Vestibular schwannoma
VSR. *See* Vestibulospinal reflex
VV. *See* Vascular vertigo

W

Walking, 71–77
    essential components of, 72t
    falls and, 557t
    gait cycle in, 72, 73f, 74t
    in hereditary ataxias, 309

Walking (*Continued*)
    kinematics of, muscle activity and,
        72–77, 75*f*, 76*f*
    kinetics, 77, 78*f*
    overground, after stroke, 163
    for people with Parkinson's, 77, 79*t*–80*t*
    spatiotemporal characteristics of,
        77, 79*t*
    stroke and, 158–159, 159*b*
Walking aids, falls and, 559
Walking disability, measurement tools for,
    115*t*–117*t*
Walking impairment, measurement tools
    for, 115*t*–117*t*
Walking speed, of clinical reasoning, 49
Walking sticks, for MND, 341
Wallerian degeneration, 585
Washing, falls and, 557*t*

Weakness, 54–55
    execution of, with bed mobility, in
        Parkinson's, 88*t*
    functional, in functional motor
        disorders, 418–419, 419*t*
    in MS, 246
    SCI, 211
    with walking in Parkinson's, 79*t*–80*t*
Weaning, in respiratory management,
    483–484
Wearable technology, for
    neurorehabilitation, 530–535, 535*b*
Weight-bearing asymmetry, in sit to stand,
    85*t*–86*t*
Weight shift, for neurorehabilitation,
    537–538
Weighting, balance and, 94
Wessex Head Injury Matrix, 650

Wheelchair
    for MND, 343–344
    for SCI, 218
Wii Fit Balance Board, 521–522, 522*f*
Wii Sports, 521, 537–538
Winging, in clinical scapular protocol, 631,
    632*f*
WizeCare system, 524–525, 525*f*
WMFT. *See* Wolf Motor Function Test
Wolf Motor Function Test (WMFT), 522
World physiotherapy (WP), 274
WP. *See* World physiotherapy
Wrist units, accelerometer data, 531,
    532*f*–533*f*

X

XR. *See* Extended reality